Saunders Tests for Self-Evaluation of Nursing Competence

Third Edition
REVISED REPRINT

DEE ANN GILLIES, R.N., B.S., M.A., M.A.T., Ed.D.

Divisional Nursing Director, Surgical Nursing
Cook County Hospital, Chicago, Illinois

IRENE BARRETT ALYN, R.N., B.A., M.S.N., Ph.D.

Professor of Nursing
University of Illinois, Chicago, Illinois

1980
W.B. SAUNDERS COMPANY   Philadelphia   London   Toronto

W. B. Saunders Company: West Washington Square
Philadelphia, PA   19105

1 St. Anne's Road
Eastbourne, East Sussex BN21 3UN, England

1 Goldthorne Avenue
Toronto, Ontario M8Z 5T9, Canada

Library of Congress Cataloging in Publication Data

Gillies, Dee Ann.

Saunders tests for self-evaluation of nursing competence.

Includes bibliographies and index.

1. Nursing—Examinations, questions, etc.   I. Alyn, Irene
   Barrett, joint author.   II. Title. [DNLM: 1. Educational
   measurement.   2. Nursing—Examination questions.
   WY18 G481s]

RT55.G5 1980   610.73′076   80–51321

ISBN 0–7216–4157–1

Saunders Tests for Self-Evaluation of Nursing Competence   ISBN   0-7216-4157-1
Revised Reprint

Last digit is the print number: 9   8   7   6   5   4   3   2   1

Dedication

For and Because of:

Minerva,
Bertha,
Fay,
and
Dana

Preface

The revised reprint of the third edition of the *Saunders Tests of Nursing Competence* has been expanded to include rationales for the answers to all test items.

As a result of recent rapid developments in medical science and increasing public demand for high quality health care, nurses have been confronted with a plethora of new knowledge from basic, medical, and/or nursing sciences. In order to function effectively, a knowledge applier must not only acquire a generous fund of pertinent scientific facts, but must combine and manipulate such facts into new configurations in order to solve clinical practice problems.

The knowledge applier in nursing will find this book an effective tool for teaching, testing, and thinking. By reviewing the enclosed clinical situations and associated test items, nurses can teach themselves the principal facts and concepts underlying nursing practice. By selecting the best from several possible answers to each item and comparing selections with those of a clinical specialist, nurses can test their grasp of nursing content. By studying the authors' rationale for each answer, each nurse can practice steps of logical thinking — isolating significant data, establishing priorities, identifying relationships, and solving problems through inductive and deductive reasoning.

This book has been helpful in preparing undergraduate nurses to take licensure examinations, and in preparing graduate nurses to enter baccalaureate and master's level nursing programs. This latest, expanded edition of the book should be helpful in stimulating the thought processes of both undergraduates and graduate nurses who embark upon a program of self-directed continuing education.

The authors thank Katherine Rose, R.N., M.S.N., who helped write rationales for Maternity nursing items, and Marcia Maurer, R.N., M.S.N., who helped write rationales for the Pediatric nursing items. Both specialists are Assistant Professors at the University of Illinois, College of Nursing.

Dee Ann Gillies
Irene Barrett Alyn

Contents

1
MATERNITY AND GYNECOLOGIC NURSING

Normal Pregnancy

Rose Christopher was 13 when she first menstruated. She had been prepared for her menarche by sex education classes at school and by her mother, who had explained menstruation and reproduction to Rose in a series of conversations during her 9th and 10th years. Rose's menstrual periods had occurred on a 28-day cycle from their onset, and she had experienced only minor and occasional discomfort during the first day of each period.

When Rose was 18 she married David Christopher, the boy next door. Rose took a job as a secretary so that David could continue his training in a two year trade school for television and radio technicians. Initially Rose took an oral contraceptive to avoid pregnancy, but dissatisfaction with the side effects of the medication led Rose to discontinue its use and she became pregnant twelve months after marriage.

Suspecting pregnancy because she had missed two menstrual periods, Rose went to her doctor. Physical examination and an H.C.G. test indicated that she was pregnant. External and internal pelvimetry indicated that Rose's pelvis was large enough to permit a normal delivery. Her V.D.R.L. test was negative and her Papanicolaou smear was interpreted as Class 1. The doctor learned that although Rose had missed only two periods, her last menstruation on January 12 had been very scant. He therefore concluded that Rose was in her third month of pregnancy and listed her last normal menstrual period as having begun on December 15.

(ANSWER BLANK ON PAGE A–1)   (CORRECT ANSWERS ON PAGE B–3)

1. The cyclic activities of the ovaries and uterine endometrium are regulated by the:
1. Cerebral cortex and the adrenal gland.
2. Hypothalamus and the anterior pituitary gland.
3. Cerebellum and the posterior pituitary gland.
4. Medulla oblongata and the thyroid gland.

2. The hormone that enhances ovarian production of estrogen during the first half of the menstrual cycle is the:
1. Growth hormone.
2. Follicle-stimulating hormone.
3. Luteinizing hormone.
4. Adrenocorticotrophic hormone.

3. During the first half of the menstrual cycle estrogen is produced by:
1. Eosinophilic cells of the anterior pituitary.
2. Theca cells of the ovarian follicle.
3. Granulosal cells of the corpus luteum.
4. Mucus glands of the endometrium.

4. Rupture of the ovarian follicle and release of the mature ovum probably occurred on which day of Rose's menstrual cycle?
1. 1st or 2nd day.
2. 6th or 7th day.
3. 13th or 14th day.
4. 20th or 21st day.

5. The process of reduction division by which chromosomes are reduced to their haploid number in the course of oogenesis is called:
1. Synapsis.
2. Mitosis.
3. Meiosis.
4. Replication.

6. How many chromosomes does the mature human ovum contain?
1. 46
2. 35
3. 23
4. 11

7. Of the total number of chromosomes found in the human ovum, one is:
1. An X chromosome.
2. A Y chromosome.
3. A Z chromosome.
4. An autosome.

8. The chromosomes of the human ovum are composed of:
  1. Amino acids.
  2. Ribonucleic acids.
  3. Branched-chain fatty acids.
  4. Deoxyribonucleic acid.

9. The aforementioned substance, of which chromosomes are composed, is a high molecular weight compound with a double helical structure containing repeating units composed of:
  a. A five carbon sugar.
  b. Purine-pyrimidine base pairs.
  c. Long-chain fatty acids.
  d. Phosphoric acid.
    1. a only.
    2. a and b.
    3. a, b, and d.
    4. All the above.

10. It is thought that the genes, or character determinants, are carried by chromosomes in the form of a:
  1. Small, kidney-shaped body with a membranous, labyrinthine interior.
  2. Code determined by the sequence of purine and pyrimidine bases.
  3. Narrow membrane-walled tube containing electrolyte solutions.
  4. Molecule containing numerous high energy phosphate bonds.

11. Rose frequently experienced slight abdominal tenderness for a few hours at the midpoint of each menstrual period. Such discomfort is referred to as:
  1. Ovulation.
  2. Borborygmus.
  3. Mittelschmerz.
  4. Colic.

12. At which of the following points in the normal menstrual cycle is the serum level of estrogen highest?
  1. 3rd day.
  2. 8th day.
  3. 13th day.
  4. 23rd day.

13. At which of the following points in the normal menstrual cycle is the serum level of estrogen lowest?
  1. 3rd day.
  2. 8th day.
  3. 13th day.
  4. 23rd day.

14. Estrogen has which of the following physiologic effects?
  a. Causes hypertrophy of the myometrium.
  b. Stimulates growth of the spiral arteries in the endometrium.
  c. Increases the quantity and pH of the cervical mucus.
  d. Stimulates growth of ductile structures in the breast.
  e. Inhibits secretion of pituitary follicle-stimulating hormone.
    1. a and b.
    2. a, b, and c.
    3. All but e.
    4. All the above.

15. The anterior pituitary hormone which stimulates production of progesterone during the latter half of the menstrual cycle is the:
  1. Growth hormone.
  2. Follicle-stimulating hormone.
  3. Luteinizing hormone.
  4. Adrenocorticotrophic hormone.

16. During the latter half of the menstrual period progesterone is secreted by the:
  1. Posterior pituitary gland.
  2. Ovarian follicle.
  3. Corpus luteum.
  4. Endometrial glands.

17. Progesterone has which of the following physiologic effects?
  a. Increases the tortuosity of the tubular endometrial glands.
  b. Stimulates secretion of the endometrial glands.
  c. Increases body temperature after ovulation.
  d. Facilitates transport of the fertilized ovum through the fallopian tubes.
  e. Inhibits uterine motility during pregnancy.
    1. a and c.
    2. b and d.
    3. All but e.
    4. All the above.

18. If conception fails to occur, menstruation takes place about two weeks following ovulation, as a result of:
  1. Enhanced secretion of estrogen.
  2. Inhibition of follicle-stimulating hormone.
  3. Stimulation of luteinizing hormone.
  4. Decrease in both estrogen and progesterone.

19. The desquamation of the superficial layers of endometrium that occurs during menstruation is initiated by:
  1. Contraction of the uterine musculature.

2. Increased trypsin production by the pancreas.

3. Vasoconstriction of the spiral arteries.

4. Stimulation of the parasympathetic nervous system.

20. The average amount of blood lost during a normal menstrual period is:

1. 15–25 ml.
2. 25–50 ml.
3. 50–150 ml.
4. 150–500 ml.

21. Which of the following are frequent side effects of oral contraceptives?

a. Nausea.
b. Dizziness.
c. Headache.
d. Weight gain.
e. Breast discomfort.
   1. a and b.
   2. c and d.
   3. All but e.
   4. All the above.

22. Conception usually occurs during which interval of time?

1. The first day of the menstrual period.
2. 12 hours following cessation of menstruation.
3. 12 to 24 hours following ovulation.
4. The day or two preceding menstruation.

23. In human beings fertilization of the ovum usually occurs in the:

1. Ovarian follicle.
2. Fallopian tube.
3. Uterine fundus.
4. Uterine corpus.

24. Implantation or attachment of the fertilized ovum to the endometrium usually occurs about which day of the normal menstrual cycle?

1. 15th day.
2. 20th day
3. 25th day.
4. 1st day.

25. The principal source of progesterone and estrogen during the first six to eight weeks of pregnancy is the:

1. Pituitary gland.
2. Embryonic chorion.
3. Corpus luteum.
4. Adrenal cortex.

26. In addition to amenorrhea, which of the following presumptive signs of pregnancy might Rose have experienced before consulting her doctor?

a. Morning sickness.
b. Breast tenderness.
c. Frequent urination.
d. Easy fatigability.
   1. a and b.
   2. c and d.
   3. All but d.
   4. All the above.

27. The nurse should instruct Rose that which of the following would be most apt to relieve her morning sickness?

1. Eliminating breakfast and eating a slightly larger than normal lunch.
2. Eating some dry, absorbent food such as crackers before arising.
3. Drinking copious amounts of clear fluids with and between meals.
4. Avoiding foods that are high in roughage or acidic in nature.

28. Morning sickness of pregnancy usually disappears by the end of the:

1. First month.
2. Third month.
3. Fifth month.
4. Seventh month.

29. Which of the following breast changes might Rose experience during early pregnancy?

a. Increase in the size of the breast.
b. Increased prominence of the nipple.
c. Increased pigmentation of the nipple and areola.
d. Increased prominence of the areolar sweat glands.
   1. a and c.
   2. b and d.
   3. All but d.
   4. All the above.

30. Which of the following presumptive and probable signs of pregnancy might the doctor have observed on Rose's initial physical and pelvic examinations?

a. Purplish discoloration of the vaginal mucosa.
b. Softening of the cervix.
c. Softening of the lower uterine segment.
d. Increase in the size of the uterus.
e. Palpation of the outlines of the fetus.
   1. a and b.
   2. a, b, and c.
   3. All but e.
   4. All the above.

31. Chadwick's sign, or the purplish discoloration of the vulvar, vaginal, and cervical mucosa, is thought to be caused by:
1. Circulatory changes produced by increased amounts of ovarian hormones.
2. Rapid growth of microorganisms in the increased vaginal secretions.
3. Decreased oxygen tension of maternal blood produced by fetal metabolism.
4. Obstruction of venous flow caused by pressure of the enlarged uterus.

32. Since Rose's last normal menstrual period began on December 15 and her last episode of vaginal bleeding on January 12, her expected confinement date would be:
1. September 15.
2. September 22.
3. October 12.
4. October 19.

33. Which of the following measurements and tests would probably be part of the physician's workup on Rose's initial visit?
a. Urinalysis.
b. Complete blood count.
c. Body weight.
d. Blood pressure.
e. Serology and Rh determination.
1. a and b.
2. c and d.
3. All but e.
4. All the above.

34. The H.C.G. test depends on the urinary excretion by the pregnant woman of:
1. Adrenocorticosteroids.
2. Ovarian estrogen.
3. Ovarian progesterone.
4. Chorionic gonadotropin.

35. The hormone identified in the H.C.G. test has the function of:
1. Stimulating development of the ovarian follicle.
2. Maintaining the corpus luteum of pregnancy.
3. Desensitizing maternal tissues to fetal protein.
4. Increasing secretion of pituitary growth hormone.

36. Most H.C.G. tests become positive about how long after conception?
1. 2 weeks.
2. 4 weeks.
3. 6 weeks.
4. 8 weeks.

37. Which of the following external pelvic measurements is the most useful in inferring the size of the pelvic inlet?
1. The distance between the lateral edges of the iliac crests.
2. The distance between the external aspects of the anterosuperior iliac spines.
3. The distance between the anterior of the symphysis pubis and the depression below the spine of the fifth lumbar vertebra.
4. The distance between the lateral edge of the iliac crest and the tip of the coccyx.

38. Which of the following is the chief internal measurement which the physician would take as part of Rose's pelvimetry?
1. The distance between the sacral promontory and the lower margin of the symphysis pubis.
2. The distance from the tip of the coccyx and the lower margin of the symphysis pubis.
3. The distance between the sacral promontory and the ischial tuberosity.
4. The distance between the tip of the coccyx and the ischial spine.

39. The V.D.R.L. test is used to diagnose:
1. Syphilis.
2. Choriocarcinoma.
3. Gonorrhea.
4. Erythroblastosis.

40. A class 1 Papanicolaou smear is characterized by:
1. Complete absence of malignant cells.
2. Excessive amount of cervical secretions.
3. The presence of occult blood.
4. Accumulations of inflammatory debris.

41. On her first visit to the doctor's office Rose's blood count would be apt to reveal a:
1. Greatly increased number of red blood cells.
2. Moderately increased number of white blood cells.
3. Slightly increased number of eosinophils.
4. Slightly decreased hemoglobin concentration.

42. During her first visit to the physician's office Rose should be instructed to do which of the following if she should develop slight vaginal bleeding?

    1. Ignore it as insignificant to the outcome of her pregnancy.

    2. Record the date and report it on the next visit to the doctor.

    3. Phone the doctor and describe the amount and duration of bleeding.

    4. Remain at complete bedrest until the bleeding ceases completely.

43. The office nurse should advise Rose to avoid wearing:

    1. A brassiere.

    2. A corset.

    3. Round garters.

    4. High-heeled shoes.

44. At which interval would Rose probably be scheduled to return to the doctor's office during her pregnancy?

    1. Every three months for a regular checkup and more frequently near term.

    2. Every two months throughout pregnancy as long as weight gain is moderate.

    3. Every month for the first seven months and more frequently near term

    4. Every two weeks throughout pregnancy and more often if complications arise.

45. On each of Rose's subsequent visits to his office the physician or his nurse would probably take which of the following measurements?

    a. Weight.

    b. Serology.

    c. Urinalysis.

    d. Rh determination.

    e. Blood pressure.

        1. a and b.

        2. c and d.

        3. a, c, and e.

        4. All the above.

46. Rose's physician would probably instruct her that her total weight gain during pregnancy should not be less than:

    1. 7 kg. (15 lbs.)

    2. 9 kg. (20 lbs.)

    3. 13 kg. (24 lbs.)

    4. 16 kg. (36 lbs.)

47. Nutritional inadequacy during pregnancy is thought to contribute to:

    a. Abortion.

    b. Stillbirth.

    c. Premature birth.

    d. Congenital defects.

        1. a and b.

        2. c and d.

        3. All but d.

        4. All the above.

48. Rose should be advised to eat a diet that includes a daily minimum of:

    a. One-half liter of milk.

    b One serving of meat and one egg.

    c. One raw and two green or yellow vegetables.

    d. One citrus and one other fruit.

    e. Two slices of whole grain bread with butter.

        1. a and c.

        2. b and d.

        3. All but e.

        4. All the above.

49. Rose should be advised that which of the following foods is the best source of vitamin A?

    1. Radish.

    2. Turnip.

    3. Cucumber.

    4. Spinach.

50. Which of the following foods is the best source of vitamin B_1 (thiamine)?

    1. Pork.

    2. Pear.

    3. Milk.

    4. Carrot.

51. Which of the following foods is the best source of vitamin B_2 (riboflavin)?

    1. Tapioca.

    2. Celery.

    3. Apple.

    4. Liver.

52. Rose should be told that a particularly good source of vitamin C is:

    1. Peach.

    2. Broccoli.

    3. Apple.

    4. Carrot.

53. Rose would probably be given supplemental doses of:

    1. Phosphorus.

    2. Calcium.

    3. Iron.

    4. Potassium.

54. The nurse should teach Rose that, in addition to milk, which of the following is high in calcium content?

    1. Turnip greens.

    2. Green peppers.

    3. Sweet corn.

    4. White potatoes.

55. Rose should be directed to eat which of the following as a good source of iron?
1. Corn oil.
2. Beef liver.
3. Bran flakes.
4. Tangerines.

56. It should be explained to Rose that which of the following is especially high in sodium?
1. Bouillon cube.
2. Apple cider.
3. Grape juice.
4. Coca-Cola.

57. If it should become necessary to limit Rose's sodium intake at any time during her pregnancy she should be taught to avoid:
a. Smoked or cured meats.
b. Frozen peas and lima beans.
c. Bread and bakery products.
d. Potato chips, popcorn, and nuts.
e. Relishes, catsup, pickles, and olives.
1. a and c.
2. b and d.
3. All but e.
4. All the above.

58. During pregnancy Rose might develop varicose veins of the lower extremities or vulva as a result of:
1. Systemic circulation of microorganisms harbored in vaginal secretions.
2. Compression of the abdominal veins by the progressively enlarging uterus.
3. Increased cardiac load imposed by the oxygen needs of the growing fetus.
4. Increased venous blood volume due to return of blood from the fetus.

59. Rose said to the office nurse, "I usually douche following my menstrual period. When should I douche during my pregnancy?" Which of the following would be the most appropriate answer?
1. "You must not, under any circumstances, take a douche throughout the remainder of pregnancy, for fear of inducing abortion."
2. "It will be unnecessary for you to douche during pregnancy. If you develop excessive secretions, the doctor or nurse will advise treatment."
3. "You may continue to douche once a month during pregnancy if you use a hand bulb syringe and a small quantity of a mild solution."
4. "You may need to douche more frequently now than formerly. Vaginal secretions increase during pregnancy and may be irritating."

60. Rose may complain of heartburn during pregnancy, a symptom thought to result from:
1. Excessive secretion of hydrochloric acid by the gastric mucosal glands in response to appetite increase.
2. Tendency of acid contents of the compressed and upward displaced stomach to reflux into the lower esophagus.
3. Friction of the parietal pericardium against the dome of the diaphragm elevated by the enlarging uterus.
4. Gastritis due to hyperacidity and hyperperistalsis provoked by emotional stresses of impending motherhood.

61. Rose asked her doctor's office nurse how much physical activity she could safely engage in during pregnancy. The nurse's answer should be based on which of the following principles?
1. Pregnant women should limit physical activities to necessary self-care and household tasks.
2. A greater than usual degree of physical activity will relieve emotional and physical symptoms.
3. There need be no external limitation of physical activity imposed at any point during pregnancy.
4. The amount of physical activity during pregnancy should be proportional to the amount of activity prior to pregnancy.

62. Rose should be advised to maintain skin cleanliness during pregnancy by means of:
1. Daily sponge baths using warm water and mild soap.
2. Twice daily shower baths using cool or cold water.
3. Daily tub or shower baths using tepid water.
4. Twice weekly tub baths using hot water.

63. What instruction should Rose and her husband be given regarding coitus during pregnancy?
1. Sexual intercourse should be avoided throughout the entire period of pregnancy.
2. Intercourse should be omitted during the times at which menstruation would normally have occurred.

3. Sexual intercourse in moderation is permitted until the last six weeks of pregnancy.
4. There need be no restriction on sexual intercourse during pregnancy.

64. Rose should be taught that the tendency to constipation during pregnancy can be reduced by:
   a. Establishing the habit of defecating at the same time every day.
   b. Eating an abundance of fresh fruits and vegetables every day.
   c. Drinking water on arising and retiring and at intervals between meals.
   d. Avoiding unnecessary emotional tension and worry.
   e. Obtaining a moderate amount of balanced physical exercise.
      1. a and c.
      2. b and d.
      3. All but e.
      4. All the above.

65. Rose is most apt to first perceive quickening or "feel life" between her:
   1. 10th and 12th weeks of pregnancy.
   2. 18th and 20th weeks of pregnancy.
   3. 26th and 28th weeks of pregnancy.
   4. 34th and 36th weeks of pregnancy.

66. The stresses of pregnancy are best tolerated when which of the following are true?
   a. The pregnancy was planned or happily accepted when confirmed.
   b. The parents have a mutually supportive interpersonal relationship.
   c. Both parents have a history of adapting smoothly to new situations.
   d. Both parents accept pregnancy and childbirth as natural events.
   e. Living facilities and financial resources are adequate to needs.
      1. a and b.
      2. c and d.
      3. All but e.
      4. All the above.

67. The placenta becomes distinguishable from the remaining fetal and maternal membranes at about which stage of intrauterine development?
   1. 1st week.
   2. 1st month.
   3. 3rd month.
   4. 5th month.

68. Which of the following are functions of the placenta?
   a. Passing nutrients from the mother's blood to the fetus.
   b. Excreting wastes from fetal metabolism into the maternal blood.
   c. Transmission of oxygen from the maternal to the fetal circulation.
   d. Inhibiting the passage of bacteria and large molecules to the fetus.
   e. Synthesizing substances required for the sustenance of pregnancy.
      1. a and b.
      2. a, b, and c.
      3. All but e.
      4. All the above.

69. Which of the following hormones are secreted by the placenta?
   a. Chorionic gonadotropin.
   b. Lactogen.
   c. Estrogens.
   d. Progesterone.
   e. Testosterone.
      1. a only.
      2. a, b, and d.
      3. All but e.
      4. All the above.

70. The exchange of nutrients and wastes between mother and fetus is governed by the physical laws of:
   1. Mechanics.
   2. Transport.
   3. Gravity.
   4. Electricity.

71. In the human being the membrane that mediates the exchange of nutrients and metabolic wastes between maternal and fetal circulation is the:
   1. Chorion.
   2. Amnion.
   3. Allantois.
   4. Decidua basalis.

72. Fetal membranes referred to as the "bag of waters" consist of which of the following?
   a. Amnion.
   b. Chorion.
   c. Decidua parietalis.
   d. Decidua basalis.
      1. a and b.
      2. c and d.
      3. All but d.
      4. All the above.

73. The umbilical cord is composed of:
   1. Two arteries and a vein embedded in a gelatinous substance.
   2. An artery, a vein, and a nerve surrounded by smooth muscle.
   3. An artery and two veins encased in a sheath of skin and mucosa.
   4. A network of arterioles, capillaries, and venules enclosed in fascia.

74. Which of the following best describes the normal placenta at term?
1. A thin ragged membrane which can be rolled into a mass the size of a clenched fist.
2. A thick circular disc 15–20 cm. in diameter weighing little more than 500 grams.
3. A mass of tissue of indefinite shape containing a variable amount of clotted blood.
4. A double-walled sac 40 cm. wide containing a network of large blood vessels.

75. During the first trimester of pregnancy Rose is most apt to view her baby as:
1. An unwelcome, unwanted responsibility that threatens her personal identity and freedom.
2. An undefined concept with great future implications but without tangible evidence of reality.
3. A real person with direct and demonstrable relationship to her own present existence.
4. An independent individual whose physical and personality characteristics can be imagined.

76. The doctor and the office nurse could do which of the following to decrease Rose's fear of labor and delivery?
a. Give her a tour of the hospital's labor and delivery suite.
b. Teach her the method and purpose of abdominal breathing.
c. Encourage her to verbalize her fears about labor and delivery.
d. Describe and explain the major events of normal labor.
e. Encourage Rose and David to attend prenatal instruction classes.
    1. a and b.
    2. b, c, and d.
    3. All but e.
    4. All the above.

When Rose visited the doctor during her fifth month of pregnancy, she complained of excessive vaginal discharge and pruritus. On examination the doctor discovered profuse white vaginal secretions, and a smear of the secretions revealed numerous *Candida albicans*. The doctor ordered nystatin (Mycostatin) vaginal suppositories, 100,000 units each, to be inserted twice a day. The physician told Rose on this visit that her blood had been determined to be type A, Rh positive, and her chest x-ray and Papanicolaou smear were both negative. Because her second blood count indicated a hematocrit of 36 per cent and a hemoglobin concentration of 11 grams per 100 ml., the doctor ordered ferrous sulfate 300 mg. to be taken orally two times a day.

On Rose's visit to the doctor during her seventh month of pregnancy her hematocrit and hemoglobin levels were both at the lower range of normal and her total weight gain had been 5 kg. During this visit fetal heart tones were found to be 136 per minute.

Rose related on this visit, as she had on each previous visit, various ways in which her husband had demonstrated his enthusiasm about the forthcoming child and his eagerness to assist in making plans for the baby's advent.

Rose was relatively comfortable during her last two months of pregnancy. Then, on September 19 at 1:00 P.M., she began to have regular, cramping abdominal pain. At 5:00 P.M. her husband brought her to the hospital.

77. The nurse should advise Rose to do which of the following in order to decrease her discomfort during the pelvic examination by the doctor?
1. Hold her breath and bear down against the doctor's hand.
2. Open her mouth and breathe deeply and regularly.
3. Concentrate on contracting the muscles of the pelvic floor.
4. Grip her ankles and pull them toward her hips.

78. Rose's monilial vaginitis, if untreated, would predispose her infant to the development of:
1. Milia.
2. Enteritis.
3. Thrush.
4. Omphalitis.

79. Prior to the advent of the antibiotics, gentian violet was used to treat monilial infections. The pharmacologic effect of locally applied gentian violet solution is:
1. Antiseptic.
2. Astringent.
3. Demulcent.
4. Analgesic.

80. The chief disadvantage to the use of gentian violet is that it:
1. Ulcerates mucosa.

2. Macerates skin.
3. Causes pain.
4. Stains linen.

81. Nystatin (Mycostatin) has which of the following pharmacologic effects?

1. Antipruritic.
2. Antiallergenic.
3. Antibiotic.
4. Anti-inflammatory.

82. A test was done to determine whether Rose's blood was Rh positive or negative in order to predict whether her future infants would be apt to develop:

1. Intracranial bleeding.
2. Faulty protein metabolism.
3. Acute hemolytic anemia.
4. Respiratory distress syndrome.

83. The chief disadvantage to the use of a chest x-ray in the diagnostic workup during early pregnancy is that:

1. X-ray would be no more accurate than physical examination in diagnosing tuberculosis or heart disease.
2. Negative findings would give Rose a false sense of security concerning her need for physical rest.
3. The dosage of radiation delivered during a chest x-ray may be harmful to embryonic tissues.
4. Thoracic problems provoked or accentuated by pregnancy do not become evident until the last trimester.

84. A Papanicolaou smear of vaginal secretions is used to diagnose:

1. Monilial vaginitis.
2. Cervical carcinoma.
3. Primary syphilis.
4. Chronic cervicitis.

85. Rose's anemia would probably be characterized by red blood cells of which of the following types?

1. Microcytic, hypochromic.
2. Poikilocytic, normochromic.
3. Macrocytic, hyperchromic.
4. Spherocytic, normochromic.

86. Ferrous sulfate should be administered:

1. Midway between meals.
2. Immediately before meals.
3. Immediately after meals.
4. Separately from other medications.

87. The pregnant uterus can usually be palpable at the level of the umbilicus at about the:

1. 14th week of pregnancy.
2. 20th week of pregnancy.
3. 26th week of pregnancy.
4. 32nd week of pregnancy.

88. Fetal heart tones are rarely audible before which point in pregnancy?

1. 6th week.
2. 12th week.
3. 18th week.
4. 24th week.

89. The fetal heart rate normally lies within which range?

1. 80 to 120 beats per minute.
2. 120 to 160 beats per minute.
3. 160 to 200 beats per minute.
4. 200 to 240 beats per minute.

90. In auscultation of the abdomen the fetal heart tones must often be differentiated from which of the following other sounds?

a. Funic souffle.
b. Uterine souffle.
c. Maternal pulse.
d. Fetal movements.
 1. a and b.
 2. c and d.
 3. All but d.
 4. All the above.

91. The funic souffle is best described as:

1. A faint, gurgling sound produced by movement of gas in the mother's intestines.
2. A soft, flowing sound due to passage of blood through the dilated uterine vessels.
3. A sharp, whistling sound produced by the rush of blood through the twisted umbilical vein.
4. Abnormal maternal heart sounds produced by circulatory turbulence due to increased heart load.

92. During her third trimester Rose would be apt to display which of the following attitudes toward her pregnancy?

1. Unreal fantasies concerning angelic infants and saintly mothers paired together in idealized life situations.
2. Vacillation between welcome acceptance of the coming infant and rejection of the restricting effects of impending parenthood.
3. Personal identification with a real baby about to be born, and realistic plans for future child care responsibilities.
4. Nonchalant indifference concerning all matters relating to the infant's future existence and her own relationship to him.

93. Which of the following instructions should the doctor's nurse give Rose concerning her admission to the hospital at term?

1. To wait until her contractions are of 90 seconds' duration at two minute intervals before going to the hospital.
2. To take with her enough money to pay the cost of three days of hospitalization at the time of registration.
3. To leave money, jewelry, and other valuables at home when she enters the hospital for labor and delivery.
4. To take with her a suitcase containing all clothing and belongings that she will need during hospitalization.

94. About the beginning of September Rose suddenly felt a sense of lightness or freedom in her upper abdomen. This sensation was the result of:

1. Decrease in the size of the placenta due to reduced blood flow.
2. Slow absorption of a portion of the amniotic fluid by the placenta.
3. Descent of the fetus with engagement of the presenting part in the pelvis.
4. Increased abdominal capacity due to separation of muscles of the abdominal wall.

When Rose entered the hospital at 5:00 P.M. on September 19 she was having moderate contractions at 10-minute intervals. The bag of waters was intact, the cervix was 25 per cent effaced, and the presenting part of the fetus was at 0 station. Rose's temperature was 98.9° F. orally, her pulse 96, respirations 22, blood pressure 120/70 mm. Hg, deep tendon reflexes 2+, hematocrit 38 per cent, urine negative, height 163 cm., and weight 70 kg. (weight before pregnancy had been 58 kg.). Physical examination revealed a term pregnancy with a vertex presentation in left occiput anterior position. The fetal heart tones were 140 per minute.

Rose was given a shower and a tap water enema on admission to the labor unit. At 6:00 P.M. Rose's cervix was 50 per cent effaced and 1 cm. dilated, with the presenting part at 0 station. At 7:00 P.M. Rose's cervix was 70 per cent effaced and the presenting part was at 0 station. At 9:00 P.M. the cervix was 100 per cent effaced and 3 cm. dilated and the presenting part was at 0 station. At 12:00 midnight the cervix was 6 cm. dilated and the station was +2. The physician ruptured the bag of waters, started an intravenous of 5 per cent glucose, and performed an epidural block. At 2:00 A.M. the cervix was 8 cm. dilated and the station was +3. At 3:00 A.M. a left mediolateral episiotomy was done and a 3300 gram (7.25 pound) boy was delivered. The placenta was expelled intact and methylergonovine maleate (Methergine) 0.2 mg. (1 ml.) was administered intravenously.

The infant's Apgar rating at 60 seconds after birth was 10. Fetal heart tones had varied between 140 and 144 throughout labor.

The episiotomy was repaired with absorbable 00 chromic catgut.

95. Uterine muscle differs from skeletal and other smooth muscle cells in:

1. Building up gradually to a peak of contraction.
2. Requiring lower oxygen supply for contractile efficiency.
3. Having the ability to retract between contractions.
4. Being impervious to ischemia, fatigue, and tetany.

96. The uterine musculature is most dense in the region of the:

1. Fundus.
2. Body.
3. Isthmus.
4. Cervix.

97. The fundus and upper uterine segment contain which of the following muscle types?

1. Circular smooth muscle fibers only.
2. Both circular and longitudinal smooth muscle.
3. A syncytium of interconnecting muscle fibers.
4. Oblique sheets of striated muscle fibers.

98. The lower uterine segment is that part of the uterus which lies below the level of the:

1. Fallopian tubes.
2. Isthmus.
3. Cervix.
4. Fornices.

99. The cervix and lower uterine segment are maintained in position during labor as a result of their attachment to the posterior pelvic wall by the:

1. Broad ligaments.
2. Round ligaments.
3. Uterosacral ligaments.
4. Parietal peritoneum.

100. The ridge between the upper and lower uterine segments is the:

1. Pars uterina.

2. Placental margin.
3. Contraction ring.
4. Internal os.

101. Which of the following have been suggested as contributing to the initiation of labor?

a. Drop in progesterone production.
b. Increased uterine irritability.
c. Diminution of placental blood supply.
d. Pituitary production of oxytocin.
e. Reflex contraction of the overdistended uterus.
    1. a and b.
    2. a, b, and c.
    3. All but e.
    4. All the above.

102. Since Rose's baby's position was left occiput anterior, the doctor would have observed which of the following signs on abdominal palpation to determine lie, presentation, and position?

a. A horizontal uterine ovoid.
b. A hard round mass in the lower abdomen.
c. Numerous nodular formations on the right side of the abdomen.
d. A large, soft, irregular mass in the uterine fundus.
    1. All but a.
    2. All but b.
    3. All but c.
    4. All but d.

103. Rose may experience nausea and vomiting during labor as a result of a tendency for:

1. Hydrochloric acid to be produced in excessive amounts.
2. Obstruction of bile flow into the small intestine.
3. Gastrointestinal motility and absorption to be decreased.
4. Anxiety to be expressed in oral-gastric symptoms.

104. In determining the duration and frequency of Rose's contractions the nurse should:

1. Distract Rose conversationally so that she is unaware that the contraction is being timed.
2. Measure only one contraction at a time so that Rose does not become too tired.
3. Time three consecutive contractions in any one period of time to ensure a representative sample.
4. Have a second nurse time the dura-

tion of the contractions while she times their frequency.

105. In evaluating the strength and duration of Rose's uterine contractions the nurse should:

1. Press her fingertips deeply and firmly into the soft tissues above the pubis.
2. Cup her hand over the area immediately to the left or right of the umbilicus.
3. Move her palm quickly from one point to another over the anterior abdomen.
4. Place her hand, with fingers spread, lightly over the fundus of the uterus.

106. In determining the duration of Rose's contractions the nurse should measure the time interval between:

1. The beginning of a contraction and the acme of that contraction.
2. The acme of a contraction and the end of the same contraction.
3. The beginning of a contraction and the end of the same contraction.
4. The beginning of a contraction and the beginning of the next contraction.

107. In determining the frequency of contractions the nurse should measure the time from:

1. The completion of one contraction to the beginning of the next.
2. The beginning of one contraction to the completion of the next.
3. The acme of one contraction to the beginning of the next.
4. The beginning of one contraction to the beginning of the next.

108. A tap water enema was given to Rose on her admission to the labor room in order to:

a. Increase the accuracy of rectal examinations to determine cervical effacement and dilation.
b. Facilitate labor by removing space-occupying masses which could obstruct fetal passage.
c. Prevent fecal contamination of the infant and the genital tract during delivery.
d. Reduce postpartum discomfort by decreasing or postponing strain on the episiotomy wound.
    1. a and b.
    2. c and d.
    3. All but d.
    4. All the above.

109. Which of the following cardinal movements occurs first in the mechanism of normal labor?
1. Internal rotation.
2. Flexion.
3. Descent.
4. Extension.

110. In a vertex presentation the fetal head usually enters the pelvic inlet so that the anteroposterior diameter of the head occupies which plane of the pelvic inlet?
1. Longitudinal.
2. Transverse.
3. Right oblique.
4. Left oblique.

111. The physiologic advantage to be gained by flexion of the fetal head during labor is the fact that in the flexed position:
1. Perineal pressure is less apt to be exerted on the anterior fontanel.
2. The head presents its smallest diameter to the pelvic inlet.
3. The head is able to exert greater pressure against the cervix.
4. The fetal nose and mouth are less apt to be obstructed by secretions.

112. Which of the following cardinal movements follows flexion in the mechanism of normal labor?
1. Engagement.
2. Internal rotation.
3. Extension.
4. External rotation.

113. As the first stage of labor progresses, which of the following changes occur in the uterus?
1. Both the upper and lower segments become longer and thinner.
2. Both the upper and lower segments become shorter and thicker.
3. The upper segment becomes shorter and thicker, the lower segment longer and thinner.
4. The upper segment becomes longer and thinner, the lower segment shorter and thicker.

114. At 8:00 P.M. Rose complained of being hungry. The nurse could safely give her:
1. Glucose water.
2. Custard.
3. Ice cream.
4. Dry toast.

115. During the second phase of Rose's first stage of labor (when her cervix was dilating from 3 to 7 cm. in diameter) the nurse should instruct her to:
1. Practice deep abdominal breathing during contractions and relax between them.
2. Take a deep breath, hold it, and forcefully bear down with each contraction.
3. Get out of bed, push on the side rails, and practice isometric exercises between contractions.
4. Assume the knee-chest position and practice pelvic rocking between contractions.

116. The nurse could best reduce Rose's discomfort during the third or transitional phase of her first stage of labor by:
1. Encouraging her to talk of her home and family.
2. Explaining diagrams illustrating the birth process.
3. Applying pressure to the sacral area of her back.
4. Giving her a complete bath and linen change.

117. How frequently should the nurse take fetal heart tones during Rose's first stage of labor?
1. Every 15–60 minutes.
2. Every 60–90 minutes.
3. Every 90–120 minutes.
4. Every 120–150 minutes.

118. The nurse should be aware that which of the following variations in fetal heart tones may be considered normal?
1. Decrease in volume during the second stage of labor.
2. Decrease in rate during the midportion of contraction.
3. Increase in rate following rupture of the membranes.
4. Increase in volume during internal rotation of the head.

119. During the transitional phase of the first stage of labor Rose seemed somewhat confused, discouraged, and irritable. Which of the following comments by the nurse would be most supportive at this time?
1. "This phase of your labor will last only one hour. Since you've already weathered nine hours of pain, you can surely hang on for a little longer."
2. "These are the hardest pains you

will have. Before long you'll be able to bear down with your contractions and it will be much easier for you.''

3. "I know that you're feeling great pain, but I'm sure that you can withstand this discomfort in a way that you can retain your self-control.''

4. "You have no reason to be discouraged. Your doctor is here, the nurses are all ready to help you, and the finest obstetrical equipment is available.''

120. Effacement is the process by which the cervix is:

1. Opened to its widest possible diameter.
2. Incorporated into the lower uterine segment.
3. Freed of the mucus plug occluding it.
4. Forced to invaginate into the upper vagina.

121. Cervical effacement and dilatation are brought about by:

a. Contraction of the uterine muscles.
b. Contraction of abdominal muscles.
c. Pressure from the bag of waters.
d. Lengthening of the vagina.
e. Pressure of the presenting part of the fetus.
   1. a only.
   2. a and b.
   3. a, c, or e.
   4. All the above.

122. Rose said to the nurse, "I wish the doctor hadn't ruptured my bag of waters. Now I'll have a dry birth.'' Which of the following responses by the nurse would be most appropriate?

1. "You needn't worry about that. Your doctor is very experienced in these matters and wouldn't do anything to jeopardize your welfare.''
2. "You have no need for concern. Rupturing the sac allows the baby's head to descend and labor is apt to be shortened as a result.''
3. "I understand that having a dry birth concerns you, but certain discomforts have to be borne for the sake of your baby's welfare.''
4. "We have weighed the chance of infection against the possible shortening of your labor and have decided to rupture your membranes.''

123. The physician waited until the fetal head was well engaged before he ruptured the bag of waters in order to:

1. Enable the bag of waters to rupture spontaneously if possible, thus avoiding difficult and painful instrumentation.
2. Prevent prolapse of the umbilical cord during the forceful expulsion of amniotic fluid from the sac.
3. Ensure that a small amount of amniotic fluid would be left in the upper portion of the amniotic sac.
4. Have the amniotic sac in a dependent enough position that it could be reached without difficulty.

124. The first stage of labor is considered to have terminated when:

1. Regular three-minute contractions have been established.
2. The bag of waters has been ruptured and drained.
3. The cervix has been completely effaced and dilated.
4. The presenting part is visible during contractions.

125. The cervix is considered to be completely dilated when the diameter of the os is:

1. 8 cm.
2. 10 cm.
3. 12 cm.
4. 14 cm.

126. The pain which Rose experienced during labor resulted from:

a. Contraction of uterine muscle when it is in an ischemic state.
b. Pressure on nerve ganglia in the cervix and lower uterine segment.
c. Stretching of ligaments adjacent to the uterus and in the pelvic joints.
d. Stretching and displacement of the tissues of the vulva and perineum.
   1. a and c.
   2. b and d.
   3. All but d.
   4. All the above.

127. Several times during Rose's labor the doctor performed a rectal examination in order to obtain information concerning:

a. Cervical effacement.
b. Cervical dilatation.
c. Station of the presenting part.
d. Type of presentation.
e. Position of the fetus.
   1. a and b.
   2. a, b, and d.
   3. All but e.
   4. All the above.

128. In the event that Rose had not urinated voluntarily during the late first stage and the second stage of labor, the nurse should first have:
1. Administered copious amounts of water and clear fluids at frequent intervals.
2. Poured water over her vulva in order to initiate relaxation of the urethral sphincter.
3. Exerted strong steady pressure with the palm of her hand on the lower abdomen.
4. Placed her on the bedpan and asked her to void in order to facilitate labor.

129. The nurse could have anticipated that the average length of Rose's contractions during the second stage of labor would be:
1. 30 seconds.
2. 60 seconds.
3. 2 minutes.
4. 4 minutes.

130. During the second stage of labor Rose's contractions would probably occur at approximately which interval?
1. Every 1 to 3 minutes.
2. Every 3 to 5 minutes.
3. Every 5 to 7 minutes.
4. Every 7 to 9 minutes.

131. In timing Rose's contractions the nurse should notify the physician if she detects a contraction lasting longer than:
1. 60 seconds.
2. 90 seconds.
3. 120 seconds.
4. 150 seconds.

132. The mechanics of the second stage of labor differ from those of the first in that during the second stage:
1. The lower uterine segment contracts more than the fundus.
2. The abdominal muscles assist in the expulsion of the fetus.
3. The joints of the pelvis are stretched and dislocated.
4. All muscles involved in fetal propulsion undergo tetany.

133. Station may best be defined as the:
1. Ratio of the degree of cervical dilation accomplished to the total possible dilation.
2. Relationship of the long axis of the fetus to the long axis of the mother's body.
3. Positional relationship of the furthermost part of the fetus to the maternal ischial spines.

134. The fetal head is engaged when:
1. The vertex of the skull is level with the symphysis pubis.
2. The biparietal diameter has passed the pelvic inlet.
3. The head rotates from the transverse to the anteroposterior position.
4. The head has descended beyond the external cervical os.

135. Fetal position during labor refers to the:
1. First body part of the fetus felt by the examiner upon vaginal examination.
2. Relationship of a fixed point of the fetus to the quadrants of the maternal pelvis.
3. Relationship of the furthermost fetal part to the ischial spines of the maternal pelvis.
4. Relationship of the long axis of the fetus to the long axis of the mother's body.

136. The nurse should expect to observe which of the following changes in Rose's vital signs during the second stage of labor?
1. Decrease in temperature.
2. Increase in blood pressure.
3. Decrease in pulse rate.
4. Increase in urinary output.

137. During the early second stage of Rose's labor fetal heart tones should be taken at least every:
1. 2 to 4 minutes.
2. 5 to 10 minutes.
3. 10 to 20 minutes.
4. 20 to 30 minutes.

138. The changes in shape of the infant's head which occur due to pressure from the walls of the birth canal are called:
1. Molding.
2. Cephalhematoma.
3. Microcephaly.
4. Caput succedaneum.

139. Aseptic technique during delivery includes:
a. Cleansing of the mother's vulva, thighs, and lower abdomen with an antiseptic or detergent solution.
b. Wearing of sterile gown and gloves, clean cap and mask by the attending physician and nurse.
c. Preparation of a sterile field and use of sterile equipment and supplies during delivery.
d. Covering the patient's abdomen,

thighs, legs, and feet with a sterile drape.

  e. Covering the patient's mouth and nose with a mask and her hands with gloves.
    1. a and b.
    2. a, b, and c.
    3. All but e.
    4. All the above.

140. As soon as "crowning" occurs Rose should be told to:
  1. Take a deep breath and bear down.
  2. Open her mouth and pant rapidly.
  3. Raise herself up on her elbows.
  4. Spread her thighs further apart.

141. In the event that crowning occurs when Rose is in the delivery room but her doctor is not available, the nurse should:
  1. Place a sterile towel over the infant's head and apply manual pressure until a physician arrives.
  2. Place a mask over Rose's face and administer a few drops of ether to delay delivery.
  3. Call for help, stay with Rose, and guide the slow delivery of the head between contractions.
  4. Instruct Rose to hold her knees together and leave to obtain help from an experienced nurse.

142. The most common position for the fetus at birth is the:
  1. Right occiput anterior.
  2. Left occiput anterior.
  3. Right occiput posterior.
  4. Left occiput posterior.

143. The physician performed the left mediolateral episiotomy primarily in order to:
  1. Decrease the chance of fetal aspiration.
  2. Reduce the pain due to perineal stretching.
  3. Prevent laceration of the perineum and the anal sphincter.
  4. Reduce the likelihood of fetal asphyxiation.

144. As soon as the infant's head is delivered the physician will:
  1. Examine the vulva and perineum for lacerations.
  2. Determine whether the cord encircles the neck.
  3. Exert strong steady pressure on the fundus.
  4. Rotate the shoulders to the anterolateral position.

145. After the aforementioned step had been taken, the physician would:
  1. Instill silver nitrate solution into the infant's conjunctival sacs and close his lids.
  2. Inject carbocaine locally and cut through the skin, fourchet, and urogenital septum.
  3. Clear the infant's nose and mouth of mucus, amniotic fluid, and vaginal secretions.
  4. Apply pressure to the infant's crown to dislodge the shoulder from the pubic arch.

146. The second stage of labor ends with:
  1. Complete cervical dilation.
  2. Bulging of the perineum.
  3. Delivery of the baby.
  4. Removal of the placenta.

147. Immediately after Rose's baby was delivered he was probably held or placed below the level of his mother's vulva for a few minutes so that:
  1. Blood and secretions could be removed from his face and body before his mother saw him.
  2. The blood in the placenta could enter the infant's body on the basis of gravity flow.
  3. The weight of the umbilical cord could facilitate release of the placenta.
  4. The slippery, active infant would be less apt to fall a great distance if dropped.

148. The physician would separate the infant from the placenta by:
  1. Dividing the cord midway between infant and placenta and disinfecting the cut surfaces.
  2. Ligating and severing the cord at its junction with the skin of the infant's abdomen.
  3. Double-clamping and cutting the cord at a point 2 to 3 centimeters from the infant's navel.
  4. Cutting the cord 7 to 8 centimeters from the umbilicus and cauterizing the stump with silver nitrate.

149. Immediately after birth the infant's respirations might be stimulated or assisted by:
  1. Bringing his feet to his face.
  2. Gentle slapping of his heels.
  3. Immersing him in cold water.
  4. Digital dilation of his anus.

150. Since Rose's infant was given an Apgar score of 10 at 60 seconds following delivery, one can assume that his heart rate at one minute after birth was:
1. Not discernible.
2. Between 50 and 100 per minute.
3. Exactly 100 per minute.
4. Over 100 per minute.

151. An Apgar rating of 10 at 60 seconds after birth signifies that the infant has demonstrated:
1. Lack of any type of respiratory movement.
2. Faint chest movement, with no cry.
3. Shallow chest movement, with a weak cry.
4. Good respiratory movements, with a strong cry.

152. An Apgar score of 10 indicates that at one minute after birth the infant's skin color was:
1. Blue throughout all body parts.
2. Pallid throughout all body parts.
3. Pink in the trunk, with blue extremities.
4. Completely pink throughout the body.

153. Immediate care of the newborn infant with an Apgar score of 10 should include:
a. Suctioning secretions from the nose and mouth.
b. Wrapping him in a sterile blanket.
c. Instilling drops into the eyes.
d. Placing him on his side in a heated bed.
e. Lowering the head of the crib.
   1. a and c.
   2. a, b, and d.
   3. All but e.
   4. All the above.

154. Normally, separation of the placenta occurs predominantly as a result of:
1. Tension exerted on the umbilical cord and placenta by the descent and emergence of the fetus during birth.
2. Disproportion between the size of the placenta and the reduced size of the site of placental attachment.
3. Hemodynamic changes in the placenta resulting from interrupted blood flow in the arteries and veins of the cord.
4. Exertion of external force on the uterine fundus by strenuous contraction of the abdominal muscles.

155. The physician would be able to determine when the placenta had completely separated from its uterine attachment because:
1. The placenta and cord would be spontaneously expelled through the vaginal canal.
2. The uterus would rise in the abdomen and change from discoid to globular form.
3. The mother's pulse and respiratory rate would increase and her blood pressure would decrease.
4. A sharp tug on the umbilical cord would result in prompt descent of the placenta.

156. In addition to the aforementioned change, other signs of placental separation might be:
a. Advancement of the visible section of the cord.
b. Sudden gushing of a moderate amount of blood.
c. Perception of acute abdominal pain by the mother.
d. Bulging of the perineum and distention of the vulva.
   1. a and b.
   2. c and d.
   3. All but d.
   4. All the above.

157. The third stage of labor is completed when the:
1. Umbilical cord has been clamped and cut.
2. Placenta and cord have been completely expelled.
3. Uterine fundus has contracted into a firm mass.
4. Uterus has been emptied of all blood and clots.

158. The fourth stage of labor is considered to be:
1. The interval between delivery and recovery from anesthesia.
2. The period of active vaginal bleeding following delivery.
3. The hour immediately following delivery of the placenta.
4. The time required for uterine massage and episiotomy repair.

159. The primary purpose of administering

methylergonovine maleate to Rose following delivery of the placenta was to:

1. Reduce postpartum infection.
2. Prevent postpartum hemorrhage.
3. Foster healing of lacerations.
4. Complete uterine involution.

160. The pharmacologic action of methylergonovine maleate (Methergine) is to:

1. Catalyze the formation of fibrin from fibrinogen.
2. Stimulate forceful contraction of uterine muscle.
3. Foster capillary resorption of inflammatory exudate.
4. Inhibit growth and multiplication of pathogens.

161. During the fourth stage of labor the condition of Rose's uterine fundus should be checked every:

1. 5 minutes.
2. 10 minutes.
3. 15 minutes.
4. 20 minutes.

162. During the fourth stage of labor the nurse should watch Rose closely for postpartum hemorrhage by:

a. Measuring the rate and volume of her pulse at frequent intervals.
b. Frequently noting the rate and character of her respirations.
c. Removing her perineal pads to determine the amount of blood absorbed.
d. Placing her hand under Rose's hips to check the lower linen for blood.
   1. a and b.
   2. c and d.
   3. All but d.
   4. All the above.

The physician wrote the following orders for Rose's care during the postpartum period:

1. Ferrous sulfate 300 mg. orally, b.i.d.
2. Propoxyphene hydrochloride (Darvon) 65 mg. orally, p.r.n. for pain.
3. Diazepam (Valium) 5 mg. orally, t.i.d.
4. Milk of magnesia 30 cc. orally, h.s., p.r.n.
5. General diet.
6. Shower as soon as desired.
'7. Blood pressure q.i.d.
8. Record intake and output for first 24 hours.
9. Will breast-feed.

10. If no complications, plan for discharge on third postpartum day.

163. If, on palpation of uterine fundus during Rose's fourth stage of labor, the nurse should find the fundus boggy, the nurse should:

1. Check the consistency of the fundus again after a 15 minute interval.
2. Massage the fundus firmly with the open hand until it becomes firm.
3. Grasp the fundus between thumb and fingers and pinch it forcefully.
4. Turn Rose onto her abdomen to compress her fundus against the mattress.

164. The nurse should expect that Rose would completely saturate a perineal pad within which interval of time following delivery?

1. 10 minutes.
2. 30 minutes.
3. 60 minutes.
4. 120 minutes.

165. The chief purpose for instilling silver nitrate solution into the newborn infant's eyes immediately after delivery is to prevent infection by:

1. *Streptococcus pyogenes.*
2. *Staphylococcus aureus.*
3. *Escherichia coli.*
4. *Neisseria gonorrhoeae.*

166. The method of choice for official identification of newborn infants would be the immediate postnatal:

1. Recording of footprints.
2. Recording of palmprints.
3. Attachment of proper identification band.
4. Description of ear lobe configuration.

167. The procedure for identification of the newborn infant should be carried out:

1. After the infant is delivered and aspirated but before the umbilical cord is clamped and cut.
2. As soon as possible after birth and while mother and infant are together in the delivery room.
3. After the mother has been taken to the ward and before the infant has been taken to the nursery.
4. Immediately upon the infant's arrival in the receiving area of the nursery and before his admission bath.

168. In addition to the recording of footprints, which further step should be taken in the delivery room to ensure proper identification of Rose's son?

    1. Securing a sample of his blood for typing procedures.
    2. Taking full face and profile photographs of his head.
    3. Affixing a nameband to two of his extremities.
    4. Recording specific descriptive identifying data on his chart.

169. Rose's care during the few days following delivery should be directed toward:

    a. Preventing puerperal infection.
    b. Fostering involutional changes.
    c. Providing physical and mental rest.
    d. Teaching self-care and baby care.
    e. Facilitating emotional solidarity of new family.
        1. a and b.
        2. a, b, and c.
        3. All but e.
        4. All the above.

170. During Rose's first postpartum day, displacement of her uterus to the right of the midline of the abdomen would probably indicate:

    1. Distention of the bladder.
    2. Retention of feces.
    3. Leiomyoma of the uterus.
    4. Postpartum endometritis.

171. How soon should Rose be able to get out of bed to go to the bathroom following delivery?

    1. Within 1 hour.
    2. Within 24 hours.
    3. Within 48 hours.
    4. Within 72 hours.

172. During Rose's second postpartum day palpation of her uterine fundus should reveal its consistency to be:

    1. Soft and boggy.
    2. Spongy and elastic.
    3. Nodular and crepitant.
    4. Smooth and hard.

173. During the first two or three days following delivery Rose may be expected to show:

    a. Increased need for sleep.
    b. Heightened interest in food.
    c. Concern for her own needs.
    d. Distrust of doctors and nurses.
    e. Marked interest in socialization.
        1. a and b.

        2. a, b, and c.
        3. c, d, and e.
        4. All the above.

174. The nurse should expect Rose to exhibit which of the following attitudes during the first two or three days after delivery?

    1. Passive and dependent.
    2. Anxious and fearful.
    3. Hostile and critical.
    4. Aggressive and independent.

175. By Rose's third postpartum day the fundus of her uterus should be palpated at which of the following levels?

    1. At the xiphoid process of the sternum.
    2. Four fingerbreadths above the umbilicus.
    3. At the umbilicus or at waist level.
    4. Four fingerbreadths below the umbilicus.

176. If Rose develops afterpains the nurse should explain to her that such pains are the result of:

    1. Reflex dilation of vessels of the endometrium.
    2. Progressive contraction of the uterine muscles.
    3. Release of tension on the uterine ligaments.
    4. Distention of the graafian follicle with fluid.

177. If, during the early postpartum period, Rose should complain of pain in her perineal region, which of the following measures might be employed to relieve her discomfort?

    a. Focusing a heat lamp on the perineal area.
    b. Application of topical analgesics in spray form.
    c. Administration of a mild analgesic by mouth.
    d. Provision of warm sitz baths twice daily.
        1. a and b.
        2. c and d.
        3. All but d.
        4. All the above.

178. During the first week following delivery Rose might be expected to experience a temporary emotional depression for a few days, which is thought to result from:

    1. Delayed reaction to the pain and discomfort of labor.
    2. Hormonal changes taking place during the puerperium.

3. Fearful anticipation of the responsibility of motherhood.
4. Jealousy of her husband's attentions to the child.

179. At about the time that Rose is discharged from the hospital, her lochia might be expected to change from:

1. Bright red to dark red blood.
2. Dark red to dark brown discharge.
3. Dark brown to faintly pink discharge.
4. Faint pink to colorless discharge.

180. Rose's chances of acquiring a puerperal infection could be greatly reduced by teaching her to:

a. Wash her perineum daily with a clean cloth, soap, and warm water.
b. Cleanse her vulva from front to back following each defecation.
c. Change perineal pads at least as frequently as every four hours.
d. Refrain from sexual intercourse and vaginal douching for two weeks.
   1. a and c.
   2. b and d.
   3. All but d.
   4. All the above.

181. Which of the following factors frequently predispose to puerperal infection?

a. Premature rupture of membranes.
b. Prolonged and difficult labor.
c. Hemorrhage following delivery.
d. Retention of placental fragments.
e. Manual removal of the placenta.
   1. a and b.
   2. c and d.
   3. All but d.
   4. All the above.

182. Which of the following is the usual mode of transmitting organisms that cause puerperal infection?

1. Droplet infection from nose and throat secretions of the doctor or nurse during delivery.
2. Coitus occurring late in pregnancy, particularly if the bag of waters has ruptured.
3. Transmission of vaginal organisms into the uterus during vaginal examination or operative manipulations.
4. Use of contaminated needles and syringes in administering parenteral medications during labor.

183. Diagnosis of puerperal infection is made on the basis of:

a. Temperature of 40° C. or above on any two of the first ten postpartum days, excluding the first 24 hours.
b. Culture of secretions obtained from the uterine cavity by passage of a sterile swab through the cervical canal.
c. Persistent observation of foul-smelling and excessive lochia during the first seven days following delivery.
d. Complaints of pain or tenderness in the vulva, vagina, pelvis, or midportion of the abdomen.
   1. a and b.
   2. c and d.
   3. All but d.
   4. All the above.

184. The organism most frequently responsible for puerperal infection is:

1. Anaerobic staphylococcus.
2. Anaerobic streptococcus.
3. Anaerobic gram-negative rods.
4. Anaerobic diphtheroid organisms.

185. The most common pathological manifestation of puerperal infection is:

1. Vaginitis.
2. Endometritis.
3. Myometritis.
4. Parametritis.

186. The usual treatment for puerperal sepsis is:

1. Administration of antibiotics to which the cultured organism is susceptible.
2. Draining accumulations of purulent material in the pelvis by colpotomy.
3. Continuous irrigation of the uterine cavity with antiseptic solutions.
4. Cervical dilation and curettage of the necrotic uterine mucosal lining.

187. Possible complications of puerperal infection include:

a. Pelvic thrombophlebitis.
b. Femoral thrombophlebitis.
c. Pulmonary abscess.
d. Pelvic cellulitis.
e. Generalized peritonitis.
   1. a and b.
   2. a, b, and e.
   3. All but d.
   4. All the above.

188. In addition to the 5 to 5.5 kg. lost at delivery, Rose would probably lose another 2.5 kg. during the puerperium as a result of:

1. Decreased interest in food.
2. Loss of extracellular fluid.
3. Increased motor activity.
4. Elevated metabolic rate.

189. Rose's protein requirement would be highest during the:
1. First trimester of pregnancy.
2. Second trimester of pregnancy.
3. Third trimester of pregnancy.
4. Trimester following delivery.

190. Which of the following best explains why Rose did not lactate during pregnancy?
1. Stimulation of the breast by sucking is the factor responsible for initiating milk production.
2. Ovulation is necessary for initiating production of hormones which stimulate lactation.
3. Only a fully mature placenta is able to produce the hormones for milk stimulation.
4. Estrogen and progesterone secreted during pregnancy inhibited production of prolactin.

191. Normal breast milk differs from colostrum in that breast milk contains proportionately:
1. More protein and more salts.
2. Less sugar and more fat.
3. Less protein and more fat.
4. Less sugar and less fat.

192. Rose should be instructed that her breasts will begin to secrete milk:
1. During the 4th stage of labor.
2. During the 1st postpartum day.
3. During the 2nd postpartum day.
4. During the 3rd postpartum day.

193. Following delivery, care of Rose's breasts should consist of:
1. Daily scrubbing with strong soap and warm water.
2. Cleansing the nipples before and applying nipple cream after each breast feeding.
3. Twice daily bathing with detergent and rinsing with sterile water.
4. Washing daily with plain water during cleansing bath or shower.

194. Breast engorgement during the first few postpartum days is the result of:
1. Increased lymphatic and venous circulation.
2. Distention of the ductile system with milk.
3. Increase in the volume of interstitial fluid.
4. Obstruction of the ampulla by muscular spasm.

195. If Rose complains of pain due to breast engorgement, which of the following measures might be used to decrease her discomfort?
1. Removal of her brassiere or breast binder.
2. Application of ice packs to her breasts.
3. Encouraging her to lie on her side.
4. Deep massage of the breasts several times daily.

196. Following delivery Rose should wear a breast binder or brassiere in order to:
a. Decrease discomfort from breast engorgement.
b. Prevent contamination of nipples and areolae.
c. Prevent permanent distortion due to overdistention.
d. Reduce exposure and embarrassment during feeding.
1. a and b.
2. c and d.
3. All but d.
4. All the above.

197. During the time that she is breast-feeding Rose should ingest what quantity of milk each day?
1. One cup to one pint.
2. One pint to one quart.
3. One quart to a quart and a half.
4. A quart and a half to two quarts.

198. During the first two days of breast-feedings the nurse should encourage Rose to limit the duration of sucking at each feeding to:
1. 3 to 5 minutes.
2. 6 to 10 minutes.
3. 11 to 15 minutes.
4. 16 to 20 minutes.

199. When Rose feeds her baby for the first time the nurse should:
1. Leave the room so Rose can interact with her baby without the presence of an authority figure.
2. Assure that the infant is sucking adequately before attending to other duties in the room.
3. Remain at Rose's side throughout the feeding period in order to give needed supervision.
4. Take the infant from Rose at intervals throughout the feeding in order to bubble him.

200. Rose should be taught to take which of the following precautions in order to decrease contamination of her infant during feeding?

1. Take a complete cleansing shower each morning.
2. Wear a breast binder 24 hours a day.
3. Wash her hands preceding each feeding.
4. Lower the spread and place the infant on the upper sheet.

201. Rose should be taught that if she develops cracks in her nipples, she should:
   a. Shorten the feeding time from the affected breast for 24 to 36 hours.
   b. Bathe the nipple frequently in 70 per cent alcohol.
   c. Cover the nipple with a shield during nursing.
   d. Cover the areola with a band-aid between feedings.
   e. Expose her breast to a therapeutic lamp twice daily.
      1. a and b.
      2. b and d.
      3. a, c, and e.
      4. All but e.

202. Besides providing a clean environment, the best method for preventing infection in a newborn infant is the use of:
      1. Proper hand washing technique.
      2. Isolation of each newborn infant.
      3. Use of individual rectal thermometers.
      4. Frequent diaper and linen changes.

203. In order to evaluate the vital signs of Rose's infant the nursery nurse should know that which of the following are normal values for the newborn?
      1. Temperature 37.8° C., pulse 80 per minute, respirations 20 per minute.
      2. Temperature 37.2° C., pulse 90 per minute, respirations 30 per minute.
      3. Temperature 36.6° C., pulse 130 per minute, respirations 40 per minute.
      4. Temperature 36° C., pulse 180 per minute, respirations 60 per minute.

204. If the nursery nurse observes that Rose's infant seems to have excessive mucus drainage from the mouth she should:
   a. Gently suction the infant's mouth with a bulb syringe.
   b. Elevate the foot of the bed to allow gravitational drainage.
   c. Record her observation and check his condition frequently.
   d. Inform the doctor of her observations on his next visit.
      1. a only.
      2. a and b.

3. All but d.
4. All the above.

205. The normal newborn infant demonstrates which of the following feeding reflexes at birth?
   a. Rooting reflex.
   b. Sucking reflex.
   c. Swallowing reflex.
   d. Gag reflex.
   e. Retrusive reflex.
      1. a and c.
      2. b and d.
      3. All but e.
      4. All the above.

206. The Moro reflex, which can be elicited in the normal newborn, consists of:
      1. Sharp dorsiflexion of the great toe and fanning of the remaining toes on stimulation of the sole of the foot.
      2. Turning his head toward the direction from which a stimulus is applied to his cheek or occiput.
      3. Symmetrical abduction and extension of both arms followed by adduction of the arms with slight tremors.
      4. Reciprocal flexion and extension of the leg when the sole of the foot touches a firm surface.

207. Since silver nitrate solution often irritates the infant's eyes, the nursery nurse should:
   a. Cleanse the eyes daily with sterile water.
   b. Wash from the inner to the outer canthus of the eye.
   c. Use a clean cotton ball for the cleansing of each eye.
   d. Grasp the head firmly to prevent trauma by the dropper.
      1. a only.
      2. a and b.
      3. a, b, and c.
      4. All the above.

208. Rose's infant's first feeding, of glucose water, will be given by the nursery nurse in order to:
      1. Allow Rose a period of long, uninterrupted rest following delivery.
      2. Decrease his exposure to pathogens during his first hours of life.
      3. Enable the nurse to observe any feeding problems which may exist.
      4. Ensure that the infant's first feeding experience be a pleasant one.

209. Rose should be told to expect that following several passages of meconium her infant will excrete a transitional stool which is typically:
1. Light yellow with pasty consistency.
2. Golden yellow with firm consistency.
3. Chartreuse with watery consistency.
4. Green, containing much mucus and flatus.

210. It is important that the nurse chart the infant's first urination and first meconium stool because:
1. The passage of these excretions is the best indicator that the infant can be given milk.
2. Absence of one of these excretions may indicate that the digestive or urinary tract is obstructed.
3. The character and consistency of the stool and urine determine the infant's future fluid needs.
4. The change from meconium to normal feces indicates that bacteria have colonized the intestine.

211. Observation of a minimal degree of jaundice in Rose's infant between the third and fifth days of life would probably be interpreted as indicating:
1. Erythroblastosis fetalis.
2. Biliary tract obstruction.
3. Acute viral hepatitis.
4. Normal neonatal hemolysis.

Rose and the baby both prospered during the three days following delivery. The infant learned to breast-feed without difficulty and lost only 220 grams of weight between September 20 and September 23. Rose's temperature, which had been 37.6° C. orally on September 20, decreased to 37° C. orally on the following day and remained normal thereafter.

Rose attended demonstrations of a baby bath and of the procedure for bottle sterilization, and her husband brought the infant's clothing to the hospital on September 23, when Rose and her son were discharged. Appointments were made for Rose to bring her son to the well baby clinic two weeks later and to visit her doctor for a routine postpartum checkup six weeks later.

212. In giving predischarge instruction the nurse should tell Rose that the baby's umbilical cord stump would separate approximately:
1. 5 days after birth.
2. 10 days after birth.
3. 15 days after birth.
4. 20 days after birth.

213. In instructing Rose regarding care of her infant's umbilical cord stump the nurse should advise her to:
1. Gently wash the stump daily and keep it dry.
2. Secure a tight abdominal binder over the stump.
3. Apply moist compresses three to four times daily.
4. Cleanse the stump with hydrogen peroxide several times daily.

214. Future family harmony will be augmented if the nurse who teaches Rose to care for her infant realizes that it is most important that Rose:
1. Be able to perform each task perfectly before she is discharged from the hospital.
2. Attempt each task only after the nurse has demonstrated it repeatedly in her presence.
3. Undertake only one task at a time in order to perfect it before attempting another.
4. Experience a feeling of success and satisfaction in the performance of each new task.

215. As she was dressing to leave the hospital Rose said to the nurse, "I notice an unpleasant odor from my vaginal flow. Will it be all right for me to douche when I get home?" Which of the following responses by the nurse would be most appropriate?
1. "Yes, you may now begin to douche daily if you use a mild antiseptic and avoid force in introducing the solution."
2. "No, douching is dangerous at this time. Soap and water perineal cleansing and frequent pad changes will relieve the problem."
3. "Don't douche now as it may be painful. There are numerous deodorant powders available which will conceal the odor."
4. "The odor is unnoticeable to anyone but yourself, so ignore it. It will disappear now that you are up and about."

216. In order to give Rose adequate predischarge instruction the nurse should be aware that a lactating mother ordinarily first menstruates about:

    1. 1 month following delivery.
    2. 4 months following delivery.
    3. 8 months following delivery.
    4. 12 months following delivery.

217. During Rose's six-week postpartum checkup the physician would probably:

    a. Determine her blood pressure and weight.
    b. Examine her urine for protein and sugar.
    c. Observe the condition of her breasts and nipples.
    d. Carry out a complete pelvic examination.
    e. Palpate her uterus to evaluate involution.

        1. a and b.
        2. a, c, and e.
        3. a, b, c, and e.
        4. All the above.

Preeclampsia

Fifteen-year-old Miss Hulda Wyatt was eight months pregnant when she registered in the prenatal clinic at a large general hospital. Her last normal menstrual period had begun on December 3, and her estimated date of delivery was September 10.

Physical examination revealed a well-developed, well-nourished female with a blood pressure of 100/72 mm. Hg, a uterine gestation of 34-week size with vertex presentation, fetal heart tones of 138 per minute, and no visible edema. Her weight was 155 pounds, a 25-pound increase above her pre-pregnancy weight. Hulda's hematocrit was 34 per cent and there was a trace of albumin in her urine. The doctor scheduled Hulda to return to clinic in one week.

In a teaching conference with the nurse on her second clinic visit Hulda indicated that her mother wanted her to place the baby for adoption. An appointment was made for Hulda to talk with the social service worker from the local Family Service Association.

On the third visit, Hulda's weight was 160 pounds, her blood pressure 126/80 mm. Hg, her urine albumin 1+, the fetal heart tones 138 per minute, and there was minimal edema of Hulda's hands and feet. The doctor made a tentative diagnosis of preeclampsia, gave Hulda a sedative and advised that she obtain extra rest and return to the clinic in one week.

One week later Hulda's weight was 166 pounds, her blood pressure 136/90 mm. Hg, urine albumin 1+, hematocrit 40 per cent, platelet count 160,000 per cu. mm., and fetal heart tones 144 per minute. There was moderate edema of her eyelids, hands, and ankles and some blurring of vision. The doctor admitted Hulda to the hospital for observation and treatment.

On admission to the hospital, Hulda's temperature was 37.2° C. orally, pulse 100 per minute, respirations 18 per minute. The fundus of her uterus was located 27 cm. above the symphysis pubis, and the fetal weight was estimated to be about 2900 grams. Vaginal examination revealed an engaged vertex presentation, 80 per cent effacement of the cervix, and intact membranes. Pelvimetry indicated that Hulda's pelvis was adequate for vaginal delivery. Blood chemistries revealed blood urea nitrogen 22 mg. per 100 ml., creatinine 1.8 mg. per 100 ml., uric acid 4.2 mg. per 100 ml. The following orders were written.

1. Bedrest with bathroom privileges.
2. Record intake and output.
3. Weigh daily.
4. Determine 24-hour urinary protein and estriol.
5. Blood pressure every four hours.
6. Phenobarbital 30 mg. q.i.d. orally.
7. Secobarbital 100 mg. h.s. orally.
8. Milk of magnesia 30 ml. orally daily p.r.n.

(ANSWER BLANK ON PAGE A-3) (CORRECT ANSWERS ON PAGE B-13)

1. Preeclampsia differs from toxemia in that toxemia is:

    1. A more severe form of preeclampsia.

    2. The terminal stage of eclampsia.

    3. Preeclampsia complicated by infection.

    4. A disease category including preeclampsia.

2. Which of the following factors are thought to predispose to development of toxemia of pregnancy?

    a. Inadequate nutrition.

    b. Multiple pregnancy.

    c. Vasomotor lability.

    d. Diabetes mellitus.

    e. Inadequate blood volume.

        1. a and c.

        2. b and d.

        3. All but d.

        4. All the above.

3. Which of the following are typical manifestations of the toxemias of pregnancy?

    a. Hypertension.

    b. Edema.

    c. Proteinuria.

    d. Convulsions.

    e. Acetonuria.

        1. a and c.

        2. b and d.

        3. All but e.

        4. All the above.

4. In the pregnant female, hypertension is defined as:

    1. A systolic pressure of 150 mm. Hg or more and a diastolic pressure of 100 mm. Hg or more.

    2. Any increase in blood pressure that is accompanied by headache, irritability, or visual disturbances.

    3. An increase of 30 mm. Hg or more in the systolic pressure and 15 mm. Hg or more in the diastolic pressure.

    4. Any increase in either systolic or diastolic blood pressure above average pre-pregnancy levels.

5. The cause of preeclampsia-eclampsia is:

    1. Unknown.

    2. Allergic.

    3. Infectious.

    4. Hereditary.

6. It has been observed that which of the following is necessary for the initiation and continuation of preeclampsia?

    1. Hypertrophied myocardium.

    2. Infected renal parenchyma.

    3. Functioning trophoblast.

    4. Hyperplastic bone marrow.

7. Which of the following is known to cure preeclampsia?

    1. Section of the sympathetic ganglion.

    2. Removal of a pheochromocytoma.

    3. Early termination of pregnancy.

    4. Administration of adrenal steroids.

8. Pathophysiologic changes that have been described as underlying causes of preeclampsia-eclampsia are:

    a. Insufficient production of blood and platelets.

    b. Fibrous tissue obliteration of glomerular capillaries.

    c. Generalized vasoconstriction and associated microangiopathy.

    d. Abnormal retention of sodium and water by body tissues.

    e. Hypersecretion of pituitary and thyroid hormones.

        1. a only.

        2. a and c.

        3. a, c, and d.

        4. All the above.

9. The renal lesion which is characteristic of preeclampsia-eclampsia is:

    1. Infection of the pelvis and calices.

    2. Glomerular capillary endotheliosis.

    3. Arteriosclerotic renal artery occlusion.

    4. Fibrotic replacement of the glomerulus.

10. The basic cause for Hulda's increasing blood pressure was:

    1. Generalized spasm of peripheral arterioles.

    2. Increased force of myocardial contraction.

    3. Increase in circulating blood volume.

    4. Decreased viscosity of circulating blood.

11. Symptoms develop in preeclampsia primarily as a result of decreased blood flow to the:

    a. Cerebrum.

    b. Lung.

    c. Kidney.

    d. Pancreas.

    e. Uterus.

        1. a and b.

        2. c and d.

        3. a, c, and e.

        4. All the above.

12. Adequate and continuous prenatal care is required to prevent eclampsia in preeclamptic patients because:

1. Effective treatment of preeclampsia consists of the administration of a variety of medications.
2. Signs of preeclampsia are of a type which the patient herself is not apt to identify.
3. Continuous psychological counseling is needed to reduce the emotional stress causing pressure elevation.
4. Strong authoritarian control is required to maintain caloric intake at a reduced level throughout pregnancy.

13. It is currently thought that a possible means of preventing eclampsia in a preeclamptic patient is restriction of:

1. Fluid intake.
2. Sodium intake.
3. Caloric intake.
4. Physical exercise.

14. As a result of Hulda's preeclampsia the fetus is particularly disposed to:

1. Hydrocephalus and spina bifida.
2. Hemolysis and jaundice.
3. Infections and anemia.
4. Hypoxia and prematurity.

15. Which of the following are possible medical complications of preeclampsia-eclampsia?

a. Cerebrovascular hemorrhage.
b. Congestive heart failure.
c. Acute pulmonary edema.
d. Acute renal failure.
   1. a and c.
   2. b and d.
   3. All but d.
   4. All the above.

16. The difference between preeclampsia and eclampsia is the fact that in the latter condition the patient exhibits:

1. Headache.
2. Visual disturbances.
3. Oliguria.
4. Convulsions.

17. The increase in Hulda's hematocrit between her 32nd and 35th weeks of gestation was probably the result of:

1. Increased hematopoiesis in the red bone marrow.
2. Decreased red blood cell destruction by the spleen.
3. Decreased transmission of red cells to the fetus.

4. A shift of fluid from the vascular compartment.

18. Which manifestation indicated that Hulda's preeclampsia had become severe enough to require hospitalization?

1. Increased fetal heart tones.
2. Diastolic blood pressure of 90 mm. Hg.
3. Edema of the face and hands.
4. Systolic blood pressure of 130 mm. Hg.

19. The nurse should observe Hulda for development of which other symptoms of severe preeclampsia?

a. Severe headache.
b. Blurring of vision.
c. Persistent vomiting.
d. Pain in the epigastrium.
e. Reduced urine output.
   1. a and c.
   2. b and d.
   3. All but e.
   4. All the above.

20. Hulda should be watched carefully for which of the following signs which typically immediately precede an eclamptic convulsion?

a. Rolling the eyes to the side.
b. Staring fixedly into space.
c. Twitching of facial muscles.
d. Flushing of the skin of the face.
e. Uttering a brief sharp cry.
   1. a and b.
   2. a, b, and c.
   3. All but e.
   4. All the above.

21. On examination the doctor will be most apt to observe which of the following abnormalities in Hulda's eyegrounds?

1. Arteriolar spasms and retinal edema.
2. Aneurismal dilation of small arterioles.
3. Numerous dark granular hemorrhages.
4. Extensive "cotton-wool" exudates.

22. If Hulda's condition should become progressively more severe, the nurse might expect to see which of the following changes in Hulda's blood chemistry values?

a. Decreased plasma bicarbonate.
b. Elevation of serum uric acid level.
c. Decreased serum protein level.
d. Increased blood urea nitrogen level.
e. Increased concentration of plasma fibrinogen.
   1. a and c.

2. b and d.

3. All but e.

4. All the above.

23. Preeclampsia predisposes Hulda to which of the following obstetrical complications?

1. Placenta praevia.

2. Abruptio placenta.

3. Uterine dystocia.

4. Uterine rupture.

24. The principal purpose for accurately recording Hulda's intake and output would be to determine:

1. The efficiency of cardiac function.

2. The amount of fluid retention.

3. The onset of metabolic acidosis.

4. The advisability of intravenous feedings.

25. Hulda's 24-hour excretion of urinary protein would be considered to be abnormal if it exceeded:

1. 0.3 gram.

2. 0.3 grain.

3. 0.3 milligram.

4. 0.3 milliequivalent.

26. During Hulda's hospitalization the following diagnostic tests should be performed daily:

a. Urine protein.

b. Weight determination.

c. Serum sodium determination.

d. Deep tendon reflexes.

e. Romberg test.

  1. a and c.

  2. a, b, and d.

  3. All but e.

  4. All the above.

27. Phenobarbital was given to Hulda for which of the following effects?

1. Vasodilation.

2. Analgesic.

3. Sedative.

4. Antihistamine.

28. Sodium secobarbital was selected for use in Hulda's treatment because in hypnotic doses it:

1. Also exerts a strong analgesic effect.

2. Has little effect on uterine muscle.

3. Relaxes arteriolar smooth muscle spasm.

4. Never produces idiosyncratic effects.

29. Phenobarbital differs from sodium secobarbital in that phenobarbital:

1. Is less effective in preventing or controlling convulsions.

2. Acts only on the subcortical levels of the nervous system.

3. Is less apt to produce toxicity due to cumulative effects.

4. Acts more slowly and over a longer period of time.

30. If the physician had placed Hulda on a moderate sodium restriction diet (1 gram), Hulda should have been taught to:

1. Use only a minimal amount of salt in cooking.

2. Use only a small amount of salt at mealtime.

3. Avoid using salt in any form before or after cooking.

4. Reduce her milk intake by 50 per cent.

31. A nurse should know that which of the following foods are high in sodium content?

a. Sweet potato.

b. Canned beets.

c. Smoked fish.

d. Chipped beef.

e. Egg whites.

  1. a, c, and e.

  2. b, c, and d.

  3. All but e.

  4. All the above.

32. The nurse should understand that a considerable problem in planning an adequate diet for Hulda is the fact that:

1. Most of the animal protein foods which are high in sodium are also valuable sources of essential amino acids.

2. Dry, nonfat milk, though very low in sodium content, is also lacking in many of the essential amino acids.

3. Those fresh fruits which are low in caloric content lack important vitamins and have a high sodium content.

4. Fatty foods, the best sources of the vitamins and minerals needed in pregnancy, also yield the most calories.

On Hulda's second day of hospitalization she complained of headache and marked blurring of vision. Her blood pressure was 138/94 mm. Hg, urine albumin 2+, and facial and hand edema were obvious. The physician ordered that she be placed in a darkened private room, and be continuously attended by a nurse. Quantitative examination of Hulda's urine revealed elimination of 1 gram of protein in 24 hours. During the same 24-hour period Hulda's fluid intake was 2400 ml. and her urinary output was 1100 ml.

33. In which of the following positions should Hulda be maintained while she is on bed rest?
1. Supine.
2. Semi-Fowler's.
3. Side lying.
4. Recumbent.

34. Which of the following examinations would the doctor be apt to perform every day during Hulda's hospital stay?
1. Thoracic auscultation.
2. Retinal examination.
3. Lumbar spinal tap.
4. Biparietal diameter.

35. If her preeclampsia should become progressively more severe, Hulda might be expected to develop which of the following visual disturbances?
a. Double vision.
b. Halo vision.
c. Dimness of vision.
d. Blind spots.
e. Retinal sheen.
　　1. a and b.
　　2. c and d.
　　3. All but d.
　　4. All the above.

36. Which of the following best explains why the physician ordered that Hulda be placed in a darkened quiet room?
1. Noise or bright light may stimulate convulsions.
2. Increased blood pressure produces restlessness.
3. External stimuli prevent sleep in toxic patients.
4. Light and noise are annoying to moribund patients.

37. Which of the following statements by the nurse would be the best explanation to Hulda of the reason for placing her in a quiet, darkened private room?
1. "There's a strong possibility that you may have convulsions and this is one way to reduce the chance that they will occur."
2. "In our experience we have found that critically ill patients recover health more rapidly when environmental stimuli are reduced."
3. "It is probable that you can recover from your illness if you cooperate

with the treatment program by getting as much rest as possible."
4. "You need as much rest as possible, so we are putting you in a quiet room order that you will be able to get extra sleep."

38. In planning Hulda's care the nurse should make provision for:
1. Several periods of physical exercise scattered throughout the day.
2. Opportunities for her to visit with other patients and personnel.
3. Long, uninterrupted periods during which she may rest and sleep.
4. Taking her on directed tours of the labor–delivery unit and nursery.

39. Hulda should be closely observed for which of the following as prodromal symptoms of eclampsia?
a. Disorientation.
b. Somnolence.
c. Nausea and vomiting.
d. Hyperreflexia.
e. Focal muscle spasms.
　　1. a and c.
　　2. b and d.
　　3. All but e.
　　4. All the above.

40. The convulsions of eclampsia are of which type?
1. Tonic contractions of flexor muscles of the upper and lower extremities.
2. Fine twitching of the small muscles of the face, hands, and feet.
3. Generalized tonic and clonic contractions of muscle throughout the body.
4. Muscular spasms confined to one body part or one particular group of muscles.

41. Which of the following precautions should be undertaken to protect Hulda from injuries in case she develops convulsions?
a. Padding the head and side rails of her bed.
b. Immobilizing her arms with cloth restraints.
c. Tying a plastic airway to the bed frame.
d. Keeping her in a prone position in bed.
e. Maintaining continuous attendance by a nurse.
　　1. a, b, and d.
　　2. a, c, and e.

3. b, c, and d.

4. All the above.

42. The nurse who cares for Hulda should assist her in routine personal hygiene by:

    a. Providing the opportunity for good mouth care.

    b. Assuring that she turns every two hours.

    c. Assisting with bathing and clothing changes.

    d. Assisting with perineal cleansing following defecation.

    e. Moving her extremities through their full range of motion.

        1. a and b.

        2. a, b, and d.

        3. All but e.

        4. All the above.

43. During Hulda's first three days of hospitalization it would be important for the nurse to observe her closely for signs of labor because:

    1. The medications she is being given tend to initiate uterine contractions.

    2. Preeclampsia will predispose Hulda to rapidly progressing and shortened labor.

    3. She may be too heavily sedated to recognize and report the early signs of labor.

    4. Placental infarctions caused by preeclampsia will produce painless labor.

While performing an Oxytocin challenge test (O.C.T.), the doctor noted a fall in the fetal heart rate accompanied by a slow return to baseline after uterine contraction and assessed that there was slight fetal distress due to mild uteroplacental insufficiency. Amniocentesis revealed a lecithin-to-sphingomyelin ratio of 3 and a 24 hour urinary estriol level of 20 mg. Hulda's tendon reflexes were normal.

Since Hulda's 24-hour urinary estriol level had decreased while her proteinuria had increased for three consecutive days, the doctor ruptured her membranes in an unsuccessful attempt to initiate labor. He then began an intravenous infusion of 5 per cent Dextrose in water and induced labor by administering oxytocin, first at the rate of 1 milliunit per minute and then increasing the rate to 5 milliunits per minute, when Hul-

da's contractions became strong and occurred at a rate of three in 10 minutes. At this point Hulda experienced a grand mal seizure, which was treated by intravenous administration of magnesium sulfate, 4 grams in a 10 per cent solution over a period of 5 minutes. She was then given 1 gram of magnesium sulfate every hour throughout delivery. Ten milliliters of 10 per cent calcium gluconate were kept available to add to her intravenous infusion should her tendon reflexes or respiratory rate have become depressed. Her urinary output remained good, with a specific gravity of 1.018. Following delivery, she was given diazepam (Valium), 10 mg. I.M. q. day.

Eight hours after her contractions began, Hulda delivered a 2900 gram infant boy who had an Apgar score of 6 at one minute after birth. After his mouth and nose were suctioned, the newborn was ventilated and placed in an incubator, with the mattress head elevated. A small roll was placed under his shoulders to hyperextend his neck. He was then transferred to the neonatal intensive care unit for observation.

44. Premature induction of labor was undertaken as part of Hulda's care in order to protect her from:

    a. Convulsions.

    b. Hemorrhage.

    c. Pulmonary edema.

    d. Heart failure.

        1. a and c.

        2. b and d.

        3. All but d.

        4. All the above.

45. The pharmacologic effect of the oxytocin solution given intravenously is to:

    1. Produce rhythmic contractions of uterine muscle fibers.

    2. Relax smooth muscle fibers of the cervix of the uterus.

    3. Initiate vigorous, sustained contraction of abdominal muscles.

    4. Produce relaxation of vaginal walls and perineal muscles.

46. In addition to its use in inducing early labor, oxytocin is sometimes used in treatment of patients with:

    1. Uterine rupture.

    2. Contracted pelvis.

    3. Uterine inertia.

    4. Prolapsed cord.

47. Hulda's safety should be ensured during administration of the oxytocin solution by providing her with:

1. An adult crib bed with fully padded siderails.
2. Copious quantities of clear liquids for oral intake.
3. Constant bedside attendance by a doctor or nurse.
4. Oxygen-carbon dioxide inhalations at intervals.

48. The nurse's responsibility during Hulda's induction is to make a frequent check of the rate of:

1. Radial pulse.
2. Cervical dilation.
3. Intravenous infusion.
4. Fetal descent.

49. During Hulda's induction with oxytocin, the rate of intravenous fluid infusion should be regulated to maintain Hulda's uterine contractions at approximately which duration?

1. One minute.
2. One and one-half minutes.
3. Two minutes.
4. Two and one-half minutes.

50. The nurse should temporarily discontinue the oxytocin solution infusion if which of the following should occur?

a. Expulsion of a small plug of bloody mucus from the vagina.
b. Progressive development of severe aching pain in the sacral area.
c. Decrease in fetal heart contractions to less than 100 per minute.
d. Contractions of the uterus of a duration greater than two minutes.
   1. a and b.
   2. c and d.
   3. All but d.
   4. All the above.

51. During the intravenous administration of oxytoxin the nurse should check the monitor and observe the fetal heart rate.

1. After absorption of 250 cc. of intravenous solution.
2. Every 5 minutes during administration of the oxytocin.
3. Following the subsidence of each uterine contraction.
4. Continuously throughout the period of administration.

52. Although it is normal for the fetal heart rate to decrease during uterine contractions, fetal heart tones should return to a normal rate and rhythm within which period of time following each contraction?

1. 15 seconds.
2. 30 seconds.
3. 60 seconds.
4. 120 seconds.

53. Diazepam (Valium) was given to Hulda for which of the following effects?

a. Sedative.
b. Muscle relaxant.
c. Diuretic.
d. Decongestant.
e. Anti-inflammative.
   1. a and b.
   2. c and d.
   3. All but e.
   4. All the above.

54. Magnesium sulfate therapy is frequently initiated eight hours prior to induction of labor for which of the following pharmacologic effects?

1. Cathartic.
2. Antacid.
3. Anticonvulsant.
4. Antiemetic.

55. Hulda should be observed for which of the following side effects of magnesium sulfate?

1. Visual blurring.
2. Pulse irregularity.
3. Abdominal distention.
4. Respiratory depression.

56. Which of the following, as an antidote to magnesium sulfate, should be kept available while magnesium sulfate is given to Hulda?

1. Calcium gluconate.
2. Potassium chloride.
3. Sodium sulfate.
4. Magnesium oxide.

Following Hulda's delivery, in addition to the routine postpartum orders, the physician ordered the following.

1. Testosterone enanthate and estradiol valerate mixture (Deladumone), 2 ml. I.M. stat. only.
2. Place in a room near the nurses' station. Seizure precautions.
3. Record fluid intake and output.
4. Vital signs q. 30 minutes times 4, then q 4 h. when awake.

5. Measure urine protein and specific gravity.

57. The pharmacologic action of the testosterone–estradiol mixture given intramuscularly to Hulda is to:
1. Stimulate strong contraction of uterine muscle.
2. Prevent spasm of uterine arteries.
3. Inhibit release of lactogenic hormone.
4. Depress the sensory cerebral cortex.

58. In planning for Hulda's care during hospitalization the nurse should be aware that:
1. Delivery will result in immediate and permanent cure of the preeclampsia.
2. Hulda may continue to convulse for 48 hours after delivery.
3. Hulda's symptoms will increase immediately after delivery, then abate.
4. Hulda will be left with chronic renal impairment following delivery.

59. During the 72 hours following Hulda's delivery the nurse should observe her for development of which of the following as a positive prognostic sign?
1. Rhinorrhea.
2. Diuresis.
3. Diaphoresis.
4. Diarrhea.

Hulda's blood pressure decreased to 110/70 mm. Hg on the day following delivery. On her first and second postpartum days she had a moderate diuresis and was free of headache, visual blurring, albuminuria, and edema.

The social worker visited Hulda daily throughout her postpartum stay in the hospital, and when Hulda was discharged on her third postpartum day the social worker scheduled a meeting with her for the same day as her six week postpartum checkup.

A representative from the Family Service Association took Hulda's son from the hospital nursery to the adoption agency.

On her six week postpartum checkup Hulda was found to be in good health. That same day the social worker assisted Hulda in completing arrangements for continuing her high school education in her former school.

60. The clinic and hospital nurses should provide which of the following services to Hulda when giving her prenatal and postnatal care and instruction?
1. Reassure Hulda that her decision to give her baby up for adoption will be advantageous both to her and to him.
2. Foster Hulda's self-respect by demonstrating their regard and concern for her present and future welfare.
3. Suggest means for ensuring that she does not repeat her earlier mistakes and direct her toward worthwhile goals.
4. Lead Hulda to explore the underlying reasons for her present situation and to evaluate her behavior objectively.

61. The hospital social worker should contribute which of the following services to Hulda's prepartum and postpartum care?
1. Assist Hulda to understand her present situation, place it in its proper perspective in relation to her life goals, and make plans for the future.
2. Help Hulda to arrive at a complete understanding of the reasons underlying her pregnancy in order to prevent a future pregnancy out of wedlock.
3. Facilitate Hulda's comprehension of her relationship to the father of her child and help her decide the nature and extent of her future relationship with him.
4. Provide a sheltered, accepting environment in which Hulda may feel free to ask questions but in which no specific answers will be given and no direction suggested.

62. In order to instruct Hulda regarding self-care following hospital discharge the nurse should understand that following recovery from preeclampsia, Hulda would probably be left with:
1. Permanently obliterated capillaries in the areas of damaged renal cortex.
2. Permanent impairment of tubular ability for excretion and resorption.
3. Slightly contracted kidneys with considerably reduced blood supply.
4. No persistent changes in renal structure or function.

63. The Family Service Agency selects adoptive parents by evaluating applicants in regard to:
- a. Chronological age of both parties.
- b. State of physical and mental health of both.
- c. Presence or absence of children in the home.
- d. Motivation underlying the desire for a child.
- e. Length and stability of the marriage.
  - 1. a and b.
  - 2. c and d.
  - 3. All but d.
  - 4. All the above.

64. The general attitude of society toward the unwed mother can best be described as:
- 1. Empathic.
- 2. Apathetic.
- 3. Condemning.
- 4. Long-suffering.

65. The general attitude of society toward the unwed father can best be described as:
- 1. Empathic.
- 2. Apathetic.
- 3. Condemning.
- 4. Long-suffering.

Placenta Praevia

Thirty-five-year-old Alice Early's sixth pregnancy was uneventful until her sixth month of gestation, when she had an episode of vaginal spotting. On the following morning she awoke to find her lower bed linen soaked with blood. Her husband phoned her obstetrician and then drove her to a nearby hospital.

On admission Alice appeared pale and anxious. Her blood pressure was 110/71 mm. Hg, her pulse 96 per minute, her hematocrit 30 per cent, her hemoglobin level 10.3 G/100 ml., and her white cell count 8300/mm³. Fetal heart tones could not be heard. After typing and cross-matching, Alice was given 3 units of whole blood. Since ultrasonography was unavailable, a sterile vaginal examination performed with a double set-up revealed a complete placenta praevia. A low cervical transverse cesarean section was performed under spinal and intravenous anesthesia and a stillborn male infant weighing 750 G. was delivered. One unit of whole blood was given to Alice during the operative procedure.

Alice returned to the recovery room in good condition with a Foley catheter in place. The following orders were on her chart:

1. Meperidine hydrochloride 50 mg. I.M. q. 4 h. p.r.n. for pain.
2. Secobarbital 100 mg. I.M. p.r.n. for sleep at h.s.
3. 5 per cent dextrose in water I.V., 1000 cc. q. 8 h.
4. Nothing by mouth.

On the day following surgery Alice's Foley catheter was removed and she was ambulated and started on a clear liquid diet. Because her temperature rose to 39° C., intravenous fluids were continued and she was given Ampicillin 1 G I.V. in a rider q. 6 h. for three days, during which time her temperature gradually decreased to 37.2° C. The intravenous Ampicillin was discontinued and replaced with Ampicillin 500 mg. orally q. 6 h., which was continued until Alice's hospital discharge on her ninth postoperative day.

(ANSWER BLANK ON PAGE A–5) (CORRECT ANSWERS ON PAGE B–15)

1. Placenta praevia can best be defined as:
  1. Thrombotic occlusion of the placental blood vessels before the fetus has developed to full maturity.
  2. Separation of the placenta from its attachment in the uterine wall before the 40th week of gestation.
  3. Implantation of the placenta in the lower uterine segment, so as to overlie the internal cervical os.
  4. Proliferation of placental tissue at a rate exceeding that required for optimal fetal nourishment.

2. Which of the following conditions are thought to predispose to occurrence of placenta praevia?
  a. Numerous previous pregnancies.
  b. Inadequate maternal nutrition.
  c. Advancing maternal age.
  d. Excessive weight gain.
  e. Chronic urinary infection.
  1. a and c.
  2. b and d.
  3. All but d.
  4. All the above.

3. Placenta praevia is thought to be a frequent cause of which of the following complications of pregnancy?
  1. Ectopic pregnancy.
  2. Hydatidiform mole.
  3. Preeclampsia-eclampsia.
  4. Spontaneous abortion.

4. Which of the following obstetrical complications is an unavoidable consequence of placenta praevia?
  1. Fetal death.
  2. Postpartum infection.
  3. Perinatal hemorrhage.
  4. Subsequent sterility.

5. Alice's vaginal bleeding was initiated by:
1. Disintegration of the Wharton's jelly surrounding the umbilical arteries and vein.
2. Rupture of the amniotic sac at a point weakened by inflammatory changes.
3. Tearing of placental attachments as a consequence of dilation of the internal os.
4. Erosion of endometrial tissue due to pressure by the overlying fetus.

6. The occurrence of placenta praevia increases the probability that Alice's labor might be complicated by:
1. Premature rupture of membranes.
2. Uterine muscle atony.
3. Unusual fetal presentation.
4. Prolapse of the cord.

7. Placenta praevia predisposes Alice's infant to which of the following hazards or complications?
1. Hemorrhage.
2. Infection.
3. Anomalies.
4. Prematurity.

8. If Alice's placenta praevia had been diagnosed after her initial episode of vaginal spotting she would probably then have been treated with:
1. Bedrest and close observation.
2. Pitocin induction of labor.
3. Elective cesarean section.
4. Administration of vitamin K.

9. Alice's vaginal examination (following hospital admission) would have been performed in:
1. The emergency room.
2. The ward treatment room.
3. Her own hospital room.
4. An operating room.

10. Alice's preparation for the sterile vaginal examination should include:
1. A low tap water enema.
2. A dose of a mild cathartic.
3. An abdominoperineal skin preparation.
4. A digital rectal examination.

11. In preparing for Alice's sterile vaginal examination the nurse should assemble:
a. Sterile cotton balls.
b. Soap solution.
c. Disinfectant solution.
d. Sterile towels.
e. Sterile gloves.
   1. All but a.

2. All but b.
3. All but d.
4. All the above.

12. In addition to a vaginal examination which of the following procedures may be used to diagnose placenta praevia?
a. X-ray of the abdomen following intravenous injection of phenolsulfonphthalein.
b. Fluoroscopy of the abdomen following intra-abdominal injection of indigo carmine.
c. Placental scan following intravenous injection of radioiodinated serum albumin.
d. Aspiration of blood when a needle is inserted into the lower uterine segment.
e. Ultrasonography when the patient has a full bladder.
   1. a only.
   2. c and e.
   3. All but d.
   4. All the above.

13. Which of the following accommodations would be best suited for Alice following her return from the recovery room?
1. Three-bed room in the obstetrical ward with newly delivered mothers.
2. Four-bed room in the obstetrical unit with undelivered patients under medical observation.
3. Single room in the obstetrical ward near the central Nurses' Station.
4. Double room in the surgical ward with a posthysterectomy patient.

14. Alice should be told that her child was stillborn:
1. As soon as she has fully recovered from the anesthetic.
2. After she has been returned to her unit from the recovery room.
3. During her first visit with her husband following surgery.
4. As soon as she is able to be fully ambulatory.

15. Alice's husband should be told that their child was stillborn:
1. Immediately following completion of the operative procedure.
2. Following completion of a postmortem examination of the infant.
3. During Alice's first visit with her husband postoperatively.
4. As soon as the family's religious advisor can assume this responsibility.

16. Alice's initial reaction to the news that her baby was stillborn would probably be that of:
1. Disbelief.
2. Anger.
3. Withdrawal.
4. Guilt.

17. One day during morning care Alice gestured to a snapshot on her bedside stand, saying, "There's a picture of my five *living* children." Which of the following responses by the nurse would be most helpful?
1. "That's a nice looking group. You have a lot to be proud of."
2. "I can imagine that it must be a great responsibility to care for five children."
3. "It sounds like you've accepted the fact that you may never have six children."
4. "Perhaps during these last few days you've been thinking about your baby who died?"

18. Alice asked the nurse, "What causes placenta praevia? I did everything my doctor told me to do." Which of the following responses by the nurse would be most helpful at this time?
1. "Placenta praevia is never the result of a lack of adequate prenatal care."
2. "You're wondering whether some action of yours contributed to your baby's death?"
3. "There are a number of types of and several possible causes for placenta praevia."
4. "I'm sure that you attempted to follow your doctor's orders conscientiously."

19. One day Alice asked the nurse, "Do you think I should attempt to have more children?" Which of the following responses would be most appropriate?
1. "Do you and your husband want more children?"
2. "Placenta praevia rarely occurs twice in the same woman."
3. "Why not decide that after you have fully recovered?"
4. "If you decide not to, you will still have five children."

20. One day Alice said to the nurse, "I want to see the nursery. Will you take me down there?" In order to respond therapeutically to this request, the nurse should first:
1. Question her carefully regarding the reason for her request.
2. Ascertain the degree of her physical strength and endurance.
3. Determine in which phase of the grief cycle Alice is operating.
4. Ask Alice's husband to accompany them to the nursery.

On the day of her discharge from the hospital Alice thanked the nurse for her help during a "trying time," adding, "Maybe we'll meet again under happier circumstances."

Diabetes and Pregnancy

Thirty-seven-year-old Molly Flowers, gravida V, para IV, had been a known diabetic for three years, was controlled on two tablets of tolbutamide, and was four months pregnant when she reported to prenatal clinic for care. Her expected date of delivery was calculated to be March 21. Physical examination revealed a temperature of 37° C., pulse 96 per minute, respirations 22 per minute, blood pressure 116/80 mm. Hg, moderate obesity, a uterine gestation of 16- to 18-week size, and uterine fundus two fingerbreadths below the umbilicus. No fetal heart tones were heard. Heart size was normal and lungs were clear to percussion and auscultation. The physician admitted Molly to the hospital for diabetic regulation.

On admission to the hospital Molly's hematocrit was 32 per cent, her fasting blood glucose level was 140 mg. per 100 ml. and a two hour postprandial blood glucose was 164 mg. per 100 ml. The physician started Molly on Lente, the nurse taught her how to give her own insulin and supervised her in testing her urine four times daily, and the dietitian instructed Molly in the planning and preparation of an 1800-calorie diabetic diet. Molly was discharged five days later, well controlled on 20 units of Lente insulin a day, taking 300 mg. of ferrous sulphate t.i.d. and a vitamin-mineral supplement daily. She was advised to test her urine four times daily at home and was scheduled to report to prenatal clinic every two weeks until the seventh month of pregnancy, and then weekly.

(ANSWER BLANK ON PAGE A–7)   (CORRECT ANSWERS ON PAGE B–16)

1. In order to improve the management of diabetes in pregnancy, the nurse should ascertain which of the following while taking the health history of any pregnant woman?
   a. History of diabetes in the family.
   b. History of stillbirth in the third trimester.
   c. History of spontaneous abortions.
   d. Delivery of a large infant (over 4000 grams).
   e. Obesity or age over 35 years.
      1. a and b.
      2. a, c, and d.
      3. All but e.
      4. All the above.

2. Pregnancy is known to produce which of the following derangements in glucose metabolism in normal subjects?
   a. Increase in the quantity of glucose filtered by the renal glomerulus.
   b. Decreased rate of removal of glucose from the blood.
   c. Loss of reactivity to a given amount of insulin.
   d. Decreased ability to utilize glucose for metabolic needs.
   e. Decreased carbon dioxide combining power of the plasma.
      1. a and c.
      2. b and d.
      3. All but c.
      4. All the above.

3. It is thought that pregnancy has a diabetogenic effect due to the increased production during pregnancy of:
   a. Adrenal corticosteroids.
   b. Anterior pituitary hormones.
   c. Parathormone.
   d. Antidiuretic hormone.
   e. Thyroxine.
      1. a and c.
      2. b and d.
      3. a, b, and e.
      4. All the above.

4. Long-standing diabetes mellitus predisposes patients to development of:
   a. Atherosclerosis.
   b. Hypertension.
   c. Retinitis.
   d. Peripheral neuritis.
   e. Glomerulosclerosis.
     1. a and c.
     2. b and d.
     3. All but e.
     4. All the above.

5. The clinic nurse who cares for Molly should be aware that which of the following obstetrical complications is more common in diabetic than nondiabetic gravidas?
   a. Renal disease.
   b. Preeclampsia—eclampsia.
   c. Hypermesis gravidarium.
   d. Monilial vaginitis.
   e. Spontaneous abortion.
     1. a and c.
     2. b and d.
     3. All but d.
     4. All the above.

6. The normal fasting serum glucose level ranges from:
   1. 40 to 80 mg. per 100 ml. of blood.
   2. 80 to 120 mg. per 100 ml. of blood.
   3. 120 to 160 mg. per 100 ml. of blood.
   4. 160 to 200 mg. per 100 ml. of blood.

7. In the normal person the serum glucose concentration should not exceed which of the following levels at two hours following a glucose meal?
   1. 80 mg. per 100 ml. of blood.
   2. 110 mg. per 100 ml. of blood.
   3. 140 mg. per 100 ml. of blood.
   4. 170 mg. per 100 ml. of blood.

8. The physician was especially interested in Molly's heart size on physical examination because diabetes mellitus is known to predispose to the development of:
   1. Rheumatic heart disease.
   2. Beriberi heart disease.
   3. Arteriosclerotic heart disease.
   4. Hypertensive heart disease.

9. The pharmacologic effect of tolbutamide is to:
   1. Substitute for exogenous insulin in facilitating cellular glucose oxidation.
   2. Stimulate release of endogenous insulin from islet cells of the pancreas.
   3. Inhibit passage of glucose through endothelial cells of the glomerulus.

   4. Stimulate resorption of glucose by the epithelial cells of the renal tubule.

10. Molly's physician changed her from tolbutamide to insulin during hospitalization because:
   1. Tolbutamide does not protect against ketosis, to which complication Molly is especially predisposed by her pregnancy.
   2. Oral hypoglycemic agents tend to increase and prolong the morning sickness that commonly occurs during pregnancy.
   3. Hypoglycemic episodes are less liable to occur following administration of insulin than following ingestion of tolbutamide.
   4. Tolbutamide does not pass the placental barrier and therefore cannot affect the oxidation of glucose by the fetus.

11. The usual procedure for testing the postprandial serum glucose concentration consists in measuring the glucose content of:
   1. Venous blood withdrawn prior to, and at 1-hour, 2-hour, and 3-hour intervals following a glucose meal.
   2. A venous blood specimen obtained one hour following ingestion of an exceedingly high carbohydrate meal.
   3. Arterial blood aspirated one-half hour following intravenous injection of a measured amount of glucose.
   4. Urine specimens obtained every 15 minutes for two hours following intravenous or oral administration of glucose.

12. The amount of urinary glucose alone would be an unsatisfactory basis upon which to calculate needed insulin dosages for Molly because:
   1. Optimal management of diabetes allows for a minimal degree of glycosuria.
   2. Even nondiabetic gravidas tend to spill glucose into their urine intermittently.
   3. It would be impossible to calculate accurately the amount of fetal glycosuria.
   4. Calculations would be skewed by the increased volume of urine produced.

13. It would be even more important for Molly to restrict her weight gain during pregnancy than it is for a nondiabetic patient to do so, because diabetes predisposes Molly to:
   1. Varicose veins of the legs and vulva.
   2. Destruction of the longitudinal foot arch.
   3. Severe disturbances in water balance.
   4. Demineralization of weight-bearing bones.

14. The 1800-calorie diet ordered for Molly consisted of 150 grams of carbohydrate, 144 grams of protein, and 70 grams of fat per day. How many calories per day were to have been contributed by carbohydrates?
   1. 150
   2. 364
   3. 600
   4. 1350

15. In Molly's prescribed diabetic diet, how many calories per day were to have been contributed by fats?
   1. 70
   2. 280
   3. 560
   4. 630

16. Molly should be taught to recognize that which of the following represent one fruit exchange?
   a. One cup of raisins.
   b. One grapefruit half.
   c. Two dozen grapes.
   d. One small orange.
   e. One cup of strawberries.
      1. a and b.
      2. a, c, and d.
      3. b, d, and e.
      4. All the above.

17. Molly should be taught that one fruit exchange contains approximately:
   1. 12 grams of carbohydrate, 8 grams of protein, and 10 grams of fat.
   2. 7 grams of carbohydrate, 2 grams of protein, and negligible fat.
   3. Negligible carbohydrate, 7 grams of protein, and 5 grams of fat.
   4. 10 grams of carbohydrate, negligible protein, and negligible fat.

18. Molly should be taught that which of the following are class A vegetables?
   a. Broccoli.
   b. Carrots.
   c. Tomatoes.
   d. Peas.
   e. Spinach.
      1. a and b.
      2. a, c, and e.
      3. b, d, and e.
      4. All the above.

19. Molly should be taught that she will be allowed how many exchanges of class A vegetables each day?
   1. 1 exchange.
   2. 2 exchanges.
   3. 3 exchanges.
   4. As many as desired.

20. Molly's physician may advise that corn oil and corn oil margarine be used as the major fat sources in Molly's diet in order to:
   1. Ensure intake of adequate amounts of vitamin A.
   2. Decrease her susceptibility to fatty food intolerance.
   3. Restrict her intake of saturated fats to a minimum.
   4. Increase her feeling of satiety after meals.

21. Molly's physician would probably wish to restrict her intake of saturated fats because these substances have been found to:
   1. Yield more calories than unsaturated fats.
   2. Predispose to development of atheromatous plaques.
   3. Produce gastric irritation, nausea, and vomiting.
   4. Foster increased sodium and water retention.

22. Which of the following meats is lowest in saturated fats?
   1. Pork.
   2. Beef.
   3. Chicken.
   4. Lamb.

23. At 2:00 P.M. on Molly's third day of hospitalization she complained of nervousness, palpitation, headache, and faintness. The nurse observed that Molly's hands trembled and that she was perspiring profusely. The nurse should:
   1. Place Molly in a supine position and summon the physician.
   2. Talk quietly to Molly in order to reduce her anxiety and fear.
   3. Administer 10 grains of aspirin to relieve fever and headache.
   4. Encourage Molly to drink 120 cc. of orange juice and call the doctor.

24. Molly should be taught to test her urine at which of the following times of day?
   1. At 6:00 A.M., then every six hours around the clock.

2. At any four voidings during hours of greatest activity.
3. Upon arising and immediately following completion of each meal.
4. One half-hour before each meal and again at bedtime.

25. Molly should be taught that she is most apt to develop an insulin reaction at which interval following insulin injection?
1. 2 to 4 hours.
2. 8 to 10 hours.
3. 14 to 16 hours.
4. 20 to 22 hours.

26. On Molly's next-to-last day in the hospital she failed to eat most of her lunch. The nurse should:
1. Report Molly's lack of appetite to her physician on his next regular visit to the unit.
2. Give Molly an amount of orange juice equivalent in carbohydrate content to the uneaten food.
3. Question Molly in order to prepare a detailed list of her food likes and dislikes.
4. Identify the uneaten foods to the dietitian so that they can be omitted from future meals.

27. The physician would probably advise Molly to continue to do her own housework and engage regularly in light exercise during pregnancy in order to:
a. Improve her peripheral circulation.
b. Decrease the tendency for constipation.
c. Foster cellular glucose oxidation.
d. Prevent diabetic renal damage.
1. a and b.
2. c and d.
3. All but d.
4. All the above.

28. On each of Molly's prenatal clinic visits following her discharge from the hospital the physician or nurse would perform which of the following tests or examinations?
a. Blood pressure determination.
b. Urinalysis for albumin and acetone.
c. Visualization of the eyegrounds.
d. Measurement of weight.
1. a and c.
2. b and d.
3. All but c.
4. All the above.

29. In order to be able to answer Molly's questions regarding control of her diabetes, the clinic nurse should be aware that Molly's insulin requirement is apt to vary during pregnancy according to which of the following patterns?
1. Increase steadily and uniformly from the first through the second and third trimesters.
2. Increase during the first and second trimesters, then remain unchanged until delivery.
3. Remain unchanged during the first trimester, then rise rapidly through the second and third trimesters.
4. Increase during the first trimester, remain stable in the second, and increase during the third trimester.

Molly attended prenatal clinic weekly from her 18th to 35th weeks of pregnancy, by which time her insulin had been increased to 40 units of Lente insulin per day, and her total weight gain was 9 kg. (19.8 pounds).

During her 36th week of gestation, Molly was admitted to the hospital for stabilization of her diabetes and assessment of fetal maturity. The doctor regulated her insulin dosage to achieve a fasting serum glucose of 90 mg. per 100 ml., a two hour post-prandial serum glucose of 140 mg. per 100 ml., and a urinary excretion of glucose less than 10 grams per day.

Using ultrasonography, the sonar biparietal diameter of the fetal head was determined to be 9.3 cm. The doctor then did an amniocentesis to assess Molly's lecithin-sphingomyelin ratio, which was 2.5. The amniotic fluid was also tested for creatinine (1.5 mg. per 100 mg.) and estriol concentration (300 mg. per ml.).

The 24-hour urinary excretion of estriol was reported to be 15 mg. An oxytocin challenge test was performed and showed occasional late deceleration of the fetal heart rate.

Molly was scheduled for a cesarean section early in her 37th week of pregnancy because she had had a previous section for a transverse lie. Molly's preoperative orders were:

1. Abdominoperineal skin preparation.
2. Shower, using soap.
3. Tap water enema at 6:00 A.M. on the morning of surgery.
4. Nothing by mouth from the previous midnight.

A low transverse cesarean section was performed under spinal anesthesia and a 4310 gram male infant was delivered in fair condition with an Apgar rating of 7 at 60 seconds after birth. Molly was given 1 ml. (1/320 gr.) of ergonovine maleate solution immediately following delivery. She arrived in the recovery room in good condition with a transfusion of type A, Rh positive blood and a liter of 5 per cent dextrose in water still infusing. The following postoperative orders were written:

1. Administer within the next eight hours an intravenous infusion of 1000 ml. of 5 per cent dextrose in ¼ normal saline with 20 units regular insulin.
2. Demerol 50 mg. q. 4 h. p.r.n. for pain.
3. Chloral hydrate 500 mg. q.h.s., p.r.n.
4. Record intake and output.
5. Diet as tolerated.
6. Dangle feet over edge of bed tonight.
7. Serum glucose.
8. Urinalysis q.i.d.
9. Regular insulin to be administered on a sliding scale for urine glucose at 7 A.M., 11 A.M., 4 P.M., 9 P.M.; 0— +1 give no insulin, +2— give 5 units regular insulin, +3 give 10 units regular insulin, +4 give 15 units regular insulin.
10. Demerol 75 mg. and Phenergan 25 mg. p.r.n. for pain.
11. Seconal 100 mg. orally at h.s. tonight.

In the morning following surgery Molly was drinking fluids without difficulty and her urinary output was adequate. Her indwelling catheter and intravenous fluids were discontinued and she was allowed out of bed at will. On her second postoperative day Molly and her husband walked to the nursery to see their son, who was not removed from the incubator until the following day.

30. The week of hospitalization preceding Molly's cesarean section should have been used to:
  a. Provide Molly with an opportunity for additional mental and physical rest.
  b. Check for the presence of respiraratory, urinary, or skin infections.
  c. Determine her levels of serum and urine glucose and keto-acids.
  d. Regulate insulin dose as needed to control serum glucose level.
  e. Assess fetal maturity and test for signs of fetal distress.
    1. a and b.

    2. c and d.
    3. All but e.
    4. All the above.

31. Why did the doctor assess the biparietal diameter of the fetal head by sonar method?
  1. To obtain an indirect indication of the presenting part.
  2. To estimate the expected date of Molly's delivery.
  3. To determine whether or not the fetus is in distress.
  4. To calculate the size and adequacy of the pelvis.

32. Lecithin-sphingomyelin ratio in the amniotic fluid is a measure of which of the following?
  1. Maternal liver function.
  2. Maternal adrenal function.
  3. Fetal liver maturity.
  4. Fetal lung maturity.

33. The normal lecithin-sphingomyelin ratio (L/S ratio) at 40 weeks gestation would be:
  1. 1.
  2. 3.
  3. 5.
  4. 7.

34. The nurse should take care to make an accurate collection of the 24-hour urine output for estriol measurement because it is used as a measure of which of the following?
  a. Integrity of the fetal pituitary-adrenal axis.
  b. Functioning of the maternal pituitary-adrenal axis.
  c. Estimation of the gestational age of the fetus.
  d. Integrity of the fetoplacental unit.
  e. Estimation of the fetal lung maturity.
    1. a and b.
    2. c and d.
    3. All but e.
    4. All the above.

35. Which of the following best describes the oxytocin challenge test?
  1. A method for testing the ability of the uterus to contract.
  2. A challenge to the pituitary gland to stimulate the adrenals.
  3. An indirect measure of the degree of fetal distress.
  4. An indirect test for estimating the length of labor.

36. If the fetal heart rate (F.H.R.) consistently fails to return to baseline within 30 seconds after the end of uterine contractions, the most probable explanation of this finding would be which of the following?

1. Head compression.
2. Umbilical cord compression.
3. Uteroplacental insufficiency.
4. Normal FHR pattern.

37. Preoperative washing of the skin with soap protects against surgical wound contamination principally by:

1. Mechanical removal of bacteria.
2. Coagulation of bacterial protein.
3. Dehydration of the bacterial cell body.
4. Altering the pH of the bacterial cell membrane.

38. Molly's preoperative preparation would be most apt to include insertion of:

1. A nasogastric tube.
2. A rectal tube.
3. An indwelling catheter.
4. Sterile vaginal packing.

39. If Molly had been allowed to deliver vaginally, labor might have precipitated severe metabolic imbalances resulting from:

1. Production of acid-base imbalance by sudden fluid loss upon rupture of fetal membranes.
2. Depletion of glycogen reserve in liver and skeletal muscles by strenuous muscular exertion.
3. Massive losses of body water and salts through diaphoresis during the second stage of labor.
4. Inability to ingest food or fluids of any type throughout the entire labor period.

40. Low transverse cesarean section is preferred to incision through the uterine fundus because the lower uterine segment:

a. Has thinner walls.
b. Is less vascular.
c. Can be covered by peritoneum.
d. Heals more rapidly.
   1. a and c.
   2. b and d.
   3. All but c.
   4. All the above.

41. The operating room nurse should be aware that infants of diabetic mothers are more apt than infants of normal mothers to display:

a. Erythroblastosis fetalis.
b. Excessive birth weight.
c. Noncommunicating hydrocephalus.
d. Cardiac enlargement.

   1. a and c.
   2. b and d.
   3. All but d.
   4. All the above.

42. Babies of diabetic mothers typically develop which of the following metabolic abnormalities?

a. Acceleration of bone growth.
b. Deposition of excessive subcutaneous fat.
c. Retention of excessive interstitial fluids.
d. Massive hyperplasia of skeletal muscle.

   1. a and c.
   2. b and d.
   3. All but d.
   4. All the above.

43. Metabolic and growth abnormalities observed in the growth rate of babies of diabetic mothers are thought to be caused by:

a. Increased production of maternal pituitary growth hormone.
b. Increased production of insulin by the fetal pancreas.
c. Increased production of maternal adrenocortical hormones.
d. Fetal hyperglycemia secondary to maternal hyperglycemia.

   1. a and b.
   2. c and d.
   3. All but d.
   4. All the above.

44. Which of the following is the nonproprietary name for Demerol?

1. Meprobamate.
2. Mephenesin.
3. Mesantoin.
4. Meperidine.

45. The pharmacologic effect of Demerol is to:

1. Reduce the blood supply to the cerebral cortex.
2. Depress the sensory portion of the cerebral cortex.
3. Block transmission of impulses through the cord.
4. Inactivate pain receptors at the periphery.

46. Which of the following is the nonproprietary name for Phenergan?

1. Phenacetin.
2. Physostigmine.
3. Promethazine.
4. Phenylephrine.

47. Phenergan has which of the following pharmacologic effects?
   a. Antihistaminic.
   b. Sedative.
   c. Antiemetic.
   d. Ataractic.
   e. Antipyretic.
      1. a and b.
      2. a and c.
      3. All but e.
      4. All the above.

48. During Molly's immediate postoperative period the recovery room nurse should:
   a. Check the consistency of the uterine fundus.
   b. Check vital signs every 15 minutes until stabilized.
   c. Check abdominal dressing and perineal pads for hemorrhage.
   d. Massage the uterus frequently to keep it firm.
      1. a and b.
      2. c and d.
      3. All but d.
      4. All the above.

49. During Molly's first eight hours following surgery, the recovery room nurse should observe her particularly for symptoms of:
   a. Internal hemorrhage.
   b. Puerperal infection.
   c. Vaginal hemorrhage.
   d. Breast engorgement.
   e. Aspiration pneumonia.
      1. a and c.
      2. a, b, and c.
      3. All but e.
      4. All the above.

50. Which of the following would be typical symptoms of internal hemorrhage?
   a. Rapid weak pulse.
   b. Marked skin pallor.
   c. Increased respiratory rate.
   d. Anxiety and apprehension.
   e. Rapid temperature elevation.
      1. a and c.
      2. b and d.
      3. All but e.
      4. All the above.

51. Cesarean section predisposes Molly particularly to:
      1. Umbilical hernia.
      2. Renal lithiasis.
      3. Pelvic thrombosis.
      4. External hemorrhoids.

52. The nurse who cares for Molly following surgery should be aware that sudden wide variations in serum glucose levels occur in diabetic postpartum patients, probably as a result of:
      1. Capricious appetite and poor eating habits.
      2. Conversion of serum glucose to lactose.
      3. Fitful production and release of insulin.
      4. Rapid shifts of water in and out of vessels.

53. Molly was encouraged to be out of bed as early as her second postoperative day in order to prevent the development of:
   a. Urinary stasis.
   b. Abdominal distention.
   c. Atonic constipation.
   d. Pelvic and femoral thrombosis.
      1. a and c.
      2. b and d.
      3. All but d.
      4. All the above.

When his respirations had become well established, Molly's infant was taken in an incubator from the operating room to the nursery and the pediatrician wrote the following orders for his care.

   1. Test capillary blood with Dextrostix every hour.
   2. Respiratory assessment every hour.
   3. Vitamin K 1 mg. I.M. stat.
   4. Calcium gluconate 1 cc. I.M. stat.
   5. Oral feeding of glucose in water.

54. For which of the following reasons was Molly's infant given calcium gluconate?
      1. To prevent development of hypocalcemic tetany.
      2. To prevent hemorrhage from the cord stump.
      3. To speed mineralization of long bones of the leg.
      4. To supply nutrients during the first day of life.

55. Infants of diabetic mothers are particularly subject to cranial injury during vaginal delivery because of their:
   a. Prematurity or immaturity.
   b. Greater than usual size.
   c. Unusually thin skull bones.
   d. Completely closed fontanels.
      1. a and b.
      2. c and d.
      3. All but d.
      4. All the above.

56. Immediately after delivery the pediatrician would treat Molly's infant by:

    a. Ensuring a patent airway by removing nasopharyngeal secretions.

    b. Stimulating respirations by gentle stroking or slapping.

    c. Removing gastric content by aspirating through a nasogastric tube.

    d. Providing external warmth through the use of blankets or an incubator.

        1. a and b.
        2. a, b, and d.
        3. All but d.
        4. All the above.

57. The nursery nurse should be aware that the preoperative insulin dosage given Molly may cause her infant to develop which of the following problems during his first few hours of life?

    1. Acidosis.
    2. Dehydration.
    3. Hypoglycemia.
    4. Diuresis.

58. The nursery nurse should be aware that 6 to 8 hours after birth infants of diabetic mothers are particularly apt to develop:

    1. Nausea and vomiting.
    2. Circulatory collapse.
    3. Respiratory distress.
    4. Abdominal distention.

59. Molly's infant's first feeding would probably be:

    1. Sterile water.
    2. Glucose water.
    3. Diluted milk.
    4. Evaporated milk.

60. Common causes for neonatal death in infants of diabetic mothers are:

    a. Premature birth.
    b. Congenital defects.
    c. Respiratory distress.
    d. Birth injury.
    e. Blood dyscrasia.

        1. a and c.
        2. b and d.
        3. All but e.
        4. All the above.

Molly recovered strength rapidly following surgery. Her insulin dosage was initially 20 units, but later reduced to 10 units of Lente insulin daily and her urine remained free of glucose. Molly and her son were both discharged from the hospital seven days after delivery and both were scheduled for visits to the family physician for long term followup.

Heart Disease and Pregnancy

"Growing pains" kept Pansy Huff in bed for several weeks during her fifteenth year, and shortly thereafter she was found to have a heart murmur. Pansy remained symptom-free, except for a systolic murmur, for the next fifteen years, during which time she was married and had two children. She was given prophylactic penicillin monthly during this interval.

When she was 31 years old Pansy became pregnant for the third time. She reported to her family physician during her second month of pregnancy, was found to be in good condition, was given ferrous sulfate, multi-vitamins, and folic acid to take daily, and was directed to return to the physician at monthly intervals as long as she continued to feel well. The physician ordered that she continue to recieve Bicillin monthly. During her first trimester Pansy experienced minimal morning sickness and occasional exertional dyspnea. Her physician placed her on a sodium restriction diet and Pansy remained fairly comfortable for the next five months, although she had gained 11.8 kg. when she visited her doctor in her 34th week of pregnancy. During this visit the physician detected that Pansy was slightly dyspneic while lying in the recumbent position and that she had 1+ pedal edema, so he admitted her to the hospital for treatment of impending congestive heart failure.

On admission, Pansy's temperature was 98.2° F., pulse 120 and regular, respirations 24, and blood pressure 110/80 mm. Hg. Her red cell count was 4.5 million per cubic millimeter and her white cell count was 10,000 per cubic millimeter. Her uterine fundus was palpated three fingerbreadths below the xiphoid process. A loud harsh systolic murmur was heard in her fifth left intercostal space, 1 cm. to the left of the mid-clavicular line. Mild rales were heard in her lung bases and her heart was slightly enlarged. The physician's impression was that Pansy had inactive rheumatic heart disease, functional class II with mitral stenosis, in mild congestive failure. He wrote the following orders:

1. Complete bedrest.
2. Digoxin 0.25 mg. b.i.d. times 3 days, then 0.25 mg. q. A.M.
3. Chlorothiazide 50 mg. b.i.d.
4. KCL, grams 1 q.i.d. orally.
5. 2000-mg. Na diet.

(ANSWER BLANK ON PAGE A–9)   (CORRECT ANSWERS ON PAGE B–19)

1. The "growing pains" which Pansy experienced when she was 15 years old were probably a manifestation of:

1. Acute allergic inflammation of synovia.

2. Bone destruction by pyogenic microorganisms.

3. Muscle fatigue induced by hyperactivity.

4. Ossification of the epiphyseal cartilage.

2. Diagnosis of Pansy's cardiac problem was complicated by the fact that:

1. The heart normally hypertrophies during the latter months of pregnancy.
2. Electrocardiography during pregnancy may produce fetal developmental defects.
3. Systolic murmurs and edema are common in normal pregnancy.
4. The euphoria associated with pregnancy causes the patient to ignore her symptoms.

3. In order to be able to give Pansy helpful instructions in self-care, the doctor's office nurse should understand that Pansy's heart disease is:

1. Psychogenic.
2. Organic.
3. Functional.
4. Temporary.

4. Pansy's red cell sedimentation rate was not determined as part of her diagnostic workup because the rate:

1. Tends to rise in the normal gravida nearing term.
2. Increases only in children suffering acute rheumatic fever.
3. Does not rise until several weeks following acute infection.
4. Is prevented from rising by the administration of digitalis.

5. Pansy's heart murmur results primarily from:

1. Bubbling of inspired air through fluid forced into the alveoli as the result of pulmonary venous congestion.
2. Unusual turbulence of flow created as blood passes through a narrowed valve between the left atrium and ventricle.
3. Friction of two acutely inflamed layers of pericardium against each other in the course of cardiac contraction.
4. Movement of pericardial fluid from one part of the sac to another, with changes in pericardial pressure.

6. Which of the following frequently precipitate congestive failure in the pregnant woman with rheumatic valvular damage?

a. Acute infectious disease.
b. Excessive weight gain.
c. Elevation of blood pressure.
d. Inadequate physical exercise.

e. Maternal-fetal blood incompatibility.

1. a and b.
2. a, b, and c.
3. All but e.
4. All the above.

7. The basic principle underlying Pansy's prenatal care should be:

1. Provision of adequate rest.
2. Administration of cardiotonics.
3. Destruction of pathogenic bacteria.
4. Limitation of fetal weight gain.

8. In order to ensure that she obtains enough rest, the physician would probably advise Pansy to:

1. Sleep eight hours each night and remain seated throughout most of each day.
2. Sleep nine hours each night and take a one-hour nap whenever she experiences fatigue.
3. Sleep ten hours each night and lie down for half an hour following each meal.
4. Sleep twelve hours each night and remain in bed except for meals and toilet activities.

9. When Pansy developed dyspnea during her first trimester it is likely that her physician would have given her which of the following directions regarding her physical activity?

1. "Try to keep as active as possible, but eliminate any activity which you find tiring."
2. "Carry on all your usual activities but learn to work at a slower pace."
3. "Avoid heavy housework, shopping, stair climbing, and all unnecessary physical effort."
4. "Get someone to do your housework and stay in bed or in a wheelchair."

10. It would be especially important for Pansy to receive ferrous sulfate during pregnancy because:

1. Anemia would predispose her to heart failure by causing a compensatory increase in cardiac output.
2. Normal hepatic stores would be lost owing to passive congestion secondary to heart failure.
3. Infants of cardiac mothers are grossly overweight and require additional iron for blood building.
4. Iron is a direct stimulant of cardiac muscle, tending to increase the force of cardiac contraction.

11. Pansy should be taught to reduce her chances of upper respiratory infection by:
- a. Avoiding large gatherings of people.
- b. Segregating herself from infected persons.
- c. Protecting herself from drafts and chilling.
- d. Eating a nutritious, well balanced diet.
- e. Obtaining adequate rest and sleep.
    1. a and c.
    2. b and d.
    3. All but e.
    4. All the above.

12. In addition to sodium restriction, Pansy's physician might order that she limit her intake of:
1. Protein.
2. Potassium.
3. Calcium.
4. Fluid.

13. Pansy first evidenced symptoms of heart failure during pregnancy because:
1. Her heart was overburdened by the necessity of pumping blood through the vessels of the fetus.
2. Maximal cardiac contractile force is required to produce amniotic fluid as a transudate of maternal blood.
3. The increase of blood volume coincident with pregnancy constituted an excessive load for her damaged heart.
4. Symptoms of which she was unaware because they had developed insidiously were detected on prenatal examination.

14. Pansy's mitral stenosis constituted an especially severe problem during pregnancy because the narrowed valve:
1. Prevented the increase in cardiac output called for by increased total blood volume and uterine blood flow.
2. Became immobilized by deposition of calcium circulating in high concentration during early fetal growth.
3. Served as a focus for reactions between antigens of fetal origin and antibodies produced by maternal tissues.
4. Was invaded by pyogenic organisms carried in the blood from primary infections in the urinary tract.

15. It is probable that Pansy's dyspnea during her 34th week of gestation was principally the result of:
1. Collapse of pulmonary alveoli because of pressure on her lung by an enlarged heart.
2. Reduction of cross-sectional area for gas exchange because of fluid in her alveoli.
3. Inadequate aeration of alveoli due to bronchial constriction and excessive secretions.
4. Interference with diaphragmatic descent by her greatly enlarged uterine fundus.

16. Pansy's pedal edema during her 34th week of pregnancy was probably indicative of:
1. Venous dilation and circulatory obstruction caused by the enlarged uterus.
2. Decreased osmotic pressure of the blood resulting from inadequate nutrition.
3. Increased pressure in the systemic venous circulation caused by cardiac inefficiency.
4. Decreased glomerular filtration resulting from increased abdominal pressure on the kidney.

17. Careful history-taking on Pansy's visit to the doctor during her 34th week of pregnancy would be apt to reveal that she had experienced which other symptoms of cardiac failure?
1. Chest pain.
2. Frequent palpitations.
3. Moist cough.
4. Dizziness on exertion.

18. Pansy's vital signs and laboratory tests on admission to the hospital were most consistent with which of the following conclusions?
1. A chronic, low-grade, localized infection was releasing pathogens into her general circulation.
2. A recently resolved acute infection had reactivated acute rheumatic inflammatory tissue changes.
3. Her damaged cardiac valve was infected and was seeding pyogenic bacteria throughout her body.
4. Previous, rather than current, in-

flammatory damage caused her heart to become functionally inadequate.

19. According to criteria established by the New York Heart Association, Pansy's functional class II diagnosis indicates that she had had:

1. No limitation of ordinary activity.
2. Dyspnea on ordinary physical activity.
3. Dyspnea on even minimal exertion.
4. Symptoms of cardiac failure at rest.

20. In addition to dyspnea, Pansy should be observed closely for appearance of which other symptoms of heart failure?

a. Bubbling rales.
b. Productive cough.
c. Rapid, weak pulse.
d. Cyanosis of lips and nails.
e. Elevation of blood pressure.
   1. a and c.
   2. b and d.
   3. All but e.
   4. All the above.

21. The physician ordered that Pansy be kept at complete bedrest in order to:

1. Increase the volume of venous blood flow to the heart.
2. Decrease the nutrient and oxygen needs of muscle tissue.
3. Increase the volume of both tidal and residual air.
4. Decrease protein catabolism and urinary protein excretion.

22. The nurse should interpret "complete" bedrest as meaning that she should perform which of the following services for Pansy?

1. Washing her face, hands, and teeth.
b. Brushing, combing, and grooming her hair.
c. Giving a daily bath and making the bed.
d. Feeding her all meals and snacks.
e. Assisting her to move about in bed.
f. Assisting her on and off the bedpan or commode.
   1. a, c, and e.
   2. b, d, and f.
   3. All but d and e.
   4. All the above.

23. During Pansy's first few days in the hospital she would probably be most comfortable in which of the following positions?

1. Sitting.
2. Supine.
3. Left lateral.
4. Right lateral.

24. In order to evaluate Pansy's response to therapy the nurse should know that the effects of a therapeutic dose of digitalis include:

a. Increasing the force of myocardial contraction.
b. Increasing the electrical excitability of the myocardium.
c. Increasing impulse conduction by the vagus nerve.
d. Increasing impulse conduction by the accelerator nerve.
e. Decreasing conduction velocity in Purkinje fibers.
   1. a and c.
   2. b and d.
   3. All but d.
   4. All the above.

25. The pharmacologic effect of chlorothiazide is to:

1. Improve the force of myocardial contraction.
2. Decrease the irritability of cardiac muscle fibers.
3. Increase renal excretion of sodium, chloride, and water.
4. Depress the cells of the sensory cerebral cortex.

26. Potassium chloride was ordered for Pansy in order to:

1. Liquefy lung secretions and stimulate the cough reflex.
2. Increase the acidity of the gastric secretions.
3. Replace potassium lost owing to chlorothiazide therapy.
4. Offset potassium deficiencies produced by her diet.

27. Which of the following foods should the nurse instruct Pansy to avoid in following a 2000-mg. sodium restriction diet?

a. Butter, peanut butter, and cheese.
b. Canned meats and vegetables.
c. Condiments and leavening agents.
d. Sauerkraut, pickles, and olives.
e. Bread and bakery products.
   1. a, b, and e.
   2. b, c, and e.
   3. All but e.
   4. All the above.

28. One morning during her bath Pansy said to the nurse, "I've never had trouble with my heart before. What did I do to make my heart fail?" Which of the following responses by the nurse would be most appropriate?

   1. "You have probably been working or exercising more strenuously than formerly and have outstripped your energy reserves."

   2. "You have perhaps been getting less rest than you need and have finally used up your reserve strength."

   3. "You have, undoubtedly, been eating unwisely, selecting foods which cause you to retain fluid and gain weight."

   4. "You've done nothing wrong. Your previously weakened heart was unable to meet the increased circulatory demands of pregnancy."

29. The nurse should observe Pansy carefully for which of the following as symptoms of digitalis intoxication?

   a. Anorexia or nausea and vomiting.

   b. Coupling or irregularity of the pulse.

   c. Headache, drowsiness, or disorientation.

   d. Blurring, diplopia, or halo vision.

     1. a and c.

     2. b and d.

     3. All but d.

     4. All the above.

Following a week of treatment Pansy's dyspnea and pedal edema disappeared. During this time her pulse rate decreased to 80 per minute and her respirations to 20 per minute. Her lungs were clear to auscultation and her heart was found to be of normal size on thoracic percussion. Pansy was maintained on digoxin but was allowed up to the bathroom during her second and third weeks of hospitalization. At the end of her 38th week of gestation Pansy spontaneously went into labor. She was given epidural anesthesia. Pansy delivered a 3150 gram daughter whose Apgar score was 10 at 60 seconds after birth. Pansy required neither episiotomy nor forceps to facilitate delivery.

In addition to routine postpartum medications and procedures Pansy was given procaine penicillin 600,000 units I.M. q. 12 h. and a testosterone-estradiol mixture I.M. to suppress lactation. After remaining in bed for the first two days postpartum, Pansy was permitted out of bed as desired. She remained free of symptoms of congestive failure and both digitalis and potassium chloride were discontinued.

Pansy was hospitalized for 10 days following delivery, during which time her physician advised Pansy and her husband to avoid having more children. He suggested that her husband have a vasectomy performed. On hospital discharge Pansy was referred to an internist for cardiac followup and arrangements were made for a visiting nurse to provide health supervision in the Huff home.

30. Pansy's care during labor should differ from that of the noncardiac gravida in that Pansy would be:

   1. Given continuous intravenous infusion of a 10 per cent glucose solution in water throughout labor.

   2. Denied both solid and liquid feedings from the beginning of the first stage of labor.

   3. Encouraged to drink small quantities of liquid at frequent intervals throughout labor.

   4. Given a strong saline enema early in labor to withdraw tissue fluid by osmotic effect.

31. During the first stage of her labor, which of Pansy's vital signs would be the most sensitive and reliable indicator of impending congestive heart failure?

   1. Temperature.

   2. Pulse rate.

   3. Respiratory rate.

   4. Blood pressure.

32. During labor Pansy should be maintained in which position?

   1. Supine.

   2. Semirecumbent.

   3. Side-lying.

   4. Sitting.

33. Epidural anesthesia is best described as:

   1. Introduction of medication directly into the spinal canal in the coccygeal region.

   2. Injection of anesthetic external to the dura mater in the lumbar area.

   3. Injection of local anesthetic directly into nerves supplying the perineum.

4. Dilution of spinal fluid with a weak Lidocaine solution.

34. Throughout Pansy's entire labor the nurse should take frequent measurements of her:

1. Urinary pH and specific gravity.
2. Fluid intake and output.
3. Pulse and respiratory rates.
4. Calf and thigh circumferences.

35. During the second stage of labor the nurse should instruct Pansy to:

1. Avoid prolonged bearing down.
2. Breathe shallowly and rapidly.
3. Sit on the side of the bed.
4. Sleep between contractions.

36. Procaine penicillin was ordered for Pansy chiefly to protect her against:

1. Bacterial endocarditis.
2. Bronchial pneumonia.
3. Chronic pyelonephritis.
4. Femoral thrombophlebitis.

37. Which of the following factors contribute to making the early postpartum period a critical phase for Pansy?

a. Occurrence of major circulatory adjustments.
b. Sudden decrease in abdominal pressure.
c. Engorgement of splanchnic vessels.
d. Fatigue produced by labor and delivery.
e. Marked blood loss during delivery.

    1. a and b.
    2. a, c, and d.
    3. All but e.
    4. All the above.

38. The physician advised Pansy to use some means of contraception because:

1. Her hospitalization experience during this confinement would predispose her to emotional lability.
2. She would be increasingly predisposed to cardiac failure with each subsequent pregnancy.
3. Her present illness indicates that additional pregnancies would result in abortion or maternal death.
4. She will probably soon require cardiac catheterization and reconstructive cardiac surgery.

39. In Pansy's case estrogen-progesterone pills were contraindicated as a means of contraception because that medicinal combination:

1. Might produce the troublesome side effect of excessive retention of extracellular fluid.
2. Necessitates physically taxing monthly trips to the doctor's office for prescription refills.
3. Would be subconsciously rejected because of its identification with cardiac medications.
4. Is often omitted by a patient with the repressed need to incur discomfort and illness.

40. Which of the following best describes the procedure of vasectomy?

1. Excision of the testes.
2. Ligation of the epididymis.
3. Excision of the seminal vesicle.
4. Ligation of the vas deferens.

Hemolytic Disease of the Newborn

Corrine Perry had type A, Rh negative blood. Her husband, Paul, had type B, Rh positive blood. Their first child, Percy, had type AB, Rh positive blood, and, though normal at birth, died of pneumonia at the age of one year. The Perrys' second child, Philip, blood type A, Rh positive, had a positive direct Coombs' test at birth and cord blood bilirubin level of 3.2 mg. per 100 ml. rising to 5.8 mg./100 ml. in 48 hours. Although Philip developed slight jaundice in his second day of life, no exchange transfusion was performed and the infant demonstrated no sequelae of hemolytic disease. Mrs. Perry was not given an injection of immunoglobulin after delivery of her children.

During Corinne's third pregnancy, her indirect Coombs' test was positive and her Rh antibody titers rose steadily during gestation. During the third trimester amniocentesis was done and the amniotic fluid was subjected to spectrophotometric analysis. Because spectrophotometry revealed hemolytic disease of the fetus, Corrine was admitted to the hospital in her 36th week of gestation and labor was induced by amniotomy and intravenous administration of oxytocin. After a three-hour labor an icteric and edematous 2700 gram girl infant was delivered without anesthesia or episiotomy. Cord blood revealed type A, Rh positive blood, a positive Coombs' test, bilirubin level of 7.2 mg. per 100 ml., and hemoglobin concentration of 13.2 mg. per 100 ml. At three hours after birth the infant's serum bilirubin level was 11.4 mg. per 100 ml., and her liver and spleen were markedly enlarged. The doctor initiated fetal heart monitoring, started a glucose infusion, and performed an exchange transfusion of 300 ml. of type A, Rh negative blood, resulting in a postexchange bilirubin of 5.2 mg. per 100 ml. The doctor wrote the following order for her infant:

1. *Place in isolette or radiant heater.*
2. *Continuous cardiac and respiratory monitoring.*
3. *Central blood pressure q.h.*
4. *Dextrose in 10 per cent water — q. ml. q.h. through umbilical artery line.*
5. *Serum electrolytes, Ca^{++}, and glucose q. 12 h.*
6. *Serum bilirubin q. 6 h.*
7. *Dextrostix q. 4 h.*
8. *Continuous phototherapy, protect eyes with shield.*
9. *Weigh q. 8.*
10. *Intake and output.*
11. *Specific gravity q. voiding.*

(ANSWER BLANK ON PAGE A-11) (CORRECT ANSWERS ON PAGE B-21)

1. At the time of Corrine's and Paul's marriage it would have been impossible for their physician to predict that any of their children would develop hemorrhagic disease because:
1. The Rh trait is not in any way genetically determined.
2. The Rh type of either parent may change with time.
3. Not all children of Rh positive fathers are Rh positive.
4. The Rh trait of a fetus may change during gestation.

2. Corrine's genotype for ABO antigens on her red blood cells could be:

a. AA
b. AO
c. AB
d. BO
e. BB

    1. a only.
    2. a or b.
    3. a, b, or c.
    4. All the above.

3. If it could be determined that both Corrine's father and her mother had had type A blood, then it would be obvious that Corrine's genotype for ABO type blood was:

1. Homozygous.
2. Isogamous.
3. Heterozygous.
4. Phenotypic.

4. Corrine Perry's blood serum contains which of the following antibodies?

1. Anti A.
2. Anti B.
3. Anti A and anti B.
4. No antibodies.

5. Paul Perry's blood serum contains which of the following antibodies?

1. Anti A.
2. Anti B.
3. Anti A and anti B.
4. No antibodies.

6. Isoimmunization can best be defined as:

1. The production of antibodies against an antigen originating from an individual of the same species.
2. The development of antibodies that react against cells, tissues, or secretions of one's own body.
3. The presence of antibodies against an antigen with which the body has had no prior contact.
4. A reaction in which all antigen molecules have been nullified by an equivalent number of antibody molecules.

7. An antigen is best defined as:

1. A substance that mechanically inactivates foreign proteins introduced into sensitized tissue by direct or hematogenous routes.
2. A protein or carbohydrate substance that will stimulate formation of antibodies when introduced into the body of a susceptible person.
3. A microorganism which is capable of surviving and multiplying in human tissues and elaborating toxic metabolites.
4. A normal byproduct of bacterial metabolism which is capable of adversely influencing human cellular function.

8. An antibody can be best defined as:

1. A globulin produced by the body in response to a specific antigen.
2. A glucoprotein resulting from combination of endogenous and exogenous metabolites.
3. A toxin produced by a bacterium and released only on its dissolution.
4. A large phagocytic cell produced by reticuloendothelial cells in the liver.

9. Percy Perry, Corrine's first son, had which of the following naturally occurring antibodies in his blood serum?

1. Anti A.
2. Anti B.
3. Both anti A and anti B.
4. No antibodies.

10. The nurse may assume that Corrine's first pregnancy contributed to her second child's hemolytic disease in that during the first pregnancy:

1. A small amount of fetal blood passed through the placenta, stimulating maternal tissues to produce anti-Rh antibodies.
2. The uterus suffered mechanical trauma which permitted passage of fetal blood across the placenta during later pregnancies.
3. Faulty placental separation created uterine vascular anomalies, facilitating later transfer of maternal cells to the fetus.
4. Corrine suffered an intercurrent bacterial infection in response to which her reticuloendothelial system produced antibodies.

11. Philip Perry, Corrine's second child, developed mild hemolytic disease as a result of:

1. Faulty implantation of placental tissues, with resulting free communication between the fetal and maternal circulations.
2. Passage of maternally produced anti-Rh antibodies across the placenta into the systemic circulation of the fetus.
3. Hyperactivity of fetal reticuloendothelial cells in sequestering and hemolyzing both red and white blood cells.
4. Antibodies developed by fetal tissues against A and B antigens deposited in the endometrium during the first pregnancy.

12. An injection of Rh immunoglobulin within 72 hours after the birth of each of her first two children would have had which of the following effects?

1. Inactivation of maternal antibodies before they stimulated antigen production in another fetus.
2. Inactivation of fetal antibodies before they stimulated antigen production in the mother.
3. Inactivation of maternal antigens before they stimulated antibody production in another fetus.
4. Inactivation of fetal antigens before they stimulated antibody production in the mother.

13. In the normal infant the cord blood hemoglobin level typically falls within which range?

1. 7.6 to 13.6 grams per 100 ml.
2. 15.6 to 19.6 grams per 100 ml.
3. 19.6 to 25.6 grams per 100 ml.
4. 25.6 to 31.6 grams per 100 ml.

14. The direct Coombs' test was used to detect in Corrine's infant the presence of:

1. Maternal chromosomes in the infant's blood.
2. Maternal red cells in the infant's serum.
3. Maternal antibodies on the infant's red cells.
4. Maternal serum in the infant's blood serum.

15. A positive reaction to the Coombs' test can most accurately be interpreted as signifying that:

1. Isoantibodies are adsorbed to the surface of red cells.
2. The concentration of serum bilirubin is markedly increased.
3. Increased hemolysis has resulted from splenic hypertrophy.
4. The serum contains excessive amounts of immune globulin.

16. Bilirubin can best be defined as:

1. An intermediary compound in fat catabolism.
2. A normal breakdown product of hemoglobin.
3. A crystalline precipitate of bile salts.
4. The protein constituent of intestinal chyme.

17. Which of the following are common causes of hyperbilirubinemia?

a. Increased hemolysis of fragile red blood cells.
b. Interference with binding of bilirubin to albumin.
c. Inadequate supply of glucuronyl transferase.
d. Increased excretion of water-soluble stercobilin.
e. Interference with bilirubin excretion from the intestines.
   1. a and b.
   2. a and c.
   3. a, c, and e.
   4. All the above.

18. Which of the following substances compete with bilirubin for binding sites on the albumin molecule?

a. Free fatty acids.
b. Sulfonamides.
c. Sodium benzoate.
d. Vitamin C.
e. Phospholipids.
   1. a only.
   2. a, b, and c.
   3. All but e.
   4. All the above.

19. Which of the following are measures to lower the blood level of bilirubin?

a. Phototherapy.
b. Exchange transfusion.
c. Thermoneutral environment.
d. Adequate oxygenation.
   1. a and b.
   2. a, b, and c.
   3. All but a.
   4. All the above.

20. Phototherapy used to decrease serum bilirubin has which of the following mechanisms of action?

1. Converts bilirubin to less toxic metabolic products.
2. Allows substrates required for bilirubin metabolism to evaporate.
3. Causes hyperthermia which accelerates the excretion of bilirubin.
4. Increases skin concentration of the vitamin D, which detoxifies bilirubin.

21. The normal range for total serum bilirubin in the newborn at one day of age is:

1. 2 to 6 mg. per 100 ml. of blood.
2. 6 to 10 mg. per 100 ml. of blood.
3. 10 to 14 mg. per 100 ml. of blood.
4. 14 to 18 mg. per 100 ml. of blood.

22. The increased serum bilirubin concentration noted at birth in Corrine's second and third infants was the result of:

1. Interruption in normal bile flow with regurgitation of pigments through the liver cell into the venous circulation.
2. Destruction of large numbers of erythrocytes with release of excessive quantities of bilirubin into the circulation.
3. Inability of the functionally immature renal glomeruli to filter large pigment molecules from the circulating blood.
4. Failure of the mechanically abnormal placenta to permit diffusion of fetal metabolic wastes into the maternal circulation.

23. Kernicterus is apt to occur in Corrine's premature infant when the serum bilirubin level exceeds:

1. 6 mg. per 100 ml.
2. 10 mg. per 100 ml.
3. 14 mg. per 100 ml.
4. 18 mg. per 100 ml.

24. In addition to Rh sensitization, which of the following situations is a frequent cause of hemolytic disease of the newborn?

1. Heavy metal intoxication.
2. Iron deficiency anemia.
3. ABO factor incompatibility.
4. Intrapartal cranial trauma.

25. Hemolytic disease of the newborn is sometimes given the name erythroblastosis, which signifies that:

1. Multiple minute hemorrhages occur in all body tissues, owing to widespread damage to capillary endothelium.
2. The red cells are hemolyzed, owing to rupture of the overdistended cell following imbibition of water.
3. Large numbers of immature red cell precursors are released into the blood from hyperactive bone marrow.
4. The infant displays a plethoric appearance due to increases in red cell numbers and blood volume.

26. Analysis of amniotic fluid obtained by amniocentesis can be used to obtain information concerning:

a. Degree of fetal maturity.
b. Sex of the fetus.
c. Fetal chromosomal abnormalities.
d. Fetal gastrointestinal malformations.
e. Fetal enzyme deficiency diseases.
1. a and b.
2. a, b, and c.
3. All but d.
4. All the above.

27. If the amniotic fluid specimen obtained by amniocentesis could not be subjected to spectrophotometric analysis as soon as it was obtained, the specimen should have been:

1. Mixed with an equal amount of saline solution and agitated gently.
2. Placed in an opaque container and stored in the ward refrigerator.
3. Injected into a sealed sterile glass bottle with a rubber top.
4. Poured into a Petri dish with an equal quantity of melted agar.

28. The amniotic fluid is chiefly derived from which of the following?

a. Maternal lymph.
b. Maternal serum.
c. Fetal urine.
d. Fetal serum.
e. Uteroplacental unit.
1. a and d.
2. b and c.
3. All but e.
4. All the above.

29. The nurse should know that which of the following most accurately reflects the rate of amniotic fluid exchange (amount of time it takes for total fluid replacement) at 40 week gestation?

1. 3 minutes.
2. 3 hours.
3. 3 days.
4. 3 weeks.

30. The degree of fetal maturity can be assessed by chemical analysis of which of the following in the amniotic fluid?

a. Lecithin.
b. Sphingomyelin.
c. Creatinine.
d. Oxytocinase.
e. Lactogen.
1. a and b.
2. a, b, and d.
3. a, b, and c.
4. All the above.

31. Which of the following are nursing responsibilities when giving care to an immature infant?
- a. Maintaining biochemical homeostasis.
- b. Fulfilling nutritional and fluid needs.
- c. Stabilizing the body temperature.
- d. Protecting the brain from hypoxia.
- e. Preventing respiratory distress syndrome.
    1. a, c, and d.
    2. a, b, and e.
    3. All but e.
    4. All the above.

32. Following amniocentesis Corrine asked the nurse, "Will sticking that needle into my abdomen hurt my baby?" Which response by the nurse would be most appropriate?
1. "You must place your faith in your doctor and assume that he is operating in your own and the baby's best interests."
2. "The slight risk from inserting the needle is more than outweighed by the value of the information obtained in protecting the baby."
3. "There is no chance whatsoever that this procedure could in any way harm either you or your baby. Don't give it another thought."
4. "It is impossible to predict all the possible effects of the procedure since it has been developed so recently."

33. In the event that amniocentesis had revealed severe erythroblastosis prior to the 32nd week of gestation, which of the following procedures could have been performed to decrease the probability of fetal death?
1. Administration of type O, Rh, positive blood transfusion to Corrine.
2. Intraperitoneal transfusion of the fetus with O-negative packed red cells.
3. Replacement of Corrine's blood with type A, Rh positive whole blood.
4. Introduction of anti-antibodies into the amniotic sac by infusion.

34. Corrine's infant's accelerated hemolysis resulted from:
1. Coating of her red blood cells by an agglutinin transmitted across the placenta from the maternal circulation.
2. Production in the fetal liver, spleen, and marrow cavities of red blood cells with mechanically defective stroma.
3. Production by the fetal liver of a substance which increases the permeability of the red blood cell membrane.
4. Sequestration of fetal red cells by hyperplastic and hyperactive elements of the fetal reticuloendothelial system.

35. Corrine's physician elected to induce her labor prematurely in order to:
1. Prevent difficult labor due to fetal hydrops.
2. Reduce maternal discomfort due to polyhydramnios.
3. Shorten fetal exposure to maternally produced antibodies.
4. Minimize the possibility of maternal hypertension.

36. Having diagnosed the fetus as having hemolytic disease, Corrine's physician would probably make which of the following adjustments in her care during labor and delivery?
- a. Giving analgesics liberally throughout the first two stages of labor.
- b. Clamping the cord promptly following birth of the infant.
- c. Cutting the cord so as to leave at least a four inch stump.
- d. Administering large and repeated doses of vitamin K during labor.
    1. a and b.
    2. b and c.
    3. All but d.
    4. All the above.

37. The nursery nurse should employ which of the following as the most sensitive technique for detecting mild jaundice in a newborn infant?
1. Immersing white filter paper in the infant's urine and observing the color of the moistened paper.
2. Observing the color of the infant's skin, sclerae, and conjunctivae under ultraviolet illumination.
3. Exerting finger pressure on the thorax and observing the color of the blanched skin in natural light.
4. Determining the color of the nailbeds when the fingertip is transilluminated with high intensity light.

38. The nursery nurse should be aware that

in erythroblastosis fetalis jaundice usually appears within what interval following birth?
1. 1–24 hours.
2. 36–60 hours.
3. 72–96 hours.
4. 108–132 hours.

39. Corrine's baby is subject to which of the following complications of his hemolytic disease?
a. Severe anemia.
b. Heart failure.
c. Massive edema.
d. Atelectasis.
1. a and c.
2. b and d.
3. All but d.
4. All the above.

40. Kernicterus, a possible complication of severe hemolytic disease of the newborn, is characterized by:
1. Obstruction of intrahepatic bile ducts by stones composed of precipitated bile salts.
2. Permanent injury to basal ganglia of the brain through intracellular deposition of bile.
3. Weakening of the intestinal wall by submucosal disposition of pigment granules.
4. Skin excoriation and infection by repeated scratching of pruritic, bile-stained tissues.

41. In kernicterus, bile pigments interfere with normal functioning of brain tissue in that they:
1. Destroy cellular energy stores by rapidly breaking down adenosine triphosphate.
2. Saponify fat globules dispersed throughout the cytoplasm of nerve cell bodies.
3. Depress cellular oxidation by inhibiting cytochrome C in the electron transfer system.
4. Render the nerve cell membrane impermeable to active transport of glucose and water.

42. The nurse should be aware that which of the following are symptoms of impending kernicterus?
a. Decreased response to stimuli.
b. Weak, high-pitched cry.
c. Loss of the Moro reflex.
d. Arching of the back.
1. a and c.
2. b and d.

3. All but c.
4. All the above.

43. Which of the following are possible effects of kernicterus?
a. Mental retardation.
b. Emotional lability.
c. Nerve deafness.
d. Muscle spasticity.
e. Athetoid movement.
1. a and b.
2. c and d.
3. All but d.
4. All the above.

44. The infant's hepatomegaly and splenomegaly are probably due to:
1. Foci of extramedullary erythropoiesis in both organs.
2. Heart failure and resulting venous congestion.
3. Deposition of iron liberated from lysed red cells.
4. Inflammatory changes associated with viral infection.

45. The nursery nurse should be aware that the Perry infant's prematurity accentuated his physiologic problems primarily because of the:
1. Lack of polymorphonuclear leukocytes normally transferred from mother to infant during the final month of gestation.
2. Inability of the immature liver cells to conjugate bilirubin in preparation for its removal from the body.
3. Greatly increased oxygen need provoked by the marked motor hyperactivity of the premature infant.
4. Tendency toward hyperthermia which would increase the rate of hemolysis by accelerating metabolic reactions.

46. The primary objective in performing an exchange transfusion is to:
1. Elevate the infant's intrahepatic iron stores in preparation for increased erythropoiesis.
2. Elevate the infant's blood pressure by increasing the viscosity of the circulating blood.
3. Provide exogenous antibodies to combat those obtained from the maternal circulation.
4. Provide compatible RBC's and increased protein to alleviate anemia and kernicterus; and remove excess bilirubin from the infant's blood stream.

47. The physician would probably take which of the following precautions in preparation for the Perry infant's exchange transfusion?
   a. Maintaining the infant N.P.O. for 3 hours prior to transfusion.
   b. Crossmatching the blood to be given against the infant's blood.
   c. Inserting a catheter to monitor the central venous pressure.
   d. Anesthetizing the infant with a small dose of ethyl ether.
      1. a only.
      2. a and c.
      3. a, b, and c.
      4. All the above.

48. The blood used for the exchange transfusion had been preserved with an acid-citrate-dextrose mixture (ACD blood). The nurse should assume which of the following responsibilities during the exchange procedure?
   a. Monitor the serum glucose during and after the exchange.
   b. Assess the PaO_2 and serum hydrogen ion concentration.
   c. Observe for muscle twitching or signs of hypocalcemia.
   d. Observe the EKG pattern for signs of hyperkalemia.
   e. Infuse protamine sulfate to neutralize the heparin added to the blood.
      1. a and c.
      2. a, b, and d.
      3. All but e.
      4. All the above.

49. Which of the following complications may occur from the exchange transfusion?
   a. Cardiac overloading.
   b. Electrolyte imbalances.
   c. Hypoglycemia.
   d. Hypothermia.
   e. Formation of air emboli.
      1. a, b, and c.
      2. a, c, and d.
      3. All but e.
      4. All the above.

50. The usual method for exchange transfusion is to:
   1. Remove a total quantity of 200 ml. of infant's blood rapidly and inject 200 ml of heparinized blood slowly.
   2. Follow serial withdrawals of 100 ml. aliquots of infant's blood with rapid administration of donor blood.
   3. Withdraw serial 15–20 ml. aliquots

of infant blood, replacing each with an equal amount of donor blood until 400 ml. have been exchanged.
   4. Administer the donor's blood slowly over a period of several hours, flushing the tubing frequently with saline solution.

51. In preparing for and carrying out the exchange transfusion, the physician would ensure that the donor blood was at 37° C. during administration in order to prevent:
   1. Cellular rupture.
   2. Bacterial growth.
   3. Cellular sedimentation.
   4. Cardiac arrest.

52. During exchange transfusion it is customary to inject 1 ml. of which of the following solutions after administration of each 100–200 ml. of donor blood?
   1. Potassium chloride.
   2. Sodium phenobarbital.
   3. Calcium gluconate.
   4. Ammonium citrate.

53. The purpose for injecting the above substance at intervals throughout the exchange transfusion is to:
   1. Prevent clotting of blood in the tubing and needle.
   2. Stimulate the rate and depth of respirations.
   3. Provide a source of ready energy for cardiac muscle.
   4. Replace ions depleted by citration of donor blood.

54. Failure to administer the aforementioned substance during the exchange transfusion would be apt to cause:
   1. Edema and ascites.
   2. Tetany and convulsions.
   3. Diuresis and diarrhea.
   4. Acidosis and coma.

55. The physician probably would take which of the following measurements at frequent intervals throughout the exchange transfusion?
   1. Rectal temperature.
   2. Tidal volume.
   3. Venous pressure.
   4. Red cell count.

56. Following the exchange transfusion the nursery nurse should observe Corrine's infant closely for:
   a. Dyspnea.
   b. Cyanosis.
   c. Bleeding.
   d. Hypoglycemia.

e. Listlessness.
   1. a and b.
   2. c and d.
   3. a, c, and e.
   4. All the above.

57. If Corrine should require blood transfusion as a result of postpartum hemorrhage, she could safely be given which of the following blood types?
   1. Type B, Rh negative.
   2. Type AB, Rh positive.
   3. Type A, Rh negative.
   4. Type A, Rh positive.

Although she was reluctant to go home without her baby, Corrine was discharged on her fifth postpartum day. For the first five days following the exchange transfusion her infant appeared to be in good condition and serial tests revealed that her hemoglobin concentration varied between 13.8 and 15 grams per 100 ml. and that her serum bilirubin level ranged between 2.2 and 6.8 mg. per 100 ml. On the seventh day following transfusion the infant's hemoglobin concentration was 11 grams per 100 ml. and her serum bilirubin was 5.8 gm. per 100 ml. The baby was discharged from the hospital and referred to the pediatric clinic for followup.

58. The Perry infant's hemoglobin concentration fell between his fifth and fourteenth postnatal day probably as a result of:
   1. Depression of hematopoiesis by bilirubin deposited in bone marrow.
   2. Sequestering of large numbers of red blood cells by the spleen.
   3. Continuing hemolysis by maternal antibodies remaining in his tissues.
   4. Exhaustion of the infant's liver stores of iron salts.

59. The Perry infant's prematurity makes it advisable that the nursery nurse provide him with:
   a. Controlled external heat.
   b. Highly humidified air.
   c. Segregation from infections.
   d. Small, frequent feedings.
      1. a and b.
      2. c and d.
      3. All but b.
      4. All the above.

Hysterectomy

Dolores Grayling confided to her neighbor that for several months she had been troubled with excessive menstrual bleeding and occasional vaginal spotting between menstrual periods. She hadn't told her husband or her two teen-age-daughters about the bleeding because she didn't want to worry them. She hadn't consulted her doctor because she dreaded the vaginal examination.

The neighbor, who had recently seen a movie about cancer detection at a woman's club meeting, insisted that Mrs. Grayling visit her doctor immediately and offered to accompany her to the office.

Mrs. Grayling agreed to her friend's proposal, insisting that they go that very afternoon to see the doctor rather than phoning for an appointment sometime in the future, saying "Now that I've decided to go, I want to get it over with."

(ANSWER BLANK ON PAGE A–13) (CORRECT ANSWERS ON PAGE B–24)

1. The neighbor's insistence that Mrs. Grayling consult her doctor immediately was probably the result of her having learned which of the following facts from the American Cancer Society movie?
1. Positive diagnosis of uterine cancer requires several weeks.
2. Beginning carcinoma can be treated with hormonal medication.
3. Malignant tumors are curable during their early stages.
4. Unusual uterine bleeding almost always signifies malignancy.

2. The most common malignancy of the female reproductive tract is carcinoma of the:
1. Vulva.
2. Cervix.
3. Fundus.
4. Ovary.

3. Customarily the physician gauges whether menstrual bleeding has been excessive, average, or scanty in amount by asking:
1. The usual duration of the menstrual period.
2. The number of pads used and their saturation.
3. Whether menstrual fluid is bright or dark.
4. The usual interval between successive periods.

4. Which of the following considerations probably contributed to Mrs. Grayling's delay in consulting her doctor about her menorrhagia and spotting?
   a. Aversion to exposure.
   b. Anxiety concerning femininity.
   c. Fear of malignancy.
   d. Dread of mutilation.
   1. a only.
   2. a and c.
   3. b and d.
   4. All the above.

On questioning Mrs. Grayling, the doctor learned that she was 38 years old, that she had two daughters, one 13 and one 14, and that she had noticed unusual fatigue for the past several weeks.

A vaginal examination revealed an apparently normal cervix, from which a Papanicolaou test was taken. A bimanual pelvic examination revealed several large, firm masses in the body of the uterus, which were interpreted as being fibroid tumors. A blood count revealed marked hypochromic anemia.

5. In preparing Mrs. Grayling for the vaginal examination, the doctor's office nurse should:

1. Instruct her to void.
2. Scrub the external genitalia.
3. Administer a vinegar douche.
4. Shave the perineal area.

60

6. In order that Mrs. Grayling's vaginal examination cause her as little distress as possible, the nurse should instruct her to do which of the following during the procedure?

1. Hold her breath and bear down firmly.
2. Breathe deeply with her mouth open.
3. Consciously tighten her abdominal muscles.
4. Lift her hips slightly off the table.

7. Which of the following is the office nurse's responsibility in assisting with Mrs. Grayling's vaginal examination?

1. Place Mrs. Grayling in lithotomy position and leave the room before the examination is begun.
2. Stand beside Mrs. Grayling and reassure her until the speculum is inserted, and then leave.
3. Stay with Mrs. Grayling during the entire time that the examination is being performed.
4. Remain in another room until the examination is completed, then enter and help Mrs. Grayling to dress.

8. During the pelvic examination the physician will:

a. Observe the vulva for skin lesions, structural abnormalities, and condition of the vaginal outlet.
b. Check for the presence of purulent exudate in the urethra and in the ducts of adjacent glands.
c. Palpate the cervix, fornices, uterine body and fundus, pelvic walls, and the ovaries.
d. Observe the cervix and vaginal walls and obtain secretions to be used for cytologic studies.
e. Palpate and observe the anal sphincter and rectal mucosa for vascular and mucosal lesions.
   1. a and b.
   2. c and d.
   3. All but e.
   4. All the above.

9. A Papanicolaou test is:
1. A culture of vaginal secretions.
2. An x-ray of the reproductive tract.
3. A stained smear of cervical cells.
4. An air insufflation of the uterus.

10. A fibroid tumor or leiomyoma arises from:
1. Mucous membrane.

2. Fatty tissue.
3. Smooth muscle tissue.
4. Connective tissue.

11. Which of the following is thought to stimulate the growth of fibroid tumors of the uterus?
1. Estrogen.
2. Moniliasis.
3. Avitaminosis.
4. Menopause.

12. Which of the following is the most likely explanation for Mrs. Grayling's unusual fatigue?

1. Nervous tissue depression by toxic substances elaborated by the uterine tumor.
2. Psychological exhaustion produced by continuous worry about the cause of her illness.
3. Interference with normal carbohydrate absorption due to pressure on the small bowel.
4. Decreased oxygen-carrying capacity of the blood due to chronic loss of body iron stores.

13. The nurse should understand that hypochromic anemia is characterized by:

1. Replacement of bone marrow by malignant cells.
2. Inadequate amount of hemoglobin in each red cell.
3. Unusual increase in the number of white cells.
4. Too rapid destruction of blood by the spleen.

14. In addition to menorrhagia, Mrs. Grayling might also demonstrate which of the following as a consequence of her uterine tumors?

a. Dysmenorrhea.
b. Urinary retention.
c. Constipation.
d. Easy fatigability.
   1. a and c.
   2. b and d.
   3. All but d.
   4. All the above.

15. A complaint by Mrs. Grayling of sudden severe pelvic pain would suggest that her fibroid tumor had:

1. Occluded the fallopian tube openings.
2. Undergone necrotic or malignant change.
3. Become twisted or bent upon its pedicle.
4. Contracted in response to intrinsic stimuli.

Because Mrs. Grayling had multiple large fibroids, had been bleeding for many months, and might not reach menopause for several years, the doctor advised that she have a hysterectomy. Mrs. Grayling was initially reluctant to undergo such an operation and gave her consent only after deliberating the matter for a week.

16. In explaining to Mrs. Grayling the consequences of undergoing a hysterectomy, the doctor would inform her that following recovery from the operation she:

1. Would be completely incapable of both sexual intercourse and child bearing.
2. Might resume sexual intercourse but would never again bear children.
3. Would be capable of intercourse but would lose desire for sexual activity.
4. Would be fully capable of both sexual intercourse and normal child bearing.

Mrs. Grayling decided to have the hysterectomy performed and was admitted to the hospital for a three-day presurgical workup. Physical examination, routine blood work, blood typing and crossmatching, urinalysis, and chest x-rays were done. She was given two units of whole blood and a high protein, high vitamin diet. She spent most of her time catching up on lost sleep, doing a little hand sewing, and visiting with her family, her minister, and two close female friends. On the night before surgery, she was given a vaginal douche, a cleansing enema, a preoperative skin preparation, and a sedative. She was given nothing by mouth after midnight and a preanesthetic medication 15 minutes before being taken to the operating room at 8:00 A.M.

17. Proteins contain which elements that are *not* found in carbohydrates and fats?

 a. Oxygen.
 b. Sulfur.
 c. Hydrogen.
 d. Phosphorus.
 e. Nitrogen.
  1. a only.
  2. a and c.
  3. b and d.
  4. b, d, and e.

18. Mrs. Grayling was given a high protein diet preoperatively in order to:

 a. Provide material for red blood cell production.
 b. Maintain normal concentrations of serum albumin.
 c. Facilitate optimum healing of the surgical incision.
 d. Compensate for immediate postoperative food lack.
  1. a only.
  2. a and c.
  3. b and d.
  4. All the above.

19. A high quality or complete protein differs from an incomplete protein in that the complete protein:

1. Contains a greater quantity of nitrogen.
2. Supplies all the essential amino acids.
3. Is never combusted as an energy source.
4. Yields a greater number of calories.

20. Which of the following foods contains protein of the highest quality?

1. Wheat cereal.
2. Lima beans.
3. Hickory nuts.
4. Whole eggs.

21. Vitamins are essential to proper nutrition because they:

1. Provide a reliable source of energy.
2. Form the chief constituent of protoplasm.
3. Flavor food substances, making them appetizing.
4. Enter into the production of cellular enzymes.

22. Which of the following vitamins is especially important in the formation of blood cells in the bone marrow?

1. Vitamin A.
2. Vitamin B_1.
3. Vitamin C.
4. Vitamin D.

23. Adequate vitamin C intake would be important for Mrs. Grayling at this time because ascorbic acid is essential for:

1. Rapid blood clotting.
2. Carbohydrate metabolism.
3. Stimulation of appetite.
4. Optimal wound healing.

24. Which of the following foods is the best source of vitamin C?

1. Cantaloupe.
2. Cottage cheese.
3. Wheat cereal.
4. Lima beans.

25. Which of the following foods are fairly good sources of vitamin A?
   a. Whole grains.
   b. Animal livers.
   c. Citrus fruits.
   d. Milk fat.
   e. Beef steak.
      1. a and c.
      2. b and d.
      3. c and e.
      4. All the above.

26. Another name for vitamin B_2 is:
   1. Niacin.
   2. Thiamine.
   3. Pyridoxine.
   4. Riboflavin.

27. Both vitamin B_1 and vitamin B_2 are involved in:
   1. Acid-base balance.
   2. Antibody formation.
   3. Tissue oxidation.
   4. Blood clotting.

28. Which of the following are fairly good sources of the B complex vitamins?
   a. Yeast.
   b. Legumes.
   c. Organ meats.
   d. Citrus fruits.
   e. Vegetable fat.
      1. a and b.
      2. a, b, and c.
      3. c and d.
      4. d and e.

29. In preparing to give Mrs. Grayling her preoperative douche, the nurse should ensure that which of the following items is sterile?
   a. Irrigating solution.
   b. Douche tip.
   c. Connecting tubing.
   d. Douche can.
      1. a only.
      2. a and b.
      3. a, b, and c.
      4. All the above.

30. The nurse should include which of the following in Mrs. Grayling's preoperative skin preparation?
   a. Scrub and shave the entire abdominal wall.
   b. Cleanse the umbilicus with soap and water.

   c. Cover the abdomen with a sterile towel.
   d. Shave the pubic and perineal regions.
   e. Paint the perineum with an antiseptic solution.
      1. a only.
      2. a and c.
      3. a, b, and d.
      4. All the above.

An abdominal hysterectomy was performed under general anesthesia and Mrs. Grayling was returned to the recovery room with an indwelling catheter in place. Both legs were encased in full-length elastic stockings. An intravenous infusion of 5 per cent dextrose in distilled water containing 20 milliequivalents of potassium chloride was started. An order was written to follow the current flask of intravenous fluid with another liter of 5 per cent dextrose in water and to give thiamine hydrochloride, 50 mg. I.M. daily.

31. A hysterectomy consists of removal of the:
   a. Uterine fundus and body.
   b. Uterine cervix.
   c. Fallopian tubes.
   d. Ovaries.
   e. Vagina.
      1. a only.
      2. a and b.
      3. All but e.
      4. All the above.

32. In checking Mrs. Grayling's vital signs during the immediate postoperative period, the nurse should be aware that which of the following would tend to depress her respiratory rate and depth:
   a. Anxiety concerning the outcome of surgery.
   b. Morphine sulfate administered preoperatively.
   c. Pentothal and ether used as anesthetics.
   d. Postoperative pain caused by nerve injury.
   e. Shock produced by operative tissue injury.
      1. a and c.
      2. b and d.
      3. b, c, and e.
      4. All the above.

33. The recovery room nurse should check Mrs. Grayling for postoperative hemorrhage by:

    a. Observing the abdominal dressing.
    b. Checking the perineal pad.
    c. Counting her radial pulse.
    d. Evaluating her skin color.
    e. Measuring her blood pressure.
        1. a and b.
        2. b and c.
        3. c and d.
        4. All the above.

34. In reviewing the information on Mrs. Grayling's chart, the recovery room nurse should be aware that which of the following conditions would greatly increase the possibility that Mrs. Grayling would develop postoperative pneumonia?

    a. Deviated nasal septum.
    b. Dietary obesity.
    c. Heavy smoking habit.
    d. Chronic bronchitis.
    e. Calcified Ghon tubercle.
        1. a and c.
        2. b and d.
        3. b, c, and d.
        4. All the above.

35. Until she recovers completely from the anesthetic given her, Mrs. Grayling should be kept in a side-lying position in order to:

    1. Facilitate drainage of nasopharyngeal secretions.
    2. Maximize the extent of thoracic expansion.
    3. Minimize tension of the abdominal suture line.
    4. Simplify the changing of lower bed linen.

36. Mrs. Grayling was given thiamine hydrochloride postoperatively in order to:

    1. Foster clotting of the blood in vessels ligated during surgery.
    2. Facilitate proper metabolism of glucose given intravenously.
    3. Stimulate capillary formation around the surgical wound.
    4. Enhance bone marrow production of new red blood cells.

37. During the immediate postoperative period, the nurse should frequently check the amount and character of Mrs. Grayling's urinary output because of the possibility of:

    1. Injury to her ureter during surgery.
    2. Kidney damage due to transfusion reaction.
    3. Introduction of bacteria through the catheter.
    4. Obstruction to urinary drainage by the perineal pad.

38. If Mrs. Grayling should develop "gas pains" postoperatively, her physician would probably order:

    1. Insertion of a rectal tube.
    2. Massage of her lower abdomen.
    3. Hypodermic injection of a narcotic.
    4. Intramuscular injection of neostigmine.

39. In planning postoperative care, the nurse should be aware that Mrs. Grayling is particularly subject to which of the following vascular complications?

    1. Varicose veins.
    2. Cerebral embolism.
    3. Aortic aneurism.
    4. Thrombophlebitis.

40. The recovery room nurse should employ which of the following measures to prevent Mrs. Grayling from developing postoperative vascular complications?

    a. Elevate the knee gatch to drain the lower extremities.
    b. Encourage her to exercise her legs and feet every hour.
    c. Massage her lower legs in the direction of her heart.
    d. Turn her frequently from side to side or from side to back.
        1. a only.
        2. a and c.
        3. b and d.
        4. All the above.

On Mrs. Grayling's first postoperative day, the doctor ordered that an abdominal binder be applied and she be allowed to sit up on the edge of the bed for a brief period of time. When she did this Mrs. Grayling complained of slight dizziness, but seemed encouraged by the opportunity to change her position in bed.

On the following day the indwelling catheter was removed and Mrs. Grayling was allowed to sit up in a chair at the side of the bed. The nurse noted that despite the fact that she was pain-free and was visited by her family, Mrs. Grayling seemed somewhat withdrawn and depressed.

41. Mrs. Grayling is particularly apt to develop which of the following gastrointestinal complications following her operation?

1. Intestinal distention.
2. Infectious diarrhea.
3. Strangulated hernia.
4. Rectovaginal fistula.

42. In preparing to turn Mrs. Grayling from a dorsal recumbent position to her right side, the nurse should first:
  1. Turn her head toward the right at a right angle to the body.
  2. Move her head and trunk to the left side of the bed.
  3. Elevate the left bed rail and pad it full length with pillows.
  4. Pull her hips and legs toward the right side of the bed.

43. The nurse should employ which of the following measures to keep Mrs. Grayling in good body alignment while she is lying on her side?
  1. Remove all pillows from beneath her head.
  2. Elevate both head and knee gatches 15 degrees.
  3. Insert a bedboard under the mattress.
  4. Support the upper arm and leg on pillows.

44. Postoperatively, Mrs. Grayling's surgeon would probably not remove her nasogastric tube until he noted the appearance of which of the following physical signs?
  1. Excessive salivation.
  2. Hunger pangs.
  3. Bowel sounds.
  4. Passage of stool.

45. Mrs. Grayling's postoperative depression was probably a result of:
  a. Hormonal changes resulting from her surgery.
  b. Cerebral ischemia following acute blood loss.
  c. Psychological reaction to loss of the uterus.
  d. Nerve tissue injury by the anesthetic agent.
  e. Concern over her family's future reaction to her.
    1. a and b.
    2. c and d.
    3. a, c, and e.
    4. All the above.

46. Which of the following would be most supportive to Mrs. Grayling postoperatively?
  1. Having her doctor assure her that the uterine tumors had been benign.
  2. Having the nurse tell her that her reaction to hysterectomy was normal.

3. Having her husband reassure her of his continued love and understanding.
4. Having her daughters say that they miss her and want her to come home.

On her second postoperative day Mrs. Grayling's intravenous was discontinued and she was given a clear liquid diet. Because she experienced no nausea, vomiting, or intestinal distention, she was rapidly advanced to a soft and then a regular high-protein diet.

Her abdominal wound healed without complication, and on her tenth postoperative day she was discharged to her home on estrogen replacement therapy. Her doctor made arrangements for her to receive follow-up care in the hospital outpatient department.

47. Mrs. Grayling was given a high-protein diet postoperatively in order to:
  a. Promote wound healing.
  b. Prevent weight gain.
  c. Facilitate blood formation.
  d. Satisfy oral cravings.
  e. Decrease fecal mass.
    1. a and c.
    2. b and d.
    3. All but e.
    4. All the above.

48. In preparing her for discharge from the hospital, the nurse should instruct Mrs. Grayling to avoid which of the following activities until her doctor specifically approves their resumption?
  a. Heavy lifting.
  b. Vaginal douching.
  c. Sexual intercourse.
  d. Tub bathing.
  e. Ballroom dancing.
    1. a and b.
    2. a, b, and c.
    3. All but d.
    4. All the above.

49. In order to increase her physical comfort following hospital discharge, Mrs. Grayling's surgeon may advise her to:
  1. Apply elastic stockings on arising for several days.
  2. Douche the perineum following defecation for a week or so.
  3. Wear a girdle or abdominal support for several weeks.
  4. Sleep with her legs elevated for several months.

Carcinoma of the Cervix

Garnet Hearn, a 46-year-old mother of five grown children, had ceased to menstruate one year before, but was admitted to the hospital with heavy vaginal bleeding of two days' duration. She told the examining physician that she had been troubled with a thick, yellow, foul-smelling discharge for the past several months and that during this same interval she had noted frequent vaginal spotting. Physical examination revealed her temperature to be 99.2° F., pulse 110 per minute, respirations 20 per minute, blood pressure 120/80 mm. Hg. The vaginal vault was filled with blood clots, the cervix was indurated with a small ulceration of the external os, and the uterus was of normal size. Rectal examination revealed bilateral parametrial induration which did not reach the pelvic wall on either side. A Papanicolaou smear and colposcopy of the cervix revealed histologic stage 3 epidermoid carcinoma of the cervix. Garnet's hematocrit was 36 per cent, her hemoglobin concentration 10 grams per 100 ml., white blood cell count 5000 per cu. mm. with a normal differential, and reticulocyte count 1.4 per cent. An intravenous pyelogram, a cystogram, proctoscopy, bone survey, and liver profile all yielded normal findings.

Following a radioactive lymphogram, Garnet was discharged from the hospital and given a series of 10 betatron treatments on an outpatient basis. One week following the last betatron treatment she was readmitted to the hospital and transfused with two units of packed cells. On the following day Garnet was given a low residue diet, a soapsuds enema, a vaginal douche, a perineal surgical preparation and was taken to the operating room for placement of radium applicators. After Garnet returned to her room the radiologist inserted radium, which was left in place for 48 hours. Since Garnet tolerated the radium application well and her hemoglobin level had risen to 12 grams per 100 ml., she was discharged to her home and scheduled for another series of 10 betatron treatments.

(ANSWER BLANK ON PAGE A–15)   (CORRECT ANSWERS ON PAGE B–27)

1. The most common early symptom of carcinoma of the cervix is:
1. Dysmenorrhea.
2. Metrorrhagia.
3. Menorrhagia.
4. Polymenorrhea.

2. Careful history-taking would probably reveal that Garnet's vaginal spotting usually occurred:
1. On arising.
2. While sitting.
3. After intercourse.
4. On stair climbing.

3. Garnet's cervix was described as indurated, meaning that the tissue was:
1. Malignant.
2. Hardened.
3. Ischemic.
4. Necrotic.

4. The parametrium is the tissue:
1. Lateral to the vagina.
2. Behind the bladder.
3. In front of the anus.
4. Surrounding the uterus.

5. The thick, yellow, foul-smelling vaginal discharge that Garnet noted during the two months preceding her hospital admission was probably the result of:
1. Overproduction of uterine secretions due to irritation.
2. Secondary infection of her ulcerated cervical neoplasm.
3. Overgrowth of yeasts which normally inhabit the vagina.
4. Desquamation of hyperemic vaginal mucosal lining.

6. Garnet's low hemoglobin concentration on hospital admission was probably the result of:
  1. Malnutrition.
  2. Infection.
  3. Bleeding.
  4. Toxicity.

7. Garnet's temperature elevation on hospital admission was probably the result of:
  1. Anxiety.
  2. Dehydration.
  3. Infection.
  4. Hyperthyroidism.

8. Which of the following factors are thought to predispose to development of cervical carcinoma?
  a. Chronic urinary cystitis.
  b. Chronic local irritation.
  c. Too frequent douching.
  d. Early and active sex life.
  e. Circumcision of the sexual partner.
    1. a and c.
    2. b and d.
    3. All but c.
    4. All the above.

9. In preparing equipment for the doctor's use in obtaining a Papanicolaou smear, the nurse should assemble:
  a. Vaginal speculum.
  b. 2 wooden spatulas.
  c. 2 clean glass slides.
  d. 2 long cotton-tipped applicators.
  e. Mixture of absolute alcohol and ether.
    1. a and b.
    2. c and d.
    3. All but d.
    4. All the above.

10. The Papanicolaou smear is usually prepared using cells obtained from the:
  a. Squamous-columnar junction of the cervix.
  b. Posterior fornix of the vagina.
  c. Anterior fornix of the vagina.
  d. Tubular glands of the uterine cavity.
    1. a and b.
    2. c and d.
    3. All but d.
    4. All the above.

11. The use of the Papanicolaou smear as an aid in diagnosing cervical carcinoma depends upon the tendency for:
  1. Malignant cells to show unusual structure and growth characteristics.
  2. Healthy cells to absorb hemoglobin pigments on exposure to free blood.
  3. Undifferentiated cells to continue to divide after removal from the body.
  4. Specific antibodies to agglutinate cells that have undergone malignant change.

12. Probably many women fail to have Papanicolaou tests performed regularly because of:
  1. Modesty.
  2. Complacency.
  3. Fear.
  4. Ignorance.

13. A class 3 Papanicolaou smear is one that reveals:
  1. No atypical or malignant cells.
  2. Apparently benign but atypical cells.
  3. Atypical but not definitely malignant cells.
  4. Clearly malignant neoplastic cells.

14. Schiller's iodine test is sometimes used as an aid in diagnosing cervical carcinoma. A positive test result, which indicates the need for cervical biopsy, consists of:
  1. Bluish discoloration of the cervix following administration of an iodine solution douche.
  2. Failure of portions of the cervix to stain when treated with a solution containing iodine.
  3. Immediate excretion in the urine of a complete dose of radioactive iodine given orally.
  4. Brownish discoloration of vaginal secretions after intravenous injection of iodine dye.

15. Colposcopy's greatest values as a diagnostic tool derives from the fact that it:
  1. Permits visualization of the cul-de-sac and allows the sampling of fluid without performing abdominal surgery.
  2. Allows direct access to the fallopian tube for purposes of tubal ligation and prevents unnecessary abdominal surgery.
  3. Makes possible biopsy of those areas of cervical tissue which are most likely to reveal significant histological change.
  4. Facilitates conization of the cervix in order to biopsy all portions of the cervix which might yield significant histological findings.

16. Epidermoid carcinoma of the cervix is a tumor arising from malignant change of:

1. Cuboidal cells lining the upper portion of the vagina.
2. Squamous cells covering the vaginal portion of the cervix.
3. Columnar cells lining the walls of the cervical canal.
4. Tubular glands located in the body of the uterus.

17. The physician classified Garnet's carcinoma as International Stage II, which indicated that her tumor had:

1. Remained confined within the cervix without invading surrounding tissue.
2. Infiltrated the parametrium without extending to the pelvic side wall.
3. Invaded the connective tissues located in the walls of the pelvis.
4. Spread beyond the limits of the pelvis to distant nodes and organs.

18. Which of the following systemic symptoms of malignancy would Garnet be apt to demonstrate?

a. Anemia.
b. Anorexia.
c. Weight loss.
d. Weakness.
    1. a and c.
    2. b and d.
    3. All but d.
    4. All the above.

19. Malignant cells differ from normal cells in that malignant cells:

a. Grow rapidly without the control of normal restraining mechanisms.
b. Possess enzyme systems yielding greater ability for anaerobic glycolysis.
c. Are easily transplanted from one part of the body to another.
d. Tend to rapidly outgrow their arterial blood supply.
    1. a and b.
    2. c and d.
    3. All but d.
    4. All the above.

20. Malignant tumors are capable of spreading from their site of origin to other tissues and organs by:

a. Direct extension of the tumor into surrounding tissue.
b. Dissemination of tumor emboli through the circulating blood.
c. Transmission of malignant cells through the lymph channels.
d. Fragments of tumor tissue breaking off in body cavities.
    1. a and b.
    2. c and d.
    3. All but d.
    4. All the above.

21. Intravenous pyelogram and cystogram were included in Garnet's workup in order to determine whether:

1. Radium could be used without injury to surrounding tissue.
2. Metastatic tumors had developed within the urinary tract.
3. Her foul-smelling discharge derived from a urinary infection.
4. Renal function was adequate to withstand radiation therapy.

22. When surgical removal is not feasible, ionizing radiation may often be used to treat malignant tumors in deep tissues because:

1. Healthy cells are completely unaffected by ionizing radiation.
2. Blood supply to normal tissue nullifies radiation effects.
3. Immature cells are the most susceptible to radiation injury.
4. Ionization converts abnormal cellular growth substances to normal ones.

23. The effect desired from Garnet's betatron and radium treatments was:

1. Conversion of the carcinomatous epithelial cells to normal.
2. Degeneration and necrosis of the malignant tumor cells.
3. Increase in blood flow through the tumor tissue.
4. Coagulation of eroded bleeding areas on the cervix.

24. In calculating the dosage of radiation to be given Garnet during her betatron treatments, the radiologist will take into consideration:

a. The rate of gamma ray emission per unit of time.
b. The length of time radiation impinges upon her tissues.
c. The distance of Garnet's tissues from the origin of radiation.
d. The type and amount of shielding used to limit the exposed area.
    1. a and c.
    2. b and d.
    3. All but d.
    4. All the above.

25. It is important that the nurse help Garnet understand which of the following facts concerning the betatron treatments ordered for her?

    a. Treatments will not be painful, but some irritability of the bladder and bowel may result.

    b. None of the large, foreboding pieces of equipment will touch her during the treatments.

    c. During the time that she is alone in the treatment room she can be seen and heard by the radiologist.

    d. A local skin reaction is a not uncommon consequence of the irradiation treatment series.

    e. The combination of radiation therapies is the most effective means of treating her illness.

        1. a, b, and c.
        2. b, c, and e.
        3. All but e.
        4. All the above.

26. Garnet said to the nurse, "I've heard that some patients get sick to their stomachs from these betatron treatments. If I do, should I stop coming for the treatments?" Which of the following would be the best answer to her question?

    1. "Don't worry about that now. If it happens, we can do something about it at that time."

    2. "I doubt that you will experience radiation sickness because only a few patients develop that reaction."

    3. "If you do get sick, stay at home for a day or two and then come back to resume treatment."

    4. "You should keep all your radiation clinic appointments even if you experience nausea or discomfort."

27. If Garnet should become nauseated during radiation therapy, her physician would be apt to order which of the following drugs for its antiemetic effect?

    1. Chloral hydrate.
    2. Chlordiazepoxide.
    3. Chlorpromazine.
    4. Chlormerodrin.

28. Garnet was given a vaginal douche prior to radium insertion in order to:

    1. Increase the volume of blood flow to the cervix and vagina.

    2. Prevent itching and burning during insertion of the radium.

    3. Dislodge friable tissue from the surface of the cervical tumor.

    4. Remove secretions that might obscure placement of the radium.

29. Garnet was given a low-residue diet immediately preceding, during, and immediately following radium insertion in order to:

    1. Prevent occurrence of vomiting as a manifestation of radiation illness.

    2. Eliminate abdominal distention due to intestinal putrefaction.

    3. Decrease the degree of bowel irritation resulting from irradiation.

    4. Reduce the metabolic work required for complete digestion of foods.

30. The surgeon will insert medicated gauze packing into Garnet's vagina following placement of the radium applicators primarily in order to:

    1. Reduce the odor of vaginal drainage.

    2. Prevent infection of the cervical ulcer.

    3. Maintain the radium in desired position.

    4. Decrease discomfort from the applicator.

31. Garnet was assigned to a private room during the period of radium application. The nurse should arrange the furniture in Garnet's room so that:

    1. Garnet's bed and bedside stand are just inside the room, one on either side of the hall door.

    2. Garnet's bed is just inside the hall door and her stand on the far side of the room.

    3. Garnet's bed and stand are parallel with a wall dividing hers from the next patient's room.

    4. Both Garnet's bed and bedside stand are as far from the hall door as possible.

32. The nurse should expect to find which of the following in place after Garnet's radium insertion?

    1. Nasogastric tube.
    2. Vaginal tampon.
    3. Indwelling catheter.
    4. Rectal tube.

33. Which of the following are important aspects of Garnet's nursing care during radium treatment?
    a. Taking her vital signs frequently in order to identify any infectious process present.
    b. Determining whether applicators are in proper position and informing the physician of any deviation.
    c. Evaluating whether or not she needs medication for relief of pain, nausea, or insomnia.
    d. Checking her position in bed and assisting her to maintain the prescribed position.
    e. Supporting her by explaining activity restrictions and telling her when treatment will be completed.
        1. a and b.
        2. b, c, and e.
        3. a, d, and e.
        4. All the above.

34. In order to protect Garnet from iatrogenic injury during the period of radium implantation the nurse should ensure that Garnet's:
    1. Hands are restrained with cloth ties.
    2. Urinary bladder remains decompressed.
    3. Eyes are shielded from direct light.
    4. Legs are abducted and restrained.

35. The nurse should instruct Garnet to maintain which of the following bed positions during the 48 hours of radium application?
    1. Recumbent, with the lower extremities fully extended.
    2. Supine, with both hips and knees slightly flexed.
    3. Side-lying, with the upper leg flexed sharply.
    4. Prone, with the hips elevated over the foot gatch.

36. The nurse should know that she will be protected from overexposure to radiation if she executes Garnet's nursing care in such a manner that she remains:
    1. In proximity to Garnet for no longer than 30 minutes at a time.
    2. At a distance of three feet from Garnet's pelvis at all times.
    3. In Garnet's room only long enough to deliver food and medicines.
    4. Behind a lead shield or apron while in Garnet's presence.

37. On the nurse's first visit to Garnet's room following the insertion of radium Garnet asked, "Are you afraid of getting too close to me?" Which response by the nurse would be most appropriate?
    1. "No. There really is no possibility that I could be dangerously irradiated from the radium implanted in your vagina."
    2. "No. I'll limit my contact with you to a safe time and distance while providing you with the care that you need."
    3. "Yes, I am a little afraid of radiation exposure, but my concern for your welfare overrides those considerations"
    4. "Why do you ask about my fear of radiation? Are you really expressing your own fear of radium treatment?"

38. During the period of radium implantation, which aspect of Garnet's nursing care should be given greatest priority?
    1. Complete bed bath.
    2. Frequent back care.
    3. Range of motion exercises.
    4. Pushing oral fluid intake.

39. While she was being given morning care on the day following radium insertion, Garnet asked the nurse, "How long will I be radioactive?" Which response by the nurse would be most suitable?
    1. "Radium has a half-life of about two days, so the degree of your radioactivity will fall off to a negligible quantity within a few days."
    2. "The vaginal and cervical tissues in contact with the radium will become radioactive, but radioactivity will cease when these tissues have sloughed."
    3. "The radium in your vagina is the source of radiation. From the time that the capsule is removed tomorrow you will be free of radioactivity."
    4. "You will remain reactive to some degree for the remainder of your life, since rays emitted by the radium will make your own tissues unstable."

40. Which of the following best describes the proper care of Garnet's bed linen during and following the period of radium implantation?
    1. No special handling techniques are required.

2. Special radiation resistant linen should be used.
3. After brief storage, the linen may be reused.
4. All exposed linen must be destroyed after use.

41. Following radium implantation Garnet might develop which of the following complications?
   1. Vaginal stenosis.
   2. Ovulation bleeding.
   3. Ureteral atrophy.
   4. Uterine prolapse.

42. If Garnet should develop a local reaction to external radiation, her skin care should include:
   a. Avoiding the use of alcohol, creams, and lotions.
   b. Avoiding constricting or irritating clothing.
   c. Air-drying the area twice daily for 20 minutes.
   d. Cleansing the area by patting with a water-moistened cloth.
   e. Taking a tub bath or shower several times each day.
      1. a and c.
      2. b and d.
      3. All but e.
      4. All the above.

43. Which of the following should be taken to Garnet's room in preparation for radium removal?

   a. Sterile glove.
   b. Sterile long-bladed forceps.
   c. Lead shield bottle or box.
   d. Sterile curved scissors.
   e. Sterile catgut suture.
      1. a and b.
      2. a, b, and c.
      3. All but e.
      4. All the above.

44. The nurse's responsibility for removal of Garnet's radium consists of:
   1. Notifying the surgeon that it is time for radium removal.
   2. Withdrawing the gauze packing from the vagina.
   3. Removing the radium application from the vagina.
   4. Returning the radium to the radiotherapy department.

On her discharge from the hospital the physician told Mr. and Mrs. Hearn that Garnet's chances for survival would be enhanced by continuous medical followup. Accordingly, Garnet returned to the doctor's office monthly for six months, then every three months for a year, then every six months. Three months after her last betatron treatment Garnet's Papanicolaou smear had reverted to class 2 and five years following treatment Garnet was still living, without evidence of metastasis from her cervical malignancy.

Postpartum Adjustment

Karla Newton, who had been an only child, had been described as a "good" girl and a "good" wife. She anticipated becoming a "good" mother.

Karla began to menstruate at 12 years of age. During her college years she referred to her menstrual periods as "the curse" because they were usually accompanied by extreme discomfort. She met her husband, Lennie, while both were waiting in the Student Health Center. She was seeking relief for dysmenorrhea and he was being treated for gastritis. They married the summer after college graduation, when Karla was 21 and Lennie 22 years of age.

Karla and Lennie's wedding ceremony was an extravaganza, and their honeymoon consisted of a month of "sun and fun." During the rest of their first summer together they lived with Lennie's family. In the fall, Lennie entered graduate school and Karla began to teach in a public intercity elementary school. Her teaching career was soon interrupted when she developed hyperemesis gravidarum. The principal reluctantly allowed her to break her teaching contract.

At first, Lennie was angry at Karla for allowing herself to become pregnant, but he soon adjusted to the idea of parenthood and began to look for an apartment to rent. When Karla was 6 months pregnant they moved from Lennie's parents' home to an apartment of their own.

Throughout the next few months they argued occasionally about money and Karla's desire to resume work after the baby was born, but each seemed to have adjusted to what he imagined his own role would be in parenting. The obstetrician commended Karla for following his orders for prenatal care.

Although her labor and delivery were neither long nor complicated, Karla complained about the pain of delivery and episiotomy. She also felt that her lochia was "excessive" in amount and duration. Lennie wanted to help Karla but was bewildered as to what was expected of him in the situation.

Karla developed insomnia and, rather than being a "good" patient, she became extremely demanding and irritable, cried frequently, and was noticeably aloof. She talked with a staff nurse, who reassured her that she was experiencing normal postpartum blues. The nurse observed that Karla avoided close contact with her baby, only touching the infant when absolutely necessary in the course of bottle feeding.

While Karla was still in the hospital her mother came to live with the Newtons to "help out" until Karla could regain her full strength. When Karla and the baby went home from the hospital her mother took care of the baby, Lennie studied for his mid-semester examination, and Karla rested.

One week after delivery, Karla asked to be taken back to the hospital because she had difficulty breathing in a sitting position. Blood gas analysis, physical examination, and chest x-ray conducted in the emergency room yielded normal results, so the examining physician sent Karla home to rest. Shortly thereafter, Karla stopped eating and sleeping. Two weeks later she became withdrawn and incoherent. Lennie and Karla's mother took her back to the obstetrician, who immediately referred her to a psychiatrist. At the time of admission to the Mental Health Center, Karla was hallucinating and relating intricate delusional ideation.

(ANSWER BLANK ON PAGE A–17) (CORRECT ANSWERS ON PAGE B–29)

1. Which of the following is true of most new mothers?
  1. They deal well with the psychological stresses of pregnancy and delivery.
  2. They are unable to cope with the exigencies of pregnancy and delivery.
  3. They feel that labor was an ordeal foisted on them unfairly by fate.
  4. They love their infants immediately and initiate taking-hold behavior in the child's care.

2. During the early postpartum period most mothers tend toward which of the following responses?
  a. Crying.
  b. Regression.
  c. Irritability.
  d. Neuroticism.
  e. Feeling blue.
    1. a and e.
    2. b and d.
    3. a, c, and e.
    4. All the above.

3. The symptoms which most mothers experience during the early postpartum period are often mislabeled as which of the following?
  1. Normal behavior of women.
  2. Indices of poor mental health.
  3. Lack of hormone secretions.
  4. Symptoms of puerperal infection.

4. Which of the following demographic variables are of no causal significance in development of postpartum illness?
  a. Age.
  b. Race.
  c. Education.
  d. Income.
  e. Parity.
    1. a only.
    2. b, c, and d.
    3. All but d.
    4. All the above.

5. Statistics show that the highest incidence of mental illness is typically found during which phase of the childbearing period?
  1. First trimester of pregnancy.
  2. Last trimester of pregnancy.
  3. Birth of child to three months postpartum.
  4. Six to nine months postpartum.

6. Those psychological symptoms observed in most women shortly after delivery could best be classified as which of the following?
  1. Postpartum anxiety reaction.
  2. Postpartum neurotic depression.
  3. Postpartum psychotic depression.
  4. Paranoid schizophrenic reaction.

7. Which of the following are typical objective components of maternal behavior during early mother-infant interaction?
  a. Physical exploration of the infant.
  b. Verbal identification of the baby.
  c. Manner of holding the infant.
  d. Amount of eye-to-eye contact.
  e. Type and amount of touching the infant.
    1. a only.
    2. a, c, and e.
    3. All but e.
    4. All the above.

8. Which of the following would indicate that the mother-infant attachment is progressing normally?
  a. Progression of the mother from fingertip to palm touching of the infant
  b. Referring to the infant through use of the masculine or feminine rather than the neuter pronoun.
  c. Touching the trunk of the baby rather than only the extremities.
  d. Positioning the baby's trunk in contact with the mother's during feeding.
  e. Frequent establishment of eye contact between mother and child.
    1. a and b.
    2. a, b, and e.
    3. All but e.
    4. All the above.

9. Which of the following factors have been found to determine the nature and degree of the mother's attachment to her infant?
  a. Early experiences with her own mother.
  b. Cultural background of the mother.
  c. Degree of health experienced in pregnancy.
  d. Time elapsed before initial contact with the infant.
  e. Behavior of the infant during initial contacts.
    1. a and c.
    2. b, c, and d.
    3. All but e.
    4. All the above.

10. Paschall and Newton found that mothers in the postpartum period scored significantly higher than national norms in which of the following variables?
1. Tendermindedness.
2. Depressiveness.
3. Submissiveness.
4. Anxiety.

11. Tendermindedness refers to the tendency to be:
1. Overprotective and cultured.
2. Inhibited, sober, and serious.
3. Suggestible and dependent.
4. Worried and emotionally immature.

12. Submissiveness refers to the tendency to be:
1. Overprotected and cultured.
2. Inhibited, sober and serious.
3. Suggestible and dependent.
4. Worried and emotionally immature.

13. Postpartum women who score high on submissiveness may also be suggestible and dependent. If the nurse had assessed Karla as suggestible and dependent during the postpartum period, the nurse should have:
1. Taken complete care of the infant encouraged Karla to read about child care.
2. Acted firmly in telling Karla that she needed to control her feelings.
3. Encouraged Karla to rest, because rest would cause her symptoms to abate.
4. Scheduled Karla for teaching classes and assigned her to share a room with an experienced mother.

14. Which of the following factors have been found to be correlated with difficulty in postpartum emotional adjustment?
1. Premarital sex.
2. Illegitimacy.
3. Venereal disease.
4. Dysmenorrhea.

15. While taking Karla's health history, the nurse should assess which of the following aspects of Karla's psychological makeup?
a. Her initial reaction to pregnancy.
b. Her assessment of her physical strength.
c. Her attitude toward herself as a woman.
d. Her attitudes toward sex and child rearing.
e. Her opinion of her own mother's child rearing ability.

1. a and c.
2. a, b, and d.
3. All but e.
4. All the above.

16. Which of the following probably made pregnancy most threatening to Karla?
1. Changing family organization and assuming new roles.
2. Evaluating whether or not mother knows best.
3. Having to give up her career as a teacher.
4. Losing the non-pregnant, childless state.

17. Which of the following probably contributed most strongly to Karla's initial disinclination toward mothering?
a. Depression due to change in body image.
b. Anxiety concerning assumption of responsibility.
c. Feeling that she had inadequate emotional support.
d. Denial of her repressed sexual urges.
e. Feeling guilty because she rejected her baby.

1. a and b.
2. b and c.
3. c and d.
4. d and e.

18. The shortness of breath which Karla experienced was probably caused by which of the following?
1. Thrombi.
2. Emboli.
3. Anxiety.
4. Emphoria.

19. Sullivan has defined anxiety as:
1. A sign that the self-esteem had been threatened.
2. An inevitable part of every interpersonal relationship.
3. A phenomenon evoked by the need for autonomy.
4. Disguised guilt arising from the use of security operations.

20. The nurse should recognize which of the following events as factors which may have contributed to Karla's illness?
a. Lennie's initial reaction to her pregnancy.
b. Karla's life style prior to marriage.
c. Change of family residence during pregnancy.
d. Lack of recognition of early symptoms of illness.

e. Lennie's inability to support her following labor.
    1. a and b.
    2. a, c, and d.
    3. All but e.
    4. All the above.

21. Which of the following were early signs of Karla's impending illness that the hospital nurses should have identified following delivery?
a. Insomnia.
b. Crying.
c. Mood change.
d. Fatigue.
e. "Excessive" lochia.
    1. b and d.
    2. a, c, and e.
    3. All but e.
    4. All the above.

22. After Karla's discharge from the hospital, her mother took over complete care of the baby. Probably Karla's interests would have been better served if her mother had:
1. Returned to her own home after Karla came home from the hospital.
2. Taken over the household chores and guided Karla in caring for her baby.
3. Spent time in entertaining Lennie so he would not feel "left out."
4. Insisted that a nurse be hired to care for the baby.

Karla responded rapidly to Stelazine and supportive therapy. She was discharged in five days and given an appointment for the crisis intervention program conducted by the nurse practitioner. Lennie was helped in understanding his reactions to being a father and husband.

During the subsequent year Karla grew in the mothering role. When her daughter was 18 months old Karla again, with Lennie's approval, resumed her teaching job.

23. The nurse practitioner should assess which of the following in her interactions with Lennie?
a. His level of anxiety and selfishness.
b. The amount of assertive behavior he exhibits.
c. His view of his fathering role.
d. His opinion of the factors precipitating Karla's illness.
e. His attitude toward his mother-in-law.

    1. a and c.
    2. a, b, and c.
    3. All but e.
    4. All the above.

24. In attempting to predict the outcome of Karla's therapy, the nurse practitioner who conducts her crisis intervention therapy sessions should be most strongly influenced by which of the following principles?
1. Karla's response to treatment is dependent upon her premorbid personality.
2. Karla's response to treatment will be most influenced by what Lennie does.
3. Karla's response to treatment is dependent upon her feeling toward the baby.
4. It is impossible to predict the outcome of most cases of postpartum illness.

25. The incidence of postpartum mental illness has been observed to be especially high in mothers of which of the following types of children?
a. Failure to thrive children.
b. Accident-prone children.
c. Children with congenital anomalies.
d. Battered children.
e. Mentally retarded children.
    1. b only.
    2. a and c.
    3. All but e.
    4. All the above.

26. Crisis is best defined as:
1. An emotional illness which is precipitated by stress.
2. An event which threatens the life style of an individual.
3. Behavior which paradoxically increases anxiety.
4. An aggressive reaction in which feelings are acted out.

27. The nurse practitioner should help Karla to initiate which of the following coping mechanisms?
a. Strengthen problem solving.
b. Redefine the event.
c. Achieve higher need satisfaction.
d. Relinquish unrealistic goals.
e. Talk about thoughts and feelings.
    1. a and c.
    2. a, b, and d.
    3. All but d.
    4. All the above.

BIBLIOGRAPHY   MATERNITY AND GYNECOLOGIC NURSING

Ackerman, N.: Psychodynamics of Family Life. New York, Basic Books, 1958.

Adamkiewicz, V. W.: What are the bonds between the fetus and the uterus? Canadian Nurse, 72:26–28 (February), 1976.

Aguilera, D. C., and Messick, J. M.: Crisis Intervention: Theory and Methodology, 2nd ed. St. Louis, C. V. Mosby Co., 1974.

American College of Obstetricians and Gynecologists, Committee on Mental Health: National study of maternity care. Chicago, American College of Obstetricians and Gynecologists, 1970.

Anthony, E. J., and Benedek, T., eds.: Parenthood: Its Psychology and Psychopathology. Boston, Little, Brown and Company, 1970.

Apgar, V.: Resuscitation of the newborn: when and how to do it. Hospital Topics, 44:105, November 1966.

Applebaum, R. M.: The modern management of successful breast feeding. Pediatric Clinics of North America, 17:203, February 1970.

Arey, L. B.: Developmental Anatomy. 7th ed. Philadelphia, W. B. Saunders, 1974.

Avery, G. B. (ed.): Neonatology: Pathophysiology and Management of the Newborn. Philadelphia, J. B. Lippincott, 1975.

Auger, J. R.: Behavioral Systems and Nursing. Englewood Cliffs, New Jersey, Prentice-Hall, 1976.

Auld, P. A.: Resuscitation of the Newborn Infant. American Journal of Nursing, 74:68–70, 1974.

Babikian, H., and Goldman, A.: A study of teenage pregnancy. American Journal of Psychiatry, 128:755–760, December 1971.

Baker, A.: Psychiatric Disorders in Obstetrics. Oxford, Blackwell Scientific, 1967.

Bardwick, J. M.: Psychology of Woman: A Study of Bio-cultural Conflicts. New York, Harper and Row, 1971.

Benson, L.: Fatherhood: A Sociological Perspective. New York, Random House, 1968.

Bergersen, B., and Krug, E.: Pharmacology in Nursing. 13th ed. St. Louis, C. V. Mosby Co., 1976.

Billingsley, A., et al.: Illegitimacy: Changing Services for Changing Times. New York, National Council on Illegitimacy, 1970.

Bondy, P. K., and Rosenberg, L. E. (eds.): Duncan's Diseases of Metabolism, 7th ed. Philadelphia, W. B. Saunders Co., 1974.

Brandt, P. A., Chinn, P. L., and Smith, M. E.: Current Practices in Pediatric Nursing. St. Louis, C. V. Mosby, 1976.

Carter, A. B.: Hypertension: its causes and treatment. Nursing Times, 67:531–533, May 6, 1971.

Chesley, L. C.: Hypertensive disorders in pregnancy. Drug Therapy, 7:10–16, 1977.

Cochran, L., ed.: Symposium on care of the newborn. Nursing Clinics of North America, 6:1–112, March 1971.

Crawford, C. O.: Health and the Family, a Medical Sociological Analysis. New York, Macmillan, 1971.

Davis, E. M., and Rubin, R.: De Lee's Obstetrics for Nurses. 18th ed. Philadelphia, W. B. Saunders Co., 1966.

Deutsch, H.: Psychology of Women, Vols. I and II. New York, Grune and Stratton, 1945.

Dick-Read, G.: Childbirth without Fear. 2nd ed. New York, Harper and Row, 1959.

Douglas, R. G., and Stromma, W. B.: Operative Obstetrics, 3rd ed. New York, Appleton-Century-Crofts, 1976.

Dunn, L. J.: The legal aspects of the controversy over sex education in the public schools. Obstetrics and Gynecology, 38:771–774, November 1971.

Eastman, N., and Hellman, L.: Williams Obstetrics. 14th ed. New York, Appleton-Century-Crofts, 1971.

Fast, J.: Body Language. New York, M. Evans and Co., 1970.

Fitzpatrick, E., and Reeder, S. R.: Maternity Nursing, 13th ed. Philadelphia, J. B. Lippincott Co., 1976.

Freeman, Ruth B.: Community Health Nursing Practice. Philadelphia, W. B. Saunders Co., 1970.

Freeman, R. K.: The use of the oxytocin challenge test for antepartum clinical evaluation of uteroplacental respiratory function. American Journal of Obstetrics and Gynecology, 121:481, 1975.

Fuch, F., and Klopper, A.: Endocrinology of Pregnancy, 2nd ed. New York, Harper and Row, 1977.

Garrett, A.: Interviewing: Its Principles and Methods, 2nd ed. New York, Family Welfare Association of America, 1972.

Goerzen, J. L., and Chinn, P. L.: Review of Maternal and Child Nursing. St. Louis, C. V. Mosby Co., 1975.

Grad, R. K., and Woodside, J.: Obstetrical analgesia and anesthesia: methods of relief for the patient in labor. American Journal of Nursing, 77:242–245, 1977.

Greiss, F. C.: Obstetric anesthesia. American Journal of Nursing, 71:67–69, January 1971.

Group for the Advancement of Psychiatry: The Right to Abortion: A Psychiatric View. New York, C. Scribner's Sons, 1970.

Grunebaum, H. U., et al.: The family planning attitudes, practices, and motivations of mental patients. American Journal of Psychiatry, 128:740–744, December 1971.

Guyton, A.: Textbook of Medical Physiology. 5th ed. Philadelphia, W. B. Saunders Co., 1976.

Hardin, G.: The history and future of birth control. Perspectives in Biology and Medicine, 10:1–18, 1966.

Hodnett, E.: Fetal monitoring—why bother? Canadian Nurse, 73:44–47 (March), 1977.

Holder, A. R.: Legal Issues in Pediatric and Adolescent Medicine. New York, John Wiley and Sons, 1977.

Ingalls, A. J., and Salerno, M. C.: Maternal and Child Health Nursing. 3rd ed. St. Louis, C. V. Mosby Co., 1975.

Keller, C., and Copeland, P.: Counseling the abortion patient is more than talk. American Journal of Nursing, 72:102–106, January 1972.

Klaus, M. M., et al.: Human maternal behavior at the first contact with her young. Pediatrics, 46:187, August 1970.

Krause, M., and Hunscher, M.: Food, Nutrition and Diet Therapy, 5th ed. Philadelphia, W. B. Saunders Co., 1972.

Kriesberg, L.: Mothers in Poverty: A Study of Fatherless Families. Chicago, Aldine, 1970.

Laurance, B., Creey, D., and Stroud, E.: Feeding babies in the 70's. Nursing Times, 73: i–iv (March), 1977.

McNall, L. K., and Galcener, J. I.: Current Practice in Obstetric and Gynecologic Nursing. St. Louis, C. V. Mosby, 1976.

Moulton, R.: Some effects of the new feminism. American Journal of Psychiatry, 134: 1–6, 1977.

Nalepka, C. D.; Understanding Thermoregulation in newborns. Journal of Obstetric, Gynecologic, and Neonatal Nursing, 5:17–19, 1976.

Newton, N.: Maternal Emotions. New York, Paul B. Hoeber, Inc., 1955.

Novak, E. R., Jones, G. S., Jones, H. W.: Novak's Textbook of Gynecology. 9th ed. Baltimore, Williams and Wilkins, 1975.

Page, E., Villee, C. A., and Villee, D. B.: Human Reproduction: The Core Content of Obstetrics, Gynecology, and Perinatal Medicine, 2nd ed. Philadelphia, W. B. Saunders, 1976.

Parad, H., ed.: Crisis Intervention: Selected Readings. New York, Family Service Association of America, 1965.

Paschall, N., and Newton, N.: Personality factors and postpartum adjustment. Primary Care, 3:741–750 (December), 1976.

Peplau, H.: Interpersonal Relations in Nursing. New York, G. P. Putnam's Sons, 1952.

Roberts, F. B.: Perinatal Nursing Care of Newborns and Their Families. New York, McGraw-Hill Book Co., 1977.

Roberts, J. E.: Suctioning the Newborn. American Journal of Nursing, 73:63–65, 1973.

Romney, S. L., Gray, M. J., Little, A. B., Merrill, J. A., Quillegun, E. J., and Strander, R.: Gynecology and Obstetrics: The Health Care of Women. New York, McGraw-Hill Book Co., 1975.

Rubin, R.: Cognitive style in pregnancy. American Journal of Nursing, 70:502–508, March 1970.

Rudolph, A. M.: The changes in circulation after birth. Circulation, 41:343, February 1970.

Schaffer, A. J., and Avery, M. E.: Diseases of the Newborn. 3rd ed. Philadelphia, W. B. Saunders Co., 1971.

Semmens, J. P.: Female sexuality and life situations: an etiologic psycho-socio-sexual profile of weight gain and nausea and vomiting in pregnancy. Obstetrics and Gynecology, 38:555–563, 1971.

Shank, R. E.: A chink in our armour. Nutrition Today, 5:2, Summer 1970.

Sodeman, W. A., and Sodeman, W. A. Jr.: Pathologic Physiology. 5th ed. Philadelphia, W. B. Saunders Co., 1974.

Sorensen, K. M., and Amis, D. B.: Understanding the world of the chronically ill. American Journal of Nursing, 67:811–817, April, 1967.

Spellacy, W. N., Buhi, W. L., and Birk, S. A.: Vitamin B_6 treatment of gestational diabetes mellitus. American Journal of Obstetrics and Gynecology, 127:299–302, 1977.

Spellacy, W. N. (ed.): Management of the High-Risk Pregnancy. Baltimore, University Park Press, 1976.

Spellacy, W. N., and Buhi, W. C.: The usefulness of amniotic fluid lecithin-sphingomyelin ratio in predicting neonatal respiratory problems. Southern Medical Journal, *66*:1090, 1973.

Taylor, K. W.: The secretion of insulin. Postgraduate Medical Journal, *47*:57–61, January 1971.

Tyson, J. E. (ed.): Symposium on Pregnancy. The Medical Clinics of North America, *61*: 3–199, 1977.

Veland, K., and Metcalfe, J.: Heart disease in pregnancy. Clinics in Perinatology, *1*: 349–367 (September), 1974.

Veland, K.: Pregnancy and Cardiovascular Disease. The Medical Clinics of North America, *61*:17–41, 1977.

Wahl, T. R., and Blythe, J.: Chemotherapy in gynecological malignancies and its nursing aspects. Journal of Obstetric, Gynecologic, and Neonatal Nursing, *5*:9–14, 1976.

Wallace, H. M.: Factors associated with perinatal mortality and morbidity. Clinical Obstetrics and Gynecology, *13*:13, March 1970.

Wohl, M., and Goodhart, R.: Modern Nutrition in Health and Disease. 5th ed. Philadelphia, Lea and Febiger, 1973.

Zamasky, H., and Strobel, K.: Care of the critically ill newborn. American Journal of Nursing, *76*:566–569 (April), 1976.

2
PEDIATRIC NURSING

Premature Infant

(ANSWER BLANK ON PAGE A–19) *(CORRECT ANSWERS ON PAGE B–31)*

The nurse in the Premature Nursery recorded the following on Francis Newberry's chart:

"June 19, 2:45 A.M.: 1170-gram male infant born after 35-week gestation period to a 21-year-old primigravida was admitted with slight respiratory distress, nasal flaring, grunting, intercostal retractions, and slight cyanosis. Apgar scores of 4 and 6 at 1 minute and 5 minutes after birth. Apical pulse 164, respirations 44, axillary temperature 96° F. Marked hypotonia. Placed in a radiant heat bed under an oxygen hood with an FI O_2 of .40. Five per cent dextrose in water started at 25 cc. Q.8 H. via scalp vein.

June 19, 7:00 A.M.: 13 cc. of intravenous fluid mixture absorbed, 12 cc. remaining in the burette. Color pink. Occasional jittery movements. Apical pulse 146, respirations 48."

1. A diagnosis of prematurity is made on the basis of which of the following criteria?
- a. Birth weight.
- b. Body length.
- c. Motor behavior.
- d. Length of gestation.
- e. Pulse rate.
    - 1. a and b.
    - 2. c and d.
    - 3. All but e.
    - 4. All the above.

2. Which of the following maternal factors are thought to be frequent causes for premature birth?
- a. Inadequate prenatal care.
- b. Multiple births.
- c. Toxemia of pregnancy.
- d. Placenta praevia.
- e. Malnutrition and debilitation.
    - 1. a and b.
    - 2. c and d.
    - 3. a, c, d, and e.
    - 4. All the above.

3. Francis' weight, converted to the avoirdupois system, is:

1. 1 pound, 2 ounces.
2. 1 pound, 9 ounces.
3. 2 pounds, 5 ounces.
4. 2 pounds, 9 ounces.

4. Which of the following signs are evaluated in computing an Apgar score for the condition of a newborn infant?
- a. Skin color.
- b. Respiratory effort.
- c. Heart rate.
- d. Muscle tone.
- e. Reflex irritability.
    - 1. a and b.
    - 2. c and d.
    - 3. All but e.
    - 4. All the above.

5. Thirty (30) cc. of a dilute solution of sodium bicarbonate was administered by IV push to Francis on his admission to the premature nursery in order to:
1. Counteract pulmonary vascular constriction produced by acidosis.
2. Increase general hydration by elevating serum sodium levels.
3. Relieve edema by decreasing water resorption from the renal tubule.
4. Facilitate digestion of protein by decreasing gastric hyperacidity.

6. Immediately on Francis' arrival in the premature nursery, the nurse should do which of the following in addition to supplying external heat?
1. Take temperature rectally.
2. Examine for anomalies.
3. Check airway for patency.
4. Cleanse skin of vernix.

7. Francis' cyanosis on admission to the nursery was evidence of:
1. Increased serum concentration of bilirubin.
2. Inadequate oxygenation of arterial blood.
3. Excessive number of red blood cells.
4. Lack of subcutaneous fatty tissue.

8. At birth Francis probably displayed which of the following physical signs of prematurity?

    a. Paucity of skin creases on the sole of the foot.

    b. Absence of hair on the crown of the head.

    c. Lack of cartilage in the lobe of the ear.

    d. Scant amounts of vernix caseosa in skin creases.

    e. Obstruction of sebaceous glands on face and chest.

        1. a and c.

        2. b and d.

        3. All but d.

        4. All the above.

9. At birth Francis is apt to display a weakened form of which of the following reflexes?

    a. Rooting reflex.

    b. Sucking reflex.

    c. Moro reflex.

    d. Walking reflex.

    e. Babinski reflex.

        1. a only.

        2. b and c only.

        3. All but e.

        4. All the above.

10. Francis' temperature, like that of most premature infants, is apt to be labile because of:

    a. Incomplete development of the temperature-regulating center in the hypothalamus.

    b. Excessive heat loss through radiation due to lack of subcutaneous fat.

    c. Rapid heat loss by radiation due to high ratio of surface area to body weight.

    d. Inefficient heat transmission by circulating blood due to weak heart action.

        1. a and b.

        2. c and d.

        3. a, b, and c.

        4. All the above.

11. If the temperature of the air surrounding Francis should drop to several degrees below his body temperature, which of the following physiological adjustments would be most effective in increasing his body heat?

    1. Rapid constriction of superficial blood vessels.

    2. Combustion of fatty acids in brown adipose tissue.

    3. Cessation of urine and sweat production.

    4. Decreased rate and depth of respiration.

12. A significant decrease in Francis' temperature below the normal level would be apt to produce which of the following effects?

    a. Extreme lethargy.

    b. Bright red skin color.

    c. Slow, shallow respirations.

    d. Diminished reflexes.

    e. Edema of face and extremities.

        1. a and c only.

        2. b and d only.

        3. All but e.

        4. All the above.

13. A sustained decrease in Francis' body temperature would predispose him to which of the following metabolic derangements?

    a. Acidosis.

    b. Hypoglycemia.

    c. Hyperkalemia.

    d. Azotemia.

    e. Hypercholesterolemia.

        1. a and b only.

        2. a, b, and c only.

        3. All but e.

        4. All the above.

14. Francis' respiratory functioning is apt to be compromised by:

    a. Decreased tone and weak contractions of the diaphragm and intercostal muscles.

    b. Failure of alveoli in large areas of the bases of both lungs to expand fully.

    c. Inability of the cartilaginous rib cage to remain rigid during inspiration.

    d. Failure of weak gag and cough reflexes to clear the airway if it becomes obstructed.

        1. a only.

        2. a and b.

        3. a, b, and d.

        4. All the above.

15. Francis must be handled gently to avoid trauma as he is more susceptible than the full-term infant to:

    a. Infection.

    b. Hemorrhage.

    c. Shock.

    d. Convulsions.

        1. a and b.

        2. c and d.

        3. All but d.

        4. All the above.

16. Which of the following characteristics of prematurity make Francis more prone to hemorrhage than a full-term infant?
- a. Increased fragility of capillary walls.
- b. Lack of subcutaneous fat padding.
- c. Decreased serum prothrombin levels.
- d. Elevated systolic blood pressure.
    1. a and c.
    2. b and d.
    3. All but d.
    4. All the above.

17. Which of the following would be the best indicator of Francis' need for oxygen?
1. Respiratory rate.
2. Skin color.
3. Pulse rate.
4. Arterial pO_2.

18. After Francis' cyanosis is relieved, extremely high oxygen concentration in his head hood would predispose him to:
1. Hypocalcemic tetany.
2. Intracranial hemorrhage.
3. Retrolental fibroplasia.
4. Pulmonary hyaline membrane disease.

19. Warming and humidification of air within the head hood is desirable in order to:
- a. Prevent drying of the bronchial secretions.
- b. Decrease fluid loss through respiration.
- c. Impair growth of microorganisms.
- d. Decrease the rate of respiration.
    1. a and b.
    2. c and d.
    3. All but d.
    4. All the above.

20. Francis will be more susceptible to infection than a full-term infant because of:
- a. Deficient placental transmission of maternal antibodies.
- b. Impaired ability to manufacture immune globulins.
- c. Inability of immature white blood cells to phagocytose bacteria.
- d. Decreased resistance of immature skin to ingress of microorganisms.
    1. a and c.
    2. b and d.
    3. a, b, and d.
    4. All the above.

21. An increased rate of tissue oxidation such as that accompanying infections would compromise Francis' metabolic balance principally by:
1. Increasing his oxygen need.
2. Decreasing liver glycogen stores.
3. Increasing blood bicarbonate levels.
4. Decreasing glomerular filtration rate.

22. Which of the following precautions should be taken by the nursery staff to protect Francis from infection?
- a. Permit only infection-free, regularly assigned personnel to enter the premature nursery.
- b. Wash hands with a germicidal preparation when leaving one infant to go to another.
- c. Place only clean objects at the head of the crib while working in the Isolette.
- d. Remove soiled diapers and linen through only the designated porthole.
- e. Damp mop and damp dust the nursery and nursery furniture daily.
    1. a and b.
    2. c and d.
    3. All but d.
    4. All the above.

23. Francis is more liable than a full-term infant to develop anemia shortly after birth because of:
- a. Unusual fragility of immature red blood cells.
- b. Deficient liver stores of iron and vitamins.
- c. Failure of hemoglobin formation to match increased blood volume.
- d. Greater than usual amounts of fetal type hemoglobin.
- e. Tendency to hemorrhage from rupture of fragile capillaries.
    1. a and b.
    2. c and d.
    3. All but e.
    4. All the above.

24. The nurse should plan Francis' care so that he is handled as little as possible, since handling subjects him to:
- a. Infection.
- b. Trauma.
- c. Exhaustion.
- d. Kernicterus.
    1. a and b.
    2. c and d.
    3. All but d.
    4. All the above.

25. Which of the following precautions should be taken by the nursing staff to conserve Francis' energy?
- a. Combine diaper changing, bed making, cleansing, and temperature taking whenever possible.
- b. Adjust the radiant heat bed to maintain a constant body temperature of 98° F.
- c. Eliminate as many as possible of the usual causes of crying and restlessness.
- d. Avoid loud noises in the nursery and prevent jostling of the Isolette.
    1. a and b.
    2. c and d.
    3. All but d.
    4. All the above.

On June 20th 10 cc. of 5 per cent dextrose in half-strength normal saline solution were given intravenously over a period of 24 hours, as ordered by the doctor. In addition, 4 cc. of 10 per cent dextrose in water were given orally every three hours for four feedings and were retained. Then intravenous infusions were discontinued and Francis was started on 6 cc. of Similac, 20 calories Q 3 H by nasojejunal tube. The doctor ordered a multivitamin mixture, kanamycin, and penicillin to be given daily. On the evening of June 20 Francis was observed to be icteric, so he was exposed to blue light.

26. Francis' jaundice was probably caused by:
1. Rupture of a great number of fragile red cells in a short period of time.
2. Inflammatory obstruction of hepatic bile ducts and resorption of pigments.
3. Extravasation of blood from ruptured capillaries into subcutaneous tissue.
4. Faulty melanin metabolism due to absence of enzymes for normal protein synthesis.

27. Excessively high concentration of bilirubin in the blood serum may cause:
1. Depression of blood-producing cells in the red bone marrow.
2. Staining and degeneration of cells in the basal ganglia.
3. Precipitation of pigment in the tubules of the kidney.
4. Obstruction of small bile ducts by precipitated pigments.

28. The purpose of the blue light to which Francis was exposed on his second day was to:
1. Stimulate increased formation of vitamin K in the skin.
2. Enhance pigment breakdown by increasing body temperature.
3. Convert indirect bilirubin to a less toxic compound.
4. Increase brain electrical activity by stimulating the optic nerve.

29. Francis was not given oral feedings during the initial hours of his first day of life so that he might:
- a. Stabilize his respiratory rate and depth.
- b. Become accustomed to the Isolette.
- c. Be observed for gag and swallow reflexes.
- d. Obtain several hours of uninterrupted sleep.
    1. a and c.
    2. b and d.
    3. a, c, and d.
    4. All the above.

30. The optimum formula for a premature infant is:
1. Average in carbohydrate, high in protein, low in fat content.
2. High in carbohydrate, low in protein, average in fat content.
3. Low in carbohydrate, moderate in protein, high in fat content.
4. Average in carbohydrate, average in protein, high in fat content.

31. The formula to which Francis was introduced on his third day of life was made of commercially prepared Similac rather than whole cow's milk because:
1. Whole milk is more apt to produce allergies than Similac.
2. Inadequacy of Francis' digestive enzymes would make fat digestion difficult.
3. Too rapid weight gain would severely compromise his small skeleton.
4. High fat intake would slow stomach emptying and cause gastric dilation.

32. Francis would have more difficulty taking oral feedings than a full-term infant because his:
- a. Sucking ability is weak.
- b. Stomach is small and atonic.
- c. Muscles are weaker and more easily fatigued.
- d. Respirations are more easily embarrassed.

1. a and b.
2. c and d.
3. a, b, and d.
4. All the above.

33. While giving Francis the oral feedings the nurse should employ which of the following adjustments?
   a. Use a soft nipple with a larger than usual opening.
   b. Administer very small quantities of glucose water at each feeding.
   c. Give more numerous feedings at shorter than usual intervals.
   d. Provide frequent opportunities for rest and bubbling.
      1. a and b.
      2. c and d.
      3. All but d.
      4. All the above.

34. Nursing care of the infant with a naso-jejunal tube includes:
   a. Measuring his abdominal circumference every eight hours.
   b. Performing hematest and reducing substance tests on stools every shift.
   c. Changing the tube every 24 hours.
   d. Irrigating the tube with normal saline every six hours.
      1. a and b only.
      2. b and c only.
      3. c and d only.
      4. All but b.

35. What is the usual frequency of stools in the typical premature infant?
   1. One every other day.
   2. One a day.
   3. Four to five a day.
   4. Eight to ten a day.

36. Francis' stools are apt to be foul-smelling because of:
   1. Lack of intestinal bacteria.
   2. High fat content of feces.
   3. Excessive intestinal mucus secretion.
   4. Increased amounts of stercobilin.

37. The immaturity of Francis' gastrointestinal tract predisposes him particularly to deficient intake of:
   a. Vitamin A.
   b. Vitamin B_1.
   c. Vitamin C.
   d. Vitamin D.
   e. Vitamin K.
      1. a and c.
      2. b, c, and d.
      3. a, d, and e.
      4. All the above.

38. Which of the following would be given to decrease Francis' bleeding tendencies?
   1. Vitamin A.
   2. Vitamin B_1.
   3. Vitamin D.
   4. Vitamin K.

39. Penicillin and kanamycin were ordered for Francis on his second day of life in order to:
   1. Inhibit overgrowth of normal inhabitants of the intestine.
   2. Destroy organisms inhabiting the urinary tract.
   3. Kill molds and yeasts in the upper digestive tract.
   4. Inhibit growth of organisms causing skin and respiratory infections.

40. Kanamycin inhibits the growth and multiplication of:
   a. *Staphylococcus aureus.*
   b. *Escherichia coli.*
   c. *Aerobacter aerogenes.*
   d. *Proteus vulgaris.*
   e. *Streptococcus pyogenes.*
      1. a and b.
      2. c and d.
      3. All but e.
      4. All the above.

41. Penicillin inhibits the growth and multiplication of:
   a. *Diplococcus pneumoniae.*
   b. *Streptococcus pyogenes.*
   c. *Neisseria meningitidis.*
   d. *Escherichia coli.*
   e. *Proteus vulgaris.*
      1. a and b.
      2. c and d.
      3. a, b, and c.
      4. All the above.

42. Ferrous sulfate was ordered for Francis because:
   1. Premature infants are deprived of the liver stores of iron deposited in the latter part of pregnancy.
   2. Iron stimulates the hematopoietic cells in the bone marrow to produce red blood cells.
   3. Increased metabolic rate requires additional iron for use in the cytochrome system.
   4. An excessive number of stools during the neonatal period caused excessive loss of iron.

When Francis was nine weeks old he weighed 2385 grams, was in an open crib, and tolerated 2 to 3 ounces of a standard commercial formula with iron every four hours. The doctor ordered Francis to be discharged, continue the current feeding routine, take multivitamin mixture 0.3 cc. daily, and return to the pediatric clinic in two weeks. He also arranged for a public health nurse to supervise Francis' care through a series of home visits.

43. Before discharging Francis the nurse should arrange for Mrs. Newberry to spend some time in the premature nursery classroom so that:

1. Mrs. Newberry may be given an opportunity to ask any questions she may have concerning Francis' growth.
2. The nurse may demonstrate detailed bath and feeding procedures to Mrs. Newberry.
3. The nurse may give her written instructions concerning feeding, cleansing, and dressing Francis.
4. Mrs. Newberry may be given an op-

portunity to handle Francis and care for him in a supportive atmosphere.

44. Mrs. Newberry asked the nurse, "Will Francis be retarded?" Which of the following would be the most appropriate response?

1. "Francis' slow start in life will undoubtedly handicap him both physically and mentally throughout his life, but the degree of retardation may be minimal."
2. "It is too soon to give an answer to that question. Any evaluation of his intellectual ability will have to wait until he has begun to talk."
3. "Francis' rate of development will be slower than that of a full-term baby, but he may be able to overcome most of his initial disability."
4. "You have no cause for concern. Francis has now survived the critical period of his life. Just offer extra inducements to stimulate him to higher achievements."

Cleft Lip and Palate

Mr. and Mrs. Heber Griffin's first child, Homer, was born with a unilateral cleft lip and cleft palate. The lip defect extended through the floor of the nostril and communicated with the defect in the anterior palate. Since the infant was in good physical condition, the surgeon advised Mr. and Mrs. Griffin that the cleft lip repair should be done immediately. The cleft palate repair would, he explained, be postponed until Homer's second or third year in order not to interfere with normal tooth development.

(ANSWER BLANK ON PAGE A–21) (CORRECT ANSWERS ON PAGE B–33)

1. After several conversations with the floor nurse, Mr. and Mrs. Griffin asked her, "What caused our baby to be deformed?" Which of the following would be the best response to their question?

1. "The fact that your child has a congenital anomaly seems to bother you a great deal."
2. "I wouldn't call it a deformity. It is only a minor defect, which is fully correctable."

3. "It's good that you are able to express your guilt feelings about the baby's deformity."
4. "Your question sounds as if you are concerned about your own responsibility in this situation."

2. For Homer's parents, the most painful aspect of his deformity is probably the fact that it:

1. Interferes with feeding.
2. Affects his face.

3. Can't be wholly corrected.

4. Requires lengthy treatment.

3. In informing Mr. and Mrs. Griffin about the etiology and significance of cleft lip and palate, the nurse should particularly emphasize which fact?

1. The two defects constitute the genetic expression of a Mendelian recessive trait.

2. It is unlikely that their later children would suffer the same deformity.

3. It is possible that their later children could experience a similar deformity.

4. Homer will probably demonstrate retarded physical and psychological development.

4. It is thought that when parents are informed that their child has been born with a disfiguring anomaly they respond with a grief reaction. What is the first stage in the normal grief reaction?

1. Acceptance.

2. Shock-denial.

3. Withdrawal.

4. Planning.

5. Which response by Mrs. Griffin would best exemplify the first stage in the normal grief reaction?

1. Sitting for long periods of time in a corner of the lounge weeping quietly.

2. Insisting on breast-feeding Homer despite explanations that dropper feeding will be necessary.

3. Accusing her husband of full responsibility for the deformity because of venereal infection.

4. Questioning one nurse after another as to whether or not surgery can correct the deformity.

6. Which reaction by Mrs. Griffin would best indicate that she has reached the acceptance phase of the grief cycle?

1. Crying as she holds the baby in her arms and lightly runs her fingers over the defect in his lip.

2. Having asked that the baby be brought to her, directing that he be returned immediately to the nursery.

3. Insisting on taking the child home rather than leaving him at the hospital for the cleft lip repair.

4. Expressing her willingness to go along with any plan for Homer's care designed by her personal physician.

7. Homer's deformity would be upsetting to his parents for which of the following reasons?

a. One usually establishes visual contact first with the face of another in close and meaningful interpersonal communication.

b. A parent's view of his child's face affects his own body-image, since the child is seen as an extension of himself.

c. It detracts from the parents' natural pride in creation and weakens their trust in the predictability of natural phenomena.

d. There is a universal but largely unconscious expectation that the newborn infant will be beautiful, whole, and unmarked.

1. a and b.

2. c and d.

3. All but d.

4. All the above.

8. For which reason would it be advisable for Homer's cleft lip to be repaired as soon as possible after birth?

1. To facilitate normal feeding and improve nutrition.

2. To eliminate the danger of aspirating secretions.

3. To increase his parents' acceptance of his defect.

4. To prevent speech impairment and voice problems.

9. Before repair of his lip and palate defects the physician will probably order that Homer be fed by:

1. Breast-feeding.

2. Intravenous fluids.

3. Metal spout cup.

4. Large, soft nipples with large holes.

10. Homer should be placed in which position during his feedings?

1. Supine.

2. Side-lying.

3. Upright.

4. Prone.

11. As a result of his deformity Homer will require which of the following adjustments of his feeding procedure?

1. Thickened bottle feedings to facilitate sucking.

2. Larger quantities of formula than the normal baby.

3. More frequent bubbling than the normal baby.

4. Less time between feedings than the normal baby.

12. Homer's cleft lip predisposes him to infection primarily as a result of:
1. Accumulation of dried milk in the skin folds of the defect.
2. Disruption of normal circulation to the circumoral tissues.
3. Faulty general nutrition resulting from difficulty in sucking.
4. Mouth breathing and consequent drying of the oral mucosa.

13. Which of the following steps may have to be taken preoperatively to protect Homer's lip defect from irritation?
1. Covering the lip defect with a gauze dressing.
2. Keeping the lip defect lubricated with petroleum jelly.
3. Extending Homer's arms and restraining them at his side.
4. Placing a gauze wick in the side of his mouth.

Since Homer gained weight steadily from birth and was free of infection, his lip defect was surgically repaired on his seventh day of life. He survived the anesthetic and operation in good condition and returned to his room with a Logan bar over the wound. He was restrained to prevent injury to the suture line. The surgeon ordered that the incision be kept free of crusting and that Homer's crying be kept to a minimum. He was given water as soon as he wakened and formula feedings eight hours postoperatively, since the water feeding was retained.

14. The purpose for placing the Logan bar over Homer's lip wound postoperatively was to:
1. Prevent stretching and separation of the suture line during crying.
2. Prevent deformity by immobilizing the two halves of the mandible.
3. Extending Homer's arms and restraining them at his side.
4. Apply gentle traction to the skin sutures closing the wound.

15. For the first 48 hours postoperatively Homer should be watched very carefully for evidence of:
1. Respiratory difficulty.
2. Circulatory failure.
3. Hypoglycemic shock.
4. Abdominal distention.

16. By which of the following means could the nurse best restrain Homer from traumatizing the lip suture line?
1. Wrap each of Homer's hands with several layers of gauze so as to construct a thick mitten and attach firmly to the wrist with tape.
2. Attach a soft cloth restraint to each wrist and tie to the bed frame so as to extend Homer's arms along his sides.
3. Secure a splint made of cloth with narrow pockets filled with tongue blades around each elbow so as to prevent elbow flexion.
4. Extent Homer's arms at his sides, place a rolled draw sheet over his waist, and tuck it under the mattress on both sides.

17. The nurse could best prevent crusting of the lip suture line by:
1. Frequent patting with sterile saline-moistened applicators.
2. Cleansing with cotton balls and green soap twice daily.
3. Application of several layers of collodion over the suture line.
4. Coating the area daily with petroleum jelly.

18. Prevention of crusting is particularly important in Homer's care in order to prevent:
1. Hypopigmentation.
2. Infection.
3. Pain.
4. Scarring.

19. Which of the following measures could the nurse use to minimize Homer's crying during the postoperative period?
a. Changing his diaper immediately after each soiling or wetting.
b. Administration of formula in several small feedings given slowly.
c. Frequent changes of position and passive exercise of his arms.
d. Provision of additional cuddling, rocking, and other pleasurable stimuli.
e. Arranging for his parents to assist in comforting him.
  1. a and b.
  2. c and d.
  3. All but e.
  4. All the above.

20. Because of the requirements of his immediate postoperative care, Homer is particularly liable to:

1. Pneumonia.
2. Hemorrhage.
3. Dehydration.
4. Acidosis.

21. Since Homer was given endotracheal anesthesia, he must be carefully observed postoperatively for evidence of:
    1. Deviated nasal septum.
    2. Laryngeal edema.
    3. Pulmonary embolism.
    4. Spontaneous pneumothorax.

22. Which of the following would be most helpful in reducing mucosal irritation resulting from endotracheal intubation?
    1. Alkaline mouth wash.
    2. Cold liquids to drink.
    3. High humidity tent.
    4. Oxygen administration.

23. In feeding Homer postoperatively the nurse should:
    a. Place him in an upright position for feeding.
    b. Administer the same formula which was given him preoperatively.
    c. Administer the formula in small amounts and slowly.
    d. Cleanse his mouth with water when the feeding is completed.
        1. a and c.
        2. b and d.
        3. All but d.
        4. All the above.

Homer recuperated from the surgical procedure without complications. The sutures were removed on the seventh postoperative day and the incision healed without infection or scarring. Homer was discharged after the nurse had instructed his parents about the care he would require at home. The surgeon arranged for Homer to be under close supervision by the cleft palate clinic and informed Mr. and Mrs. Griffin that palate repair would not be done until Homer's second or third year.

24. In deciding how Mr. and Mrs. Griffin are to feed Homer at home the doctor will be guided by which of the following facts?
    1. The surgical lip repair will have destroyed all sensory nerve endings, thus depriving Homer of most pleasurable sensations normally associated with feeding.

    2. The palate defect will interfere with creation of a vacuum in the mouth and will permit regurgitation of fluid from the mouth into the nose.
    3. A palatal prosthesis can be immediately installed which will occlude the defect in the roof of the mouth and make normal sucking possible.
    4. Repair of the lip defect will prevent food loss from the mouth, enabling Homer to be fed by those methods normally employed for any infant of the same age.

25. In instructing the Griffins concerning Homer's home care the nurse should emphasize that he is more susceptible than a normal infant to:
    1. Food allergies.
    2. Respiratory infections.
    3. Infectious diarrhea.
    4. Gastric dilatation.

26. The treatment team responsible for Homer's health supervision in the cleft palate clinic will probably include which of the following specialists?
    a. Social worker.
    b. Nurse.
    c. Surgeon.
    d. Dentist.
    e. Speech therapist.
        1. a and c.
        2. b and c.
        3. All but d.
        4. All the above.

27. Part of Homer's medical follow-up in the cleft palate clinic will probably include tests of his:
    1. Vision.
    2. Hearing.
    3. Taste.
    4. Reflexes.

28. The cleft palate clinic personnel will probably observe that Mr. and Mrs. Griffin's attitude toward Homer tends to be one of:
    1. Overprotection.
    2. Rigid discipline.
    3. Casual neglect.
    4. Inconsistency in affection.

29. As soon as Homer has acquired enough teeth to hold a palate prosthesis, one will be provided him in order to prevent:
    1. Development of chronic sinus infection.
    2. Distorted growth of facial bones.
    3. Fixation of improper speech habits.
    4. Loss of the senses of taste and smell.

Pyloric Stenosis

Rexford Glick, who weighed seven pounds at birth, was discharged from the hospital on his third day of life. During the next two weeks at home he developed severe vomiting and weight loss, although his appetite remained good. Finally Rexford's mother brought the infant to the hospital emergency room for treatment.

Rexford's physical examination revealed severe dehydration, epigastric distention, and a palpable olive-sized mass in the right upper abdomen. The physician admitted the infant to the hospital, ordered upper gastrointestinal tract x-rays, complete blood count, blood chemistries, and urinalysis. The physician interpreted the physical, laboratory, and x-ray findings as indicating pyloric stenosis.

(ANSWER BLANK ON PAGE A–23)   (CORRECT ANSWERS ON PAGE B–34)

1. Persistent vomiting in an infant is apt to produce:
   a. Decreased skin turgor.
   b. Metabolic alkalosis.
   c. Decreased blood volume.
   d. Progressive starvation.
   e. Increased urine output.
      1. a and b.
      2. c and d.
      3. All but e.
      4. All the above.

2. Vomiting due to pyloric obstruction is typically characterized as:
   a. Bile-stained and scanty.
   b. Initiated with great force.
   c. Decreasing in severity with time.
   d. Unaccompanied by nausea.
      1. a and b.
      2. a and c.
      3. b and c.
      4. b and d.

3. Careful history-taking may reveal that Rexford had developed which gastrointestinal symptom besides vomiting?
   1. Excessive salivation.
   2. Noisy eructations.
   3. Decreased frequency of stools.
   4. Fresh blood in the stools.

4. The tissue change characteristic of pyloric obstruction in infants is:
   1. Neoplastic obstruction of the opening between the stomach and small bowel.
   2. Edema of the mucosal lining of the stomach.
   3. Hypertrophy of the circular muscle fibers at the lower end of the stomach.
   4. Scarring of the semilunar valve between the stomach and small bowel.

5. Mrs. Glick will probably have observed which of the following immediately after each of Rexford's feedings?
   a. Marked distention of the epigastric region.
   b. Peristaltic waves traversing the epigastrium.
   c. Severe engorgement of periumbilical veins.
   d. Loud and high-pitched bowel sounds.
   e. Sudden expulsion of diarrhea stool.
      1. a and b.
      2. b and c.
      3. c and d.
      4. d and e.

6. Rexford could be expected to demonstrate which of the following signs of dehydration?
   a. Dry oral mucosa.
   b. Sunken eyeballs.
   c. Wrinkled skin.
   d. Concentrated urine.
      1. a and c.
      2. b and d.
      3. All but d.
      4. All the above.

7. Which of the following blood chemistry findings would Rexford be most apt to demonstrate?
   a. Low serum chloride.
   b. Low serum potassium.
   c. Low serum calcium.

d. Low serum pH.
e. Low serum bicarbonate.
    1. a, b, and c.
    2. c and d.
    3. All but e.
    4. All the above.

Rexford was given phenobarbital sedation, 5 per cent glucose in saline intravenously, and parenteral preparations of vitamins B_1, D, and K for three days in order to improve his physical condition prior to surgical repair of his pyloric obstruction. During these three days Rexford was given small amounts of a thickened formula slowly by gavage feeding, and a small quantity of food was absorbed in this fashion.

On the morning of surgery a nasogastric tube was inserted to empty his stomach and the tube was left in place. Atropine was given preoperatively and ether anesthesia was used during the procedure.

8. Vigorous preoperative treatment was needed for Rexford because his weakened condition made him particularly susceptible to which of the following complications during surgery?
    1. Circulatory shock.
    2. Acute asphyxiation.
    3. Systemic infection.
    4. Intestinal distention.

9. Which of the following is the pharmacologic effect of vitamin K that explains its administration to Rexford at this time?
    1. It is utilized in the synthesis of prothrombin by the liver.
    2. It stimulates proliferation of capillaries in granulation tissue.
    3. It increases the resistance of epithelial tissues to injury.
    4. It accelerates the rate of oxidative reactions in tissue cells.

10. With which of the following functions is vitamin K utilization primarily associated?
    1. Blood clotting.
    2. Wound healing.
    3. Respiratory gas exchange.
    4. Protein anabolism.

11. Vitamin K deficiency is frequently observed in the newborn because:
    1. The typical infant diet is poor in foods serving as a natural source of the vitamin.
    2. The liver has not yet had time to store adequate quantities of vitamin K.
    3. The intestinal bacteria that synthe-size vitamin K have not yet been colonized.
    4. Intestinal peristalsis is too rapid to permit absorption from the small bowel.

12. The pharmacologic effect of vitamin C that accounts for its preoperative administration to Rexford is its ability to:
    1. Stimulate hematopoiesis in red bone marrow.
    2. Enhance serum protein formation in the liver.
    3. Stimulate fibroblasts and capillary proliferation.
    4. Increase prothrombin production by liver parenchyma.

13. Vitamin B_1 is especially important to Rexford's preoperative fluid therapy in that thiamin facilitates:
    1. Glycolysis and glucose utilization.
    2. Fluid filtration by renal glomeruli.
    3. Maintenance of serum osmotic pressure.
    4. Oxygen adsorption by red blood cells.

14. In addition to thiamin, what other vitamins are included in the B complex group?
    a. Cyanocobalamine.
    b. Riboflavin.
    c. Ascorbic acid.
    d. Pyridoxine.
    e. Viosterol.
        1. a and c.
        2. b and d.
        3. a, b, and d.
        4. All the above.

15. The purpose of giving Rexford a thickened formula preoperatively was to:
    1. Supply increased calories in a smaller quantity of liquid.
    2. Delay the emptying time of the stomach.
    3. Provide him greater satiety value during his feeding periods.
    4. Provide a stimulus for increased intestinal peristalsis.

16. During gavage it would be advisable for the nurse to place Rexford in which position?
    1. Supine on a well-padded treatment table.
    2. Cradled in her arms or in an assistant's lap.
    3. Lying on his right side, propped by a pillow.
    4. Head elevated 45 degrees on rolled blankets or pads.

17. Which of the following substances would best serve to lubricate the catheter to be used during gavage?
1. Sterile normal saline.
2. Petroleum jelly.
3. Mineral oil.
4. Ordered formula.

18. How should the nurse determine the distance to which the catheter should be inserted during gavage?
1. Insert the catheter slowly until it will no longer advance with gentle pressure.
2. Measure the distance from the ear lobe to the nose to the distal end of the sternum.
3. Double the distance between the tip of the nose and the lobe of the ear.
4. Introduce the catheter slowly, applying suction at serial stages until liquid is aspirated.

19. In gavage, the nurse should consider which of the following as normal reactions to passage of the tube through the nasopharynx and esophagus?
a. Coughing.
b. Cyanosis.
c. Gagging.
d. Flushing.
e. Apnea.
   1. a and b.
   2. c and d.
   3. a, c, and d.
   4. All the above.

20. By what means should the nurse ensure that the catheter has been inserted into the stomach rather than into the lung?
1. Pour a small quantity of the formula into the tube and listen for rales.
2. Inject 3–5 ml. air into the tube while auscultating the stomach.
3. Inject a syringe full of air into the tube and watch for gastric distention.
4. Apply strong suction to the tube and note the character of aspirated fluid.

21. Before removing the gavage tube, what precaution should be taken?
1. Pinch the tube tightly to prevent leakage during withdrawal.
2. Inject 5 cc. of air through the tube to empty it.
3. Siphon off a small quantity of formula to observe its consistency.
4. Press gently on the epigastrium to facilitate eructation.

22. In assisting the physician to insert the nasogastric tube preoperatively the nurse could best immobilize Rexford by:
1. Wrapping a sheet around his trunk and then over his arms extended along his sides.
2. Pinning Rexford's night shirt to the bed linen so as to extend his arms perpendicularly.
3. Holding the infant's arms above his head with one hand and extending his legs with the other.
4. Attaching a soft cloth belt around his waist and tying it to the frame of the bed.

23. The surgical treatment of choice for pyloric stenosis is:
1. Excision of the pylorus with an anastomosis of the gastric fundus to the duodenum.
2. Gastroenterostomy with a side-to-side anastomosis of the stomach and jejunum.
3. Incision through the hypertrophied muscle of the pylorus down to the mucosa.
4. Undermining and removal of the mucosa of the pylorus and upper portion of the duodenum.

24. The nurse should observe Rexford closely for which of the following as possible signs of atropine overdosage?
a. Dry, flushed skin.
b. Dilated pupils.
c. Decreased respirations.
d. Increased temperature.
   1. a and b.
   2. c and d.
   3. a, b, and d.
   4. All the above.

On his return to the recovery room following the operation Rexford's pulse was 140 per minute, respirations 30 per minute, and blood pressure 80/60 mm. Hg. One hundred ml. of 5 per cent glucose in saline were administered intravenously. On the first postoperative day the intravenous infusion was discontinued and the nasogastric tube was removed. One-half ounce of 5 per cent dextrose solution was given by bottle and retained. At two hour intervals throughout the remainder of the day slightly increased amounts of dextrose solution were administered. Since Rexford retained all the glucose solution feedings, he was advanced to a dilute evaporated milk formula on the second postoperative day and to a full formula on the day following.

25. Immediately following his return from the operating room Rexford should be placed in which of the following positions?
1. Supine with his head on a small pillow.
2. On his side with his back supported.
3. On his stomach with his head turned to the side.
4. Sitting upright by means of a jacket restraint.

26. The surgeon ordered that the dextrose in saline intravenous solution given postoperatively should run for a period of six hours. Using a microdrop apparatus, the nurse should regulate the solution flow at:
1. 4 microdrops per minute.
2. 16 microdrops per minute.
3. 32 microdrops per minute.
4. 48 microdrops per minute.

27. The principal reason for careful regulation of the intravenous infusion is to protect Rexford against:
1. Metabolic acidosis.
2. Acute thrombophlebitis.
3. Heart failure.
4. Abdominal distention.

28. For as long as the nasogastric tube is left in place following surgery, which of the following precautions should be taken by the nurse?
1. Rexford should be kept in an upright sitting position.
2. Rexford's arms should be kept restrained.
3. Rexford should be given water at frequent intervals.
4. Rexford should be held by the nurse or his mother.

29. On the first few occasions that Rexford is given a formula following his operation he should be fed by:
1. Medicine dropper.
2. Bulb syringe.
3. Nasogastric tube.
4. Spout cup.

30. Which of the following measures should the nurse take to decrease vomiting when regular feeding is resumed postoperatively?
1. Rock Rexford's crib for 15 minutes before and after each feeding.
2. Elevate the foot of his bed before and after each feeding.
3. Use nipples with larger than usual openings to prevent air ingestion.
4. Hold Rexford in a sitting or upright position during and after feeding.

31. The nurse should take which of the following precautions postoperatively in order to prevent contamination of Rexford's surgical wound?
1. Apply his diaper low, below the dressing.
2. Keep a pediatric urine collector in place.
3. Keep him in a supine position continuously.
4. Seal the gauze dressing with plastic wrap.

32. Mrs. Glick asked the nurse, "Since the doctor didn't actually remove Rexford's tumor, might it not cause trouble later?" Which of the following would be the most appropriate response?
1. "Why don't you explain to the doctor your uncertainties and fears about Rexford's future? He'll answer all your questions."
2. "Yes, it is possible that he might develop obstructive symptoms later. If so, take him immediately to your doctor."
3. "He will not have symptoms again in childhood, but should be warned to watch for digestive difficulties in his adult life."
4. "There is no reason to expect either recurrence of the obstruction or repetition of the surgical procedure."

Rexford experienced an uneventful postoperative period and was discharged one week after surgery.

Whooping Cough

Eight-week-old Sidney Kaufman had a mild unproductive cough that got worse and became paroxysmal within ten days. His parents brought him to the hospital when he developed cyanosis during and vomiting following the paroxysms. On admission Sidney's temperature was 99.4° F. rectally, pulse 128 per minute, respirations 46 per minute, hemoglobin 11.4 grams per 100 ml., hematocrit 33 per cent, white blood cell count 29,000 per cu. mm. with 73 per cent lymphocytes, 18 per cent segmented neutrophils, 3 per cent eosinophils, and 6 per cent monocytes. He weighed 8 pounds, 13 ounces (having weighed 6 pounds, 2 ounces at birth), and Mrs. Kaufman revealed that he had not had any of his baby shots.

Physical examination revealed a well-developed, well-nourished infant with injection of the pharyngeal mucosa and conjunctivae. Chest examination revealed diffuse inspiratory rales and tracheal rhonchi. Chest x-ray revealed increased markings in the right hilar region. During the examination Sidney suffered a paroxysm consisting of several short expiratory bursts followed by a long inspiratory whooping cough. His face was deeply flushed during the paroxysms, he perspired profusely, and afterward he vomited a moderate quantity of a coagulated milk and mucus mixture. A pharyngeal swab and a Bordet-Gengou cough plate was taken for cultures and Sidney was tentatively diagnosed as having whooping cough with diffuse pneumonitis. The following orders were written:

1. Erythromycin 40 mg./kg. orally q. 6 h. for five days.
2. Isolation.
3. Croupette with oxygen and cold humidity.
4. Nasopharyngeal suction p.r.n.
5. Oral feedings of 4 ounces of 5 per cent dextrose in ¼ N. saline q. 4 h. today. Tomorrow begin formula of evaporated milk and water, 1:2, 4 ounces q. 4 h.

(ANSWER BLANK ON PAGE A–25) (CORRECT ANSWERS ON PAGE B–36)

1. The causative organism for whooping cough is:
   1. *Histoplasma capsulatum.*
   2. *Bordetella pertussis.*
   3. *Klebsiella pneumoniae.*
   4. *Beta-hemolytic Streptococcus.*

2. Sidney probably contracted whooping cough by means of:
   1. Ingestion of food inoculated with the causative organism.
   2. Imbibing water contaminated by body secretions from an infected person.
   3. Direct contact with or droplet spray from an infected person.
   4. Ingestion of unpasteurized milk obtained from infected cows.

3. The incubation period of an infectious disease is the interval between:
   1. Exposure to the etiological organism and the appearance of the first symptom.
   2. The appearance of the earliest symptom and the development of an elevated temperature.
   3. The appearance of major definitive symptoms and subsidence of symptoms with beginning recovery.
   4. The introduction of the causative agent and the production of specific antibodies.

4. The incubation period for whooping cough is commonly:

1. 1 to 3 days.
2. 2 to 4 days.
3. 7 to 10 days.
4. 14 to 40 days.

5. Whooping cough differs from measles in that:

1. The causative organisms of pertussis enter the body through the upper respiratory tract.
2. There is little transfer of pertussis antibodies from the mother to the fetus.
3. The initial phase of pertussis is characterized by symptoms of upper respiratory infection.
4. Bronchopneumonia is apt to occur as a result of secondary infection in pertussis.

6. Artificial active immunization against pertussis could be given Sidney at the appropriate age by administration of:

1. Gamma globulin.
2. An antitoxin.
3. A convalescent serum.
4. A vaccine.

7. Pertussis immunization is usually given in combination with immunization for which of the following?

a. Tetanus.
b. Diphtheria.
c. Measles.
d. Smallpox.
e. Poliomyelitis.
   1. a only.
   2. a and b.
   3. a, b, c, and e.
   4. All the above.

8. The preferred age for initial immunization against pertussis is:

1. One to two weeks.
2. Two to three months.
3. Three to four months.
4. One year.

9. The pathophysiologic changes underlying symptoms in whooping cough are:

1. Inflammation of bronchial and bronchiolar mucosa with obstruction of passageways by mucus plugs and mucopurulent exudate.
2. Ischemic necrosis of alveolar walls with exudation of blood serum from pulmonary capillaries into air sacs and terminal bronchioles.
3. Histamine-induced constriction of smooth muscle fibers encircling the lumina of the bronchi, bronchioles, and alveolar ducts.
4. Accumulation in the basilar alveoli of inflammatory exudate, which subsequently solidifies and is replaced by fibrous tissue.

10. The nurse should explain to the Kaufmans that Sidney's disease can be communicated to susceptible persons from one week before development of paroxysms to:

1. Appearance of the whooping cough.
2. One week after symptoms develop.
3. Two weeks after symptoms develop.
4. Three weeks after symptoms develop.

11. In helping Mrs. Kaufman to understand and accept Sidney's symptoms the nurse should strive to convey which of the following concepts?

1. Vomiting reduces cardiac work load by decreasing the volume of vascular fluid.
2. Paroxysms, though frightening and exhausting, are useful in removing secretions.
3. Profuse sweating during spasms decreases the fever accompanying the infection.
4. Facial flushing during coughing results from temperature spikes preceding paroxysms.

12. In planning nursing care for Sidney in the hospital the nurse should be aware that his paroxysms are most apt to occur:

1. In the morning.
2. At midday.
3. In the late afternoon.
4. At night.

13. If Sidney demonstrates severe and frequent paroxysms, he will be prone to:

1. Cerebral hemorrhage.
2. Severe malnutrition.
3. Diaphragmatic hernia.
4. Aortic aneurysm.

14. In order to decrease the chance of Sidney's developing malnutrition the nurse should:

a. Hold him during feedings.
b. Weigh him twice weekly.
c. Plan his care to provide rest periods.
d. Record frequency of vomiting.
e. Record his intake of formula.
   1. a and b.
   2. a, b, and c.
   3. c, d, and e.
   4. All the above.

15. If Sidney should vomit his formula immediately after feeding the nurse should:

1. Withhold oral feedings for two hours.
2. Measure the amount of vomitus.
3. Place him flat on his abdomen.
4. Give him another 3 ounces of formula.

16. Which of the following actions by the nurse would be the most supportive to Sidney during a paroxysm?

1. Go to him, support his abdomen, and stay with him until the paroxysm subsides.
2. Elevate the head of the bed and then gently rock it back and forth.
3. Increase the rate of oxygen administration and direct it toward his face.
4. Wipe his face free of perspiration and place a cool cloth on his forehead.

17. Sidney's explosive coughing would be apt to cause:

1. Subconjunctival hemorrhage.
2. Ruptured tympanic membrane.
3. Perforation of the trachea.
4. Spontaneous pneumothorax.

18. Erythromycin is better suited for Sidney's treatment than penicillin because *Bordetella pertussis* is which of the following types of organisms?

1. Intracellular diplococcus.
2. Acid-fast bacillus.
3. Gram-negative bacillus.
4. Anaerobic spore-former.

19. Sidney's illness especially predisposes him to pneumonia because of the fact that his:

1. Respiratory cilia are unable to remove foreign material from his lung parenchyma.
2. Pulmonary arterial blood supply is decreased in volume, speed, and quality.
3. Overwhelming septicemia will rapidly exhaust his normal body defenses.
4. Extreme weakness will render him bedridden and immobile for some time.

20. Which of the following are frequent pulmonary complications of whooping cough?

a. Pneumonia.
b. Bronchitis.
c. Atelectasis.
d. Emphysema.
e. Bronchiectasis.
1. a and b.
2. c and d.
3. All but e.
4. All the above.

21. Which of the following nursing measures will decrease Sidney's susceptibility to pulmonary complications?

a. Nasopharyngeal suctioning.
b. Prone positioning.
c. Postural drainage.
d. Protection against chilling.
1. a and b.
2. a, b, and c.
3. All but d.
4. All the above.

22. Sidney should be observed for signs of which of the following gastrointestinal complications frequently occurring in patients with whooping cough?

a. Umbilical hernia.
b. Rectal prolapse.
c. Gastric ulcer.
d. Ulcerative colitis.
e. Pylorospasm.
1. a only.
2. a and b.
3. a, b, and d.
4. All the above.

23. In carrying out concurrent disinfection of Sidney's equipment, supplies, and excreta, the nurse should:

a. Encase his linen in a bag marked "Isolation" to be laundered separately.
b. Place disposable diapers in a plastic garbage bag and tie it shut.
c. Wear a gown while giving direct nursing care to Sidney.
d. Provide Sidney with his own thermometer, bedpan, and urinal.
e. Serve Sidney's food on paper or plastic disposable containers.
1. a and b.
2. a, b, and c.
3. a, c, d, and e.
4. All the above.

The initial cough plate cultures were negative but subsequent cultures made from swabs of Sidney's nasopharynx were positive for *Bordetella pertussis*. After ten days of erythromycin, oxygen, and high-humidity therapy, Sidney's paroxysms and vomiting were much decreased in severity and frequency and his vital signs were normal. He was maintained in isolation but his parents were notified that he could be discharged in another week.

24. In teaching Mrs. Kaufman to care for Sidney at home, the nurse should advise her to do which of the following in order to reduce Sidney's paroxysms?

  a. Provide a quiet and restful environment.

  b. Protect against rapid changes in temperature.

  c. Give small, thickened feedings frequently.

  d. Provide an adequate supply of fresh, warm air.

  e. Give him extra attention between paroxysms.

    1. a and b.

    2. a, c, and d.

    3. All but e.

    4. All the above.

25. In instructing Mrs. Kaufman about Sidney's home care it is especially important that the nurse tell her that:

  1. All feedings should be diluted with water.

  2. Paroxysms of coughing may continue for several weeks.

  3. A steam humidifier should be used continuously.

  4. Baths should be omitted until coughing ceases.

After two weeks of hospitalization Sidney was discharged, having lost 7 ounces of weight during his illness. A referral was made to the public health nursing agency for home care follow-up. Mrs. Kaufman was instructed to take Sidney to the family pediatrician for further medical supervision.

Meningomyelocele and Hydrocephalus

Dolores Sommersett had a normal delivery but was born with a 3 by 3 inch meningomyelocele covered by a thin membrane over the lower lumbar and sacral regions. Although her head was only slightly larger than normal at birth, a progressive and abnormal increase in head circumference became noticeable within a few weeks. Therefore, when she was two months old Dolores was prepared for a ventriculoperitoneal shunt to prevent excessive head enlargement.

On admission Dolores was found to be malnourished but in no apparent distress. Her extremities were normal except for absent sensation in both feet. Blood tests and urinalysis revealed no abnormal findings. Mrs. Sommersett indicated that Dolores did not eat well and seemed fretful. The physician ordered cranial and spinal x-rays and scheduled Dolores for a ventriculogram and tracer dye studies.

(ANSWER BLANK ON PAGE A–27)   (CORRECT ANSWERS ON PAGE B–37)

1. A meningomyelocele may best be defined as:

1. A soft fluctuant sac, containing portions of meninges, nerve roots, spinal cord, and cerebrospinal fluid, which protrudes through a defect in the bony spine.
2. A cyst containing elements of hair, teeth, and skin, which derives from an embryonic nest and is usually located in the lower region of the back.
3. A dilated sacculated meningeal blood vessel with weakened walls containing mural thrombi and tending to rupture when subjected to elevated blood pressure.
4. A localized aggregation of inflammatory debris, surrounded by a membrane and located in the cancellous bone of the vertebral bodies.

2. Spina bifida may best be defined as:

1. The formation of a membranous septum through the middle of the spinal canal.
2. Rupture of the cartilaginous disc separating the bodies of two adjacent vertebrae.
3. A defect in fusion of the posterior neural arch of one or more vertebrae.
4. Traumatic separation of a spinal nerve root from its normal attachment with the cord.

3. Before repair of the meningomyelocele Dolores should, for the most part, be kept in which position?

1. Prone.
2. Side-lying.
3. Sitting.
4. Semi-Fowler's.

4. Hydrocephalus can be most accurately defined as:

1. Greatly increased head diameter due to spreading of the sutures by massive cerebral edema.
2. Progressive enlargement of the head due to excessive accumulation of cerebrospinal fluid.
3. Elevation of the dome of the skull by a hematoma secondary to skull fracture.
4. Distention of the frontal, maxillary, and ethmoid sinuses with inflammatory exudate.

5. Hydrocephalus is caused by:

1. Excessive production or impaired absorption of cerebrospinal fluid.
2. Massive exudation of fluid from overdistended cerebral capillaries.
3. Slow persistent hemorrhage from lacerated cranial arterioles.
4. Cerebral destruction by a progressively enlarged serous cyst.

6. The nurse should carefully observe the nature and frequency of Dolores' voiding in order to determine whether:

1. Nervous control of bladder function has been impaired.
2. Fluid intake has been adequate to meet metabolic needs.
3. Restricted mobility has produced urinary stasis and infection.
4. There is a coincident inborn error of protein metabolism.

7. Cerebrospinal fluid is produced by the:

1. Arachnoid layer of the meninges.
2. Arteries in the circle of Willis.
3. Choroid plexuses of the lateral ventricles.
4. Vital centers in the medulla oblongata.

8. Cerebrospinal fluid is found normally in the:

1. Epidural space.
2. Subdural space.
3. Subarachnoid space.
4. Subpial space.

9. The chief function of cerebrospinal fluid is to:

a. Distribute antibodies to cells of the brain and spinal cord.
b. Buffer the brain and cord against mechanical trauma.
c. Remove metabolic wastes from nerve cell metabolism.
d. Facilitate expansion and contraction of brain tissue.
   1. a and b.
   2. b and c.
   3. c and d.
   4. All the above.

10. Which of the following are frequent causes of obstruction to normal cerebrospinal fluid circulation?

a. Tumor obstructing a ventricle.
b. Congenital stenosis of the aqueduct.
c. Meningeal adhesions following meningitis.
d. Pressure from a depressed skull fracture.
   1. a and b.

2. c and d.
3. All but d.
4. All the above.

11. Which of the following are characteristic signs and symptoms of hydrocephalus?
 a. Progressive abnormal increase in head circumference.
 b. Downward and outward deflection of the eyeballs.
 c. Separation of the sutures and widening of the fontanels.
 d. Some degree of impairment of brain function.
  1. a and b.
  2. a, b, and c.
  3. All but d.
  4. All the above.

12. The sites at which obstructions to cerebrospinal fluid flow most often occur are:
 a. Aqueduct of Sylvius.
 b. Foramen of Monro.
 c. Foramen of Magendie.
 d. Circle of Willis.
  1. a and b.
  2. c and d.
  3. a, b, and c.
  4. All the above.

13. In making a specific diagnosis of hydrocephalus, the physician may have to rule out which of the following conditions?
 a. Prematurity.
 b. Subdural hematoma.
 c. Intracranial tumor.
 d. Achondroplastic dwarfism.
  1. a and c.
  2. b and d.
  3. All but d.
  4. All the above.

14. The pathophysiologic defect underlying the production of symptoms in hydrocephalus is:
 1. Unusually increased intracranial pressure.
 2. Inadequate oxygenation of the cerebral cortex.
 3. Accumulation of toxic cellular metabolites.
 4. Lack of myelin insulation of nerve fibers.

15. Hydrocephalus, if untreated, may be expected to cause mental retardation because:
 1. Hypertonic cerebrospinal fluid draws vital nutrients and minerals out of nerve cells, disturbing their function.
 2. The gradually dilating ventricles compress the brain against the cranial vault, causing pressure atrophy of nerve cells.
 3. Anoxic cerebral nerve cells gradually die and are liquefied by enzymes released from the dying cells.
 4. Interruption of cerebral blood supply results in distribution of inadequate nutrients to brain tissue.

16. Dolores' malnourished appearance is probably the result of:
 1. Anorexia and nausea.
 2. Pyloric obstruction.
 3. Hyperactive peristalsis.
 4. Intestinal malabsorption.

17. The nurse should employ which of the following measures to improve Dolores' nutrition?
 a. Plan care so as to avoid moving her following feeding.
 b. Hold her while administering each feeding.
 c. Feed slowly and bubble at frequent intervals.
 d. Place her on the right side following each feeding.
  1. a only.
  2. a and b.
  3. All but d.
  4. All the above.

18. Which of the following adaptations should be made in Dolores' clothing?
 1. Construct shirts and gowns to open all the way down the back.
 2. Provide larger than usual neck openings in all garments.
 3. Use only skirts and shirts made of cotton flannel.
 4. Use extra large diapers, applying them over the meningomyelocele.

19. A ventriculogram is a procedure in which:
 1. Air is introduced into the ventricles as an aid to x-ray visualization.
 2. A radiopaque dye is injected into a ventricle and its circulation traced by fluoroscopy.
 3. Electrical impulses generated by the cerebral cortex overlying a ventricle are recorded.
 4. A radioactive substance is injected into the spinal canal and the ventricular radioactivity measured.

20. Which of the following are common untoward effects following a ventriculogram?
- a. Headache.
- b. Hyperpyrexia.
- c. Nausea.
- d. Tinnitus.
- e. Blurred vision.
  - 1. a and c.
  - 2. b and d.
  - 3. All but e.
  - 4. All the above.

21. Dolores' care following the ventriculogram should include:
- a. Keeping her flat in bed.
- b. Checking for signs of increased intracranial pressure.
- c. Administration of oxygen hourly for 8 hours.
- d. Forcing the rapid ingestion of large amounts of fluids.
  - 1. a and b.
  - 2. c and d.
  - 3. All but d.
  - 4. All the above.

22. Which of the following dyes would be suitable for the tracer studies done in conjunction with Dolores' ventriculogram?
1. Barium sulfate.
2. Pantopaque.
3. Lipiodol.
4. Phenolsulfonphthalein.

23. Which of the following findings on dye tracer studies would indicate obstructive hydrocephalus?
1. Forceful reflux of dye and cerebral fluid through the needle and syringe immediately following dye injection.
2. Aspiration of deeply dye-stained cerebral tissue by punch biopsy technique two days after dye injection.
3. Failure of dye to appear in the lumbar spinal fluid 15 to 20 minutes after its introduction into the ventricle.
4. X-ray observation that all dye injected into the lateral ventricle is retained in that chamber.

Dolores' ventriculogram and dye studies indicated a noncommunicating or obstructive type of hydrocephalus. A ventriculoperitoneal shunt was performed, using a catheter to drain excessive fluid from the ventricle through the internal jugular vein to the superior vena cava. A Pudenz valve was inserted into the catheter where it lay in the superficial tissue behind the right ear.

When Dolores was returned to the recovery room after the operation the following orders were written:

1. Keep flat.
2. Glucose water feedings as soon as tolerated. If retained, may be followed by house formula.
3. Ampicillin oral suspension 50 mg. q.i.d.
4. Multivitamin mixture 0.6 cc. orally daily.

24. The purpose of the Pudenz valve employed in Dolores' operation is to:
1. Filter pathogenic microorganisms from the cerebral spinal fluid.
2. Accelerate the movement of cerebrospinal fluid from the cranium to the spine.
3. Permit the painless introduction of antibiotics into the subarachnoid space.
4. Facilitate the one-way flow of cerebrospinal fluid from the ventricle to the peritoneal cavity.

25. Complications that frequently develop following the formation of a ventriculoperitoneal shunt using a Pudenz valve are:
- a. Thrombotic occlusion of the ventricular catheter at some point.
- b. Dislodging of the catheter from one or both of its terminal attachments.
- c. Failure of the valve to open and close at the desired pressure.
- d. Growth of microorganisms in the valve.
  - 1. a and b.
  - 2. c and d.
  - 3. All but d.
  - 4. All the above.

26. It is important that Dolores be kept flat in bed following surgery because:
1. Too rapid depression of the anterior fontanel might cause a subdural hematoma.
2. Head elevation together with decreased intracranial pressure might cause hypotension.
3. Elevating the head would increase the rate of cerebrospinal fluid production.
4. Maintaining a supine position decreases the tendency for postoperative vomiting.

27. It is important that an accurate record of Dolores' fluid intake and output be kept during the first few days postoperatively in order to:
1. Provide information for calculating her need for intravenous or oral fluid intake.
2. Estimate the amount of cerebrospinal fluid shunted from ventricle to vena cava.
3. Check for symptoms of circulatory shock and congestive heart failure.
4. Determine whether reduction in intracranial pressure has relieved earlier urinary incontinence.

28. Following Dolores' operation the nurse should observe the tenseness of the anterior fontanel in order to determine:
1. The general level of body hydration.
2. The adequacy of drainage of cerebrospinal fluid.
3. The approximate level of systolic blood pressure.
4. The degree of skin turgor and elasticity.

29. Ampicillin was ordered for Dolores primarily in order to:
1. Reduce the possibility of septicemia from infection in the shunt.
2. Prevent ascending urinary infections due to incontinence.
3. Decrease intestinal bacteria, which overgrow on glucose water diet.
4. Eliminate skin bacteria to prevent infection of the meningomyelocele.

30. Which of the following are common untoward gastrointestinal effects of ampicillin therapy?
a. Nausea.
b. Vomiting.
c. Diarrhea.
d. Mucosal irritation.
e. Reduction of normal intestinal flora.
   1. a and b.
   2. a, b, and e.
   3. All but e.
   4. All the above.

31. Before the meningomyelocele repair the nurse should do which of the following in feeding Dolores?
1. Hold her during feedings, gently covering the sac with a sterile gauze square.
2. Place her on her side with her back supported and hold the bottle while she nurses.
3. Maintain her in a prone position and administer the formula with a rubber-tipped dropper.
4. Place her in a supine position with the meningomyelocele between pillows and hold the bottle.

32. During this period of Dolores' care Mrs. Sommersett should be invited to come regularly to the hospital in order to assist with Dolores':
1. Feeding.
2. Bathing.
3. Dressing.
4. Back care.

33. Frequent and meticulous skin care is especially important in Dolores' treatment because:
a. Fecal and urinary incontinence will cause frequent soiling.
b. Her neurological problems will limit motor activity somewhat.
c. Inadequate nutritional intake has predisposed her to tissue breakdown.
d. The covering of the meningomyelocele is subject to pressure injury.
   1. a and b.
   2. c and d.
   3. All but d.
   4. All the above.

Although Dolores recuperated from the operation, the shunt functioned only sporadically. Therefore, three weeks later she underwent surgery for replacement of the Pudenz valve and attached tubing, which were found to be blocked. Two weeks after the second operation she was taken to surgery for repair of the meningomyelocele. Under general anesthesia the sac was trimmed of excess tissue, fascia and skin flaps were rotated to cover the defect, and the reinforcing tissues were sutured in place. The physician wrote the following postoperative orders:

1. Measure head circumference daily.
2. Keep on abdomen.
3. Vital signs until stable, then q.i.d.
4. Observe for signs of increased intracranial pressure.
5. Glucose water when fully responsive and house formula as soon as tolerated.
6. Ampicillin oral suspension 50 mg. q.i.d.
7. Reinstitute multivitamin mixture 0.6 cc. orally, daily.

34. Dolores' meningomyelocele was repaired during infancy primarily to prevent:
1. Neurologic deficit due to infection, adhesions, and mechanical trauma.
2. Spontaneous rupture or ulceration of the sac with subsequent meningitis.
3. Extrusion of additional spinal cord or nerve tissue into the sac during movement.
4. Massive hemorrhage from spinal blood vessels exposed at the edge of the defect.

35. The major objective of surgical repair of the meningomyelocele was to:
1. Prevent loss of spinal fluid and consequent dehydration.
2. Improve Dolores' appearance and ensure her acceptance.
3. Enable Dolores to lie supine and to wear normal clothing.
4. Close the surface defect and preserve functioning nerve tissue.

36. Dolores' head circumference should be measured regularly in order to:
1. Determine whether the rate of head growth is normal.
2. Calculate the level of intracranial pressure.
3. Ascertain when the cranial sutures are completely fused.
4. Estimate the amount of cerebrospinal fluid retained.

37. Signs of increased intracranial pressure are:
a. Bulging fontanels.
b. Irritability.
c. Lethargy.
d. Vomiting.
e. Slow pulse rate.
   1. a and b.
   2. c and d.
   3. All but e.
   4. All the above.

38. Following meningomyelocele repair the nurse should do which of the following when feeding Dolores?
a. Keep her in the prone position.
b. Elevate her head slightly.
c. Withdraw the nipple frequently.
d. Pick her up to bubble her.
   1. a and b.
   2. c and d.
   3. All but d.
   4. All the above.

Dolores recovered slowly following repair of the meningomyelocele. Mrs. Sommersett came to the hospital daily to feed her. The ventriculoperitoneal shunt continued to function satisfactorily and her rate of head growth decreased, so that her head was more nearly proportionate in size than it had been on hospital admission.

The physician estimated that Dolores' mental retardation, if any, would be minimal. He explained to the Sommersetts that they should obtain help from the physiotherapist in toilet-training Dolores. Dolores was discharged after a total of four months of hospitalization.

39. In teaching Mr. and Mrs. Sommersett about the care that Dolores would require at home the nurse should instruct them concerning:
a. The need for bladder training to establish some degree of urinary control before Dolores begins school.
b. The possibility that mental ability has been impaired to some degree by increased intracranial pressure.
c. Recognition and reporting of signs and symptoms which would indicate an increase in intracranial pressure.
d. The necessity for continuous medical supervision to ensure operation of the ventriculoperitoneal shunt.
e. The need to compensate for sensory loss in protecting Dolores' feet from thermal and mechanical trauma.
   1. a and b.
   2. a, c, and d.
   3. All but e.
   4. All the above.

40. Since the physician estimated that Dolores would probably be mildly retarded, her intelligence quotient would be within which of the following ranges?
1. 60 to 80.
2. 40 to 60.
3. 20 to 40.
4. 0 to 20.

41. Mr. and Mrs. Sommersett should be helped to understand that if Dolores proves to be mildly retarded she will have the most difficulty with:
1. Symbol recognition.
2. Abstract reasoning.
3. Controlling impulses.
4. Remembering facts.

Cystic Fibrosis

Sonya Schreckengost weighed seven pounds at the time of her birth. Two months later her mother noted that the infant was having three to four loose greenish-brown stools a day. She also noted that the stools were frequently foul-smelling and frothy. During the next few months Sonya failed to gain weight so her mother took her to the pediatric clinic at the age of nine months.

The examining physician found Sonya to be poorly developed, underweight, and suffering from bronchitis with frequent nonproductive coughing. Her temperature was 101.4° F. rectally. Because the physician suspected cystic fibrosis and bacterial bronchitis or bronchopneumonia, he admitted Sonya to the hospital and ordered routine blood tests, quantitative sweat test, stool analysis, and chest x-ray. Sonya's family health history revealed that she had no siblings, but one of her first cousins had cystic fibrosis.

(ANSWER BLANK ON PAGE A–29) (CORRECT ANSWERS ON PAGE B–39)

1. Another name for the disease cystic fibrosis is:
 1. Histoplasmosis.
 2. Lipoid pneumonia.
 3. Pulmonary stenosis.
 4. Mucoviscidosis.

2. It would be advisable to explain to Mr. and Mrs. Schreckengost that cystic fibrosis is what type of disease?
 1. Congenital.
 2. Malignant.
 3. Hereditary.
 4. Developmental.

3. Since cystic fibrosis is transmitted as a mendelian recessive trait, and since both Mr. and Mrs. Schreckengost have always been in good health, it may be assumed that:
 1. Neither parent carries the gene for the disease.
 2. Only one of the two parents carries the determining gene.
 3. Both parents are heterozygous carriers of the trait.
 4. Both parents have the disease in mild form.

4. The probability is that which percentage of Mr. and Mrs. Schreckengost's children will develop cystic fibrosis?
 1. 25 per cent.
 2. 50 per cent.
 3. 75 per cent.
 4. 100 per cent.

5. The pathophysiologic problem underlying the symptoms of cystic fibrosis is:
 1. Sluggish lymph circulation due to increased tortuosity of vessels.
 2. Hypertrophy of smooth muscle fibers surrounding tubular structures.
 3. Production of abnormally tenacious secretions by the exocrine glands.
 4. Obstruction of glandular ducts by uric acid crystals or calcium stones.

6. Sonya's small stature was probably primarily due to:
 1. Poor appetite and ingestion of less than normal quantities of food.
 2. Failure to absorb nutrients because of a lack of pancreatic enzymes.
 3. Secretion of less than normal amounts of pituitary growth hormone.
 4. Development of muscular and bony atrophy from lack of motor activity.

7. In what way would cystic fibrosis have predisposed Sonya to bronchitis?
 1. Tenacious secretions obstruct bronchial lumina and normal bacterial inhabitants multiply in accumulated secretions.
 2. Increased neuromotor irritability causes constriction of the bronchial lumen, interfering with normal drainage.
 3. Her general malnutrition is followed by impaired serum globulin formation, which lowers resistance to infection.
 4. Increased secretion of saliva predisposes to aspiration of bacteria-laden oral and nasal secretions.

8. Cystic fibrosis would also predispose Sonya to later development of which of the following lung disorders?
1. Pleural effusion.
2. Spontaneous pneumothorax.
3. Obstructive emphysema.
4. Cavitary tuberculosis.

9. Sonya's elevated temperature on admission to the hospital is probably the result of:
1. Failure of the temperature regulating mechanism because of decreased circulating blood volume.
2. Increased production of body heat due to elevated basal metabolic rate.
3. Inability to dissipate body heat by evaporation, owing to severe dehydration.
4. Resetting of the temperature-regulating center to a higher level by pyrogens.

10. Since Sonya had an acute bacterial bronchial infection on admission to the hospital, one would expect her to have which of the following blood findings?
1. Increased erythrocytes.
2. Increased neutrophils.
3. Increased lymphocytes.
4. Increased monocytes.

11. The chronic lung infections, emphysematous changes, and pulmonary fibrosis characteristic of cystic fibrosis would predispose Sonya to which of the following circulatory disorders?
1. Constrictive pericarditis.
2. Systemic hypertension.
3. Cardiac arrhythmias.
4. Cor pulmonale.

12. The foul-smelling, frothy character of Sonya's stools resulted from the presence in the stool of large amounts of:
1. Hydrochloric acid.
2. Bile salts.
3. Undigested fat.
4. Sodium and chloride.

13. Obstruction of ducts by thickened tenacious secretions might cause Sonya to develop which liver complication?
1. Infectious hepatitis.
2. Liver abscess.
3. Biliary cirrhosis.
4. Primary hepatoma.

14. The impairment of pancreatic function in cystic fibrosis can be demonstrated by:
a. Testing duodenal juice for proteo-
lytic, lipolytic, and amylolytic enzymes.
b. Determining the presence of trypsin in a stool specimen.
c. Measuring the level of insulin activity in the circulating blood.
d. Roentgenography of the pancreatic duct system using radiopaque dye.
1. a and b.
2. c and d.
3. All but d.
4. All the above.

15. For the quantitative sweat test a sample of Sonya's sweat would be obtained by iontophoresis of:
1. Atropine.
2. Pilocarpine.
3. Scopolamine.
4. Neostigmine.

16. From which of the following sites would a sample of Sonya's sweat be taken for the quantitative sweat test?
a. The forehead or brow.
b. Flexor surface of the forearm.
c. The folds of the axilla.
d. Extensor surface of the thigh.
e. The inguinal region.
1. a and c.
2. b and d.
3. All but d.
4. All the above.

17. In preparing the selected site for sweat collection the nurse should:
1. Dust the skin with a fine layer of talcum powder.
2. Cleanse the area with warm soapy water and pat dry.
3. Wash the skin with distilled water and dry thoroughly.
4. Disinfect the skin carefully with 70 per cent alcohol solution.

18. In cystic fibrosis, frequent stools and lack of lubricating mucus often produce:
1. Intussusception.
2. Volvulus.
3. Anal fissure.
4. Rectal prolapse.

19. Which finding on Sonya's sweat test would support a diagnosis of cystic fibrosis?
1. Presence of small amounts of trypsin.
2. Increased levels of sodium and chloride.
3. High concentration of uric acid crystals.
4. Failure of sweat production during hyperpyrexia.

Sonya's blood count revealed a hemoglobin level of 11 grams, and a white cell count of 12,000 with 54 per cent neutrophils. The sweat test showed chloride level of 120 mEq. and sodium level of 137 mEq. per liter. Chest x-ray showed patchy consolidation and increased bronchial markings consistent with chronic lung infection. Sputum culture revealed normal respiratory flora and the presence of *Staphylococcus aureus*. The doctor confirmed the diagnosis of cystic fibrosis and ordered Viokase, a pancreatic extract, 150 mg. three times a day and an evaporated milk and water formula with Karo and banana powder added. Parenteral gentamicin and methicillin were given to control the pulmonary infection. A mixture of propylene glycol and half-molar sodium chloride was administered in aerosol form. Supplemental vitamin therapy was ordered.

20. Gentamicin is effective against which of the following organisms?
    a. *Escherichia coli*.
    b. *Klebsiella pneumoniae*.
    c. *Aerobacter aerogenes*.
    d. *Pseudomonas aeruginosa*.
    e. *Corynebacterium diphtheriae*.
        1. a only.
        2. a, b, and c.
        3. All but e.
        4. All the above.

21. Sonya should be observed for which of the following as possible symptoms of gentamicin toxicity?
    a. Vomiting.
    b. Headache.
    c. Dizziness.
    d. Skin eruption.
    e. Proteinuria.
        1. a and b.
        2. c and d.
        3. All but e.
        4. All the above.

22. Methicillin differs from regular penicillin in that the former:
    1. Is effective against staphylococci which produce penicillinase.
    2. Is unaltered by contact with gastric or intestinal juices.
    3. Produces no pain on administration by the intramuscular route.
    4. Exerts its strongest bacteriostatic effect against streptococci.

23. The purpose for administering propylene glycol by aerosol method was to:

    1. Liquefy and loosen bronchial secretions.
    2. Inhibit the growth of pathological bacteria.
    3. Relax spasm of bronchial smooth muscles.
    4. Foster absorption of product of inflammation.

24. Which of the following vitamins would Sonya be most apt to need on a supplemental basis?
    a. Vitamin A.
    b. Vitamin B_1.
    c. Vitamin C.
    d. Vitamin D.
    e. Vitamin K.
        1. a and b.
        2. c and d.
        3. b, c, and e.
        4. a, d, and e.

25. The nurse should observe Sonya carefully for evidence of bleeding tendencies which, if present, would probably be the result of:
    1. Increased capillary permeability.
    2. Failure to absorb vitamin K.
    3. Decreased thrombocyte levels.
    4. Impaired fibrinogen production.

26. In selecting a patient unit for Sonya the nurse should consider which of the following as being *least* suitable for meeting Sonya's needs?
    1. A single room next to the nurses' station.
    2. A double room with a child who has pneumonia.
    3. A triple room with two diabetic children.
    4. A ward of children with orthopedic problems.

27. Sonya would be in need of excellent skin care during hospitalization for which of the following reasons?
    a. Malnutrition and dehydration reduce tissue resistance to injury and infection.
    b. Weight loss increases the danger of pressure injury over bony prominences.
    c. Frequent stools increase the possibility of skin excoriation on the buttocks.
    d. Elevated sweat electrolyte predispose the skin to irritation.
        1. a and b.
        2. c and d.
        3. All but d.
        4. All the above.

28. Since Sonya had no cardiac distress, in which of the following positions should the nurse place Sonya to effect postural drainage?

    1. Prone, with the foot end of the crib elevated several inches.

    2. On her left side with a large pillow behind her back.

    3. Lying across the bed with her head hanging over the side.

    4. Sitting upright tied to the head of the bed with a jacket restraint.

29. It is especially important that the nurse do which of the following when giving Sonya methicillin?

    1. Stretch the skin before injecting.

    2. Introduce the needle at a 90-degree angle.

    3. Inject the antibiotic deep I.M.

    4. Rotate the site of injection.

During one month of hospitalization Sonya's stools decreased in number to two per day and lost their foul odor. She adjusted to the high caloric, high protein, low fat diet with supplemental pancreatic extract and vitamin therapy, gaining four pounds. X-ray revealed resolution of her bronchopulmonary infection. Sonya was discharged after her parents were instructed in the treatment regimen to be followed at home and the importance of followup medical supervision.

30. In planning for Sonya's long-term care the physician would be most conscientious in ensuring that the child receives immunization against which of the following?

    a. Pertussis.

    b. Smallpox.

    c. Rubeola.

    d. Diphtheria.

    e. Influenza.

        1. a only.

        2. a and b.

        3. c and d.

        4. a, c, and e.

31. Mr. and Mrs. Schreckengost should be taught that Sonya's disease renders her particularly susceptible to which complication during midsummer weather?

    1. Severe sunburn.

    2. Infectious diarrhea.

    3. Heat prostration.

    4. Respiratory allergies.

32. The Schreckengosts should be advised to protect Sonya during hot weather by taking which of the following precautions?

    a. Preventing excessive physical activity.

    b. Replacing milk intake with fruit juice.

    c. Administering additional sodium chloride.

    d. Avoiding cream pies and raw fruit.

    e. Eliminating all outdoor activity.

        1. a and c.

        2. b and d.

        3. a, c, and e.

        4. All the above.

33. The physician will probably advise Mr. and Mrs. Schreckengost to secure which of the following pieces of equipment for Sonya's use at home following hospital discharge?

    1. Gatch bed.

    2. IPPB respirator.

    3. Rocking bed.

    4. Mist tent.

34. Which of the following procedures should Mr. and Mrs. Schreckengost be taught for removing Sonya's excessive pulmonary secretions at home?

    a. Aspiration using an aseptic syringe.

    b. Aerosol administration of a wetting agent.

    c. Intermittent positive pressure breathing.

    d. Postural drainage technique.

    e. Mouth to mouth breathing.

        1. a and c.

        2. b and d.

        3. a, c, and e.

        4. All the above.

35. Which of the following foods could safely be included in Sonya's diet following her discharge from the hospital?

    a. Bananas.

    b. Vegetables.

    c. Cottage cheese.

    d. Lean meat.

    e. Whole milk.

        1. a and b.

        2. a, b, and c.

        3. All but e.

        4. All the above.

36. While the nurse was giving the Schreckengosts home care instruction Sonya's mother said, "Sonya will be ready to walk soon. Should I discourage that in order to conserve her strength?" Which of the following responses by the nurse would be most appropriate?

    1. "Yes. You should keep her from walking as long as possible. She is

too weak and underdeveloped to undertake normal toddler activities.''

2. "You may allow her to try to walk but stay with her continuously so that if she falls you can stop the activity and put her to bed.''

3. "As a matter of fact you should encourage her in physical activity since movement is very helpful in preventing accumulation of lung secretions.''

4. "It's really too soon to worry about that now. Wait until she attempts to walk and then let the doctor decide whether she's able.''

Eczema

Although he was a full-term infant, Victor Skinner weighed only 5 pounds, 12 ounces at birth. During his first four months he was breast-fed and gained weight steadily. Victor was weaned suddenly when his mother was hospitalized for acute pyelonephritis. He was put on a Similac formula and was given cereals and fruits. Several times from his 6th to his 12th months his mother noted reddened, flaking areas on his cheeks.

When Victor was one year old the family acquired a puppy. Shortly thereafter Victor developed a severe erythematous papulovesicular rash on his face, neck, trunk, antecubital and popliteal areas, which he scratched to the point of bleeding. The family physician advised getting rid of the dog and treated the rash, which he diagnosed as eczema, with Benadryl syrup and steroid salve. The rash improved but never completely disappeared. The physician postponed Victor's routine immunizations.

(ANSWER BLANK ON PAGE A–31) (CORRECT ANSWERS ON PAGE B–40)

1. The average birth weight of a normal full-term male infant is:
1. 6 pounds to 6 pounds, 2 ounces.
2. 6 pounds, 6 ounces to 6 pounds, 8 ounces.
3. 6 pounds, 12 ounces to 6 pounds, 14 ounces.
4. 7 pounds, 2 ounces to 7 pounds, 4 ounces.

2. How does the time of Victor's weaning from the breast compare with typical practice?
1. Much earlier than usual.
2. Somewhat earlier than usual.
3. About the same as usual.
4. Somewhat later than usual.

3. Victor's weaning at the age of four months can be assumed to have been difficult primarily because he was:
1. Forced to accept unfamiliar solid foods at the same time that he was denied breast milk.
2. Deprived of his mother's presence at the same time that he was changed to bottle feeding.
3. Switched from sweet-tasting breast milk to a commercial preparation with little flavor.
4. Distracted from feeding by the discomfort of teething, which occurs at about the same time.

4. Eczema is classified as which type of disease?
1. Nutritional.
2. Metabolic.
3. Infectious.
4. Allergic.

5. Psychological studies have shown that in their relationship to their child, mothers of eczematous infants are often excessively:
1. Neglectful.
2. Permissive.
3. Punitive.
4. Controlling.

6. Which of the following have frequently been identified as offending allergens in infants with eczema?
  a. Eggs.
  b. Dust.
  c. Wool.
  d. Animal dander.
  e. Cow's milk.
    1. a and b.
    2. a, b, and c.
    3. All but e.
    4. All the above.

7. Which effect of adrenocorticosteroids explains their use in the treatment of Victor's skin rash?
  1. Elevation of blood glucose levels by glycogenolysis.
  2. Increased hydration by decreasing renal sodium excretion.
  3. Suppression of tissue changes of the inflammatory reaction.
  4. Creation of euphoria by increasing motor and mental activity.

8. Diphenhydramine (Benadryl) was used in treating Victor's skin rash for which of the following effects?
  1. Antibiotic.
  2. Demulcent.
  3. Antihistamine.
  4. Analgesic.

9. The family physician decided that Victor's prophylactic immunizations should not be given as originally scheduled because:
  1. His hyperactive immune mechanisms render him secure against common childhood infections.
  2. The protein constituents of vaccines would be apt to cause exacerbation of his skin rash.
  3. His heightened sensory perception would make the immunizations exceptionally painful.
  4. Taking him out of doors immediately following an illness would lower his resistance to infection.

10. In addition to withholding Victor's immunizations, it would be important for the doctor to tell the Skinners to keep Victor from contact with any child having had a smallpox vaccination in order to protect Victor against:
  1. Contact dermatitis.
  2. Generalized vaccinia.
  3. Anaphylactic shock.
  4. Id reaction.

When Victor was 18 months old he suffered a severe exacerbation of his skin rash, which his mother associated with his having recently eaten pancakes, and Victor was hospitalized for treatment. The rash covered large areas of his face, chest, and extremities, was primarily vesicular, and was excoriated, bleeding, and crusted. His temperature was 103° F. rectally. The physician ordered:

  1. Acetaminophen (Tylenol) 100 mg. orally q. 4 h. for temperature over 101° F. rectally.
  2. Apply Lassar paste with 1 per cent tar to the skin lesions.

11. In obtaining Victor's health history from Mr. and Mrs. Skinner, which information should the admitting nurse chart as potentially helpful in diagnosing and treating his skin problem?
  a. Types of soaps and dusting powders used in his daily care.
  b. Lotions, creams, and emollients previously used to treat his rash.
  c. Fabric content of clothing, bed linen, and furnishings in his room.
  d. The date on which all foods in his present diet were introduced.
    1. a and c.
    2. b and d.
    3. All but b.
    4. All the above.

12. For which pharmacologic effect was acetaminophen (Tylenol) given to Victor at this time?
  1. Antipyretic.
  2. Hypnotic.
  3. Antipruritic.
  4. Bacteriostatic.

13. Which of the following methods would be best suited for removing the encrustations from Victor's skin lesions?
  1. Washing with mild soapy water and a soft cloth.
  2. Rubbing with a soft brush soaked in warm water.
  3. Continuous application of gauze soaked in normal saline.
  4. Gently lifting the crust free with sterile thumb forceps.

14. Which of the following is the active ingredient in Lassar's paste?
  1. Penicillin.
  2. Glycerine.

3. Trypsin.

4. Zinc oxide.

15. The local effect of Lassar's paste on the skin is:

1. Demulcent.

2. Enzymatic.

3. Astringent.

4. Bacteriostatic.

16. In order to ensure maximum therapeutic effect from the application of Lassar's paste to Victor's facial lesions the nurse should:

1. Apply ointment to his face only after he has fallen asleep for the night.

2. Immobilize his head with halter and sandbags after application of the paste.

3. Apply a stockinette face mask to keep the paste in contact with his skin.

4. Apply paste to the facial lesions immediately before his bathing and feeding.

17. Why would it be especially important to reduce Victor's temperature to normal as soon as possible?

1. The temperature elevation will make him irritable and uncooperative with treatment.

2. The diaphoresis which accompanies temperature elevation increases itching and scratching.

3. Elevated temperature accelerates cellular metabolism and increases caloric needs.

4. Increased temperature renders body tissues and fluids more suitable for bacterial growth.

18. Which of the following are possible complications of acute eczema, against which Victor's nursing care should protect him?

a. Infection.

b. Hemorrhage.

c. Scarring.

d. Contractures.

    1. a and c.

    2. b and d.

    3. a, b, and c.

    4. All the above.

19. Victor's itching could best be relieved by bathing him in a weak solution of:

1. Sodium hypochlorite.

2. Starch and sodium bicarbonate.

3. Hydrogen peroxide.

4. Potassium permanganate.

20. In order to prevent Victor from scratching himself during his bath procedure the nurse should:

a. Bathe him in cold water containing a few drops of glycerine.

b. Place several floating toys in the bathtub to divert his attention.

c. Give him several brief partial baths rather than one full bath daily.

d. Remove only one of his extremities from restraints at a time.

e. Arrange for a second nurse to hold both his hands during the bath.

    1. a and c.

    2. b and d.

    3. All but d.

    4. All the above.

21. In making Victor's bed the nurse should:

1. Place a large piece of plastic over the bed linens or make the bed per the usual hospital procedure.

2. Secure the upper bed linen by tucking it in along the sides of the mattress rather than at the bottom.

3. Suspend the upper bed linen from the crib sides to permit the free circulation of air.

4. Place small, cotton, flannel-covered pillows between his legs and between arms and trunk.

22. If skin cultures reveal that Victor's lesions are not secondarily infected, which of the following would be best suited for use as a skin cleanser?

1. Mineral oil.

2. Ivory soap.

3. Aqueous Zephiran chloride solution.

4. Hydrogen peroxide.

23. If, however, Victor's skin lesions should become infected, which of the following would be best suited for use as a skin cleanser?

1. Normal saline.

2. Hexachlorophene.

3. Sodium bicarbonate.

4. Milled oatmeal soap.

24. Which organism is most apt to be responsible for secondary infection of eczematous lesions?

1. *Staphylococcus aureus.*

2. *Diplococcus pneumoniae.*

3. *Candida albicans.*

4. *Escherichia coli.*

25. Which types of restraint should be used to prevent Victor from scratching his rash?

    a. Place gauze or stocking mittens over both hands and secure with wrist ties.

    b. Splint elbows with tongue blades inserted into a pocketed muslin band.

    c. Apply a Posey belt to his waist and tie it to the frame at the bed sides.

    d. Secure his wrists with a clove hitch and tie the attached gauze to the bed frame.

        1. a and b.

        2. b and c.

        3. b and d.

        4. c and d.

26. The nurse should not rely on Victor's crying as a signal to restrain him from scratching because:

    1. He would come to interpret the application of restraints as a punishment for crying.

    2. Eczematous babies tend to scratch rather than to cry in response to frustration.

    3. It would be difficult for her to be within earshot of his voice at all times.

    4. The procedure would spoil him by demonstrating that his cry would always be responded to.

27. It would be advisable for the nurse to plan Victor's care so that she can take him from the crib and hold him at frequent intervals throughout the day in order to:

    a. Offset the danger of hypostatic pneumonia.

    b. Reduce the frustration of physical restraint.

    c. Demonstrate acceptance through physical contact.

    d. Hasten linen changing and bed making.

        1. a and b.

        2. c and d.

        3. All but d.

        4. All the above.

Because Victor's skin lesions improved greatly during two weeks of hospitalization, he was discharged. The physician decided to wait until some time in the future to do sensitivity skin testing and ordered that, for the present, the following foods be eliminated from Victor's diet: cow's milk, eggs, citrus fruits, tomatoes, wheat breads, and cereals.

28. Why was Victor not skin tested at this time to identify the allergens responsible for his eczema?

    1. A child's immune mechanisms are not mature enough to yield reliable skin hypersensitivity reactions until his third year.

    2. Application of even minute quantities of allergens in skin testing could seriously aggravate his present skin lesions.

    3. A small child could not sit still for long enough periods of time to permit satisfactory application of test doses.

    4. The cost of skin testing is so great that Victor's family could not undertake it together with payment of hospital fees.

29. Which therapeutic adjustment would the physician probably advise as a consequence of Victor's dietary restrictions?

    1. Administration of synthetic vitamins.

    2. Addition of chocolate-flavored goat's milk.

    3. Serving all food in plastic containers.

    4. Pushing quantities of water after feedings.

30. In teaching Mr. and Mrs. Skinner about the care Victor will need at home the nurse should strive to convey which of the following concepts?

    a. There is no way of achieving a complete and permanent cure for eczema.

    b. An eczematous infant is more than usually susceptible to skin and respiratory infections.

    c. With time, Victor's skin problems will disappear and be replaced with respiratory problems.

    d. Victor needs evidence of warm affection freely given but without overprotection.

        1. a and c.

        2. b and d.

        3. a, b, and d.

        4. All the above.

31. Before Victor's discharge from the hospital, Mrs. Skinner should be given an opportunity to:

1. Compute the caloric and nutritive values of the foods permitted in Victor's restricted diet.
2. Observe the nurse preparing and applying restraints to prevent Victor from scratching his lesions.
3. Bathe Victor and apply skin cream to the lesions with help and supervision by the nurse.
4. Talk with parents of eczematous infants who are being successfully managed in the outpatient clinic.

32. In instructing Mrs. Skinner regarding the best way to dress Victor following hospital discharge, the nurse should advise her to:
   a. Change his diapers as soon as they become wet or soiled.
   b. Wash his clothing in a bland soap and rinse it thoroughly.
   c. Dress him in garments made only of undyed cotton.
   d. Dress him in as little clothing as possible to avoid overheating.
   e. Dress him in paper gowns which can be sterilized before use.
      1. a and b.
      2. a, b, and c.
      3. All but e.
      4. All the above.

33. In the long-term supervision of Victor's health, the family physician will be especially alert for the possible development of:
   1. Duodenal ulcer.
   2. Bronchial asthma.
   3. Ulcerative colitis.
   4. Cardiac arrhythmia.

Laryngotracheo-bronchitis

When two-year-old Lena Barcus was admitted to the pediatric hospital at 6:00 p.m. on New Year's Day, she had been ill for two days with an upper respiratory infection that had progressed rapidly from rhinorrhea to dyspnea, cough, and noisy respirations.

The examining physician noted that Lena's temperature was 103.4° F. rectally, pulse 140 per minute, respirations 36 per minute with inspiratory stridor. Her lungs were clear to auscultation and chest x-ray showed no pulmonary consolidation. During physical examination Lena was restless and experienced frequent spasms of brassy, unproductive coughing.

Bronchoscopic examination was negative. Blood tests indicated normal hemoglobin concentration and red cell count, a white cell count of 15,000 per cu. mm. with a normal differential. The physician diagnosed Lena's illness as laryngotracheobronchitis and wrote the following orders:

1. Throat smear and culture. Antibiotic sensitivity tests of isolated organisms.
2. Blood culture.
3. Place in ultrasonic mist tent.
4. Encourage oral fluid intake.
5. Tetracycline 100 mg. I.M. q. 6 h.
6. Ampicillin 250 mg. I.M. q. 6 h.

(ANSWER BLANK ON PAGE A–33) (CORRECT ANSWERS ON PAGE B–41)

1. A bronchoscopic examination was performed as part of Lena's diagnostic workup in order to rule out the possibility of:

    1. Aspiration of a foreign body.
    2. Perforation of the trachea.
    3. Tumor of the bronchus.
    4. Tracheo-esophageal fistula.

2. Diagnostic tests included direct smear and culture of Lena's pharyngeal secretions in order to rule out a diagnosis of:

    1. Parotitis.
    2. Allergy.
    3. Tuberculosis.
    4. Diphtheria.

3. The primary objective in Lena's care should be to:

    1. Prevent secondary infection.
    2. Conserve her physical strength.
    3. Maintain a patent airway.
    4. Ensure adequate nutrition.

4. Which of the following organisms have frequently been implicated in the cause of laryngotracheobronchitis?

    a. *Streptococcus viridans.*
    b. *Staphylococcus albus.*
    c. *Diplococcus pneumoniae.*
    d. *Hemophilus influenzae.*
    e. *Influenza virus.*
        1. a and c.
        2. b and d.
        3. All but e.
        4. All the above.

5. The pathophysiologic change underlying Lena's respiratory difficulty on hospital admission was:

    1. Obliteration of pulmonary alveoli by coagulated inflammatory exudate.
    2. Obstruction of respiratory passages by mucosal edema and tenacious exudate.
    3. Narrowing of bronchial lumen by prolonged smooth muscle contraction.
    4. Desquamation of respiratory epithelium due to an allergic hypersensitivity.

6. Stridor is best defined as a:

    1. Harsh, high-pitched sound during respiration due to obstruction of air passages.
    2. Soft tissue depression of the supraclavicular and intercostal areas during inspiration.
    3. Series of explosive coughs occurring in rapid succession during a single respiration.
    4. Combination of mouth breathing, nasal flaring, and grunting respirations.

7. Lena's respiratory difficulty on hospital admission was probably due to obstruction of her:

    1. Pharynx.
    2. Larynx.
    3. Trachea.
    4. Bronchi.

8. Probably Lena's cough was unproductive on her admission to the hospital because:

    1. It was due simply to drying of the lower respiratory mucosa.
    2. The alveolar inflammatory material was in the form of a coagulum.
    3. Extreme smooth muscle spasm had completely constricted the bronchi.
    4. Tracheobronchial secretions were too thick and tenacious to be lifted.

9. The nurse should do which of the following to decrease Lena's apprehension concerning hospitalization?

    a. Have the parents accompany Lena to her room before leaving to give admission data to the clerk.
    b. Introduce Lena to the nurses and aides who will be responsible for providing her care.
    c. Reassure Lena's parents that she will be given close supervision and care suited to her needs.
    d. Obtain information from Lena's parents concerning her eating, sleeping, and toilet habits.
        1. a and b.
        2. a, c, and d.
        3. b, c, and d.
        4. All the above.

10. Which of the following are apt to be among Lena's reactions to hospitalization?

    a. Crying each time her mother leaves the ward.
    b. Throwing her toys from the bed to the floor.
    c. Responding to her mother's fear with increased anxiety.
    d. Demonstrating fear of being separated or abandoned.
    e. Wetting her bed, especially at night.
        1. a only.

2. a and b.
3. a, b, and d.
4. All the above.

11. For which of the following reasons is it imperative that Lena be constantly attended during the initial period of hospitalization?
   a. To provide reassurance and a feeling of security.
   b. To observe signs of impending laryngeal obstruction.
   c. To force small amounts of liquids every few minutes.
   d. To maintain the temperature of the croupette at 98° F.
      1. a and b.
      2. c and d.
      3. All but d.
      4. All the above.

12. What adjustment should the nurse make to facilitate observation of Lena's symptom progression?
   1. Leave Lena's gown open in front to expose her chest.
   2. Position a bright floor lamp directly over the croupette.
   3. Place the croupette by the desk in the nurses' station.
   4. Examine her glottis frequently, using a flashlight and mirror.

13. Continuing and progressive inflammation of Lena's laryngeal mucosa is apt to produce:
   1. Yawning and hiccoughs.
   2. Nausea and vomiting.
   3. Hoarseness and aphonia.
   4. Ulceration and hemorrhage.

14. In which position will Lena probably be most comfortable?
   1. Prone.
   2. Supine.
   3. Side-lying.
   4. Sitting.

15. If Lena's temperature continues to rise, the nurse should be alert to the development of:
   1. Hemorrhage.
   2. Pneumothorax.
   3. Convulsions.
   4. Projectile vomiting.

16. The nurse should encourage Lena to drink copious amounts of liquids in order to assist in:
   a. Lowering her temperature.
   b. Liquefying bronchial secretions.
   c. Preventing generalized dehydration.
   d. Diluting bacterial toxins.
      1. a only.
      2. a and b.
      3. All but d.
      4. All the above.

17. Ampicillin differs from penicillin in that the former:
   1. Is more rapidly absorbed from muscle tissue.
   2. Suppresses growth of gram-negative bacteria.
   3. Is not inactivated by the enzyme penicillinase.
   4. Never provokes allergic tissue reactions.

18. Cold humidification rather than steam is preferred for Lena's treatment because:
   1. A steam humidifier is a potential safety hazard.
   2. Cold humidity loosens secretions to a greater degree.
   3. Cold humidity would tend to reduce mucosal edema.
   4. Cool water vapor is more readily absorbed by the mucosa.

19. Lena's restlessness was probably the result of:
   1. Anoxia.
   2. Acidosis.
   3. Dehydration.
   4. Toxemia.

20. To which of the following complications would Lena's illness predispose her?
   a. Atelectasis.
   b. Pneumonia.
   c. Otitis media.
   d. Convulsions.
   e. Cardiac failure.
      1. a and c.
      2. b and d.
      3. All but e.
      4. All the above.

21. If while caring for Lena the nurse should detect unequal chest expansion, she should report her observation, since it would suggest:
   1. Restriction of the inflammatory process to only one lung.
   2. Atelectasis following complete occlusion of a large bronchus.
   3. Cardiac enlargement due to congestive heart failure.
   4. Phrenic nerve paralysis by bacterial exotoxins.

22. In order to correctly assess Lena's condition the nurse should be aware that a period of quiet following a period of extreme restlessness would probably signify:
1. Resolution of the inflammatory coagulum.
2. Decreased production of bronchial exudate.
3. Approach of physical exhaustion or asphyxia.
4. Relaxation of spasm of bronchial muscles.

23. Appearance of which of the following symptoms should alert the nurse to possible development of laryngeal obstruction?
  a. Restlessness and apprehension.
  b. Pallid or gray skin color.
  c. Suprasternal and infrasternal retractions.
  d. Visible inspiratory effort.
1. a only.
2. a and b.
3. All but c.
4. All the above.

Throat culture revealed beta-hemolytic streptococci and pneumococci. Pneumococci were isolated from the blood culture. On the basis of sensitivity tests, ampicillin 500 mg. orally was ordered to be given q. 6 h.

During the next few hours Lena's respirations became more labored and noisy and her cough increased in frequency and severity. Her skin was ashen and she developed suprasternal and intercostal retractions. The nurse notified the physician, who performed a tracheostomy and ordered that Lena be placed in an oxygen tent with high humidity. Lena's color improved and her respirations became less labored.

24. Ampicillin is effective against which of the following organisms?
  a. *Streptococcus pyogenes.*
  b. *Diplococcus pneumoniae.*
  c. *Staphylococcus aureus.*
  d. *Escherichia coli.*
1. a and c.
2. b and d.
3. All but d.
4. All the above.

25. High humidification was ordered as part of Lena's care in order to prevent:
1. Bacterial growth in her respiratory passages.

2. Further rise in her temperature and pulse rate.
3. Drying and crusting of her laryngeal exudate.
4. Loss of body fluid by rapid evaporation.

26. Following the tracheostomy, it would be even more important that Lena be constantly attended by a nurse because:
  a. Continuous reassurance is needed to counteract anxiety evoked by the tracheostomy tube.
  b. Lena would no longer cry to summon help when she experienced respiratory distress.
  c. The tracheostomy tube would have to be suctioned frequently to remain unobstructed.
  d. Lena might need to be discouraged from dislodging the tracheostomy tube.
1. a only.
2. a and b.
3. All but d.
4. All the above.

27. Which of the following pieces of equipment should be kept in Lena's room following tracheostomy?
  a. Sterile obturator.
  b. Sterile duplicate tracheostomy tube.
  c. Suction machine.
  d. Cool vapor humidifier.
1. a and c.
2. b and d.
3. All but d.
4. All the above.

28. Immediately following the tracheostomy procedure, Lena's tracheostomy should be aspirated every:
1. 15 minutes.
2. 30 minutes.
3. Hour.
4. 2 hours.

29. In order to prevent secondary infection of Lena's tracheal secretions, the nurse should take which of the following precautions in giving her tracheostomy care?
1. Cleanse the skin surrounding the tracheostomy with antiseptic solution.
2. Use a fresh sterile, disposable catheter for each tracheal aspiration.
3. Soak the inner cannula in a hydrogen peroxide solution every four hours.

4. Place a sterile gauze dressing around the edge of the tracheostomy.

30. In aspirating Lena's tracheostomy the nurse should:

1. Apply suction to the catheter only while withdrawing it.
2. Remove both inner and outer cannula before inserting the catheter.
3. Untie the twill neck tapes while cleansing the skin edges of the wound.
4. Twirl the catheter rapidly while withdrawing it slowly during removal.

31. By which of the following means should the nurse loosen Lena's tracheal secretions before aspirating her tracheostomy?

1. Give her three or four forceful slaps on the back.
2. Place a few drops of sterile saline into the inner cannula.
3. Spray her posterior pharynx with sterile distilled water.
4. Encourage her to rapidly drink a full glass of water.

32. The inner cannula of the tracheostomy tube should be removed and cleansed at least every:

1. 4 hours.
2. 8 hours.
3. 12 hours.
4. 24 hours.

33. Which of the following would be best suited for use in cleansing the inner cannula of the tracheostomy tube?

1. Narrow roller gauze and normal saline.
2. Toothbrush and warm soapy water.
3. Pipe cleaners and hydrogen peroxide.
4. 2-cc. syringe and sterile distilled water.

34. If the outer cannula of the tracheostomy tube should accidentally be dislodged from the trachea during care, the nurse should:

1. Reinsert the tracheostomy tube with the aid of the sterile obturator.
2. Cover the wound with a sterile gauze square and secure with adhesive tape strips.
3. Insert the inner cannula and hold it in place until help is available.
4. Apply manual traction to skin areas surrounding the tracheostomy to hold it open.

Five days after the tracheostomy was performed Lena's respirations had decreased to 26 per minute and cough and stridor were absent. Her temperature was 100° F. rectally and she was taking a soft diet and drinking liquids freely. When the lumen of the tracheostomy tube was plugged with a cork, Lena was able to breathe through her nose and mouth, so on the following day the tube was removed and a sterile dressing was applied to the incision.

On the day after the tube was removed Lena was allowed to spend time in the playroom with other children. She continued to improve, gaining appetite and strength, and she was discharged two weeks after her admission.

35. At the time of her hospitalization Lena would be expected to have acquired the ability to:

a. Walk up and down stairs alone.
b. Drink out of a cup without spilling.
c. Jump from a low object to the floor.
d. Build a tower of six blocks.
e. Ride a tricycle with ease.
    1. a and b.
    2. a, b, and c.
    3. a, b, c, and d.
    4. All the above.

36. Which of the following best describes Lena's probable behavior in her play activities?

1. Playing alongside but not with her peers.
2. Preferring group play activities with other toddlers.
3. Enjoying a game of hop-scotch with an older child.
4. Selecting only girls of the same age for playmates.

37. In disciplining Lena during hospitalization the nurse should be aware that the chief psychological task of the two year old is to:

1. Distinguish herself as a being separate from her mother.
2. Identify and assume traits of the parent of the opposite sex.
3. Develop an awareness that she controls her own life situation.
4. Gain control of instinctual drives without losing self-esteem.

38. Which of the following might be residual effects following an episode of laryngotracheobronchitis?

   a. Chronic bronchitis.
   b. Bronchiectasis.
   c. Emphysema.
   d. Lung abscess.
   e. Pleural adhesions.
   1. a and c.
   2. b and d.
   3. All but e.
   4. All the above.

39. Mrs. Barcus should be advised that humidification can be provided at home, if it should be needed, by which of the following means?

   a. Placing wide, flat pans of water on the radiators.
   b. Keeping the windows of Lena's room wide open.
   c. Allowing the hot water to run in the shower.
   d. Placing a pan of water on a hot plate.
   1. a only.
   2. a and c.
   3. a, c, and d.
   4. All the above.

Bronchial Asthma

Maria Sanchez was four and her mother had been dead for two months when she suffered her first asthmatic attack. Her aunt, with whom she lived, brought her to the hospital examining room in acute respiratory distress. She indicated that Maria had had a bad cold for three days, during which period she had frequently awakened during the night with paroxysms of coughing and wheezing.

On admission Maria was coughing, anxious, and perspiring freely. Her temperature was 100.8° F. rectally, her pulse was 112 per minute, and her respirations were 40 per minute. Chest auscultation revealed hyperresonance, expiratory wheezing, and rhonchi. Her neck veins were distended and there was flaring of her alae nasi.

The physician diagnosed Maria's illness as an acute attack of asthma and administered 0.2 ml. of a 1:1000 solution of epinephrine subcutaneously. Because epinephrine did not relieve Maria's dyspnea, the physician admitted her to the pediatric ward and ordered the following:

1. Oxygen tent with high humidity.
2. Aminophylline 50 mg. rectally q. 6 h.
3. Ephedrine sulfate 8 mg. orally t.i.d.
4. Phenobarbital 25 mg. orally t.i.d.
5. Potassium iodide 2 gr. orally t.i.d.

Under this treatment Maria's dyspnea subsided within two days, at which time the physician discontinued the aminophylline and potassium iodide. Because her condition continued to improve, Maria was discharged on her fifth day of hospitalization to the Pediatric Allergy Clinic for sensitivity testing and follow-up. Her aunt was taught to control Maria's asthmatic attacks with aminophylline rectal suppositories.

(ANSWER BLANK ON PAGE A–35)   (CORRECT ANSWERS ON PAGE B–43)

1. The pathophysiology of bronchial asthma includes:
   a. Spasm of bronchial muscles.
   b. Edema of bronchial mucosa.
   c. Production of abnormal respiratory secretions.
   d. Dilation of terminal bronchioles.
   e. Filling of alveoli with exudate.
       1. a only.
       2. a, b, and c.
       3. All but d.
       4. All the above.

2. It has been observed that the onset of asthma is often triggered by:
   1. Sudden change in climate.
   2. Alteration in dietary regimen.
   3. Exposure to new surroundings.
   4. Separation from a loved person.

3. Which of the following allergens may provoke an asthmatic attack?
   a. Eggs.
   b. Milk.
   c. House dust.
   d. Pollens.
   e. Molds.
       1. a only.
       2. a and b.
       3. a, b, and c.
       4. All the above.

4. During an asthmatic attack Maria's bronchial secretions would differ from those of a well person in that they would be:
   1. Thinner and more copious.
   2. Thicker and more tenacious.
   3. Frothy and blood streaked.
   4. Purulent and foul-smelling.

5. The hyperresonance of Maria's chest detected on her admission to the hospital was a manifestation of:
   1. Constriction of bronchi.
   2. Consolidation of air sacs.
   3. Overdistention of alveoli.
   4. Distention of the pleural sac.

6. At the time of her admission to the hospital Maria's respirations would probably be characterized by:
   1. Absence of breath sounds in one lung.
   2. Paradoxic movements of the chest wall.
   3. Prolongation of the expiratory phase of breathing.
   4. Continuous changes in respiratory rate and depth.

7. The flaring of Maria's alae nasi was probably a manifestation of:
   1. Acute anxiety.
   2. Inspiratory difficulty.
   3. Physical exhaustion.
   4. Respiratory acidosis.

8. Maria would probably not be given oxygen unless she were to develop:
   1. Dyspnea.
   2. Cyanosis.
   3. Acidosis.
   4. Hemoptysis.

9. In planning care for Maria the nurse should assume that, during the three days preceding hospital admission, Maria had probably received inadequate:
   a. Sleep.
   b. Hydration.
   c. Nutrition.
   d. Attention.
   e. Stimulation.
       1. a and b.
       2. a and c.
       3. b and d.
       4. b and e.

10. Immediately following her admission to the hospital Maria would probably be most comfortable in which position?
   1. Lying flat on her back.
   2. Sitting upright in bed.
   3. Lying on her abdomen.
   4. Reclining on her left side.

11. The emergency room nurse should make which of the following available for possible use in caring for Maria on admission?
   1. Emesis basin.
   2. Nasogastric tube.
   3. Endotracheal tube.
   4. Tracheostomy set.

12. On her admission to the hospital Maria would be apt to demonstrate which of the following unusual blood findings?
   1. Thrombocytopenia.
   2. Hypochromia.
   3. Lymphocytosis.
   4. Eosinophilia.

13. Which of the following laboratory values would indicate that Maria had developed respiratory failure?
   a. Arterial $_pCO_2$ above 55 mm. Hg.
   b. Blood pH below 7.32.
   c. Hematocrit below 30 per cent.
   d. Serum K below 4 mEq./liter.
   e. Arterial $_pO_2$ above 100 mm. Hg.
       1. a and b.
       2. a, b, and c.
       3. All but d.
       4. All the above.

14. If Maria's asthmatic attacks are somehow related to interpersonal tensions, it would be her relationship with which of the following persons which should be most carefully investigated?

    1. Her aunt.
    2. Her uncle.
    3. Her female cousin.
    4. Her male cousin.

15. In the human, epinephrine is produced by the:

    1. Anterior pituitary.
    2. Posterior pituitary.
    3. Adrenal cortex.
    4. Adrenal medulla.

16. Epinephrine was given to Maria in order to produce which of the following effects?

    1. Relaxation of bronchial spasm.
    2. Acceleration of pulmonary circulation.
    3. Liquefaction of respiratory secretions.
    4. Increased formation of antibodies.

17. If Maria should become "epinephrine-fast" as a result of prolonged use of the drug, the physician might treat her acute asthmatic attacks with:

    1. Aminophylline.
    2. Atropine.
    3. Papaverine.
    4. Physostigmine.

18. Ephedrine is a member of which drug group?

    1. Sympathomimetic.
    2. Adrenergic blocker.
    3. Parasympathomimetic.
    4. Parasympathetic blocker.

19. Ephedrine was ordered for Maria in order to:

    1. Decrease respiratory secretions.
    2. Relax bronchial muscles.
    3. Constrict alveolar capillaries.
    4. Increase serum glucose level.

20. Maria should be observed for development of which of the following as a possible toxic effect of ephedrine?

    1. Tinnitus.
    2. Diarrhea.
    3. Nervousness.
    4. Purpura.

21. Phenobarbital exerts which of the following types of action?

    1. Depression of the central nervous system.
    2. Stimulation of the sympathetic nervous system.
    3. Depression of the parasympathetic nervous system.
    4. Blockade of transmission at the myoneural junction.

22. Potassium iodide was ordered for Maria in order to:

    1. Improve tone of respiratory muscles.
    2. Prevent development of respiratory acidosis.
    3. Inhibit growth of pathogenic organisms.
    4. Liquefy tracheobronchial secretions.

23. Which of the following is a possible toxic effect of prolonged administration of potassium iodide?

    1. Coryza.
    2. Gastritis.
    3. Dizziness.
    4. Singultus.

24. In addition to rest and drug therapy, which of the following treatments would be apt to alleviate Maria's respiratory discomfort?

    a. Postural drainage.
    b. Mist tent.
    c. Oxygen administration.
    d. Intermittent positive pressure breathing.
    e. Tracheostomy tube.
        1. a and b.
        2. a, b, and c.
        3. All but e.
        4. All the above.

25. In caring for Maria during her first day in the hospital the nurse should take particular pains to provide Maria with:

    1. Additional warm bedcovers.
    2. Generous fluid intake.
    3. Frequent linen changes.
    4. Darkened, quiet environment.

26. In her interactions with Maria the nurse should be especially careful to avoid displaying which of the following feelings toward the child?

    1. Affection.
    2. Protectiveness.
    3. Concern.
    4. Irritation.

27. Maria's aunt should be advised to protect the child from which of the following, as possible precipitants of an asthmatic attack?

    a. Exposure to extreme cold.
    b. Strenuous physical exercise.

c. Sudden intense emotion.

d. Ingestion of gas-forming foods.

e. Change in sleep schedule.

    1. a and b.

    2. a, b, and c.

    3. All but d.

    4. All the above.

28. Maria's aunt should be advised to protect Maria from contact with which of the following on her return to her home?

a. Dogs and cats.

b. Stuffed toys.

c. Feather pillows.

d. Cigarette smoke.

e. Paint fumes.

    1. a and c.

    2. b and d.

    3. All but d.

    4. All the above.

29. Aminophylline is a member of which of the following drug groups?

    1. Central nervous system stimulants.

    2. Cardiac glycosides.

    3. Xanthine diuretics.

    4. Sympathetic stimulants.

30. Aminophylline was ordered for Maria for which of the following effects?

    1. Vasopressor.

    2. Bronchodilator.

    3. Anti-inflammatory.

    4. Myocardiotonic.

31. Maria's aunt should be instructed to observe the child for which of the following as toxic effects from overuse of aminophylline suppositories?

a. Flushing.

b. Headache.

c. Nervousness.

d. Vomiting.

e. Pruritus.

    1. a, b, and c.

    2. a, b, c, and d.

    3. c, d, and e.

    4. All the above.

32. Isoproterenol is a member of which of the following drug groups?

    1. Alpha adrenergic.

    2. Beta adrenergic.

    3. Cholinergic.

    4. Anticholinergic.

33. Isoproterenol was given to Maria for which of the following effects?

    1. Vasoconstrictor.

    2. Vasodilator.

    3. Bronchodilator.

    4. Myocardial stimulant.

34. The nurse who cares for Maria in the Allergy Clinic should take a careful medical history in an attempt to relate Maria's incidence of asthmatic attacks to:

a. Food or liquids ingested.

b. Time of the day, week, or year.

c. Places inside or outside the home.

d. Presence of concomitant infections.

e. Interaction with significant persons.

    1. a and b.

    2. a, b, and c.

    3. All but d.

    4. All the above.

35. In seeking to identify possible inhalant allergens responsible for Maria's attacks, consideration should first be given to which of the following aspects of Maria's home environment?

    1. Maria's bedroom.

    2. The kitchen.

    3. The living room.

    4. The bathroom.

36. In testing Maria for sensitivity to possible allergens, the suspected irritant will probably be administered:

a. Over a skin scratch.

b. Intracutaneously.

c. By patch test.

d. By application to mucosa.

e. By inhalation.

    1. a or b only.

    2. a or c only.

    3. Any but e.

    4. Any of the above.

37. In giving Maria skin scratch sensitivity tests it would be desirable to take into account the overall reactivity of her skin on the day of the test by:

    1. Observing the degree of skin discoloration by pinching the skin.

    2. Checking the speed of capillary filling in the nail following a blanch test.

    3. Measuring the skin temperature of the test area before and after the test.

    4. Making a control scratch to which no allergen is applied, in the test area.

38. Which of the following drugs should be kept at hand when intracutaneous skin tests are being performed?

    1. Epinephrine.

    2. Aminophylline.

    3. Diphenhydramine.

    4. Isoproterenol.

39. In the event that Maria is found to be sensitive to house dust, her aunt should be advised to render the child's room as dust free as possible by:

a. Stripping the room of all furniture but a bed, table, wooden chair, and dresser.
b. Covering box springs, mattress, and foam pillow with heavy plastic covers.
c. Eliminating all rugs, curtains, drap-eries, Venetian blinds, bookcases, and stuffed toys.
d. Utilizing only cotton bedclothes and sleeping garments and washing them frequently.
e. Keeping windows and doors closed and damp dusting the room every day.
  1. a and b.
  2. c and d.
  3. All but d.
  4. All the above.

Cerebral Palsy

Buddy English was born following 36 weeks of gestation and suffered mild jaundice during his first few days of life due to Rh incompatibility. His jaundice was never extreme and he was not given an exchange transfusion. When Buddy was two years old his mother was concerned because he was not able to stand or walk, so she took him to the family physician. Finding Buddy to be a frail child, with poor balance when sitting and marked spasticity of muscles of the lower extremities, the doctor made a diagnosis of cerebral palsy with spastic diplegia and referred Buddy to the pediatric neurology clinic at the local university medical center.

The clinic team found that Buddy demonstrated some mental retardation, hearing loss in both ears, marked adduction of the thighs with spasticity of the gracilis, rectus femoris, hamstrings, soleus, and gastrocnemius, a 20-degree flexion contracture of the hip, and ankle clonus. Medical history revealed no family member with a similar disorder.

(ANSWER BLANK ON PAGE A–37)   **(CORRECT ANSWERS ON PAGE B–44)**

1. Cerebral palsy can best be defined as a:
  1. Congenital paralysis of voluntary muscles due to hereditary factors.
  2. Permanent loss of sensation resulting from a birth injury.
  3. Muscle weakness and incoordination caused by severe emotional stress.
  4. Difficulty in controlling voluntary muscles due to brain damage.

2. Diplegia is best defined as a condition in which:
  1. Only two of the four extremities evidence symptoms of dysfunction.
  2. Both legs are paralyzed to an equal degree and the arms to a lesser extent.
  3. Similar parts on both sides of the body evidence motor paralysis.
  4. There is paralysis of both the upper and lower extremities on one side.

3. Which of the following are thought to be possible causes of cerebral palsies?
a. Premature birth.
b. Intracranial hemorrhage.
c. Asphyxia neonatorum.
d. Measles encephalitis.
  1. a and b.
  2. c and d.
  3. All but d.
  4. All the above.

4. In addition to the above, erythroblastosis fetalis is thought to contribute to development of cerebral palsy by:

1. Causing damage to nerve cells especially sensitive to oxygen lack.
2. Inactivating a chemical mediator liberated at interneuronal synapses.
3. Interfering with production of an enzyme needed in protein metabolism.
4. Producing cerebral edema and consequent pressure atrophy of the cerebral cortex.

5. Generally, cerebral palsies are characterized by pathologic changes in the:
1. Arterial circle at the base of the brain.
2. Third, fourth, and lateral ventricles.
3. Pyramidal tracts of the central nervous system.
4. Dura mater or arachnoid layer of the meninges.

6. The nurse who admits Buddy to the hospital should spend a prolonged period of time with Mrs. and Mrs. English for the primary purpose of:
1. Outlining in detail the various types of therapy which may be employed in treating a spastic child.
2. Finding out as many details as possible about Buddy's abilities, habits, interests, and responses to people.
3. Reassuring them that the hospital team can and will provide Buddy with the care that he needs.
4. Encouraging them to express fully their thoughts and feelings about Buddy's illness and hospitalization.

7. Intelligence testing of children with cerebral palsy is apt to be invalid because they:
a. May have some degree of visual or hearing defects.
b. Tend to have difficulty in speech, gesture, and manipulation.
c. Are apt to lack the social skills required to cooperate with the examiner.
d. Become anxious under pressure and perform less well than they are capable of doing.
e. Lack attention span of sufficient length to complete the examination.
1. a only.
2. b and c.
3. All but e.
4. All the above.

8. The increased tension of Buddy's hip adductors, hip internal rotators and calf muscles will tend to produce:
1. Scissoring and toe pointing.
2. Marked bowing of the legs.
3. Knock-knee deformity.
4. Dislocation of the hip.

9. A contracture can best be defined as:
1. A temporary decrease in the muscle contractile force due to ischemia.
2. A permanent contraction of a muscle due to spasm or paralysis.
3. A decrease in muscle mass due to atrophy from disuse.
4. An increase in muscle size due to hyperplasia of muscle fibers.

10. Clonus can best be defined as:
1. Spasmodic alteration of contraction and relaxation.
2. Slow, irregular writhing movement of an extremity.
3. Sustained contraction of major skeletal muscles.
4. Twitching of the fibers in a single muscle unit.

11. The basis of Buddy's treatment should be:
1. Continuous sedation.
2. Muscle training.
3. Tremor prevention.
4. Social seclusion.

12. It is especially important for the nurse to obtain detailed information about the pattern of Buddy's life at home and the nature of his interactions with others because:
1. His slow speech and the pressure of time in the hospital situation will make it impossible to obtain such information from him.
2. It is desirable that the nurse reverse at once any bad habits or unhealthy influences engendered by his guilt-ridden parents.
3. It is imperative that the hospital routines and relationships exactly parallel those of his home in order for him to be comfortable.
4. Subjecting him to expectations beyond his abilities would make him apprehensive, decrease his motivation and courage, and hinder his achievement.

13. The success of Buddy's treatment program will depend upon whether:
  a. He has sufficient capacity to make rehabilitation of permanent value.
  b. His parents understand and are committed to the goals of the program.
  c. Family and community resources exist to make continuing care possible.
  d. Effective communication occurs among all persons and agencies involved in his care.
  e. The work of each therapist is so oriented as to permit positive gain from contributions of other team members.
    1. a and b.
    2. c and d.
    3. All but e.
    4. All the above.

14. The nurse may expect Buddy to demonstrate which of the following manifestations of his organic brain damage?
  a. Irritability.
  b. Overactivity.
  c. Impulsiveness.
  d. Short attention span.
  e. Mood swings.
    1. a and b.
    2. c and d.
    3. All but e.
    4. All the above.

15. Buddy is apt to have which of the following perceptual difficulties?
  a. Poor eye-hand coordination.
  b. Distorted spatial sense.
  c. Impaired ability to differentiate textures.
  d. Impairment of body-image.
    1. a and b.
    2. c and d.
    3. All but d.
    4. All the above.

A complete muscle evaluation was made by a physiotherapist. Buddy was found to have almost complete range of motion of the lower extremities with gravity eliminated. The doctor ordered:

  1. Physiotherapy for stretching of hamstrings, knees, and foot joints. Practice walking with parallel bars.
  2. Occupational therapy for practice in self-help skills regarding feeding, toilet, and dressing.

16. The nurse can maximize the effectiveness of Buddy's physiotherapy sessions by:
  1. Providing a period of quiet relaxation before his physiotherapy session.
  2. Repeating his prescribed exercises before putting him to bed.
  3. Praising him unqualifiedly for every new motor activity attempted.
  4. Urging him to higher levels of performance in each exercise period.

17. The nurse should arrange for Buddy's afternoon rest periods to be longer than those for other patients his age because:
  1. His home pattern has accustomed him to long periods of withdrawal from others.
  2. He will require additional time to relax before he will be able to fall asleep.
  3. He will need more time to ruminate over his experiences and feelings than other children.
  4. He should spend considerable time away from the nurse to counteract his tendency toward dependence.

18. The nurse can best assist Buddy to sleep during afternoon rest periods by:
  1. Holding his hand throughout the nap period.
  2. Keeping his environment calm and pleasant.
  3. Encouraging him in strenuous activity beforehand.
  4. Giving him a cookie before putting him to bed.

19. The nurse may find that Buddy is poorly motivated to learn new motor skills because of:
  1. Lack of desire to acquire the abilities of other children of his acquaintance.
  2. Failure of the treatment team to determine his interest in the new skills offered.
  3. A series of past failures to master muscular activities despite strong effort.
  4. His parents' having neglected to provide tangible rewards for previous achievements.

20. Which of the following adjustments should be made by the nurse in helping Buddy to feed himself?
  a. Build up utensil handles to make them easier to grasp.

b. Use a U-shaped table to provide him elbow support.

c. Create table depressions to stabilize his bowl, cup, and glass.

d. Provide additional time and a relaxed environment for his meals.

e. Provide training in eating skills apart from mealtimes.
   1. a only.
   2. a and b.
   3. a, b, and c.
   4. All the above.

21. Buddy's feeding problems are apt to be complicated by:
   1. Secretion of saliva inadequate in quantity as well as mucin and enzyme content.
   2. Hypertonicity and spasm of the involuntary muscles of the pharynx and esophagus.
   3. A tendency for his tongue to push food forward rather than backward.
   4. A considerable delay in the eruption of the lower bicuspid and molar teeth.

22. Which of the following foods would be particularly well-suited for use in training Buddy in self-feeding skills?
   1. Spaghetti.
   2. Applesauce.
   3. Green peas.
   4. Canned peaches.

23. Which of the following devices might the nurse use to establish a hand to mouth pattern for Buddy which would serve as a basis for beginning self-feeding?
   a. Giving him Safetipops to suck for between-meal treats.
   b. Playing games that call for pointing out his mouth, nose, and eyes.
   c. Encouraging him to eat such finger foods as celery and carrot sticks.
   d. Having him practice raising an empty glass to his mouth and setting it down again.
      1. a only.
      2. a and b.
      3. All but d.
      4. All the above.

24. Over-reliance on soft foods in Buddy's diet may have predisposed him to:
   1. Gastric hypoacidity.
   2. Dental caries.

   3. Vitamin deficiency.
   4. Intestinal flatulence.

25. What should be the first step in Buddy's bladder training?
   1. Place him on the toilet seat for 15 minutes after he wets his diaper.
   2. Keep a record for several days of the time of each voiding throughout the day.
   3. Have him sit on the toilet for half an hour following each meal and before bedtime.
   4. Have him touch his wet diaper and then drop it into the toilet bowl while he observes.

26. Which of the following would facilitate Buddy's successful bowel training?
   a. Nutritious and varied diet.
   b. Adequate fluid intake.
   c. Moderate physical exercise.
   d. Daily tap water enemas.
      1. a and c.
      2. b and d.
      3. All but d.
      4. All the above.

27. Which of the following adjustments of Buddy's clothing would assist him in developing skill in dressing himself?
   a. Using elastic thread to sew buttons on shirts, jackets, and coats.
   b. Employing Velcro fasteners on waistbands, shirtfronts, and cuffs.
   c. Sewing a leather or cloth tab to the backs of shoes and slippers.
   d. Attaching key chains or light pull chains to zipper pulls.
      1. a only.
      2. a and b.
      3. All but d.
      4. All the above.

28. Buddy's training should *not* parallel that of a normal child in which of the following respects?
   1. Disciplining for disobedience, destructiveness, and lack of respect for others.
   2. Giving him increasing amounts of responsibility for self-care and self-direction.
   3. Encouraging him to compete with other children in mastery of language skills.
   4. Allowing him to accept the consequences of his mistakes, misdeeds, and carelessness.

29. Buddy will probably not have experienced normal opportunities for emotional growth because he will have had:
- a. Decreased independent locomotion.
- b. Limited ability to care for himself.
- c. Difficulty in talking with other people.
- d. Infrequent opportunities to demonstrate personal worth.
- e. Little responsibility for decision making.
    1. a only.
    2. a and b.
    3. a, b, and c.
    4. All the above.

Buddy remained in the hospital for two months, during which time he made rapid progress in learning to feed himself. Bladder and bowel training were begun and Mrs. English was taught how to carry on the training at home following Buddy's hospital discharge. She was also taught to give Buddy stretching exercises for his feet and knees, and was shown how to assist him in muscle relaxation. Buddy was fitted with short leg braces and learned to stand with the support of parallel bars. Mrs. English was advised to keep Buddy in his braces during his waking hours and at his standing table four hours a day. She was also advised to keep his legs in aluminum posterior splints at night.

Buddy was registered at the local United Cerebral Palsy center where he would receive educational and speech therapy twice a week. Arrangements were made for a public health nurse to give instruction and assistance to Buddy and his parents in their home, and Buddy was scheduled to return regularly to the outpatient clinic for medical followup and re-evaluation.

30. In order to plan for Buddy's long term care the nurse must understand that:
1. Permanent care will require months or years of expensive treatment.
2. The basic defect underlying Buddy's disorder cannot be eliminated.
3. None of the available therapies can improve his motor abilities.
4. Children with combined physical and mental handicaps eventually require institutionalization.

31. On one of her visits to the hospital Mrs. English asked the nurse, "Will Buddy become even more helpless as he gets older?" What would be the most informative response?
1. "No. If any change at all occurs in his condition, there will be a marked gain in motor ability occurring in the next few years."
2. "Well, I don't expect that he will. However, there have been instances in which children with this disease did regress with time."
3. "There is no reason to expect that his motor difficulties will increase if the program of muscle re-education is carried out."
4. "I see that this concerns you a great deal, but I am unable to answer your question. No one can predict what Buddy's future will be."

32. The nurse should guide Mr. and Mrs. English toward which method of coping with society's attitudes of rejection toward cerebral palsy sufferers?
1. Confining Buddy to his own home and permitting contact only with relatives and a few close family friends.
2. Informing Buddy that he will spend most of his life in special institutions with other handicapped persons.
3. Gradually enlarging Buddy's social world so that he develops friendships with both normal and handicapped children.
4. Ignoring society's rejection and encouraging Buddy to be outgoing by exposing him to a variety of social situations.

33. The public health nurse should provide which of the following services to the English family?
- a. Advise Mr. and Mrs. English concerning Buddy's nutritional requirements and health needs.
- b. Interpret Buddy's progress in growth and development to Mr. and Mrs. English.
- c. Encourage the entire family to maintain optimum physical and mental health.
- d. Help the family to make the home situation as quiet and relaxing as possible.
- e. Act as liaison person in keeping parents, physicians, nurses, and therapists informed of each other's activities.

1. a and b.
2. c and d.
3. All but e.
4. All the above.

34. One of the primary responsibilities of the public health nurse toward Buddy's parents is:

1. Providing the type and amount of emotional support that will enable Mr. and Mrs. English to carry out the demanding program for Buddy's care without sacrificing their own mental or physical health.
2. Informing Mr. and Mrs. English of the several sources from which they may obtain financial assistance in meeting the expenses caused by Buddy's lengthy hospitalization and medical followup.
3. Assisting the Englishes by carrying out, on a regular basis, those techniques and procedures in Buddy's care which they find physically taxing, esthetically unpleasant, or unduly time-consuming.
4. Advising them in the purchase of special furniture, equipment, and supplies or in the adaptation of their existing facilities to achieve the most efficient provision of Buddy's daily care.

Burn

Rudy Simmers spilled a pot of hot coffee over his left trunk and thigh while his mother went next door to borrow two eggs. His shrieks brought back his mother, who rushed him to the emergency room of a nearby hospital.

The examining physician noted that three-year-old Rudy was frightened and irritable, weighed 34 pounds, and had suffered large second degree burns of the left trunk and several smaller third degree burns of the left thigh. He estimated that Rudy's burns covered 15 per cent of his body. Rudy's temperature was 99.8° F. rectally, pulse 120 per minute, and respirations 30 per minute. Because Mrs. Simmers indicated that Rudy had received a complete series of diphtheria-pertussis-tetanus immunizations, the doctor gave him a booster dose of tetanus toxoid. Rudy's red blood cell count was 4.8 million per cu. mm., his hematocrit 37 per cent, his hemoglobin 13 grams per 100 ml. of blood, and his white blood cell count was 8,300 per cu. mm. with a normal differential.

Rudy was admitted to the pediatric division, a plasma transfusion was started in a saphenous vein cutdown at the medial malleolus, clinical photographs were taken of Rudy's burns, and an indwelling catheter was inserted. The doctor wrote the following orders:

1. Place in isolation (burns are to be treated by the open method).
2. Morphine sulfate 15 mg. I.V. p.r.n. for pain.
3. Type and crossmatch.
4. Intake and output record (record hourly output for first 48 hours).
5. Notify doctor if urinary output is less than 25 cc. per hour.
6. Nothing by mouth for 48 hours.
7. Capillary hematocrit determination q. 4 h.
8. Serum electrolyte determination q. 8 h.
9. Fluid therapy during the first 24 hours to include:

a. Plasma 120 cc.
b. Normal saline 350 cc.
c. 5 per cent dextrose in distilled water 1100 cc.

half of which is to be given in the first 8 hours, and one-fourth of which is to be given both in the second and the third 8 hours.

10. Fluid therapy during the second 24 hours to include:
   a. Plasma 60 cc.
   b. Normal saline 175 cc.
   c. 5 per cent dextrose in distilled water.
11. Apply 10 per cent Sulfamylon cream (mafenide acetate) to burn wounds every four hours.

(ANSWER BLANK ON PAGE A–39) (CORRECT ANSWERS ON PAGE B–46)

---

1. In estimating the extent of Rudy's burns, the physician would have considered the skin of his anterior trunk to constitute what percentage of his total skin area?
  1. 4.5 per cent.
  2. 9.0 per cent.
  3. 18.0 per cent.
  4. 36.0 per cent.

2. Each of Rudy's lower extremities would account for what percentage of his total skin surface?
  1. 7 per cent.
  2. 15 per cent.
  3. 30 per cent.
  4. 60 per cent.

3. Which of the following is most characteristic of a second degree burn?
  1. Reddening of the skin with a moderate degree of pain.
  2. Destruction of the upper layer of the skin with blistering.
  3. Destruction of superficial and deep skin layers with severe pain.
  4. Complete destruction of skin and underlying tissue with charring.

4. The primary objective in treatment of Rudy's secondary burns will be to prevent:
  1. Blistering.
  2. Discoloration.
  3. Infection.
  4. Hemorrhage.

5. Which of the following skin structures are destroyed in a third degree burn?
  a. Nerve fibers.
  b. Sweat glands.
  c. Hair follicles.
  d. Sebaceous glands.
     1. a and b.
     2. b and c.
     3. c and d.
     4. All the above.

6. Rudy's third degree burns will differ from his second degree burns in which of the following respects?
  a. They must be grafted, and heal with some scarring.
  b. They will be less painful initially.
  c. They will exude a smaller amount of serum.
  d. They will less readily become infected.
     1. a only.
     2. a and b.
     3. a, b, and c.
     4. All the above.

7. The initial medical care of Rudy's burns should include:
  a. Removal of adherent foreign material from the burned surface.
  b. Gentle washing of the burned area with iodine-based solution.
  c. Thorough rinsing of the burned area with normal saline.
  d. Shaving hair from the burned area and from the area immediately surrounding it.
  e. Excision of fragments of dead and devitalized tissue.
     1. a and c.
     2. a, b, and c.
     3. All but e.
     4. All the above.

8. Why did the examining physician take time to weigh Rudy when he was admitted in such extreme discomfort?
1. To have information from which to determine Rudy's general level of physical development.
2. To provide a basis for calculating the amount of intravenous fluid he should receive.
3. To facilitate later recognition of symptoms of impending congestive heart failure.
4. To serve as a guide for dietary management in the convalescent phase of his illness.

9. It was advisable to give Rudy a booster dose of tetanus toxoid because:
1. Circulatory shock prevents mobilization of antibodies to areas of infection.
2. Necrotic tissue in a burn supports growth and multiplication of bacteria.
3. Parents cannot be relied upon to report immunizations correctly in emergencies.
4. Excessive fluid administration will dilute already existing antibodies.

10. *Clostridium tetani* is characterized by its ability to:
a. Grow and multiply in the absence of atmospheric oxygen.
b. Elaborate an exotoxin especially harmful to nerve tissue.
c. Utilize dead organic matter as a source of energy.
d. Produce highly resistant spores in unfavorable environments.
   1. a and b.
   2. b and c.
   3. c and d.
   4. All the above.

11. The nurse should be aware that Rudy is susceptible to which of the following as complications either of his injury or his prescribed treatment?
a. Cardiac failure.
b. Septic shock.
c. Peptic ulcer.
d. Hip contracture.
e. Renal failure.
   1. a and b.
   2. a, b, and c.
   3. All but e.
   4. All the above.

12. Upon admitting Rudy to his unit the nurse should:

1. Place him between sterile sheets and place a reverse isolation sign on his door.
2. Apply unmedicated gauze pressure dressings to both second and third degree burns.
3. Cover his third degree burns with Vaseline gauze strips secured with roller bandages.
4. Scrub burned surfaces briskly to remove dead tissue and rinse with sterile saline solution.

13. What is the pharmacologic effect of morphine?
1. Analgesic.
2. Antispasmodic.
3. Ataractic.
4. Antiemetic.

14. Which of the following is a possible side effect of morphine?
1. Tinnitus.
2. Constipation.
3. Gingivitis.
4. Nasal stuffiness.

15. There is some risk involved in using morphine to relieve chronic pain in that prolonged use is apt to cause:
1. Delayed healing.
2. Cumulative effects.
3. Physical dependence.
4. Allergic reaction.

16. Rudy should be closely observed for symptoms of circulatory shock, which include:
a. Increased pulse rate and decreased pulse force.
b. Fall in systolic and diastolic blood pressure.
c. Pallor or mottling of the skin.
d. Decreased skin temperature in the extremities.
   1. a only.
   2. a and b.
   3. c and d.
   4. All the above.

17. Which of the following are essential to protect Rudy from development of shock?
a. Replacing fluid loss.
b. Relieving burn pain.
c. Maintaining body heat.
d. Reducing fear and apprehension.
   1. a and b.
   2. b and c.
   3. c and d.
   4. All the above.

18. Rudy will need large quantities of intravenous fluid during the acute phase of his illness to compensate for:
   a. Oozing of serum from the surface of the burned area.
   b. Extravasation of fluid into the burned area and surrounding tissue.
   c. Reduced oral fluid intake during the first 48 hours following injury.
   d. Massive diuresis following the burn, due to renal tubular damage.
      1. a only.
      2. a and b.
      3. a, b, and c.
      4. All the above.

19. Rudy's fluid loss during his first two days in the hospital will be proportional to:
      1. His body weight before injury.
      2. The increase in protein catabolism.
      3. The surface area of the burn.
      4. The amount of plasma administered.

20. Which of the following findings would indicate that Rudy was receiving less than adequate fluid replacement?
      1. Stable measurements of both hematocrit and urine volume.
      2. Rising hematocrit value and decreasing urine volume.
      3. Falling values of both hematocrit and urine volume.
      4. Decreasing hematocrit value and increasing urine volume.

21. During the first 48 hours of hospitalization a reduction in Rudy's urinary output to below 25 cc. per hour might be interpreted to indicate which of the following?
   a. Inadequate fluid replacement.
   b. Hypovolemic circulatory shock.
   c. Impending renal failure.
   d. Ascending urinary infection.
      1. a only.
      2. a or b only.
      3. a, b, or c only.
      4. Any of the above.

22. To prevent accidental inaccuracies in reporting urinary output the nurse should make sure that:
   a. The indwelling catheter is patent and the drainage tubing is uncompressed.
   b. The urine specimens are obtained at exactly one hour intervals.
   c. Urine does not leak around the catheter or at tubing connections.
   d. Urine collection bottles are carefully labelled, capped, and removed.
      1. a and c.
      2. b and d.
      3. All but d.
      4. All the above.

23. Morphine was administered to Rudy intravenously rather than hypodermically in order to avoid which of the following problems?
      1. Secondary contamination of the burn wound.
      2. Faulty absorption of the drug.
      3. Fibrosis of possible skin donor sites.
      4. Hypersensitivity reaction to the drug.

24. Oral fluids were withheld during the acute stage of Rudy's illness because he would be particularly prone to:
      1. Aspiration and pneumonia.
      2. Gagging and strangulation.
      3. Vomiting and abdominal distention.
      4. Hyperperistalsis and diarrhea.

25. Which of the following are possible symptoms of overhydration from administration of excessive intravenous fluids?
   a. Temperature elevation.
   b. Bubbling rales.
   c. Nausea and vomiting.
   d. Muscle twitching.
      1. a and c.
      2. b and d.
      3. All but d.
      4. All the above.

26. Which of the following is a possible complication of fluid therapy for which Rudy should be carefully observed during the first 72 hours of treatment?
      1. Thrombophlebitis.
      2. Cerebral edema.
      3. Heart failure.
      4. Urinary retention.

27. Which of the following symptom complexes should cause the nurse to suspect impending toxemia due to absorption of cellular debris from the burned area?
      1. Increase in temperature, pulse, and respiration, with a drop in blood pressure and urine output.
      2. Steady decrease in temperature, pulse rate, and motor activity, with increased hematocrit and blood pressure.

3. Development of slow regular bounding pulse and deep blowing respirations, with output of copious urine.
4. Rapid weak irregular pulse and rapid difficult respirations, with subnormal temperature, cyanosis, and anxiety.

28. Sulfamylon cream (mafenide acetate) was applied to Rudy's burn wounds in order to:

1. Stimulate growth of granulation tissure.
2. Inhibit growth of pathogenic bacteria.
3. Prevent loss of tissue fluid.
4. Depress transmission of pain impulses.

29. Rudy's care will include daily removal of the dried Sulfamylon cream (mafenide acetate) from previous applications by:

1. Rinsing with tepid tap water.
2. Wiping with saline moistened gauze.
3. Scraping with sterile tongue blades.
4. Soaking in a whirlpool tub.

On Rudy's fourth hospital day his temperature was 100.6° F. rectally, his pulse was 112 per minute, respirations 30 per minute, hematocrit 33 per cent and hemoglobin 11 grams per 100 ml. The physician gave a transfusion of 250 cc. of O positive blood. For the next few days Rudy was fretful, anorexic, and incontinent of feces. An eschar formed over the burn wounds of the trunk and thigh, which the physician first debrided on Rudy's eighth hospital day, using codeine analgesia. Rudy's wounds were debrided every three days thereafter with gradual replacement of necrotic tissue by granulation tissue.

During this time the physician and social worker talked several times with Mrs. Simmers in an effort to help her understand and accept Rudy's current problems and plan realistically for his future care.

30. Which of the following could have contributed to Rudy's temperature elevation on the fourth day of illness?

a. Underhydration.
b. Burn toxemia.

c. Local infection.
d. Decreased heat radiation.
   1. a only.
   2. a and b.
   3. a, b, and c.
   4. All the above.

31. Rudy's anemia probably developed initially as a result of:

1. Blood loss from the surface of third degree burns.
2. Marrow depression by circulating bacterial toxins.
3. Hemolysis of red cells due to heat injury.
4. Nutritional inadequacy of iron, protein, and vitamins.

32. Rudy's anorexia was probably the result of:

1. Regression.
2. Toxemia.
3. Gastritis.
4. Avitaminosis.

33. Rudy's fecal incontinence was probably a manifestation of:

1. Shock.
2. Diarrhea.
3. Regression.
4. Hypermetabolism.

34. An eschar may best be defined as:

1. A thickened, roughened line of skin which is elevated above surrounding tissue.
2. A tough coagulum of necrotic tissue that develops over a burned area.
3. An aggregation of suppurative material developing within dead tissue.
4. A band of contracted scar tissue that causes deformity by shortening.

35. In preparing Rudy for debridement of his burned areas the nurse should strive to convey which of the following concepts?

1. He will be given enough analgesic before debridement that he will feel no physical pain.
2. Debridement causes considerable pain, but since the discomfort is brief, it can be withstood.
3. Debridement is an absolutely necessary though unpleasant experience, and she will be there to help him.
4. He will experience little pain or discomfort if he will refrain from watching the procedure.

36. The nurse should help Rudy to express his negative feelings concerning his injury by:

1. Permitting him to cry loudly and move freely on the treatment table during the wound cleansing and debridement procedures.
2. Allowing him to control his hospital situation by refusing to eat, drink, sleep, and have wounds dressed from time to time.
3. Encouraging him to verbalize in detail his guilt about having touched something on the stove after having been told not to do so.
4. Providing him with an opportunity to act out his guilt concerning the accident by playing house.

37. Which of the following actions by the nurse would provide Rudy the greatest degree of support concerning his self-concept?

1. Discouraging him from looking at his burn wounds during cleansing and debridement.
2. Pointing out to him each evidence of healing of various burn wounds.
3. Showing him photographs illustrating progressive healing of other children's burns.
4. Reassuring him repeatedly that the burns will heal quickly, leaving no disfiguration.

38. Which of the following adjustments should be made in order to improve Rudy's nutrition?

1. Arrange for a nurse, an aide, or Mrs. Simmers to feed all foods served to him.
2. Serve only those foods which he has eaten at home and prepare them in a similar manner.
3. Plan with the doctor to debride wounds at a point midway between mealtimes.
4. Allow Rudy to eat or drink anything he desires at whatever time he requests it.

39. It would be advisable to serve Rudy between-meal snacks of foods rich in:

1. Carbohydrates.
2. Proteins.
3. Fats.
4. Minerals.

40. From the standpoint of the healing of his burn wounds, which of the following bed positions would be most therapeutic for Rudy?

1. Side-lying with the left arm and leg uppermost.
2. Fowler's position, with arms supported on pillows at his sides.
3. Lying flat on his back with his legs fully extended.
4. Supine, with hip and knees flexed at a 15-degree angle.

41. Which of the following microorganisms is most apt to contaminate Rudy's burn wounds?

a. *Staphylococcus aureus.*
b. *Pseudomonas aeruginosa.*
c. *Proteus vulgaris.*
d. *Bacillus subtilis.*
    1. a and b.
    2. a, b, and c.
    3. a, c, and d.
    4. All the above.

42. In addition to using sterile bed linen, the nurse should do which of the following to reduce the possibility that Rudy's burns will become infected?

a. Wear a mask while caring for him and change it every hour.
b. Wear a sterile gown while working in his room and change it when necessary.
c. Direct Mr. and Mrs. Simmers to wear gowns and masks when visiting.
d. Wash her hands before and after Rudy's care and after handling soiled articles.
    1. a only.
    2. a and b.
    3. a, b, and c.
    4. All the above.

On Rudy's 21st day of hospitalization his third degree thigh wounds were covered with patch grafts obtained from the anterior aspect of his right thigh. Rudy required morphine to relieve pain in the grafted and donor sites for several days following surgery. The graft was covered with sterile mesh gauze, which was kept moist with Dakin's solution. Two weeks after surgery was performed the grafts had fused together fairly well. Rudy was given daily tub bath soaks to remove the dressings and a week later was discharged. He was to return to the burn clinic monthly.

43. The purpose of grafting skin over Rudy's thigh burns was to:
1. Foster healing and decrease infection.
2. Prevent discoloration of the burned area.
3. Reduce his pain and discomfort from the burn.
4. Facilitate greater movement in bed.

44. Grafting of Rudy's third degree burns was delayed until three weeks after the injury in order to permit:
1. Restoration of normal fluid and electrolyte balance.
2. Removal of eschar and formation of granulation tissue.
3. Improvement of general nutritional and psychological status.
4. Gradually decreasing awareness of skin sensations of pain.

45. The chief advantage of an autograft over a homograft is the fact that autografts:
1. Are less likely to slough.
2. Are less likely to become infected.
3. More nearly match the skin of the area.
4. Need not be stored before using.

46. Which of the following adjustments in the bed making procedure would most decrease Rudy's discomfort following the skin grafting?
1. Elevating the knee gatch of the bed to relieve tension on the skin of the thighs.
2. Using a bed cradle to prevent the sterile upper sheet from touching his body.
3. Leaving off the upper sheet until the wounds on both thighs have ceased to weep.
4. Placing a large plastic square over the grafted area to protect it against drafts.

47. Following skin grafting Rudy's diet should be:
1. High in carbohydrate and calories, low in protein.
2. High in roughage and fluid, low in calories.
3. High in calories, protein, vitamins, and minerals.
4. High in fat, low in carbohydrate, protein, and fluid.

48. In order to offset some of Rudy's feelings of loneliness, the nurse should:

a. Wrap him in a sterile sheet and hold him in her lap twice a day.
b. Place his bed where he can see other patients and personnel.
c. Use television, radio, and stories to divert his attention.
d. Accompany him during debridement, skin grafting, and tub soaks.
   1. a only.
   2. a and b.
   3. a, b, and c.
   4. All the above.

49. The active ingredient of Dakin's solution is:
1. Hydrogen peroxide.
2. Boric acid.
3. Sodium hypochlorite.
4. Silver nitrate.

50. Dakin's solution was applied to Rudy's skin graft dressings in order to:
1. Prevent blood loss by fostering fibrinous occlusion of the capillaries.
2. Disinfect the wound by disrupting the enzyme systems of bacteria.
3. Decrease discomfort by anesthetizing sensory nerve and organs.
4. Toughen and harden the tissue by precipitating cellular proteins.

51. The nurse could somewhat decrease Rudy's discomfort during removal of the dressings from the grafted area by:
1. Using cold water in the tub to decrease skin sensation of pain.
2. Having Rudy assist by easing the dressing free with a sterile cloth.
3. Shortening the procedure by pulling the gauze free rapidly and without warning.
4. Talking rapidly and animatedly throughout the procedure and ignoring his cries.

52. In preparing Mr. and Mrs. Simmers for Rudy's return to his home the nurse should emphasize the importance of their continuing daily:
1. Doses of morphine to relieve discomfort in the burn wound and graft donor sites.
2. Exercise of the joints of his lower extremities through full range of motion.
3. Dressing of the burn and donor areas with wide strips of Vaseline gauze.
4. Abrasive scrubbing of the burned areas with green soap and a rough washcloth.

Juvenile Diabetes Mellitus

Mrs. Rumbaugh was 40 years old when her sixth child, Sylvia, was born. Sylvia was a full-term baby, weighing 8 pounds, 10 ounces. When Sylvia was four years old, Mrs. Rumbaugh consulted the family physician because the child was drinking large quantities of water, urinating frequently, and was enuretic. On the basis of urinalysis, blood glucose determination, and a glucose tolerance test, Sylvia was diagnosed as having diabetes mellitus. For several months she was well-controlled with 12 units of Lente insulin daily, but a year and a half later she was admitted in comatose condition to the pediatric unit of a large city hospital.

Mrs. Rumbaugh told the examining physician that four days before Sylvia had developed the "flu," then had progressed from headache and vomiting to drowsiness and, finally, to deep sleep.

Physical examination revealed soft eyeballs, acetone breath odor, deep noisy respirations of 30 per minute, rales in the bases of both lungs, and decreased skin turgor. Laboratory tests revealed a blood glucose concentration of 460 mg. per 100 ml., blood urea nitrogen 20 mg. per 100 ml., serum chloride 100 mEq. per liter, $_pCO_2$ 30 mm. Hg, pH 7.2, serum sodium 130 mEq. per liter, serum potassium 5.4 mEq. per liter. Blood tests revealed a white cell count of 15,000 per cu. mm., with 75 per cent polymorphonuclear neutrophils, 15 per cent lymphocytes, and 7 per cent monocytes. Urinalysis revealed 4+ glucose and 4+ acetone.

(ANSWER BLANK ON PAGE A–41)   (CORRECT ANSWERS ON PAGE B–48)

Sylvia's physician wrote the following orders:

1. Insulin (crystalline zinc) 30 units stat.
2. Ringer's lactate 300 ml. I.V. to be given in one hour. Then administer Ringer's lactate with 10 mEq. potassium I.V. 300 ml. over the next 8 hours.
3. Urinalysis for sugar, acetone, specific gravity every hour for the first 8 hours.
4. Ampicillin 250 mg. I.V. q.i.d. for four doses then 250 mg. orally q.i.d.
5. Repeat blood chemistries and blood gases.
6. Oral fluids on second hospital day as tolerated. Then give regular diet of 1440 calories (CHO – 190 gm., PRO – 50 gm., FAT – 60 gm.). Intake of fluid to total 1800 ml.

1. The physiologic defect underlying symptom production in diabetes mellitus is:

1. Increased absorption of glucose from the intestine.
2. Decreased electrolyte absorption from renal tubule.
3. Increased rate of respiration in the tissue cells.
4. Decreased production of insulin by the pancreas.

2. In order to understand the production of symptoms in the diabetic child, the nurse should know that insulin has which of the following metabolic effects?

a. Speeds the transport of glucose through the cell membrane.
b. Assists the conversion of glucose to glycogen and then its storage in the liver.
c. Facilitates the synthesis of fats from intermediates of carbohydrate breakdown.

d. Increases resorption of water molecules from the kidney tubule.

e. Promotes the sliding of actin and myocin molecules in muscle.
1. a and b.
2. c and d.
3. a, b, and c.
4. All the above.

3. Diabetes mellitus is which of the following types of disease?
1. Degenerative.
2. Collagen.
3. Hereditary.
4. Auto-immune.

4. Since neither Mr. nor Mrs. Rumbaugh has symptoms of diabetes, one may assume that:
1. Sylvia developed the disease due to a gene mutation.
2. Both parents are carriers of the recessive gene for diabetes.
3. Sylvia's disease is secondary to a chronic pancreatitis.
4. Sylvia's disorder is purely functional and can be cured.

5. In addition to polydipsia, polyuria, and glycosuria, Sylvia might have experienced which other symptoms of diabetes at the age of four years?
a. Muscular weakness.
b. Weight loss.
c. Increased appetite.
d. Increased pulse pressure.
e. Increased skin discoloration.
1. a and b.
2. a, b, and c.
3. All but d.
4. All the above.

6. The normal fasting venous serum glucose level is:
1. 40 to 70 mg. per 100 ml. of blood.
2. 70 to 100 mg. per 100 ml. of blood.
3. 100 to 130 mg. per 100 ml. of blood.
4. 130 to 160 mg. per 100 ml. of blood.

7. The glucose tolerance test consists of:
1. Giving a high carbohydrate and high liquid diet for three days, then obtaining blood sugar levels before and after a 12 hour fast.
2. Taking a blood and a urine sample following an 8 hour fast. Then a standard oral dose of glucose is given, and hourly blood and urine samples are obtained.
3. Administering 50 ml. of 50 per cent glucose solution intravenously, and then immediately determining blood glucose levels at one, two, and three hour intervals.
4. After a twelve hour fast, determining blood glucose levels before and two hours after the subcutaneous administration of a standard dose of regular insulin.

8. Sylvia's findings on the glucose tolerance test would probably differ from those of a nondiabetic child in that Sylvia's:
1. Serum glucose level would rise above normal within one hour following glucose administration.
2. Serum glucose level would not decrease to normal following a dose of regular insulin.
3. Serum glucose would not return to normal levels within three hours following glucose administration.
4. Serum glucose level would not decrease following a prolonged period of fasting.

9. Sylvia's blood chemistry tests would be most apt to reveal elevation of:
1. Uric acid.
2. Total cholesterol.
3. Serum globulin.
4. Creatinine.

10. Glycosuria develops in diabetes as a result of:
1. Bacterial injury to the epithelial cells of the glomerular capillary, which permits molecules of larger than usual size to pass into the tubule.
2. Elevation of serum glucose above the level at which it can, after filtration through the glomerulus, be completely resorbed from the tubule.
3. Toxic paralysis of renal tubular cells with consequent inability to resorb glucose from the tubular lumen into the efferent tubule.
4. Concentration of the traces of glucose present in normal urine into a smaller quantity of liquid, due to decreased excretion of water.

11. The serum glucose concentration above which glucose is usually excreted in the urine is:
1. 80 mg. per 100 ml. of blood.
2. 120 mg. per 100 ml. of blood.
3. 180 mg. per 100 ml. of blood.
4. 220 mg. per 100 ml. of blood.

12. The frequency of urination which Sylvia developed at the age of four years as probably the result of:
   1. Ascending infection of the urinary tract.
   2. Hyperactive bladder emptying reflex.
   3. Osmotic effect of glucose excreted by the kidney.
   4. Nervousness and anxiety due to illness.

13. Sylvia's enuresis at the age of four was probably a result of:
   1. Irritation of the bladder mucosa by high concentrations of glucose.
   2. Degenerative changes in the nerves controlling bladder function.
   3. Bladder overdistention due to secretion of excessive amounts of urine.
   4. Regression provoked by the discomfort associated with illness.

14. Lente insulin differs from crystalline or regular insulin in that Lente insulin:
   1. Acts over a longer period of time.
   2. Less often causes insulin shock.
   3. Acts more rapidly after administration.
   4. Is more highly purified.

15. While she is acidotic, the concentration of hydrogen ions in Sylvia's serum will be:
   1. Slightly less than normal.
   2. Within normal range.
   3. Slightly higher than normal.
   4. Greatly increased above normal.

16. The decrease in Sylvia's serum pH during acidosis was primarily the result of:
   1. Utilization of base bicarbonate to buffer ketones.
   2. Neutralization of chloride ions by blood proteins.
   3. Conversion of carbonic acid to carbon dioxide and water.
   4. Combustion of acetone to fatty acids and glycerol.

17. The normal range for serum pH level is:
   1. 7.15 to 7.22.
   2. 7.25 to 7.32.
   3. 7.35 and 7.42.
   4. 7.45 to 7.52.

18. Which of the following are symptoms of diabetic acidosis?
   a. Excessive urination.
   b. Dry, flushed skin.
   c. Mental dullness.
   d. Rapid, weak pulse.
   e. Extreme hunger.
      1. a and b.

2. c and d.
3. All but e.
4. All the above.

19. Careful questioning of Mrs. Rumbaugh would be apt to reveal that Sylvia had experienced which of the following symptoms during the 2 or 3 days preceding onset of coma?
   a. Nausea and vomiting.
   b. Shortness of breath.
   c. Abdominal pain.
   d. Dependent edema.
   e. Muscle twitching.
      1. a and c.
      2. b and d.
      3. All but e.
      4. All the above.

20. In order to appreciate the multiplicity of Sylvia's problems upon hospital admission, the nurse should know that the metabolic disturbances occurring in diabetic acidosis include:
   a. Loss of water from intracellular and extracellular compartments.
   b. Rapid and excessive breakdown of tissue protein and fat.
   c. Movement of phosphates and potassium out of tissue cells.
   d. Accumulation of beta-hydroxybutyric and acetoacetic acids in the blood.
   e. Decrease in concentration of serum bicarbonate and sodium ions.
      1. a and b.
      2. c and d.
      3. All but e.
      4. All the above.

21. Which of the following is the most definitive test for diabetes mellitus?
   1. Quantitative urine glucose concentration.
   2. Fasting blood glucose level.
   3. Glucose tolerance test.
   4. Carbon dioxide combining power of serum.

22. What probably precipitated Sylvia's present episode of acidosis?
   1. Increased motor activity.
   2. High intake of carbohydrates.
   3. Desensitization to Lente insulin.
   4. Body response to infection.

23. In which way did Sylvia's response to the pulmonary infection contribute toward her acidosis?
   1. Toxins produced by the causative organisms nullified the insulin she had been given.
   2. Insulin was lost in the increased

urine, perspiration, and sputum associated with the infection.

3. Fever produced by the infection increased the metabolic rate, increasing insulin use.

4. Pulmonary consolidation interfered with respiratory gas exchange, elevating serum carbon dioxide level.

24. Sylvia's comatose condition at the time of her hospital admission was the result of:

1. Depression of cerebral activity by toxic metabolites.

2. Cerebral anoxia due to rapidly decreasing arterial pressure.

3. Cerebral ischemia due to thrombotic occlusion of cranial vessels.

4. Cerebral hypotension secondary to severe dehydration.

25. On physical examination Sylvia's eyeballs were found to be unusually soft. This phenomenon is the result of:

1. Inadequate nutrition.

2. General dehydration.

3. Cerebral dysfunction.

4. Muscular flaccidity.

26. In obtaining a sample of Sylvia's urine for analysis the nurse should:

1. Save all of Sylvia's urine in a large jug, mix, and remove small aliquots for testing.

2. Have Sylvia partially empty her bladder into the bedpan, then collect the remaining urine for the test.

3. Instruct Sylvia to void on arising and discard that urine. Collect a specimen 30 minutes later for testing.

4. Direct Sylvia to void fifteen minutes both before and after giving her 300 ml. of fluid to drink rapidly.

27. Ketone bodies eliminated in Sylvia's urine and present in her blood serum derive from:

1. Intermediate breakdown products of the injected insulin.

2. Precipitation of excess glucose in the circulating blood.

3. Increased breakdown of body fat to supply energy.

4. Catabolic end-products of damaged tissue proteins.

28. While Sylvia remains in a diabetic coma, the nurse should test her urine for glucose and acetone every:

1. 1 to 2 hours.

2. 3 to 4 hours.

3. 5 to 6 hours.

4. 7 to 8 hours.

29. The severe hyperpnea which Sylvia evidenced on hospital admission is referred to as:

1. Cheyne-Stokes respirations.

2. Paradoxical respirations.

3. Kussmaul breathing.

4. Respiratory stridor.

30. The deep respirations characteristic of diabetic acidosis constitute a physiologic adaptation directed toward:

1. Increasing the oxygen intake per unit of time.

2. Speeding blood flow through the pulmonary circuit.

3. Eliminating increased amounts of carbon dioxide.

4. Decreasing pressures in the ascending vena cava.

31. The carbon dioxide combining power of the plasma is an indirect measurement of the serum concentration of:

1. Insulin.

2. Bicarbonate ions.

3. Oxyhemoglobin.

4. Glucose.

32. Crystalline rather than Lente insulin was used to treat Sylvia during acidosis because:

1. Crystalline insulin acts within a much shorter period of time and can be given intravenously.

2. Occurrence of acidosis indicates that she had become resistant to the effects of Lente insulin.

3. Sylvia would be less apt to develop hyperinsulinism when being treated with crystalline insulin.

4. Crystalline insulin exerts, per unit, a greater carbohydrate-regulating effect than does Lente insulin.

33. After the initial expansion of the vascular volume, the physician ordered that Sylvia be given 250 ml. of fluid intravenously in eight hours. Using a 60 drop per milliliter microdrip apparatus the fluid should be infused at which rate?

1. 10 microdrops per minute.

2. 20 microdrops per minute.

3. 30 microdrops per minute.

4. 40 microdrops per minute.

Sixteen hours after treatment was initiated Sylvia regained consciousness. Her indwelling catheter was removed. She was given and retained small quantities of clear liquids, so she was started on a regular diet and was given crystalline insulin four times a day, the insulin dose being calculated according to the results of serial urinalyses.

34. After Sylvia's acidosis had been relieved by treatment, maintenance of which of the following urinary findings would indicate satisfactory metabolic control?

    1. Negative glucose, negative acetone.
    2. Trace of glucose, negative acetone.
    3. One plus glucose, trace of acetone.
    4. Negative glucose, one plus acetone.

On her third hospital day Sylvia was allowed to be up in a wheel chair. Three days later she was allowed up and about at will. At this time she was changed from crystalline insulin to 17 units of Lente insulin every day. The nurse then made the first of several appointments for Mr. and Mrs. Rumbaugh to meet with her and Sylvia for instruction regarding urinalysis, insulin administration, dietary management, personal hygiene, and exercise needs.

35. In order to provide needed health instruction for Sylvia's parents, the nurse should be aware that which of the following factors would tend to increase the severity of Sylvia's diabetes?

    a. Excessive exercise.
    b. Nervous exhaustion.
    c. Repeated infections.
    d. Excessive carbohydrate intake.
    e. Change of climate.
        1. a and c.
        2. b and d.
        3. All but e.
        4. All the above.

36. The nurse should help Mr. and Mrs. Rumbaugh to understand and accept which of the following concepts in order to ensure optimal care for Sylvia in the future?

    a. Diabetes is a permanent condition for which control rather than cure is possible.
    b. The daily care which Sylvia needs should be established as routine aspects of family life.
    c. Diabetes, when accepted and controlled, need not interfere with normal growth and development.
    d. Sylvia's mother should be responsible for managing Sylvia's care until she reaches adulthood.
        1. a and b.
        2. b and c.
        3. a, b, and c.
        4. All the above.

37. Which of the following statements most accurately describes the relationship between psychic and physiologic factors in diabetes mellitus?

    1. Diabetes mellitus is caused by the unconscious expression of hostility through the endocrine system.
    2. Changes in the emotional state of the diabetic patient vary the character of his glucose tolerance curve.
    3. The ritual followed in calculating and preparing a rigidly controlled diet leads to compulsive behavior.
    4. Biochemical abnormalities on a cellular level cause impaired nerve impulse transmission and produce personality changes.

38. Mr. and Mrs. Rumbaugh asked the nurse, "Why has Sylvia's insulin dosage been increased since last year? Is she getting worse?" Which response would be most appropriate?

    1. "It may not be that she is deteriorating. Diabetes which begins in childhood is always more severe and harder to regulate."
    2. "Since insulin is used in energy production and tissue building, insulin needs will tend to increase continuously during the growth period."
    3. "Her insulin requirement has increased only because of her infection. When that is completely resolved she'll go back to her previous dosage."
    4. "Her underlying problem is no more severe than formerly, but probably you have not controlled her nutritional intake rigidly enough."

39. When instructing the Rumbaughs concerning Sylvia's dietary needs, the nurse should indicate that Sylvia should receive:

    1. Two cups of milk, one serving of the meat group, three servings of the vegetable-fruit group and four servings of the bread-cereal group daily.
    2. Five cups of milk, three servings of the meat group, two servings of the vegetable-fruit group, and two servings of the bread-cereal group daily.
    3. Three cups of milk, one serving of meat, three servings of the vegetable-fruit group, and four servings of the bread-cereal group daily.
    4. Four cups of milk, two servings of the meat group, four servings of the vegetable-fruit group, and four servings of the bread-cereal group daily.

40. In order to discuss dietary regulation

with Sylvia's parents, the nurse should be aware that one gram of fat yields:

1. Half as many calories as one gram of protein.
2. Exactly as many calories as one gram of protein.
3. About twice as many calories as one gram of carbohydrate.
4. Approximately as many calories as one gram of carbohydrate.

41. How frequently should Mr. and Mrs. Rumbaugh be instructed to test Sylvia's urine at home?

1. Every other day.
2. Every morning.
3. Twice a day.
4. Four times a day.

42. Mr. and Mrs. Rumbaugh should be taught that insulin shock is apt to result from:

a. Accidental administration of an overdose of insulin.
b. Ingestion of less than the usual quantity of food.
c. Greater than usual amounts of physical activity.
d. Development of a chronic skin or respiratory infection.
   1. a and b.
   2. c and d.
   3. All but d.
   4. All the above.

43. Mr. and Mrs. Rumbaugh should know that symptoms of hyperinsulinism are:

a. Extreme weakness.
b. Pale, moist skin.
c. Nervousness and tremor.
d. Hunger pangs.
e. Rapid, deep respirations.
   1. a and c.
   2. b and d.
   3. All but e.
   4. All the above.

44. The nurse should inform Sylvia's parents that Sylvia is most apt to develop a reaction to Lente insulin:

1. One hour after administration.
2. 3 to 4 hours after administration.
3. 5 to 6 hours after administration.
4. 8 to 12 hours after administration.

45. Mr. Rumbaugh said to the nurse, "My boss has diabetes and he takes pills to control it. Why can't we give Sylvia pills instead of the shots?" Which answer would be most appropriate?

1. "The pills work by stimulating sluggish cells to increase their insulin output. Sylvia's cells have lost the ability to respond to stimulation."
2. "Children are prone to stomach upsets. If Sylvia should vomit you would have no way of knowing how much medicine she had absorbed."
3. "Children's metabolism and peristalsis is so accelerated that they don't have time to absorb the drug when it is given by mouth."
4. "It will be easier to teach Sylvia the importance of close diabetic control when the drug is given by injection than when it is given orally."

46. It is important that Sylvia and her parents be given detailed health instruction because inadequate control of Sylvia's diabetes would predispose her to:

a. Stunting of growth.
b. Iron deficiency anemia.
c. Lack of sexual development.
d. Contracture deformities.
e. Mental retardation.
   1. a and c.
   2. b and d.
   3. All but d.
   4. All the above.

47. Mr. and Mrs. Rumbaugh should be taught to protect Sylvia from exposure to persons with infections because:

a. Sylvia is more apt to acquire an infection than a nondiabetic child.
b. Infection would tend to upset Sylvia's diet, insulin, and activity control.
c. Infections in diabetic children are often followed by complications.
d. Sylvia is incapable of producing antibodies against microorganisms.
   1. a and b.
   2. c and d.
   3. All but d.
   4. All the above.

48. What special guideline should the nurse give the Rumbaughs concerning Sylvia's clothing needs?

1. Dress her in lighter weight clothing than usual to prevent sweating.
2. Buy well-fitting shoes and discard them as soon as she outgrows them.
3. Insist that she wear a sweater at all times to avoid chilling.
4. Avoid woolen clothing of any type to ensure against skin irritation.

Because Sylvia remained well-controlled with Lente insulin while on a regimen of full activity in the hospital, she was discharged and scheduled to return for continuing health supervision in the diabetic clinic.

Nephrosis

Otto Barnum had been well except for a succession of upper respiratory infections when at the age of four years, following a severe pharyngitis, he developed edema of his eyelids, feet, and thighs.

Mrs. Barnum took Otto to the family physician who detected firm, nonpitting edema of the lower extremities and marked proteinuria, and admitted the child to the hospital.

The examining physician found Otto apparently well-developed and well-nourished, with a blood pressure of 120/80 mm. Hg, pulse 120 per minute, respirations 28 per minute and shallow, and temperature 100° F. orally. His pharyngeal mucosa was slightly reddened, and scattered cervical lymph nodes were palpable. His heart was of normal size, his abdomen was protuberant, an abdominal fluid wave was left on percussion, and his scrotum was markedly edematous.

Laboratory tests revealed normal red blood cell count, hemoglobin, hematocrit, and urine specific gravity. Abnormal findings included a white cell count of 13,600 per cu. mm., with 87 per cent polymorphonuclear cells and 10 per cent lymphocytes, a red blood cell sedimentation rate of 37 mm. per hour, total plasma protein 4.8 grams per 100 ml., serum albumin 7.8 grams per 100 ml., serum cholesterol 306 mg. per 100 ml., and 4+ albuminuria with a moderate number of casts. Throat culture revealed a moderate number of pneumococci. Antistreptolysin-O titer was 12. Otto's illness was diagnosed as nephrotic syndrome. The physician ordered the following:

1. Bedrest.
2. Penicillin orally 200,000 units q. 6 h.
3. Prednisone 15 mg. q.i.d.
4. Hydrochlorothiazide 12.5 mg. orally t.i.d.
5. Record intake and output and save urine for a 24-hour quantitative albumin determination.
6. Regular diet.
7. Weigh daily.

(ANSWER BLANK ON PAGE A–43) (CORRECT ANSWERS ON PAGE B–49)

1. Although the cause of childhood nephrosis is unknown, it has been demonstrated that exacerbations of nephrosis are often precipitated by:
1. Psychic stress.
2. Acute infections.
3. Mechanical trauma.
4. Dietary indiscretions.

2. Childhood nephrosis itself is believed to be the forerunner of:
1. Urinary calculi.
2. Acute pyelonephritis.
3. Chronic glomerulonephritis.
4. Polycystic kidney.

3. Otto's medical history would probably reveal that, in addition to generalized edema, he has suffered which other symptoms of the nephrotic syndrome?
a. Pallor.
b. Lassitude.
c. Irritability.
d. Anorexia.
e. Diarrhea.

1. a and b.
2. c and d.
3. All but d.
4. All the above.

4. Which of the following symptoms are generally less characteristic of nephrosis than of acute glomerulonephritis in children?
   a. Hematuria.
   b. Cylindruria.
   c. Hypertension.
   d. Proteinuria.
   e. Azotemia.
      1. a and b.
      2. c and d.
      3. a, c, and e.
      4. All the above.

5. The pathologic tissue change which is generally associated with childhood nephrosis is:
   1. Decreased volume of arterial blood flow to the kidney.
   2. Fibrinoid degeneration of epithelial cells of the basement membrane.
   3. Obstruction of urine flow through the renal collecting tubules.
   4. Destruction of renal cortex by large confluent abscesses.

6. Otto's rapid shallow respirations were probably caused by:
   1. Pneumonia.
   2. Acidosis.
   3. Anemia.
   4. Ascites.

7. Otto's edema resulted primarily from:
   1. Increased hydrostatic pressure in his veins.
   2. Decreased force of left ventricular contraction.
   3. Increased permeability of capillary walls.
   4. Decreased osmotic pressure of the blood.

8. Edema due to nephrosis differs from that due to congestive heart failure in that nephrotic edema:
   1. Never becomes generalized in distribution.
   2. Develops first in the periorbital tissues.
   3. Is invariably relieved by rest in bed.
   4. Does not shift with changes in position.

9. Otto's enlarged abdomen was probably the result of:
   1. Infiltration of the liver with large fat-filled cells.

2. Distention of the large intestine with flatus.
3. Accumulation of transudate in the peritoneal cavity.
4. Increase in the thickness of subcutaneous fat.

10. Otto's elevated white blood cell count was probably the result of:
   1. Bone marrow stimulation by accumulated nitrogenous wastes.
   2. Increased leukocyte production provoked by his pharyngitis.
   3. Generalized hyperplasia and hyperactivity of lymphoid tissue.
   4. The relative effect of an absolute decrease in red blood cells.

11. Polymorphonuclear leukocytes typically constitute what portion of the total white blood cell count in the well four-year-old child?
   1. 10 per cent.
   2. 30 per cent.
   3. 50 per cent.
   4. 70 per cent.

12. Which of the following conclusions can justifiably be drawn from Otto's increased red cell sedimentation rate?
   1. His red bone marrow activity is depressed.
   2. The cells are unusually large and hyperchromic.
   3. An inflammatory process is present in his body.
   4. Increased fragility has caused marked lysis of cells.

13. Which of the following are included in the total plasma protein measurement?
   a. Albumin.
   b. Creatinine.
   c. Globulin.
   d. Phenylalanine.
   e. Fibrinogen.
      1. a and b.
      2. c and d.
      3. a, c, and e.
      4. All the above.

14. Cholesterol is:
   1. A monatomic alcohol which is a component of animal fats and oils.
   2. A sterol which, when subjected to ultraviolet rays, yields vitamin A.
   3. An organic compound with hormonal functions produced by the adrenal gland.
   4. A pigment released from the hemoglobin which is excreted in the bile.

15. Which of the following types of casts are most characteristic of childhood nephrotic syndrome?
  a. Granular.
  b. Hyaline.
  c. Erythrocytic.
  d. Leukocytic.
  e. Waxy.
      1. a and b.
      2. c and d.
      3. All but e.
      4. All the above.

16. The upper limit of the normal antistreptolysin-O titer is 250 units. Otto's titer indicates that:
      1. He is currently suffering from an overwhelming streptococcal infection.
      2. He has recovered from a streptococcal infection in the recent past.
      3. He had long ago developed immunity against all strains of streptococci.
      4. His throat infection was caused by an organism other than streptococcus.

17. Prednisone was ordered for Otto primarily to:
      1. Provide him with a sense of well-being.
      2. Prevent development of skin and respiratory infections.
      3. Stimulate vascular resorption of edema and ascites.
      4. Decrease inflammatory changes in his glomeruli.

18. The administration of prednisone creates which of the following problems in protecting Otto from complications of nephrosis?
      1. The drug will markedly increase his edema.
      2. The drug will depress him mentally and physically.
      3. The drug masks the symptoms of infection.
      4. The drug will produce intolerance for protein foods.

19. Which of the following are possible untoward side effects of adrenal steroid therapy?
  a. Gastric ulcer.
  b. Cushing's syndrome.
  c. Delayed healing.
  d. Emotional disturbance.
  e. Activation of healed tuberculosis.
      1. a and b.
      2. a, b, and c.
      3. All but e.
      4. All the above.

20. Cushing's syndrome includes which of the following symptoms?
  a. Moon face.
  b. Muscle weakness.
  c. Abdominal striae.
  d. Facial hirsutism.
  e. Osteoporosis.
      1. a and b.
      2. c and d.
      3. All but d.
      4. All the above.

21. Penicillin exerts a bacteriostatic effect on susceptible organisms by virtue of its ability to:
      1. Suppress the formation of the bacterial cell wall.
      2. Coagulate the protein of the bacterial protoplasm.
      3. Prevent normal replication of desoxyribonucleic acid.
      4. Destroy enzymes regulating cellular oxidation of nutrients.

22. While he is being treated with prednisone, Otto should be very carefully observed for symptoms of:
      1. Dehydration.
      2. Hemorrhage.
      3. Infection.
      4. Shock.

23. The physician would be apt to decrease or discontinue Otto's prednisone dosage if he were to develop:
      1. Lassitude.
      2. Hypertension.
      3. Hematuria.
      4. Anorexia.

24. Hydrochlorothiazide was given to Otto in order to:
      1. Block inflammatory response.
      2. Decrease cholesterol formation.
      3. Eliminate retained fluid.
      4. Relieve anxiety and discomfort.

25. While he is being treated with hydrochlorothiazide, Otto should be closely observed for which of the following symptoms of electrolyte disturbance?
      1. Muscle weakness.
      2. Tetanic seizures.
      3. "Blowing" respirations.
      4. "Flapping" tremor.

26. An accurate record of fluid intake and output is especially important in Otto's care because:

1. It is a reliable index of adequacy of infection control.
2. It is a subtle way of determining his nutritional status.
3. It provides data for assessing kidney function.
4. It serves as a basis for determining intravenous fluid needs.

27. The objective of weighing Otto daily is to:

1. Measure the adequacy of his nutritional intake.
2. Check the accuracy of the fluid intake record.
3. Determine changes in the amount of edema and transudate.
4. Impress Otto with the importance of eating well.

28. To be of maximum diagnostic significance, Otto's daily weight measurement should be taken:

1. By the same nurse or attendant.
2. Immediately after he has voided.
3. At the same time every day.
4. When he is completely disrobed.

29. Otto's edema is apt to obscure symptoms of:

1. Infection.
2. Malnutrition.
3. Anemia.
4. Obstruction.

Because Otto's condition failed to improve after two weeks of prescribed therapy, hydrochlorothiazide was discontinued and furosemide, 40 mg. orally, was given daily.

30. Furosemide was given to Otto in order to produce:

1. Diuresis.
2. Bacteriostasis.
3. Sedation.
4. Catharsis.

31. The onset of the pharmacologic effect of furosemide occurs approximately:

1. 5 minutes after administration.
2. 30 minutes after administration.
3. 3 hours after administration.
4. 18 hours after administration.

32. Which of the following are possible toxic effects of furosemide?

a. Skin rash.
b. Paresthesias.
c. Nausea and vomiting.
d. Thrombocytopenia.
e. Hyperglycemia.

1. a and c.
2. b and d.
3. All but d.
4. All the above.

33. What type of diet would the doctor probably order for Otto?

1. Normal diet with increased protein and slightly restricted salt.
2. Low protein diet with no restriction of salt intake.
3. Normal diet with slightly reduced carbohydrate content.
4. Elimination diet similar to that used for allergic patients.

34. Since Otto is apt to be anorexic, which of the following might encourage him to eat?

1. Permitting a second serving of any food which he especially likes.
2. Providing double quantities of every food served on his meal tray.
3. Offering food to him on every occasion that a nurse enters his room.
4. Waiting until Otto makes a specific request for a particular food and then providing it promptly.

35. Otto is particularly prone to develop skin infections because of:

a. Susceptibility of his edematous skin to pressure injury.
b. Deficiency of protein and vitamins due to anorexia.
c. Decreased production of gamma globulin by lymphatic tissue.
d. Marked decrease in numbers of neutrophilic white cells.

1. a and b.
2. c and d.
3. All but d.
4. All the above.

36. What measures should be taken by the nurse in order to protect Otto's skin from infection and injury?

a. Scrubbing with germicidal soap twice daily.
b. Providing for frequent changes of position.
c. Eliminating friction between opposing skin surfaces.
d. Avoiding use of adhesive tape on his skin.
e. Improving his general nutritional status.

1. a and b.
2. a, b, and c.
3. b, c, and d.
4. b, c, d, and e.

37. Otto's daily skin care should include:
   a. Frequent bathing of the genitalia and application of cornstarch.
   b. Supporting the scrotum with a soft dressing and T-binder.
   c. Separation of opposing skin surfaces with cotton material.
   d. Massaging pressure points gently with lanolin-containing lotion.
   e. Placing sheepskin padding under his hips, elbows, and heels.
      1. a and b.
      2. c and d.
      3. All but e.
      4. All the above.

38. Optimal care of Otto's edematous periorbital tissues would include:
   a. Applying warm compresses daily.
   b. Irrigating his eyes with normal saline.
   c. Darkening the room with shades.
   d. Elevating his head during the day.
      1. a and c.
      2. b and d.
      3. a, b, and c.
      4. All the above.

39. What precaution should be taken by the nurse to ensure the accuracy of the 24-hour urine collection?
   a. Teach Otto the necessity of using the urinal to save all his urine, rather than voiding in the lavatory.
   b. Pour the urine from each voiding during the collection period into a gallon jug containing a small amount of disinfectant.
   c. When beginning the collection, have Otto void and discard the urine, but save the specimen voided at the end of the collection period.
   d. After all urine has been collected for 24 hours, mix it well, record the total, and send 200 cc. to the laboratory.
      1. a and c.
      2. b and d.
      3. a, b, and c.
      4. All the above.

40. During Otto's hospitalization which of the following determinations will be made at frequent intervals in order to follow the progress of his recovery?
   a. Urine albumin content.
   b. Serum albumin level.
   c. Serum cholesterol level.
   d. Blood clotting time.
   e. Glucose tolerance test.
      1. a and b.
      2. a, b, and c.
      3. All but e.
      4. All the above.

41. Since Otto would probably experience only moderate discomfort during his two-month hospital stay, play and diversional activity are necessary. Which of the following would be suitable for him?
   1. Playing games of checkers with the nurse while remaining completely supine in bed.
   2. Participating in such role-playing activities as playing "house," "doctor," and "cowboy."
   3. Skipping rope, playing hopscotch, and shooting marbles in the playroom with a boy of his own age.
   4. Reading comic books, coloring pictures, and watching television for one hour at a time.

42. To which of the following levels of motor skill should Otto have advanced by the time of his hospitalization?
   1. Walking fast but running stiffly.
   2. Walking up and down stairs alone.
   3. Beginning ability to ride a tricycle.
   4. Talking, jumping, and climbing well.

43. Otto will probably have which teeth?
   1. The central and lateral incisors only.
   2. The cuspids and the central incisors.
   3. The cuspids and first molars.
   4. All of the primary or deciduous teeth.

44. If his edema does not restrict motion or respiration Otto could be allowed out of bed. What precaution should be taken by the nurse before taking Otto to the playroom?
   1. Make certain that all sharp objects are removed from the room.
   2. Close all windows and shades to eliminate drafts and strong light.
   3. Remove or cover all shiny objects in which he could observe his image.
   4. Remove all children from the playroom who have infections.

45. Otto is most likely to demonstrate which of the following psychological reactions to his massive edema?
   1. Acting-out behavior.
   2. Temper tantrums.
   3. Moderate depression.
   4. Body-image changes.

Otto's edema persisted until his third week of hospitalization, then gradually subsided. During his fourth week in the hospital a renal biopsy was done, revealing dilated glomerular capillaries, slightly thickened basement membranes, and a few local areas of cellular proliferation throughout the glomeruli.

Because Otto responded to steroid therapy he was discharged after six weeks of hospitalization. Mr. and Mrs. Barnum were informed of the probable course and treatment for Otto's illness, the home care required, the dosage of prednisone to be administered, and the date on which Otto was to return to the physician's office.

46. Nursing care for Otto following the renal biopsy should include:
1. Keeping him in bed in a prone position for twelve hours.
2. Directing him to sit on the edge of the bed and dangle his feet.
3. Putting him in a wheel chair and placing him near the nurses' station.
4. Allowing him to walk from the treatment room to his unit.

47. Which of the following complications is most apt to occur following a renal biopsy?
1. Pulmonary embolus.
2. Hemorrhage and shock.
3. Thrombus formation.
4. Increased edema.

48. Otto's parents should be given predischarge instructions concerning which of the following?

a. Need for continued medical supervision.
b. Dosage and frequency of ordered medication.
c. Symptoms of adrenal corticoid overdosage.
d. Means for protecting Otto from infections.
   1. a and b.
   2. c and d.
   3. All but c.
   4. All the above.

49. Mr. and Mrs. Barnum should be taught to administer Otto's prednisone:
1. Between meals.
2. Immediately before meals.
3. During meals.
4. Early in the morning.

50. It should be explained to Mr. and Mrs. Barnum that it is especially important to protect Otto from infectious contacts since:
1. Kidney damage will have caused him to lose most of his serum immune globulins.
2. Adrenocorticosteroids tend to mask symptoms of infection and delay healing.
3. His antistreptolysin-O titer revealed that he is unusually susceptible to streptococcal infections.
4. Massive edema impairs the liver's ability to manufacture antibodies against bacteria.

Tetralogy of Fallot

Timothy Wilt was a full-term baby delivered without complication who was found to have a heart murmur during an early well baby checkup. The physician told Mrs. Wilt that the murmur indicated a possible cardiac defect, and Timothy was referred to the pediatric cardiac clinic for follow-up and a complete cardiac workup at a later date.

Between his second and fourth years Timothy experienced two episodes of cyanosis in conjunction with upper respiratory infections. Between his fourth and fifth years his mother noted that he fatigued easily, was dyspneic on exertion, and squatted during strenuous play. During the same interval the clinic physician noted that Timothy had developed mild finger clubbing and cyanosis.

(ANSWER BLANK ON PAGE A-45)   (CORRECT ANSWERS ON PAGE B-51)

1. Which of the following maternal factors has been implicated as a possible cause of congenital cardiac defects?

1. Rubella during the first trimester of pregnancy.
2. Excessive and rapid weight gain during pregnancy.
3. Hypertension associated with preeclampsia.
4. Metabolic acidosis due to diabetes mellitus.

2. The differentiation of the heart and great vessels occurs during which part of fetal life?

1. Between the 2nd and 10th weeks.
2. Between the 12th and 20th weeks.
3. Between the 22nd and 30th weeks.
4. Between the 32nd and 40th weeks.

3. Cyanosis is caused by:

1. A partial pressure of oxygen in arterial blood of less than 100 mg. Hg.
2. A decrease in red blood cells below 4 million per cu. mm.
3. The presence of more than 3 to 4 grams per 100 ml. of deoxygenated hemoglobin in arterial blood.
4. A relatively greater decrease in white blood cells than in red blood cells.

4. The clinic physician noticed Timothy's cyanosis before Mr. and Mrs. Wilt did because:

1. The cyanosis in tetralogy is so slight that it requires special instruments for detection.
2. Cyanosis is usually caused by emotional stress, like that engendered by exposure to unfamiliar situations.
3. It is difficult to detect fine changes in a person whom one sees daily in familiar situations.
4. Cyanosis is first detected in the conjunctivae and oral mucosa, sites that parents do not usually examine.

5. The club-like appearance of Timothy's fingers derives from:

1. Edema and fibrous tissue proliferation due to peripheral hypoxia.
2. Increased amounts of red bone marrow in the terminal phalanges.
3. Scar tissue repair of infarctions produced by thrombosed capillaries.
4. Exudation of serum proteins through necrotic blood vessel walls.

6. Timothy's easy fatigability was probably due to:

1. Deficient intake of high caloric and high vitamin containing foods.
2. Inadequate development and decreased tone of skeletal muscles.
3. Low blood pressure associated with decreased numbers of red blood cells.
4. Inadequate oxygen to support tissue glucose oxidation for energy.

7. Mrs. Wilt should be taught to make which adjustment to facilitate Timothy's comfort in play activities during the years before cardiac surgery is done?

1. Select adults and sedate older children for play companions.
2. Chaperone him throughout all play to check undue exertion.
3. Provide toys which are light and easy to manipulate.
4. Limit his play to purely intellectual or sensory diversion.

8. The Wilts should be instructed to operate on which of the following principles in disciplining Timothy?

1. Avoid all forms of both physical and verbal discipline.
2. Employ disciplinary measures only when needed to ensure his safety.
3. Refrain from the use of any corporal discipline, such as spanking.
4. Discipline him as they would any of their other children.

When he was five years old and weighed 42 pounds, Timothy was admitted to the hospital for cardiac catheterization, angiocardiography, and possible cardiac surgery. Timothy's blood examination revealed a red cell count of 6 million per cu. mm., hemoglobin concentration of 18 grams per 100 ml., hematocrit of 60 per cent, white cell count of 6300 per cu. mm., with 63 per cent segmented neutrophils, 22 per cent lymphocytes, 5 per cent monocytes, and 10 per cent eosinophils. His urine was normal. Chest x-ray revealed cardiac enlargement, especially of the right ventricle, and decreased pulmonary blood flow. Auscultation of the chest revealed a loud systolic murmur over the precordium. The electrocardiogram was interpreted as indicating right ventricular hypertrophy. The doctor ordered procaine penicillin G 150,000 units I.M. twice a day. On the night before cardiac catheterization the nurse spent extra time with Timothy prior to his bedtime. At 7:00 A.M. on the day of catheterization he was given promethazine hydrochloride (Phenergan) 10 mg. I.M., meperidine hydrochloride (Demerol) 30 mg. I.M., and chlorpromazine (Thorazine) 10 mg. I.M.

9. Timothy's polycythemia can best be understood as an adjustment evoked by his:
1. Cardiac enlargement.
2. Poor dietary intake.
3. Low blood pressure.
4. Tissue oxygen need.

10. Timothy's higher than normal hematocrit was probably a result of his:
1. Dehydration.
2. Polycythemia.
3. Leukocytosis.
4. Hyperproteinemia.

11. The x-ray findings of right ventricular hypertrophy combined with decreased pulmonary blood flow are suggestive of:
1. Tricuspid insufficiency.
2. Pulmonary stenosis.
3. Mitral stenosis.
4. Aortic insufficiency.

12. Hypertrophy of Timothy's myocardium was caused by:
1. Increase in the number of cardiac muscle fibers.
2. Infiltration of inflammatory cells between muscle fibers.
3. Increase in the size of each individual muscle fiber.
4. Distention of the coronary vessels by unusually viscous blood.

13. The systolic murmur heard on auscultation of Timothy's chest was probably caused by:
1. Marked friction of the visceral pericardium against the surface of the heart during the contraction phase of the cardiac cycle.
2. Vibrations produced by blood jetting through the septal defect when pressure is increased by contraction of the ventricles.
3. Abrasion of the parietal pleura of the right lung by the movement of the greatly enlarged right ventricle.
4. Marked sliding of myocardial fibers on one another in contracting forcefully enough to empty the overloaded right heart.

14. It is important for the admitting nurse to learn what information Timothy has been given concerning the proposed hospitalization and surgery in order to:
1. Avoid wasting time and boring Timothy by needless repetition of information already transmitted.
2. Evaluate the intelligence and sensitivity of the Wilt's as a basis for her interactions with them.
3. Predict Timothy's response to certain hospital experiences and to evaluate his responses to care.
4. Duplicate the Wilts' pattern of conveying information, attitudes, and plans for the future to Timothy.

15. In planning Timothy's care in the hospital the nurse should realize that Timothy may be unable to handle the usual frustrations of childhood gracefully because:
a. He lacks self-confidence in his motor and social abilities.
b. He feels anxious concerning his physical welfare and future.
c. His parents have tended to shield him from frustration.
d. His defect has made him overdependent on his parents.
e. Adults have usually capitulated to his requests and demands.
   1. a and b.
   2. c and d.
   3. All but e.
   4. All the above.

16. What is the nurse's responsibility regarding consent for Timothy's cardiac catheterization procedure?
1. Explaining the procedure in detail to Timothy and his parents.
2. Securing Mr. and Mrs. Wilt's verbal approval for the procedure.
3. Ascertaining that the Wilts understand the risks of catheterization.
4. Obtaining the signature of one of the parents signifying informed consent.

17. Which of the following measures might be helpful in reducing Timothy's anxiety concerning the cardiac catheterization procedure?

    a. Giving a clear, simple explanation of the procedure, using a play hospital; doctor, nurse, and patient dolls; and some of the equipment used for the catheterization.

    b. Allowing him to have free and guided play with dolls and selected equipment to display his understanding of the explanation and any evidence of anxiety.

    c. Taking Timothy and his parents on a visit to the catheterization room to see the "machine" and "table" and to meet the staff and technicians.

    d. Encouraging him to talk with another patient who has undergone catheterization in order to preview the situation through another's experience.

        1. a and b.
        2. c and d.
        3. All but d.
        4. All the above.

18. After the cardiac catheterization procedure was described to Timothy he asked the nurse, "Will it hurt?" How should she respond?

    1. "No aspect of the procedure will be in any way painful for you."
    2. "No. It will not be painful but you may be frightened by the equipment."
    3. "I don't really know because this is a procedure which I've never experienced."
    4. "Yes, your leg will hurt for a short time near the beginning of the procedure."

19. Which of the following is the pharmacologic effect of sodium phenobarbital?

    1. Analgesic.
    2. Antispasmodic.
    3. Sedative.
    4. Anticonvulsant.

20. The average adult hypodermic dose of sodium phenobarbital is 100 milligrams. What is a suitable dosage for Timothy?

    1. 15 milligrams.
    2. 30 milligrams.
    3. 45 milligrams.
    4. 60 milligrams.

21. Promethazine hydrochloride (Phenergan) has which of the following pharmacologic effects?

    a. Antihistaminic.
    b. Antiemetic.
    c. Ataractic.
    d. Narcotic potentiator.

        1. a only.
        2. a and b.
        3. All but d.
        4. All the above.

22. For which of the following purposes might promethazine hydrochloride's pharmacologic action be helpful in Timothy's preparation for cardiac catheterization?

    1. To prevent the occurrence of upper respiratory irritation and infection.
    2. To offset hypersensitivity reactions to the intravenous dyes used.
    3. To eliminate arterial spasm in response to catheter insertion.
    4. To decrease bronchial constriction caused by meperidine hydrochloride.

23. Meperidine hydrochloride (Demerol) was given to Timothy for its effect as a:

    1. General anesthetic.
    2. Narcotic antagonist.
    3. Moderate analgesic.
    4. Sympathomimetic.

24. Chlorpromazine (Thorazine) has which of the following pharmacologic effects?

    a. Analgesic.
    b. Antiemetic.
    c. Anticonvulsant.
    d. Tranquilizing.

        1. a and c.
        2. b and d.
        3. a, b, and c.
        4. All the above.

25. Penicillin and streptomycin were given to Timothy before and after cardiac catheterization in order to prevent:

    1. Rhinitis and pharyngitis.
    2. Thrombophlebitis and endocarditis.
    3. Bronchitis and pneumonia.
    4. Gastritis and enteritis.

26. A local anesthetic would be preferred to a general anesthetic for Timothy's cardiac catheterization because the local anesthetic would be:

    1. Less likely to alter cardiac dynamics by depression of respirations.
    2. More effective in alleviating anxiety evoked by the procedure.
    3. Less apt to raise blood pressure to dangerously high levels.
    4. Less painful to administer than a general anesthetic.

27. In Timothy's case the cardiac catheter would probably be introduced through the:

1. Left basilic vein.
2. Left main bronchus.
3. Posterior chest wall.
4. Femoral vein.

28. Nonradiopaque dyes, like Evan's blue or indocyanine green, may be used during cardiac catheterization in order to:

1. Outline cardiac chambers and large thoracic vessels prior to structural identification under fluoroscopic examination.
2. Provide a means of measuring the speed and volume of blood flow through the heart and great vessels.
3. Test the ability of the reticuloendothelial system to remove foreign substances from the circulation.
4. Determine whether large molecules carried in the blood stream are capable of crossing the alveolar membrane.

29. The nurse should observe Timothy carefully for which of the following symptoms of hypersensitivity reaction to the dyes used during the cardiac catheterization?

a. Nausea.
b. Flushing of the skin.
c. Respiratory distress.
d. Pain in the chest.
    1. a only.
    2. a and b.
    3. a, b, and c.
    4. All the above.

30. Angiocardiography can best be described as:

1. A set of chest x-rays taken from various angles with the patient in different positions to reveal the surface contour of the heart.
2. A graphed curve of the oxygen saturation of a series of blood samples obtained from each cardiac chamber and great vessel in sequence.
3. A series of x-ray films illustrating the blood flow through the heart and great vessels, which are outlined by a radiopaque dye.
4. A record of the passage of electrical impulses accompanying contraction from the sino-atrial node to all parts of the myocardium.

31. Timothy's care following cardiac catheterization should include:

a. Frequent check of vital signs.
b. Observation of catheter insertion site for bleeding.
c. Check of pedal and popliteal pulses every 30 minutes.
d. Provision of food and fluid as soon as tolerated.
e. Ambulatory privileges 24 hours after catheterization.
    1. a and b.
    2. c and d.
    3. All but d.
    4. All the above.

32. The nurse should be alert to development of which of the following as possible complications of right heart catheterization?

a. Bacterial infection of the endocardium.
b. Thrombophlebitis of veins traversed by the catheter.
c. Cardiac arrhythmias • of various types and severity.
d. Compression of the heart by hemopericardium.
    1. a and b.
    2. c and d.
    3. All but d.
    4. All the above.

Timothy's catheterization data were interpreted as indicating tetralogy of Fallot with right to left shunt at the ventricular level and increased pressure in the right ventricle. It was decided to attempt surgical repair of Timothy's cardiac defects. One week later, in an open heart procedure using hypothermia and the heart-lung machine, Timothy's ventricular defect was sealed with a Teflon patch, and a pulmonary valvotomy was done.

Upon his arrival in the recovery room Timothy was in good condition with a central venous catheter in place and a blood transfusion running. The doctor connected drainage tubes from the pericardial cavity and from both right and left pleural cavities to water-sealed suction drainage and placed him on a volume controlled respirator with 45 per cent oxygen and high humidification. An intra-arterial line was inserted. The physician ordered:

1. Nothing by mouth.
2. Reinstitute preoperative penicillin.
3. Determine central venous pressure q. h.
4. Vital signs q. 15 minutes until stable.
5. Follow blood transfusion with 5 per cent dextrose in one-quarter strength normal saline I.V.
6. Aspirate nasopharynx q. 2 h. and p.r.n.
7. Determine blood gases q. 4 h.
8. Foley catheter.

33. Tetralogy of Fallot is a syndrome consisting of which of the following combinations of defects?

   1. Right atrial and left atrial hypertrophy, interatrial and interventricular septal defects.

   2. Right ventricular hypertrophy, stenosis of the pulmonary artery, interventricular septal defect, and overriding of the aorta.

   3. Persistence of the embryonic vessel connecting the pulmonary artery to the descending aorta, with hypertrophy of the left ventricle.

   4. Origination of the aorta from the right ventricle and origination of the pulmonary artery from the left ventricle.

34. Preparation of Timothy for surgery should include giving him experience in:

   a. Use of the intermittent positive pressure breathing mask.

   b. Spending some time in an oxygen tent.

   c. Turning from side to side, deep breathing, and coughing.

   d. Passive movement of his extremities through full range of motion.

     1. a and b.

     2. c and d.

     3. All but d.

     4. All the above.

35. What method should the nurse use to inform Timothy about what he will experience in the recovery room following surgery?

   1. Tell him which symptoms he will experience and describe the treatments he will receive.

   2. Show him pictures of the recovery room and the equipment used in the unit.

   3. Show him a movie or filmstrip of a child being cared for in a recovery unit.

   4. Have him turn, cough, and deep breathe a doll to which chest tubes have been attached.

36. In preparing the Wilts to understand Timothy's immediate postoperative care, the nurse should try to warn them of:

   1. The possibility that the surgical procedure might have no effect whatever on his symptoms.

   2. The chance that he might not survive the physiologic stresses of the postoperative period.

   3. The presence of a large number of complex and unfamiliar pieces of equipment at his bedside.

   4. The surgeon's inability to judge the success of the operation immediately after surgery.

37. The nurse could most effectively provide Timothy emotional support concerning his impending surgical operation by conveying to him which of the following ideas?

   1. He will feel no pain or fear during the immediate preoperative or operative period.

   2. A team of highly skilled surgeons will be responsible for doing his surgery.

   3. She will be waiting in the recovery room to care for him when he returns from surgery.

   4. Many other children with similar problems have faced cardiac operations bravely.

38. The purpose for inducing hypothermia before beginning Timothy's operation was to:

   1. Decrease his pain perception by impeding sensory impulse transmission.

   2. Induce sleep by decreasing oxygen and glucose supply to the cerebral cortex.

   3. Decrease tissue oxygen need by lowering the rate of cellular metabolism.

   4. Reduce operative blood loss by causing forceful and prolonged vasoconstriction.

39. The advantage of using a heart-lung machine for Timothy's operation is the fact that the machine:

   1. Eliminates problems involved in administering oxygen concomitantly with an inhalation anesthetic.

   2. Makes possible a bloodless field in which to execute the intricate surgical repairs required.

   3. Enables more effective monitoring of cardiopulmonary functioning during the operation.

   4. Prevents respiratory tract trauma and irritation by avoiding the use of endotracheal intubation.

40. Which of the following pieces of equipment should be kept in Timothy's unit during his immediate postoperative period?

   a. Tracheostomy set.

   b. Thoracentesis set.

   c. Cardiac defibrillator.

   d. Electrocardiography machine.

e. Intermittent positive pressure breathing machine.
   1. a and b.
   2. c, d, and e.
   3. All but e.
   4. All the above.

41. The nurse should check and record Timothy's pulse rates at which of the following points?
   a. Radial artery.
   b. Brachial artery.
   c. Femoral artery.
   d. Dorsalis pedis artery.
      1. a only.
      2. a and b.
      3. a, c, and d.
      4. All the above.

42. In checking to determine whether there is any bleeding from Timothy's thoracic incision the nurse should:
   1. Observe the outer layer of the dressing only, taking pains not to disturb Timothy.
   2. Remove the chest dressing entirely without exerting any tension on the chest tubes.
   3. Raise the lower edge of the dressing in order to visualize the full length of the suture line.
   4. Turn Timothy to his right side to determine whether the lower bed linen is bloody.

43. What precautions should the nurse take in order to prevent interruption of thoracic suction and drainage?
   a. Tape all connections between chest tubes, glass adaptors, and flexible tubing.
   b. Maintain drainage collection receptacle below the level of the mattress at all times.
   c. Check equipment frequently to ascertain whether the fluid level fluctuates in the drainage apparatus.
   d. Keep heavy clamps available at the bedside to occlude the chest tube if it is accidentally disconnected from the drainage tubing.
   e. Tape or pin the drainage tubing to the lower bed linen so as to permit movement without tension on the tubing.
      1. a and c.
      2. b and d.
      3. All but e.
      4. All the above.

44. It is important that Timothy's urinary output be measured hourly during the immediate postoperative period in order to detect any sign of:
   1. Metabolic acidosis.
   2. Bacterial cystitis.
   3. Electrolyte imbalance.
   4. Renal shutdown.

45. If the nurse observes Timothy sucking his thumb she should:
   1. Recognize the action as needed regression and permit him to continue.
   2. Gently remove his thumb from his mouth while diverting him conversationally.
   3. Request permission to offer him ice chips or sips of water by mouth.
   4. Ask the doctor for advice concerning means for breaking the habit.

46. It is important to suction Timothy's nasopharynx at frequent intervals during the immediate postoperative period in order to:
   1. Hasten his recovery from anesthetic depression.
   2. Prevent lung infection by aspirated secretions.
   3. Stimulate the rate and depth of respirations.
   4. Obtain a completely accurate record of fluid output.

47. High humidification of the air Timothy breathes will assist his recovery by:
   1. Soothing irritated laryngeal and tracheal mucosa.
   2. Decreasing his sensation of thirst postoperatively.
   3. Inhibiting the growth of pulmonary pathogens.
   4. Dilating his severely constricted bronchial tree.

48. In order to interpret the significance of Timothy's blood gas concentrations during the first few hours postoperatively, the nurse should know that the normal partial pressure of oxygen in venous blood is:
   1. 15 to 20 mm. Hg.
   2. 25 to 30 mm. Hg.
   3. 35 to 40 mm. Hg.
   4. 45 to 50 mm. Hg.

49. Which of the following would be apt to produce a decrease in venous PO_2?
   a. Inadequate gas exchange.
   b. Loss of blood volume.
   c. Impaired tissue perfusion.
   d. Elevation of blood pressure.
   e. Increase in blood pH.
      1. a and b.
      2. a, b, and c.
      3. All but d.
      4. All the above.

50. The normal partial pressure of oxygen in arterial blood is approximately:
1. 40 mm. Hg.
2. 60 mm. Hg.
3. 80 mm. Hg.
4. 100 mm. Hg.

51. Which of the following symptoms might indicate the development of laryngeal and tracheal edema resulting from trauma by the endotracheal intubation procedure?
a. Wheezy breathing.
b. Croupy cough.
c. Intercostal retractions.
d. Shortness of breath.
e. Cyanosis of the lips and nails.
1. a and b.
2. c and d.
3. All but e.
4. All the above.

52. Timothy's hands may need to be restrained when he is first brought to the recovery room in order to:
1. Give him a sense of physical security against subjective feelings of nausea and vertigo.
2. Keep him from slowing the flow rate of the transfusion by flexing his elbow.
3. Reduce the chance that he might remove the chest tubes either willfully or accidentally.
4. Ensure absolute bedrest by making it impossible for him to move about in bed.

53. The chief danger from overhydrating Timothy postoperatively is the possibility of provoking:
1. Cerebral edema.
2. Congestive heart failure.
3. High blood pressure.
4. Urinary bladder distention.

54 The normal range for central venous pressure is:
1. 5–10 cm. H_2O.
2. 10–15 mm. Hg.
3. 15–20 mg. %.
4. 20–25 mEq./L.

55. The chief danger from underhydrating Timothy postoperatively is the possibility of provoking:
1. Decubitus ulcers.
2. Urinary retention.
3. Intravascular clotting.
4. Kidney stone formation.

56. It is important that Timothy's temperature be kept from increasing postoperatively because hyperthermia:
1. Increases water need to a level requiring oral intake.
2. Raises cellular metabolic rate, oxygen need, and heart rate.
3. Produces irreversible brain damage in patients with poor circulation.
4. Provokes electrolyte imbalance due to salt and water loss in sweat.

57. Portable x-ray equipment will be used to take chest films several times during Timothy's first few postoperative days principally to determine whether:
1. The tips of the thoracic drainage tubes have moved.
2. The Teflon patch remains attached to the ventricular septum.
3. The left lung is gradually re-expanding to normal size.
4. Surgical manipulation of the lung has caused pleurisy.

58. During his first few postoperative days the nurse should observe Timothy closely for symptoms of:
a. Heart failure.
b. Ventricular fibrillation.
c. Circulatory shock.
d. Thoracic hemorrhage.
e. Peripheral emboli.
1. a and b.
2. c and d.
3. All but d.
4. All the above.

59. In instructing the Wilts concerning the care they are to give Timothy following hospital discharge, the nurse must realize that they will have a tendency to:
1. Disbelieve that Timothy is now capable of gradual increase in physical activity.
2. Encourage him in too rapid increase of independence in self-care.
3. Ignore him now that his need for protection has been dramatically reduced.
4. Consider him more vigorous than his undeveloped musculature will permit him to be.

Timothy weathered the immediate postoperative period without complication. His bowel sounds reappeared on the third postoperative day, the respirator was discontinued, and he was given clear liquids to drink. Since his left lung was fully expanded on the fifth postoperative day, the chest tubes were removed. On his seventh postoperative day he was up in a wheel chair for brief periods. On the next day, half the sutures were removed from his thoracic incision. Two days later the remaining sutures were removed and Timothy was permitted to be up at will. Seventeen days after surgery he was discharged and referred back to the pediatric cardiac clinic.

Tonsillectomy

Quincy Howard, a five-year-old boy, had suffered repeated bouts of acute tonsillitis and pharyngitis since the age of two years. He had been given penicillin by the family doctor during several of the more serious of these episodes. Quincy's mother wanted his tonsils removed so he wouldn't miss school the following year. Because the frequency of the infections had increased and because both the tonsils and adenoids were markedly hypertrophied, the family doctor ordered Quincy to the local hospital for a tonsillectomy and adenoidectomy.

(ANSWER BLANK ON PAGE A–47)   (CORRECT ANSWERS ON PAGE B–54)

1. In advising surgical treatment for Quincy at this time the doctor should explain to Mrs. Howard that hypertrophy of the tonsils and adenoids tends to produce:
   a. Mouth breathing.
   b. Chronic pyorrhea.
   c. Otitis media.
   d. Recurrent epistaxis.
   e. Dental caries.
      1. a and c.
      2. a and d.
      3. a, b, c, and e.
      4. All the above.

2. It is also thought that chronically infected tonsils and adenoids may predispose to which of the following diseases in susceptible individuals?
   1. Chronic hypothyroidism.
   2. Rheumatic fever.
   3. Myelogenous leukemia.
   4. Acute appendicitis.

3. Before scheduling Quincy's operation for late summer or early fall the surgeon would check to see whether Quincy has been immunized against:
   1. Influenza.
   2. Tuberculosis.
   3. Poliomyelitis.
   4. Tetanus.

4. When and by whom should Quincy be told about his forthcoming operation?
   1. By the family physician in the doctor's office.
   2. By his parents before admission to the hospital.
   3. By the nurse during the hospital admission procedure.
   4. By his mother on the morning of the operation.

In order to minimize the time that Quincy must spend in the hospital, the doctor arranged for Quincy to be admitted early in the morning on the day of surgery, and the operation was scheduled for 11:00 A.M. Mr. and Mrs. Howard were advised that if no problems developed Quincy would be discharged during the evening of that same day or on the following morning. Routine laboratory tests were done in the doctor's office and the test results were phoned to the hospital.

5. Which of the following explanations of the operation would be best suited to Quincy's need to understand what is going to happen to him?
1. "You will be put into a deep sleep and a surgeon will snip out the infected tissue from your throat. This operation will keep you from having any sore throats which will cause you to miss school."
2. "You will be given a medicine for sleep and your tonsils will be removed. Afterward, your throat will be sore, so you'll be given ice cream to eat. When you're awake and feeling better, you'll go home again."
3. "A doctor will put a mask over your face and give you an anesthetic. While you're unconscious your tonsils will be cut out. When you awaken you will be unable to talk or eat solid food for a while."
4. "You'll be taken on a cart to the operating room, a large, bright room filled with a lot of shiny and interesting equipment. The nurse there will talk to you and the doctor will take care of you."

6. The family doctor or his office nurse should advise Mr. and Mrs. Howard to do which of the following in preparing Quincy for surgery?
1. Withhold all food and liquids from the previous supper and give a cleansing enema early on the day of operation.
2. Withhold only solid food after the previous supper and give a liquid breakfast early on the day of surgery.
3. Give a sedative the evening before surgery and bring Quincy to the hospital next morning without waking him.
4. Carry out feeding and sleeping routines entirely as usual, but push fluids during the twelve hours before surgery.

7. Which of the following laboratory tests should be included as part of Quincy's preoperative work up?
   a. Routine urinalysis.
   b. Complete blood cell count.
   c. Bleeding time determination.
   d. Clotting time determination.
   e. Red cell sedimentation rate.

1. a and b.
2. c and d.
3. All but e.
4. All the above.

8. In order to interpret the significance of Quincy's laboratory test results, the nurse should know that the red blood cell count for a healthy five year old boy is:
1. 6.0 million per cu. mm.
2. 5.4 million per cu. mm.
3. 4.7 million per cu. mm.
4. 4.0 million per cu. mm.

9. The nurse should also know that the normal clotting time, by capillary tube method, is:
1. 1 to 3 minutes.
2. 3 to 6 minutes.
3. 6 to 12 minutes.
4. 12 to 18 minutes.

10. The normal bleeding time is:
1. 1 to 3 minutes.
2. 3 to 6 minutes.
3. 6 to 9 minutes.
4. 9 to 12 minutes.

11. A routine urinalysis includes examination of the urine for which of the following substances?
   a. Glucose.
   b. Albumin.
   c. Casts.
   d. Blood cells.
   e. Phenylketones.
      1. a and b.
      2. b and d.
      3. All but e.
      4. All the above.

12. The value of the red cell sedimentation rate determination as a diagnostic aid derives from the fact that:
1. The presence of increased or abnormal plasma proteins during infectious processes causes agglutination of red blood cells.
2. The increase in numbers of white blood cells coincident with infection results in phagocytosis of erythrocytes.
3. Dehydration produced by febrile diseases causes increased blood viscosity and decreased speed of blood flow through vessels.
4. Bacterial toxins cause premature lysis of circulating red blood cells and release excessive bilirubin into blood serum.

13. The nurse who admits Quincy to the hospital should examine him especially carefully for the presence of which of the following anesthetic hazards?
  1. Loose teeth.
  2. Deviated nasal septum.
  3. Elongated uvula.
  4. Excessive oral secretions.

14. To be prepared to answer Mr. and Mrs. Howard's question concerning the forthcoming operation, the nurse should know that the chief function of tonsillar and adenoidal tissue is:
  1. Manufacture of agranulocytic white blood cells.
  2. Removal of pathogens from the respiratory tract.
  3. Warming and humidification of inspired air.
  4. Improving the volume and resonance of the voice.

According to the doctor's orders, at 10:45 A.M. the floor nurse gave Quincy atropine as a preanesthetic medication and took him to the operating room where he was given an ether anesthetic. His tonsils and adenoids were removed and Quincy was returned unconscious to the recovery room. His doctor left the following postoperative orders:

  1. May have Kool-aid or a popsicle when fully awake if nausea not present.
  2. Aspirin rectal suppository .125 gram q. 4 h. p.r.n. for throat pain.
  3. Ice collar if desired.
  4. May be discharged at 7:00 P.M., if temperature is normal and surgical resident approves release.

15. The average adult dose of atropine given intramuscularly is 0.4 mg. What would be the approximate dose for a five-year-old child? Quincy is 44 inches tall and weighs 42 pounds.
  1. 0.03 to 0.1 mg.
  2. 0.1 to 0.3 mg.
  3. 0.3 to 0.5 mg.
  4. 0.5 to 0.9 mg.

16. The pharmacologic action of atropine which explains its use as a preanesthetic medication for Quincy is its ability to:
  1. Relax spasm of circular smooth muscle fibers.
  2. Decrease production of mucus secretions.
  3. Depress motor and sensory motor cortex.
  4. Decrease the intensity of pain perception.

17. In spite of the fact that the operation had been explained to Quincy, the floor nurse observed that he seemed apprehensive concerning the care he was to receive. What adjustment would it be advisable that the nurse make in administering his preanesthetic medication?
  1. Administer the injection without telling him in advance that he is to receive it.
  2. Take another person into the room to immobilize Quincy while the medication is given.
  3. After entering the room, set the medication down and explain the injection procedure in detail.
  4. Refrain from administering the medication until Quincy reaches the operating room.

18. To provide the greatest possible safety and comfort for Quincy on the way to the operating room the nurse should:
  a. Secure him to the cart with a sheet restraint or strap placed over the abdomen.
  b. Place him on the cart so that his head faces in the direction that the cart moves.
  c. Cover him with a warm, light blanket which is tucked in over his feet, arms, and shoulders.
  d. Stand at the head end of the cart when pushing it through the hall and entering and leaving elevators.
  e. Maintain a running conversation with Quincy throughout the trip to the operating room.
     1. a and b.
     2. b, c, and d.
     3. All but e.
     4. All the above.

19. The recovery room nurse should place Quincy in which position immediately following his return from the operating room?
  1. Supine, with head turned toward the left side.
  2. Supine, with head lowered and knees flexed.
  3. Sitting, with head supported on the over-bed table.
  4. Prone, with head turned to one side.

20. Which of the following observations by the recovery room nurse during the immediate postoperative period should cause her to suspect hemorrhage from the operative site?
- a. Unusual restlessness.
- b. Slow, bounding pulse.
- c. Pale, cool skin.
- d. Greatly constricted pupils.
- e. Frequent swallowing.
    1. a and b.
    2. b and d.
    3. a, c, and e.
    4. All the above.

21. If the recovery room nurse notes the presence of copious quantities of serosanguinous secretions in Quincy's mouth, she should remove them by gentle suctioning in order to:
1. Decrease foul mouth odor and taste.
2. Hasten recovery from the anesthetic.
3. Prevent aspiration of secretions.
4. Aid clot formation in tonsillar fossae.

22. When Quincy awakened he complained of severe throat pain. Which adaptation should the nurse make to minimize the discomfort of aspirin administration?
1. Follow the aspirin suppository with 500 ml. of a prewarmed oily suspension.
2. Crush the suppository and allow it to melt prior to insertion through the tube.
3. Help Quincy to assume the knee-chest position before suppository insertion.
4. Tell Quincy that insertion of the suppository is similar to having his rectal temperature taken.

23. Which of the following effects of cold explain why the application of an ice collar might be expected to reduce Quincy's postoperative discomfort?
- a. Construction of vessels dilated as part of the inflammatory reaction.
- b. Decreased transmission of impulses along sensory nerve fibers.
- c. Improved tone and increased tension of striated muscle fibers.

- d. Prevention of bacterial multiplication in the nasopharynx.
    1. a and b.
    2. c and d.
    3. a, b, and d.
    4. All the above.

Quincy awakened quickly from the anesthetic and recuperated throughout the remainder of the day without evidencing any complications. He was checked by the house staff physician and discharged at 7:30 P.M. on the operative day.

24. Which of the following instructions should the nurse give Mrs. Howard concerning the care that Quincy would need at home during the next few days?
1. Give a high protein, high calorie diet, allow him out of bed, but confine him to his own room.
2. Provide additional rest periods and protect him from exposure to upper respiratory infections.
3. Administer only liquid food and maintain strict bedrest except for bathroom privileges.
4. Return him immediately to full regular feeding, rest, play and social routines.

25. Mrs. Howard said to the nurse, "Quincy has taken this operation real hard. Do you suppose he'll be awhile getting over it?" In order to respond appropriately the nurse should know that the normal five-year-old is:
- a. Physically active, with much aggressive play and fantasy.
- b. Apt to alternate between aggressive and regressive behavior.
- c. Especially fearful of physical pain and physical injury.
- d. Desirous of doing what is expected of him by significant adults.
    1. a only.
    2. a and b.
    3. a, b, and c.
    4. All the above.

Epilepsy

Mrs. Manuel C. de Baca, 30, brought her eight-year-old daughter, Socorro, to the university hospital pediatric clinic for an examination. Mrs. C. de Baca explained, "Socorro acts funny. She drops things, rolls her eyes, and shakes her head sometimes for no reason. I think maybe she has spells."

The clinic nurse who weighed Socorro and took her temperature noted that the child seemed shy and frightened.

(ANSWER BLANK ON PAGE A–49)   (CORRECT ANSWERS ON PAGE B–55)

1. Which approach by the nurse would be most likely to reduce Socorro's discomfort at this time?

1. Directing her conversation to Mrs. C. de Baca alone, relieving Socorro of the need to talk.
2. Guiding Socorro through the weight and temperature taking with gestures rather than words.
3. Drawing Socorro aside for a brief conversation that does not include Mrs. C. de Baca.
4. Inviting Mrs. C. de Baca to accompany Socorro to the small examining room where weight and temperature are taken.

2. In recording a history of Socorro's growth and development on the chart for the clinic doctor's later reference, the nurse should include which of the following points of information relevant to Socorro's present problem?

a. Duration and character of delivery.
b. Age at which breast-feeding ceased.
c. Familial incidence of neurological disease.
d. Number of older siblings in the family.
e. Food idiosyncrasies and intolerances.
   1. a and c.
   2. b and d.
   3. All but e.
   4. All the above.

3. Which of the following disorders in infancy may produce organic brain changes of the type responsible for epilepsy?

a. Intracranial hemorrhage.
b. Cerebral laceration.
c. Asphyxia neonatorum.
d. Bacterial meningitis.
e. Lead encephalopathy.
   1. a and b.
   2. a, b, and c.
   3. All but e.
   4. All the above.

4. The nurse recorded Socorro's height as 48 inches and her weight as 45 pounds. How do Socorro's measurements compare with those of other eight-year-old girls?

1. Much taller than average.
2. Somewhat heavier than average.
3. About average in both measurements.
4. Shorter and smaller than expected.

5. In order to evaluate Socorro's social and psychological level of development the nurse should know that the principal task for the child during the latency period is:

1. Exploring and manipulating his own body parts.
2. Tolerating frustration in small doses.
3. Winning recognition by learning and producing.
4. Beginning separation from his family.

6. Which question by the nurse would probably be most successful in stimulating Socorro to describe her school activities?

1. "Now we need some information about your education. What are you learning in school?"
2. "You've told me that you are in the second grade, Socorro. What kind of things do you do there?"
3. "Socorro, tell me all about your school. I'll bet you like school a lot, don't you?"
4. "How does it happen that you are eight years old and only in the second grade, Socorro?"

In his conversation with Socorro and her mother, the doctor learned that Socorro had two older brothers and three younger sisters, all apparently in good health. Mrs. C. de Baca said, "Socorro's brothers and sisters tease her."

The doctor did a complete physical examination, finding no abnormalities. He then directed Socorro to breathe rapidly in and out for a minute and then hold her breath. A few minutes later Socorro stiffened in her chair, rolling her eyes, hyperextending her neck, and moving her lips soundlessly. A few seconds later, when she again responded to the doctor's questioning, she had no memory of the episode. An electroencephalogram done on the following day revealed a three per second spike and wave pattern typical of petit mal epilepsy.

The physician informed Mrs. C. de Baca that Socorro had a mild seizure disorder. He ordered trimethadione (Tridione) to be given three times a day and asked the nurse to give the needed health instruction. He indicated that Socorro should return to the clinic in two weeks.

7. In understanding the brothers' and sisters' reaction to Socorro's illness the nurse should be aware that:

a. Parents tend to overprotect and indulge their sick or handicapped children.
b. People generally view seizures as a frightening and ominous type of behavior.
c. Lack of sophistication causes children to be more accepting of seizures than adults.
d. Children recognize that humorous treatment of a serious subject renders it less painful.
e. Relatives would not be embarrassed

by Socorro's seizures, though non-relatives might be.

1. a and b.
2. c and d.
3. a, c, and e.
4. b, c, and d.

8. Following a seizure Socorro is likely to be:

1. Confused.
2. Hostile.
3. Hyperactive.
4. Euphoric.

9. The physician's objective in having Socorro breathe rapidly in and out for a minute was to:

1. Produce generalized muscular relaxation.
2. Determine her respiratory reserve.
3. Test her cardiovascular functioning.
4. Precipitate a petit mal seizure.

10. The physiologic effect of Socorro's breathing rapidly in and out for a minute was to:

1. Increase her blood hydrogen ion concentration.
2. Increase her arteriolar blood pressure.
3. Reduce her blood carbon dioxide level.
4. Reduce her cerebral blood volume.

11. The effect of such hyperventilation would be to produce a brief:

1. Cardiac compensation.
2. Cerebral anoxia.
3. Metabolic acidosis.
4. Respiratory alkalosis.

12. When Mrs. C. de Baca learned that Socorro was to have an electroencephalogram done, she asked the nurse, "What is it, the encephalogram?" Which response would be most helpful?

1. "A procedure by which electrodes are attached to Socorro's scalp to pick up and amplify the electrical potential generated by her cerebral cortex."
2. "A test to determine whether the pattern of electrical current generated by Socorro's brain tissue is similar to that of known epileptics."
3. "A painless diagnostic test in which metal plates are attached to Socorro's head and connected to a machine to record the electrical activity in her brain."
4. "A procedure which will enable the physician to determine the exact nature and cause of these spells

which Socorro has been having the past few months."

13. The pharmacologic action of trimethadione explains its use in Socorro's treatment in its ability to:

1. Slow transmission of ascending impulses in the spinal cord.
2. Decrease the excitability of the motor area of the cerebral cortex.
3. Block transmission of impulses through peripheral motor nerves.
4. Inhibit production of acetylcholine at peripheral nerve endings.

14. Trimethadione is preferred to phenobarbital for control of petit mal seizures chiefly because trimethadione:

1. Produces less hypnotic effect.
2. Is considerably less expensive.
3. Never causes toxic manifestations.
4. Exerts strong mood ameliorating effects.

15. Which of the following are possible toxic effects of trimethadione?

a. Nausea.
b. Photophobia.
c. Skin rash.
d. Agranulocytosis.
e. Jaundice.
    1. a only.
    2. b and c.
    3. All but d.
    4. All the above.

16. What should the nurse teach Mrs. C. de Baca about administering trimethadione to Socorro?

1. To pulverize the medication tablet and dissolve it in water before administration.
2. To administer the drug before meals and follow it with large quantities of milk.
3. To refrain from giving the drug when Socorro has upper respiratory infections.
4. To make arrangements with the school nurse to give Socorro the midday dose of medication.

17. If trimethadione should prove ineffective in Socorro's treatment, the physician would be apt to order which of the following drugs to control her seizures?

1. Chlorpromazine.
2. Diphenylhydantoin.
3. Paramethadione.
4. Meprobamate.

18. In order to answer Mrs. C. de Baca's and Socorro's questions concerning the child's illness, the nurse should know that

which of the following statements are true?

a. There is evidence to suggest familial susceptibility to epilepsy.
b. Meningitis and encephalitis may predispose a child to seizures.
c. Traumatic laceration of brain tissue may provoke convulsions.
d. Anoxia of cerebral tissue may institute convulsive episodes.
    1. a and b.
    2. c and d.
    3. a, b, and d.
    4. All the above.

19. What principle should guide the nurse in giving Socorro and her mother instruction concerning needed home care?

1. Transmission of the greatest possible amount of information about epilepsy during the first clinic visit will prevent treatment errors at home.
2. Avoidance of the terms epilepsy, convulsion, and seizure will enable the family to accept Socorro's illness without anxiety.
3. Needed information should be given them in small amounts in each of several successive clinic visits to facilitate assimilation.
4. Socorro and her mother will accept only that information which they request from the nurse by means of direct questioning.

20. Mrs. C. de Baca should be warned that petit mal seizures could be induced by Socorro's exposure to:

1. A blinking light.
2. High humidity.
3. Loud noises.
4. Temperature extremes.

21. Which of the following instructions to Socorro and Mrs. C. de Baca would be most helpful in preventing Socorro's seizures?

1. "On those occasions when Socorro is unusually tired or suffering an infection of some kind, give her a double dose of medicine."
2. "Since extreme fatigue causes seizures in sensitive children, be sure that Socorro has at least ten hours of sleep every night."
3. "If, for some reason, Socorro must be subjected to excitement, encourage her to breathe slowly and deeply in order to relax."
4. "Stimulate Socorro to higher interest levels and greater activity by encouraging physical exercise and increased social activities."

22. What information should be given to Socorro and her mother to ensure Socorro's safety regarding her seizures?

    1. After they have made a record of the pattern of the attacks they will be able to predict the exact time of day the seizure will occur.

    2. Socorro can be helped to identify a group of motor or sensory signs that will precede each attack and warn her to take precautions.

    3. Specially constructed and padded utensils and toys should be used to prevent Socorro's being seriously injured during a seizure.

    4. Socorro need be dissuaded only from those physical activities that would require absolute and continuous mental alertness.

23. The nurse explained to Mrs. C. de Baca that, with the prescribed diet and medication, Socorro's seizures would probably be controlled. However, as a safety precaution she described a typical grand mal convulsion and outlined the care which Socorro would need if she should ever have such an episode. Which of the following are characteristic of a grand mal seizure?

    a. Sudden occurrence of unconsciousness.

    b. Tonic then clonic muscle spasms.

    c. Upward or sideward deviation of the eyes.

    d. Facial pallor or cyanosis.

    e. Urinary or fecal incontinence.

        1. a and b.

        2. a, b, and c.

        3. All but e.

        4. All the above.

24. If Socorro should have a grand mal seizure, the person with her should:

    a. Loosen the clothing about her neck and waist.

    b. Turn her head to the side to facilitate drainage of secretions.

    c. Place a small pillow or folded garment beneath her head.

    d. Remove nearby objects to protect her extremities from injury.

    e. Force a small stick or rag between her clenched teeth.

        1. a and b.

        2. a, b, and c.

        3. All but e.

        4. All the above.

25. Mrs. C. de Baca asked the nurse, "Will this trouble make Socorro slow in school?" Which response by the nurse would be most appropriate?

    1. "Absolutely not. Socorro's disease has nothing to do with her intelligence. Please don't give the matter another thought."

    2. "So long as she has only small seizures they will have no effect on her brain. Therefore she must be treated to prevent big seizures."

    3. "There is no reason to expect the disease to decrease Socorro's ability to learn. Therefore, it is important to treat her as a normal child."

    4. "Because Socorro may become mentally retarded due to brain damage suffered during convulsions, it is important to give the medicine regularly."

Socorro was well controlled on Tridione, having only rare petit mal seizures during the next two years. She came regularly to clinic and, as time passed, seemed to look forward to her bimonthly visits with the clinic doctor and nurse. Because Mrs. C. de Baca and the other family members began to treat Socorro more as a normal child, Socorro came to adopt a matter-of-fact attitude toward her illness, speaking of it rarely, but appropriately.

Leukemia

Mr. and Mrs. MacLeod were shocked to learn that their eight-year-old son, Mike, had leukemia. Mike had been treated for otitis media with antibiotics, but had to be taken back to the doctor because he remained pale and listless. The physician found that Mike had a hemoglobin concentration of 6 grams per 100 ml., a hematocrit of 22 per cent, 62,000 platelets per cu. mm. of blood, and a white blood cell count of 12,500 per cu. mm. with 70 per cent lymphocytes, 12 per cent monocytes, 16 per cent polymorphonuclear neutrophils, and 2 per cent eosinophils.

Suspecting leukemia, the doctor hospitalized Mike. A bone marrow biopsy revealed acute stem cell leukemia, with 50 per cent blasts, 29 per cent promyelocytes, 5 per cent myelocytes, 9 per cent metamyelocytes, 3 per cent bands, and 4 per cent lymphocytes. The admitting nurse learned that during the past year Mike had developed a vesicular rash accompanying each of several upper respiratory infections, and for the past two months had seemed to bruise easily. Mike's admission temperature was 101.6° rectally, pulse 120, respirations 24, and blood pressure 100/60 mm. Hg. He had a small retinal hemorrhage, soggy, bleeding gums, an enlarged liver, several large cervical and inguinal lymph nodes, and petechiae on both lower legs.

(ANSWER BLANK ON PAGE A–51)   (CORRECT ANSWERS ON PAGE B–56)

1. Leukemia is classified as which of the following types of disease?
1. Nutritional.
2. Neoplastic.
3. Infectious.
4. Allergic.

2. The pathophysiologic change underlying the production of symptoms in leukemia is:
1. Progressive replacement of red bone marrow with fibrous connective tissue cells.
2. Phagocytosis of red cells and platelets by overlarge and hyperactive leukocytes.
3. Proliferation and release of immature white blood cells into the circulating blood.
4. Excessive destruction of leukocytes in the liver, spleen, and lymph nodes.

3. In order to interpret the significance of Mike's laboratory test findings, the nurse should know that the normal hemoglobin concentration for an eight-year-old boy is:
1. 6 grams per 100 ml. of blood.
2. 9 grams per 100 ml. of blood.
3. 11 grams per 100 ml. of blood.
4. 14 grams per 100 ml. of blood.

4. Mike's pallor following his recovery from otitis media was a manifestation of:
1. Malnutrition.
2. Infection.
3. Anemia.
4. Hemolysis.

5. The primary cause of Mike's anemia was:

1. Excessive loss of red cells by hemorrhage.
2. Accelerated breakdown of erythrocytes in the spleen.
3. Deficient production of normal red cells by the marrow.
4. Inability of the liver to store iron and vitamins.

6. The hematocrit is a measurement of the:
1. Average size of red cells in the circulating blood.
2. Relative amount of hemoglobin per red blood cell.
3. Percentage of the blood which consists of cellular elements.
4. Ratio of circulating red blood cells to leukocytes.

7. The average hematocrit for a normal eight-year-old is:
1. 10 per cent.
2. 25 per cent.
3. 40 per cent.
4. 55 per cent.

8. How did Mike's anemia contribute to his listlessness?
1. Insufficient oxygen reached tissue cells for proper oxidation of foodstuffs.
2. Lowered blood pressure caused reduced glucose transport to tissue cells.
3. Palpitations and pain consumed inordinate amounts of his available energy.
4. Decreased blood velocity permitted accumulation of toxic cellular wastes.

9. The chief function of neutrophilic granulocytes is:
 1. Initiating fibrous tissue infiltration of tissue defects.
 2. Phagocytosing infectious bacteria and inflammatory debris.
 3. Catalyzing the transition of soluble fibrinogen to fibrin.
 4. Transporting oxygen and foodstuffs to tissue cells.

10. At the time of hospital admission, which of Mike's white blood cell types was most severely reduced in number?
 1. Lymphocytes.
 2. Monocytes.
 3. Neutrophils.
 4. Eosinophils.

11. Mike's retinal hemorrhage and petechiae were probably the result of:
 1. Decreased fibrinogen concentration.
 2. Inadequate blood calcium.
 3. Faulty prothrombin production.
 4. Insufficient numbers of platelets.

12. Mike's elevated temperature on hospital admission was probably the result of:
 1. Dehydration.
 2. Brain damage.
 3. Penicillin sensitivity.
 4. Hypermetabolism.

13. Careful history-taking may reveal that Mike has demonstrated which other symptoms of acute leukemia?
 a. Weight loss.
 b. Bone pain.
 c. Chronic constipation.
 d. Circumoral cyanosis.
 e. Urinary frequency.
   1. a and b.
   2. c and d.
   3. All but e.
   4. All the above.

14. In order to plan Mike's nursing care, the nurse should understand that he would be especially susceptible to infection because:
 1. Anoxic tissues are excessively vulnerable to bacterial ingress.
 2. Enlarged lymph nodes discharge sequestered pathogens into the blood.
 3. Immature leukocytes are unable to phagocytose bacteria normally.
 4. Hypersensitivity reactions make him a poor candidate for antibiotic therapy.

15. Mike's hepatomegaly and lymphadenopathy are probably due to:

1. Infiltration by abnormal leukocytes.
2. Infection by bacteria and viruses.
3. Rapid accumulation of edema fluid.
4. Hemorrhage from fragile capillaries.

16. The sites commonly used for bone marrow biopsies are:
 a. A vertebra.
 b. Radius.
 c. Iliac crest.
 d. Femur.
 e. Skull.
   1. a and c.
   2. b and d.
   3. All but e.
   4. All the above.

The doctor ordered the following:

1. Type and crossmatch.
2. Transfuse with one unit of packed cells.
3. May ambulate 24 hours after transfusion.
4. Diet as tolerated.
5. Chloral hydrate 300 mg. orally H.S., p.r.n.
6. Weigh three times a week.
7. Ampicillin 250 mg. orally, q. 6 h.
8. 6-Mercaptopurine 50 mg. orally, daily.
9. Prednisone 2 mg. orally daily.

17. Mike was given a transfusion of packed cells rather than whole blood in order to:
 1. Provide maximum hemoglobin in minimum additional blood volume.
 2. Avoid administration of antigens responsible for hypersensitivity reactions.
 3. Reduce the time required for completion of the transfusion procedure.
 4. Decrease the expense of treatment by reducing the number of transfusions needed.

18. Administration of large quantities of fluid intravenously might cause Mike to develop high output cardiac failure as a result of his:
 1. Hypermetabolism.
 2. Malnutrition.
 3. Hepatomegaly.
 4. Anemia.

19. Care should be taken to transfuse Mike with blood that has been typed and crossmatched to his own in order to prevent:
 1. Infection.
 2. Agglutination.
 3. Overhydration.
 4. Hemorrhage.

20. Which of the following would be most apt to result from transfusing Mike with incompatible blood?

1. Cerebral hemorrhage.
2. Coronary occlusion.
3. Acute renal failure.
4. Thrombophlebitis.

21. While the transfusion is being administered the nurse should observe Mike for:

  a. Apprehensiveness.
  b. Urticaria.
  c. Chilling.
  d. Backache.
  e. Headache.
    1. a and b.
    2. c and d.
    3. a, c, and e.
    4. All the above.

22. If Mike should develop symptoms of a transfusion reaction the nurse should:

  1. Clamp off the blood and administer normal saline rapidly through the same tubing.
  2. Continue to observe Mike and chart symptoms in the sequence in which they occur.
  3. Slow the rate of the transfusion, give an analgesic, and take his vital signs.
  4. Stop the transfusion, let normal saline run slowly, and notify the physician.

23. In the early stages of Mike's disease, complete bedrest was not ordered. What limitations, if any, should be placed on the amount of his activity?

  1. Enforce long intervals of rest in bed but allow him bathroom privileges.
  2. Encourage him in all but the most physically active games and pastimes.
  3. Allow him to govern his own exercise according to his interest and ability.
  4. Keep him out of bed but in a wheel chair or cart throughout his waking hours.

24. The type of diet that would best meet Mike's nutritional requirements is:

  1. High protein, no fat.
  2. High carbohydrate, low fluid.
  3. High caloric, liquid.
  4. Well-balanced, soft.

25. In order to ensure optimum nutrition for Mike, the nurse might have to circumvent difficulties created by his:

  a. Anorexia.
  b. Gastric hyperacidity.
  c. Buccal ulceration.
  d. Intestinal hypomotility.
  e. Hypermetabolism.

    1. a and c.
    2. b and d.
    3. a, c, and e.
    4. All the above.

26. The principal effect of chloral hydrate is:

  1. Analgesic.
  2. Hypnotic.
  3. Anticonvulsant.
  4. Antihistaminic.

27. Mike should be observed for which of the following as a possible toxic effect of chloral hydrate?

  1. Gastric irritation.
  2. Gingival hypertrophy.
  3. Bronchial spasm.
  4. Clonic convulsions.

28. The nurse should expect to find which of the following on examination of Mike's weight chart over a period of several weeks?

  1. A rapid, steady increase in weight due to increasing amounts of edema formation.
  2. Violent fluctuations in weight due to alternating diuresis and fluid retention.
  3. Gradual decline in weight due to a combination of anorexia and hypermetabolism.
  4. Rapid, excessive weight loss due to diarrhea, vomiting, and glycosuria.

29. Ampicillin differs from penicillin G in that ampicillin:

  1. Disrupts the nucleus rather than inhibiting cell wall formation.
  2. Inhibits certain gram-negative as well as gram-positive organisms.
  3. Is excreted in the feces rather than in the urine.
  4. Will not deteriorate upon standing in solution.

30. The principal effect of 6-mercaptopurine (Purinethol) is to:

  1. Block nucleic acid synthesis in rapidly dividing cells.
  2. Hasten the process of differentiation of blood stem cells.
  3. Foster the lysis of immature leukocytes in the spleen.
  4. Sequester immature white cells in the marrow for a longer period of time.

31. During treatment with 6-mercaptopurine, Mike might be expected to develop:

  1. Hyperglycemia.
  2. Hypercholesterolemia.
  3. Hyperuricemia.
  4. Hypernatremia.

32. Which of the following actions of 6-mercaptopurine render it a potentially dangerous drug?
1. Constriction of smooth muscles of the bronchi.
2. Depression of the vital centers in the medulla.
3. Production of acute ventricular fibrillation.
4. Inhibition of mitosis in normal body cells.

33. Signs of toxicity that may indicate an overdosage of 6-mercaptopurine are:
a. Nausea and vomiting.
b. Tinnitus or deafness.
c. Bloody diarrhea.
d. Motor ataxia.
e. Mucosal ulcerations.
   1. a and b.
   2. c and d.
   3. a, c, and e.
   4. All the above.

34. Which of the following blood findings would cause the physician to temporarily discontinue Mike's daily dosage of 6-mercaptopurine?
1. Lymphocytosis.
2. Leukopenia.
3. Poikilocytosis.
4. Polycythemia.

35. Prednisone was given to Mike in order to produce which of the following effects?
1. Decreased excretion of sodium.
2. Increased liver glycogenolysis.
3. Lysis of abnormal lymphocytes.
4. Enhanced protein anabolism.

During four days of hospitalization Mike's hemoglobin increased from 6 grams to 10 grams per 100 ml., but he ate poorly and complained of homesickness. Mrs. MacLeod, who had visited Mike twice daily in the hospital, was taught the importance of administering the ordered 6-mercaptopurine regularly at home and was directed to bring Mike to the hematology clinic two weeks after hospital discharge.

During the next four months the clinic doctor observed that Mike had brief periods of comparative comfort and well-being, but that his blood picture and general condition seemed to be steadily deteriorating, despite alternating courses of 6-mercaptopurine and cyclophosphamide, and monthly transfusions given on an outpatient basis. Finally Mike developed profound nausea and anorexia, generalized petechiae and mucosal hemorrhages. He was brought to the hospital in critical condition. On admission Mike's hemoglobin was 5 grams per 100 ml., his hematocrit was 18 per cent, and his white blood count was 3500 per cu. mm. with 65 per cent lymphocytes, 8 per cent monocytes, 20 per cent polymorphonuclear leukocytes, and 7 per cent immature forms. A transfusion of packed cells was given and orders were written for tetracycline 200 mg. intramuscularly q.i.d. and vincristine 0.05 mg. per Kg. weekly. The physician told Mr. and Mrs. MacLeod that Mike's condition was hopeless. He died quietly the following evening.

36. The physician arranged for Mike's first period of hospitalization to be kept to a minimum length because:
1. Daily trips to and from the hospital would have been fatiguing and discouraging to his parents.
2. Prolonged hospitalization at that point would have confirmed his parents' fear of his inevitable death.
3. Hospitalization throughout his entire illness would have encouraged undue emotional dependence on others.
4. Early in his illness Mike would be most comfortable and happy in his own home with his parents.

37. Which of the following is a common toxic effect of cyclophosphamide?
1. Urticaria.
2. Alopecia.
3. Jaundice.
4. Convulsions.

38. In order to appreciate Mr. and Mrs. MacLeod's shock at being told that Mike's prognosis was hopeless, the nurse should realize that they had probably interpreted his brief remissions as:
1. Evidence that they had misunderstood the significance of the diagnosis.
2. Fulfillment of their wishes for his complete recovery from leukemia.
3. Resulting from the superior therapeutic abilities of the doctor.
4. Temporary respite from their overwhelming grief and concern.

39. Mrs. MacLeod asked the admitting nurse, "What if I had brought him to the hospital when he first developed an earache? Would that have saved him?" Which of the following would be the most appropriate response?

   1. "No, Mike's ear infection was probably the result and not the cause of his leukemia."

   2. "It's impossible to answer that question. We know almost nothing about the cause of leukemia."

   3. "Don't think about that now. It is too late to wonder what might have been."

   4. "Perhaps later when he has taken care of Mike the doctor will answer your question."

40. Mrs. MacLeod continued, saying, "Well I've got to blame someone or something and I can't blame my husband or God, so I've got to blame myself!" Which response should the nurse use?

   1. "It's hard for me to understand why you say you must blame yourself for Mike's illness. Could you tell me more about that?"

   2. "Look at it this way. Is it any more logical for you to blame yourself for Mike's illness than to blame God or your husband?"

   3. "Don't add to your own or your husband's grief by attributing Mike's illness to your own or his imagined short-comings."

   4. "You don't really mean what you say. It is inconceivable to me that you could blame anyone for a tragedy of this type."

41. Which of the following are essential aspects of Mike's physical care during the terminal phase of his illness?

   a. Gentle turning as required to prevent pneumonia and decubiti.

   b. Isolating him from infectious contacts by reverse isolation technique.

   c. Promoting rest by giving medicines and feedings during waking periods.

   d. Administering mouth care to remove food, blood, and microorganisms.

   e. Encouraging socialization with others to distract him from his symptoms.

     1. a and b.
     2. c and d.
     3. All but e.
     4. All the above.

42. Which of the following means should the nurse avoid when providing mouth care for Mike?

   1. Frequent brushing of his teeth using a soft brush and saline solution.

   2. Encouraging him to rinse out his mouth after meals with a mild mouthwash.

   3. Removing food particles, dried blood, and secretions with cotton-tipped applicators.

   4. Swabbing his buccal cavity, palate, and tongue with a peroxide-soaked gauze square.

43. Which of the following methods would most effectively protect Mike from infection?

   1. Gowning and masking all persons entering his room.

   2. Assigning the same three nurses to care for him day after day.

   3. Limiting his visitors to members of his immediate family.

   4. Administering large doses of several different antibiotics.

44. Teamwork is advisable in providing care for Mike during his fatal illness because:

   1. It would be unwise to burden a single doctor and nurse with so depressing a situation even for a short period of time.

   2. Different personnel from those needed to meet Mike's need must be available to meet the parents' needs.

   3. The complexity of the problems presented requires cooperation among various specialists with common aims but different skills.

   4. The child should be given opportunity to relate to as many persons as possible in the little time left to him.

45. Which of the following is a possible toxic effect of vincristine?

   a. Alopecia.
   b. Constipation.
   c. Foot drop.
   d. Paresthesias.
   e. Bladder atonia.

     1. a and b.
     2. c and d.
     3. All but e.
     4. All the above.

46. Which of the following is the most common cause of death in acute childhood leukemia?

   1. Intracranial hemorrhage.
   2. Spontaneous pneumothorax.
   3. Heart failure.
   4. Acute peritonitis.

47. Why might Mr. and Mrs. MacLeod demonstrate greater difficulty in accepting the idea of Mike's impending death than would Mike himself?
  a. Parents would be apt to feel responsibility for this aspect of their child's life in the same way that they have assumed responsibility for other aspects of his life.
  b. When facing death, children adopt a complacent and accepting attitude toward their impending demise, which constitutes repression of their overwhelming anxiety.
  c. The thought of death is more painful to those who are to be left behind than to the person who is dying, because the survivors anticipate how the loss will alter their lives.
  d. Because children tend to view life on a daily or weekly basis, Mike would be able to maintain his usual view of the future during his terminal illness, though his parents would not.
    1. a and b.
    2. c and d.
    3. a, b, and d.
    4. All the above.

48. Which of the following actions by the MacLeods would most help them to accept the fact of Mike's imminent death?
  a. Expressing their fear and grief.
  b. Describing omissions of needed care.
  c. Remembering family experiences involving Mike.
  d. Attributing Mike's illness to past events.
  e. Expressing their resentment and anger.
    1. a only.
    2. b and d.
    3. a, c, and e.
    4. All the above.

49 The fact that there was a period of time between the establishment of a diagnosis and Mike's death was probably helpful to the MacLeods because:
    1. They had an opportunity to explore the possibility that the diagnosis was inaccurate by reading medical literature and seeking consultation.
    2. Separation occurred over a period of time, allowing a substantial part of the mourning process to take place before Mike's death.
    3. They were able to enlist the help of family and friends in supporting Mike, thus decreasing emotional stresses impinging upon themselves.
    4. There was time to make burial arrangements before Mike's death, relieving them of decisions at the time of their greatest bereavement.

50. Mike himself would be apt to demonstrate which of the following attitudes toward the outcome of his illness?
    1. Extreme irritation and anger.
    2. Strong denial of discomfort.
    3. Passive acceptance and resignation.
    4. Excessive and lachrymose grieving.

51. The nurse may unconsciously avoid Mike when she realizes that he is dying because:
    1. She feels that her time would be more effectively spent in caring for patients who have a chance of recovering.
    2. Dying patients reveal by word and action that they need time alone to confront the threat of imminent death.
    3. Members of the health professions tend to view a patient's death as a thwarting of their occupational aims.
    4. She wishes to relinquish her relationship with him so that he may strengthen his bond with his parents.

52. When dying, Mike is apt to be fearful and feel helpless. Which of the following actions by the nurse would be most supportive to him?
    1. Allowing him to control as many aspects of care as is feasible.
    2. Exploring with him the probable reason for his fearfulness.
    3. Discussing with him the usual feelings of dying children.
    4. Keeping him from making any decisions about his daily care.

53. When it becomes apparent that Mike is moribund the nurse should plan his care so that she:
    1. Withdraws from the room on every possible occasion in order that Mike and his parents may be alone.
    2. May be in the room with Mike and

his parents nearly continuously during the last hours of his life.

3. Can frequently be relieved of her duties on his behalf by other personnel assigned to the unit.

4. Spends no more time in his room than she has on previous occasions when his condition was less severe.

54. In order to be able to effectively assist Mike and his parents to cope with the fact of his death, the nurse must first have:

1. Acquired a deep and unshakable belief in a deity and a life after death.

2. Worked out her own personal philosophy concerning the meaning of life and death.

3. Identified a friend or counselor to whom she can vent her own grief after his death.

4. Reached the conclusion that Mike and his parents will both be benefited by his early death.

Rheumatic Fever

Clifford Wirth thought that his ankle was swollen because he had sprained it playing baseball. When on the following day the other ankle began to swell and both became quite painful, his mother took him to the hospital. The examining physician learned that 13-year-old Clifford had complained of a sore throat two weeks before and that his knees, wrists, and finger joints were swollen and painful, but less so than his ankles. He had a rash on his trunk and thighs. His temperature was 102° F., pulse 136, respirations 24, and blood pressure 115/70 mm. Hg. On physical examination the doctor found Clifford's heart normal in size with a grade two systolic murmur at the apex. His cardiac rhythm was irregular with frequent extrasystoles.

Laboratory tests revealed a hematocrit of 30 per cent, hemoglobin 10.1 grams per 100 ml., white blood cell count 15,000 per cu. mm. with a normal differential, red cell sedimentation rate of 50 mm. per hour, C-reactive protein 4+, antistreptolysin-O titer 625. A throat culture later revealed growth of group A beta-hemolytic streptococci. The physician made a diagnosis of acute rheumatic fever and ordered:

1. Complete bedrest.
2. Footboard.
3. Bed cradle.
4. Acetylsalicylic acid, 20 grains, q.i.d.
5. Benzathine penicillin G (Bicillin), 1.2 million units I.M. stat.

(ANSWER BLANK ON PAGE A–53) (CORRECT ANSWERS ON PAGE B–58)

1. Rheumatic fever is which of the following types of disease?
1. Nutritional.
2. Endocrine.
3. Infectious.
4. Collagen.

2. It is thought that the tissue changes of rheumatic fever occur as a result of:

1. Destruction of body cells by pathogenic bacteria.
2. Hypersensitive reaction to a bacterial antigen.
3. Failure of tissue differentiation due to avitaminosis.
4. Decreased cellular metabolism due to hormonal imbalance.

3. The pathology of rheumatic fever chiefly involves changes in which basic type of tissue?
1. Muscular.
2. Nervous.
3. Connective.
4. Epithelial.

4. Which of the following structures is apt to be involved in acute rheumatic fever?
a. Synovia.
b. Endocardium.
c. Myocardium.
d. Pericardium.
1. a only.
2. a and b.
3. a, b, c.
4. All the above.

5. In obtaining Clifford's health history the nurse should be alert to the mention of which of the following as evidence of previous episodes of rheumatic fever?
a. Watery diarrhea.
b. Growing pains.
c. Frequent epistaxis.
d. Episodic vertigo.
1. a and b.
2. b and c.
3. c and d.
4. All the above.

6. In order to be able to explain Clifford's illness to his parents, the nurse should understand that his joint pathology includes the presence of:
1. Large numbers of rapidly multiplying streptococci.
2. Numerous dead bacteria and polymorphonuclear cells.
3. Massive blood clots and some fresh blood.
4. Excessive synovial fluid and inflammatory cells.

7. Clifford's temperature and pulse rate are characteristic of acute rheumatic fever in that:
1. Both are elevated to a greater degree than would be typical in infection.
2. The pulse elevation is disproportionately greater than the temperature increase.
3. Both are less elevated than would be expected in a seriously ill child.
4. The temperature is elevated to a far greater degree than is the pulse rate.

8. Clifford's skin rash is most apt to be:
1. Erythematous.
2. Maculopapular.
3. Pustular.
4. Vesicular.

9. The level of Clifford's antistreptolysin-O titer indicates that he has:
1. Recently suffered a streptococcic infection.
2. Acquired immunity to streptococcal toxins.
3. Never been exposed to the streptococcus.
4. No body defenses against streptococci.

10. The nurse should observe Clifford carefully for development of which of the following other symptoms of rheumatic fever?
a. Nausea and vomiting.
b. Subcutaneous nodules.
c. Urinary frequency.
d. Choreiform movements.
1. a and c.
2. b and d.
3. All but d.
4. All the above.

11. Clifford's therapeutic program will be directed primarily toward the prevention of which possible complication of his illness?
1. Progressive joint ankylosis.
2. Skeletal muscle contraction.
3. Congestive heart failure.
4. Cerebrovascular hemorrhage.

12. In order to assist in realizing the primary objective of Clifford's hospitalization, the nurse should plan his care so that:
1. He may have long periods of uninterrupted rest during which he is not disturbed for care.
2. She will continuously attend him by going in and out of his room at frequent intervals.
3. Different members of the hospital team are with him at staggered intervals throughout the day.
4. He rapidly assumes responsibility for one after another of the several aspects of his care.

13. The doctor's purpose in giving Clifford benzathine penicillin G (Bicillin) was to:
1. Reverse the tissue changes causing joint symptoms.
2. Destroy bacteria inhabiting the myocardium.
3. Prevent streptococcal infection and rheumatic reactivation.
4. Sterilize the joint effusion and facilitate healing.

14. Which of the following are expected pharmacologic effects of the salicylates?
    a. Analgesic.
    b. Antipyretic.
    c. Antibiotic.
    d. Anticonvulsant.
    e. Antispasmodic.
        1. a and b.
        2. c and d.
        3. All but e.
        4. All the above.

15. Which of the following results may be expected from the administration of salicylates?
    a. Reduction of joint swelling.
    b. Alleviation of joint pain.
    c. Decrease in body temperature.
    d. Decrease in antistreptolysin-O titer.
    e. Increase in hematocrit.
        1. a only.
        2. a, b, and c.
        3. b, c, and d.
        4. All the above.

16. Possible toxic effects of acetylsalicylic acid are:
    a. Headache.
    b. Nausea.
    c. Tinnitus.
    d. Purpura.
    e. Gingival hypertrophy.
        1. a and c.
        2. b and d.
        3. All but e.
        4. All the above.

17. The physician ordered the bed cradle in order to:
    1. Protect Clifford's painful joints from the weight of the bed covers.
    2. Facilitate greater exercise and mobility during Clifford's bedrest.
    3. Suspend a lamp for the application of external heat to the limbs.
    4. Prevent foot drop due to malposition and contracture deformities.

18. In order to minimize Clifford's joint pain the nurse should:
    1. Put all joints through full range of motion twice daily.
    2. Massage the joints briskly with lotion or liniment frequently.
    3. Immobilize the joints in functional position.
    4. Apply warm water bottles or heating pads over involved joints.

19. Clifford would require frequent and scrupulous skin care because he would:
    a. Spend considerable time in a supine or sitting position during hospitalization.
    b. Cooperate with the order for physical immobility only so long as he is comfortable.
    c. Be apt to perspire profusely during the febrile period of his illness.
    d. Excrete increased quantities of salt through the skin due to renal impairment.
        1. a only.
        2. a and b.
        3. a, b, and c.
        4. All the above.

Clifford's joint pain was quickly and dramatically relieved by salicylate therapy. His temperature decreased to normal by his third hospital day, but his pulse only decreased to 104 during the same period. One week after admission, joint pain, heat, and swelling had completely disappeared and the C-reactive protein had decreased to 2+, but the erythrocyte sedimentation rate remained at 50 mm. per hour.

The doctor continued to maintain Clifford on bedrest and was successful in doing so, despite Clifford's natural adolescent resentment of restraint by authoritative adults.

20. The decrease in Clifford's C-reactive protein from 4+ to 2+ can be interpreted to mean that:
    1. He is losing the ability to produce antibodies.
    2. The rheumatic process is decreasing in severity.
    3. Increased numbers of streptococci are being destroyed.
    4. Damaging inflammatory changes are occurring in his liver.

21. Clifford's erythrocyte sedimentation rate is chiefly helpful to the physician in indicating:
    1. Whether or not the streptococci are sensitive to penicillin.
    2. The concentration of streptococci in circulating blood.
    3. The presence of an inflammatory process in the body.
    4. The adequacy of erythrocytes in numbers and size.

22. The nurse should anticipate that after Clifford's joint pain is relieved he will be:
1. Afraid to do anything for himself.
2. Unwilling to remain at complete bedrest.
3. Inclined to develop pain at another site.
4. Disappointed to be symptom-free and independent.

23. Clifford asked the nurse, "Why do I have to stay in bed? I feel okay." What would be the most appropriate response?
1. "You have to stay in bed because the doctor ordered you to. I'm enforcing the rule to protect you from complications."
2. "Rheumatic fever is capable of causing serious heart damage. Unless you remain absolutely still you may develop cardiac disease."
3. "Rheumatic fever causes damage to joint tissue. You must refrain from movement in order to prevent deforming arthritis."
4. "I know it's difficult to remain inactive when you feel well, but rest will ensure your recovery from this temporary illness."

24. The nurse should observe Clifford carefully for indications of congestive heart failure, which include:
a. Dyspnea.
b. Cough.
c. Edema.
d. Cyanosis.
e. Weak pulse.
   1. a only.
   2. a and b.
   3. c and d.
   4. All the above.

25. Which of the following physical changes could be expected to develop with Clifford's pubescence?
a. Increase in size of the genitals.
b. Swelling of breast tissue.
c. Growth of pubic, axillary, facial, and chest hair.
d. Deepening of the voice.
e. Production of spermatozoa.
   1. a and c.
   2. b, d, and e.
   3. a, c, d, and e.
   4. All the above.

26. Since Clifford had experienced normal psychosocial growth up to this point in his life, he should already have developed which of the following?

a. A sense of trust, in that he feels he can count on others to meet his needs.
b. A sense of autonomy, in that he knows he has a mind and will of his own.
c. A sense of initiative, in that he wants to learn to do what he sees others doing.
d. A sense of industry, duty, or accomplishment toward real tasks that he can complete.
e. A sense of identity, in that he has firmly established who he is and what his role in society will be.
   1. a and b.
   2. a, b, and c.
   3. All but e.
   4. All the above.

27. Clifford's primary task during adolescence will be to develop a:
1. Degree of self-discipline.
2. Sense of right and wrong.
3. Lasting sense of well-being.
4. Firm sense of self.

28. Which of the following will Clifford have accomplished if, in fact, he does successfully complete the tasks associated with adolescence?
a. Creation of a satisfactory relationship with girls.
b. Separation from parents and family.
c. Acceptance of his new body image.
d. Integration of his personality toward responsibility.
e. Decision concerning what vocation he will follow.
   1. a and b.
   2. a, b, and c.
   3. All but e.
   4. All the above.

29. During his hospitalization Clifford developed an attitude of detachment, boredom, and negativism, which was probably an attempt to:
1. Call attention to his newly developed masculinity.
2. Mask his anxiety about his illness and future.
3. Act out one aspect of adolescent ambivalence.
4. Cover up his feelings of inferiority and guilt.

30. Clifford asked the nurse, "How important am I to anyone?" Which of the following responses would be most appropriate?

1. "I wonder what prompts you to ask this question now, when you are sick in a hospital and away from home?"
2. "You don't need to worry about your importance to others. I'll stay with you a while to show you that I care for you."
3. "If you are worried about your parents' feelings toward you, you needn't. Today they cried after leaving your room."
4. "It shocks me that you ask this question. You get along well here and are well-liked by everyone."

On Clifford's fifteenth hospital day his pulse rate again increased to 132 and the nurse noticed that he was short of breath. Physical examination revealed an enlarged heart and a grade two systolic murmur at the apex. Chest x-ray with a barium swallow indicated slight enlargement of the left ventricle and left atrium, and marked enlargement of the right ventricle. Electrocardiography also revealed right ventricular enlargement. The doctor made a diagnosis of mitral stenosis with congestive heart failure. He digitalized Clifford and ordered:

1. Absolute bedrest.
2. Digitoxin 0.1 mg. orally, daily.
3. Low sodium diet.
4. Furosemide (Lasix) 40 mg. "O" daily.

31. Clifford's shortness of breath was probably the result of:
1. Obstruction of the glottis due to edema of the mucosa.
2. Compression of the trachea by an enlarged right atrium.
3. Transudation of fluid from the capillaries into the alveoli.
4. Sudden decrease in the number of circulating erythrocytes.

32. A cardiac murmur can best be defined as:
1. An additional heart tone, produced by the rubbing together of inflamed pericardial surfaces.
2. An abnormal heart sound, produced by irregularities in blood flow and valve closure.
3. A dull hum produced by the splashing of increased quantities of pericardial fluid.

4. A rasping noise caused by friction of an enlarged heart against the sternum.

33. Which of the following explanations by the nurse would best meet Clifford's need for understanding the purpose of and procedure for electrocardiography?
1. "The electrocardiogram illustrates transmission of the excitatory impulse across the myocardium, giving information about heart functioning."
2. "The electrocardiogram is a picture of the heart that indicates abnormality in size and shape of the heart and great vessels."
3. "This electrocardiogram is a painless measurement of heart action which will yield information helpful in deciding your treatment."
4. "The electrocardiogram is a highly complex technical procedure which is used in studying the dynamics of various heart disorders."

34. The pharmacologic effect of digitoxin is to increase:
1. The rate of nerve impulse conduction.
2. The force of myocardial contraction.
3. The diameter of coronary arterioles.
4. The number of cardiac muscle fibers.

35. Toxic effects of digitalis are facilitated by a tendency for it to exhibit which of the following effects within the body?
1. Accumulation.
2. Deterioration.
3. Precipitation.
4. Inhibition.

36. Typical symptoms of digitoxin toxicity are:
a. Nausea.
b. Blurred vision.
c. Diarrhea.
d. Disorientation.
  1. a and c.
  2. b and d.
  3. All but d.
  4. All the above.

37. The nurse should be aware that the myocardial depressant effect of digitalis is increased in which of the following conditions?
1. Hypertension.
2. Hypokalemia.
3. Hypothermia.
4. Hyperglycemia.

38. A low sodium diet was ordered for Clifford because:
1. Sodium ions depress impulse transmission across the myocardium.
2. Lowered sodium intake results in improved appetite.
3. Retention of sodium in heart failure increases edema.
4. Sodium antagonizes the cardiotonic effect of digitalis.

39. The pharmacologic effect of furosemide (Lasix) is to:
1. Increase the strength and decrease the rate of myocardial contractions.
2. Block resorption of sodium and water from the renal tubule.
3. Enhance capillary absorption of water from the interstitial spaces.
4. Increase the aperture of cardiac valves by relaxing the chordae tendineae.

After two weeks of digitoxin therapy and continued bedrest, Clifford's heart rate decreased to 86 per minute, and chest x-rays and electrocardiography indicated that his heart size had returned to normal. His sedimentation rate decreased to 20 mm. per hour but the systolic murmur remained unchanged.

Because Mr. and Mrs. Wirth were concerned about the amount of the hospital bill and because Clifford begged to be allowed to go home, the doctor discharged him on a regular daily dosage of digitoxin, listed him with the city's rheumatic fever registry, and scheduled him to return to cardiac clinic monthly for benzathine penicillin G injections and medical followup.

40. Clifford and his parents need information about which of the following as important aspects of his home care program?
a. Protection from infectious contacts.
b. Maintenance of optimal nutrition.
c. Recognition of rheumatic symptoms.
d. Avoidance of physical exercise.
e. Technique for urine analysis.
  1. a only.
  2. a and b.
  3. a, b, and c.
  4. All the above.

41. Clifford and his parents should be taught that it is extremely important for him to avoid future streptococcal infections because:
1. His leukocytes will become progressively less able to phagocytose bacteria.
2. Each subsequent streptococcal infection increases his chances of cardiac damage.
3. His sensitization to streptococci predisposes him to anaphylaxis during subsequent infections.
4. Later streptococcic infections can expected to produce glomerulonephritis.

42. Clifford and his parents should be taught how to take his pulse in order to:
1. Graph daily pulse variations.
2. Determine need for penicillin.
3. Detect digitoxin overdosage.
4. Check effects of exercise.

43. Why did the doctor elect to use monthly benzathine penicillin G injections rather than daily oral penicillin tablets to protect Clifford from subsequent streptococcal infections?
1. The single dose of benzathine penicillin is less expensive than daily doses of oral penicillin.
2. It is less traumatic psychologically for males to take medications parenterally than orally.
3. Rheumatic fever victims feel so well between attacks that they often discontinue prophylactic medications.
4. Clifford will be forced to return to clinic because parenteral medications must be given by a nurse.

Lead Poisoning

Eighteen-month-old Peter Plummer was apparently sleeping when he was brought by his mother to the Emergency Room of a large pediatric hospital. His mother told the nurse that Peter had been ill for several days with nausea, irritability, poor appetite, and muscular incoordination. She said that the child had vomited his breakfast approximately an hour before and had shortly thereafter fallen to the floor "in a fit."

During the intake interview Peter's mother revealed that, prior to this illness, Peter had been an active, apparently healthy child but had frequently been observed to eat non-food items which he had found on the floor. Mrs. Plummer also revealed that she was separated from her husband, was receiving support from Aid to Dependent Children, and was living with her five small children (18 months, 3 years, 4 years, 5 years, and 7 months of age) in a badly run down old tenement building in which there were several areas of chipped paint and falling plaster.

Peter's physical examination revealed a pale, frail child weighing 24 pounds, with a fast pulse, muscle weakness, hyperactive reflexes, and joint pain on movement. Initial laboratory tests revealed a serum lead concentration of 102 mcg.%, a hematocrit of 27%, hemoglobin concentration of 7.6 G.%, white blood cell count of 7000/mm.³, and a platelet count of 120,000/mm.³ His serum glucose, blood urea nitrogen, and serum electrolytes were all within normal limits. X-rays of his long bones revealed a faintly visible "lead line" on Peter's humerus and femur. A flat plate of the abdomen revealed no opacities within the lumen of the gastrointestinal tract. A diagnosis of lead poisoning was made and the following orders were written:

1. B.A.L. (British Anti-Lewisite) 4 mg./Kg. "IM" q. 4 h. for 24 hours.
2. 4 hours after the last dose of B.A.L. start E.D.T.A. (calcium ethylene diamine tetraacetate) 12.5 mg./Kg. "IM" q. 4 h. for 4 days.
3. On the third hospital day start ferrous sulfate gr. 15 "O" t.i.d.
4. Save all urine and test it daily for lead, albumin, and blood.
5. Following 4 days of E.D.T.A. therapy start on penicillamine 100 mg./Kg. per day for 5 days, then
6. Reduce penicillamine to 50 mg./Kg. per day.
7. Diazepam (Valium) 1 mg. "IM" t.i.d.

(ANSWER BLANK ON PAGE A–55)   (CORRECT ANSWERS ON PAGE B–59)

1. Which of the following is the most likely source of Peter's lead intoxication?
1. Inhalation of automobile exhaust fumes.
2. Ingestion of paint and plaster chips.
3. Contact of lead toys with open skin lesions.
4. Ingestion of fruit covered with insect spray.

2. In addition to the foregoing, which of the following are potential sources of lead intoxication?
a. Transmission of water through lead pipes
b. Food storage in lead glazed earthenware.
c. Storage of drinking water in lead lined cisterns.
d. Use of lead soldered vessels for cooking.
e. Inhalation of dust from slum demolition sites.
   1. a only.
   2. a and b only.
   3. All but d.
   4. All the above.

3. Which of the following are thought to be causes of pica (the repetitive search for and ingestion of non-food substances)?
- a. Nutritional inadequacy.
- b. Physiological stress.
- c. Familial predisposition.
- d. Cultural conditioning.
- e. Inadequate mothering.
  1. a and c only.
  2. b and d only.
  3. a, b, and e only.
  4. All the above.

4. The pathophysiology of lead intoxication typically includes:
1. Myocardial ischemia.
2. Hepatic necrosis.
3. Renal calculi.
4. Cerebral edema.

5. Lead is toxic to body tissues as a result of its tendency to:
1. Destroy cell wall structure.
2. Produce chromosomal injury.
3. Coagulate cellular protoplasm.
4. Inactivate cellular enzymes.

6. There is research evidence suggesting that the absorption, retention, and toxicity of lead are increased by:
1. Dietary deficiency of iron and calcium.
2. Imbalance between animal and plant protein.
3. Inadequate intake of oral fluids.
4. Excessive intake of carbohydrates.

7. Peter's nervous irritability during the period preceding hospital admission was probably the result of:
1. Increased rate of cellular metabolism.
2. Frustration of oral dependency needs.
3. Lowering of serum glucose concentration.
4. Increased intracranial pressure.

8. Peter's anemia is most likely the result of:
1. Impaired absorption of iron from the bowel.
2. Inadequate storage of vitamins by the liver.
3. Chronic gastrointestinal tract bleeding.
4. Increased fragility of red blood cells.

9. Which of the following ocular findings would be compatible with the pathophysiology of lead intoxication?
1. Lid lag.
2. Papilledema.
3. Exophthalmos.
4. Conjunctivitis.

10. A more detailed medical history might reveal that Peter had demonstrated which other symptoms of chronic lead intoxication?
- a. Weakness.
- b. Anorexia.
- c. Colic.
- d. Cyanosis.
- e. Muscle incoordination.
  1. a and b only.
  2. c and d only.
  3. All but d.
  4. All the above.

11. The "lead line" seen in Peter's leg and arm bones is the result of:
1. Absorption of lead sulfate into the medullary bone marrow.
2. Fibrotic obliteration of lymphatics which filter lead from the blood.
3. Deposition of lead phosphate along the epiphyseal line.
4. Deposition of additional compact bone along articular surfaces.

12. An x-ray of Peter's abdomen was ordered to check for the presence of:
1. Paint chips.
2. Pyloric obstruction.
3. Intestinal distention.
4. Perforated viscus.

13. During the first few hours following his admission to the hospital, Peter should be carefully observed for the occurrence of:
1. Laryngeal obstruction.
2. Generalized convulsions.
3. Gastric hemorrhage.
4. Urinary suppression.

14. In informing Mrs. Plummer about the effects of lead poisoning, the nurse should explain that his present toxic state will probably cause Peter to demonstrate which of the following during hospitalization?
1. Diminution of visual and auditory acuity.
2. Loss of recently acquired developmental skills.
3. Greatly increased hunger and thirst.
4. Symptoms of psychotic or neurotic withdrawal.

15. As soon as the diagnosis of Peter's illness is confirmed, Mrs. Plummer should be advised to:
1. Move from her present apartment to a dwelling which is in better condition.

2. Bring in the rest of her children for measurement of serum lead levels.

3. Make application to place Peter in an institution for retarded children.

4. Consult a lawyer to initiate suit against her current landlord.

16. When Mrs. Plummer leaves the hospital to go home on the evening of Peter's first day in the hospital, Peter's reaction is most apt to consist of:

1. Stunned disbelief.
2. Panicky crying.
3. Motionless withdrawal.
4. Quiet resignation.

17. The nurse should use which of the following measures to facilitate Peter's getting to sleep when he is put to bed at night?

1. Leave the room lights on and the hall door open until he falls asleep.
2. Give him a cookie to eat or a pacifier to suck on until he becomes drowsy.
3. Sit beside his bed and tell him a story after the lights have been put out.
4. Hold and rock him until he becomes sleepy and put him to bed with a favorite toy.

18. A typical eighteen-month-old child should be able to perform which of the following actions?

a. Sit unaided with head erect.
b. Grasp object by opposing the thumb and fingers.
c. Walk unaided on a flat surface.
d. Engage in cooperative play with other children.
e. Maintain complete bowel and bladder control.
   1. a only.
   2. a and b only.
   3. a, b, and c only.
   4. All the above.

19. Peter can be expected to display which of the following as normal or expected reactions to hospitalization?

a. Grief.
b. Anger.
c. Depression.
d. Anxiety.
e. Regression.
   1. All but b.
   2. All but c.
   3. All but e.
   4. All the above.

20. During his hospitalization Peter would be apt to interpret his mother's absence as:

1. A welcome respite from parental control.
2. Abandonment for previous wrongdoing.
3. An indication that she is also ill.
4. A temporary departure from established routines.

21. In caring for Peter the nurse should employ which of the following measures in order to prevent complications of his illness?

1. Push oral fluids.
2. Avoid unnecessary handling.
3. Apply wrist restraints.
4. Change position frequently.

22. The primary objective of Peter's treatment would be to:

1. Hasten the absorption of lead salts from the intestine.
2. Prevent pathological fractures of lead impregnated bones.
3. Decrease the concentration of lead in blood and nervous tissue.
4. Facilitate storage of lead salts in liver and muscle.

23. Which of the following is a common sequela of inadequately treated chronic lead intoxication?

1. Mental retardation.
2. Cardiac failure.
3. Chronic colitis.
4. Deforming arthritis.

24. Lead is eliminated from the body chiefly by way of the:

1. Skin.
2. Lungs.
3. Intestine.
4. Kidney.

25. The pharmacological effect of calcium ethylene-diamine-tetra-acetate (E.D.T.A.), which explains its use in Peter's treatment, is its tendency to:

1. Produce constriction of small arteries and arterioles.
2. Increase the permeability of glomerular capillaries.
3. Form a non-ionizable compound with lead.
4. Draw interstitial fluid into the intestinal lumen.

26. During treatment with E.D.T.A. Peter should be observed carefully for which symptom of drug toxicity?

1. Jaundice.
2. Purpura.
3. Diarrhea.
4. Albuminuria.

27. Following administration of B.A.L. (British Anti-Lewisite) the nurse should be alert for development of which of the following as an undesirable side effect of the drug?
1. Hypertension.
2. Hyperthyroidism.
3. Hyperpyrexia.
4. Hyperreflexia.

28. The pharmacological effect of penicillamine, which explains its use in Peter's treatment, is its tendency to:
1. Inhibit the mitosis of bacterial cells.
2. Reverse the binding of lead to cellular compounds.
3. Block the deposition of lead in bones.
4. Decrease the energy needs of tissue cells.

29. The action of diazepam, which explains its use in Peter's treatment, is its ability to:
1. Block transmission of pain impulses to the cerebral cortex.
2. Block impulse transmission through the limbic system.
3. Inhibit the motor arm of lower spinal reflexes.
4. Prevent impulse transmission through sympathetic ganglia.

30. Which of the following are possible side effects of diazepam (Valium)?
a. Drowsiness.
b. Ataxia.
c. Dermatitis.
d. Jaundice.
e. Blood dyscrasias.
  1. a and c only.
  2. b and d only.
  3. All but d.
  4. All the above.

31. On his third day in the hospital Peter sent his breakfast back to the kitchen untouched, refused his morning bath, and turned his face to the wall when the nurse attempted to talk to him. His actions were most likely the result of:
1. Toxic effects of medication.
2. Withdrawal and regression.
3. Increasing cerebral edema.
4. Previous social isolation.

32. Peter's serum lead level and his lethargy decreased steadily under E.D.T.A. treatment. On his fifth day of hospitalization Peter was sufficiently improved to be sitting up and playing in his crib when his mother visited. On seeing Mrs. Plummer,

Peter began to cry loudly and threw blocks at her. Distraught, Mrs. Plummer asked the nurse, "What shall I do? He doesn't want me to come near him." Which of the following responses by the nurse would be most helpful to Mrs. Plummer?
1. "He's rejecting you because he feels you abandoned him. Sit on the other side of the room until he gets adjusted to seeing you again."
2. "He acts the same way toward the nurses and doctors. His anger is probably due to nervous tissue irritability."
3. "He's trying to provoke you to anger so he can tell whether you can still love him when he's ill and irritable."
4. "He's angry because he's been separated from you. It's good that he can rid himself of these feelings by expressing them."

On the eleventh day following his admission to the hospital Peter's blood lead level was 32 mcg.%, his hemoglobin was 35 G.%, and his appetite was good. An appointment was made for his mother to bring him to the Pediatric Outpatient Clinic in two weeks, and he was discharged to his home on maintenance doses of penicillamine and ferrous sulfate.

33. In teaching Mrs. Plummer about Peter's nutritional needs after hospital discharge, the nurse should take into account the fact that which of the following is common in the feeding behavior of the normal 18-month-old child?
1. Anorexia.
2. Dysphagia.
3. Regurgitation.
4. Eructations.

34. The best means for increasing Peter's pleasure in eating would be to:
1. Serve him his meals at a different time and place than that of other family members.
2. Encourage him to eat with his fingers rather than with regular utensils and dishes.
3. Allow him to determine the sequence in which he will eat the different foods served him.
4. Permit him to eat as much as he likes of whatever he likes whenever he wants to.

35. Which of the following should be avoided in Peter's diet following hospital discharge?

    a. Coffee.

    b. Nuts.

    c. Chocolate.

    d. Candy.

        1. a and b only.

        2. b and c only.

        3. c and d only.

        4. All the above.

36. In preparing Mrs. Plummer to care for Peter at home, she should be told that the medication he is receiving will cause his stools to become:

    1. Clay colored.

    2. Bright yellow.

    3. Red tinged.

    4. Dark green.

37. Maximum absorption of iron containing medications occurs when the medication is given:

    1. Immediately before a meal.

    2. In conjunction with a meal.

    3. Immediately following a meal.

    4. Midway between meals.

38. In preparing Mrs. Plummer to care for Peter following discharge, the nurse should advise her of the need to supervise his activities more closely so as to prevent his:

    1. Climbing up on furniture.

    2. Putting things into his mouth.

    3. Drinking carbonated beverages.

    4. Becoming chilled or overheated.

39. In order to facilitate Peter's long-term care, a referral should be made to the local health department for:

    1. Assignment of a homemaker to the Plummer family.

    2. Provision of basic nutrition instruction to Mrs. Plummer.

    3. Correction of any building violations in the Plummer apartment.

    4. Increasing the amount of financial support given the Plummer family.

40. In teaching Mrs. Plummer about Peter's postdischarge care, the nurse should stress his need for followup clinic visits, since his disease and the long-term treatment which it requires make him susceptible to:

    a. Decalcification of bones.

    b. Increased red cell fragility.

    c. Episodic cardiac arrhythmias.

    d. Pulmonary infarction and abscess.

    e. Diffuse intravascular clotting.

        1. a and b only.

        2. a, b, and c only.

        3. All but e.

        4. All the above.

41. When she came to get Peter on the day of his discharge from the hospital, Mrs. Plummer told the nurse, "I'll see he doesn't eat any more paint—if I have to hold him on my lap all day!" The nurse should caution Mrs. Plummer against overconfining and overprotecting Peter, since he needs normal play activities in order to:

    a. Develop manual dexterity.

    b. Explore his environment.

    c. Acquire space perception.

    d. Learn problem solving skills.

    e. Handle aggression constructively.

        1. a and b only.

        2. a, b, and c only.

        3. All but e.

        4. All the above.

42. As part of a problem of prophylaxis against lead poisoning, laws have been passed which:

    1. Require the removal of lead water pipes from older buildings.

    2. Prevent the addition of lead to internal combustion fuels.

    3. Prevent the use of lead containing paint on children's toys.

    4. Require labelling of interior paints as to their lead content.

Failure To Thrive

Patty Skelly was nine months old when she was admitted to a pediatric medical unit for weakness and failure to gain weight. Patty's mother, a harried twenty-three year old whose husband had abandoned her six months before with four small children, had brought the child to the hospital at the insistence of a Board of Health nurse, who had given Patty her poliomyelitis vaccine. Mrs. Skelly told the admitting nurse that Patty had been a full term baby, had been 50 cm. long, and had weighed 3.2 kg. at birth. She had gained weight slowly during her first six months; her weight had then held constant for a month or so, and she had lost a pound or two during the month preceding hospitalization. Patty was being fed an Enfamil formula and occasional bites of table food, but had always been a "poor eater" and had frequent "colds" and colic. Patty's health problems had increased in severity during the past three months when Mrs. Skelly had started to work part time as a waitress and had left the children in the care of a high school girl who lived next door. During the admission interview, it became apparent that none of Mrs. Skelly's children had been eating a well-rounded diet, as Mrs. Skelly's financial difficulties frequently made it impossible for her to buy meat, fresh fruit, and milk in sufficient quantity to feed her family.

Physical examination revealed that Patty was 62 cm. long and weighed 6 kg. Her temperature and respirations were normal, her skin was sallow and wrinkled, and her muscles were hypotonic. Her clavicles, ribs, elbows, wrists, sacrum, knees, and ankles were unusually prominent. Her eyes were sunken and her facial features pinched and expressionless. She was apathetic throughout much of the examination, but when lifted and turned, she emitted a thin piercing cry. When allowed to lie undisturbed on the examining table she turned her head rapidly from one side to the other. Mrs. Skelly pointed out a bald spot on Patty's head, which she said was the result of such to and fro motion of the head.

Since physical examination revealed no evidence of a systemic disorder which would account for a feeding difficulty, for impaired intestinal absorption, for impaired food utilization, or for increased caloric expenditure, the physician made a tentative diagnosis of "failure to thrive" and admitted the infant to the hospital for further testing and observation. He ordered that Patty be given a formula and feeding schedule to provide 900 calories and 1000 cc. of fluid per day in four feedings.

(ANSWER BLANK ON PAGE A–57)   (CORRECT ANSWERS ON PAGE B–61)

1. In evaluating the adequacy of Patty's present weight the nurse should know that the usual pattern of weight gain for a normal infant is to:

1. Weigh twice as much as the end of the first year as he did at the time of birth.
2. Double his weight by the end of the sixth month and treble it by the end of the year.
3. Gain weight at much slower than normal rate if the birth weight was lower than normal.
4. Gain weight for the first six months, lose weight for the next three, and gain for the next three.

2. It is generally agreed that the primary cause of the "failure to thrive" syndrome is:

1. Inadequate intake of B complex vitamins.
2. Genetically determined deficiency of digestive enzymes.
3. Inefficient intestinal absorption due to hypermotility.
4. Severely disturbed mother-child relationship.

3. Which of the following mistakes or omissions by Mrs. Skelly has probably contributed most to Patty's failure to thrive?

1. Neglecting to arrange for a quiet environment during rest and sleep periods.
2. Placing undue stress on the need for early bowel and bladder control.
3. Failure to provide sufficient sensory, verbal, and play stimulation.
4. Disregard of Patty's need for supplemental vitamins and minerals.

4. Differential diagnosis of "failure to thrive" syndrome may require ruling out which other causes of malnutrition and/or retarded development?

   a. Thyroid or pituitary deficiency.
   b. Cystic fibrosis.
   c. Congenital heart disease.
   d. Chronic glomerulonephritis.
   e. Certain chromosomal abnormalities.
     1. a and c only.
     2. b and d only.
     3. All but d.
     4. All the above.

5. Which of the following tests would probably be used to rule out urinary tract causes for Patty's malnutrition?

   a. Urinalysis.
   b. Blood urea nitrogen.
   c. Urine specific gravity.
   d. Intravenous pyelogram.
   e. Phenylsulfonphthalein excretion test.
     1. a and b only.
     2. a, b, and c only.
     3. All but e.
     4. All the above.

6. Which of the following are chromosomal abnormalities which may give rise to retarded mental and physical development?

   a. Down's syndrome.
   b. 18 trisomy syndrome.
   c. Hurler's syndrome.
   d. Cushing's syndrome.
   e. Adrenogenital syndrome.
     1. a and b only.
     2. a, b, and c only.
     3. All but d.
     4. All the above.

7. Which of the following childhood diseases would produce increased caloric expenditure?

   a. Parasitic infestation.
   b. Tuberculosis.
   c. Hyperthyroidism.
   d. Diabetes mellitus.
   e. Rickets.
     1. a and b only.
     2. a, b, and c only.
     3. All but e.
     4. All the above.

8. Which of the following childhood diseases results in impaired absorption of nutrients from the small intestine?

   a. Cystic fibrosis.
   b. Disaccharidase deficiency.
   c. Celiac sprue.
   d. Pylorospasm.
   e. Peptic ulcer.
     1. a and b only.
     2. a, b, and c only.
     3. All but e.
     4. All the above.

9. In addition to perverted social response, infants deprived of adequate maternal support often demonstrate which other symptoms of psychological stress?

   a. Abnormal appetite.
   b. Intestinal colic.
   c. Head banging.
   d. Body rocking.
   e. Sleep disturbances.
     1. a and b only.
     2. c and d only.
     3. All but e.
     4. All the above.

10. In evaluating the nature of Patty's illness and determining its cause, members of the health team should observe Mrs. Skelly for evidence of pyschological maladjustment, since it is known that mothers of "failure to thrive" infants are frequently:

   a. Immature.
   b. Insecure.
   c. Depressed.
   d. Withdrawn.
   e. Socially isolated.
     1. a or b only.
     2. c or d only.
     3. Any but e.
     4. Any of the above.

11. In interviewing Patty's mother the physician, nurse, and social worker should be alert for revelation of stress in Mrs. Skelly's life, which could account for difficulty in mothering Patty. Typical examples of such stress would be:

   a. History of early maternal loss.
   b. Conflicts precipitated by separation from parents.
   c. Ambivalence concerning sexual identity.
   d. History of dystocia or postpartum depression.
   e. Doubts concerning her adequacy as a mother.
     1. a and c only.
     2. b and d only.
     3. All but e.
     4. All the above.

12. Which of the following comments by Mrs. Skelly during the admission interview might indicate an inadequate maternal response toward Patty?

1. "I haven't felt very strong for some time now. I guess I had too many babies too close together."
2. "Patty is the smallest of my kids, and the quietest, and the slowest to develop. She's not as strong as the rest."
3. "It's hard to raise kids by yourself. My husband left me with no money and four kids to take care of."
4. "I can't give in and feed her every time she begins to whimper. After all, I don't want to spoil her."

13. In seeking information from Mrs. Skelly concerning the cause of Patty's failure to thrive, it would be most important to investigate Mrs. Skelly's:

1. Long-range plans for Patty's education and upbringing.
2. Memories of the illnesses of her other children.
3. Opinion as to Patty's temperament and personality.
4. Interest in cooking, sewing, and other housewifely activities.

14. Infantile colic is best described as:

1. Passage of frequent liquid stools containing blood and mucus.
2. Invagination of a segment of bowel into an adjacent portion.
3. Paroxysms of abdominal distention and pain accompanied by severe crying.
4. Reverse peristalsis and projectile vomiting due to gastric obstruction.

15. It is thought that infantile colic may be caused or aggravated by:

a. Excessive air swallowing during feedings or crying.
b. Overdistention of bowel with too great volume of formula.
c. Parental anxiety and insecurity regarding child handling.
d. Intestinal allergy to cow's milk.
e. Excessive intake of carbohydrate.
   1. a and b only.
   2. c and d only.
   3. All but d.
   4. All the above.

16. Patty's numerous "colds" were probably the result of:

1. Hypersensitivity reaction to the modified protein of the Enfamil formula.
2. Impaired production of immune globulins due to protein deficiency.
3. Lowered resistance of endothelium to infection due to vitamin A deficiency.
4. Decreased production of white blood cells due to delayed bone growth.

17. Which of the following would be the best way for the admitting room nurse to approach Patty on their first meeting?

1. Immediately pick Patty up and rock her back and forth while talking to her in a quiet tone of voice.
2. Allow Patty to observe her and initiate investigative advances before picking the child up or examining her.
3. Engage Patty in a game of "peek-a-boo" or "pat-a-cake" to relax her and pave the way for the examination.
4. Put Patty on the examining table and hold her arm gently while directing conversation toward Mrs. Skelly.

18. The head rolling movements which the nurse observed Patty engaging in should be interpreted as:

1. A type of stylized ritualistic behavior resulting from mental retardation.
2. A means for physical expression or discharge of overwhelming anxiety.
3. A type of self stimulation which results from sensory deprivation.
4. Jacksonian type seizures resulting from foci of cerebral irritation.

19. Which of the following signs are characteristically seen in malnourished infants?

a. Decreased pulse.
b. Decreased blood pressure.
c. Subnormal temperature.
d. Decreased skin turgor.
e. Disproportionately large head.
   1. a and b only.
   2. a, b, and c only.
   3. All but e.
   4. All the above.

20. On the basis of standard growth curves determined for large numbers of normal infants, a girl weighing seven pounds at birth would be expected to reach what weight within the first nine months of life?

1. 13 to 15 pounds.
2. 15 to 17 pounds.

3. 17 to 19 pounds.

4. 19 to 21 pounds.

21. On the basis of standard growth curves determined for large numbers of normal infants, a girl measuring 50 cm. in length at birth could be expected to reach what length within the first nine months of life?

1. 56–60 cm.

2. 60–64 cm.

3. 64–68 cm.

4. 68–72 cm.

22. In order to evaluate the level of Patty's physical development, the nurse would need to know that by nine months of age the normal infant should be able to:

1. Creep with trunk parallel to the floor, using hands and knees to propel himself forward.

2. Make beginning stepping motions with both legs when held erect so that his feet touch the floor.

3. Walk sideways around furniture or from one chair to another while holding on with one hand.

4. Pull himself to his feet from a sitting position by holding a crib rail for support.

23. According to Erickson, the chief psychological task during the first year of life is the development of a sense of:

1. Trust.

2. Autonomy.

3. Initiative.

4. Industry.

24. In order to evaluate Patty's vocal and social development the nurse must know that by nine months of age the normal infant can be expected to:

1. Recognize adult anger and cry when scolded.

2. Speak one or two words while imitating adult inflection.

3. Repeat a performance which brings an approving response.

4. Play "bye-bye," "pat-a-cake," and similar games.

25. Patty's loss of weight during the month prior to admission was most likely chiefly due to inadequate intake of:

1. Vitamin C.

2. Iron.

3. Protein.

4. Fat.

26. Which of the following is the most likely cause for Patty's discomfort when handled by the nurse?

1. Peripheral polyneuritis due to lack of vitamin B_1.

2. Thinning of skin and subcutaneous tissues due to lack of vitamin A.

3. Decalcification of bones as a result of lack of vitamin D.

4. Subperiosteal hemorrhages due to lack of vitamin C.

27. In observing Patty for clinical evidence of avitaminosis, the nurse should be aware that the milk formula which Patty has been fed is apt to be most deficient in:

1. Vitamin A.

2. Vitamin B complex.

3. Vitamin C.

4. Vitamin D.

28. Patty's irritability on admission to the hospital would be most apt to result from inadequate intake of:

1. Vitamin A.

2. Vitamin B complex.

3. Vitamin C.

4. Vitamin D.

29. The customary milk formula can be expected to meet the infant's daily need for which of the following minerals?

a. Calcium.

b. Sodium.

c. Phosphorus.

d. Iron.

e. Potassium.

1. a and c only.

2. b and d only.

3. All but d.

4. All the above.

30. In order to evaluate the physiological effects of Patty's malnutrition, the nurse should know that typical symptoms of thiamine deficiency are:

a. Tachycardia.

b. Absent knee and ankle jerks.

c. Apathy.

d. Muscle atrophy.

e. Anorexia.

1. a and b only.

2. c and d only.

3. All but e.

4. All the above.

31. The wrinkled condition of Patty's skin on admission was indicative of:

1. Dehydration.

2. Acidosis.

3. Hypoproteinemia.

4. Hypoglycemia.

32. At the time of hospital admission Patty's eyes appeared to be sunken as a result of:

1. Periorbital edema.
2. Loss of retrobulbar fat.
3. Decreased intraocular tension.
4. Decreased thyroid secretion.

33. In planning Patty's nursing care the nurse should take into consideration the fact that the infant learns to recognize and fear strangers at which age?

1. 5–6 months of age.
2. 7–8 months of age.
3. 9–10 months of age.
4. 11–12 months of age.

34. In planning for Patty's care in the hospital, the nurse should take into consideration the fact that at nine months of age the normal infant begins to:

1. Develop temper tantrums when frustrated.
2. Demonstrate a desire for independence in feeding.
3. Fear going to bed and being left alone.
4. Strive for autonomy through negativistic behavior.

35. Careful observation of Patty over a period of time would probably reveal which of the following indications of abnormal social response?

a. Rigid facial expression.
b. No evidence of distress when her mother leaves the room.
c. Intense preoccupation with inanimate objects with neglect of humans.
d. Refusing eye contact by dropping her head or holding her hands over her eyes.
e. Turning away when approached by the nurse or the doctor.
  1. a and b only.
  2. d and e only.
  3. All but c.
  4. All the above.

36. In helping to counteract the negative effects of Patty's sensory deprivation during recent months, the nurse should:

a. Hold and cuddle her at frequent intervals.
b. Give her frequent changes of position and changes of view.
c. Place colorful pictures and mobiles around her crib.
d. Offer her toys presenting a variety of colors, contours, textures, and sounds.
e. Talk and sing to her while giving care and feeding her.
  1. a only.
  2. a, b, and c only.
  3. All but e.
  4. All the above.

37. In watching Mrs. Skelly's interactions with Patty in the hospital the nurse will probably observe that, when Mrs. Skelly feeds her daughter,

1. Patty eats with greater relish than when fed by the nurse.
2. There is little or no eye contact between the two.
3. Mrs. Skelly holds the bottle awkwardly and at the wrong angle.
4. Mrs. Skelly fails to burp the infant at intervals throughout feeding.

38. The nurse should teach Mrs. Skelly that which of the following "table foods" would be suitable additions to Patty's diet following hospital discharge?

a. Cooked wheat cereal.
b. Hard cooked egg yolk.
c. Cooked carrots.
d. Raw ripe banana.
e. Applesauce.
  1. a and c only.
  2. b and d only.
  3. All but e.
  4. All the above.

39. The primary goal of the nurse in dealing with Mrs. Skelly should be to:

1. Instruct her in the principles of optimum nutrition.
2. Encourage her to seek psychological counseling for her problems.
3. Identify social agencies to assist her with financial and social problems.
4. Assist her to find greater satisfaction in mothering Patty.

40. It would be important to provide emotional support and counseling for Mrs. Skelly, both to facilitate correction of Patty's malnutrition and to decrease the chances that Mrs. Skelly will later:

1. Overnourish Patty by too frequent feedings.
2. Compensate for her guilt by overprotecting Patty.
3. Spoil Patty by giving her preferential treatment.
4. Express her rejection of Patty by physical abuse.

41. Which of the following actions by the nurse would be most helpful in improving the quality of the relationship between Mrs. Skelly and Patty?
1. Giving Mrs. Skelly books and pamphlets describing the long-range satisfactions to be derived from child rearing.
2. Providing opportunity for Mrs. Skelly to confide her personal problems and worries in some detail.
3. Showing Mrs. Skelly a movie which depicts pleasurable interplay between a mother and child at feeding time.
4. Arranging for Mrs. Skelly to meet other low income mothers who live in her neighborhood and have similar problems.

Patty ate well and gained weight steadily during the next week. She was quiet, responding slowly to friendly overtures by the ward personnel. Mrs. Skelly visited her daughter for brief periods each afternoon and evening and seemed pleased by Patty's gain in weight. On the tenth day following Patty's admission to the hospital she was discharged to her home with an appointment to be seen in Pediatric Clinic during the following week.

42. Which of the following actions by the nurse would be most effective in providing psychological support for Mrs. Skelly following Patty's discharge from the hospital?
1. Give her a card indicating the address and telephone number of a physician to whom she should bring Patty if problems develop.
2. Invite her to stop by with Patty to visit the ward nursing staff whenever she is in the neighborhood of the hospital.
3. Arrange for a public health nurse who has been given a resumé of Patty's case to visit the home weekly for follow-up care and supervision.
4. Encourage her to join the local block club, P.T.A. or Sunday School in her neighborhood and to become friendly with other women of her own age.

BIBLIOGRAPHY   PEDIATRIC NURSING

Alfonso, D., and Harris, T.: Continuous positive airway pressure. American Journal of Nursing, 76:570–573, April, 1976.

Altshuler, A.: Complete transposition of the great arteries. American Journal of Nursing, 71:96–98, January 1971.

Asperheim, M., and Eisenhauer, L.: The Pharmacologic Basis of Patient Care. Philadelphia, W. B. Saunders Company, 1977.

Avery, G. B.: Neonatology—Pathophysiology and Management of the Newborn. Philadelphia, J. B. Lippincott Co., 1975.

Behrman, R. E.: Neonatal-Perinatal Medicine—Diseases of the Fetus and Infant, 2nd ed. St. Louis, C. V. Mosby Co., 1977.

Bellam, G.: The first year of life. American Journal of Nursing, 69:1244–1246, June 1969.

Bergersen, B., and Krug, E.: Pharmacology in Nursing. 11th ed. St. Louis, C. V. Mosby Co., 1969.

Betson, C., Valoon, P., and Soika, C.: Cardiac surgery on neonates: a change for life. American Journal of Nursing, 69:69–73, January 1969.

Bowlby, J.: Separation anxiety. International Journal of Psychoanalysis, 41:89–113, March-June 1960.

Breckenridge, M., and Murphy, M.: Growth and Development of the Young Child, 8th ed. Philadelphia, W. B. Saunders Company, 1969.

Brody, E.: Minority Group Adolescents in the United States. Baltimore, Williams and Wilkins, 1968.

Brown, J., and Hepler, R.: Stimulation, a corollary to physical care. American Journal of Nursing, 76:578–581, April, 1976.

Campbell, J.: Nursing children with hydrocephalus. Nursing Times, September 13, 1965, pp. 1139–1140.

Campbell, L.: Special behavioral problems of the burned child. American Journal of Nursing, 76:220–224, January, 1976.

Caplan, G.: Patterns of parental response to the crisis of premature birth. Psychiatry, 23:365–374, 1960.

Caplan, G., Mason, E., and Kaplan, D.: Four studies in crisis in parents of prematures. Community Mental Health Journal, 1:149–161, Summer 1965.

Cardwell, V. E.: Cerebral Palsy. Springfield, Illinois, Charles C Thomas, 1965.

Carlson, C. E., ed.: Behavioral Concepts and Nursing Intervention. Philadelphia, J. B. Lippincott Co., 1970.

Caskey, K., Blaylock, E., and Wauson, B.: The school nurse and drug abusers. Nursing Outlook, 18:27–30, December 1970.

Chodoff, P.: Understanding and management of the chronically ill. I. American Practitioner, 13:136–144, February 1962.

Chodoff, P.: Understanding and management of the chronically ill. II. American Practitioner, 13:165–170, March 1962.

Chodoff, P., et al.: Stress, defenses and coping behavior: observations in parents of children with malignant disease. American Journal of Psychiatry, 120:743–749, 1964.

Coffin, M. A.: Nursing Observations of the Young Patient. Dubuque, Iowa, William C. Brown, 1970.

Conn, H., ed.: Current Therapy 1977. Philadelphia, W. B. Saunders Company, 1977.

Conway, A., and Williams, T.: Parenteral alimentation. American Journal of Nursing, 76:574–577, April 1976.

Cornfeld, D., and Schwartz, M. W.: Nephrosis: a long term study of children treated with corticosteroids. Journal of Pediatrics, 68:507–515, April 1966.

Davidsohn, I., and Henry, J. B., eds.: Todd-Sanford Clinical Diagnosis by Laboratory Methods. 15th ed. Philadelphia, W. B. Saunders Co., 1974.

Debuskey, M., ed.: The Chronically Ill Child and His Family. Springfield, Illinois, Charles C Thomas, 1971.

Dewey, J.: Eighteen ways to live with asthma. Nursing, 75:48–51, April 1975.

Dlin, B. M., Fischer, H., and Huddel, B.: Psychologic adaptation to pacemaker and open heart surgery. Archives of General Psychiatry, 19:599, 1968.

Dobrin, R. S., Larsen, C. D., and Holliday, M.: The critically ill child: acute renal failure. Pediatrics, 48:286–293, August 1971.

Drillen, C. M.: The small-for-date infant: etiology and prognosis. Pediatric Clinics of North America, 17:9, February 1970.

Duc, G.: Assessment of hypoxia in the newborn. Pediatrics, 48:469–481, September 1971.

Duncan, G., ed.: Diseases of Metabolism, 6th ed. Philadelphia, W. B. Saunders Co., 1969.

Eason, W. M.: The Dying Child. Springfield, Illinois, Charles C Thomas, 1970.

Eckstein, H.: Congenital pyloric stenosis. Nursing Mirror, 29:v–vi, July 1966.

Engel, G.: Grief and grieving. American Journal of Nursing, 64:93–98, September 1964.

Erikson, E. H.: Childhood and Society. 2nd ed. New York, W. W. Norton Co., 1963.

Evans, F. M.: Psychosocial Nursing. New York, The Macmillan Co., 1971.

Falconer, M. et al.: The Drug, the Nurse, the Patient, 5th ed. Philadelphia, W. B. Saunders Company, 1974.

Farson, R., Hauser, P., Stroup, H., and Wiener, A.: The Future of the Family. New York, Family Service Association, 1969.

Feifel, H., ed.: The Meaning of Death. New York, McGraw-Hill Book Co., 1959.

Finnie, N.: Handling the Young Cerebral Palsied Child at Home. Ed. by Una Haynes. New York, E. P. Dutton, 1970.

Goffman, E.: Stigma. Englewood Cliffs, N. J., Prentice Hall Inc., 1963.

Goldfarb, A.: Puberty. Clinical Obstetrics and Gynecology, 11:769, September 1968.

Goldfogel, L.: Working with the parent of a dying child. American Journal of Nursing, 70:1675–1679, August 1970.

Goldman, L., and Gilman, A., eds.: The Pharmacological Basis of Therapeutics. 4th ed. New York, The Macmillan Co., 1970.

Goodman, L. S., and Gilman, A.: The Pharmacological Basis of Therapeutics, 5th ed. New York, Macmillan Co., 1975.

Goodwin, J. W., Gooden, J. O., and Chance, G. W.: Perinatal Medicine – the Basic Science Underlying Clinical Practice. Baltimore, Williams and Wilkins Co., 1976.

Grant, J., Moir, E., and Fago, M.: Parenteral hyperalimentation. American Journal of Nursing, 69:2392–2395, November 1969.

Group for the Advancement of Psychiatry: Normal Adolescence: Its Dynamics and Impact. New York, Charles Scribner's Sons, 1968.

Guyton, A. C.: Textbook of Medical Physiology. 4th ed. Philadelphia, W. B. Saunders Co., 1971.

Hammar, S., and Holterman, V.: Interviewing and counseling adolescent patients. Clinical Pediatrics, 9:47, January 1970.

Hamovith, M.: The Parent and the Fatally Ill Child. Los Angeles, Delmar, 1968.

Hazan, S. J.: Psychiatric complications following cardiac surgery. I. Journal of Thoracic Cardiovascular Surgery, 51:307, 1966.

Hirt, M., ed.: Psychological and Allergic Aspects of Asthma. Springfield, Illinois, Charles C Thomas, 1965.

Hoffman-LaRoche, Inc.: Aspects of Anxiety, 2nd ed. Philadelphia, J. B. Lippincott Co., 1971.

Holt, K. S.: Assessment of Cerebral Palsy. London, Lloyd-Luke, Ltd., 1965.

Hunn, V. K.: Cardiac pacemakers. American Journal of Nursing, 69:749–754, April 1969.

James, E. E.: The nursing care of the open heart patient. Nursing Clinics of North America, 2:543–558, September 1967.

Johnson, M., and Fassett, B.: Bronchopulmonary hygiene in cystic fibrosis. American Journal of Nursing, 69:320–324, February 1969.

Keats, S.: Cerebral Palsy. Springfield, Illinois. Charles C Thomas, 1965.

Khurana, R., and White, P.: Juvenile onset diabetes. Postgraduate Medicine, 49:118–123, April 1971.

Klaus, M., and Fanaroff, A.: Care of the High Risk Neonate. Philadelphia, W. B. Saunders Company, 1973.

Klaus, M. H., and Kennell, J. H.: Maternal-Infant Bonding. St. Louis, C. V. Mosby Co., 1976.

Krause, M., and Hunscher, M.: Food, Nutrition and Diet Therapy. 5th ed. Philadelphia, W. B. Saunders Co., 1972.

Laing, J.: The Management and Nursing of Burns. London, English University Press, 1967.

Larsen, V.: Stresses of the childbearing years. American Journal of Public Health, 56:32, January 1966.

Larson, D., and Gaston, R.: Current trends in the care of burned patients. The American Journal of Nursing, 67:319–327, February 1967.

Lederer, H.: How the sick view their world. Journal of Social Issues, 8:4–10, 1952.

Lesser, A.: Health of Children of School Age. Washington, D. C., U. S. Department of Health, Education, and Welfare. Children's Bureau Publication No. 427, 1964.

Levesque, L.: Nurse's role in croup management. Hospital Topics, 39:66–67, November 1961.

Lightwood, R.: Paterson's Sick Children. 9th ed. Philadelphia, J. B. Lippincott Co., 1971.

Lindeman, E.: Symptomatology and management of acute grief. American Journal of Psychiatry, 101:141–148, September 1944.

Lovelock, P.: Sick children at home. The Canadian Nurse, 61:623–627, August 1965.

Lubchenco, L. O.: Assessment of gestational age and development at birth. Pediatric Clinics of North America, 17:125–145, 1970.

Lyons, L. M.: Repair of cleft lip. Nursing Times, 62:563–564, April 29, 1966.

MacBryde, C., ed.: Signs and Symptoms: Applied Pathologic Physiology and Clinical Interpretation. 4th ed. Philadelphia, J. B. Lippincott Co., 1964.

Marlow, D. R.: Textbook of Pediatric Nursing. 5th ed. Philadelphia, W. B. Saunders Co., 1977.

Masoro, E., and Siegel, P. D.: Acid Base Regulation: Its Physiology and Pathophysiology. Philadelphia, W. B. Saunders Co., 1971.

Matthews, L., Doershuk, C., and Spector, S.: Mist tent therapy of the obstructive pulmonary lesion of cystic fibrosis. Pediatrics, 39:176–185, February 1967.

Maxwell, P., Linss, M., McDonnough, P., and Kinder, J.: Routines on the burn ward. American Journal of Nursing, 66:522–525, March 1966.

Merritt, H. H.: A Textbook of Neurology. 4th ed. Philadelphia, Lea and Febiger, 1967.

Minckley, B. B.: Expert nursing care for burned patients. American Journal of Nursing, 67:104–107, January 1967.

Moore, M.: Diabetes in children. The American Journal of Nursing, 67:104–107, January 1967.

Morrissey, J.: Death anxiety in children with a fatal illness. American Journal of Psychotherapy, 18:606–615, 1964.

Mussen, P. H., ed.: Carmichael's Manual of Child Psychology. Vols. 1 and 2. 3rd ed. New York, J. Wiley and Sons, 1971.

Nyhan, W.: The treatment of acute lymphocytic leukemia. Journal of Pediatrics, 68:969–970, June 1966.

Ollstein, R., et al.: Burns and their treatment: management of burned patients—a demanding form of nursing care. Hospital Management, 111:1, 22–39, January 1971.

Ollstein, R., et al.: The burn center concept: total patient care is the keystone of an effective burn center. Hospital Management, 111:1, 22–26, February-March 1971.

Osofsky, H. J.: Somatic, hormonal changes during adolescence. Hospital Topics, 46:95, April 1968.

Pendleton, T., and Simonson, J.: Training children with cerebral palsy. American Journal of Nursing, *64*:126–129, May 1964.

Peplau, H.: Interpersonal Relations in Nursing. New York. G. P. Putnam's Sons, 1952.

Reed, A.: Lead poisoning: silent epidemic and social crime. American Journal of Nursing, *72*:2181–2184, December, 1972.

Robinson, C. N.: Fundamentals of Normal Nutrition. New York, The Macmillan Co., 1968.

Rogenes, P., and Moylan, J.: Restoring fluid balance in the patient with severe burns. American Journal of Nursing, *76*:1952–1957, December 1976.

Ross, E. K.: What is it like to be dying? American Journal of Nursing, *71*:54–61, January 1971.

Rubin, M.: Balm for burned children. American Journal of Nursing, *66*:297–302, February 1966.

Rudolph, A. M., Barnett, H. L., and Einhorn, A. H.: Pediatrics, 16th ed. New York, Appleton-Century-Crofts, 1977.

Ruess, A. L.: Behavioral aspects of the physically handicapped child. Journal of the American Physical Therapy Association, *42*:163–167, March 1962.

Schaffer, A.: Diseases of the Newborn, 4th ed. Philadelphia, W. B. Saunders Company, 1977.

Schneer, H. I.: The Asthmatic Child. New York, Harper and Row, 1963.

Schonfeld, W. A.: Body image in adolescents: a psychological concept for the pediatrician. Pediatrics, *31*:845–855, May 1963.

Schwab, L., Callison, C., and Frank, M.: Cystic fibrosis. American Journal of Nursing, *63*:62–69, February 1963.

Shrand, H.: Hydrocephalus. Nursing Times, *59*:1136–1138, September 13, 1963.

Smith, D., and Bierman, E.: The Biologic Ages of Man. Philadelphia, W. B. Saunders Company, 1973.

Smith, D. T., Conant, N. F., and Overman, J. R.: Zinsser Microbiology. 13th ed. New York, Appleton-Century-Crofts, 1964.

Sodeman, W., and Sodeman, W., Jr.: Pathologic Physiology. 4th ed. Philadelphia, W. B. Saunders Co., 1967.

Sutow, W., Sullivan, M., and Taylor, G.: Status of present treatment for acute leukemia in children. Cancer Research, *25*:1481–1490, October 1965.

Tait, B.: Diet therapy in renal failure. Journal of Practical Nursing, *26*:23–25, February, 1976.

Thomas, J., and Ulpis, E.: A seasonal hazard: laryngotracheobronchitis. American Journal of Nursing, *61*:52–54, March 1961.

Traisman, H., and Newcomb, A.: Management of Juvenile Diabetes Mellitus. St. Louis, C. V. Mosby Co., 1965.

Ujhely, G. B.: Grief and depression: implications for preventive and therapeutic nursing care. Nursing Forum, *5*:28, 1966.

Varvaro, F.: Teaching the patient about open heart surgery. American Journal of Nursing, *65*:111–115, October 1965.

Vaughn, V. C., and McKay, R. J.: Nelson Textbook of Pediatrics, 10th ed. Philadelphia, W. B. Saunders Company, 1975.

Verwoerdt, A.: Communication with the fatally ill. Ca: A Cancer Journal for Clinicians, *15*:105–111, May-June 1965.

Waechter, E., and Blake, F.: Nursing Care of Children. 9th ed. New York, J. B. Lippincott, 1976.

Waring, W., Brunt, C. H., and Helman, B.: Mucoid impaction of the bronchi in cystic fibrosis. Pediatrics, *39*:166–175, February 1967.

Waters, W. R.: The patient with severe burns. The Canadian Nurse, *61*:367–371, May 1965.

Whaley, L. F., and Wong, D. L.: Nursing Care of Infants and Children. St. Louis, C. V. Mosby Co., 1979.

Willman, V.: Anatomy and physiology of the heart in congenital heart disease. American Journal of Nursing, *60*:190–193, February 1960.

Willson, M.: Multidisciplinary problems of meningomyelocele and hydrocephalus. Journal of the American Physical Therapy Association, *45*:1139–1146, December 1965.

Wilson, A., et al.: Whooping cough: difficulties in diagnosis and ineffectiveness of immunization. British Medical Journal, *2*:623–626, September 11, 1965.

Wintrobe, M. M., et al.: Harrison's Principles of Internal Medicine. 6th ed. New York, McGraw-Hill Book Co., 1970.

Yashon, D., and Sugar, O.: Today's problems in hydrocephalus. Archives of Diseases in Childhood, *39*:58–60, 1964.

Young, D. S., and Hicks, J. M.: The Neonate. New York, J. Wiley and Sons, 1976.

3
MEDICAL-SURGICAL NURSING

Coronary Heart Disease

Mr. John Powers, a portly 55-year-old businessman, consulted his private physician concerning episodes of pressing, choking chest pain. On the basis of a medical history and a complete physical examination, the physician made a diagnosis of arteriosclerotic heart disease with angina pectoris.

(ANSWER BLANK ON PAGE A–59)   (CORRECT ANSWERS ON PAGE B–63)

1. Characteristically, the onset of angina pectoris causes a person to:
  1. Breathe deeply.
  2. Bend forward.
  3. Become immobile.
  4. Lose balance.

2. Angina pectoris is caused by:
  1. Friction between the visceral and parietal pericardia.
  2. A decrease in the alveolar surface for gas exchange.
  3. Increased blood pressure in the pulmonary circulation.
  4. An inadequate supply of oxygen to the myocardium.

3. Which of the following would be most apt to precipitate Mr. Powers' anginal attacks?
  1. Alcoholic intake.
  2. Psychological depression.
  3. Change of position.
  4. Physical exertion.

4. In addition to the foregoing, which of the following often provoke angina pectoris?
  a. Strong emotion.
  b. Eating a heavy meal.
  c. Exposure to cold.
  d. Recumbent position.
  e. Exposure to sunlight.
    1. a and b.
    2. a, b, and c.
    3. All but d.
    4. All the above.

5. Mr. Powers' chest pain would be apt to radiate toward the:
  a. Right axilla.
  b. Left shoulder.
  c. Neck.
  d. Left fifth finger.
  e. Umbilicus.
    1. a, b, and c.
    2. b, c, and d.
    3. c, d, and e.
    4. All the above.

6. Mr. Powers did not consult his physician when he first began to experience angina. Probably this delay resulted from his:
  1. High threshold for physical pain and discomfort.
  2. Denial of the significance of the pain.
  3. Disinclination to react quickly to changed circumstances.
  4. Fear that the symptom was psychosomatic in origin.

In addition the doctor wrote a prescription for nitroglycerin and instructed Mr. Powers to use the medication as often as necessary to relieve chest pain. He advised Mr. Powers to decrease his physical activities and to obtain more rest. The office nurse instructed Mr. Powers in administration of the nitroglycerin.

7. In advising Mr. Powers to decrease his physical activities, the doctor would probably instruct him to especially avoid:
  1. Driving a car.
  2. Shoveling snow.
  3. Carrying groceries.
  4. Climbing stairs.

8. The chief pharmacologic action of nitroglycerin is to:
  1. Constrict cardiac chambers.
  2. Stimulate myocardial fibers.
  3. Accelerate cardiac contraction.
  4. Dilate coronary arteries.

9. The usual dose of nitroglycerin is:
  1. 60 mg.
  2. 6.0 mg.
  3. 0.6 mg.
  4. 0.06 mg.

10. Mr. Powers should be instructed to take the ordered dose of nitroglycerin:
   a. Whenever he begins to experience chest pain.
   b. Before each meal and before going to bed.
   c. Whenever he can foresee stress which may cause angina.
   d. At approximately three-hour intervals throughout the day.
   e. When he is unable to relieve chest pain by resting.
      1. a and c.
      2. b and d.
      3. c and e.
      4. All the above.

11. Following her instruction regarding administration of nitroglycerin, Mr. Powers told the office nurse, "I'll try not to take too many of the pills." Which response by the nurse would be most helpful at this point?
   1. "There is some danger of addiction to nitroglycerin, so take a pill only when you have severe chest pain."
   2. "You should restrict yourself to no more than 5 pills each day in order to prevent drug overdose."
   3. "Allow at least a four hour interval between doses of nitroglycerin. More frequent doses may produce a toxic reaction."
   4. "Nitroglycerin is nonhabituating. You will be safe in taking a pill whenever you feel the onset of chest pain."

12. Mr. Powers should be instructed to protect his nitroglycerin pills from deterioration by keeping them:
   a. In a dark environment.
   b. In an airtight container.
   c. In a cool place.
   d. In a metal box.
   e. In a plastic envelope.
      1. a only.
      2. a, b, and c.
      3. All but e.
      4. All the above.

13. When taking his nitroglycerin tablets, Mr. Powers should be taught to:
   1. Hold the tablet under his tongue and refrain from swallowing until the tablet is dissolved.
   2. Crush the tablet and dissolve it in a copious amount of water before swallowing it.
   3. Swallow the tablet quickly, using a minimum of liquid to facilitate its ingestion.
   4. Imbed the tablet in food before ingestion and follow it with a drink of milk.

14. The nurse should explain to Mr. Powers that after taking nitroglycerin he may expect pain relief in approximately:
   1. 2 to 3 seconds.
   2. 20 to 30 seconds.
   3. 2 to 3 minutes.
   4. 20 to 30 minutes.

15. During her conversation with Mr. Powers, the nurse should explain that a possible untoward reaction to nitroglycerin is:
   1. Nausea.
   2. Headache.
   3. Drowsiness.
   4. Tinnitus.

16. Mr. Powers should be instructed that, if administration of a nitroglycerin tablet fails to bring relief of anginal pain in 5 to 10 minutes:
   1. The physician should be notified.
   2. The dosage should be repeated.
   3. Ten grains of aspirin should be taken.
   4. He should be taken to a hospital.

17. Which of the following is a long-acting nitrate medication which is occasionally given to prevent anginal attacks?
   1. Amyl nitrate.
   2. Pentaerythritol tetranitrate.
   3. Silver nitrate.
   4. Nitrofurantoin.

18. The physician will probably advise Mr. Powers to:
   a. Lose weight.
   b. Avoid alcohol.
   c. Stop smoking.
   d. Stop golfing.
   e. Avoid salt.
      1. a and c.
      2. b and d.
      3. c and e.
      4. All the above.

19. Mr. Powers asked the office nurse why he must avoid strenuous outdoor activity. To answer his question the nurse must understand that:
   1. External cold produces cutaneous vasodilation.
   2. Exercise increases skeletal muscle oxygen need.

3. Lowered temperature accelerates chemical reactions.
4. Physical exertion increases peristaltic activity.

20. It is thought that regular mild exercise may be beneficial to a patient with ischemic heart disease by:
1. Increasing the thickness of the cardiac muscle.
2. Causing dilation of the lower cardiac chambers.
3. Accelerating development of myocardial collateral circulation.
4. Decreasing glycogen stores in the myocardium.

21. The physician and nurse should advise Mr. Powers to:
1. Avoid any physical activity other than that essential to his family and work roles.
2. Pace himself so the degree of his physical discomfort is less than that which provokes chest pain.
3. Gradually increase his activities to to the point that he finally resumes his premorbid life pattern.
4. Relinquish as many as possible of his household and employment activities to other persons.

One month after consulting his physician Mr. Powers was awakened from sleep by agonizing substernal pain. He continued to have chest pain throughout the next day. Because his usual dose of nitroglycerin did not afford relief, Mrs. Powers finally called the doctor to report her husband's condition. The physician made a tentative diagnosis of coronary occlusion and ordered an ambulance to take Mr. Powers to the local hospital immediately.

22. Typically, the pain of coronary occlusion differs from that of angina pectoris in that the former is:
1. Intermittent in nature.
2. More apt to radiate.
3. More responsive to rest.
4. Less often provoked by exertion.

23. Mr. Powers should be observed for development of which of the following symptoms, which often follow myocardial infarction?
a. Pallor.
b. Diaphoresis.
c. Anxiety.
d. Breathlessness.
e. Vomiting.
   1. a and c.
   2. b and d.
   3. All but e.
   4. All the above.

When Mr. Powers arrived at the hospital, he was admitted to a private room. His own physician performed a physical examination and an electrocardiogram, confirming the diagnosis of myocardial infarction. Mr. Powers' temperature was 99.4° F. orally, pulse 92 per minute, respirations 22 per minute, blood pressure 110/70 mm. Hg. (His doctor recalled that Mr. Powers' usual blood pressure was approximately 130/86 mm. Hg.) His white blood cell count was 12,000 per cubic millimeter.

24. An electrocardiogram is a recording of the:
1. Difference between systolic and diastolic pressures.
2. Transmission of nervous impulses over the myocardium.
3. Vibrations created by closure of the cardiac valves.
4. Volume of coronary artery blood flow.

25. Mr. Powers asked the nurse the purpose of the electrocardiogram. Which of the following replies would be most appropriate?
1. "This tracing of heart action will help guide us in caring for you."
2. "This measure of cardiac efficiency will enable the doctor to predict your recovery rate."
3. "This test of heart impairment will indicate the degree of permanent damage to your heart."
4. "This record of heart damage will identify the cause of your cardiac disorder."

26. A myocardial infarction consists of:
1. Dilation of heart chambers.
2. Irritation of heart covering.
3. Necrosis of heart muscle.
4. Destruction of a heart valve.

27. Myocardial infarction usually results from a:
1. Critical reduction in blood supply.
2. Marked increase in muscle metabolism.
3. Sudden irregularity of cardiac contraction.
4. Gradual reversal of impulse conduction.

28. In planning long-term care for Mr. Powers, the nurse should be aware that which of the following are possible complications of a myocardial infarction?
  a. Congestive failure.
  b. Hypertensive crisis.
  c. Ventricular fibrillation.
  d. Hemopericardium.
  e. Cardiac arrest.
      1. a and b.
      2. c and d.
      3. All but b.
      4. All the above.

29. Mrs. Powers asked the nurse the reason for Mr. Powers' heart attack. In order to reply helpfully, the nurse should know that coronary occlusion is usually the result of:
  1. Increased viscosity of the blood.
  2. Deceleration of the blood flow.
  3. Bacterial irritation of the endothelium.
  4. Atheromatous vessel wall plaques.

30. Mr. Powers' myocardial infarction may unconsciously represent which of the following to him?
  a. A threat of castration.
  b. A shameful weakness.
  c. A state of helplessness.
  d. A form of punishment.
  e. An escape from competition.
      1. a and c.
      2. b and d.
      3. All but e.
      4. All the above.

The doctor wrote the following orders for Mr. Powers:

1. Attach to cardiac monitor.
2. Morphine sulfate 10 mg. H. stat. and q. 4 h. p.r.n.
3. Oxygen by nasal catheter.
4. Absolute bedrest. No visitors but Mrs. Powers.
5. Heparin sodium 50 mg. I.V. stat. and again in 6 hours.
6. Warfarin (Coumadin) 50 mg. orally tomorrow morning.
7. Coagulation time determination stat. and q. 6 h. times 6.
8. Prothrombin time determination 24 hours after first dose of Coumadin and q. A.M. thereafter.
9. Serum C.P.K. determination stat. and q.d.
10. Serum G.O.T. determination stat. and q.d.
11. Serum G.P.T. determination stat. and q.d.
12. Serum L.D.H. determination stat. and q.d.
13. Vital signs q. 4 h., apical-radial pulse determinations q. 4 h.
14. No hot or cold liquids.
15. Phenobarbital 30 mg. orally q.i.d.
16. Milk of magnesia 30 cc. q. h.s.

31. Morphine was given to Mr. Powers in order to:
  1. Reduce his pulse rate to a normal level.
  2. Prevent reflex coronary spasm due to pain.
  3. Increase the force of cardiac contraction.
  4. Relax smooth muscle in blood vessel walls.

32. The pharmacologic effect of morphine is to:
  1. Relieve pain locally by reversing inflammatory tissue changes.
  2. Inactivate neural transmitters released at the myoneural junction.
  3. Block transmission of sensory impulses through the spinal cord.
  4. Raise the threshold of the cerebral cortex to pain signals.

33. In observing Mr. Powers, the nurse should know that which of the following symptoms would be most suggestive of an idiosyncratic reaction to morphine?
  1. Decreased respirations.
  2. Progressive drowsiness.
  3. Generalized pruritus.
  4. Constriction of pupils.

34. Before administering each dose of morphine sulfate to Mr. Powers the nurse should:
  1. Check his pulse.
  2. Count his respirations.
  3. Note his skin color.
  4. Offer oral fluids.

35. Mr. Powers was given several doses of morphine during the first three days of his hospitalization. Which of the following symptoms would be most suggestive of morphine toxicity?
  1. Hot, dry skin.
  2. Rapid weak pulse.
  3. Periodic apnea.
  4. Widely dilated pupils.

36. Oxygen was ordered for Mr. Powers in an effort to:
  1. Minimize the extent of myocardial necrosis.
  2. Increase the caliber of coronary arteries.

3. Enhance the force of myocardial contraction.
4. Decrease the bulk of cardiac muscle fibers.

37. When oxygen is administered by nasal catheter, the flowmeter should be set to supply oxygen at:
1. 2 to 4 liters per minute.
2. 4 to 6 liters per minute.
3. 6 to 8 liters per minute.
4. 8 to 10 liters per minute.

38. In order to protect Mr. Powers from hazards deriving from the use of oxygen therapy, the nurse should:
1. Remove all pillows from his bed.
2. Cover his shoulders with a shawl.
3. Apply a hot water bottle to his feet.
4. Place a "No Smoking" sign on his door.

39. The nurse should interpret the order for absolute bedrest to mean that Mr. Powers may be allowed to:
a. Feed himself.
b. Brush his teeth.
c. Comb his hair.
d. Wash his face.
   1. a only.
   2. a and b.
   3. All the above.
   4. None of the above.

40. Palpation of Mr. Powers' radial artery will reveal no information about:
1. Pulse volume.
2. Pulse rate.
3. Pulse deficit.
4. Pulse rhythm.

41. Mr. Powers' apical and radial pulse rates should be counted during the same minute by two nurses because:
1. The rate of either pulse may vary from minute to minute.
2. This arrangement causes less strain for the patient.
3. This method provides a check against the counts of both nurses.
4. This procedure reduces the expenditure of nursing time.

42. A considerable difference between the apical and radial pulse rates would indicate:
1. Stronger left than right ventricular muscle.
2. Numerous weak ineffectual cardiac contractions.
3. Thickened myocardium and large heart chambers.

4. Increased pressure in the systemic arteries.

43. The pharmacologic effect of heparin is to:
1. Bind ionized calcium in the serum.
2. Prevent release of platelets from the marrow.
3. Inhibit prothrombin formation by the liver.
4. Prevent conversion of fibrinogen to fibrin.

44. In addition to the foregoing, heparin produces which other effect which would be helpful to Mr. Powers?
1. Relieves spasm of smooth muscle fibers.
2. Decreases lipid concentration in the serum.
3. Increases the permeability of capillary endothelium.
4. Improves the oxygen-binding capacity of hemoglobin.

45. Warfarin (Coumadin) was ordered for Mr. Powers in order to:
1. Relieve pain from myocardial damage.
2. Increase the caliber of coronary vessels.
3. Improve the strength of heart contraction.
4. Prevent extension of the coronary thrombus.

46. The pharmacologic effect of warfarin (Coumadin) is to:
1. Inhibit cholinesterase production.
2. Interfere with prothrombin formation.
3. Liquefy the necrotic area of myocardium.
4. Block conversion of fibrinogen to fibrin.

47. The physician will order future doses of warfarin on the basis of measurements of Mr. Powers':
1. Clotting time.
2. Prothrombin time.
3. Bleeding time.
4. Capillary fragility.

48. In observing Mr. Powers for untoward effects of continued use of warfarin, the nurse should be particularly alert to the occurrence of:
1. Headache.
2. Vomiting.
3. Cloudy urine.
4. Pruritus.

49. In assessing Mr. Powers' illness, his serum enzyme concentrations would be used to determine whether or not:

1. Microcirculation had been impeded as a result of a systemic coagulation defect.
2. Metabolic acidosis had developed as a consequence of impaired tissue perfusion.
3. Coronary flow had been sufficiently reduced to cause death of heart muscle fibers.
4. Renal tubular damage had resulted from decreased arterial blood pressure.

50. Which of the following positions would be least taxing to Mr. Powers' damaged heart?

1. Supine, with his head raised 20 degrees and his arms supported on pillows.
2. Flat on his back with the foot of the bed slightly elevated.
3. Lying on his left side with his right arm supported on pillows.
4. Lying on his right side with his left leg elevated on pillows.

Mr. Powers slept at intervals during his first night in the hospital. On the morning following admission he required morphine to relieve substernal pain. He then slept soundly until noon when, despite the nurse's objections, he insisted that he be brought water with which to bathe himself.

51. Which of the following mental mechanisms probably prompted Mr. Powers' insistence that he bathe himself?

1. Suppression.
2. Denial.
3. Projection.
4. Sublimation.

52. What comment by the nurse would be most helpful to Mr. Powers at this time?

1. "Your doctor left orders that you must not exert yourself at all."
2. "Your condition is so serious that any activity would be dangerous."
3. "Don't worry about my bathing you. It's a regular routine for me."
4. "I realize that you'd rather bathe yourself, but you may not do so today."

53. On the morning following his admission to the hospital, the nurse should determine Mr. Powers' temperature by:

1. Placing the thermometer under the tongue for five minutes.
2. Holding a thermometer in his axilla for five minutes.
3. Inserting a thermometer into the rectum for five minutes.
4. Laying her hand on his forehead for a few seconds.

54. Which of the following nursing measures would be of greatest importance in treating Mr. Powers during his first few days in the hospital?

1. Giving the prescribed warfarin.
2. Providing absolute rest.
3. Restriction of fluid intake.
4. Provision of low sodium diet.

Serum enzyme concentrations immediately following Mr. Powers' admission were only minimally elevated, but by the third hospital day his serum G.O.T. and L.D.H. levels were 149 and 1070 units per ml. of blood, respectively. An electrocardiogram taken on the third day revealed inversion of T waves and ST complex depression. Prothrombin time varied but was stabilized at 28 seconds after one and one-half weeks of treatment. During his first week of hospitalization Mr. Powers was given passive exercise and was directed to flex and extend his toes, fingers, and hands. During his second week of hospitalization he was allowed to sit up in a chair and walk around his room.

55. On Mr. Powers' fourth hospital day the nurse's aide who had assisted in making the bed said to the nurse, "Mr. Powers hasn't had any pain today and says that he feels all right. Why must he still stay in bed?" Which of the following answers would be most accurate?

1. "He has recovered from that attack but is prone to others. Therefore he must remain in the hospital while he is taught how to reduce his activities and conserve his energy."
2. "A part of his heart muscle has died because its blood supply was shut off. The dead tissue will liquefy and be removed. It will take several weeks for scar tissue to close the defect."
3. "We can't be sure that he has recovered from the attack until his doctor takes another electrocardiogram. Perhaps then he will be allowed to care for himself at home."

4. "His heart has recovered, but he was left apprehensive by the attack. It will take some time before he feels confident enough to begin to do things for himself again."

56. During the first week of his illness, Mr. Powers' diet is apt to be:
1. General diet without coffee or tea.
2. High calorie, high protein, low fat diet.
3. Small, soft, bland feedings five times daily.
4. Alkaline ash diet with increased liquids.

At 7:00 a.m. on the eighth day after admission the nurse found Mr. Powers slumped against the bed siderail, coughing and gasping for breath. His pulse was 120 and irregular, respirations were 26 and shallow, and his lips and nailbeds were cyanotic. The doctor was notified. Auscultation of Mr. Powers' chest revealed moist rales and weak heart tones. His blood pressure was 90/60 mm. Hg, and chest x-ray revealed cardiac dilation. An electrocardiogram indicated strain patterns. The doctor gave Mr. Powers morphine sulfate 10 mg. "IV," digitalized him using deslanoside (Cedilanid-D) parenterally, and placed him on Digoxin 0.5 mg. "O" and Lasix 40 mg. "O" Q day. Continuous cardiac monitoring was resumed, and a catheter was inserted for measuring central venous pressure.

57. The most likely explanation for Mr. Powers' present symptoms is that he has:
1. Become resistant to warfarin.
2. Been incorrectly positioned.
3. Developed congestive failure.
4. Contracted bronchial pneumonia.

58. Which of the following would the doctor be able to detect on physical examination?
a. Increase in heart size.
b. Impairment of valvular function.
c. Disturbance of heart rhythm.
d. Presence of pulmonary edema.
e. Weakness of cardiac contraction.
    1. a and c.
    2. b and d.
    3. All but e.
    4. All the above.

59. Mr. Powers' current blood pressure level probably results from the fact that:
1. Physical inactivity has decreased smooth muscle tone.

2. Administration of morphine has eliminated psychic stress.
3. The damaged myocardium is unable to contract forcefully.
4. Warfarin has produced generalized dilation of vessels.

60. Mr. Powers' dyspnea is primarily due to:
1. Accumulation of serous fluid in alveolar spaces.
2. Obstruction of bronchi by mucoid secretions.
3. Compression of lung tissue by a dilated heart.
4. Restriction of respiratory movement by ascites.

61. The physician instituted continuous cardiac monitoring for Mr. Powers chiefly to detect indications of impending:
1. Digitalis toxicity.
2. Cardiac recompensation.
3. Ventricular fibrillation.
4. Myocardial rupture.

62. As a consequence of his myocardial infarction Mr. Powers might develop which of the following arrhythmias?
a. Atrial flutter.
b. Atrial fibrillation.
c. Nodal rhythm.
d. Heart block.
e. Premature ventricular contractions.
    1. a and b.
    2. a, b, and c.
    3. All but d.
    4. All the above.

63. Which of the following electrocardiographic characteristics is typical of atrial flutter?
1. No P wave preceding every other QRS complex.
2. Many more P waves than QRS complexes.
3. Widening and distortion of QRS complex.
4. T waves directed oppositely to QRS complex.

64. Which of the following electrocardiographic characteristics is typical of first degree heart block?
1. PR interval longer than 0.2 seconds.
2. Inversion of the T wave.
3. Widening of QRS complex.
4. Twice as many P waves as QRS complexes.

65. Which of the following electrocardiographic characteristics is typical of second degree heart block?
1. PR interval longer than 0.2 seconds.
2. Inversion of the T waves.
3. Widening of QRS complex.
4. Twice as many P waves as QRS complexes.

66. Which of the following electrocardiographic features is characteristic of premature ventricular contractions?
a. No preceding P wave.
b. Widened, distorted QRS complex.
c. Compensatory pause following the PVC.
d. PR interval longer than 0.2 seconds.
e. 2 to 3 times as many P waves as QRS complexes.
1. a and b.
2. a, b, and c.
3. All but e.
4. All the above.

67. In the event that Mr. Powers should develop cardiac arrest when the nurse is alone in the room with him, she should:
a. Clear the airway of secretions and dentures.
b. Institute mouth to mouth respirations.
c. Give him a strong blow on the chest.
d. Begin external cardiac compression.
e. Summon help and notify the doctor.
1. a and c.
2. b and d.
3. All but d.
4. All the above.

68. Mr. Powers' cyanosis was the result of:
1. Decreased speed of blood flow.
2. Increased amount of reduced hemoglobin.
3. Decreased venous blood pressure.
4. Increased viscosity of the blood.

69. It is thought that edema develops in congestive heart failure as a consequence of:
a. Elevated hydrostatic pressure in capillaries distal to distended veins.
b. Inability of the congested liver to produce an adequate quantity of albumin.
c. Retention of sodium and water by the inadequately perfused kidney.
d. Decreased osmotic pressure of the blood secondary to anemia.
1. a and c.
2. b and d.
3. All but d.
4. All the above.

70. Edema due to cardiac failure tends to be:
1. Painful.
2. Non-pitting.
3. Dependent.
4. Periorbital.

71. Mr. Powers' edema would render him especially prone to:
1. Dorsiflexion of the feet.
2. Muscle hyperirritability.
3. Saphenous thrombosis.
4. Decubiti in the sacral area.

72. Which of the following signs would suggest development of digitalis intoxication?
1. Orthostatic hypotension.
2. Exfoliative dermatitis.
3. Pulsus bigeminus.
4. Intention tremor.

73. Which of the following is thought to be the site of action of furosemide (Lasix)?
1. Proximal tubule.
2. Ascending loop of Henle.
3. Distal tubule.
4. Collecting duct.

74. Furosemide (Lasix) is classified as a diuretic of which type?
1. Osmotic.
2. Aldosterone antagonist.
3. Carbonic anhydrase inhibitor.
4. Potassium sparing.

75. Which of the following is a possible adverse side effect of furosemide?
1. Arrhythmia.
2. Deafness.
3. Orthostatic hypotension.
4. Paresthesias.

76. Measurement of which of the following would provide the best indicator of the therapeutic effectiveness of furosemide administration?
1. 24-hour urine output.
2. Decrease in diastolic blood pressure.
3. Concentration of sodium in the urine.
4. Change in urine specific gravity.

77. When properly positioned, the tip of the central venous pressure catheter should be located in the:
1. External jugular vein.
2. Right atrium.
3. Right ventricle.
4. Pulmonary artery.

Mr. Powers made a slow but steady recovery from cardiac failure. Following a week of intensive treatment, oxygen and continuous monitoring were discontinued and he was gradually permitted to assume minimal self-care activities. During his fourth week of hospitalization Mr. Powers participated more actively in physical therapy. Serum enzymes had dropped to within the normal range by the end of his fourth week of illness.

78. In measuring Mr. Powers' central venous pressure it would be important to place the zero line of the manometer at the level of his:
  1. Carotid bifurcation.
  2. Suprasternal notch.
  3. Angle of Louis.
  4. Right atrium.

79. The normal range for central venous pressure is from:
  1. 4 to 10 cm. H_2O.
  2. 10 to 30 mm. Hg.
  3. 50 to 70 cm. H_2O.
  4. 90 to 110 mm. Hg.

80. Central venous pressure readings would be most helpful in making inferences concerning:
  1. Right heart efficiency.
  2. Myocardial impulse conduction.
  3. Coronary blood flow.
  4. Perfusion of peripheral tissues.

81. In preparing Mr. Powers for sleep during his convalescence, the following nursing measures should be executed in which order?
  a. Administer the ordered sedative.
  b. Extinguish the room lights.
  c. Give an alcohol back rub.
  d. Change and tighten the linen.
  e. Offer the bedpan and urinal.
    1. e, c, d, a, b.
    2. a, d, c, e, b.
    3. a, e, d, b, c.
    4. d, e, c, b, a.

82. Which of the following physiologic changes would tend to predispose Mr. Powers to the formation of venous thrombi?
  a. Slowing of the flow of blood.
  b. Inflammation of the venous wall.
  c. Decreased viscosity of blood.
  d. Constriction of the venous lumen.
    1. a and b.
    2. c and d.

  3. All but c.
  4. All the above.

83. Thrombophlebitis is characterized by:
  1. Deposition of calcium salts beneath the intima.
  2. Constriction of the vessel by external pressure.
  3. Destruction of elastic and muscle fibers in the wall.
  4. Formation of a clot on an inflamed vessel lining.

84. Which of the following comfort devices would be contraindicated for use in caring for Mr. Powers?
  1. Overbed table.
  2. Knee roll.
  3. Linen cradle.
  4. Foot board.

85. The nurse should instruct Mr. Powers to prevent phlebothrombosis by:
  1. Massaging the calves of his legs briskly three times daily.
  2. Dangling his legs over the edge of the bed once daily.
  3. Keeping his legs extended with his toes pointing up.
  4. Tightening and relaxing his leg muscles several times daily.

86. Which of the following nutritional factors is thought to contribute to development of coronary artery disease?
  1. Excessive intake of cholesterol.
  2. Inadequate intake of vitamins.
  3. Excessive ingestion of alcohol.
  4. Inadequate intake of protein.

Mr. Powers continued to make an uneventful recovery. Prior to his hospital discharge, Mr. Powers and his wife received instruction from the nurse concerning his care at home.

87. In discussing his future diet, the nurse should make sure that Mr. Powers understands that he should avoid foods with heavy amounts of:
  a. Cholesterol.
  b. Purines.
  c. Calories.
  d. Potassium.
  e. Sodium.
    1. a and b.
    2. a, c, and e.
    3. c and d.
    4. All the above.

88. Which of the following questions by the nurse would be most appropriate in helping Mr. Powers to consider the need for modification of his family and business responsibilities?
1. "Do you think you will be able to avoid doing as much work as before the attack?"
2. "What interests and hobbies do you plan to pursue after your retirement from work?"
3. "What changes have you thought about making in regard to your various activities?"
4. "Do you suppose that it would be a good idea for you to find a less demanding job?"

89. In her last conversation with Mr. Powers the nurse discussed with him the need for future medical followup. Which of the following would be the best approach in opening the subject?
1. "Remember to go back to see your doctor twice a month."
2. "If you develop any further trouble, call your doctor."
3. "I guess you know what to do about seeing your doctor again?"
4. "Have you discussed with your doctor how often you're to see him?"

Rheumatoid Arthritis

Mrs. Emma Turk was 40 years old when she was admitted to the hospital for treatment of acute arthritis. Mrs. Turk had first noticed pain and swelling in her hands, knees, and ankle joints three years before, immediately following the death of her mother. On that occasion her family doctor had treated her with bedrest and salicylates and the symptoms had subsided, leaving only slight stiffness in her hands and knees.

The present attack of acute joint pain and swelling had begun suddenly and was related, Mrs. Turk felt, to the fact that she had been working unusually long hours in the restaurant owned and operated by her husband.

(ANSWER BLANK ON PAGE A–61)   (CORRECT ANSWERS ON PAGE B–69)

1. Salicylates belong to which of the following drug groups?
1. Peripheral nerve fiber stimulants.
2. Parasympathetic nervous system depressants.
3. Sympathetic nervous system stimulants.
4. Central nervous system depressants.

2. Sodium salicylate was given to Mrs. Turk during her previous illness for which of the following effects?
1. Antipyretic.
2. Antibiotic.
3. Anti-inflammatory.
4. Antiseptic.

To the nurse who admitted her, Mrs. Turk expressed concern lest her present illness interfere with her daughter Nora's college plans. Mr. Turk felt that Nora should postpone her schooling in order to take over her mother's position as restaurant cashier.

3. The nurse should consider Mrs. Turk's comments about Nora's college plans as:
1. Conversational small talk of a social nature, having no relationship to her illness.
2. Evidence of typical intrafamilial tension with which the nurse should not be concerned.

3. Privileged communication between patient and nurse, which the nurse must never reveal.
4. Information about family problems which may influence Mrs. Turk's welfare and should be charted.

The nurse took Mrs. Turk's vital signs. Temperature was 100.2° F. orally; pulse, 92 per minute, respirations 22 per minute, and blood pressure 96/60 mm. Hg.

4. The elevation of Mrs. Turk's temperature, pulse, and respiratory rate are probably manifestations of:
 1. Anxiety concerning hospitalization.
 2. Chronic physical exhaustion.
 3. Prolonged salicylate therapy.
 4. Inflammatory joint reaction.

5. The nurse can most accurately interpret Mrs. Turk's blood pressure as being:
 1. Temporarily reduced below her normal level.
 2. Low owing to overwork and consequent fatigue.
 3. Evidence of inadequate mobilization of body defenses.
 4. Lower than usual for a woman 40 years of age.

6. Mrs. Turk may demonstrate which of the following as additional symptoms of rheumatoid arthritis?
 a. Rough brittle nails.
 b. Joint crepitation.
 c. Hypertrophied lymph nodes.
 d. Subcutaneous nodules.
 e. Splenomegaly.
   1. a and b.
   2. c and d.
   3. All but d.
   4. All the above.

7. Which of the following devices should the nurse use in preparing Mrs. Turk's bed?
 1. Overhead frame.
 2. Bed board.
 2. Side rails.
 4. Rubber pillow.

8. In planning Mrs. Turk's care, the nurse should know that treatment during the acute phase of her illness will be aimed at preventing or minimizing later:
 1. Cardiac damage.
 2. Joint deformity.
 3. Kidney obstruction.
 4. Systemic infection.

The physician's physical examination and Mrs. Turk's history indicated the following:

1. Wasted and fatigued appearance, anxious facial expression.
2. Edema, erythema, and increased skin temperature of the elbows, wrists, proximal interphalangeal joints, knees, and ankles. Considerable restriction of motion in all involved joints.
3. Skin and conjunctival pallor.
4. Poor oral hygiene and evidence of dental caries.
5. Poor appetite.
6. Frequent insomnia.

A tentative diagnosis was made of acute rheumatoid arthritis.

9. Which of the following factors probably have contributed to Mrs. Turk's physical appearance?
 a. Poor nutrition.
 b. Weight loss.
 c. Overwork.
 d. Joint pain.
   1. a only.
   2. a and b.
   3. a, b, and c.
   4. All the above.

10. The swelling of Mrs. Turk's finger joints is probably due to:
 1. Infiltration of pus into muscles and fibrous tissue surrounding the joint.
 2. Extravasation of blood from skin capillaries into the subcutaneous tissue.
 3. Formation of bony spurs on the edges of articulating surfaces in the joint.
 4. Distention of the joint capsule by an increased amount of synovial fluid.

11. Mrs. Turk's present difficulty in moving her hand, foot, and ankle joints is most likely the result of:
 1. Muscle spasm.
 2. Nerve paralysis.
 3. Circulatory impairment.
 4. Bony displacement.

12. Mrs. Turk's pallor is probably indicative of:
 1. Shock.
 2. Infection.
 3. Anemia.
 4. Malnutrition.

13. The finding of dental caries in Mrs. Turk's physical examination is of particular significance because it is thought that dental caries may:
1. Indicate inadequate intake of proper nutrients over a prolonged period of time.
2. Constitute a focus of infection which distributes toxic substances to sensitive joint tissue.
3. Contraindicate the use of cortico-steroids for the interruption of joint inflammation.
4. Signify a widespread systemic disturbance of calcium metabolism as a cause of arthritis.

14. Mrs. Turk's history of insomnia should motivate the nurse to:
1. Investigate the psychosomatic origins of her arthritis.
2. Place her in a room that will be quiet at night.
3. Request a sedative to be administered at bedtime.
4. Restrict visitors during evening visiting hours.

15. Rheumatoid arthritis is thought to be which of the following types of disease?
1. Malignant.
2. Nutritional.
3. Collagen.
4. Metabolic.

16. Which of the following is the usual end result of progressive joint damage in untreated rheumatoid arthritis?
1. Bony ankylosis.
2. Chronic osteomyelitis.
3. Pathological fractures.
4. Joint hypermobility.

The doctor wrote the following orders:

1. Complete blood count, hematocrit, and hemoglobin level.
2. Differential white blood cell count.
3. Red blood cell sedimentation rate.
4. Latex fixation test.
5. X-rays of chest, hands, arms, feet, legs, and spine.
6. Absolute bedrest.
7. Aspirin 900 mg. orally q. 4 h.
8. Prednisone 2.5 mg. orally a.c. and h.s.
9. Ascorbic acid 100 mg. t.i.d. orally.
10. Diazepam (Valium) 5 mg. orally t.i.d.
11. High calorie, high protein, high vitamin diet.
12. Ferrous sulfate 300 mg. orally q.i.d.

17. The hematocrit is a measurement of the:
1. Quantity of blood ejected by each cardiac contraction.
2. Ratio of hemoglobin concentration to the number of red cells.
3. Level of maturation of circulating red blood cells.
4. Volume of blood cells per unit of circulating blood.

18. A differential white cell count is a measurement of the:
1. Ratio of white blood cells to red cells and platelets.
2. Volume of white cells in a given quantity of blood.
3. Number of each of the various types of white cells.
4. Time required for white cell production in the marrow.

19. Which of the following types of white blood cell is most apt to be increased in a patient with an acute inflammation?
1. Neutrophil.
2. Eosinophil.
3. Lymphocyte.
4. Monocyte.

20. The red cell sedimentation rate is a measurement of the:
1. Frequency with which red cells are filtered through the glomerular arterioles.
2. Time required for a red cell to be removed from the circulation by the liver or spleen.
3. Speed at which red cells will settle to the bottom of a calibrated tube of blood.
4. Degree to which red cells tend to adhere to the endothelial linings of arteries and veins.

21. Which of the following pathologic changes are most apt to have occurred in Mrs. Turk's diseased joints?
a. Erosion of articular cartilage.
b. Resorption of osseous tissue.
c. Deposition of uric acid crystals.
d. Increased density of compact bone.
1. a and b.
2. a and c.
3. a, b, and c.
4. All the above.

22. Which of the following x-ray findings would best support a diagnosis of rheumatoid arthritis?

1. Large, asymmetrical soft tissue tophi.
2. Marked narrowing of the joint space.
3. Bony excrescences on the joint margin.
4. Increased thickness of the bony cortex.

23. Absolute bedrest was ordered for Mrs. Turk at this time in order to:
1. Prevent damage to acutely inflamed joint surfaces.
2. Reduce the metabolic activities of muscles and nerves.
3. Decrease caloric demands during the period of anorexia.
4. Foster blood cell, antibody, and globulin manufacture.

24. Cortisone is normally produced by the:
1. Pituitary gland.
2. Pancreas.
3. Adrenal cortex.
4. Ovarian follicle.

25. Prednisone was ordered for Mrs. Turk for which of the following pharmacologic effects?
1. Maintenance of sodium and potassium balance.
2. Improvement of carbohydrate metabolism.
3. Production of androgen-like effects.
4. Interference with inflammatory reactions.

26. In caring for Mrs. Turk, the nurse should be alert to which of the following as a possible symptom of prednisone toxicity?
1. Edema.
2. Diaphoresis.
3. Tinnitus.
4. Pruritus.

27. Another name for ascorbic acid is:
1. Vitamin C.
2. Aspirin.
3. Colchicine.
4. Hydrochloric acid.

28. Ascorbic acid was probably ordered for Mrs. Turk in order to:
1. Denature the protein of the cell membranes of bacteria.
2. Promote normal formation and function of connective tissue.
3. Stimulate increased flow of digestive juice and improve appetite.
4. Neutralize the histamine in the joint tissue causing the inflammation.

29. In addition to its tranquilizing effect diazepam (Valium) was given to Mrs. Turk in order to:
1. Counteract the inflammatory response.
2. Block pain impulse transmission.
3. Relax spasms of skeletal muscles.
4. Prevent drug hypersensitivity reactions.

30. Which of the following is a possible side effect of diazepam (Valium)?
1. Cyanosis.
2. Drowsiness.
3. Polyuria.
4. Hiccoughs.

31. Ferrous sulfate was given to Mrs. Turk to facilitate:
1. Synthesis of hemoglobin.
2. Formation of collagen.
3. Migration of lymphocytes.
4. Secretion of enzymes.

32. Which of the following are possible toxic effects of ferrous sulfate?
a. Headache.
b. Anorexia.
c. Nausea.
d. Constipation.
e. Diarrhea.
　1. a and c.
　2. b and d.
　3. All but e.
　4. All but a.

33. The doctor ordered a high caloric, high protein, high vitamin diet for Mrs. Turk in order to:
a. Facilitate a gain in weight.
b. Improve appetite and digestion.
c. Foster resolution of inflammation.
d. Provide material for tissue replacement.
　1. a only.
　2. a and b.
　3. a, b, and c.
　4. All the above.

34. If aspirin and prednisone should be ineffective in reducing Mrs. Turk's symptoms, her physician may order that she be given:
a. Chloroquine.
b. Phenylbutazone.
c. Indomethacin.
d. Colchicine.
e. Gold sodium thiomalate.
　1. a or b only.
　2. a, b, or c only.
　3. Any but d.
　4. All the above.

The diagnostic tests indicated the following:

1. Red blood cells 4 million per cu. mm.
2. Hematocrit 40 per cent.
3. Hemoglobin 70 per cent.
4. Increased red cell sedimentation rate.
5. White blood cell count 13,000 per cu. mm.
6. Neutrophils 74 per cent, eosinophils 2 per cent, basophils 0.5 per cent, lymphocytes 20 per cent, monocytes 3 per cent.
7. Positive Latex fixation test.

35. The findings from Mrs. Turk's blood tests indicated:
1. A proportional reduction in both red blood cells and hemoglobin concentration.
2. A proportionately greater decrease in numbers of red cells than in hemoglobin.
3. A proportionately greater decrease in hemoglobin concentration than in red cells.
4. A proportionate increase in both the hemoglobin concentration and in hematocrit level.

36. Mrs. Turk's elevated red blood cell sedimentation rate can most accurately be interpreted to indicate:
1. An infectious basis for her arthritic symptoms.
2. An unfavorable prognosis for her joint disease.
3. Adequate circulating antibodies against infection.
4. The presence of inflammation somewhere in the body.

37. Mrs. Turk's white blood cell count is:
1. Less than normal.
2. Within normal range.
3. Moderately increased.
4. Considerably above normal.

38. Which of Mrs. Turk's white blood cells shows a proportionately greater increase than the others?
1. Neutrophils.
2. Eosinophils.
3. Lymphocytes.
4. Monocytes.

39. The Latex fixation test is used to identify the presence in the blood serum of a rheumatoid factor, or:
1. Virus.
2. Phagocyte.
3. Enzyme.
4. Macroglobulin.

The doctor constructed posterior plaster splints for Mrs. Turk's legs and feet and directed that they be removed only during bathing and bed making.

40. Mrs. Turk's feet should be given special care and attention because the muscles, skin, and subcutaneous tissues over her inflamed joints are apt to be:
1. Atrophic.
2. Hemorrhagic.
3. Callused.
4. Scaling.

41. During the acute phase of her illness, Mrs. Turk will be particularly susceptible to:
1. Convulsions.
2. Urticaria.
3. Cystitis.
4. Decubiti.

42. Without treatment, Mrs. Turk would be most apt to develop which of the following hand deformities?
a. Ulnar deviation of the fingers.
b. Hyperextension of the wrists.
c. "Swan neck" deformity of the fingers.
d. Hyperextension of metacarpophalangeal joints.
e. Subluxation of interphalangeal joints.
  1. a and b.
  2. a, c, and e.
  3. All but e.
  4. All the above.

43. During her first few days of hospitalization, which of the following nursing measures would contribute most in protecting Mrs. Turk against the development of later postural deformities?
1. Frequent massage of inflamed joints.
2. Maintenance of optimum body alignment.
3. Application of warm packs to extremities.
4. Provision of active and passive exercise.

44. In order to provide proper body alignment, the nurse should position Mrs. Turk so that:
1. Every joint is maintained in an absolutely neutral position.
2. All hinge joints are immobilized by posterior splinting.

3. Each joint is placed in position of maximum function.
4. Only ball and socket joints remain in any degree of flexion.

45. Mrs. Turk's arm and hand should be maintained in the position normally assumed when:
1. Operating a typewriter.
2. Holding a glass of water.
3. Fastening a brassiere.
4. Having the palm read.

46. Which of the following contracture deformities would Mrs. Turk be most apt to develop if she were not given effective nursing care?
1. Flexion of metacarpophalangeal joints.
2. Hyperextension of the knee joints.
3. External rotation of the upper arm.
4. Dorsiflexion of the foot at the ankle.

47. Mrs. Turk is more apt to develop wrist drop than hyperextension because:
1. Attention to personal hygiene more often requires wrist flexion than extension.
2. The flexor muscles of the wrist are stronger than the wrist extensors.
3. The dorsal blood supply of the arm is more rich than the volar blood supply.
4. Bony spurs on the articulating bony surfaces prevent extension and favor flexion.

48. Which of the following are psychosocial factors which will influence Mrs. Turk's adjustment to her disease?
a. Her relationship with her mother.
b. The socioeconomic status of her family.
c. Her sexual identification and adjustment.
d. The length of her formal education.
e. Her methods of emotional expression.
1. a, b, and d.
2. a, c, and e.
3. All but e.
4. All the above.

On her second hospital day Mrs. Turk complained of severe joint pain while the nurse was bathing her and making the bed.

49. The nurse could most suitably and safely reduce Mrs. Turk's joint discomfort by:
1. Applying ice bags to the swollen joints.
2. Using a cradle to support the bed linen.
3. Moving her extremities through full range of motion.
4. Elevating the head and foot gatches of the bed.

After one week of hospitalization, Mrs. Turk's joint symptoms had subsided remarkably. The joint swelling, redness, and heat had disappeared, but voluntary motion in the involved joints was still considerably less than normal.

The doctor ordered that Mrs. Turk be sent daily to physiotherapy for paraffin hand soaks and Hubbard Tank exercise under water. He also ordered that the nurse institute passive and active exercises of Mrs. Turk's hands, elbows, knees, and feet.

50. Which of the following approaches by her nurse would be most helpful to Mrs. Turk?
1. Confrontation of anger.
2. Firm and directive.
3. Nondirective and passive.
4. Permissive and easygoing.

51. Paraffin soaks were ordered for Mrs. Turk's hands in order to:
1. Constrict dilated vessels.
2. Toughen skin tissue.
3. Relieve muscle spasm.
4. Stimulate bone growth.

52. The purpose of passively exercising Mrs. Turk's arms, hands, legs, and feet is to:
a. Increase blood flow to the part.
b. Prevent muscle atrophy.
c. Preserve range of joint motion.
d. Prevent shortening of muscles.
1. a only.
2. a and b.
3. a, b, and c.
4. All the above.

53. Which of the following would be the most reliable index of the proper amount and duration of exercise for Mrs. Turk?
1. Color and temperature of the skin.
2. Variation in pulse rate and rhythm.
3. Rate and depth of respirations.
4. Incidence and duration of pain.

54. On the first occasion that the nurse carried out passive exercises, Mrs. Turk complained of discomfort. She asked, "Why must I be put through this punishment?" Which of the following responses by the nurse would be most appropriate?

1. "The doctor wants to learn how much damage you have incurred during this attack."
2. "These exercises will retard loss of muscle strength and minimize stiffness of your joints."
3. "I'll tell the doctor about your discomfort. Perhaps he will cancel the order for exercise."
4. "Exercises are not punishment. They are an important part of the treatment given for arthritis."

55. Mrs. Turk controlled her emotions well and seldom overtly expressed hostility toward others. Which of the following are suggestive of covert hostility?

a. Denying joint pain.
b. Demanding repeated explanations.
c. Refusing to eat certain foods.
d. Resisting suggested treatment.
e. Failing to perform active exercises.
   1. a, c, and d.
   2. b, d, and e.
   3. All but e.
   4. All the above.

56. Which of the following measures would be of the greatest help in providing Mrs. Turk with proper nourishment while she is in the hospital?

1. Plan for a nurse or a relative to be available to feed her at every mealtime.
2. Arrange for her to have a longer than usual mealtime to avoid being hurried.
3. Have the dietitian visit daily to explain the necessity for eating her entire meal.
4. Request the family to prepare her favorite dishes; bring them in, and feed them to her.

Mrs. Turk's joint symptoms abated considerably after three weeks of hospital care, but she was bored and unhappy in the hospital. Her doctor decided that she should be discharged to her home, where she would be in more close contact with family affairs.

57. In teaching Mrs. Turk's daughter, Nora, how to prepare paraffin soaks for Mrs. Turk at home, which of the following points should be stressed?

1. Paraffin should be heated with care over a flame because it is inflammable.
2. Used paraffin should be immediately discarded so that it is not reused.
3. A nylon stocking should be used to cover the part before applying the paraffin.
4. Only two coats of paraffin should be applied at one time, to avoid burning the skin.

58. In teaching Mrs. Turk how to care for herself at home the nurse should advise her to:

1. Support her arms in slings when sitting in a chair.
2. Lie flat on her back when resting or sleeping.
3. Wear an abdominal binder when getting out of bed.
4. Wear soft-soled rather than hard-soled slippers for walking.

59. In teaching Mrs. Turk concerning self-care after hospital discharge, the nurse should know that which of the following are possible untoward effects of cortisone dosage?

a. Impaired wound healing.
b. Peptic ulcer.
c. Psychotic states.
d. Diabetes mellitus.
   1. a and b.
   2. b and c.
   3. c and d.
   4. All the above.

60. With the passage of time and in spite of treatment, Mrs. Turk suffered increasing limitations of joint motion. The clinic nurse could help Mrs. Turk to remain self-sufficient by making which of the following devices available for her use?

a. Long-handled shoehorn.
b. Bathtub chair.
c. Long-handled reaching tongs.
d. Built-up toilet seat.
e. Four-legged walker.
   1. a and c.
   2. b and d.
   3. All but e.
   4. All the above.

Bronchiectasis and Segmental Lung Resection

Throughout his lifetime, Ben Kaufman had weathered a succession of respiratory diseases. His mother often related that he had developed pneumonia following several childhood infections. In adolescence he developed hay fever, and as a young adult he suffered from chronic sinusitis and bronchitis. At the age of 35 he was diagnosed as having bronchiectasis. In spite of close medical supervision, his symptoms became worse during the next five years, and he was finally hospitalized for a complete medical workup and surgical removal of the diseased portions of his lung.

(ANSWER BLANK ON PAGE A–63)   (CORRECT ANSWERS ON PAGE B–73)

1. To which of the following allergens was Mr. Kaufman probably sensitive as an adolescent?

1. Strawberries.
2. Ragweed pollen.
3. Penicillin.
4. Horse serum.

2. It is thought that the symptoms of hay fever develop when antigen and antibody combine in the tissues, causing liberation of:

1. Adrenalin.
2. Acetylcholine.
3. Histamine.
4. Cholinesterase.

3. Which of the following is the most accurate definition of bronchiectasis?

1. Encapsulated collection of pus in the lung.
2. Fibrotic obliteration of the terminal bronchi.
3. Saclike or tubular dilation of the bronchi.
4. Traumatic rupture of the bronchiolar wall.

4. Which of the following is thought to predispose to development of bronchiectasis?

1. Right heart failure.
2. Inhalation of coal dust.
3. Bronchial pneumonia.
4. Acute pleural effusion.

5. Which of the following cause development of bronchiectasis?

a. Decreased bronchial blood supply.
b. Prolonged bronchial obstruction.
c. Increased pulmonary artery pressure.
d. Chronic bronchial infection.
e. Immobility of costochondral junction.

1. a and c.
2. b and d.
3. All but d.
4. All the above.

On arriving at the hospital, Mr. Kaufman was admitted to a private room on the medical-surgical floor. He told the nurse who admitted him that his chief complaints were chronic productive cough, anorexia, and dyspnea on exertion.

6. Mr. Kaufman probably has which of the following pathologic changes in his bronchi?
  a. Replacement of ciliated columnar epithelium with nonciliated cuboidal epithelium.
  b. Distortion of bronchial wall by bands of fibrous scar tissue.
  c. Destruction of smooth muscle and elastic tissue fibers in bronchial wall.
  d. Obliteration of bronchial lumen by pedunculated polyps arising from the bronchial wall.
  e. Anastomotic connections between branches of the bronchial artery and pulmonary artery.
      1. a and b.
      2. a, b, and c.
      3. All but d.
      4. All the above.

7. The nurse found that Mr. Kaufman's pulse was regular. She should therefore count Mr. Kaufman's pulse for what period of time?
  1. 15 seconds.
  2. 30 seconds.
  3. 60 seconds.
  4. 120 seconds.

8. In addition to rate, what other characteristics should the nurse note concerning Mr. Kaufman's respirations?
  a. Depth to which air is drawn into the lung.
  b. Sounds produced by movement of air in and out.
  c. Rhythmicity or pattern of respiratory movement.
  d. Magnitude of chest and abdominal movements.
  e. Length of inspiration in comparison to expiration.
      1. a and b.
      2. b and c.
      3. c and d.
      4. All the above.

9. Mr. Kaufman's sputum would be apt to be:
  1. Thin and watery.
  2. Scant and rusty.
  3. Mucopurulent.
  4. Serosanguineous.

10. The nurse will probably observe that Mr. Kaufman's sputum tends to:
  1. Increase in quantity as the day progresses.
  2. Settle into three layers on standing.
  3. Change in color from one day to the next.
  4. Contain large amounts of dark red blood.

11. At which of the following times would Mr. Kaufman's cough probably have been most troublesome and his sputum most copious?
  1. On arising.
  2. At midday.
  3. At meal times.
  4. On retiring.

12. During severe paroxysms of coughing Mr. Kaufman is apt to experience:
  a. Hiccoughs.
  b. Emesis.
  c. Asphyxia.
  d. Syncope.
  e. Convulsion.
      1. a and c.
      2. b and d.
      3. All but d.
      4. All the above.

13. Mr. Kaufman should be observed for symptoms of which of the following as possible complications of bronchiectasis?
  a. Pneumonitis.
  b. Empyema.
  c. Hemoptysis.
  d. Tuberculosis.
  e. Cor pulmonale.
      1. a and b.
      2. a, c, and e.
      3. All but d.
      4. All the above.

14. In planning care for Mr. Kaufman, the nurse should know that his paroxysms of coughing would most often be precipitated by:
  1. Decreasing temperature.
  2. Increasing humidity.
  3. Changing position.
  4. Ingesting food.

15. The nurse should instruct Mr. Kaufman that when he coughs he should:
  1. Turn his head to the side if he is in the company of others.
  2. Place his hand over his mouth to prevent dispersal of droplets.
  3. Expectorate directly into a paper bag attached to the bedside.
  4. Cover his mouth and nose with several thicknesses of paper tissues.

16. Mr. Kaufman's anorexia was predominantly the result of his:
  1. Disinclination for physical exercise.

2. Frequent expectoration of foul sputum.
3. Decreased basal metabolic rate.
4. Increased vertical diameter of the thorax.

17. Which of the following is the best definition of dyspnea?
1. Awareness of the necessity for respiratory effort.
2. Sensation of sharp pain on taking a deep breath.
3. Deficient oxygenation of blood in the lung alveoli.
4. Insufficient supply of oxygen to the body tissues.

18. In which of the following positions would Mr. Kaufman probably be most comfortable?
1. Sitting upright with his head and arms resting on an overbed table.
2. Resting in a semi-upright sitting position with arms supported by pillows.
3. Reclining on his left side with right arm and leg supported on pillows.
4. Lying flat on his back with a small pillow placed under his shoulders.

19. Mr. Kaufman told the nurse that he was still required to take pills to control his hay fever symptoms during the late summer and fall. The pills were probably:
1. Sympathomimetics.
2. Bronchodilators.
3. Antihistamines.
4. Sedatives.

20. When she discovered that Mr. Kaufman had taken medications during the hay fever season, the nurse should determine whether he understood that these drugs tend to produce:
1. Nausea.
2. Urticaria.
3. Anemia.
4. Drowsiness.

21. Mr. Kaufman should have been instructed that while taking medications for hay fever he should avoid:
1. Eating rich food.
2. Driving a car.
3. Ingesting alcohol.
4. Exposure to sun.

Mr. Kaufman's physical examination revealed:

1. Temperature 99.4° F. orally, pulse 88 per minute, respirations 26 per minute.

2. General muscle wasting and evidence of weight loss.
3. Pale, boggy nasal mucosa and heavy postnasal drainage.
4. Increased anterior-posterior diameter of the chest.
5. Areas of decreased resonance in the right lung base.
6. Moist rales in the lower right lung.
7. Clubbing of the fingers.

22. The most probable cause for Mr. Kaufman's temperature elevation was:
1. Hypersecretion of thyroxin.
2. Decreased fluid intake.
3. Increased tissue catabolism.
4. Infection of pooled secretions.

23. Which of the following was probably chiefly responsible for Mr. Kaufman's loss of weight?
1. Increased metabolic rate.
2. Poor intestinal absorption.
3. Decreased food intake.
4. Impaired protein metabolism.

24. Mr. Kaufman's pale, boggy nasal mucosa was indicative of:
1. Virus infection.
2. Heart failure.
3. Chronic anemia.
4. Allergic rhinitis.

25. Mr. Kaufman's increased anterior-posterior diameter of the chest was suggestive of:
1. Osteoarthritis.
2. Heart failure.
3. Emphysema.
4. Mediastinitis.

26. The decreased resonance noted in Mr. Kaufman's right lung base was probably due to:
1. Accumulation of fluid in the pleural space.
2. Increase in the diameter of the bronchioles.
3. Filling of the alveoli with inflammatory exudate.
4. Formation of fibrous adhesions between the pleurae.

27. The rales in Mr. Kaufman's right lower lung probably resulted from:
1. Fibrous tissue obliteration of alveoli damaged by chronic infection.
2. Formation of fistulae between lung parenchyma and the pleural space.
3. Accumulation of secretions in sacs formed by the coalescing of alveoli.
4. Increased blood flow through dilated and anastomosed blood vessels.

28. Which of the following is thought to be the cause of finger clubbing in patients with bronchiectasis?
  1. Anoxia of peripheral tissues.
  2. Edema of dependent parts.
  3. Spasm of digital vessels.
  4. Chronic vitamin deficiency.

The doctor made a diagnosis of chronic sinusitis and bronchiectasis of the right lower lung. The following orders were written for a presurgical workup:

  1. Complete blood count and hemoglobin determination.
  2. Urinalysis.
  3. Chest x-ray.
  4. Pulmonary function studies.
  5. Bronchoscopy.
  6. Bronchogram.
  7. Electrocardiogram.
  8. Blood and sputum cultures.

29. Mr. Kaufman's chronic sinusitis had contributed to his development of bronchiectasis by:
  1. Extension of infection along the mucosal lining of the respiratory tract.
  2. Sensitizing the alveolar lining to inhalant allergens causing sinusitis.
  3. Drainage of secretions through the posterior pharynx to the lung bases.
  4. Lowering the body's resistance to infectious and degenerative diseases.

30. In order to determine Mr. Kaufman's blood cell count, the laboratory technician would probably obtain a blood sample from Mr. Kaufman's:
  1. Ear lobe capillary.
  2. Basilic vein.
  3. Radial artery.
  4. Sternal marrow.

31. In obtaining blood for a cell count, sterile disposable lancets are preferred to those which are chemically sterilized because the latter may permit transmission of:
  1. Hemolytic anemia.
  2. Myelogenous leukemia.
  3. Homologous serum hepatitis.
  4. Miliary tuberculosis.

32. Routine urinalysis would include determination of which of the following characteristics of Mr. Kaufman's urine?
  a. Acidity or alkalinity.
  b. Specific gravity.
  c. Presence of sugar.
  d. Presence of albumin.
  e. Presence of blood cells.
    1. a only.
    2. a and b.
    3. a, b, and c.
    4. All the above.

33. Which of the following precautions should the nurse observe in obtaining a specimen of Mr. Kaufman's urine for analysis?
  1. Administer a large amount of fluid orally before obtaining the sample of urine.
  2. Collect the urine specimen in a sterile bottle with a screw top and a volume scale.
  3. Obtain the urine for examination by means of catheterization using sterile technique.
  4. Prepare a urine specimen of sufficient quantity to be able to measure specific gravity.

34. In preparing Mr. Kaufman to cooperate in the taking of his chest x-ray, the nurse should know that the x-ray technician will instruct him to do which of the following before taking the picture?
  1. Pant rapidly with his mouth open.
  2. Breathe deeply and cough several times.
  3. Take a deep breath and hold it.
  4. Elevate his arms over his head.

35. Mr. Kaufman asked the nurse, "What is a vital capacity determination?" What response would be most appropriate?
  1. "A test to determine how much air you exhale after the deepest possible inhalation."
  2. "A measurement of the amount of oxygen utilized by the body during a specified time."
  3. "An estimation of the volume of lung tissue that is capable of being fully expanded."
  4. "A calculation of lung volume from the measurement of anteroposterior and lateral chest x-rays."

36. In order to inform Mr. Kaufman about the purpose of bronchoscopy, the nurse should know that which of the following can be accomplished by the procedure?
  a. Observation of bronchial mucous membrane.
  b. Injection of dye into pulmonary air passages.
  c. Removal of fluid from the pleural cavity.

d. Evacuation of bronchiectatic cavities.
1. a only.
2. b and c.
3. a, b, and d.
4. All the above.

37. In planning care for Mr. Kaufman during his diagnostic workup, the nurse should know that which of the following complications is particularly apt to occur following bronchoscopy, due to the mechanical trauma caused by the procedure?
1. Pharyngeal perforation.
2. Laryngeal obstruction.
3. Tracheal stenosis.
4. Pleural laceration.

38. The nurse should withhold solid food for four hours following Mr. Kaufman's return from bronchoscopy in order to prevent:
1. Projectile vomiting.
2. Aspiration of food.
3. Abdominal distention.
4. Acid eructation.

39. In preparing Mr. Kaufman for bronchoscopy and bronchogram, the nurse should encourage him to practice:
1. Splinting his abdominal muscles while he coughs deeply.
2. Swallowing while pinching the nose to occlude the nostrils.
3. Breathing in and out through the nose with the mouth open.
4. Hyperextending the neck and moving the head from side to side.

40. Which of the following treatments would be ordered as part of Mr. Kaufman's preparation for the bronchogram?
1. Steam inhalation.
2. Postural drainage.
3. Ice collar.
4. Throat irrigation.

41. Which of the following precautions should the nurse observe before sending Mr. Kaufman to x-ray for a bronchogram?
1. Record his apical and radial pulse rates.
2. Place a mask over both his mouth and nose.
3. Remove any false teeth or bridges he may have.
4. Aspirate his pharyngeal secretions with a syringe.

The following orders were written for Mr. Kaufman's treatment:

1. Procaine penicillin 1.2 million units I.M. b.i.d.
2. Saturated solution of potassium iodide 5 minims q.i.d.
3. Pentobarbital (Nembutal) 90 mg. h.s., p.r.n.
4. High protein, high vitamin, high calorie diet.
5. Push fluids.
6. Postural drainage for 15 minutes t.i.d.

42. Penicillin was ordered for Mr. Kaufman primarily in order to:
1. Kill bacteria present in the nose, mouth, throat, and trachea.
2. Arrest coryza, sinusitis, and chronic posterior pharyngeal drainage.
3. Inhibit growth of organisms in secretions accumulated in the lung.
4. Prevent hematogenous spread of infectious organisms throughout the body.

43. Which of the following precautions should the nurse observe before giving Mr. Kaufman his initial dose of penicillin?
1. Record his repiratory and pulse rates.
2. Inject a few minims of the drug intradermally.
3. Administer large amounts of fluids orally.
4. Ask him whether he is allergic to penicillin.

44. Saturated solution of potassium iodide was given to Mr. Kaufman in order to:
1. Depress the medullary cough center.
2. Inhibit the action of histamine.
3. Relax bronchial muscles.
4. Increase bronchial secretions.

45. Saturated solution of potassium iodide should be administered by:
1. Placing it on a spoon and giving it undiluted.
2. Mixing it with water and administering it orally.
3. Placing it in a nebulizer and giving it by inhalation.
4. Pouring it over ice chips, to be sipped slowly.

46. Pentobarbital (Nembutal) was ordered for Mr. Kaufman in order to:
1. Prevent cough by depressing the cough center.
2. Relieve pain due to pleural inflammation.
3. Allay apprehension and induce restful sleep.
4. Decrease the rate and depth of respiration.

47. Which of the following nursing measures should be carried out before giving Mr. Kaufman his dose of pentobarbital at bedtime?
    a. Offer the urinal.
    b. Administer oral hygiene.
    c. Massage his back.
    d. Straighten his linen.
    e. Turn out the room light.
        1. a and b.
        2. c and d.
        3. a, b, c, and d.
        4. All the above.

48. The doctor ordered a high protein diet for Mr. Kaufman primarily in order to:
    1. Replace tissue protein destroyed by bacterial infection.
    2. Provide materials for increased blood cell production.
    3. Increase the liver stores of iron, copper, and vitamins.
    4. Supplement carbohydrates as a source of metabolic energy.

49. A high caloric diet was ordered for Mr. Kaufman primarily because he had:
    1. Little subcutaneous fat to serve as insulation.
    2. Lowered general resistance to infection.
    3. Impaired ability to store glycogen in the liver.
    4. Increased rate of cellular metabolism.

50. Which of the following food servings is the best source of protein?
    1. 3 ounces canned tuna.
    2. 1 cup canned red beans.
    3. 1 cup creamed cottage cheese.
    4. 1 cup whole milk.

51. Which of the following vegetable servings contains the greatest amount of protein?
    1. $\frac{1}{2}$ cup canned sweet potatoes.
    2. $\frac{1}{2}$ cup canned green beans.
    3. $\frac{1}{2}$ cup canned peas.
    4. $\frac{1}{2}$ cup canned corn.

52. Which of the following food servings contains the greatest number of calories?
    1. $\frac{1}{2}$ cup canned sweet potatoes.
    2. $\frac{1}{2}$ cup cooked green beans.
    3. $\frac{1}{2}$ cup canned peas.
    4. $\frac{1}{2}$ cup canned corn.

53. Which of the following food servings contains the most calories?
    1. 1 cup whole milk.
    2. 2 slices fried bacon.
    3. 3 ounces broiled hamburger.
    4. 1 medium baked potato.

54. Which of the following foods is the best source of both calories and protein?
    1. 1 boiled frankfurter.
    2. $\frac{1}{2}$ cup cottage cheese.
    3. 1 cup baked custard.
    4. 1 poached egg.

55. Which of the following measures should the nurse employ to stimulate Mr. Kaufman to eat as much as possible of the food served to him?
    a. Give oral hygiene before meals.
    b. Remove the sputum cup from view.
    c. Serve smaller meals at greater frequency.
    d. Assist with feeding when dyspneic.
        1. a only.
        2. a and b.
        3. a, b, and c.
        4. All the above.

56. Mr. Kaufman should be encouraged to drink large quantities of fluids in order to:
    a. Prevent crystallization of penicillin in the kidney.
    b. Liquefy lung secretions and facilitate their removal.
    c. Reduce body temperature and decrease metabolic rate.
    d. Increase blood volume and systolic pressure.
        1. a only.
        2. a and b.
        3. b and c.
        4. All the above.

57. Thoracentesis is to empyema as which of the following is to bronchiectasis?
    1. Lobectomy.
    2. Postural drainage.
    3. Aerosol penicillin.
    4. Breathing exercises.

58. Postural drainage was ordered for Mr. Kaufman in order to:
    1. Empty the sinus cavities.
    2. Stimulate ciliary action.
    3. Improve pulmonary circulation.
    4. Remove pooled secretions.

59. In planning care for Mr. Kaufman, the nurse should know that the most common hazards of postural drainage are:
    1. Nausea and vomiting.
    2. Aspiration and asphyxia.
    3. Dizziness and falling.
    4. Headache and tinnitus.

60. At which of the following times should the nurse institute postural drainage for Mr. Kaufman?
    1. 15 minutes before meals.
    2. One hour before meals.

3. 15 minutes after meals.

4. One hour after meals.

61. If he can tolerate it, the nurse should place Mr. Kaufman in which of the following positions for postural drainage?

1. Lying face down in bed with the foot of the bed frame elevated on shock blocks.

2. In the knee-chest position on a firm, flat surface, with the head turned to one side.

3. Lying across the bed on his abdomen with his head and trunk over the side of the bed.

4. Sitting in a chair with his forearms braced on his thighs and his head between his knees.

62. While Mr. Kaufman is in postural drainage position the nurse should provide him with:

a. A glass of water.

b. Tissue wipes.

c. Sputum cup.

d. Small pillow.

e. Call bell.

   1. a and b.

   2. c and d.

   3. b, c, and e.

   4. All the above.

63. In order to increase the benefit of postural drainage, the nurse should tell Mr. Kaufman that while he is in postural drainage position, he should:

1. Take short, shallow breaths to reduce the danger of coughing.

2. Swallow forcefully and frequently to prevent regurgitation of food.

3. Compress one nostril at a time and exhale to open his sinuses.

4. Breathe deeply and cough in order to stimulate removal of sputum.

64. On the first few occasions that Mr. Kaufman performs postural drainage, the nurse should:

a. Help him assume the correct position.

b. Pound his back to encourage drainage.

c. Discourage coughing as being too exhausting.

d. Remain with him throughout the procedure.

e. Help him to resume a normal position afterward.

   1. a only.

   2. a and b.

   3. b and c.

   4. a, d, and e.

65. In planning long-term care and health teaching for Mr. Kaufman, the nurse should know that bronchiectasis predisposes him to:

1. Pleural adhesions.

2. Hiatus hernia.

3. Systemic hypertension.

4. Cardiac failure.

66. Mr. Kaufman told the nurse that he had on several occasions expectorated blood during severe paroxysms of coughing. Severe hemoptysis could give rise to which complication?

1. Pulmonary abscess.

2. Aspiration pneumonia.

3. Spontaneous pneumothorax.

4. Air embolism.

67. What is the most effective treatment for bronchiectasis?

1. Inhalation of aerosol decongestants.

2. Parenteral administration of antibiotics.

3. Bronchoscopic drainage of lung cavities.

4. Surgical removal of diseased tissue.

Surprisingly, Mr. Kaufman's chest x-ray and bronchogram revealed bronchiectatic cavities in the right lower lung only. His red blood cell count was 5,300,000 per cu. mm., his white cell count was 11,000 per cu. mm., and his hemoglobin was 88 per cent. His urinalysis, electrocardiogram, and blood culture and sputum revealed no abnormal findings.

It was decided to surgically remove the diseased portions of Mr. Kaufman's right lung. He was given atropine sulfate 0.4 mg. and meperidine hydrochloride 100 mg. H. preoperatively, and a right lower lobe segmentectomy was performed under general anesthesia given by endotracheal tube. Before closure of the incision, a catheter was placed in the chest cavity and connected to a water-seal drainage system.

Mr. Kaufman was unconscious when he was returned to the recovery room. The surgeon checked the operation of the chest drainage apparatus, started oxygen administration by nasal catheter, and wrote the following orders:

1. Meperidine hydrochloride, 50 mg. H. p.r.n. for pain.

2. 1000 cc. 5 per cent dextrose in distilled water q. 12 h. for two days.

3. Ampicillin Gm. 1 I.M. q.i.d.
4. Secobarbital 10 mg. q.h.s.
5. Intermittent positive pressure breathing, 15 minutes t.i.d. at 15 mm. water pressure and with isoproterenol hydrochloride (Isuprel) 1:200 solution 1 cc. and normal saline 10 cc. in the nebulizer.
6. Turn frequently and encourage coughing and deep breathing.

68. Which of the following solutions is usually placed in the drainage collection bottle in preparing the water-seal drainage apparatus?
1. Sterile water.
2. Ammonium carbonate.
3. Hexachlorophene.
4. Sodium citrate.

69. Mr. Kaufman's chest catheter and attached water-seal drainage apparatus were intended to:
a. Drain blood and serum from the pleural space.
b. Facilitate gradual re-expansion of the right lung.
c. Prevent drying and irritation of bronchial mucosa.
d. Liquefy bronchial secretions and stimulate coughing.
1. a only.
2. a and b.
3. a, b, and c.
4. All the above.

70. What is the purpose of the fluid in the drainage collection bottle?
1. To facilitate removal of bloody drainage from the bottle.
2. To foster removal of chest secretions by capillarity.
3. To prevent entrance of air into the interpleural space.
4. To decrease the danger that bacteria may ascend the tubing.

71. Immediately following Mr. Kaufman's arrival in the recovery room, the nurse should undertake which of the following measures concerning the chest drainage apparatus?
1. Secure the chest catheter to the wound dressing with a sterile safety pin.
2. Mark the time and the fluid level on the side of the collection bottle.
3. Agitate the collection bottle to prevent clotting of blood in the glass tube.
4. Raise the collection bottle to bed level to check patency of the system.

72. Which of the following observations should the nurse interpret as indications that the water-seal drainage apparatus is functioning properly?
a. Fluctuation of the fluid level in the long glass rod with respiration.
b. Steady decrease in the level of fluid in the drainage collection bottle.
c. Moderate bubbling of air from the glass rod through the fluid.
d. Maintenance of a solid column of fluid in the long glass rod.
1. a and b.
2. a and c.
3. b and c.
4. b and d.

73. The nurse should check the chest drainage apparatus frequently in order to decrease the possibility of:
a. Removal of the catheter from the chest incision.
b. Separation of the catheter from the drainage tubing.
c. Disconnection of the drainage tubing from the bottle.
d. Breakage of the floor drainage collection bottle.
1. a only.
2. a and b.
3. c and d.
4. All the above.

74. Which of the following pieces of equipment should be kept in plain sight at Mr. Kaufman's bedside to prevent complications arising from breakage of the drainage bottle or disconnection of the catheter from the drainage tubing?
1. Two large forceps.
2. Roll of adhesive tape.
3. Chest binder.
4. Tracheostomy tube.

75. What position would be most suitable for Mr. Kaufman after his blood pressure has stabilized postoperatively?
1. Prone.
2. Supine.
3. Right Sims'.
4. Fowler's.

76. During the immediate postoperative period it would be important for Mr. Kaufman to be given his prescribed analgesic in order to:
1. Compensate for his unusually low threshold for pain.
2. Reduce respiratory rate and depth until the incision heals.

3. Facilitate deep coughing to remove bronchial secretions.

4. Decrease his awareness of oxygen and suction apparatus.

77. An intermittent positive pressure breathing device was used in treating Mr. Kaufman postoperatively in order to:

1. Provide more adequate lung aeration than could be achieved by unassisted respiration.

2. Encourage respiration at a faster rate than that established by respiratory center control.

3. Force air through the infected secretions which had accumulated in the lung bases.

4. Foster increased contractile strength of the diaphragm, abdominal muscles, and thoracic muscles.

78. Isoproterenol hydrochloride (Isuprel) was given to Mr. Kaufman in order to:

1. Increase the systolic blood pressure.

2. Decrease spasm of bronchial muscles.

3. Stimulate the medullary respiratory center.

4. Inhibit growth of pathogens in the lung.

Mr. Kaufman was able to drink clear liquids on the day following the operation and progressed to a general diet within a few days. He was helped to sit on the edge of the bed on the second postoperative day but refused to get out of bed into a chair until two days later because, he said, "I'm too weak and tired to churn around like that."

79. Which of the following measures would be most helpful in protecting Mr. Kaufman from development of postural deformities following his operation?

1. Elevation of his right arm on several thick pillows.

2. Tying his right hand to the frame at the head of the bed.

3. Passive and active exercises of his right arm and shoulder.

4. Advising him to rest and sleep only on his right side.

80. Which of the following are probably responsible for Mr. Kaufman's pronounced feeling of weakness postoperatively?

a. Blood loss during surgery.

b. Depressant effect of analgesics.

c. Decrease in nutritional intake.

d. Reduction in vital capacity.

1. a only.

2. a and b.

3. a, b, and c.

4. All the above.

On the fourth postoperative day, x-ray indicated that Mr. Kaufman's right lung had fully expanded, so the chest drainage tube was removed.

Mr. Kaufman recuperated slowly from his operation, gradually increasing in strength and optimism until he was discharged from the hospital on his seventeenth postoperative day. He received long-term medical followup from his private physician and was eventually able to return to his job as a furniture salesman.

Appendicitis and Appendectomy

Don Sharp, a 17-year-old Catholic college student, was stricken with periumbilical pain while playing baseball. Because the pain increased rapidly in intensity during the next few hours, his fraternity brothers took him to the dispensary. The nurse put Don to bed and called the school physician.

Before the physician arrived the nurse took Don's medical history and vital signs, obtained a blood sample for a complete blood count, and did a routine urinalysis. Don complained of constipation, abdominal pain, and nausea. His temperature was 100.6° F. orally, his pulse 92 per minute, respi-

rations 22 per minute, and blood pressure 104/76 mm. Hg. Don's blood count revealed 15,000 white cells per cu. mm., of which 80 per cent were poly-morphonuclear leukocytes. His hemoglobin concentration was 15 grams per 100 ml. of blood, hematocrit 50 per cent. Urinalysis revealed no abnormal findings.

When the physician arrived he found Don to be pale, sweating, and vomiting. His pain was then localized in the right lower abdomen, midway between the umbilicus and the anterior-superior spine of the ileum, and his abdominal wall was rigid to palpation. The doctor made a diagnosis of acute appendici-tis and ordered that Don be admitted to the university hospital immediately, that gastric siphonage be instituted, and that he be prepared for an emer-gency appendectomy.

(ANSWER BLANK ON PAGE A–65)   (CORRECT ANSWERS ON PAGE B–79)

1. While waiting for the examining physician to arrive, the dispensary nurse could safely grant Don's request for:
   1. A drink of water.
   2. A cleansing enema.
   3. A medication for pain.
   4. Elevation of the bed head.

2. Instead of periumbilical and right lower quadrant pain, Don's appendicitis might have produced:
   a. Pain on rectal examination.
   b. Pain in the lumbar region.
   c. Pain on defecation.
   d. Pain on micturition.
   e. Pain in the hip.
      1. a only.
      2. a, b, and c.
      3. All but e.
      4. All the above.

3. It would be helpful for the nurse in the university hospital to obtain which of the following information about Don as a basis upon which to plan his later nursing care?
   a. His understanding of his symptoms, diagnosis, and proposed treatment.
   b. The location of his family and their apparent importance to him.
   c. His previous experience with hospitalization and surgical treatment.
   d. His smoking, drinking, and eating habits and allergies, if any.
   e. His religious and social affiliations and his attitudes toward both.
      1. a and b.
      2. a, b, and c.
      3. All but e.
      4. All the above.

4. Why is it important for the nurse to explain to Don what she is about to do before taking his blood pressure?
   1. Muscle tension interferes with sound transmission.
   2. Questions during the procedure distract the nurse.
   3. Anxiety produces an elevation in blood pressure.
   4. Opportunity is created to ask his normal pressure.

5. Don's vomiting was probably the result of:
   1. Reflex response to the functional intestinal obstruction produced by appendiceal inflammation.
   2. Stimulation of the emetic center in the medulla oblongata by the sudden development of hyperthermia.
   3. Psychosomatic disturbance of gastrointestinal motility in response to marked fear and anxiety.
   4. Hypersecretion of gastric acid following parasympathetic overstimulation during stress.

6. Neutrophils usually comprise what per cent of the total white blood cell count?
   1. 5 per cent.
   2. 20 per cent.
   3. 45 per cent.
   4. 70 per cent.

7. What is the chief function of neutrophils in an acute infection?
   1. Supplying needed nutrients to damaged tissue.
   2. Engulfing and destroying bacteria in an infected area.
   3. Neutralizing exotoxins produced by pathogenic bacteria.

4. Generating the production of fibrous scar tissue.

8. Don's physical examination on hospital admission would be apt to reveal:
   a. Rebound tenderness in the right lower quadrant.
   b. Absence of normal bowel sounds.
   c. Absence of superficial abdominal reflexes.
   d. Dilation and engorgement of peri-umbilical vein.
   e. Enlargement of lymph nodes in the inguinal region.
      1. a and b.
      2. a, b, and c.
      3. All but d.
      4. All the above.

9. In which of the following positions would Don probably be most comfortable on his admission to the hospital unit?
   1. Sitting upright in a chair.
   2. Lying absolutely flat on his back.
   3. On his side, with right knee bent.
   4. Prone, with his head turned to one side.

10. In order to provide Don the needed psychological support preoperatively, the nurse should realize that he may express his fear of surgery through which of the following behaviors?
   a. Persistently changing the subject whenever the impending operation is referred to.
   b. Repeatedly asking for information previously given him by the physician or nurse.
   c. Failure to look at the nurse or to respond verbally to her conversation.
   d. Talking rapidly and in uninterrupted fashion of trivial matters unrelated to his illness.
   e. Making numerous unnecessary demands on the nurse for physical care and attention.
      1. a and b.
      2. a, b, and c.
      3. All but c.
      4. All the above.

The following preoperative orders were written:

1. Abdominal skin preparation.
2. Aqueous penicillin 600,000 units I.M. stat.
3. Empty urinary bladder immediately before surgery.
4. Meperidine hydrochloride 75 mg. H. and atropine sulfate 0.5 mg. H. 15 minutes before going to the operating room.

11. In preparing for Don's preoperative skin preparation, the nurse should assemble which of the following?
   a. Safety razor.
   b. Sterile basin.
   c. Sterile gauze pledgets.
   d. Small hand brush.
   e. Bottle of soap.
      1. a and b.
      2. a, b, and d.
      3. All but d.
      4. All the above.

12. Which of the following indicates the extent of Don's skin area that should be cleansed and shaved prior to the appendectomy?
   1. From the umbilicus to the groin on the right side of the abdomen.
   2. From the umbilicus to the groin from bedline to bedline.
   3. From the nipple line to the groin on the right side of the body.
   4. From the nipple line to the groin, from bedline to bedline.

13. The skin of Don's abdomen should be shaved before the operation in order to:
   1. Facilitate skin incision.
   2. Indicate the site to be draped.
   3. Prevent infection of the wound.
   4. Reduce postoperative scarring.

14. Which of the following organisms is most frequently an inhabitant of normal skin?
   1. *Aerobacter aerogenes.*
   2. *Clostridium perfringens.*
   3. *Micrococcus pyogenes.*
   4. *Streptococcus pyogenes.*

15. Don should void immediately before the operation in order to:
   1. Permit better visualization of the appendix.
   2. Facilitate operative handling of other viscera.
   3. Prevent injury to the bladder during surgery.
   4. Eliminate one source of postoperative discomfort.

16. What precaution should the nurse take before giving Don aqueous penicillin?
1. Ascertain that his urine is free of albumin.
2. Measure his blood pressure in standing position.
3. Ask him whether he is allergic to penicillin.
4. Inject a few minims of procaine into the injection site.

17. Don's preoperative preparation should include teaching him to:
a. Take in a deep breath slowly and exhale slowly.
b. Inhale deeply, splint his abdomen, and cough explosively.
c. Turn from side to side, assuming Sims' position.
d. Alternately flex and extend his hips and knees.
e. Plantar flex, dorsiflex, and circumduct his feet.
   1. a and c.
   2. b and d.
   3. All but e.
   4. All the above.

18. Don's preoperative preparation should include telling him that he may expect which of the following on recovering from the anesthetic?
a. Pain in his operative site.
b. Nausea and epigastric distress.
c. Intravenous infusion of fluid.
d. Expectoration of copious sputum.
e. Intermittent use of IPPB respirator.
   1. a and b.
   2. a, c, and e.
   3. All but e.
   4. All the above.

19. Who should give the consent for Don's operation?
1. Don Sharp.
2. Don's father.
3. The president of Don's fraternity.
4. The president of the university.

20. Who is legally responsible for securing written consent for a surgical operation?
1. The surgeon.
2. The head nurse.
3. The director of nurses.
4. The hospital administrator.

21. Which of the following conditions must be met to ensure the legality of a consent for surgical operation?

1. The patient must have detailed knowledge of the procedure to be done.
2. The patient must write out his consent and sign it.
3. The agreement must be witnessed by a licensed professional worker.
4. Consent must be obtained at least an hour before surgery is begun.

22. Since Don's operation was scheduled as an emergency procedure, it would be particularly important for the nurse to:
1. Reassure him that the operation is a common procedure.
2. Build his confidence in the surgeon performing the operation.
3. Call a priest to administer the sacrament of extreme unction.
4. Administer a complete bath and shampoo using hexachlorophene soap.

23. Meperidine is similar to morphine in its tendency to:
a. Alter the affective reaction to pain.
b. Produce spasm of intestinal muscles.
c. Depress the medullary respiratory center.
d. Produce psychic dependency and addiction.
   1. a and c.
   2. b and d.
   3. All but d.
   4. All the above.

24. Meperidine was given to Don preoperatively in order to:
a. Allay anxiety and apprehension about surgery.
b. Reduce the volume of intestinal secretions.
c. Decrease the required dose of anesthetic.
d. Constrict the rectal and urinary sphincters.
e. Prevent postoperative nausea and vomiting.
   1. a and c.
   2. b and d.
   3. All but d.
   4. All the above.

25. The principal reason for administering atropine sulfate preoperatively was to:
1. Depress the sensory cortex.
2. Improve cardiac contraction.

3. Decrease respiratory secretions.

4. Increase sphincter tone.

26. After Don has been given his preoperative medications, the nurse should:

1. Remove his head pillow.

2. Elevate the bed head.

3. Apply extra blankets.

4. Apply bed siderails.

27. Which of the following precautions is it most important that the nurse take in transporting Don to the operating room?

1. Cover his eyes with a small hand towel.

2. Pull the covers well up over his shoulders.

3. Elevate the side rails or secure cloth restraints.

4. Avoid transporting him on crowded elevators.

On being moved from the stretcher to the operating table, Don said to the nurse, "I'll feel a lot better when this ordeal is all over."

28. Probably Don fears his impending operation in part because it is natural to equate anesthesia with:

1. Amnesia.

2. Intoxication.

3. Insanity.

4. Death.

The operation was performed under cyclopropane anesthesia given by way of an endotracheal tube. During surgery a swollen, fluid-filled appendix was removed.

29. The chief advantage of administering an anesthetic agent by endotracheal tube rather than by face mask is the fact that the former method:

1. Prevents respiratory obstruction.

2. Permits use of less anesthetic.

3. Produces less postoperative discomfort.

4. Facilitates concomitant oxygen administration.

30. Cyclopropane is suitable as a general anesthetic for major surgery because:

a. The anesthetic dose is much less than the toxic dose.

b. It does not produce irritation of respiratory mucosa.

c. It is capable of producing a good degree of muscle relaxation.

d. It causes rapid and pleasant induction and recovery.

1. a and c.

2. b and d.

3. All but d.

4. All the above.

31. Which of the following are possible toxic effects of cyclopropane anesthesia?

a. Decreased respiratory rate.

b. Bronchial spasm.

c. Cardiac arrhythmias.

d. Increased salivation.

e. Hepatocellular failure.

1. a only.

2. a, b, and c.

3. All but d.

4. All the above.

32. The first stage of anesthesia is known as the stage of:

1. Excitement.

2. Analgesia.

3. Medullary paralysis.

4. Surgical anesthesia.

33. Which part of the central nervous system is depressed first by cyclopropane?

1. Cerebrum.

2. Cerebellum.

3. Medulla oblongata.

4. Spinal cord.

34. During the second stage of anesthesia Don is apt to demonstrate:

1. Weak, thready pulse.

2. Shallow respirations.

3. Constricted pupils.

4. Struggling movements.

35. Which of the following abilities would Don lose last during induction of anesthesia?

1. Movement.

2. Feeling.

3. Hearing.

4. Speech.

36. The chief risk incurred in the use of cyclopropane as an anesthetic is:

1. Danger of an explosion.

2. Possibility of anoxemia.

3. Irritation of lung tissue.

4. Postoperative vomiting.

37. The final stage of anesthesia is known as the stage of:

1. Excitement.

2. Analgesia.

3. Medullary paralysis.

4. Surgical anesthesia.

38. The fourth stage of anesthesia is characterized by:

1. Uncontrolled movement.
2. Flushed skin.
3. Nonreactive pupils.
4. Elevated blood pressure.

39. Which of the following are thought to predispose to development of acute appendicitis?

a. Kinking of the appendix.
b. Presence of a fecalith.
c. Repeated throat infections.
d. Inadequate food intake.
   1. a and b.
   2. c and d.
   3. a, b, and c.
   4. All the above.

40. Which of the following is the most common precipitating cause of acute appendicitis?

1. Ingestion of foods containing chemical toxins.
2. Mechanical obstruction of the ileocecal valve.
3. Mechanical irritation by overlying pelvic viscera.
4. Invasion of appendiceal wall by intestinal bacteria.

41. An acutely infected appendix is apt to rupture due to:

1. Tissue necrosis produced by constriction of vessels in the wall of the organ.
2. Friction of the dilated organ against surrounding loops of peristalsing intestine.
3. Inability of the organ to drain due to blockage by inflammatory debris.
4. The large quantity of proteolytic enzymes contained in purulent material.

42. Peritonitis resulting from rupture of an inflamed appendix is primarily due to:

1. Chemical irritation by digestive juices.
2. Bacterial invasion by intestinal organisms.
3. Mechanical pressure by distended bowel.
4. Ischemic damage from mesenteric thrombosis.

Following surgery Don was taken to the recovery room. The doctor ordered:

1. 1000 cc. 5 per cent dextrose in normal saline I.V. to run for 8 hours.
2. Meperidine hydrochloride 50 mg. H. p.r.n. for pain.
3. Tetracycline 500 mg. I.V. q. 6 h. for two days, then tetracycline 200 mg. I.M. b.i.d.

On the evening of the operative day Don suffered extreme nausea and had difficulty voiding. Gastric siphonage was initiated by the doctor.

43. Which of the following pieces of equipment should be available in the postanesthetic unit?

a. Oxygen flowmeter.
b. Suction machine.
c. Mechanical airway.
d. Positive pressure respirator.
e. Cardiopulmonary resuscitation cart.
   1. a and b.
   2. a, b, and c.
   3. a, b, c, and d.
   4. All the above.

44. Which of the following would be most helpful in maintaining Don's airway while he is still unconscious in the recovery room?

1. Leaving the oropharyngeal airway in place.
2. Placing a pillow under his shoulders.
3. Raising his arms over his head.
4. Elevating the foot of the bedframe.

45. The recovery room nurse should remain with Don postoperatively until she observes that:

a. His pharyngeal reflexes have returned.
b. He is oriented to his general surroundings.
c. His vital signs have become stabilized.
d. He is moving about freely in bed.
   1. a only.
   2. a and b.
   3. a, b, and c.
   4. All the above.

46. Don may suffer which of the following complications as a result of endotracheal intubation during surgery?

a. Sore throat.
b. Hoarseness.
c. Laryngeal or tracheal edema.
d. Tracheal collapse.
e. Laryngospasm.

1. a and b.
2. a, b, and c.
3. All but e.
4. All the above.

47. As soon as Don recovers from his anesthetic he should be placed in which of the following positions?
1. Trendelenburg.
2. Low Fowler's.
3. Right Sims'.
4. Left Sims'.

48. Since the physician did not specify the rate at which Don's intravenous infusion should run, the nurse should regulate its flow to approximately:
1. 5 drops per minute.
2. 30 drops per minute.
3. 60 drops per minute.
4. 90 drops per minute.

49. Which of the following concentrations of saline solution would be isotonic with the blood?
1. 9 per cent.
2. 0.9 per cent.
3. 0.09 per cent.
4. 0.009 per cent.

50. What is the probable cause of Don's inability to void postoperatively?
1. Edema of the urethral mucosa.
2. Spasm of the bladder sphincter.
3. Atony of the bladder muscle.
4. Pressure of the bladder against the pubes.

51. The nurse could best stimulate Don to void by:
1. Applying manual pressure to the supra-pubic region.
2. Placing a warm water bottle on the lower abdomen.
3. Assisting him to a sitting position on the edge of the bed.
4. Encouraging the ingestion of large amounts of fluid.

52. The average daily urinary output for a normal adult is approximately:
1. 6000 cc.
2. 3000 cc.
3. 1500 cc.
4. 750 cc.

53. Which of the following measures would contribute most to minimizing Don's discomfort in having the gastric suction tube inserted?
1. Cover his eyes throughout the entire procedure.
2. Have him drink water before beginning tubation.
3. Immerse the tube in chipped ice before insertion.
4. Place him on his left side as the tube is advanced.

54. It is important for Don to walk soon after his operation in order to produce:
a. Increased respiratory exchange of gases.
b. Improved tone of smooth muscle of the bowel.
c. Enhanced perception of sensory stimuli.
d. Accelerated blood flow in the extremities.
1. a and c.
2. b and d.
3. a, b, and d.
4. All the above.

55. Healing of Don's surgical wound is most apt to be retarded by inadequate intake of:
1. Carbohydrate.
2. Protein.
3. Fat.
4. Minerals.

56. In order to promote capillary proliferation and formation of scar tissue, Don may be given a supplementary dose of:
1. Vitamin A.
2. Vitamin B_1.
3. Vitamin C.
4. Vitamin D.

57. During the afternoon of the third postoperative day, Don's dressing was changed. In preparing to change his dressing, which of the following items should the nurse assemble?
a. Clean masks.
b. Sterile tissue forceps.
c. Sterile gauze pads.
d. Sterile gloves.
1. All but a.
2. All but c.
3. All but d.
4. All the above.

58. Which of the following will most effectively remove adhesive from the skin?
1. Soap and water.
2. Hydrogen peroxide.
3. Ethyl alcohol.
4. Ethyl ether.

59. At midnight on his third postoperative day, Don complained that he was unable to sleep. The nurse noted that his vital signs were normal, his wound was in good condition, and he was not in pain. Which of the following measures should she employ first?

1. Change his position and give him a backrub.
2. Repeat the pentobarbital given at bedtime.
3. Administer the meperidine ordered postoperatively.
4. Call the house physician to examine him.

Six days after surgery, Don had recovered sufficiently to have his wound sutures removed and to be discharged from the hospital to his room at the fraternity house. A week later he was given permission to return to classes.

60. In instructing student patients at the school dispensary, the nurse should emphasize which of the following points in order to help in reducing deaths from appendicitis?

1. Importance of complete annual physical examinations.
2. Dangers from indiscriminate use of cathartics.
3. Inadvisability of self-medication with antibiotics.
4. Contribution of the various food groups to health.

Peptic Ulcer and Gastric Resection

John Gunderson, 43-year-old owner of a small, neighborhood grocery store, developed chronic dyspepsia when his business failed and he was forced to declare bankruptcy. He consulted his doctor when nausea and vomiting caused him to lose sleep at night, and was admitted to the local hospital for a complete workup. Mr. Gunderson told the admitting room nurse that his chief complaints were burning epigastric pain, nausea, and vomiting. Questioning by the nurse revealed that he did not smoke or drink alcoholic beverages, but drank coffee in large quantities.

(ANSWER BLANK ON PAGE A-67)   (CORRECT ANSWERS ON PAGE B-85)

1. Which of the following emotional factors is thought to contribute to the production of a peptic ulcer?
1. Threat of separation from the mother figure.
2. Anxiety relating to identification of the sexual role.
3. Strong unconscious passive-dependent oral needs.
4. Chronic inhibition of strong hostile-aggressive drives.

2. It is thought that emotional stress and conflict contribute to ulcer formation through:

1. Disorganization of cerebral cortex appetite controls.
2. Loss of pituitary control of endocrine functioning.
3. Excessive stimulation of the parasympathetic system.
4. Increased activity of the sympathetic nervous system.

3. Increased parasympathetic activity predisposes to peptic ulcer by effecting gastric:
a. Hypersecretion.
b. Hypertrophy.
c. Hypermotility.

d. Hyperplasia.
e. Hypertonia.
   1. a and b.
   2. c and d.
   3. a, c, and e.
   4. All the above.

The physician's physical examination of Mr. Gunderson revealed skin and mucosal pallor, poor tissue turgor, and slight abdominal tenderness. The following diagnostic tests were ordered:

1. Complete blood count.
2. Stool guaiac test.
3. Complete gastrointestinal tract x-rays.
4. Gastric analysis with Ewald test meal.

A tentative diagnosis was made of gastric or duodenal peptic ulcer.

4. The tissue change most characteristic of peptic ulcer is:
   1. A ragged erosion of mucosa covered with purulent exudate.
   2. A sharp excavation of surface membrane with a clean base.
   3. A lumpy mass of necrotic tissue with surface bleeding.
   4. An elevated ridge of fibrous tissue with wrinkled margins.

5. When interpreting the history of Mr. Gunderson's illness, the nurse should be aware that pain due to peptic ulcer usually develops:
   1. Immediately before meals.
   2. While eating or drinking.
   3. Immediately after eating.
   4. Two to three hours after meals.

6. Careful questioning of Mr. Gunderson by the nurse would probably reveal that his epigastric pain had been most often relieved by:
   1. Avoidance of food and drink.
   2. Massage of the upper abdomen.
   3. Ingestion of milk and crackers.
   4. Purging with a high enema.

7. Pallor due to anemia is usually most easily detected in the:
   1. Lips.
   2. Gums.
   3. Ear lobe.
   4. Nail beds.

8. Mr. Gunderson's poor tissue turgor is probably related to his:
   1. Psychological stress.
   2. Recent vomiting.

3. Cellular hypoxia.
4. Loss of sleep.

9. Which of the following results of Mr. Gunderson's blood count would best support a diagnosis of peptic ulcer?
   1. Neutrophilic leukocytes.
   2. Hypochromic anemia.
   3. Marked thrombocytopenia.
   4. Blast cell proliferation.

10. The stool guaiac test was ordered to detect the presence of:
   1. Hydrochloric acid.
   2. Undigested food.
   3. Occult blood.
   4. Inflammatory cells.

11. In order to ensure the validity of the guaiac test, the nurse should prepare Mr. Gunderson by:
   1. Restricting all food and fluids on the day before the test is done.
   2. Forcing fluids in large quantities on the day of the test.
   3. Withholding red meat for 72 hours before securing the stool specimen.
   4. Administering a tap water enema to obtain a diarrheal stool sample.

12. Which of the following means would be used to facilitate the x-ray visualization of Mr. Gunderson's stomach and duodenum?
   1. Administering barium sulfate solution orally.
   2. Insufflating air through a gastric drainage tube.
   3. Serving a light meal with a high fat content.
   4. Injecting an iodine containing dye intravenously.

13. In order to inform Mr. Gunderson accurately concerning the nature of a barium meal, the nurse should know that the flavor of barium sulfate is:
   1. Sour.
   2. Bitter.
   3. Salty.
   4. Chalky.

14. In preparing Mr. Gunderson for his upper gastrointestinal tract x-rays, the nurse should tell him to expect the examination to include:
   1. Ingestion of numerous liquid and semi-soft meals in quick succession.
   2. Removal of stomach secretions through a nasogastric drainage tube.
   3. Administration of radiopaque drugs intramuscularly or intravenously.
   4. Taking serial pictures as he assumes various positions on the table.

15. Which of the following nursing activities would be essential in preparing Mr. Gunderson for gastric analysis?
    1. Pushing fluids for 24 hours preceding the test.
    2. Administering enemas on the preceding evening.
    3. Withholding food on the morning of analysis.
    4. Recording the pulse rate when beginning the test.

16. An Ewald test meal consists of:
    1. 4 arrowroot cookies and 1½ cups of weak tea.
    2. 200 ml. broth and 200 grams broiled steak.
    3. 1 cup milk and 1 ounce cream.
    4. 1 boiled egg and 1 cup of strong coffee.

17. Which of the following findings on gastric analysis would best support a diagnosis of peptic ulcer?
    1. Absence of gastric secretions.
    2. Increased hydrochloric acid.
    3. Lack of intrinsic factor.
    4. Decreased gastric motility.

The diagnostic tests yielded the following data:

    1. Red blood cell count 5,100,000 per cu. mm. of blood.
    2. Hemoglobin 64 grams per 100 ml.
    3. Positive reaction of stool to guaiac test.
    4. Radiographic evidence of an ulcer crater on the superior aspect of the duodenal bulb.
    5. Increased volume of both free and total hydrochloric acid in gastric secretions.

18. Hypochromic anemia is characterized by red blood cells that differ from normal cells by being:
    1. Grossly irregular in shape.
    2. Less filled with hemoglobin.
    3. Larger in total volume.
    4. Without nuclear chromatin.

19. Mr. Gunderson developed hypochromic microcytic anemia as a consequence of:
    1. Inadequate intake of vitamins and protein.
    2. Depletion of the body's store of iron.
    3. Toxic interference with red cell function.
    4. Excessive destruction of cells in the spleen.

The doctor indicated on Mr. Gunderson's chart that the diagnosis of duodenal peptic ulcer had been confirmed by diagnostic tests, and ordered:

    1. Sippy No. 1 diet.
    2. Aluminum hydroxide gel (Amphogel), drams 1 every hour.
    3. Propantheline bromide (Pro-Banthine) 15 mg. orally t.i.d.
    4. Phenobarbital 30 mg. orally t.i.d.

20. Which of the following physiologic changes may have contributed to the development of Mr. Gunderson's ulcer?
    a. Increased secretion of hydrochloric acid.
    b. Decreased production of gastric mucus.
    c. Increased production of pancreatic enzymes.
    d. Local ischemia of gastric mucosa.
       1. a only.
       2. b and c.
       3. All but c.
       4. All the above.

21. Which of the following are possible complications of duodenal ulcer?
    a. Acute hemorrhage.
    b. Macrocytic anemia.
    c. Pyloric obstruction.
    d. Gallstones.
    e. Bowel perforation.
       1. a and b.
       2. a, c, and e.
       3. All but e.
       4. All the above.

22. The Sippy No. 1 diet ordered for Mr. Gunderson consisted of:
    1. A small quantity of a milk and cream mixture every hour.
    2. Frequent feedings of thin soups and clear meat broths.
    3. Five meals a day of puréed vegetables and ground meat.
    4. Three light meals of bland foods containing no roughage.

23. The Sippy diet will not be given to Mr. Gunderson over a long period of time because prolonged administration would predispose him to development of:
    1. Atherosclerosis.
    2. Anorexia.
    3. Regression.
    4. Constipation.

24. Aluminum hydroxide gel (Amphogel) would be preferred to sodium bicarbonate in treating Mr. Gunderson's hyperacidity because, unlike sodium bicarbonate, aluminum hydroxide gel:
    1. Is not absorbed from the bowel.

2. Does not predispose to constipation.
3. Rapidly dissolves in all body fluids.
4. Has no effect on phosphorus excretion.

25. In addition to its antacid effects, aluminum hydroxide gel is locally:
   1. Depressant.
   2. Cleansing.
   3. Astringent.
   4. Irritating.

26. The pharmacologic effect of propantheline bromide (Pro-Banthine) is to:
   1. Neutralize hydrochloric acid.
   2. Inhibit gastrointestinal motility.
   3. Depress the cerebral cortex.
   4. Coat and soothe mucous membranes.

27. Which of the following are frequent side effects of propantheline bromide (Pro-Banthine)?
   a. Dry mouth.
   b. Hiccoughs.
   c. Visual blurring.
   d. Urinary retention.
      1. a and b.
      2. b and c.
      3. a, c, and d.
      4. All the above.

28. The pharmacologic effect of phenobarbital is to:
   1. Block impulse transmission over sensory nerve tracts.
   2. Decrease hydrochloric acid formation in the stomach.
   3. Depress neurons of ascending reticular formation.
   4. Interfere with the normal action of acetylcholine.

29. Phenobarbital is normally detoxified by the:
   1. Stomach.
   2. Liver.
   3. Pancreas.
   4. Spleen.

30. In planning long-term care for Mr. Gunderson, the nurse might be aware that a common result of barbiturate intoxication is:
   1. Gingival hypertrophy.
   2. Respiratory depression.
   3. Clonic convulsions.
   4. Aplastic anemia.

31. In talking with Mr. Gunderson regarding ways in which he might reduce his psychological stress the nurse made the following comment, "You expect too much of yourself." What was the therapeutic intent of this statement?

   1. To persuade him to allow the nurses to execute his total care.
   2. To help him to develop a fastidious approach to self-care.
   3. To provoke him to vocalization of his personal concerns and hostilities.
   4. To give him permission to relax his demands upon himself.

32. In order to help Mr. Gunderson to learn to decrease the emotional stress associated with his daily routines, the nurse should guide her conversation with him to enable him to:
   a. Set priorities in regard to daily activities.
   b. Improve the level of his problem solving.
   c. Express concerns about his economic status.
   d. Plan opportunities for daily relaxation.
   e. Recognize the relationship between stress and symptoms.
      1. a, b, and c.
      2. a, b, and d.
      3. All but e.
      4. All the above.

Mr. Gunderson was continued on this regimen for three weeks with only minimal relief of his symptoms. At the end of that time he signed himself out of the hospital against his physician's advice, saying that he could no longer leave his business unattended. Just before Mr. Gunderson left the unit, a dietician gave him a written copy of a strict ulcer diet and explained how to prepare the included foods.

33. The Sippy diet prescribed for Mr. Gunderson was probably lacking in:
   1. Cooked cereal.
   2. Fried foods.
   3. Lean meats.
   4. Boiled eggs.

34. Which of the following foods might be included on a strict ulcer diet?
   a. Cooked rice.
   b. Stewed tomatoes.
   c. Cream of pea soup.
   d. Ground beef.
   e. Cottage cheese.
      1. a and c.
      2. b and d.
      3. a, c, and e.
      4. All the above.

35. Which of the following foods might be included on a liberal ulcer diet?
  a. Cream of Wheat cereal.
  b. Baked potato.
  c. Applesauce.
  d. Strained spinach.
  e. Roast chicken.
      1. a and c.
      2. b and d.
      3. All the above.
      4. None of the above.

36. The nurse reasoned that Mr. Gunderson would probably not adhere to his prescribed diet because the dietary instruction was:
  a. Too brief to be meaningful.
  b. Given at an inopportune time.
  c. Unsupported by followup.
  d. Not given to his wife as well.
      1. a only.
      2. a and b.
      3. All but d.
      4. All the above.

For the next twelve months Mr. Gunderson was treated by his family physician with antacids and antispasmodics, but he continued to suffer epigastric pain, nausea, and vomiting. He did not follow the prescribed ulcer diet, nor did he abstain from drinking coffee despite constant reminders from his doctor to do so. Finally he was admitted one night to the hospital emergency room after having vomited a large quantity of bright red blood.

37. Mr. Gunderson had been advised by his doctor not to drink coffee because it:
      1. Increases mental activity.
      2. Stimulates gastric secretions.
      3. Increases smooth muscle tone.
      4. Elevates systolic blood pressure.

38. Probably Mr. Gunderson's failure to follow his prescribed ulcer treatment was a manifestation of his:
      1. Inability to accept what he considers to be a health deficiency in himself.
      2. Acting out the medical staff's expectation of his failure to follow orders.
      3. Lack of understanding of the complications which might result from his ulcer.
      4. Attempt to control the behavior of his family and friends.

On physical examination Mr. Gunderson was found to have a temperature of 97.8° F. orally, pulse 124 per minute, respirations 26 per minute, and blood pressure 90/60 mm. Hg. The doctor noted that he was pale and anxious, and that his skin was moist and clammy. Gastric suction siphonage was begun and the gastric drainage was observed to contain both bright red blood and material resembling coffee grounds.

39. In relating Mr. Gunderson's present symptoms to the history of his illness, the nurse should have concluded that his pallor, pulse rate, and blood pressure could best be accounted for on the basis of his:
      1. Longstanding malnutrition.
      2. Serum electrolyte imbalance.
      3. Gastrointestinal hemorrhage.
      4. Continued use of propantheline bromide.

40. The nurse could best allay Mr. Gunderson's anxiety immediately following his admission to the hospital by:
  a. Remaining with him throughout his emergency room examination and transfer to the ward.
  b. Telling him that his gastric hemorrhage, which had been minimal, had now ceased.
  c. Placing the gastric drainage bottle so that it is not in his direct line of vision.
  d. Inviting his wife to remain with him throughout the examination and gastric evacuation.
  e. Giving a brief explanation of each step in the admission and treatment procedures.
      1. a and b.
      2. c and d.
      3. a, c, and e.
      4. All the above.

41. Which of the following could be responsible for the fact that Mr. Gunderson's respiratory rate is above normal?
  a. Epigastric pain.
  b. Anxiety feelings.
  c. Recent hemorrhage.
  d. Metabolic acidosis.
      1. a and b.
      2. a and d.
      3. All but d.
      4. All the above.

42. Continuous gastrointestinal decompression is particularly apt to produce:
1. Hemorrhage.
2. Constipation.
3. Hiccoughs.
4. Alkalosis.

Following three days of treatment, Mr. Gunderson's bleeding had ceased and upper gastrointestinal x-rays were done, revealing a large ulcer crater on the anterior wall of the duodenum and narrowing of the pylorus. The doctor ordered that Mr. Gunderson be given two units of blood and scheduled him to have a subtotal gastrectomy, vagotomy, and gastrojejunostomy.

43. Which of the following factors probably contributed to the doctor's decision that Mr. Gunderson should have a subtotal gastrectomy?
  a. His age and general physical condition.
  b. His unsatisfactory response to medical therapy.
  c. The probability that the ulcer was malignant.
  d. The danger that phenobarbital addiction might occur.
   1. a only.
   2. b only.
   3. All but d.
   4. All the above.

44. The rationale for removing the lower 40 to 50 per cent of the stomach as part of Mr. Gunderson's treatment is the fact that:
1. Hydrochloric acid is chiefly secreted by glands in the lower half of the stomach.
2. Ulcers in the lower portion of the stomach are particularly subject to malignant degeneration.
3. A hormone produced in the lower stomach wall is capable of stimulating acid secretion.
4. Interruption of vagal stimulation will render the pylorus incapable of opening and closing.

45. Which of the following anatomic facts explains why Mr. Gunderson's duodenum was not totally removed?
1. The head of the pancreas is adherent to the duodenal wall.
2. The common bile duct empties into the duodenal lumen.
3. The wall of the jejunum contains no intestinal villi.
4. The jejunum receives its blood supply through the duodenum.

On the following day Mr. Gunderson was given 50 mg. of meperidine hydrochloride, 25 mg. of promethazine, and 0.4 mg. of atropine and was then taken to the operating room where a subtotal gastrectomy, a gastrojejunostomy, and a vagotomy were done under cyclopropane anesthesia. Mr. Gunderson tolerated the surgical procedure well and was still unconscious when taken to the recovery room. His nasogastric tube was attached to low suction for three days. He was given an intravenous infusion of 5 per cent dextrose in $1/4$ normal saline containing a multivitamin preparation and 20 mEq. KCl.

46. A vagotomy was done as part of Mr. Gunderson's surgical treatment in order to:
1. Decrease the secretion of hydrochloric acid.
2. Improve the tone of gastrointestinal muscles.
3. Increase the blood supply to the jejunum.
4. Prevent the transmission of pain impulses.

47. In Mr. Gunderson's immediate postoperative care, the nurse must be particularly conscientious in encouraging him to cough and breathe deeply at frequent intervals because:
1. Marked changes in intrathoracic pressure will stimulate gastric drainage.
2. The high abdominal incision will lead to shallow breathing to avoid pain.
3. The phrenic nerve will have been destroyed during the surgical procedure.
4. Deep breathing will prevent postoperative vomiting and intestinal distention.

48. The nurse should expect that for the first few hours postoperatively, the drainage from Mr. Gunderson's nasogastric tube will be:
1. Clear and colorless.
2. Bright red.
3. Dark red.
4. Yellow-green.

49. In irrigating the nasogastric tube following surgery, the nurse should be particularly careful to avoid:
1. Exerting undue pressure on the gastric suture line.
2. Injecting irrigating solution into the lung air sacs.
3. Advancing the nasogastric tube into the duodenum.
4. Touching the gastric incision with irrigating solution.

50. The nasogastric tube is left in place for the first few postoperative days in order to:
  a. Keep the suture lines clean.
  b. Watch for postoperative bleeding.
  c. Prevent strain on the incision.
  d. Block bile flow to the intestine.
1. a only.
2. a and b.
3. All but d.
4. All the above.

51. Which of the following substances would be most suitable for use in administering mouth care to Mr. Gunderson while the nasogastric tube is in place?
1. Cold tap water.
2. Normal saline solution.
3. Thin starch solution.
4. Glycerine and lemon juice.

52. Mr. Gunderson would probably be most comfortable in which of the following positions during his immediate postoperative period?
1. Supine.
2. Left Sims' position.
3. Low Fowler's position.
4. Trendelenburg's position.

53. Whenever his nurse was unable to spend time talking with Mr. Gunderson he loudly demanded service, using abusive language and accusing her of not giving him proper care. This behavior on his part is probably the result of his:
1. Unresolved need to be dependent, which he fears and denies.
2. Inability to communicate meaningfully with other people.
3. Shame at having developed what he knows is a psychosomatic illness.
4. Feelings of superiority in regard to members of the nursing team.

On the third postoperative day, Mr. Gunderson's nasogastric tube was removed and he was given sips of water to drink. Within the next few days he progressed from a clear liquid to a soft diet, then to a general diet, served in six small meals daily.

54. Which of the following findings probably caused the doctor to remove Mr. Gunderson's nasogastric tube on the third postoperative day?
1. Inflammation of the pharyngeal mucosa.
2. Absence of bile in the gastric drainage.
3. Return of bowel sounds to normal.
4. Passage of numerous diarrheal stools.

55. Which of the following foods might be included in a clear liquid diet?
  a. Tea.
  b. Milk.
  c. Gelatin.
  d. Ice cream.
  e. Bouillon.
1. a only.
2. b and d.
3. a, c, and e.
4. All the above.

56. Milk is omitted from a clear liquid diet because it:
1. Produces gas.
2. Contains calories.
3. Produces nausea.
4. Coats the mucosa.

57. Which of the following foods might be included in a soft diet?
  a. Baked custard.
  b. Macaroni and cheese.
  c. Poached egg.
  d. Cooked farina.
  e. Mashed potato.
1. a only.
2. a and c.
3. b and d.
4. All the above.

On his fourteenth postoperative day Mr. Gunderson complained of feeling weak, clammy, and light-headed immediately after lunch. His doctor was summoned, and after examining Mr. Gunderson, he diagnosed the distress as a manifestation of the "dumping syndrome."

58. In order to give Mr. Gunderson needed dietary instruction, the nurse must understand that the dumping syndrome is the result of:

1. The body's absorption of toxins produced by liquefaction of dead tissue.
2. Too rapid emptying of food and fluid from the stomach into the jejunum.
3. Formation of an ulcer at the margin of the gastrojejunal anastomosis.
4. Obstruction of venous blood flow from the stomach into the portal system.

59. Which of the following instructions should be given Mr. Gunderson at this time?

a. Eat frequent and small meals.
b. Avoid drinking fluids with meals.
c. Eliminate sweet foods and drinks.

d. Lie down briefly after each meal.
1. a and c.
2. b and d.
3. All the above.
4. None of the above.

Following nutrition instruction and adjustment of Mr. Gunderson's diet, he experienced no further symptoms of the dumping syndrome. Mr. Gunderson continued to recover, increasing in both weight and strength until he was discharged from the hospital on his 21st postoperative day. Arrangements were made for him to receive regular medical and nutritional followup in the hospital's outpatient clinic.

Pernicious Anemia

Mrs. Nettie White's landlady brought her to the hospital because she was unable to care for herself any more. Mrs. White was 60 years old and had lived in a furnished room since she had been widowed seven years before. During the past several months she had become progressively more weak and confused and had complained of numbness and tingling in her legs and feet. For several days she had not left her room at all and had subsisted on tidbits of food brought to her by other residents of the rooming house.

(ANSWER BLANK ON PAGE A-69)   (CORRECT ANSWERS ON PAGE B-90)

During Mrs. White's physical examination the physician observed:

1. Marked skin pallor, with a pale yellow tinge.
2. Smooth, beefy red tongue.
3. Temperature 98° F. orally, pulse 96 per minute, respirations 24 per minute.
4. Loss of vibratory and position sense in the lower extremities.

A complete blood count, a bone marrow biopsy, a gastric analysis, and a Schilling test revealed:

1. Red blood cell count 1,200,000 per cu. mm., with great variety in shape and size.

2. White blood cell count 4000 per cu. mm.
3. Hemoglobin concentration 6 grams per 100 ml.
4. Hyperplastic bone marrow with numerous megaloblasts.
5. Absence of hydrochloric acid on tests of gastric secretions.
6. Defective absorption of vitamin B_{12}.

A diagnosis was made of pernicious anemia and the following orders were written:

1. Vitamin B_{12}, 30 micrograms I.M. daily.
2. Complete bedrest.
3. Diet as tolerated.
4. Dilute hydrochloric acid 2 cc. t.i.d. with meals.

1. Through careful questioning of Mrs. White and her landlady, the physician might learn that Mrs. White had experienced which other symptoms of pernicious anemia?
   a. Palpitation. *Flatulence*
   b. Orthopnea.
   c. Chest pain. *Constipation*
   d. Indigestion.
   e. Pedal edema. *Hair loss*
      1. a and b.
      2. c and d.
      3. All but e.
      4. All the above.

2. Which of the following should be used in the preparation of Mrs. White's hospital bed?
   a. Footboard.
   b. Plastic covered pillow.
   c. Extra blankets.
   d. Rubber ring.
      1. a only.
      2. a and b.
      3. a and c.
      4. All the above.

3. While assisting Mrs. White from the wheel chair to the bed, the nurse noted that Mrs. White seemed short of breath. Her dyspnea was probably the result of:
      1. Anoxia. *Hypoxia*
      2. Anxiety.
      3. Heart failure.
      4. Pneumonia. *Polycythemia*

4. Which of the following foods would be most suitable for Mrs. White's dinner on the day of admission?
      1. Barbecued ribs.
      2. Creamed chicken.
      3. Fried perch.
      4. Polish sausage.

5. On Mrs. White's admission to the hospital, tests of her serum would be most apt to reveal increased:
      1. Plasma protein.
      2. Icteric index.
      3. Cholesterol esters.
      4. Lactose dehydrogenase.

6. Mrs. White's pale yellow skin color probably resulted from:
      1. Chronic malnutrition.
      2. Excessive hemolysis.
      3. Intrahepatic obstruction.
      4. Mild hypotension.

7. Slight jaundice would be most easily observed in the:
      1. Skin of the abdomen.
      2. Beds of the fingernails.
      3. Mucosa of the mouth.
      4. Sclera of the eye.

8. The smooth, beefy red appearance of Mrs. White's tongue is probably the result of:
      1. Low-grade infection.
      2. Chemical irritations.
      3. Mechanical trauma.
      4. Vitamin deficiency.

9. Any delay in instituting treatment for Mrs. White's pernicious anemia would be most apt to result in irreversibility of her:
      1. Blood cell irregularities.
      2. Digestive difficulties.
      3. Neurological disturbances.
      4. Skin color changes.

10. Mrs. White could be expected to display which of the following types of behavior as a result of her illness?
   a. Depression.
   b. Irritability.
   c. Amnesia.
   d. Paranoid ideas.
   e. Delirium.
      1. a and c.
      2. b and d.
      3. All but d.
      4. All the above.

11. Which of the following would be most suitable for administering mouth care to Mrs. White?
      1. Long, cotton-tipped applicators.
      2. A tissue forceps and cotton balls.
      3. A toothbrush with firm bristles.
      4. A tongue blade wrapped with gauze.

12. Mrs. White's tachycardia is probably the result of:
      1. A chronic low-grade bacterial infection.
      2. Atheromatous narrowing of coronary arteries.
      3. Reflex response to chronic tissue anoxia.
      4. Anxiety produced by the physical examination. *assessment*

13. Mrs. White's complaint of numbness and tingling of the feet was probably the result of:
      1. Decreased arterial blood flow.
      2. Skeletal muscle fatigue.
      3. Spinal cord degeneration.
      4. Peripheral nerve irritation.

14. Which of the following presumably contributed to Mrs. White's poor eating habits in recent weeks?
   a. Sore mouth and tongue.
   b. Impairment of taste and smell.

c. Difficulty in handling utensils.

d. Lack of physical activity.

    1. a only.

    2. a and b.

    3. All but d.

    4. All the above.

15. In which of the following sites are red blood cells produced in the greatest number in the adult?

    1. Liver.

    2. Spleen.

    3. Lymph nodes.

    4. Bone marrow.

16. How does a mature red blood cell differ from a mature white blood cell?

    1. The red cell lacks a cell membrane.

    2. The red cell is larger than the white.

    3. The red cell has lost its nucleus.

    4. The red cell has cytoplasmic granules.

17. Hemoglobin is composed of a protein joined to:

    1. A phosphorus compound.

    2. An iron compound.

    3. A copper compound.

    4. A calcium compound.

18. The average life span of a normal red blood cell is:

    1. One week.

    2. One month.

    3. Four months.

    4. One year.

19. Red blood cells are normally broken down in the:

    1. Heart.

    2. Lung.

    3. Kidney.

    4. Spleen.

20. Which of the following is most characteristic of all types of anemia?

    1. Decreased number of red blood cells.

    2. Decreased amount of hemoglobin per cell.

    3. Decreased volume of circulating blood.

    4. Decreased oxygen-carrying capacity of the blood.

21. Which of the following mechanisms is the underlying cause of pernicious anemia?

    1. Acute blood loss.

    2. Chronic blood loss.

    3. Defective blood production.

    4. Bone marrow replacement.

22. Which of the following blood findings would be most characteristic of pernicious anemia?

    1. Microcytosis.

    2. Normocytosis.

    3. Macrocytosis.

    4. Spherocytosis.

23. Mrs. White's blood count is apt to reveal:

    1. Greater than normal number of thrombocytes.

    2. Relative decrease in the number of lymphocytes.

    3. Decreased number of granulocytic white cells.

    4. Reduction in the number of monocytes.

24. From which of the following sites would the doctor be most apt to obtain a sample of Mrs. White's bone marrow for biopsy?

    1. Cranium.

    2. Sternum.

    3. Vertebra.

    4. Radius.

25. Mrs. White asked the nurse what a marrow biopsy was (having overheard the doctor use the term). Which of the following explanations would be most helpful to Mrs. White at this time?

    1. "A biopsy is an examination of tissue taken from a living subject. A biopsy, is therefore, an examination of bone marrow from a living patient."

    2. "The examination of the bone marrow is carried out by a specially trained hematologist. I'm sure that your doctor would be happy to explain it to you."

    3. "The examination consists of staining a specimen of red marrow and counting the numbers of the different types of red and white blood cells in it."

    4. "The doctor takes a small sample of marrow from the breastbone and examines it under a microscope to determine how new blood cells are being produced."

26. Mrs. White's bone marrow was most likely hyperplastic for which of the following reasons?

    1. As a result of a chronic infection.

    2. In response to cellular oxygen lack.

    3. As a consequence of marrow replacement.

    4. As a result of malignant tissue changes.

27. Which of the following explanations of gastric analysis would be most helpful to Mrs. White?
   1. "The doctor will insert a tube down your throat into your stomach, remove some digestive juice, and test it to obtain information about the cause of your symptoms."
   2. "A Levin tube will be used to aspirate gastric secretions, which will then be analyzed for hydrochloric acid to determine the efficiency of gastric functioning."
   3. "There is nothing to worry about. This is a minor, painless procedure, performed routinely as part of the diagnostic workup of many patients with symptoms like yours."
   4. "Examination of gastric secretions indicates the ability of the mucosa to secrete substances necessary for the absorption and use of vitamins in blood formation."

28. Which of the following pieces of equipment should the nurse assemble for the doctor's use in doing the gastric analysis?
   a. Nasogastric tube.
   b. Small metal basin.
   c. Bulb syringe.
   d. Hypodermic syringe and needle.
   e. Electric suction machine.
      1. a and b.
      2. a and e.
      3. a, b, and c.
      4. All but e.

29. One pharmacologic action of histamine is to:
   1. Inhibit the flow of digestive juices.
   2. Decrease gastrointestinal motility.
   3. Stimulate the secretion of hydrochloric acid.
   4. Depress the sensory cerebral cortex.

30. Through what route is histamine phosphate administered?
   1. Oral.
   2. Hypodermic.
   3. Intramuscular.
   4. Intravenous.

31. Analysis of Mrs. White's gastric secretions following injection of histamine will probably reveal:
   1. Lack of free hydrochloric acid.
   2. Increase in gastric activity.
   3. Delayed gastric evacuation.
   4. Decrease in volume of secretions.

32. The Schilling test was used to determine Mrs. White's ability to absorb vitamin B_{12} by:

1. Counting the number of dividing cells in a bone marrow specimen obtained 24 hours after a dose of vitamin B_{12} is given orally.
2. Measuring the urinary excretion of an oral dose of radioactive B_{12} both with and without a concomitant dose of intrinsic factor.
3. Ascertaining the amount of B_{12} eliminated in the stool during the second 24-hour period following an oral dose of vitamin B_{12}.
4. Calculating the amount of radioactive B_{12} in a blood sample drawn 24 hours after administration of an intramuscular dose of vitamin B_{12}.

33. While giving morning care to Mrs. White the nurse should:
   1. Allow her to rest at intervals throughout the procedure.
   2. Encourage her to carry out active exercises of the extremities.
   3. Keep her as immobile as possible in order to conserve her strength.
   4. Assume the full burden of conversation so Mrs. White need not talk.

34. While giving her daily care, the nurse should observe Mrs. White for which of the following as a possible complication of her disease?
   1. Alopecia.
   2. Decubitus.
   3. Tetany.
   4. Ecchymoses.

35. To which of the following circulatory disorders would Mrs. White be particularly susceptible before antianemic therapy begins to take effect?
   1. Peripheral thrombophlebitis.
   2. Pulmonary embolism.
   3. Congestive heart failure.
   4. Cerebrovascular hemorrhage.

36. Which of the following emotional states is Mrs. White most apt to display during the early period of her hospitalization?
   1. Apathy.
   2. Euphoria.
   3. Hysteria.
   4. Irritability.

37. As the nurse was preparing her for sleep on her first hospital day, Mrs. White complained that her feet were cold. Which of the following would not be suitable in relieving Mrs. White's complaint of cold feet?
   1. Wool stockings.
   2. Extra blankets.
   3. Hot water bottle.
   4. Heat cradle.

38. In preparing Mrs. White for sleep each evening the nurse should:

1. Massage her hands and feet briskly.
2. Offer her warm tea and toast.
3. Raise the side rails of the bed.
4. Immobilize her legs with sandbags.

39. Nurses should be alerted to check Mrs. White frequently during the night because she is especially liable to develop:

1. Insomnia.
2. Disorientation.
3. Convulsions.
4. Nosebleed.

40. Which of the following is thought to be the cause of pernicious anemia?

1. Insufficient intake of meat, eggs, and grain.
2. Decreased permeability of the intestinal wall.
3. Failure of the stomach to secrete an intrinsic factor.
4. Toxic depression of hemopoietic cells in the marrow.

41. Vitamin B_{12} would not be given orally to Mrs. White because it would:

1. Further irritate her sore tongue.
2. Produce indigestion and nausea.
3. Not be absorbed from the intestine.
4. Produce severe constipation.

42. Administration of vitamin B_{12} may be expected to completely relieve all but which of Mrs. White's symptoms?

1. Weakness and vertigo.
2. Soreness of the tongue.
3. Lack of appetite.
4. Loss of position sense.

43. While Mrs. White is confined to bed the nurse should provide for active and passive motion of her extremities in order to:

a. Improve morale.
b. Prevent muscle atrophy.
c. Prevent vascular thrombosis.
d. Discourage postural deformities.
e. Increase physical endurance.

1. a and b.
2. a, b, and c.
3. All but e.
4. All the above.

44. In long-term planning for Mrs. White's care, the nurse should anticipate that Mrs. White may frequently:

1. Refuse to eat.
2. Crave sour foods.
3. Drink excess liquid.
4. Request extra snacks.

45. On Mrs. White's second hospital day the nurse noted that Mrs. White had eaten very little of her lunch. When the nurse questioned her about her appetite, Mrs. White told the nurse that she was too tired to eat. Which of the following responses by the nurse would be most helpful to Mrs. White?

1. "You should be able to feed yourself without any trouble. Lifting a spoon to your mouth requires very little energy."
2. "I understand how worn out you feel, but eating a good diet will help to relieve the cause of your fatigue."
3. "Don't bother to eat just now. In a few days you will be strong enough to really enjoy the food given you."
4. "You cannot be so tired as all that. Perhaps you magnify your symptoms because you are feeling depressed."

46. If Mrs. White continues to refuse to eat, the nurse should:

1. Threaten to report her refusal to the doctor.
2. Explore further her reasons for not eating.
3. Serve her meals in the cafeteria or dining room.
4. Ignore the matter and serve the prescribed diet.

47. The physician ordered that Mrs. White be given dilute hydrochloric acid for the primary purpose of:

1. Inhibiting the growth of bacteria in the oropharynx.
2. Providing satiety by stimulation of the taste buds.
3. Facilitating optimum digestion of protein foodstuffs.
4. Reversing a tendency toward metabolic alkalosis.

48. What precaution should the nurse take in administering dilute hydrochloric acid to Mrs. White?

1. Mix the drug with milk and advise that it be drunk at intervals throughout the meal.
2. Dilute the drug in half a glass of water and administer it slowly through a drinking tube.
3. Give the drug undiluted and direct that it be drunk rapidly immediately before the meal.
4. Examine Mrs. White's mouth and withhold the drug if her tongue appears to be irritated.

49. Mrs. White's landlady confided to the nurse that other residents of her building had collected money to buy Mrs. White a gift. The landlady asked the nurse to suggest a suitable present. The nurse might best propose:
   1. A box of chocolate candy.
   2. A cotton flannel bedjacket.
   3. A tablecloth to embroider.
   4. A pair of house slippers.

50. Which of the following consequences of her illness particularly predispose Mrs. White to the development of foot drop?
   1. Deterioration of elastic fibers.
   2. Diminished caloric intake.
   3. Loss of position sense.
   4. Decreased attention span.

51. In order to protect Mrs. White against development of foot drop, several times each day the nurse should:
   1. Remind her to move both ankle joints through their full range of motion.
   2. Instruct her to sit on the edge of the bed and dangle her feet for a few minutes.
   3. Align her feet and have her press them alternately against the footboard.
   4. Assist her in standing briefly at the side of the bed or in walking around the bed.

52. Which of the following laboratory findings would indicate that Mrs. White was responding favorably to treatment?
   1. Increased reticulocyte count.
   2. Decreased gastric acidity.
   3. Increased color index.
   4. Increased marrow cellularity.

Three weeks after treatment was begun Mrs. White's red blood cell count had risen to 2,400,000 per cu. mm. and she was no longer confused. Her doctor ordered that she be allowed to ambulate three times each day.

53. The nurse must be particularly alert to protect Mrs. White against which of the following when she is first given ambulatory privileges?
   1. Chilling.
   2. Fainting.
   3. Falling.
   4. Infection.

54. Mrs. White's diet should be especially high in:
   1. Leafy vegetables.
   2. Citrus fruits.
   3. Whole grain cereals.
   4. Muscle meats.

55. In giving nutrition instruction to Mrs. White the nurse should explain in detail the:
   1. Chief sources of each of the B complex vitamins.
   2. Constituents of an adequate basic diet.
   3. Foods containing large quantities of iron and copper.
   4. Differences between essential and non-essential amino acids.

56. Before Mrs. White is discharged from the hospital, she should be taught that she will need to be treated for pernicious anemia:
   1. Until her blood count is normal.
   2. Until all symptoms have disappeared.
   3. Throughout her entire hospital stay.
   4. For the remainder of her life.

After five weeks of hospitalization Mrs. White's red blood cell count and hemoglobin concentration had both risen to the lower limit of the normal range. Her appetite was greatly improved, she seemed more alert and interested in her surroundings, and she had ceased to complain of paresthesias and cold feet. Following discharge she returned to her room in the boarding house, as arranged through predischarge communication between the hospital social service worker and Mrs. White's landlady. A public health nurse provided followup care for Mrs. White, consisting of first bimonthly and then monthly visits during which the nurse administered vitamin B_{12}, 100 micrograms intramuscularly, and supervised her personal hygiene, activity, and nutrition.

Cholelithiasis and Cholecystectomy

Mrs. Cora Peach was a good cook who enjoyed rich food and was considerably overweight. One evening she was brought into the hospital emergency room, writhing with pain. She was accompanied by her four teen-age daughters and her distraught husband. They informed the doctor and nurse that two days before, Mrs. Peach had developed severe sharp pain in her right upper abdomen and right shoulder area and had vomited a moderate quantity of semidigested food after eating a large meal. Her vomiting and pain persisted, although she had eaten no solid food in two days. Physical examination and diagnostic tests revealed:

1. Slight scleral icterus.
2. Muscle guarding and tenderness of the right upper abdomen. Abdomen not distended.
3. Hard, pear-shaped mass palpated in the right upper quadrant.
4. Temperature 101.6° F. orally, pulse 92 per minute, respirations 24 per minute, and blood pressure 140/100 mm. Hg.
5. 4,500,000 red blood cells and 13,000 white blood cells per cu. mm. of blood and hemoglobin concentration 13 grams per 100 ml.
6. Urine contained 2+ bile, no urobilinogen.
7. Clay-colored stool obtained on rectal examination.
8. Serum alkaline phosphatase, 32 King Armstrong units; serum amylase, 62 units per ml.
9. Normal electrocardiogram.

(ANSWER BLANK ON PAGE A–71)   (CORRECT ANSWERS ON PAGE B–95)

1. Which of the following pieces of equipment would the technician or physican use in doing Mrs. Peach's blood tests?
   a. Pipettes.
   b. Microscope.
   c. Centrifuge.
   d. Hemoglobinometer.
     1. All but a.
     2. All but b.
     3. All but c.
     4. All but d.

2. The nurse should interpret Mrs. Peach's temperature elevation and white blood cell count as probably indicative of:
   1. Shock.
   2. Hemorrhage.
   3. Inflammation.
   4. Dehydration.

The doctor made a diagnosis of biliary colic, admitted Mrs. Peach to a private room on the surgical unit, and wrote the following orders:

1. Nothing by mouth.
2. Insert nasogastric tube and attach to low intermittent suction.
3. Meperidine hydrochloride 100 mg. H. stat. and q. 4 h. p.r.n. for pain.
4. Atropine 0.5 mg. H. stat, and q. 6 h.
5. 1000 cc. of 5 per cent dextrose in distilled water intravenously.
6. Keflin 1 Gram "I.V. piggyback" Q. 6 H.
7. X-ray of the abdomen.
8. Intravenous cholangiogram.

3. The function of the normal gallbladder is to:
1. Manufacture bile from blood pigments.
2. Remove bacteria and toxins from bile.
3. Concentrate and store bile for later use.
4. Transmit liver bile to the duodenum.

4. In addition to right upper quadrant pain, which of the following symptoms of gallbladder disease might Mrs. Peach have had?
   a. Eructation after eating.
   b. Vomiting of coffee ground material.
   c. Abdominal distention after meals.
   d. Diarrheal stools containing mucus.
       1. a and b.
       2. a and c.
       3. b and c.
       4. b and d.

5. Normal urine contains which of the following?
1. 4+ bile and no urobilinogen.
2. 2+ bile and 2+ urobilinogen.
3. No bile and 4+ urobilinogen.
4. No bile and a trace of urobilinogen.

6. Urobilinogen is produced by:
1. Refinement of blood pigments by the liver.
2. Concentration of bile by the gallbladder.
3. Crystallization of bile salts in the kidney.
4. Action of intestinal bacteria on bilirubin.

7. Urine that contains bile is typically what color?
1. Red.
2. Yellow.
3. Brown.
4. Black.

8. The presence of bile in Mrs. Peach's urine results from:
1. Absorption of bile pigments by the blood, following obstruction of bile flow to the duodenum.
2. Destruction of glomerular walls by bacteria disseminated from the infected gallbladder.
3. Absorption of excessive urobilinogen from the small intestine into the mesenteric blood vessels.
4. Excessive hemolysis of red blood cells as a result of fever, bacteremia, and septicemia.

9. Biliary colic is a result of:
1. Strong episodic wringing contractions of the gallbladder and bile ducts.
2. Toxic paralysis of the smooth muscle fibers of the biliary tree.
3. Development of abnormal eddy currents in bile stored in the gallbladder.
4. Abnormal distention of the fibrous capsule of the liver or gallbladder.

10. Meperidine is classified in which of the following drug groups?
1. Central nervous system depressants.
2. Peripheral nervous system depressants.
3. Sympathetic nervous system depressants.
4. Parasympathetic nervous system depressants.

11. Before administering the stat. dose of meperidine, the nurse should identify Mrs. Peach by:
1. Checking the room number with the medication card.
2. Reading her name aloud from the medication card.
3. Asking her to state her first and last name.
4. Reading her name on the tag affixed to the bed.

12. Atropine belongs to which of the following groups?
1. Sympathetic stimulants.
2. Sympathetic depressants.
3. Parasympathetic stimulants.
4. Parasympathetic depressants.

13. Which of the following sites would be best suited for injection of the ordered dose of atropine?
1. Upper arm.
2. Buttocks.
3. Anterior thigh.
4. Lateral thigh.

14. Prior to administration of the hypodermic medication, the tissues of the injection site should be pinched and lifted slightly in order to:
   a. Provide a firm surface through which to insert the needle.
   b. Decrease discomfort by numbing the sensory receptors.
   c. Reduce the danger of striking underlying bone with the needle.

d. Retard absorption of the drug from the injection site.
    1. a only.
    2. a and b.
    3. c and d.
    4. All but d.

15. After withdrawing the hypodermic needle from the tissues, the nurse should rub the injection site with an alcohol pledget in order to:
1. Remove microorganisms from the skin.
2. Decrease transmission of pain impulses.
3. Relieve itching caused by the injection.
4. Foster absorption of the medication.

16. In giving a hypodermic injection to Mrs. Peach, at what angle should the needle be inserted?
1. 15 degrees.
2. 45 degrees.
3. 60 degrees.
4. 90 degrees.

17. Atropine was ordered for Mrs. Peach in order to:
1. Decrease gastrointestinal secretions.
2. Relieve spasm of smooth muscle fibers.
3. Increase gallbladder peristalsis.
4. Depress pain impulses from the viscera.

18. In order to detect atropine overdosage and toxicity, the nurse should be particularly alert to the development of:
a. Dry mouth.
b. Skin pallor.
c. Dilated pupils.
d. Tinnitus.
    1. a only.
    2. a and c.
    3. b and d.
    4. All the above.

19. The pharmacologic antidote to atropine is:
1. Epinephrine.
2. Scopolamine.
3. Phentolamine.
4. Physostigmine.

20. Mr. Peach asked the nurse, "What's the matter with my wife? Is it something serious? What's being done for her?" Which of the following responses would be most appropriate?
1. "Why don't you go sit down in the waiting room? I'll be sure to call you if her condition changes."
2. "No, there's nothing seriously wrong with your wife. She is being treated for gallbladder disease."
3. "I'm not permitted to give you that information. The doctor will have to answer your questions later."
4. "We are still investigating the cause for her illness. She has been given a medication to relieve her pain."

21. Intravenous infusion of dextrose solution was ordered for Mrs. Peach primarily in order to:
1. Increase the blood volume.
2. Flush out the renal tubules.
3. Dilute toxins in the blood.
4. Build up liver glycogen stores.

22. Which of the following should the nurse assemble for the doctor's use in starting Mrs. Peach's intravenous infusion?
a. Adhesive tape.
b. Container of sterile pledgets.
c. Armboard.
d. Sphygmomanometer.
e. Small basin.
    1. All but b.
    2. All but c.
    3. All but d.
    4. All the above.

23. The nurse should check Mrs. Peach's intravenous infusion frequently for any indication of:
a. Extravasation of the solution.
b. Accidental removal of the needle.
c. Obstruction of the needle.
d. Compression of the tubing.
e. Too rapid infusion of fluid.
    1. a and b.
    2. c and d.
    3. All but e.
    4. All the above.

24. Keflin was ordered for Mrs. Peach in order to:
1. Prevent hypostatic pneumonia.
2. Combat gallbladder infection.
3. Prevent infection of the infusion site.
4. Destroy bacteria in the bowel.

25. Which of the following is a frequent complication of the intravenous administration of antibiotics?
1. Anaphylactic shock.
2. Segmental phlebitis.
3. Cardiac arrhythmia.
4. Arteriovenous fistula.

26. Mrs. Peach should be in which of the following positions to receive an injection of tetracycline?
1. Lying on her side with the upper leg flexed.
2. Lying on her abdomen with toes pointed in.
3. Standing beside the bed, bent forward at the hips.
4. Lying supine with one knee flexed and inverted.

27. At what angle with the skin surface should the needle be inserted for injection of the tetracycline ordered for Mrs. Peach?
1. 15 degrees.
2. 45 degrees.
3. 60 degrees.
4. 90 degrees.

28. After the needle has been inserted into the tissue, what precautions should the nurse observe before injecting the medication?
1. Decrease the angle of the needle with the skin.
2. Draw back on the plunger to aspirate fluid.
3. Lift up the tissue surrounding the injection site.
4. Check the attachment of the needle to the syringe.

29. Tetracycline is effective against which of the following organisms?
a. *Streptococcus pyogenes.*
b. *Staphylococcus aureus.*
c. *Escherichia coli.*
d. *Proteus vulgaris.*
  1. a only.
  2. a and b.
  3. All but d.
  4. All the above.

30. Under what condition will gallstones be visible on ordinary flat plate x-ray of the abdomen?
1. When there are numerous stones.
2. When stones fill the entire organ.
3. When the stones are composed of calcium.
4. When the cystic duct is obstructed.

On careful questioning by the doctor, Mrs. Peach recalled that on several occasions during the past year she had experienced indigestion following the ingestion of fatty, fried, and gas-forming foods. She also remembered that her stools had been light-colored and her skin had been yellow on one of these occasions.

31. The ingestion of fatty food had usually precipitated Mrs. Peach's episodes of upper abdominal pain because:
1. Fatty foods contain higher amounts of cholesterol than do carbohydrates.
2. Fatty foods tend, more than others, to generate gas and cause bowel distention.
3. Fat in the duodenal contents initiates the reaction that causes gallbladder contraction.
4. Fat in the stomach increases the rate and amplitude of peristaltic contractions.

32. Which of the following foods tend to be gas-forming?
a. Lima beans.
b. Cabbage.
c. Onions.
d. Cantaloupe.
e. Raw apple.
  1. a and b.
  2. a, b, and c.
  3. All but e.
  4. All the above.

33. Why did Mrs. Peach have clay-colored stools?
1. Decrease in red blood cell breakdown.
2. Obstruction of bile flow to the bowel.
3. Interference with absorption of nutrients.
4. Loss of normal bacterial flora of the bowel.

34. Mrs. Peach's acholic stools suggested that:
1. The gallstones were confined to the gallbladder alone.
2. Stones were present in both the gallbladder and the cystic duct.
3. A stone had passed into and lodged in the common duct.
4. A gallstone had migrated into the duct of the pancreas.

Mrs. Peach's abdominal x-ray revealed multiple irregular opacities in the right upper abdominal quadrant, which the doctor interpreted as stones in the gallbladder. Her total serum bilirubin was 3 mg. per 100 ml.

35. Gallstones may be composed of:
a. Cholesterol crystals.
b. Bile salts.
c. Calcium salts.

d. Uric acid crystals.
    1. a only.
    2. a and b.
    3. c and d.
    4. All but d.

36. Which of the following factors are most apt to have contributed to the formation of Mrs. Peach's gallstones?
    a. Hypercholesterolemia.
    b. Biliary stasis.
    c. Hepatic cirrhosis.
    d. Kidney stones.
        1. a and b.
        2. c and d.
        3. All but d.
        4. All the above.

37. Excessive intake of which of the following foods may predispose a person to gallstone formation?
    a. Eggs.
    b. Corn oil.
    c. Margarine.
    d. Milk.
    e. Pork.
        1. a and b.
        2. b and c.
        3. a, d, and e.
        4. All the above.

38. Biliary stasis is thought to predispose to gallbladder disease by:
    1. Facilitating precipitation of bile salts.
    2. Producing diverticulae of the gallbladder.
    3. Causing reflux of chyme from the intestine.
    4. Attracting fibroblasts from surrounding tissue.

39. Infection is thought to predispose to formation of gallstones by:
    1. Dehydrating bile, rendering it more viscous and subject to stasis.
    2. Producing proteinaceous debris which serves as a nidus for stone formation.
    3. Stimulating formation of antibodies which agglutinate and precipitate bile salts.
    4. Causing increased hemolysis and increased production of bile pigments.

40. Which of the following is the upper limit of normal for total serum bilirubin concentration?
    1. 0.01 mg. per 100 ml. of plasma.
    2. 0.1 mg. per 100 ml. of plasma.
    3. 1.5 mg. per 100 ml. of plasma.
    4. 15.0 mg. per 100 ml. of plasma.

41. Jaundice does not usually become visible until the serum bilirubin concentration exceeds:
    1. 1 mg. per 100 ml.
    2. 4 mg. per 100 ml.
    3. 8 mg. per 100 ml.
    4. 12 mg. per 100 ml.

42. Mrs. Peach's jaundice is which of the following types?
    1. Hemolytic.
    2. Hepatogenous.
    3. Obstructive.
    4. Catarrhal.

43. Mrs. Peach complained of pruritus of the arms and legs. Which of the following nursing measures might be most helpful in relieving her discomfort?
    1. Bathing in weak sodium bicarbonate solution.
    2. Dusting with liberal amounts of talcum powder.
    3. Moistening the skin with isopropyl alcohol.
    4. Rubbing the skin briskly with a coarse piece of cloth.

Within 24 hours Mrs. Peach's pain had subsided. Three days later her temperature was 98.6° F. orally, her stool was brown, and her urine was free of bile. Her serum bilirubin had decreased to 2.0 mg. per 100 ml. and her serum amylase was normal. Although she still experienced some tenderness in the right upper abdomen, Mrs. Peach was allowed to leave the hospital. She was instructed to remain on a low fat diet and to visit her family physician weekly for followup care.

44. Intermittent jaundice is most common in which of the following conditions?
    1. Cirrhosis of the liver.
    2. Acute cholecystitis.
    3. Common duct stone.
    4. Carcinoma of the pancreas.

45. Which of the following foods should be omitted from a low fat diet?
    a. Cottage cheese.
    b. Chocolate.
    c. Nuts.
    d. Bacon.
    e. Chicken.
        1. a only.
        2. a and b.
        3. b, c, and d.
        4. All the above.

46. Mrs. Peach asked the nurse, "Why must I see my doctor every week? I've recovered, haven't I?" Which of the following replies would be most appropriate?
1. "You've recovered from this attack, but you still have gallstones. The doctor wishes to keep a close check on your condition through frequent office visits."
2. "Yes, you have fully recovered, but the doctor feels that you require constant health supervision to protect you from developing other illnesses in the future."
3. "No, you haven't recovered. You are still in danger of developing complications that could prove to be much more serious than your recent illness."
4. "I'm sure that the doctor has a good reason for asking you to come to his office weekly. Are you worried about the expense involved in such care?"

Mrs. Peach was supervised closely by her family physician for two months. Then, because she continued to experience indigestion despite strict adherence to a low fat diet, she was readmitted to the hospital for a cholecystectomy.

47. Which of the following might be possible complications of recurrent bouts of untreated cholecystitis?
a. Viral hepatitis.
b. Carcinoma of the pancreas.
c. Rupture of the gallbladder.
d. Acute peritonitis.
e. Biliary cirrhosis.
   1. a and b.
   2. b and c.
   3. c, d, and e.
   4. All the above.

The doctor ordered the following:

1. Cholecystogram.
2. Liver function tests.
3. Chest x-ray.
4. Bleeding and clotting time determination.
5. Type and crossmatch.
6. Vitamin K, 20 mg. I.M. daily.
7. Electrocardiogram.

48. The cholecystogram was ordered to:
1. Facilitate visualization of stones in the gallbladder and bile ducts.
2. Determine the bacterial agent responsible for gallbladder infections.
3. Estimate the degree of liver damage produced by obstructive jaundice.
4. Differentiate between cholesterol-containing and pigment-containing stones.

49. The contrast medium used in making a cholecystogram is:
1. Barium sulfate.
2. Iodoalphionic acid.
3. Calcium sulfate.
4. Radioactive gold.

50. For oral cholecystography the dye will be administered to Mrs. Peach how long before the x-ray films are taken?
1. 10 to 15 minutes.
2. 1 to 2 hours.
3. 4 to 6 hours.
4. 10 to 12 hours.

51. To ensure the validity of the gallbladder visualization studies following oral administration of dye, the nurse should check to see that Mrs. Peach:
1. Has a gastric tube inserted.
2. Drinks copious amounts of fluids.
3. Does not vomit the dye.
4. Receives serial enemas.

52. After the first two x-rays were taken of her gallbladder region, Mrs. Peach was given a high fat meal in order to:
1. Increase the rate of peristalsis.
2. Restore her blood sugar level.
3. Soothe the duodenal mucosa.
4. Cause the gallbladder to empty.

53. In caring for Mrs. Peach following the gallbladder visualization studies, the nurse should know that urinary excretion of the dye may be accompanied by:
1. Slight hematuria.
2. Urinary frequency.
3. Temporary pain.
4. Severe chills.

54. Mrs. Peach's gallbladder did not appear on x-ray following oral administration of dye, so intravenous cholangiography was attempted. Mrs. Peach's oral cholangiography may have been unsuccessful because of:
a. Decreased intestinal absorption of the dye.
b. Inability of the liver to excrete the dye.
c. Inability of x-ray to penetrate abdominal fat.
d. Hypersensitivity of body tissues to the dye.

e. Obstruction of the common bile duct by stones.
 1. a or b.
 2. c or d.
 3. All but e.
 4. All the above.

55. The contrast medium used for intravenous cholecystography is:
 1. Phenosulfonphthalein.
 2. Sodium iodipamide.
 3. Decholin sodium.
 4. Fluorescein sodium.

56. For intravenous cholecystography the dye will be administered to Mrs. Peach how long before taking the x-ray films?
 1. 10 minutes.
 2. 60 minutes.
 3. 6 hours.
 4. 10 hours.

57. Which of the following is a possible toxic effect of the dye used in intravenous cholangiography?
 1. Headache.
 2. Hypotension.
 3. Hiccoughs.
 4. Flushing.

58. Liver function tests were ordered as part of Mrs. Peach's preoperative workup because:
 1. The chances are good that she had hepatitis as well as gallstones.
 2. Liver damage would greatly increase her risk in undergoing surgery.
 3. Inhalation anesthetic agents are eliminated from the body by the liver.
 4. All obese persons may be assumed to have some degree of hepatic dysfunction.

59. Which of the following are liver function tests?
 a. Total and direct serum bilirubin concentration.
 b. Alkaline phosphatase concentration.
 c. Albumin to globulin ratio.
 d. Determination of prothrombin level.
 e. Cephalin-cholesterol flocculation test.
 1. a and b.
 2. c and d.
 3. All but e.
 4. All the above.

60. A van den Bergh test is a measurement of the:
 1. Ability of the liver to remove dye from the blood.

2. Capacity of the liver to manufacture glycogen.
 3. Amount of bilirubin in the circulating blood.
 4. Pressure of blood in the portal circulation.

61. Serum alkaline phosphatase is typically elevated in which of the following conditions?
 1. Primary hepatoma.
 2. Biliary obstruction.
 3. Liver abscess.
 4. Chronic malnutrition.

62. The normal ratio of albumin to globulin in the blood serum is:
 1. 4 : 1
 2. 2 : 1
 3. 1 : 2
 4. 1 : 4

63. Patients with liver damage tend to show changes in the albumin/globulin ratio because:
 1. Diseased hepatic cells cannot produce normal amounts of albumin.
 2. Hyperactive phagocytic cells destroy the albumin produced by the liver.
 3. Distorted sinusoids impair the absorption of albumin into the blood.
 4. Hyperplastic lymphoid tissue manufactures excessive amounts of globulin.

64. Prothrombin is a blood protein that is concerned with:
 1. Immune reactions.
 2. Blood clotting.
 3. Tissue building.
 4. Blood cell formation.

65. The cephalin-cholesterol flocculation test is used to determine the:
 1. Concentration of bile in the blood.
 2. Presence of abnormal serum proteins.
 3. Efficiency of pigment metabolism.
 4. Amount of fatty acid in portal blood.

66. A chest x-ray was ordered primarily to determine whether Mrs. Peach had:
 1. Evidence of an old, primary healed tuberculous lesion.
 2. Cardiac changes characteristic of congestive failure.
 3. Lung pathology contraindicating inhalation anesthetic.
 4. Osteoarthritic changes in the thoracic spinal vertebrae.

On cholecystogram, the dye outlined several irregular masses in the gallbladder, which were interpreted to be stones. Mrs. Peach's liver function tests were normal except for the prothrombin level, which was slightly decreased. Her clotting time had increased to 10 minutes, but the bleeding time was roughly normal. She was found to have type A, Rh positive blood. Neither the electrocardiogram nor the chest x-ray revealed any abnormal findings.

67. Mrs. Peach's prolonged clotting time was probably the result of:
   1. Decreased viscosity of peripheral blood.
   2. Depressed marrow production of platelets.
   3. Inadequate absorption of vitamin K.
   4. Impaired elasticity of blood vessels.

68. The purpose of giving Mrs. Peach large doses of vitamin K was to:
   1. Stimulate increased thrombocyte production.
   2. Prevent operative and postoperative hemorrhage.
   3. Foster resolution of ecchymotic skin lesions.
   4. Encourage a return of normal appetite controls.

69. Vitamin K is used in the formation of:
   1. Bilirubin.
   2. Prothrombin.
   3. Cholecystokinin.
   4. Albumin.

70. Which of the following aspects of Mrs. Peach's illness is responsible for her difficulty in absorbing vitamin K from food?
   1. Obstruction of bile flow to the intestine.
   2. Distention of the small bowel with gas.
   3. Circulation of bilirubin in the blood.
   4. Increased tone of smooth muscle fibers.

71. An electrocardiogram was included in Mrs. Peach's preoperative workup because she would be particularly liable to develop what type of heart disease?
   1. Rheumatic heart disease.
   2. Acute bacterial endocarditis.
   3. Arteriosclerotic heart disease.
   4. Cor pulmonale.

72. Which of the following might the nurse do to prepare Mrs. Peach for the electrocardiographic examination?

   a. Explain the nature and purpose of the test.
   b. Make her comfortable in a supine bed position.
   c. Apply electrode jelly to the selected skin sites.
   d. Elevate the side rails of the bed.
   e. Apply a sphygmomanometer cuff to the arm.
      1. a and b.
      2. a, b, and c.
      3. a, b, and d.
      4. a, b, and e.

Mrs. Peach's gallbladder, which was filled with small stones, was removed under cyclopropane anesthesia. A Penrose drain was placed near the cystic duct stump and brought out through a stab wound. Then a stone was removed from the common bile duct and a T-tube was left in the duct with the long end of the tube brought out through the wound and sutured to the skin. Mrs. Peach received one unit of blood during the operation and was returned to the recovery room unconscious, with a nasogastric tube attached to low intermittent suction and an intravenous infusion of 5 per cent dextrose in distilled water running. I.P.P.B. treatments were ordered to be given t.i.d.

73. As soon as Mrs. Peach was returned from the operating room, the recovery room nurse should have checked her chart to determine:
   1. Her history of past and present illnesses.
   2. The total blood loss during the operation.
   3. The anesthetic used and drugs given during surgery.
   4. The sponge and instrument counts taken postoperatively.

74. The blood given Mrs. Peach during surgery would have served to:
   a. Replace blood loss.
   b. Maintain blood pressure.
   c. Restore electrolyte imbalance.
   d. Protect liver cells from anoxia.
      1. a only.
      2. a and b.
      3. All but c.
      4. All the above.

75. The Penrose drain was placed near the cystic duct stump in order to:
   1. Permit irrigation of the gallbladder bed.

2. Prevent bile flow through the common duct.
3. Remove bile and blood spilled during surgery.
4. Facilitate aspiration of pus from the wound.

76. The function of the T-tube was to:
1. Drain blood and serum from the operative site.
2. Prevent bile contamination of the cystic duct stump.
3. Reroute bile flow to the reconstructed cystic duct.
4. Provide bile drainage while the common duct is edematous.

77. The nasogastric tube was left in place following surgery in order to:
1. Administer high caloric liquid feedings.
2. Simplify administration of medications.
3. Facilitate collection of bile specimens.
4. Prevent postoperative nausea and vomiting.

78. Which of the following solutions would be most satisfactory for use in irrigating Mrs. Peach's gastric tube?
1. Tap water.
2. Normal saline.
3. Hydrogen peroxide.
4. Soda water.

79. In planning Mrs. Peach's postoperative care, the nurse should consider that the nature of the operation has particularly disposed Mrs. Peach to:
1. Pulmonary embolus.
2. Bronchopneumonia.
3. Wound evisceration.
4. Intestinal obstruction.

80. In which of the following positions would Mrs. Peach be most comfortable on her return from the operating room?
1. Trendelenburg.
2. Right Sims'.
3. Low Fowler's.
4. Supine.

81. The purpose of placing Mrs. Peach in low Fowler's position following surgery was to:
1. Reduce the work load of the heart.
2. Decrease blood flow to the head.
3. Encourage normal bladder function.
4. Facilitate drainage from the tubes.

82. Immediately following surgery the recovery room nurse should check Mrs. Peach's

wound dressing for excessive blood and bile every:
1. 5 minutes.
2. 15 minutes.
3. 30 minutes.
4. 60 minutes.

83. During the first twenty-four hours after surgery, Mrs. Peach may require several doses of the prescribed analgesic in order that she does not:
1. Move about too freely and dislodge the tube.
2. Irritate her throat by excessive coughing.
2. Develop gas pains from increased peristalsis.
4. Limit respiratory excursion to avoid pain.

84. Which of the following nursing measures should be instituted to protect Mrs. Peach from developing postoperative pneumonia?
a. Administer oral hygiene frequently.
b. Change bed position periodically.
c. Encourage coughing and deep breathing.
d. Monitor respiratory function frequently.
   1. a and b.
   2. b and c.
   3. All but d.
   4. All the above.

85. On her third postoperative day Mrs. Peach's intravenous needle was accidentally dislodged from the vein and some dextrose solution infiltrated into the tissues of her arm. After disconnecting the infusion, which of the following measures might the nurse employ to reduce pain at the site of infiltration?
1. Elevate her arm over her head.
2. Wrap the arm with a circular bandage.
3. Apply warm moist packs to overlying skin.
4. Massage the tissues with an alcohol sponge.

86. The physician ordered that the bile drainage from Mrs. Peach's T-tube be saved and administered to her through the gastric tube in order to:
1. Re-establish electrolyte balance.
2. Test the success of the operation.
3. Improve efficiency of digestion.
4. Provide readily available nutrients.

87. Which of the following measures should be undertaken to make the administration of bile by gastric tube as pleasant as possible for Mrs. Peach?

    1. The bile should be chilled before pouring it into the tube.

    2. Sips of fruit juice should be offered at intervals during intubation.

    3. The bile should be kept from her view throughout the procedure.

    4. The tube should be held high to increase the speed of the bile flow.

88. Mrs. Peach asked the nurse, "Will I have to stay on a fat free diet for the rest of my life?" Which of the following responses would be most appropriate?

    1. "You'll have to remain on a fat free diet from now on in order to avoid a return to your previous symptoms."

    2. "It's too early to say. Later, when we see whether your operation is successful, we'll know the answer."

    3. "Only your doctor can answer that. Why don't you ask him about it before you are discharged from the hospital?"

    4. "After you have fully recovered from surgery you will probably be able to eat a normal diet, avoiding excessive fat."

Mrs. Peach quickly regained strength following her operation. She progressed rapidly from a clear liquid, to a soft, to a general low fat diet. The T-tube was removed on the tenth postoperative day and the resulting wound had healed by the fifteenth postoperative day when Mrs. Peach was discharged. She was instructed to eat a regular diet, avoiding only excessive fat intake, and was cautioned to avoid heavy lifting for another two months.

Cerebrovascular Accident

Fifty-five-year-old Mr. Oscar Crown was riding on the commuter train when he suffered a stroke. He was taken in a police ambulance to the hospital, where the examining physician noted that he was about 5 feet, 9 inches in height, weighed about 200 pounds, and was unconscious and convulsing. His temperature was 99.6° F. rectally, his pulse was 96 per minute, respirations 20 per minute, and blood pressure 260/140 mm. Hg. Fundoscopic examination revealed narrowing and tortuosity of the retinal vessels, and chest auscultation indicated a moderately enlarged heart. Lumbar puncture disclosed that the spinal fluid was bloody and under increased pressure. Cheyne-Stokes respirations developed soon after admission. The physician diagnosed Mr. Crown's illness as a cerebral hemorrhage, indicating that the right arm and leg would probably be paralyzed. The doctor inserted an indwelling catheter and administered 50 cc. of 50 per cent glucose solution intravenously.

(ANSWER BLANK ON PAGE A-73)   **(CORRECT ANSWERS ON PAGE B-103)**

    1. Questioning of Mr. Crown's fellow train passengers might reveal that, prior to lapsing into unconsciousness, Mr. Crown experienced which of the following symptoms of intracerebral hemorrhage?

    a. Severe headache.

    b. Facial asymmetry.

    c. Slurred speech.

    d. Weakness of extremities.

    e. Feeling of nausea.

1. a only.
2. a, b, and c.
3. b, c, and d.
4. All the above.

2. Which of the following factors probably contributed to Mr. Crown's intracerebral hemorrhage?
   a. Weakness of blood vessel wall.
   b. Sudden rise in blood pressure.
   c. Greatly reduced blood viscosity.
   d. Decreased number of blood platelets.
   e. Increased amount of circulating heparin.
      1. a and b.
      2. b and c.
      3. c and d.
      4. All the above.

3. Immediately following his admission to the hospital Mr. Crown's pulse would probably be:
   1. Normal in rate and volume.
   2. Fast and weak.
   3. Slow and bounding.
   4. Intermittently irregular.

4. On hospital admission Mr. Crown's skin is apt to be:
   1. Cold and damp.
   2. Hot and flushed.
   3. Pale and dry.
   4. Cyanotic and mottled.

5. In order to determine Mr. Crown's level of consciousness the admitting nurse should know that deep coma is characterized by:
   a. Lack of spontaneous, purposeful movement.
   b. Absence of corneal and pupillary reflexes.
   c. Failure to respond to external stimuli.
   d. Muscular twitching and automatic movement.
   e. Bowel and bladder incontinence.
      1. a and b.
      2. a, b, and c.
      3. All but d.
      4. All the above.

6. In preparing a unit for Mr. Crown's use, it would be of greatest importance for the admitting nurse to provide:
   1. A firm footboard.
   2. A tracheal suction machine.
   3. A bed linen cradle.
   4. Sandbags and trochanter rolls.

7. When initiating nursing care for Mr. Crown the admitting room nurse should:
   a. Raise the foot of the bed.
   b. Loosen his collar and belt.
   c. Provide padded side rails.
   d. Apply arm and leg restraints.
      1. a only.
      2. a and d.
      3. b and c.
      4. All the above.

8. Cerebral arteriosclerosis would predispose Mr. Crown to cerebral hemorrhage by:
   1. Narrowing the vessel lumen.
   2. Roughening the intimal lining.
   3. Retarding blood flow.
   4. Decreasing vascular elasticity.

9. The examining physician indicated that Mr. Crown was suffering from systemic hypertension. Which of the following are possible causes of hypertension?
   a. Inadequate arterial perfusion of the kidney cortex.
   b. Sustained overstimulation of the sympathetic nervous system.
   c. Secretion of vasopressors by a tumor of the adrenal medulla.
   d. Excessive production of the mineralocorticoids by the adrenal.
      1. a and c.
      2. b and d.
      3. All but d.
      4. All the above.

10. What would be the normal blood pressure for a man of Mr. Crown's age and weight?
   1. 200/130 mm. Hg.
   2. 140/100 mm. Hg.
   3. 130/80 mm. Hg.
   4. 110/70 mm. Hg.

11. Which of the following factors influence the level of blood pressure?
   a. Force of cardiac contraction.
   b. Elasticity of arteries.
   c. Constriction of arterioles.
   d. Total volume of blood.
      1. a and b.
      2. b and c.
      3. All but d.
      4. All the above.

12. Which of the following is of greatest importance in determining the quantity of blood flow to tissues?
   1. Systolic pressure.
   2. Diastolic pressure.
   3. Mean arterial pressure.
   4. Pulse pressure.

13. Changes in the diameter of which of the following vessels is of greatest significance in regulating peripheral resistance to blood flow?

    1. Arteries.
    2. Arterioles.
    3. Capillaries.
    4. Veins.

14. Of the following factors which was probably most responsible for Mr. Crown's extreme elevation of systolic pressure on hospital admission?

    1. Increased rate of cardiac contraction.
    2. Increased viscosity of the blood.
    3. Hypertrophy of the myocardium.
    4. Increase in relative blood volume.

15. Narrowing and tortuosity of Mr. Crown's retinal vessels indicated:

    1. Impaired visual acuity.
    2. Hypertensive damage.
    3. Massive blood loss.
    4. Damaged occipital cortex.

16. Mr. Crown's cardiac enlargement was chiefly the result of:

    1. Obesity.
    2. Hypertension.
    3. Shock.
    4. Hemorrhage.

17. The work load of the heart is the product of:

    1. The stroke volume of the heart times the rate of cardiac contraction.
    2. The total cardiac volume times the resistance offered by the cardiac valves.
    3. The cardiac output times the mean pressure against which it is pumped.
    4. The total blood volume times the linear distance of the blood circuit.

18. In obtaining Mr. Crown's medical history from his wife, the physician would be alert for any indication that Mr. Crown had experienced such symptoms of cerebrovascular disturbance as:

    a. Occasional dizziness.
    b. Syncopal attacks.
    c. Visual disturbances.
    d. Muscular weakness.
    e. Transient paralysis.
        1. a and c.
        2. b and d.
        3. All but e.
        4. All the above.

19. In which of the following positions should the nurse place Mr. Crown in preparing him for a lumbar puncture?

    1. Sitting on a stool with his elbows supported on a table before him.
    2. Lying flat on his abdomen with a large pillow under his midsection.
    3. Lying on his side with the upper leg flexed and the lower extended.
    4. Lying on his side with back arched and knees and head drawn together.

20. In order to maintain Mr. Crown in proper position during the lumbar puncture procedure, efforts should be made to:

    1. Eliminate distracting conversation among personnel.
    2. Restrain his arms in a folded position over his chest.
    3. Prevent plantar flexion of both his feet and toes.
    4. Keep his uppermost shoulder from falling forward.

21. In preparing equipment for a lumbar puncture, in what order should the nurse arrange the following on the sterile instrument tray?

    a. Water manometer.
    b. 2 cc. syringe and needle.
    c. Two-way stopcock.
    d. Sterile test tubes.
    e. Lumbar puncture needle.
        1. a, b, c, d, e.
        2. e, b, c, d, a.
        3. c, b, a, e, d.
        4. b, e, c, a, d.

22. Which of the following is the normal range for spinal fluid pressure?

    1. 0 to 180 mm. of water.
    2. 80 to 180 mm. of water.
    3. 180 to 280 mm. of water.
    4. 280 to 380 mm. of water.

23. Xanthochromia of Mr. Crown's spinal fluid would indicate:

    1. Elevated pressure.
    2. Hemoglobin pigment.
    3. Increased protein.
    4. Bacterial toxins.

24. On neurological examination the doctor observed that Mr. Crown demonstrated a positive Babinski reflex, which consists of:

    1. Flexion of the forearm when the biceps tendon is tapped.
    2. Extension of the leg when the patellar tendon is struck.
    3. Tremor of the foot following brisk, forcible dorsiflexion.
    4. Dorsiflexion of the great toe when the sole is scratched.

25. Which of the following signs may be used to determine, while Mr. Crown is still comatose, which side of his body will later be weak or paralyzed?

1. The affected cheek puffs out with respiration.
2. The affected arm appears to be slightly cyanotic.
3. The affected side has a cooler skin temperature.
4. The affected leg seems to be slightly edematous.

26. The physician administered 50 per cent glucose solution intravenously to Mr. Crown in order to:

1. Provide nourishment.
2. Foster clot resorption.
3. Increase blood volume.
4. Decrease brain edema.

27. Which of the following is the most accurate description of Cheyne-Stokes respirations?

1. High-pitched crowing sounds produced by obstruction of air passages.
2. Alternating periods of apnea and gradually accelerating respirations.
3. Progressive development of regular, slow, and stertorous breathing.
4. Bubbling, gurgling noises synchronized with respiratory movements.

28. During his first day in the hospital Mr. Crown should receive frequent mouth care because:

1. He will experience severe thirst during the time that he is unable to take liquids orally.
2. His oral mucosa will become dried and cracked owing to mouth breathing during coma.
3. His mouth will contain dried blood from having bitten his tongue during convulsions.
4. Tactile stimulation of the tongue and buccal mucosa will facilitate returning consciousness.

29. Which of the following would be best suited to cleanse Mr. Crown's teeth during his first hospital day?

1. Toothbrush and toothpaste.
2. Gauze-covered applicator and water.
3. Spout cup and antiseptic solution.
4. Cotton-tipped applicator and alkaline mouthwash.

30. During his period of unconsciousness, the nurse should talk to Mr. Crown while she is taking care of him because:

1. The habit of addressing him conversationally will stimulate her to individualize his care.
2. His family will interpret her talking to him as an indication of a positive prognosis.
3. Addressing him by name is the most reliable means of detecting his return to consciousness.
4. He may be able to hear another's conversation even though he cannot respond to it.

31. In constructing a plan for care the nurse should remember that for the first week of his hospitalization, Mr. Crown is in greatest jeopardy from:

1. Thrombophlebitis.
2. Decubitus.
3. Pneumonia.
4. Cystitis.

32. While he remains unconscious, the nurse responsible for Mr. Crown's care should make her chief priority:

1. Turning him from side to side every two hours.
2. Keeping a rolled towel under the femoral trochanter.
3. Instilling water into his mouth at hourly intervals.
4. Maintaining a small pillow in the right axilla.

33. As Mr. Crown's condition improves and his level of consciousness increases, which of the following behaviors will he exhibit first?

1. Ability to carry out simple commands.
2. Restlessness and tremulous movement.
3. Response to loud noise and bright lights.
4. Nonspecific response to painful stimuli.

Twenty-four hours after admission Mr. Crown regained consciousness. On awakening, his right arm and leg were paralyzed and he was unable to speak. He cried on recognizing his wife and son, who stood waiting and watching at the bedside. The nurse noted that his pulse was 88 per minute and his blood pressure was 210/120 mm. Hg. While changing the drawsheet she observed that the skin was reddened over his spine and coccyx.

34. The hemorrhage responsible for Mr. Crown's present symptoms probably occurred from rupture of a branch of the:
1. Anterior cerebral artery.
2. Middle cerebral artery.
3. Posterior cerebral artery.
4. Vertebral artery.

35. On awakening from coma, Mr. Crown would be most apt to demonstrate which type of paralysis?
1. Bilateral.
2. Flaccid.
3. Periodic.
4. Spastic.

36. In planning a rehabilitation program for Mr. Crown the nurse should know that with proper treatment Mr. Crown's neurological status may continue to improve for what period of time following his hemorrhage?
1. 1 month.
2. 3 months.
3. 6 months.
4. 12 months.

37. Mr. Crown's wife asked the nurse whether Mr. Crown's right arm and leg would always be completely paralyzed. In replying to Mrs. Crown, the nurse should know that Mr. Crown may be expected to regain some degree of function because:
1. New neurones will be regenerated to replace the damaged ones.
2. Much of his initial paralysis was due to edema of brain tissue.
3. Strokes are characterized by functional rather than organic changes.
4. Many of his early symptoms were part of a hysterical reaction.

38. If Mr. Crown should be left with any permanent paralysis, in which of the following regions would it be apt to be most severe?
1. Face.
2. Arm.
3. Back.
4. Leg.

39. Mr. Crown's son asked why his father hadn't been able to speak on awakening from coma. In answering his question the nurse should assume that which of the following was responsible?
1. Injury to the cortical motor speech area.
2. Paralysis of the muscles of the pharynx.
3. Severe dehydration of the oropharyngeal mucosa.
4. Hysterical interference with the ability to speak.

40. If the nurse should observe in Mr. Crown a steady rise in temperature together with a slowing of pulse and respirations, she should report these symptoms, since they suggest:
1. Absorption of the clot from the vessel.
2. Injury to vital centers in the medulla.
3. Development of cardiac failure.
4. Development of bronchial pneumonia.

41. What would be the most satisfactory means of meeting the problem of Mr. Crown's incontinence when the catheter was removed on his recovery from coma?
1. Restriction of oral fluid intake.
2. Insertion of an indwelling catheter.
3. Offering the urinal every four hours.
4. Application of disposable diapers.

42. By what means is the hospital staff most apt to prolong the period of Mr. Crown's incontinence?
1. By showing great concern for his comfort.
2. By failing to spend enough time with him.
3. By grouping him with more active patients.
4. By readily changing his soiled bed linen.

43. Each time she bathes Mr. Crown the nurse should especially observe him for:
1. Slow digital capillary refilling following pressure.
2. Distention of the epigastric or periumbilical regions.
3. Paradoxical movements of the chest during respirations.
4. Calf swelling, redness, heat, or tenderness.

44. While the nurse was bathing Mr. Crown, he suddenly shouted "no, no, no," while pointing excitedly at a glass on the bedside stand. He indicated in pantomime that he wished a drink of water. His behavior indicated:
1. Amnesic aphasia.
2. Hysterical aphasia.
3. Receptive aphasia.
4. Motor aphasia.

45. In planning for Mr. Crown's care during the next few weeks, the nurse should anticipate that his speech will be characterized by:
a. Frequent emotional outbursts of profanity and obscenity.
b. Substitution of words of the opposite meaning from that intended.

c. Gradual relapse to a condition of absolute mutism.

d. Sudden recovery of his previous level of speech skill.
   1. a and b.
   2. a and c.
   3. a and d.
   4. All the above.

46. In caring for Mr. Crown during his first weeks of illness the nurse should:
1. Anticipate his wishes so as to eliminate his need to talk.
2. Communicate by means of questions he can answer by shaking his head.
3. Keep up a steady flow of talk to make his silence less obvious.
4. Provide him opportunity to speak as frequently as possible.

47. In teaching Mr. Crown to talk again, the nurse should begin her instruction with:
1. Pictures of common objects.
2. Newspaper headlines.
3. Children's stories.
4. Popular novels.

48. By which of the following means should the nurse teach Mr. Crown the word "pencil"?
a. Show him an ordinary lead pencil.
b. Allow him to handle and use a pencil.
c. Show him a picture of a pencil.
d. Show him the printed word "pencil."
e. Enunciate the syllables of the word "pencil."
   1. a and b.
   2. b and c.
   3. c and d.
   4. All the above.

49. The preferred method of caring for the reddened area on Mr. Crown's back would be to:
1. Rub it with lotion and turn him on his side frequently.
2. Apply zinc oxide ointment and cover it with a gauze pad.
3. Powder his back and place a rubber ring under his hips.
4. Replace the rubber draw sheet with a cotton flannel pad.

50. Mr. Crown would be most apt to display which of the following attitudes during the first few days of his hospitalization?
1. Euphoria.
2. Placidity.
3. Hostility.
4. Depression.

51. In repositioning Mr. Crown following his back care, what position would most effectively protect him from the early complications of his illness?
1. Horizontal dorsal recumbent.
2. Turned toward the paralyzed side.
3. Head elevated at a 30 degree angle.
4. Foot of the bed elevated 15 degrees.

52. Which of the following activities should Mr. Crown be encouraged to try on the first or second day of hospitalization?
1. Sitting up on the side of the bed.
2. Pressing his feet against the footboard.
3. Moving from the bed to a wheel chair.
4. Raising his legs against counterforce.

53. The nurse observed that Mr. Crown could not completely close his right eye. What measure should be taken to protect the eye from injury?
1. Irrigate the eye daily with sterile saline solution.
2. Instill sterile ointment and cover the eye with a patch.
3. Apply a bland ointment to the everted lower lid.
4. Provide sunglasses and shade the lights in the room.

54. On the evening of Mr. Crown's second hospital day the doctor ordered that he be given a bland soft diet. What precaution should the nurse take before beginning to feed Mr. Crown?
1. Place pillows under his head and his right arm.
2. Assess his ability to swallow by offering ice chips.
3. Order that his food be served in unbreakable containers.
4. Allow all his food to cool to room temperature.

55. On the seventh day of his hospitalization the doctor noted that muscles in Mr. Crown's right arm and leg were no longer flaccid, but were spastic. The development of spastic paralysis would predispose Mr. Crown to:
1. Athetoid movements.
2. Decubitus ulcerations.
3. Contracture deformities.
4. Grand mal convulsions.

56. Which of the following nursing measures would be most helpful in preventing typical upper extremity deformities in Mr. Crown?

1. Movement of joints through full range of motion four times a day.
2. Immobilization of the wrist with an aluminum splint.
3. Support of the lower arm and hand in a cloth sling.
4. Diathermy and massage to muscles of the shoulder girdle.

57. The nurse could be most helpful in preventing typical lower extremity deformities in Mr. Crown by:

1. Placing a restraining sheet over his thighs.
2. Flexing his knees over a rolled blanket.
3. Supporting his feet at right angles to his legs.
4. Placing him on his abdomen for long periods.

58. Which of the following devices would be most effective in preventing Mr. Crown from developing footdrop?

1. Sandbags.
2. Pillows.
3. Footboard.
4. Bed cradle.

59. Mr. Crown should be observed for indications of fecal impaction, a common symptom of which is:

1. Severely distended abdomen.
2. Musical, high-pitched bowel sounds.
3. Frequent expulsion of flatus.
4. Numerous small liquid stools.

60. Which of the following would be most satisfactory for preventing constipation in Mr. Crown?

1. Administration of mineral oil.
2. Massage of the abdominal muscles.
3. Insertion of rectal suppositories.
4. Ingestion of fruit and vegetables.

61. Mr. Crown's paralyzed right hand and awkwardness in using his left hand made it difficult for him to manipulate dishes and silverware. Which of the following would be the best solution for this problem?

1. Providing nutrition by intravenous and gastric tube feedings.
2. Assigning nursing personnel to feed him each of his meals.
3. Arranging for his wife to be present to assist him with meals.
4. Encouraging him to feed himself using special containers and utensils.

62. Under the physician's direction the nurse instituted an exercise program to prepare Mr. Crown for later ambulation. In teaching Mr. Crown to do quadriceps-setting exercises with his left leg the nurse should tell him to:

1. Abduct his leg as far as possible from the midline while lying supine and without moving his trunk.
2. Lie on his abdomen, then raise his foot slowly until the knee is flexed at a 90° angle.
3. Push his popliteal space against the bed and lift his heel off the mattress to the count of five.
4. Dangle the leg over the side of the bed, then swing the lower leg back and forth, pendulum fashion.

Through a combination of gestures and isolated words, Mr. Crown confided to the nurse his fear that his body was shrinking in length. Then his lip began to quiver and he wept quietly for several minutes.

63. Mr. Crown's comment demonstrated his:

1. Distrust of the abilities of the professionals who serve him.
2. Lack of faith in the efficacy of his prescribed treatment program.
3. Alteration of body-image following severe sensory and motor loss.
4. Conviction that his illness will eventually terminate in death.

64. Which of the following would be most apt to impede Mr. Crown's rehabilitation following his stroke?

1. The irreversibility of the organic changes that have occurred in his brain.
2. His family's failure to encourage him toward independent activity.
3. The doctors' and nurses' inability to coordinate all aspects of his rehabilitation program.
4. Society's unwillingness to accept persons with any degree of physical incapacitation.

On his eighth hospital day Mr. Crown developed sharp inspiratory chest pain, cough, and shaking chills. His temperature was 105° F. orally, his pulse was 104 per minute and bounding, and his respirations were 28 per minute. His face was flushed and he was severely dyspneic. The doctor found decreased breath sounds and a pleural friction rub in the right chest on auscultation. He made a diagnosis of acute pneumonia, obtained blood and sputum for culture, and wrote the following orders:

1. 1000 cc. of 5 per cent dextrose in distilled water I.V.
2. Tetracycline hydrochloride 500 mg. to be added to the intravenous solution.
3. Tetracycline hydrochloride 200 mg. orally q. 6 h.
4. Oxygen tent.
5. Codeine elixir 30 mg. orally p.r.n.
6. Tepid sponges every hour to reduce temperature to 103° F.
7. Chest x-ray (portable).

65. Which of the following factors would have contributed to Mr. Crown's development of pneumonia?
   a. Pneumococci normally inhabiting the nasopharynx.
   b. Impairment of the reflex action of the epiglottis.
   c. Difficult swallowing due to pharyngeal paralysis.
   d. Pulmonary stasis due to prolonged immobility.
      1. a and b.
      2. b and c.
      3. c and d.
      4. All the above.

66. The chest x-ray revealed that Mr. Crown had bronchial pneumonia and right pleural effusion. In which position would he probably be most comfortable?
   1. Sitting in high Fowler's position.
   2. Reclining in right Sims' position.
   3. Lying supine with arms over his head.
   4. Leaning forward over the overbed table.

67. Which of the following was chiefly responsible for Mr. Crown's chest pain?
   1. Pleural inflammation.
   2. Cardiac enlargement.
   3. Intercostal muscle spasm.
   4. Irritation of the phrenic nerve.

68. The cause for Mr. Crown's shaking chills was the:
   1. Effect of bacterial protein on the hypothalamus.
   2. Decrease of glycogen stores in skeletal muscle.
   3. Heat loss due to evaporation of perspiration.
   4. Imbalance of electrolytes in the body fluids.

69. Which of the following is most characteristic of the dyspnea produced by pneumonic consolidation of the lung?

   1. Asthmatic wheezing.
   2. Expiratory grunt.
   3. Blowing respirations.
   4. Inspiratory stridor.

70. The doctor's chief reason for ordering blood and sputum cultures for Mr. Crown was to:
   1. Evaluate the quality of the body's defense against the lung infection.
   2. Obtain colonies of the causative organism for use in drug sensitivity tests.
   3. Verify the diagnosis of pneumonia made from history and physical examination.
   4. Determine the stage of the disease and the probable duration of illness.

71. Which of the following blood changes is most characteristic of pneumonia?
   1. Decreased erythrocytes.
   2. Increased neutrophils.
   3. Decreased platelets.
   4. Increased lymphocytes.

72. In observing Mr. Crown's behavior during the height of his pneumococcal infection, the nurse should be particularly alert to evidence of:
   1. Apathy.
   2. Depression.
   3. Delirium.
   4. Denial.

73. Which of the following are possible toxic effects of the tetracycline given to Mr. Crown?
   a. Dyspepsia.
   b. Diarrhea.
   c. Jaundice.
   d. Azotemia.
   e. Purpura.
      1. a and b.
      2. c and d.
      3. All but d.
      4. All the above.

74. While caring for Mr. Crown in the oxygen tent the nurse should maintain the humidity within the tent at a concentration of:
   1. 5 per cent.
   2. 20 per cent.
   3. 35 per cent.
   4. 50 per cent.

75. Codeine was ordered for Mr. Crown in order to produce:
   1. Relaxation of the bronchial muscles.
   2. Depression of the cough reflex.
   3. Increase in the coronary circulation.
   4. Stimulation of the respiratory center.

76. Thirty milligrams of codeine is equivalent to which of the following in the apothecary system of measurement?
1. 1 grain.
2. ½ grain.
3. ¼ grain.
4. ⅛ grain.

77. It would be advisable to quickly reduce Mr. Crown's greatly elevated temperature in order to:
1. Reduce the loss of body fluids.
2. Prevent severe electrolyte imbalance.
3. Decrease nutritional requirements.
4. Prevent irreversible brain damage.

78. In what sequence is Mr. Crown likely to produce the following types of sputum?
a. Purulent.
b. Bloody.
c. Watery.
d. Rusty.
    1. a, c, b, d.
    2. b, d, a, c.
    3. d, a, c, b.
    4. c, b, d, a.

79. Which of the following skin lesions is Mr. Crown likely to develop in conjunction with his pneumonia?
1. Erythema nodosum.
2. Angioneurotic edema.
3. Herpes simplex.
4. Pityriasis rosea.

80. What would indicate the occurrence of crisis in the course of Mr. Crown's pneumonia?
1. The precipitous occurrence of massive hemoptysis.
2. Sudden drop in temperature, pulse, and respirations.
3. Appearance of bacteria in the circulating blood.
4. Complete cessation of all respiratory movement.

81. Which of the following are possible complications of Mr. Crown's pneumonia?
a. Lung abscess.
b. Cardiac failure.
c. Paralytic ileus.
d. Infectious hepatitis.
    1. a and b.
    2. b and c.
    3. All but d.
    4. All the above.

82. Which action by the nurse would be most effective in protecting Mr. Crown from development of skin pressure sores?
1. Maintaining him at all times on an alternating pressure mattress with sheepskin padding over bony prominences.
2. Determining how long he can remain in one position without focal skin reddening, and then moving him accordingly.
3. Keeping the skin over pressure points scrupulously clean and dry and massaging it twice daily with lanolin ointment.
4. Changing him from the back to first one side, then the other side-lying position every two hours round the clock.

Mr. Crown recovered from pneumonia slowly, but without developing any complications. Because he had achieved only minimal return of hand function and because he required further speech re-education, Mr. Crown was referred to the local rehabilitation institute for further care.

Mammary Carcinoma and Mastectomy

Mrs. Mary Forman discovered a lump in her left breast while taking a bath. She consulted her family doctor a few days later at the insistence of her sister, who was a registered nurse. The doctor recalled that Mrs. Forman was 40, had been married for 15 years, had no children, and had always complained of breast tenderness and nodularity prior to menstruation. Physical examination revealed slight asymmetry of the breasts, with the left nipple deviated laterally and superiorly. A fixed mass, 3 cm. in diameter, was located in the upper outer quadrant of the left breast, and an enlarged lymph node was found in the left axilla.

The doctor made a tentative diagnosis of malignant breast tumor and advised Mrs. Forman that she should be admitted to the hospital immediately for a complete preoperative workup, mammography, breast biopsy, and possible mastectomy.

(ANSWER BLANK ON PAGE A–75) (CORRECT ANSWERS ON PAGE B–110)

1. As a nurse, Mrs. Forman's sister was probably aware of the fact that the incidence of breast carcinoma is highest in:
  1. Unmarried girls in their late teens.
  2. Married women in their early twenties.
  3. Multiparous women in their late thirties.
  4. Childless women of menopausal age.

2. Which of the following breast symptoms may indicate the presence of a mammary carcinoma?
  a. Retraction of the nipple.
  b. Puckering of the skin.
  c. Discharge from the nipple.
  d. Alteration of contour.
    1. a and b.
    2. b and c.
    3. c and d.
    4. All the above.

3. The breast lumps frequently observed by Mrs. Forman prior to menstruation were probably:
  1. Enlargement of lymph nodes.
  2. Thrombosis of subcutaneous veins.
  3. Degeneration of fatty tissue.
  4. Engorgement of mammary ducts.

4. A malignant tumor can best be described as one that:
  1. Is produced by an unknown cause.
  2. Tends to regress and exacerbate.
  3. Steadily increases in tissue mass.
  4. Begins slowly and insidiously.

5. Which of the following characteristics generally differentiate malignant tumors from benign tumors?
  a. Lack of a capsule.
  b. More rapid growth.
  c. Less mature cells.
  d. Spread to distant parts.
    1. a and b.
    2. b and c.
    3. c and d.
    4. All the above.

6. Positive diagnosis of malignant breast tumor can be made by which of the following means?
  a. Visual inspection of the breast.
  b. Careful manual palpation.
  c. Anterior-posterior chest x-ray.
  d. Biopsy of breast tumor tissue.
    1. c only.
    2. d only.
    3. All the above.
    4. None of the above.

7. Metastasis of a malignant tumor occurs by:
   1. Extension of tumor tissue into surrounding normal organs.
   2. Rupture of tumor capsule and extrusion of its contents.
   3. Blood and lymph transmission of cells to distant sites.
   4. Death and putrefaction of tissue deprived of nutrition.

8. Carcinoma of the breast frequently metastasizes to the:
   a. Other breast.
   b. Lung.
   c. Brain.
   d. Spine.
   e. Liver.
      1. a only.
      2. a and b.
      3. All but d.
      4. All the above.

9. The doctor would probably interpret the palpable lymph node in Mrs. Forman's axilla as evidence that:
   1. She has a breast abscess as well as a tumor.
   2. Tumor cells have not spread beyond that point.
   3. Cells have metastasized from the primary site.
   4. Inflammation has caused lymphatic hypertrophy.

10. Mammography consists of:
    1. Irradiation of the breast with low voltage x-ray to identify contrasts in soft tissue densities.
    2. X-ray of the breast following injection of a radiopaque dye into the mammary artery.
    3. Use of infrared photography to identify areas of increased blood supply in breast tissue.
    4. X-ray of the breast following injection of a radiopaque dye into the ductal system.

11. On her first day in the hospital, Mrs. Forman said to the nurse, "This lump in my breast is cancer, isn't it?" Which of the following initial responses would be most appropriate?
    1. "Of course not! Whatever gave you such a ridiculous idea?"
    2. "A positive diagnosis can't be made until surgery is done."
    3. "Yes, the doctor feels that you probably have cancer."

4. "You're worried about the outcome of your surgery, aren't you?"

12. Which of the following tests would probably be included in Mrs. Forman's preoperative workup?
    a. Complete blood count.
    b. X-ray of the chest.
    c. Liver function tests.
    d. Blood chemistries.
       1. a only.
       2. a and b.
       3. All but d.
       4. All the above.

On her second day in the hospital, after having had a preoperative workup that included, in addition to the foregoing, typing and crossmatching, blood chemistry, urinalysis, skeletal x-ray survey, and an electrocardiogram, Mrs. Forman told her nurse that she had decided not to have surgery done and wished to go home. Mrs. Forman's husband and physician were summoned and after considerable discussion with her, persuaded her to undergo the operation.

13. Mrs. Forman's blood was found to be Type A. Which of the following blood types could she safely be given by transfusion?
    a. Type A.
    b. Type B.
    c. Type AB.
    d. Type O.
       1. a only.
       2. a and c.
       3. a and d.
       4. All the above.

14. Which of the following would be most apt to occur if Mrs. Forman were given incompatible blood during the operation?
    1. The pH of Mrs. Forman's serum would be decreased.
    2. The red cells of the donor's blood would be agglutinated.
    3. The fibrinogen of Mrs. Forman's blood would be destroyed.
    4. The serum of the donor's blood would become coagulated.

15. Routine blood chemistry tests include measurement of:
    a. Prothrombin.
    b. Creatinine.
    c. Hemoglobin.
    d. Albumin.
    e. Cholesterol.
       1. a only.

2. a and c.

3. b and d.

4. b, d, and e.

16. The doctor ordered that Mrs. Forman should have skeletal x-ray survey taken in order to:

1. Stimulate production of blood cells in the marrow.

2. Irradiate the lymphoid tissue throughout the body.

3. Check for the occurrence of bony metastases.

4. Identify any arthritis which might impede rehabilitation.

17. Which of the following probably contributes most to Mrs. Forman's reluctance to undergo surgery for mastectomy?

1. Fear of postoperative discomfort.

2. Curtailment of childbearing activities.

3. Threat to feminine identification.

4. Concern over hospitalization costs.

18. In preparing Mrs. Forman for surgery, the nurse should scrub and shave which of the following skin areas?

1. Lateral aspect of the left breast and anterior aspect of the thigh.

2. Anterior chest, bedline to bedline, and both axillary regions.

3. Left thorax, front and back, to the lower border of the rib cage.

4. Neck, back and front of the left thorax to the umbilicus, and left arm.

19. Which of the following chemicals would most effectively remove polish from Mrs. Forman's fingernails?

1. Ethyl alcohol.

2. Hydrogen peroxide.

3. Tannic acid.

4. Carbon tetrachloride.

20. Which of the following should be removed before Mrs. Forman is transported to the operating room?

a. False teeth.

b. Contact lenses.

c. Pierced earrings.

d. Wedding band.

   1. a only.

   2. a and b.

   3. All but d.

   4. All the above.

The student nurse who admitted Mrs. Forman to the hospital and helped care for her during the preoperative period was allowed to accompany her to the operating room and to circulate for the operation.

21. Nurses who work in the operating room are expected to wear special shoes that will:

1. Discourage the transportation of bacteria.

2. Provide additional traction on slick floors.

3. Conduct static electricity to the floor.

4. Prevent relaxation of the longitudinal arch.

22. Which of the following safety measures should be undertaken by the circulating nurse after Mrs. Forman has been placed on the operating table?

a. Compare information on her identification bracelet with that on her chart and the schedule.

b. Secure her to the table by fastening canvas straps across her abdomen and upper legs.

c. Check her chart for a signed operative permit and a record of preoperative medication given.

d. Affix her left arm to a padded armboard securely attached to the operating table.

   1. a only.

   2. b only.

   3. c only.

   4. All the above.

23. It is inadvisable for the circulating nurse to regulate the temperature of the operating room by opening the window because this maneuver would:

a. Allow entry of dust-laden air.

b. Admit distracting street noise.

c. Expose the patient to drafts.

d. Generate an electrical spark.

   1. a only.

   2. a and b.

   3. All but d.

   4. All the above.

24. Before donning her sterile gown, the scrub nurse should cleanse her hands and arms by:

1. Washing with soap and running water for five minutes.

2. Lathering with green soap and allowing to air dry.

3. Immersing in a basin of strong disinfectant solution.

4. Scrubbing with a brush and soap for ten minutes.

25. In moving from the scrub sink into the operating room, the scrub nurse should hold her arms above her waist and her hands higher than her elbows in order to:
1. Signify to other personnel that she is scrubbed and ready to begin.
2. Keep water from running down her arms and contaminating her clean hands.
3. Reduce the temptation to touch unsterile supplies and equipment.
4. Slip into the sterile gown held up for her by the circulating nurse.

26. Before putting on her sterile gown, the scrub nurse should remove the water from her upper extremities by:
1. Waving her arms back and forth at her sides.
2. Shaking her hands briskly over a floor basin.
3. Blotting hands and arms with a paper towel.
4. Drying hands, wrists, and arms with a sterile towel.

27. Which of the following indicates the sequence in which the scrub nurse should put on the garb which she must wear while assisting the doctor with the surgical operation?
   a. Sterile gown.
   b. Rubber gloves.
   c. Head turban.
   d. Face mask.
   1. a, b, c, d.
   2. b, a, d, c.
   3. c, d, a, b.
   4. d, c, b, a.

28. To pick up her sterile gown prior to putting it on, the scrub nurse should:
1. Seize it by the neckband, lift it up and hold it at arm's length.
2. Use a sterile transfer forceps to remove the gown from the sterile pack.
3. Wrap one hand with a sterile towel and grasp the gown with that hand.
4. Don one sterile glove and use that hand to lift the gown from the table.

29. Which of the following parts of her newly donned gown should be considered to be contaminated?
   a. Neckband.
   b. Waist front.
   c. Waist back.
   d. Lower sleeve.
   1. a only.
   2. a and c.
   3. b and d.
   4. None of the above.

30. The circulating nurse may provide the scrub nurse with additional sterile equipment during the course of the operation by:
   a. Unwrapping only the outer cover of a sterile package and allowing the scrub nurse to seize the sterile inner portion.
   b. Removing a sterile object from its container with sterile transfer forceps and placing it on the sterile table.
   c. Holding out a freshly sterilized instrument on an autoclave tray, from which the scrub nurse may remove the object.
   d. Peeling back the outer cover from a sterile package and flipping the inner sterile bundle onto the sterile table.
   1. a only.
   2. b only.
   3. a, b, and c.
   4. All the above.

Since her biopsy revealed adenocarcinoma, a radical mastectomy was performed. The resulting wound was covered with skin flaps and a skin graft from the thigh, a catheter was left in place to drain the operative area, and an elastic pressure dressing was applied to the left chest. Mrs. Forman's left arm was bandaged tightly to her side and she was taken to the recovery room, where the flap catheter was attached to low suction. Mrs. Forman regained consciousness quickly. Because she experienced no nausea or vomiting, she was fed clear liquids on the evening of surgery and a soft diet the following day. The doctor ordered that she be given meperidine hydrochloride (Demerol) 75 mg. I.M. q. 4 h., p.r.n. for pain.

31. After Mrs. Forman's biopsy was performed the surgical drapes and instruments were removed, the surgical field was redraped, and a new set of instruments were obtained because:
1. The drapes and instruments would have been contaminated during the first skin incision.
2. It would be necessary to count sponges and instruments before making the second incision.
3. The second procedure required a much larger surgical site and more instruments.
4. Malignant cells might otherwise be

transferred from the biopsy site to other tissue.

32. Which of the following tissues were removed from the left side of Mrs. Forman's chest during the radical mastectomy?

    a. Breast tissue.
    b. Subcutaneous fat.
    c. Pectoral muscles.
    d. Axillary lymph nodes.
        1. a only.
        2. a and b.
        3. All but d.
        4. All the above.

33. What type of graft was probably used to cover the skin defect produced during Mrs. Forman's radical mastectomy?

    1. Pedicle.
    2. Pinch.
    3. Full thickness.
    4. Split thickness.

34. The graft donor site on Mrs. Forman's thigh could best be cared for by:

    1. Exposing it intermittently to ultraviolet light.
    2. Covering it with petroleum gauze for one week.
    3. Applying antiseptic and wrapping with an elastic bandage.
    4. Keeping it covered with warm saline-soaked dressings.

35. The nurse should frequently check both the operation of the suction apparatus attached to the flap catheter and the quantity of fluid aspirated in order to prevent:

    1. Destruction of the skin graft.
    2. Displacement of the mediastinum.
    3. Collapse of the left lung.
    4. Distention of the pleural sac.

36. The primary purpose for the pressure dressing that was applied to Mrs. Forman's chest wound was to:

    1. Decrease the volume and rate of arterial circulation into the operative area.
    2. Ensure continuous and firm contact between the skin graft and underlying tissue.
    3. Decrease the pain and itching normally associated with the healing of a skin incision.
    4. Maintain the drainage catheter immobile and in proper position under the skin graft.

37. During the immediate postoperative period, the nurse should closely observe Mrs. Forman's left arm and hand for symptoms of:

    1. Chemical dermatitis.
    2. Circulatory impairment.
    3. Subcutaneous hemorrhage.
    4. Contracture deformities.

38. The nature of Mrs. Forman's surgery especially predisposes her to:

    1. Pulmonary congestion and atelectasis.
    2. Coronary artery thrombosis.
    3. Small bowel obstruction.
    4. Peripheral thrombophlebitis.

39. During the postanesthetic period the nurse should check Mrs. Forman for wound bleeding every:

    1. 15 minutes.
    2. 30 minutes.
    3. 60 minutes.
    4. Two hours.

40. What precaution should the recovery room nurse take in checking Mrs. Forman for postoperative bleeding?

    1. Remove the wound dressing in order to inspect the entire incision line.
    2. Abduct the left arm in order to permit full visualization of the dressing.
    3. Run her hand under the patient's left side to feel the lower bed linen.
    4. Rotate the drainage catheter slightly with a sterile forceps to encourage drainage.

41. The recovery room nurse can best minimize Mrs. Forman's postoperative discomfort by:

    1. Placing an ice bag over the area of the axillary wound.
    2. Releasing the edges of the elastic pressure dressing.
    3. Supporting her left arm full length with pillows.
    4. Turning her to the left Sims' position with knees flexed.

42. The nurse should protect Mrs. Forman from postoperative pulmonary complications by:

    a. Turning her from her back to her right side every 2 hours.
    b. Supporting her left arm and chest while she coughs up secretions.
    c. Maintaining her head and shoulders in position to facilitate chest expansion.
    d. Administering ordered analgesic often enough to control chest pain.
    e. Instituting intermittent positive pressure breathing four times a day.
        1. a and b.
        2. a, b, and c.
        3. All but e.
        4. All the above.

43. In order to prevent postoperative wound dehiscence, the nurse should instruct Mrs. Forman that for the first few days after her operation:
1. She must refrain from both coughing and deep breathing.
2. Her left shoulder will be immobilized by a Velpeau bandage.
3. She will be maintained continuously in left Sims' position.
4. Her left arm will be held against her body with tape.

44. Wound dehiscence is the:
1. Overgrowth of granulation and scar tissue.
2. Bacterial infection of a skin suture line.
3. Bursting open of a closed surgical incision.
4. Formation of a freely draining sinus tract.

45. After removal of the pressure dressing, venous return flow in Mrs. Forman's left arm should be assisted by:
a. Positioning her arm so each joint is higher than the next proximal joint.
b. Changing the position of her left arm and hand at frequent intervals.
c. Encouraging her to frequently extend her fingers, wrist, and elbow.
d. Massaging her hand and arm each time that her position is changed.
e. Applying occasional pressure to her upper arm with a blood pressure cuff.
   1. a only.
   2. a, b, and c.
   3. All but e.
   4. All the above.

On her first postoperative day, Mrs. Forman's doctor ordered that she be allowed to sit in a chair at the side of her bed. On her third postoperative day the chest pressure dressing was removed and passive and active arm exercises were begun.

46. The nurse should assist Mrs. Forman the first few times she gets out of bed because Mrs. Forman would be particularly disposed to:
1. Visual impairment.
2. Postural hypotension.
3. Pulmonary embolism.
4. Loss of balance.

47. Which of the following devices would be most helpful in positioning Mrs. Forman's left arm so as to minimize discomfort when she first sits up in a chair?
1. Overbed table.
2. Airplane splint.
3. Overhead trapeze.
4. Two pillows.

48. Which of the following postural deformities is Mrs. Forman most apt to develop postoperatively?
1. Deviation of the head to the left.
2. Drooping of the left shoulder.
3. External rotation of the left arm.
4. Exaggerated thoracic spinal curve.

49. Which of the following exercises should Mrs. Forman be encouraged to begin on the third postoperative day?
a. Flexing and extending fingers of the left hand.
b. Pronation and supination of the left forearm.
c. Internal and external rotation of the left arm.
d. Circumduction of the left arm at the shoulder.
   1. a only.
   2. a and b.
   3. All but d.
   4. All the above.

50. The nurse should guide Mrs. Forman through which of the following exercises as part of her physical rehabilitation?
a. "Climbing" the wall with her fingers.
b. Twirling a rope tied to a doorknob.
c. Brushing and combing her own hair.
d. Doing pushups from the prone position.
   1. a only.
   2. a and c.
   3. All but d.
   4. All the above.

51. Mrs. Forman should be instructed to do her prescribed hand and arm exercises under which of the following conditions?
1. When no one is nearby to observe and question her activities.
2. While maintaining good normal standing or sitting posture.
3. When the exercises can be executed without causing her discomfort.
4. To the accompaniment of music of gradually increasing speed.

Mrs. Forman objected to carrying out the prescribed exercises, saying, "Why do you insist that I wear myself out with these silly routines? I feel as though I'm pulling my stitches loose."

52. Which of the following responses by the nurse would be most appropriate?
1. "I realize that the exercises may cause you discomfort, but they are necessary to keep your muscles and joints supple so you will have full range of arm motion in the future."
2. "These silly routines, as you call them, were ordered by your doctor as one part of your total physical rehabilitation. Why don't you ask him to explain their purpose?"
3. "These maneuvers have been designed by a physiotherapist to keep you from developing muscular contractions and joint ankyloses, both of which may occur if you don't exercise."
4. "Don't worry about your stitches. They are made of strong material and are well anchored and securely tied. Skin sutures rarely give way, and can easily be replaced if necessary."

The flap catheter was removed on the third postoperative day and both the chest and thigh wounds healed without difficulty. Because Mrs. Forman had expressed concern about the change in her appearance wrought by the operation, the surgeon suggested that she be fitted with a breast prosthesis. The prosthesis was secured and she was taught how to use and care for it by the nurse.

Mrs. Forman was discharged two weeks after admission with the understanding that she would receive regular followup care by her own physician.

53. Predischarge preparation for Mrs. Forman should include:
1. Instructing her to avoid doing any housework, gardening, or shopping.
2. Arranging for a public health nurse to visit her home daily.
3. Teaching her the procedure for self-examination of her right breast.
4. Advising her to limit her social activities for a few weeks.

54. When instructing Mrs. Forman concerning self-care following hospital discharge, the nurse should inform her that which of the following is a possible consequence of her operation?
1. Contractures of the thigh.
2. Lymphedema of the arm.
3. Furunculosis of the axilla.
4. Keloidosis of the scar.

55. Postoperatively Mrs. Forman was given a short course of radiotherapy in order to:
1. Stimulate the body's defense system to increased activity.
2. Facilitate scar tissue formation and wound healing.
3. Increase blood flow to the operative area.
4. Destroy malignant cells not removed by surgery.

56. Mrs. Forman should be instructed that she can minimize symptoms of radiation sickness by:
1. Pushing fluids in large quantities both before and after radiation treatment.
2. Eating a small meal of toast, jello, and tea immediately before treatments.
3. Abstaining from eating and drinking for three hours before and after treatments.
4. Avoiding fatty, gas-producing, and highly seasoned foods during the treatment series.

57. Mrs. Forman should be advised that her chest scar can be made smoother and softer by:
1. Applying warm, moist dressings to it every night.
2. Keeping it covered with a vaseline gauze dressing.
3. Massaging it gently and regularly with cocoa butter.
4. Rubbing it briskly with tincture of alcohol every day.

58. Following hospital discharge, Mrs. Forman would be most apt to demonstrate unresolved feelings concerning her operation by:
1. Incessant complaining about chest pain, shoulder discomfort, and fatigue.
2. Avoidance of usual social activities involving family and friends.
3. Hectic participation in an unusually heavy program of physical activity.
4. Sudden and unprovoked angry outbursts concerning trivial issues.

59. Which of the following measures would increase Mrs. Forman's rapid social reintegration following her operation?
  - a. Explanation by the surgeon of the full range of physical activities of which she is capable.
  - b. Demonstration by the prosthetist of the variety of wearing apparel with which the prosthesis can be worn.
  - c. Reassurance by the nurse that she is expected to return to her former life routines.
  - d. Her family's adoption of a supportive attitude about both the operation and the prosthesis.
    1. a only.
    2. a and c.
    3. b and d.
    4. All the above.

60. If Mrs. Forman should, after some months or years, develop evidence of carcinoma metastases to other organs, which of the following forms of therapy might then be helpful in improving her comfort and prolonging her life?
  - a. X-ray irradiation.
  - b. Gonadal hormones.
  - c. Bilateral oophorectomy.
  - d. Cytotoxic agents.
  - e. Adrenalectomy.
    1. a only.
    2. a and b
    3. All but c.
    4. All the above.

Prostatic Hypertrophy and Prostatectomy

Mr. Edward Ridgely, a 60-year-old widower, lived with his sister. He had been employed for 35 years as a shipping clerk with the same firm. Over a period of several months Mr. Ridgely developed gradually increasing dysuria. Finally his discomfort became so great that, despite his embarrassment, he sought help at the emergency room of the local hospital.

The examining physician listened to Mr. Ridgely's history of illness, examined a voided specimen of his urine, and performed a rectal examination. Because the examination revealed that Mr. Ridgely's prostate was enlarged, the doctor admitted Mr. Ridgely to the hospital and called a urologist to see him. On admission Mr. Ridgely's temperature was 101.6° F. orally, pulse 92 per minute, respirations 22 per minute, and blood pressure 140/90 mm. Hg.

The urologist catheterized Mr. Ridgely following urination, obtaining 500 cc. of residual urine, which was thick and foul-smelling. An indwelling catheter was inserted and connected to a decompression drainage apparatus. Urine culture, high fluid intake, and sulfisoxazole, 1 gram orally q. 4 h., were ordered.

(ANSWER BLANK ON PAGE A–77)   (CORRECT ANSWERS ON PAGE B–116)

1. It is thought that prostatic hypertrophy is the result of:
  1. Irritation of the bladder mucosa by gravel or toxic metabolites.
  2. Hyperactivity of parasympathetic nerves supplying the urethra.
  3. Chronic bacterial infection of the endothelial lining of the urethra.
  4. Endocrine imbalance between the pituitary gland and the testes.

2. The most serious possible consequence of untreated prostatic hypertrophy would be:

1. Decrease in sexual potency.
2. Formation of a vesicorectal fistula.
3. Development of hypochromic anemia.
4. Destruction of renal parenchyma.

3. In addition to dysuria, which of the following symptoms are frequently associated with prostatic hypertrophy?

a. Frequency of urination, especially at night.
b. Urgency and incontrollable urination.
c. Decreased size and force of the urinary stream.
d. Difficulty in starting the urinary flow.
e. Dribbling at the end of urination.
   1. a and c.
   2. b and d.
   3. a, d, and e.
   4. All the above.

4. In order to prevent contamination of Mr. Ridgely's voided urine specimen, the doctor would:

a. Retract the prepuce and cleanse the glans with a mild antiseptic.
b. Scrub the entire penis and perineum with green soap and sterile water.
c. Use sterile containers for collecting and transporting the specimen.
d. Have him void into first one and then another container without stopping.
   1. a only.
   2. b only.
   3. a, c, and d.
   4. All the above.

5. The doctor performed a rectal examination as part of Mr. Ridgely's workup primarily in order to:

1. Explore the condition of the rectal and anal mucosa.
2. Investigate the existence of enlarged lymph nodes.
3. Judge the size and consistency of the prostate gland.
4. Ascertain whether or not the bladder was distended.

6. Which of the following pieces of equipment should the nurse assemble for the doctor's use in performing a rectal examination?

a. Rubber glove.
b. Lubricating jelly.
c. Drape sheet.
d. Head lamp.
e. Proctoscope.
   1. a and c.
   2. a, b, and c.

3. c, d, and e.
4. All the above.

7. The enlargement of Mr. Ridgely's prostate gland is probably the result of:

1. Distention of the organ by pus.
2. Filling of the lumen with urine.
3. Hyperplasia of glandular tissue.
4. Formation of stones in the ducts.

8. An enlarged prostate gland causes symptoms of urinary obstruction because it:

1. Lies within the lumen of the middle urethra.
2. Encircles the urethra directly below the bladder.
3. Surrounds the ureteral openings into the bladder.
4. Is located on the floor of the urinary bladder.

9. The presence in Mr. Ridgely's bladder of residual urine following urination is indicative of:

1. Spinal cord damage.
2. Increased sympathetic tone.
3. Bladder decompensation.
4. Incipient uremia.

10. Which of the following are possible complications of untreated prostatic hypertrophy?

a. Cystitis.
b. Acute retention.
c. Hydroureter.
d. Hydronephrosis.
e. Pyelonephritis.
   1. a and b.
   2. c and d.
   3. All but e.
   4. All the above.

11. Mr. Ridgely's prostatic hypertrophy makes him especially prone to urinary infection because:

1. The enlarged lumen of the gland tends to harbor pathogenic bacteria.
2. Excessive prostatic secretions make his urine more strongly alkaline.
3. Stagnant urine is an excellent culture medium for bacterial growth.
4. Intestinal bacteria readily migrate into necrotic prostatic tissue.

12. Which of the following nursing measures would provide the best control against urinary tract infection?

1. Supplying additional blankets and flannel pajamas.
2. Encouraging ingestion of large quantities of fluids.
3. Advising frequent turning and deep breathing.
4. Emptying urinary drainage collection bottles frequently.

13. The amount of residual urine obtained by catheterizing Mr. Ridgely following urination enabled the doctor to determine the:
1. Efficiency of renal functioning.
2. Duration of prostatic hypertrophy.
3. Severity of urinary infection.
4. Degree of urinary obstruction.

14. The thick, foul-smelling character of Mr. Ridgely's urine suggests the existence of:
1. Bladder hemorrhage.
2. Prostatic malignancy.
3. Venereal disease.
4. Urinary infection.

15. An indwelling catheter differs from a plain catheter in having:
1. An inflatable balloon.
2. More openings at the tip.
3. A wider internal diameter.
4. Considerably greater length.

16. The doctor used decompression drainage rather than straight drainage of Mr. Ridgely's bladder in order to:
a. Prevent the possibility of acute dehydration.
b. Eliminate the problem of catheter obstruction.
c. Avoid bleeding from the chronically distended bladder.
d. Assist in maintaining the tone of the bladder muscle.
   1. a and b.
   2. c and d.
   3. All the above.
   4. None of the above.

17. To ensure proper urinary drainage for Mr. Ridgely, the nurse should check the drainage equipment frequently in order to avoid:
a. Compression of the catheter under his thigh.
b. Formation of kinks or loops in the tubing.
c. Obstruction of the tubing by clotted blood.
d. Submerging the tube in the stagnant urine.
   1. a only.
   2. a and c.
   3. b and d.
   4. All the above.

18. In the process of decompressing Mr. Ridgely's bladder, what adjustment will the doctor make in the drainage apparatus?
1. Withdraw the catheter a few mm. every day.
2. Lower the 'Y' connecter a slight distance each day.
3. Remove the catheter for gradually lengthening periods.
4. Elevate the drainage bottle on stools of increasing height.

After a week of decompression drainage the urologist performed a cystoscopic examination, which revealed enlargement of the middle lobe of Mr. Ridgely's prostate and hypertrophy of the bladder musculature with trabeculation. The results of the diagnostic tests performed during the first week were:

1. Urine culture yielded growth of *Escherichia coli* and *Streptococcus faecalis*.
2. Blood urea nitrogen: 24 mg. per 100 ml.
3. Creatinine: 1.2 mg. per 100 ml.
4. Electrocardiogram, essentially normal.
5. Chest x-ray, slightly increased anterior-posterior diameter of the chest.
6. Intravenous pyelogram, slightly dilated right ureter and right kidney pelvis.
7. Serum alkaline phosphatase: 3.0 Bodansky u.
8. Serum acid phosphatase: 1.5 Bodansky u.
9. Red blood cell count 4,800,000 per cu. mm. of blood.
10. White blood cell count 11,000 per cu. mm. of blood.
11. Hemoglobin: 85 per cent of normal.

The physician ordered that Mr. Ridgely be put on straight catheter drainage and continue with high fluid intake and sulfisoxazole in preparation for a transurethral resection of his enlarged prostate gland.

19. Mr. Ridgely's preparation for cystoscopic examination should include:
1. Scrubbing and shaving his perineum.
2. Having him sign an operative permit.
3. Forcing fluids during the preceding day.
4. Withholding food and fluids for 12 hours.

20. Which of the following types of anesthesia would probably be used during Mr. Ridgely's cystoscopic examination?
1. Instillation of lidocaine solution into the urethral meatus.
2. Injection of 10 mg. of tetracaine solution into the subarachnoid space.
3. Intravenous injection of a small dose of a short acting barbiturate.

4. Administration of a small amount of nitrous oxide by inhalation.

21. During Mr. Ridgely's cystoscopic examination it is especially important that he be positioned so as to prevent:
1. Hyperextension of joints in the cervical spine.
2. Pressure of abdominal viscera on the diaphragm.
3. Pressure on popliteal vessels and nerves.
4. Eversion and plantar flexion of the feet.

22. Mr. Ridgely's bladder muscle hypertrophy was the result of:
1. Replacement of muscle with fibrous scar tissue following infection.
2. Edema of the bladder wall due to inflammatory narrowing of blood vessels.
3. Compensating efforts to overcome obstruction of the bladder neck.
4. Direct extension of tumor tissue from the prostate to the bladder.

23. The bacteria isolated from Mr. Ridgely's urine probably entered his urinary tract by:
1. Ascending from the perineum through the urethra, bladder, and ureter.
2. Migrating to the bladder or kidney through the regional lymph nodes.
3. Transmission from distant organs to the kidney by way of the blood.
4. Direct extension from infectious processes in nearby pelvic viscera.

24. Which of the following should be provided in order for Mr. Ridgely's straight urinary drainage system to function effectively?
a. The collection catheter should be lower than the bladder.
b. The tubing should be flexible enough to fall into coils without kinking.
c. The collection container should be vented or be distendible.
d. The drainage tubing should be about five feet in length.
e. The collection bottle should be attached to the lower edge of his robe when he ambulates.
    1. a and b.
    2. a, b, and c.
    3. All but e.
    4. All the above.

25. Which of the following measures should be employed in caring for Mr.

Ridgely's urinary drainage system so as not to exacerbate his urinary tract infection?
a. Empty the urine collection container at least every eight hours.
b. Cleanse all system connections with antiseptic solution whenever they are broken.
c. Cleanse the catheter at the meatus frequently with antiseptic-soaked gauze.
d. Replace drainage tubing and collection container with a sterile set every three days.
    1. a and b.
    2. a, b, and c.
    3. All but d.
    4. All the above.

26. Which of the following diets would be most suitable for Mr. Ridgely during his preoperative period?
1. High protein diet.
2. Low roughage diet.
3. High fat diet.
4. Low purine diet.

27. The purpose of a urine culture is to:
1. Determine the duration of a urinary infection.
2. Identify the organism causing a urinary infection.
3. Locate the exact site of a urinary infection.
4. Determine the severity of a urinary infection.

28. In preparing a sample of Mr. Ridgely's urine to be sent to the laboratory for culture, the nurse should:
1. Collect the urine in a sterile container.
2. Filter the urine through gauze before bottling.
3. Centrifuge the urine and send only the sediment.
4. Add a few drops of formalin to the specimen.

29. The doctor will consider Mr. Ridgely's blood urea nitrogen level in determining whether:
1. His general nutritional state will permit safe surgical intervention.
2. There has been any decrease in the functional efficiency of the kidney.
3. There is evidence of a systemic transmission of the urinary infection.
4. The cause of the obstruction is malignant rather than benign.

30. Creatinine may be defined as:
1. An intermediate product of normal fat metabolism.
2. A pigment released by the rupture of red blood cells.
3. A product of muscle metabolism normally excreted in urine.
4. A serum protein that is important in blood clotting.

31. An electrocardiogram was ordered as part of Mr. Ridgely's presurgical workup because:
a. His is the age group with a high incidence of arteriosclerotic heart disease.
b. His blood pressure is sufficiently elevated that heart damage may be inferred.
c. A standard might be needed against which to compare a postoperative cardiogram.
d. He is uremic and should be checked for possible pericardial effusion.
  1. a and c.
  2. b and d.
  3. All the above.
  4. None of the above.

32. An intravenous pyelogram was performed chiefly in order to determine whether:
1. The renal blood vessels had been narrowed by arteriosclerotic plaques or thrombi.
2. The renal glomerulus was capable of filtering toxins from the circulating blood.
3. The tubular cells of the kidney had retained their normal powers of absorption.
4. Structural changes had occurred in the kidney and ureters as a result of obstruction.

33. Elevation of the serum alkaline phosphatase level may indicate:
1. Infection of renal parenchyma.
2. Metastatic carcinoma of bone.
3. Presence of stones in the ureter.
4. Arteriosclerotic heart disease.

34. Serum acid phosphatase level is elevated in:
1. Prolonged malnutrition.
2. Chronic infection.
3. Prostatic carcinoma.
4. Diabetic acidosis.

35. Sulfisoxazole was ordered for Mr. Ridgely in order to:
1. Dilate his internal urinary sphincter.
2. Prevent spasm of the bladder muscle.
3. Inhibit formation of essential coenzymes.
4. Relieve pain and burning on urination.

Finally, fifteen days after admission, Mr. Ridgely's intravesicular pressure and his blood urea nitrogen level had both decreased sufficiently that the doctor thought that he could withstand a surgical procedure. A transurethral resection was done under spinal anesthesia.

36. The nurse should advise Mr. Ridgely's sister that for several days following the surgery Mr. Ridgely will:
1. Be fed through a nasogastric tube.
2. Excrete urine which is blood stained.
3. Receive oxygen by mouth or catheter.
4. Be unable to sit up in bed.

37. In which of the following positions would Mr. Ridgely be placed during his operation?
1. Supine.
2. Lithotomy.
3. Genupectoral.
4. Trendelenburg.

38. In a transurethral resection the hyperplastic prostatic tissue is removed by means of:
1. A curette.
2. A scalpel.
3. An electrode.
4. A scissors.

39. During a transurethral resection, bleeding is controlled by:
1. Catgut ligatures.
2. Manual pressure.
3. Astringent chemicals.
4. Electrocoagulation.

40. It would be especially important for Mr. Ridgely to be given an adequate explanation of the surgical procedure he is to undergo because:
1. During surgery it will be necessary for him to respond to the surgeon's demands that he turn.
2. He will be expected to remain con-

tinent of urine throughout the entire surgical procedure.

3. He will be aware of the activities and conversation of operating room personnel during the procedure.
4. The nature of his symptoms and the unconscious meaning of surgery will make him fear death.

41. Five per cent dextrose in water solution was instilled into Mr. Ridgely's bladder during the surgical procedure in order to:
   a. Wash away pieces of resected prostatic tissue.
   b. Remove blood and clots from the operative area.
   c. Distend the bladder to protect it from injury.
   d. Restore the blood volume lost through bleeding.
      1. a only.
      2. a and b.
      3. All but d.
      4. All the above.

42. Dextrose solution rather than sterile water was used as an irrigating solution during the transurethral reaction because the latter would predispose Mr. Ridgely to:
   1. Edema formation.
   2. A hemolytic reaction.
   3. Renal failure.
   4. Hypertensive crisis.

43. Dextrose solution rather than normal saline solution was used to irrigate Mr. Ridgely's bladder during the transurethral resection because the latter:
   1. Hemolyzes red blood cells.
   2. Encourages bacterial growth.
   3. Corrodes metallic instruments.
   4. Transmits electrical current.

44. In addition to providing for urinary drainage, a Foley catheter was inserted during surgery to:
   a. Splint and immobilize the urethra.
   b. Exert pressure on the operative site.
   c. Dilate the internal urinary sphincter.
   d. Eliminate the impulse for micturition.
      1. a only.
      2. a and b.
      3. a, b, and c.
      4. All the above.

Mr. Ridgely was returned to his room following the operation, with an indwelling catheter in place and with an intravenous infusion of 1000 cc. of 5 per cent dextrose in distilled water running. When connected to a straight drainage apparatus the catheter yielded bloody drainage. His temperature was 98° F. orally, pulse 92 per minute, respirations 24 per minute, and blood pressure 100/70 mm. Hg.

45. Which of the following may have contributed to production of Mr. Ridgely's lowered blood pressure postoperatively?
   a. Spinal anesthesia.
   b. Loss of blood.
   c. Preoperative sedation.
   d. Abrupt handling.
      1. a only.
      2. b and c.
      3. c and d.
      4. All the above.

46. In caring for Mr. Ridgely during his immediate postoperative period the nurse should understand that he is particularly prone to:
   a. Hemorrhage.
   b. Shock.
   c. Confusion.
   d. Peritonitis.
      1. a only.
      2. a and b.
      3. All but d.
      4. All the above.

47. During Mr. Ridgely's first postoperative day his catheter should be irrigated frequently in order to:
   1. Evacuate clots from the bladder.
   2. Prevent formation of bladder stones.
   3. Restore normal bladder muscle tone.
   4. Minimize constriction of the bladder neck.

48. During Mr. Ridgely's postoperative period, what information should the nurse give him concerning his indwelling catheter?
   1. He should limit his movements in order to avoid dislodging the catheter accidentally.
   2. He will experience no pain or discomfort so long as the catheter remains in position.
   3. Pressure of the Foley bag will produce an uncomfortable feeling of urinary urgency.
   4. The catheter will be removed as soon as he is allowed to be out of bed and walking.

49. The nurse should instruct Mr. Ridgely that during his postoperative recovery period, straining at stool must be avoided because it is apt to produce:

1. Cardiac dilation and failure.
2. Cerebrovascular hemorrhage.
3. Herniation of the bladder wall.
4. Hemorrhage from the operative site.

50. Which of the following means would be most satisfactory for controlling Mr. Ridgely's bowel activity during the early postoperative period?

1. Mild cathartics.
2. Cleansing enemas.
3. High bulk diet.
4. Rectal suppositories.

51. In planning long-term care and instruction for Mr. Ridgely the nurse should be aware that a fairly frequent postoperative complication of a transurethral resection is:

1. Bladder rupture.
2. Urinary fistula.
3. Wound infection.
4. Urethral stricture.

By the fifth postoperative day Mr. Ridgely's urinary drainage was clear and the catheter was removed. His morale improved markedly and he began to talk about going home and starting back to work.

52. In preparing Mr. Ridgely to care for himself at home immediately following hospital discharge, the nurse should teach him to:

a. Drink large quantities of liquids frequently.
b. Avoid vigorous exercise and heavy lifting.
c. Take mild laxatives to prevent constipation.
d. Notify the doctor of any sign of bleeding.

    1. a and c.
    2. b and d.
    3. All but d.
    4. All the above.

53. In giving Mr. Ridgely predischarge instruction the nurse should teach him to avoid consumption of:

1. Tobacco.
2. Alcohol.
3. Aspirin.
4. Salt.

54. In planning long-term care for Mr. Ridgely, the nurse must be aware of the fact that which of the following complications may occur about two weeks after transurethral resection?

1. Severe hemorrhage.
2. Urinary retention.
3. Shaking chills.
4. Pulmonary embolus.

Diabetes Mellitus and Leg Amputation

Mrs. Rose Hershey, a 47-year-old housewife, was accompanied by her sister to a large city hospital and was admitted with a diagnosis of diabetic coma. She was unconscious, with a temperature of 100.6° F. rectally, pulse 92 per minute, respirations 22 per minute, and blood pressure 160/100 mm. Hg. Her sister reported that Mrs. Hershey had not known that she had diabetes, but that she had been complaining of weight loss, excessive thirst, and increased urination. The doctor ordered that an indwelling catheter be inserted. Urinalysis revealed 4+ sugar, 4+ acetone, numerous bacteria and pus cells, and occasional red blood cells.

(ANSWER BLANK ON PAGE A–79)   (CORRECT ANSWERS ON PAGE B–120)

1. The metabolic defect responsible for Mrs. Hershey's diabetes mellitus is:
1. Diminished production of thyroxin and triiodothyronine by the thyroid.
2. Hypofunction of the anterior lobe of the pituitary gland.
3. Inadequate secretion by the beta cells of the islets of Langerhans.
4. Decreased production of glucocorticoids by the adrenal cortex.

2. Characteristically, respirations of the patient in diabetic acidosis are:
1. Shallow and irregular.
2. Uneven in rate and depth.
3. Very deep, but unlabored.
4. Rapid and labored.

3. Mrs. Hershey's temperature elevation was probably due to:
a. Dehydration.
b. Brain damage.
c. Infection.
d. Hyperkinesis.
e. Hyperthyroidism.
   1. a and c.
   2. b and d.
   3. c and e.
   4. All the above.

4. Which of the following tests would a physician be most apt to use in differentiating diabetic acidosis from coma due to cerebral hemorrhage?
1. Testing the urine for glucose.
2. Measurement of serum glucose.
3. Determination of systolic pressure.
4. Examination of retinal vessels.

5. In obtaining a history of Mrs. Hershey's illness from her sister, the nurse should be especially alert to mention of which of the following as possible consequences of diabetes mellitus?
a. Excessive fatigue.
b. Burning on urination.
c. Increased appetite.
d. Blurring of vision.
e. Itching of the skin.
   1. a and b.
   2. c and d.
   3. a, b, c, and d.
   4. All the above.

6. Excessive thirst developed primarily as a result of:
1. Need for increased amounts of water to hydrolyze food during digestion.

2. Loss of excessive body water due to increased daily urine volume.
3. Reflex adaptation to a sustained elevation of body temperature.
4. Compensatory adjustment to decreased production of posterior pituitary hormone.

7. Mrs. Hershey's weight loss was the result of:
a. Elimination of glucose in the urine.
b. Increased rate of cellular metabolism.
c. Combustion of tissue protein for energy.
d. Anorexia due to circulating bacterial toxins.
   1. a and c.
   2. b and d.
   3. All but c.
   4. All the above.

8. Mrs. Hershey's polyuria was the result of:
1. Increased glomerular permeability due to generalized vascular damage.
2. Increased glomerular filtration due to decreased serum albumin concentration.
3. Increased volume of glomerular filtrate due to elevated blood pressure.
4. Decreased water resorption due to high tubular osmotic pressure.

9. Mrs. Hershey's coma was primarily the result of:
1. Sudden reduction in serum glucose.
2. Decreased tissue perfusion.
3. Interference with tissue oxidation.
4. Cerebral depression by ketones.

10. Which of the following metabolic defects was the cause of Mrs. Hershey's acidosis?
1. Depletion of mineral stores.
2. Increased storage of glycogen.
3. Incomplete oxidation of fats.
4. Excessive destruction of protein.

11. On her admission to the hospital, analysis of Mrs. Hershey's blood serum would have revealed higher than normal levels of:
a. Acetone.
b. Acetoacetic acid.
c. Beta-hydroxybutyric acid.
d. Acetylcholine.
e. 5-hydroxytryptamine.
   1. a and b.
   2. a, b, and c.
   3. All but d.
   4. All the above.

12. The doctor ordered that an indwelling catheter be inserted in order to:
1. Prevent ascending urinary tract infections.
2. Obtain serial urine specimens for analysis.
3. Prevent repeated soiling of skin and bed linen.
4. Ensure complete emptying of the bladder.

13. The nurse should use which of the following devices to distend the balloon of the indwelling catheter?
1. A metal funnel.
2. A hypodermic syringe.
3. An oxygen gauge.
4. A bulb syringe.

14. Which of the following would be most suitable for distending the balloon of the indwelling catheter?
1. Warm tap water.
2. Ordinary room air.
3. Oxygen under pressure.
4. Sterile water.

15. Which of the following precautions should be taken by the nurse while Mrs. Hershey has an indwelling catheter in place?
1. "Milk" the catheter and drainage tubing at frequent intervals to prevent obstruction.
2. Wash the area around the urethral orifice with soap and water several times daily.
3. Disconnect the tubing and irrigate the catheter with antiseptic solution twice daily.
4. Instill a few milliliters of antiseptic solution into the urine collection bag daily.

16. The nurse should interpret Mrs. Hershey's urinary findings as most suggestive of:
   a. Diabetic acidosis.
   b. Urinary suppression.
   c. Bladder infection.
   d. Renal arteriosclerosis.
   1. a only.
   2. a and c.
   3. b and d.
   4. All the above.

17. In planning for Mrs. Hershey's future care the nurse should anticipate her need for:
   a. Frequent catheter irrigation.
   b. Increased fluid intake.
   c. Intake and output record.
   d. Serial urine analyses.
   1. a only.
   2. a and b.
   3. b, c, and d.
   4. All the above.

18. The factor which predisposed Mrs. Hershey to bladder infection was her:
1. Polyuria.
2. Albuminuria.
3. Glycosuria.
4. Ketonuria.

19. Which of the following is within the normal range for fasting blood glucose concentration?
1. 50 mg. per 100 ml. of blood.
2. 100 mg. per 100 ml. of blood.
3. 150 mg. per 100 ml. of blood.
4. 200 mg. per 100 ml. of blood.

20. The normal renal threshold for glucose is approximately:
1. 90 mg. per 100 ml. of blood.
2. 130 mg. per 100 ml. of blood.
3. 170 mg. per 100 ml. of blood.
4. 210 mg. per 100 ml. of blood.

21. The normal carbon dioxide combining power of the plasma is approximately:
1. 5 volumes per cent.
2. 15 volumes per cent.
3. 25 volumes per cent.
4. 35 volumes per cent.

Serum glucose level was measured, indicating a concentration of 400 mg. per 100 ml. Carbon dioxide combining power of the plasma was found to be 35 volumes per 100 ml. The physician gave 100 units of regular insulin intravenously and started an intravenous infusion of 1000 cc. of 5 per cent dextrose in saline. Hourly urinalyses were done and additional doses of regular insulin and intravenous glucose were given until the urine was free of acetone and showed only a trace of glucose.

Mrs. Hershey awakened 12 hours after admission. By this time her serum glucose level had dropped to 230 mg. per 100 ml. Her physician wrote the following orders:

1. Remove the indwelling catheter.
2. Urinalysis for sugar and acetone q.i.d.
3. Sulfisoxazole, 1 gram q.i.d.

22. The doctor gave Mrs. Hershey intravenous glucose in conjunction with regular insulin in order to:
1. Facilitate proper fat metabolism.
2. Reduce edema of brain tissues.
3. Stimulate glomerular filtration.
4. Increase glycogenolysis in the liver.

23. Hourly urinalyses were done while Mrs. Hershey was being treated for acidosis in order to:

1. Estimate the amount of fluid retention.
2. Serve as a guide for further insulin dosages.
3. Identify symptoms of renal tubular damage.
4. Determine the seriousness of the bladder infection.

24. The physician ordered that Mrs. Hershey's catheter be removed as soon as she recovered from coma because:

1. She would be embarrassed to learn that she had been incontinent while comatose.
2. The catheter would become dislodged as she began to move about freely in the bed.
3. An indwelling catheter predisposes to infection by pressure injury to urinary mucosa.
4. The catheter would restrain her from movement and predispose her to pneumonia.

25. The physician ordered periodic analyses of Mrs. Hershey's urine in order to:

1. Check the accuracy of analyses done by individual nurses.
2. Teach the patient the importance of regular testing.
3. Estimate the total quantity of glucose lost daily.
4. Determine the time at which glycosuria was heaviest.

26. Which of the following precautions should be employed in order to obtain the most informative urine specimen?

1. Have the patient empty her bladder completely half an hour before the specimen is collected.
2. Instruct the patient to void at the exact time established for collection of specimens.
3. Cleanse the vulva with cotton sponges soaked with green soap before collecting the specimen.
4. Save the specimen from the first few ounces voided at the hour specified for collection.

27. Insulin exerts which of the following physiologic effects?

a. Promotes storage of blood glucose as liver glycogen.
b. Enhances transport of glucose across muscle cell membranes.
c. Blocks filtration of glucose through glomerular capillaries.
d. Fosters resorption of water by kidney tubular cells.
e. Increases basal metabolic rate of all tissue cells.
  1. a and b.
  2. c and d.
  3. All but e.
  4. All the above.

28. Mrs. Hershey's insulin was administered subcutaneously rather than orally because:

1. Intestinal absorption is impaired in the diabetic.
2. Insulin is destroyed by gastrointestinal juices.
3. Parenteral administration produces more rapid effect.
4. Hormones tend to be irritating to mucus membranes.

29. Which of the following types of insulin acts most rapidly?

1. Protamine zinc.
2. Regular.
3. Neutral protamine Hagedorn.
4. Globin.

Having regulated Mrs. Hershey on regular insulin for two days, the physician ordered that she be given N.P.H. insulin, 60 units subcutaneously, daily.

30. The peak effect of N.P.H. insulin occurs approximately how long after administration?

1. 2 hours.
2. 4 hours.
3. 10 hours.
4. 24 hours.

31. The duration of action of N.P.H. insulin is about:

1. 4 hours.
2. 10 hours.
3. 24 hours.
4. 72 hours.

32. Before withdrawing a dose of N.P.H. insulin from its container the nurse should:

1. Place the vial in a small pan of warm water.
2. Insert a sterile needle into the vial stopper.
3. Rotate the vial gently between the palms.
4. Hold the vial in one hand and shake vigorously.

33. How many minims of U. 100 insulin must be used in order to give Mrs. Hershey 60 units of insulin?

    1. 9 minims.
    2. 12 minims.
    3. 15 minims.
    4. 20 minims.

34. Which of the following symptoms would suggest that Mrs. Hershey had received an overdose of insulin?

    1. Flushed skin, nausea, and vomiting.
    2. Pallor, fatigability, dyspnea.
    3. Tremulousness, anxiety, sweating.
    4. Hyperpnea, drowsiness, and fever.

35. Emergency treatment of hyperinsulinism consists of administering:

    1. Glucose intravenously.
    2. Insulin hypodermically.
    3. Adrenalin intramuscularly.
    4. High caloric liquids by gavage.

36. In preparing her for self-care following hospital discharge, the nurse should explain to Mrs. Hershey that she will probably require insulin administration and/or dietary management for how long?

    1. For the duration of her present urinary infection.
    2. Until her weight is reduced to a normal level.
    3. Until her urine is negative for sugar and acetone.
    4. For the remainder of her lifetime.

37. Sulfisoxazole was ordered for Mrs. Hershey in order to:

    1. Impede bacterial growth.
    2. Neutralize chemical toxins.
    3. Stimulate mucosal proliferation.
    4. Enhance leukocyte formation.

38. How many tablets of sulfisoxazole would the nurse have to use in order to administer 1 gram of the drug if the container were marked: SULFISOXAZOLE: Tablet 1 = $7\frac{1}{2}$ grains?

    1. 1 tablet.
    2. 2 tablets.
    3. 4 tablets.
    4. 8 tablets.

39. The physician wrote a dietary order for Mrs. Hershey calling for 180 grams of carbohydrate, 90 grams of protein, and 80 grams of fat. How many calories would such a diet provide?

    1. 1400 calories.
    2. 1800 calories.
    3. 2100 calories.
    4. 2300 calories.

40. Mrs. Hershey's diet should be planned to provide her a midafternoon and a bedtime snack in order to:

    1. Ensure more complete satisfaction of her oral needs.
    2. Prevent formation of a peptic ulcer due to stress.
    3. Minimize fluctuation of her blood glucose level.
    4. Provide more opportunities for dietary instructions.

41. To determine the approximate caloric requirement of a diabetic patient at complete bed rest, the patient's ideal weight in pounds should be multiplied by:

    1. 7.5.
    2. 10.
    3. 12.5.
    4. 15.

42. In planning Mrs. Hershey's diet a minimum of 1 gram of carbohydrate per pound of body weight would be required to prevent:

    1. Infection.
    2. Hyperinsulinism.
    3. Acetonuria.
    4. Food cravings.

43. In planning Mrs. Hershey's diet the physician would provide her a minimum protein intake of:

    1. 0.3 gram per pound of body weight.
    2. 0.5 gram per pound of body weight.
    3. 0.7 gram per pound of body weight.
    4. 0.9 gram per pound of body weight.

44. Mrs. Hershey should be taught that one half cup of which of the following vegetables contains approximately 7 grams of carbohydrate?

    1. Green peas.
    2. Green beans.
    3. Spinach.
    4. Eggplant.

45. One half cup of which of the following vegetables contains approximately 15 grams of carbohydrate?

    1. Stewed beets.
    2. Steamed carrots.
    3. Boiled turnips.
    4. Mashed potatoes.

Several days later Mrs. Hershey's cystitis appeared to be under control and her diabetes seemed to be fairly well regulated. The nurse began to teach Mrs. Hershey to administer her own insulin.

46. Mrs. Hershey should be taught that which of the following would be a suitable food exchange for one slice of baker's bread?

1. ½ cup applesauce.
2. ½ cup winter squash.
3. ½ cup lima beans.
4. ½ cup whole milk.

47. Which of the following would be a suitable food exchange for one small orange?
1. 1 cup strawberries.
2. 8 dried prunes.
3. 1 cup applesauce.
4. 1 large banana.

48. Mrs. Hershey should be taught that which of the following is a suitable food exchange for one ounce of beefsteak?
1. 3 ounces of cheddar cheese.
2. 2 eggs.
3. 1 ounce of haddock.
4. 1 cup cottage cheese.

49. Mrs. Hershey should be taught that which of the following is a suitable food exchange for one teaspoon of butter?
1. 1 small olive.
2. 1 medium avocado.
3. ½ cup peanuts.
4. 1 teaspoon mayonnaise.

50. When the nurse brought the equipment tray to begin demonstration of insulin administration, Mrs. Hershey complained, "My sister is a diabetic, too. She takes medicine by mouth. Why can't I?" Which of the following responses by the nurse would convey the most accurate information to Mrs. Hershey?
1. "Probably you can in a few months, when your insulin dose and dietary prescription have been regulated."
2. "Some physicians prefer one medication, some another. Why don't you ask your doctor about it?"
3. "Mild diabetes can sometimes be controlled with pills, but usually newly diagnosed diabetics are regulated with insulin."
4. "You are a more severe diabetic than she. The oral form of insulin would be ineffective in your treatment."

51. For which of the following activities should Mrs. Hershey assume full responsibility after hospital discharge?
a. Injection of insulin.
b. Testing of urine.
c. Preparation of diet.
d. Care of the feet.
e. Recognition of hyperinsulinism.
  1. a and b.
  2. d and e.
  3. All but c.
  4. All the above.

52. In prescribing Mrs. Hershey's diabetic diet her physician would consider her:
a. Body size and weight.
b. Age and general condition.
c. Usual types of activity.
d. Former dietary habits.
e. Cultural background.
  1. a and c.
  2. a, b, and c.
  3. All but d.
  4. All the above.

53. Mrs. Hershey asked the nurse, "My doctor says that I can't handle sugar well. Why must I limit the amounts of fats and meat I eat?" What is the best answer to her question?
1. "Total caloric intake must be decreased so that you lose weight."
2. "Fats and meat can be changed to simple sugars by the body tissues."
3. "Weighing all food will give you additional practice with the scale."
4. "Total food intake will be decreased until your digestion improves."

54. What is the principal reason for the difficulty some diabetic patients have in adhering to a prescribed diet?
1. They have long-standing food preferences which are hard to ignore.
2. Prescribed food servings and exchanges are difficult to memorize.
3. Special diabetic foods are more expensive than ordinary foods.
4. Relatives tend to encourage departures from prescribed dietary patterns.

55. Which of the following sites should the nurse indicate to Mrs. Hershey as suitable for insulin administration?
a. Lateral aspect of the upper arm.
b. Volar surface of the lower arm.
c. Anterior abdominal wall.
d. Anterior aspect of the thigh.
  1. a only.
  2. a and b.
  3. a, c, and d.
  4. All the above.

56. Mrs. Hershey was taught to vary the site of insulin injection in order to:
1. Minimize discomfort from the injection.
2. Avoid unsightly skin discoloration.
3. Prevent subcutaneous tissue fibrosis.
4. Develop skill in handling the syringe.

57. Mrs. Hershey should be taught to sterilize her syringe and needle at home by:
1. Washing the syringe and needle in hot soapy water before and after use.
2. Immersing syringe and needle for fifteen minutes in alcohol after use.
3. Boiling the syringe and needle for 20 minutes before each use.
4. Baking the syringe and needle in a 250° F. oven for 20 minutes after use.

58. In testing urine with Clinitest tablets, which of the following color reactions would indicate a 4+ glucose concentration?
1. Violet.
2. Blue.
3. Green.
4. Orange.

59. The nurse should warn Mrs. Hershey that her diabetes will make her especially susceptible to:
1. Bleeding gums.
2. Digestive upsets.
3. Chronic constipation.
4. Skin infections.

60. Mrs. Hershey should be taught that which of the following would contribute to the development of diabetic acidosis?
a. Respiratory infection.
b. Dietary indiscretions.
c. Omission of insulin dosage.
d. Exposure to inclement weather.
e. Surgical operations.
1. a and b.
2. a, b, and c.
3. All but e.
4. All the above.

61. Mrs. Hershey should be taught that one symptom of impending diabetic coma is:
1. Listlessness and drowsiness.
2. Profuse diaphoresis.
3. Severe hunger pangs.
4. Anxiety and restlessness.

62. Mrs. Hershey should be instructed to carry which of the following articles in her purse at all times?
a. Diabetic identification card.
b. Hypodermic syringe.
c. Vial of insulin.
d. Pieces of hard candy.
1. a and b.
2. a and d.
3. b and c.
4. b and d.

63. Mrs. Hershey should be taught to include which of the following measures in the care of her feet?

a. Bathe daily with warm water and mild soap.
b. Dry by brisk rubbing with a rough towel.
c. Cut toenails straight across.
d. Anoint feet with alcohol after bathing.
e. Wear clean hose and change daily.
1. a and b.
2. a, c, and e.
3. d and e.
4. All the above.

64. Mrs. Hershey will need long-term medical followup to protect her from which of the following possible complications of diabetes mellitus?
a. Degenerative retinopathy.
b. Peripheral neuritis.
c. Gangrene of the foot.
d. Coronary heart disease.
e. Duodenal peptic ulcer.
1. a and b.
2. c and d.
3. All but e.
4. All the above.

65. During predischarge instruction Mrs. Hershey should be advised to exercise moderately every day in order to:
1. Enhance feelings of physical well-being.
2. Promote utilization of carbohydrates.
3. Improve circulation in legs and feet.
4. Preserve muscle tone and joint mobility.

After three weeks of hospitalization Mrs. Hershey was discharged to her home. She made fairly regular visits to the hospital diabetic clinic until a year later, when she developed a sore toe and was unable to walk. After she had been in bed for two weeks at home, her husband brought her back to the hospital because the toe was swollen and black. A surgeon was called to examine Mrs. Hershey. He determined that her right great toe was gangrenous, that circulation to the right leg was severely impaired, and advised her that the leg should be amputated above the knee. Mrs. Hershey consented to the operation. She talked at length with the nurse concerning her feeling about having her leg removed. After a complete preoperative workup her right leg was encased for several hours in ice, following which the amputation was performed under spinal anesthesia.

66. On her visits to Diabetic Clinic the sites used by Mrs. Hershey for insulin injection should be examined for evidence of:
1. Necrosis.
2. Thrombophlebitis.
3. Lipodystrophy.
4. Calcification.

67. An extremity with impaired arterial blood flow may be expected to demonstrate which of the following symptoms?
a. Skin pallor.
b. Cramping pain.
c. Decreased temperature.
d. Trophic changes.
1. a and b.
2. c and d.
3. All but d.
4. All the above.

68. The probable cause for development of gangrene in Mrs. Hershey's foot was:
1. Sudden obstruction of a large artery of the leg by a thrombus formed in the heart and released into the peripheral circulation.
2. Gradual occlusion of a leg vein by a thrombus formed in response to repeated mechanical trauma to the vessel wall.
3. A need for increased blood supply during an acute inflammatory reaction that exceeded the capacity of the narrowed arterial tree.
4. Distribution through the systemic circulation of pathogenic organisms from foci of infection in the urinary tract.

69. In anticipating her postoperative situation Mrs. Hershey was probably most concerned about her:
1. Physical disfiguration.
2. Wound pain.
3. Phantom sensations.
4. Dependence on others.

70. Encasing Mrs. Hershey's leg in cracked ice for some time before amputation would produce:
a. Increased arterial blood supply.
b. Inhibition of pain sensation.
c. Curtailment of infection.
d. Retardation of gangrene.
1. All but a.
2. All but b.
3. All but c.
4. All but d.

71. In preparing to receive Mrs. Hershey in the recovery room following her amputation the nurse should have ready:
1. A rubber pillow.
2. An elastic bandage.
3. A bedboard.
4. A tourniquet.

Mrs. Hershey received a blood transfusion during the operation and intravenous glucose in distilled water immediately upon her return to the recovery room. Her vital signs stabilized rapidly following her recovery from anesthesia. She suffered little postoperative pain but did experience "phantom limb" sensations, for which she had been prepared by her surgeon before the operation.

72. Which of the following elements contribute to Mrs. Hershey's body image concept?
a. Her own view of her body.
b. Her internal thoughts about her body.
c. Her physical sensations of body functioning.
d. Her family's reaction to her body's appearance.
e. Her ideal formulation of her body image.
1. a only.
2. a, b, and d.
3. All but e.
4. All the above.

73. Psychologically, Mrs. Hershey may view amputation of her leg as a threatened loss of:
a. Self.
b. Status.
c. Security.
d. Freedom.
e. Motion.
1. a and b.
2. a, b, and c.
3. All but b.
4. All the above.

74. The quality of Mrs. Hershey's body image disturbance will be chiefly related to:
1. The actual degree of her bodily alteration.
2. Her perception of her physical disfiguration.
3. The stigma attached by society to disfigurement.
4. The degree of family disturbance created by her disability.

75. The best means for reducing the edema of Mrs. Hershey's stump on the second day following her leg amputation would be to:

1. Elevate the stump on rubber covered pillows.
2. Crank up the foot gatch of the bed-frame.
3. Raise the foot of the bed frame on blocks.
4. Suspend the stump from a Balkan frame.

76. Which of the following bed exercises would contribute most to preparing Mrs. Hershey for the use of crutches?

1. Pulling herself to sitting position by a rope tied to the foot of the bed.
2. Slowly raising and lowering her good leg while keeping the knee extended.
3. Kneading a small sponge rubber ball between the palms and the fingers.
4. Using the palms of her hands to push herself up from a prone position.

77. Improper positioning of Mrs. Hershey following amputation of her right leg would be apt to produce:

1. Flexion contracture at the hip of the amputated limb.
2. Flexion contracture at the knee of the unaffected leg.
3. Adduction of the stump toward the midline of the body.
4. External rotation of the unaffected leg at the hip.

78. After Mrs. Hershey's surgical wound healed completely, which type of dressing would probably be ordered for her stump?

1. Warm moist compresses.
2. Dry fluff gauze.
3. Vaseline gauze strips.
4. Elastic pressure bandage.

Mrs. Hershey made a rapid recovery following her leg amputation. The stump healed completely, and Mrs. Hershey learned to apply the elastic bandage which had been ordered to shrink and shape the stump. She also learned to walk with the aid of crutches and, after four weeks in the hospital, was discharged to her home. Plans were made to fit her for a prosthesis at a later date.

Fractured Femur and Internal Fixation

LeRoy Marble, a 68-year-old retired farmer, had never been seriously ill in his life, when he fell on the ice and broke his leg. His son, Bob, found him lying in the icy barn lot, saw that his right leg was twisted and that he was in great pain, and summoned an ambulance.

Mr. Marble entered the hospital emergency room swearing loudly. He answered the examining physician's initial questions with, "Mind your own business, Sonny," and demanded to be taken home.

(ANSWER BLANK ON PAGE A–81)   (CORRECT ANSWERS ON PAGE B–127)

1. In addition to pain, which other symptoms might Mr. Marble be expected to develop if he had fractured his upper femur?

a. Swelling.
b. Ecchymosis.
c. Angulation.
d. Abnormal motion.
   1. a only.

2. b only.

3. All but d.

4. All the above.

2. In caring for Mr. Marble immediately following his fall in the barn lot, it would have been most important to:

1. Cover him with a blanket to prevent chilling.

2. Obstruct his view of the injured leg.

3. Apply manual traction to realign the leg.

4. Splint the injured leg before moving him.

3. The probable reason for Mr. Marble's having addressed the examining physician as "Sonny" was his wish to:

1. Relate to the doctor in the same fashion as to his own son.

2. Prove to onlookers his stoic ability to withstand great pain.

3. Establish some degree of control over a frightening situation.

4. Indicate his lack of respect for professional education.

After the doctor had untied the leg splint, the nurse removed Mr. Marble's trousers in order to facilitate physical examination. The doctor noted that Mr. Marble's right leg appeared to be shortened and externally rotated. The soft tissues in the region of the right hip were noticeably discolored and swollen. Mr. Marble was unable to move the leg and complained of severe pain in the hip and thigh. Mr. Marble was sent to x-ray for anterior-posterior and lateral x-rays of both femurs, which revealed an intertrochanteric fracture of the right femur with displacement and overriding of the fragments.

4. The preferred method for removing Mr. Marble's trousers would be to:

1. Grasp the trousers by the cuffs and pull on both pant legs simultaneously.

2. Roll him from one side to the other, removing one trouser leg at a time.

3. Roll the trousers down under his hips, grasp the pockets, and pull over both feet.

4. Split the right trouser leg to the waist and pull the pants over the left leg.

5. The soft tissues of Mr. Marble's thigh were discolored because of:

1. Decreased arterial circulation to the lower extremities.

2. Obstruction of venous blood flow from the right leg.

3. Extravasation of blood into muscle and subcutaneous tissues.

4. Damage to skin by enzymes released from the broken bone.

6. Both an anterior-posterior and a lateral x-ray were ordered of Mr. Marble's right leg in order to:

1. Investigate the extent of soft tissue damage caused by the fractured bone.

2. Determine the degree of overriding, angulation, and displacement of fragments.

3. Rule out the possibility of an associated compression fracture of the pelvis.

4. Check the adequacy of arterial circulation to the injured hip and thigh.

7. The factor most responsible for the displacement of fracture fragments in Mr. Marble's leg was probably the:

1. Force of his fall on the hip.

2. Initial attempt to move his leg.

3. Hematoma in the overlying muscle.

4. Tonic spasm of large leg muscles.

8. The most likely explanation for the shortening of Mr. Marble's right leg would be that the femoral fragments were:

1. Comminuted.

2. Impacted.

3. Rotated.

4. Overriding.

9. Which of the following factors would most predispose Mr. Marble to the development of shock during his first few hours of hospitalization?

1. Loss of a large amount of blood into the soft tissues surrounding the fracture site.

2. Pooling of blood in the right lower leg due to torsion and occlusion of the major veins.

3. Depression of the medullary vasomotor center by toxins released from injured tissues.

4. Generalized vasodilation as a reflex response to severe muscle and bone pain.

10. The symptoms of shock are:
   a. Slow pulse.
   b. Moist skin.
   c. Increased temperature.
   d. Gray pallor.
   e. Stertorous respirations.
      1. a and c.
      2. b and d.
      3. All but e.
      4. All the above.

The doctor wrote the following orders:

1. Admit to the fracture ward.
2. Apply Buck's extension traction to the right leg with 5 pounds of weight.
3. Carry out complete preoperative diagnostic workup.
4. Prepare for open reduction and fixation of the right hip with a Smith-Peterson nail and attached metal plate.

11. Which of the following nursing measures should be carried out before moving Mr. Marble to the fracture ward from the emergency room?
   1. A tourniquet should be placed under his leg.
   2. The splint should be reapplied to his right leg.
   3. An Ace bandage should be applied to his right thigh.
   4. An ice bag should be applied to the fracture site.

12. Which of the following pieces of equipment should the nurse use in preparing a bed for Mr. Marble in the fracture ward?
   1. A plastic mattress cover.
   2. A full length bedboard.
   3. A wire linen cradle.
   4. A high wooden footboard.

13. Mr. Marble's son asked the nurse, "What's Buck's extension?" What response by the nurse would be most appropriate?
   1. "It is a rather technical procedure for treating fractures and dislocations, named for the doctor who developed it."
   2. "It is a device which will be used in treating your father. Maybe the doctor will explain it to you as he applies it."
   3. "The suspension of a weight from your father's leg by means of adhesive strapping and a rope, in order to reduce his discomfort."
   4. "Why do you ask? Are you afraid that your father is not receiving the care which he requires for recovery?"

14. Buck's extension is an example of:
   1. Skin traction.
   2. Skeletal traction.
   3. Balanced traction.
   4. Intermittent traction.

15. Buck's extension traction was applied to Mr. Marble's leg primarily to:
   1. Overcome tonic muscle spasm.
   2. Prevent soft tissue swelling.
   3. Reduce the fractured femur.
   4. Maintain the fracture reduction.

16. The nurse should prepare Mr. Marble's leg for application of Buck's extension traction by:
   1. Washing and thoroughly drying the skin.
   2. Closely shaving the leg with a safety razor.
   3. Applying a coating of talcum powder.
   4. Disinfecting the leg with green soap and iodine.

17. What supplies and equipment should the nurse assemble for the doctor's use in applying Buck's extension traction?
   a. Spreader board.
   b. Plaster bandage.
   c. Moleskin.
   d. Knee sling.
   e. Pulley.
      1. a and b.
      2. c and d.
      3. a, c, and e.
      4. b, d, and e.

18. In applying Buck's extension traction to Mr. Marble's leg the physician would provide countertraction by:
   1. Applying a head halter and attached weight.
   2. Suspending the hips in a pelvic sling.
   3. Placing a sandbag across the upper thigh.
   4. Elevating the foot of the bed on blocks.

19. In caring for Mr. Marble while he is in Buck's extension traction, the nurse should be particularly alert to the development of:
   1. Excoriation of the skin of the groin.
   2. Swelling of the peripatellar tissues.
   3. Clonic spasms of calf and foot muscles.
   4. Plantar flexion and inversion of the foot.

20. The nurse should check Mr. Marble's traction equipment several times a day in order to ensure that:
- a. His right foot is braced firmly against the foot of the bed.
- b. The suspended weight is steadied against the metal bed frame.
- c. The traction rope is free from the weight of the bedlinen.
- d. The rope knots are secure and do not touch the pulley.
  1. a and b.
  2. a and d.
  3. b and c.
  4. c and d.

21. In addition to the standard tests, which of the following would probably be included in Mr. Marble's preoperative workup?
1. Liver biopsy.
2. Cranial x-rays.
3. Cystoscopy.
4. Electrocardiogram.

Two days later the preoperative workup had been completed, yielding the following findings:

1. Chest x-ray: Heart is of normal size and configuration. Lungs are free of fluid but reveal some emphysematous changes.
2. Blood count: 4,500,000 red cells per cu. mm. of blood, 10,000 white cells per cu. mm. of blood, hemoglobin 80 per cent of normal, hematocrit 40 per cent.
3. Blood type O, Rh positive.
4. Urinalysis: 1 to 2 epithelial cells and 1 to 2 casts per low power field, specific gravity 1.020.
5. Serum total protein 6.4 grams per 100 ml. of blood.
6. Fasting blood sugar 120 mg. per 100 ml. of blood.
7. Blood urea nitrogen 20 mg. per 100 ml. of blood.

22. Emphysema is characterized by:
1. Collapse of a portion of lung tissue.
2. Overdistention of pulmonary alveoli.
3. Replacement of air sacs by scar tissue.
4. Distention of the pleural sac with fluid.

23. In planning Mr. Marble's care during the operative and immediate postoperative period, the nurse should consider that his emphysematous lung changes are most apt to cause difficulty by:
1. Interfering with adequate oxygenation of the blood.
2. Seeding pathogenic bacteria to distant body parts.
3. Throwing off emboli into the general circulation.
4. Increasing the body's requirement for caloric intake.

24. The probable explanation for the epithelial cells found in Mr. Marble's urinary sediment is that they were:
1. Evidence of abnormally increased permeability of the glomeruli.
2. Symptomatic of toxic injury to the tubular portion of the nephron.
3. Indicative of a bacterial infection of the ureter or bladder.
4. Normal cells of the bladder lining, shed in the usual fashion.

25. Urinary casts consist of:
1. Abnormal concretions of minerals around clumps of bacteria or debris.
2. Precipitations of chemical substances normally held in solution.
3. Molds of the renal tubules composed of cellular or protein material.
4. Collections of layered sediment in urine left standing for a time.

26. The normal range for specific gravity of urine is from:
1. 1.000 to 1.010.
2. 1.010 to 1.020.
3. 1.020 to 1.030.
4. 1.030 to 1.040.

On the following morning, Mr. Marble was taken to surgery. He was given a spinal anesthetic, an open reduction was done of the femoral fracture, and the bone fragments were immobilized with a nail and attached plate. After the operative incision had been closed and dressed, the doctor applied lightweight boot casts to both lower legs and connected the casts at the ankle with a horizontal bar two feet long. Mr. Marble was returned to his room on the fracture ward awake, with an indwelling catheter in place, and with reduced sensation in his lower extremities. The doctor ordered that Mr. Marble be given meperidine hydrochloride (Demerol) 50 mg. 'H.' p.r.n. for pain and chloral hydrate 500 mg. orally h.s.

27. Scrupulous care should be taken that the skin is not cut during Mr. Marble's preoperative skin preparation, as such injury would increase his chances of postoperative:
1. Itching.
2. Scarring.
3. Thrombophlebitis.
4. Osteomyelitis.

28. Spinal anesthesia results from injecting an anesthetic agent into the:
1. Subdural space by way of the foramen magnum.
2. Subarachnoid space below the third lumbar vertebra.
3. Subcutaneous tissues and muscles adjacent to the vertebrae.
4. Epidural space by way of the sacro-coccygeal hiatus.

29. Chloral hydrate, rather than a barbiturate, was ordered as a sedative for Mr. Marble because a barbiturate would be apt to cause him to become:
1. Addicted.
2. Confused.
3. Euphoric.
4. Regressed.

30. The doctor applied boot casts after internal fixation of Mr. Marble's fractured femur in order to:
1. Discourage flexion of the left hip.
2. Prevent footdrop during immobilization.
3. Prevent hyperextension of the right knee.
4. Prevent adduction of the right leg.

31. In applying a plaster cast to Mr. Marble's leg, in which order should the nurse hand the following items to the physician?
a. Plaster bandage.
b. Sheet wadding.
c. Tubular stockinette.
d. Felt padding.
1. c, b, d, a.
2. b, d, c, a.
3. d, c, a, b.
4. a, b, d, c.

32. Water for moistening plaster bandage should be kept at which temperature?
1. 65° Fahrenheit.
2. 85° Fahrenheit.
3. 105° Fahrenheit.
4. 125° Fahrenheit.

33. In helping the doctor to apply the casts to Mr. Marble's leg, the nurse should hold each plaster bandage in the water until:
1. The end of the bandage falls free from the roll.
2. Plaster sediment diffuses into the surrounding water.
3. Bubbles cease to rise from the edge of the roll.
4. The core of the roll telescopes out from the center.

34. How much time is required for plaster of paris to set?
1. 10 minutes.
2. One hour.
3. Eight hours.
4. 24 hours.

35. What equipment should the nurse use in preparing Mr. Marble's unit for his return from the operating room?
a. Adjustable siderails.
b. Wooden bedboard.
c. Balkan frame.
d. Plastic covered pillows.
e. Heat lamp.
1. a and c.
2. a, b, and d.
3. All but e.
4. All the above.

36. Immediately after Mr. Marble has been returned to his room the nurse should make sure that:
1. The cast edges are bound with adhesive.
2. All toes on both feet are visible.
3. Caked plaster is washed off his skin.
4. The cast is immobilized with sandbags.

37. After Mr. Marble's return from the operating room the nurse should check for postoperative hemorrhage by:
1. Lifting the corner of the dressing to expose the suture line.
2. Running her hand under his thigh to feel the lower bed linen.
3. Exerting slight pressure over the wound while observing the dressing.
4. Observing the color of his conjunctivae, lips, fingers, and toes.

38. In observing Mr. Marble's right foot, which of the following symptoms should suggest to the nurse that circulation to the extremity has been impaired?
a. Pallor.
b. Coldness.

c. Cyanosis.

d. Edema.

   1. a only.

   2. b and c.

   3. All the above.

   4. None of the above.

39. The blanching test consists of observing the blood flow to Mr. Marble's toe after:

   1. Applying an ice bag to the toe.

   2. Immersing the toe in cold water.

   3. Momentary compression of the nail.

   4. Compression of the popliteal artery.

40. In the event that Mr. Marble should develop symptoms of circulatory embarrassment of his right lower extremity and his doctor cannot be contacted, the nurse should:

   1. Remove the sheet wadding from the cast.

   2. Cut a window in the cast.

   3. Bivalve the cast and its lining.

   4. Remove the cast entirely.

41. Mr. Marble's cast should be checked to determine that it is not compressing the peroneal nerve at which of the following points?

   1. Below the tibial tuberosity on the anterior aspect of the leg.

   2. In the popliteal space between the tendons of the gastrocnemius.

   3. Below the head of the fibula on the lateral side of the leg.

   4. Between the lateral malleolus of the fibula and the Achilles tendon.

42. Which of the following symptoms are possible indications of pressure on the peroneal nerve?

   a. Numbness and tingling of the foot.

   b. Burning sensation in leg and foot.

   c. Inability to extend the toes.

   d. A feeling of pressure on the lateral aspect of the leg.

   e. Difficulty in flexing the knee.

     1. a only.

     2. a and b.

     3. All but e.

     4. All the above.

43. Which of the following nursing measures would facilitate proper drying of Mr. Marble's newly applied casts?

   a. Handling the cast with the palms while moving him into bed.

   b. Supporting the entire cast on rubber covered pillows.

   c. Placing him on a bedboard and a firm mattress.

   d. Leaving the cast completely uncovered and exposed to air.

   e. Maintaining him in one position throughout the drying procedure.

     1. a and c.

     2. b and d.

     3. All but e.

     4. All the above.

44. The preferred method for drying Mr. Marble's casts would be to:

   1. Leave the casts uncovered in a well-heated room.

   2. Surround both casts with several hot water bottles.

   3. Place each cast under an electric heat cradle.

   4. Circulate air around the casts with an electric fan.

45. In order to increase Mr. Marble's comfort while the casts are drying the nurse should:

   1. Apply hot water bottles to his head and feet.

   2. Cover with a blanket those body parts not casted.

   3. Support the bed covers over the cast with a cradle.

   4. Open the windows and doors to facilitate air circulation.

46. About how much time would be required for complete drying of Mr. Marble's casts?

   1. 30 minutes.

   2. Two hours.

   3. Eight hours.

   4. 36 hours.

47. Which of the following might predispose to excoriation of the skin of Mr. Marble's legs?

   a. Pressure from indentations made by pressure on the wet cast.

   b. Inadequate padding of bony prominences at the ankle and heel.

   c. The presence of plaster crumbs or other objects inside the cast.

   d. Roughened, unfinished plaster margins at the top and bottom of the cast.

     1. a and c.

     2. b and d.

     3. All but d.

     4. All the above.

48. In checking Mr. Marble for skin excoriations, infection, and decubiti inside his leg casts, the nurse should be particularly alert to:

    a. Itching sensations in the skin covered by the cast.

    b. A localized area of heat on the surface of the plaster.

    c. A circumscribed area of discoloration on the cast surface.

    d. An offensive smell emanating from the inside of the cast.

        1. a and b.

        2. c and d.

        3. b and c.

        4. All the above.

49. Mr. Marble should be turned frequently from his back to his abdomen in order to prevent development of:

    a. Pneumonia.

    b. Phlebothrombosis.

    c. Decubiti.

    d. Renal stones.

        1. a only.

        2. a and b.

        3. All but d.

        4. All the above.

50. Which of the following is most apt to predispose Mr. Marble to peripheral vascular problems?

    1. Circulation in the blood of toxins released from necrotic tissue.

    2. Increased deposition of fatty substances beneath vessel linings.

    3. Decreased formation of blood cells due to bone marrow destruction.

    4. Stasis of blood in the legs due to lack of muscular contraction.

51. Bedridden older patients are particularly liable to urinary tract dysfunction as a result of:

    a. Decreased ability of the proximal tubule to resorb salts.

    b. Stasis of urine in the renal pelvis, ureters, and bladder.

    c. Mobilization of calcium from bones due to motor inactivity.

    d. Incomplete bladder emptying due to discomfort in using a urinal.

        1. a and b.

        2. a and c.

        3. b and c.

        4. c and d.

52. Which of the following nursing measures would be most helpful in protecting Mr. Marble from genitourinary problems?

    1. Offering the urinal at frequent intervals throughout the day.

    2. Keeping an accurate record of urinary output volume.

    3. Changing his position at regular intervals.

    4. Encouraging him to drink large amounts of water frequently.

53. In order to prevent atrophy of his leg muscles Mr. Marble should be encouraged to:

    1. Perform isometric muscle exercises of both the right and left leg.

    2. Move his left hip and foot through full range of motion.

    3. Massage his right thigh and foot every two hours.

    4. Move about in bed as freely and as frequently as possible.

54. During Mr. Marble's first two weeks in the hospital the nurse moved him from bed to a cart or wheelchair twice a day, in order to:

    a. Relieve pressure on the skin of the buttocks.

    b. Prevent pooling of bronchopulmonary secretions.

    c. Improve muscle tone in the lower extremities.

    d. Prevent stasis of urine in the kidney and bladder.

        1. All but a.

        2. All but b.

        3. All but c.

        4. All but d.

X-rays taken during the second week of Mr. Marble's hospitalization indicated callus formation, so the boot casts were removed, passive and active exercises of his legs were begun, and he was helped up into a wheelchair three times daily.

55. Callus may be defined as a:

    1. Thickened and hardened skin area produced by chronic friction or pressure.

    2. Liquefaction of previously clotted blood in the process of absorption.

    3. Collection of loose fatty tissue containing many immature blood cells.

    4. Semirigid preosseous tissue formed by cells in the thickened periosteum.

56. Following removal of Mr. Marble's boot casts the nurse should care for the skin of his legs and feet by:
1. Dusting liberally with talcum powder.
2. Painting with tincture of benzoin.
3. Cleansing with ether and alcohol.
4. Applying lotion or emollient salve.

After he learned to crutch walk without bearing weight on his right leg. Mr. Marble was discharged to his son's home. He was not permitted to bear weight on his right leg until after an x-ray revealed osseous union in the sixth month following his operation. The physical therapist then taught him to ambulate with the help of a walker. Mr. Marble planned to live with his son until he had recovered sufficient strength to walk without aid. As soon as possible, Mr. Marble insisted, he would go back to his bachelor existence on the farm. "Too many folks in too little space in town," he explained to the clinic nurse.

Cirrhosis of the Liver

Tom Kemper, 45, was an unemployed house painter who was known to drink heavily and to have portal cirrhosis. He had been hospitalized on four occasions for acute alcoholism and on three occasions for pneumonia during the past ten years. He was admitted to the emergency room of a large city hospital after having vomited a large quantity of bright red blood and smaller quantities of material with a coffee ground appearance.

(ANSWER BLANK ON PAGE A–83)   (CORRECT ANSWERS ON PAGE B–131)

The house physician observed the following on physical examination:

1. Ascites.
2. Splenomegaly.
3. Mild jaundice.
4. Spider angiomas on face and upper trunk.
5. Moderate gynecomastia.
6. Respirations 26 per minute and shallow.
7. Marked pallor of conjunctivae, oral mucosa, and nailbeds.
8. Edema of lower extremities.
9. Purpuric spots on arms and legs.

Laboratory tests yielded the following results:

1. Red blood cells 3,900,000 per cu. mm. of blood.
2. White blood cells 10,000 per cu. mm. of blood.
3. Prothrombin time 67.5 per cent.
4. Total bilirubin 4.67 mg. per 100 ml. of serum.
5. Serum albumin concentration 2.8 grams per 100 ml. of serum.
6. Serum globulin concentration 2.6 grams per 100 ml. of serum.
7. Serum cholesterol concentration 225 mg. per 100 ml. of serum; cholesterol esters 112 mg. per 100 ml. of serum.
8. Serum alkaline phosphatase 57.9 units.
9. Serum glutamic pyruvic transaminase 102 units per ml.
10. Serum glutamic oxalic transaminase 99 units per ml.
11. Liver biopsy: changes consistent with Laennec's or portal cirrhosis.

1. The functions of the normal liver include:
   a. Storage of reserve carbohydrate.
   b. Removal of nitrogen from amino acids.
   c. Storage of minerals and vitamins.
   d. Production of digestive enzymes.
   e. Removal of foreign particles from the blood.
      1. a and b.
      2. c and d.
      3. All but d.
      4. All the above.

2. Which of the following vitamins are stored by the normal liver?
- a. Vitamin A.
- b. Vitamin B complex.
- c. Vitamin C.
- d. Vitamin D.
- e. Vitamin K.
    1. All but a.
    2. All but c.
    3. All but e.
    4. All the above.

3. Portal cirrhosis is characterized by:
1. Catarrhal inflammation of sinusoids.
2. Purulent infection of bile ducts.
3. Fibrotic replacement of liver cells.
4. Ischemic degeneration of liver capsule.

4. The structural changes in Mr. Kemper's liver probably include:
- a. Distortion of parenchymal cells by fat globules.
- b. Distortion of lobules by connective tissue septa.
- c. Formation of nodules of proliferating liver cells.
- d. Constriction of interlobular arteries and veins.
- e. Narrowing of the lumen of interlobular canaliculi.
    1. a only.
    2. a and b.
    3. a, b, and c.
    4. All the above.

5. The most probable cause of Mr. Kemper's cirrhosis is:
1. Hypersensitivity to foreign protein.
2. Obstruction of major bile ducts.
3. Long term nutritional inadequacy.
4. Viral inflammation of liver cells.

6. Which conditions, other than chronic alcoholism, may lead to hepatic cirrhosis?
- a. Viral hepatitis.
- b. Inhalation of CCl_4.
- c. Bile regurgitation.
- d. Amoebic dysentery.
- e. Tertiary syphilis.
    1. a only.
    2. a, b, and c.
    3. All but e.
    4. All the above.

7. Careful history-taking might reveal that Mr. Kemper had experienced which other symptom of portal cirrhosis?
- a. Anorexia.
- b. Flatulence.
- c. Easy fatigability.
- d. Diarrhea.
- e. Loss of pubic hair.
    1. a and b.
    2. c and d.
    3. All but e.
    4. All the above.

8. Excessive alcoholic ingestion predisposes Mr. Kemper to which of the following diseases, as well as to portal cirrhosis?
- a. Peptic ulcer.
- b. Gallstones.
- c. Pancreatitis.
- d. Renal stones.
- e. Intestinal diverticula.
    1. a and c.
    2. b and d.
    3. All but e.
    4. All the above.

9. The most accurate conclusion the nurse could draw from the coffee ground appearance of Mr. Kemper's vomitus is that:
1. His bleeding was venous in origin.
2. His hemoglobin concentration was very low.
3. The blood had been altered by gastric juice.
4. The blood was mixed with concentrated bile.

10. Immediately following Mr. Kemper's admission to the medical ward, which of the following should the nurse provide in order to make him more comfortable?
1. Scrupulous mouth care.
2. Vigorous back rub.
3. Complete tub bath.
4. Shave and haircut.

11. Which of Mr. Kemper's symptoms can be directly related to increased pressure in the portal system?
- a. Dyspepsia.
- b. Gynecomastia.
- c. Splenomegaly.
- d. Purpura.
- e. Ascites.
    1. a and b.
    2. d and e.
    3. a, c, and e.
    4. All the above.

12. Mr. Kemper's portal hypertension is the result of:
1. Acceleration of portal blood flow secondary to severe anemia.
2. Compression of liver substance due to calcification of the liver capsule.
3. Sustained contraction of vascular muscles in response to emotional stress.
4. Twisting and constriction of intra-

lobular and interlobular blood vessels.

13. The nurse should know that Mr. Kemper's pathophysiology predisposes him to:
1. Splenic rupture.
2. Umbilical hernia.
3. Renal stones.
4. Bladder stricture.

14. As a consequence of his ascites Mr. Kemper would probably find which position most comfortable for sleep?
1. Supine.
2. Side-lying.
3. Semi-Fowler's.
4. Prone.

15. Spider angiomata are thought to be the result of:
1. Increase in the systemic blood pressure.
2. Failure of the liver to detoxify estrogens.
3. Interference with the normal healing process.
4. Increase in the permeability of capillaries.

16. Which of the following pathologic changes produced increased pressure in Mr. Kemper's portal circulation?
1. Infarction of the spleen and replacement with scar tissue.
2. Proliferation of fibrous tissue around blood vessels in the liver.
3. Pressure of ascitic fluid against vessels in the intestinal wall.
4. Obstruction of the portal vein by thrombi formed of bile pigments.

17. While bathing Mr. Kemper's lower extremities the nurse might expect to observe evidence of:
1. Arterial occlusion.
2. Acute arthritis.
3. Contracture deformities.
4. Peripheral neuritis.

18. Mr. Kemper would have been particularly predisposed to the aforementioned disorder by:
1. Inadequate intake of vitamins.
2. High blood level of alcohol.
3. Bilirubin deposition in tissues.
4. Decreased oxygen tension of blood.

19. If Mr. Kemper's jaundice should increase markedly in severity he might be expected to develop:
1. Hiccoughs.
2. Pruritus.
3. Anuria.
4. Diarrhea.

20. Which of the following is thought to be the cause of Mr. Kemper's gynecomastia?
1. Inadequate intake of vitamin B_1.
2. Excessive blood levels of estrogens.
3. Decreased urinary excretion of sodium.
4. Increased intake of unneeded calories.

21. Mr. Kemper's shortness of breath probably derived from:
a. Anemia.
b. Angina.
c. Ascites.
d. Acidosis.
1. a and c.
2. b and d.
3. All the above.
4. None of the above.

22. The alteration of Mr. Kemper's serum albumin/serum globulin ratio from normal resulted from the fact that his:
1. Diseased liver was unable to produce serum albumin at the normal rate.
2. Biliary obstruction caused excessive retention of globulin in the serum.
3. Increased metabolic rate stimulated increased production of albumin by the liver.
4. Biliary tract infection caused mobilization of globulins from the serum into the tissues.

23. Which of the following represents the normal value of serum cholesterol concentration?
1. 25 to 120 mg. per 100 ml. blood.
2. 150 to 250 mg. per 100 ml. blood.
3. 275 to 375 mg. per 100 ml. blood.
4. 400 to 500 mg. per 100 ml. blood.

24. In the normal person cholesterol esters constitute what percentage of the total serum cholesterol?
1. 45 to 50 per cent.
2. 55 to 60 per cent.
3. 65 to 70 per cent.
4. 75 to 80 per cent.

25. Which of the following blood findings would be consistent with Mr. Kemper's diagnosis of advanced cirrhosis?
a. Decreased red blood cells.
b. Decreased clotting time.
c. Decreased cholesterol esters.
d. Decreased serum bilirubin.
1. a and b.
2. a and c.
3. All but d.
4. All the above.

26. Which of the following might be expected to have contributed to Mr. Kemper's anemia?
  a. Inability of the liver to store vitamin B_{12}.
  b. Long term lack of adequate nutrition.
  c. Loss of iron through gastrointestinal bleeding.
  d. Fatty infiltration of the red bone marrow.
  e. Failure to excrete intrinsic factor.
      1. a and d.
      2. b and c.
      3. a, b, and c.
      4. All the above.

27. Mr. Kemper's pedal edema was probably caused by:
  a. Increased urinary excretion of sodium.
  b. Increased systemic venous pressure.
  c. Decreased serum albumin concentration.
  d. Decreased permeability of the capillaries.
  e. Decreased renal tubular resorption.
      1. a and d.
      2. b and c.
      3. All but e.
      4. All the above.

28. The nurse should observe Mr. Kemper for what symptoms of impaired prothrombin production?
  a. Fever.
  b. Petechiae.
  c. Epistaxis.
  d. Edema.
      1. a and d.
      2. b and c.
      3. All the above.
      4. None of the above.

29. Mr. Kemper's purpuric spots were the result of:
      1. Decreased prothrombin level of the serum.
      2. Increased pressure in the portal system.
      3. Toxic injury to blood vessel walls.
      4. Excessive trauma following sensory loss.

30. In addition to esophageal varices Mr. Kemper would be prone to develop varicose veins in the:
      1. Pharynx.
      2. Appendix.
      3. Bladder.
      4. Rectum.

31. The factor responsible for Mr. Kemper's development of esophageal varices was:
      1. Acceleration of arterial blood flow to the liver parenchyma.
      2. Retardation of lymphatic circulation from the epigastrium.
      3. Establishment of venous collateral circulation circumventing the liver.
      4. Stagnation of bile flow to the gastrointestinal tract.

32. The nurse should check Mr. Kemper frequently for which of the following as symptoms of recurring hemorrhage?
  a. Tachycardia.
  b. Hypotension.
  c. Thirst.
  d. Listlessness.
      1. a and b.
      2. c and d.
      3. All but d.
      4. All the above.

33. Hemorrhage from esophageal varices predisposes Mr. Kemper to development of:
      1. Liver abscess.
      2. Biliary calculi.
      3. Hepatic coma.
      4. Portal thrombosis.

34. If Mr. Kemper should develop hypovolemic shock, blood transfusions would be needed to prevent acute:
      1. Cholecystitis.
      2. Peptic ulcer.
      3. Pancreatitis.
      4. Hepatic necrosis.

A Sengstaken-Blakemore tube was inserted and the following orders were written for Mr. Kemper's care:

  1. Bedrest.
  2. Give nothing by mouth.
  3. Type and crossmatch. Transfuse with 2 units of whole blood.
  4. Administer cleansing enemas until return fluid is clear.
  5. Vitamin K, 10 mg. I.M. b.i.d.
  6. Thiamine hydrochloride 50 mg. I.M. daily.

35. Which of the following would most effectively reduce the metabolic work load of Mr. Kemper's diseased liver?
      1. Keeping him at absolute bedrest.
      2. Giving vitamins by parenteral route.
      3. Restricting fluid intake to a minimum.
      4. Giving high protein tube feedings.

36. In which of the following positions should Mr. Kemper be maintained following insertion of the Sengstaken-Blakemore tube?
   1. Supine.
   2. Lateral.
   3. Trendelenburg.
   4. Low Fowler.

37. The primary purpose of the balloon that was inserted into Mr. Kemper's esophagus was to:
   1. Prevent vomiting.
   2. Control bleeding.
   3. Reduce peristalsis.
   4. Obtain tissue specimens.

38. To maintain proper functioning of the esophageal balloon, it is the nurse's responsibility to:
   1. Remove the tube daily and replace it with a freshly sterilized apparatus.
   2. Check the manometer regularly to determine the pressure in the balloon.
   3. Offer ice chips periodically to decrease discomfort from the tube.
   4. Release the nasal tape and advance the tube a slight distance every day.

39. In observing Mr. Kemper following insertion of the esophageal balloon, the nurse should know that a possible complication from use of the balloon is:
   1. Interference with the patient's normal appetite controls.
   2. Production of acidosis through excessive loss of fluid.
   3. Creation of a mucosal ulcer from pressure by the balloon.
   4. Stimulation of vomiting by interference with peristalsis.

40. The use of the esophageal balloon in treating Mr. Kemper necessitates which of the following nursing measures?
   1. Encouragement of coughing and deep breathing.
   2. Administration of warm saline throat irrigations.
   3. Application of an ice collar to the neck.
   4. Aspiration of saliva from the posterior pharynx.

41. The nurse should leave which of the following pieces of equipment at Mr. Kemper's bedside while the esophageal balloon is in place:
   1. Padded tongue blade.
   2. Emesis basin.
   3. Head lamp.
   4. Humidifier.

42. If the physician should order that Mr. Kemper be given feedings through the Sengstaken-Blakemore tube, the nurse should:
   1. Chill the liquid to the point that ice crystals form on its surface before administration.
   2. Advance the tube a few millimeters before injecting the liquid in order to avoid trauma to varices.
   3. Administer the fluid slowly and in small quantities in order to avoid regurgitation of the tube.
   4. Deflate the esophageal balloon completely in order to facilitate passage of fluid into the stomach.

43. Why were serial enemas ordered for Mr. Kemper?
   1. To facilitate removal of edema fluid.
   2. To relieve paralysis of the small bowel.
   3. To prevent absorption of blood proteins.
   4. To stimulate evacuation of excess gas.

44. Which of the following symptoms frequently indicate the development of hepatic coma?
   a. Nausea and vomiting.
   b. Low-grade fever.
   c. Diarrheal stool.
   d. Abdominal pain.
   e. Increased serum transaminase.
      1. a and c.
      2. b and d.
      3. All but e.
      4. All the above.

Although his esophageal bleeding stopped and the esophageal balloon was removed, Mr. Kemper's condition became worse during his first week in the hospital. He became progressively more drowsy and icteric, developed an offensive breath odor, a flapping tremor, elevated serum sodium, and decreased serum potassium. The physician felt that Mr. Kemper was in impending hepatic coma and electrolyte imbalance. He ordered blood transfusions, intravenous glucose, neomycin, and prednisone.

45. The doctor ordered that prednisone be given to Mr. Kemper in order to:
   1. Block allergic tissue responses.
   2. Facilitate normal excretion of bile.
   3. Foster localization of infection.
   4. Mobilize body responses to stress.

46. Which of the following terms applies to Mr. Kemper's unpleasant breath odor?
1. Kussmaul's respirations.
2. Hepar lobatum.
3. Putrefactive miasma.
4. Fetor hepaticus.

47. The tremor Mr. Kemper developed was probably a result of:
1. Muscular weakness due to low caloric intake.
2. Peripheral neuritis due to lack of vitamin B_1.
3. Increased metabolic rate due to infection.
4. Irritation of nervous tissue by toxic metabolites.

48. In a healthy individual, the normal daily intake of fluid is within which range?
1. 1000 to 1500 ml. per day.
2. 1500 to 2000 ml. per day.
3. 2000 to 2500 ml. per day.
4. 2500 to 3000 ml. per day.

49. Which of the following are cations?
a. Sodium ion.
b. Chloride ion.
c. Potassium ion.
d. Bicarbonate ion.
e. Calcium ion.
 1. a and b.
 2. a, c, and e.
 3. b and d.
 4. All the above.

50. Which of the following is the normal range for serum sodium?
1. 125 to 130 mEq. per liter.
2. 135 to 145 mEq. per liter.
3. 155 to 165 mEq. per liter.
4. 175 to 185 mEq. per liter.

51. Which of the following are symptoms of hypernatremia?
a. Flushed skin.
b. Intense thirst.
c. Oliguria.
d. Elevated temperature.
e. Dry mucous membranes.
 1. a and c.
 2. b and d.
 3. All but e.
 4. All the above.

52. Sodium retention is most apt to result from:
1. Hypopituitarism.
2. Hyperthyroidism.
3. Hypoparathyroidism.
4. Hyperaldosteronism.

53. The normal range for serum chloride concentration is:
1. 95 to 105 mEq. per liter.
2. 115 to 125 mEq. per liter.
3. 135 to 145 mEq. per liter.
4. 155 to 165 mEq. per liter.

54. Which of the following is the normal range for serum potassium concentration?
1. 1.5 to 3 mEq. per liter.
2. 3.5 to 5 mEq. per liter.
3. 5.5 to 7 mEq. per liter.
4. 7.5 to 9 mEq. per liter.

55. The nurse should observe Mr. Kemper for which of the following, as symptoms of potassium depletion?
a. Nausea and vomiting.
b. Weak, irregular pulse.
c. Muscular weakness.
d. Shallow respirations.
e. Intestinal distention.
 1. a and b.
 2. a, b, and c.
 3. All but e.
 4. All the above.

56. Which of the following foods would be best suited to increase Mr. Kemper's intake of potassium?
a. Orange juice.
b. Whole milk.
c. Dried raisins.
d. Cheddar cheese.
e. Coca-Cola.
 1. a and b.
 2. a, c, and e.
 3. All but e.
 4. All the above.

57. Which of the following predispose Mr. Kemper to development of decubitus ulcers?
a. Chronic nutritional deficiency.
b. Presence of subcutaneous edema.
c. General muscle wasting.
d. Relative immobility in bed.
 1. a and b.
 2. c and d.
 3. All but d.
 4. All the above.

58. Mr. Kemper was given glucose intravenously in order to:
1. Withdraw fluid from tissues into blood vessels.
2. Foster deposition of glycogen in the liver.
3. Increase the excretion of fluid by the kidney.
4. Decrease the appetite for oral feedings.

59. Neomycin is effective against which of the following?
- a. Gram-negative bacteria.
- b. Gram-positive bacteria.
- c. Rickettsiae.
- d. Viruses.
  1. a and b.
  2. b and c.
  3. c and d.
  4. All the above.

60. Neomycin is administered by which route?
1. Orally.
2. Subcutaneously.
3. Intramuscularly.
4. Intravenously.

61. Neomycin was ordered for Mr. Kemper in order to:
1. Prevent the development of bacterial bronchitis and pneumonia.
2. Control secondary infection in the intrahepatic bile ducts.
3. Destroy intestinal organisms that break down proteins to ammonia.
4. Eliminate microorganisms from the kidney, ureters, and bladder.

62. If Mr. Kemper should become comatose he would probably be nourished by means of:
1. Gastric tube feeding of milk and cream.
2. Gastrostomy tube feedings of egg nog.
3. Intravenous infusions of 10 to 15 per cent glucose.
4. Intravenous infusions of protein hydrolysates and vitamins.

63. Mr. Kemper should be carefully observed for the development of:
- a. Pneumonia.
- b. Cholelithiasis.
- c. Abdominal hernia.
- d. Peptic ulcer.
- e. Pulmonary embolus.
  1. a only.
  2. a and b.
  3. a, c, and d.
  4. All the above.

Following two weeks of intensive treatment, Mr. Kemper began to show signs of improvement. He became more alert, less icteric, and was able to take a high caloric, low sodium diet. He then began to complain of pruritus, insomnia, dyspepsia, and dyspnea. The physician decided that Mr. Kemper's dyspepsia and dyspnea were a result of his severe ascites and prepared to do a paracentesis.

64. What is the chief disadvantage of performing a paracentesis to relieve Mr. Kemper's ascites?
1. Reduction of blood pressure.
2. Loss of body proteins.
3. Contamination of the peritoneum.
4. Decrease in renal filtration.

65. Which of the following would be most apt to relieve Mr. Kemper's anxiety concerning the paracentesis?
1. Cover his eyes throughout the entire experience.
2. Distract him with talk about neutral subjects.
3. Describe what he will experience during the procedure.
4. Allow him to handle the paracentesis equipment.

66. In setting up the sterile tray of paracentesis equipment, the nurse should consider that the physician will use the equipment in which order?
- a. Trocar and cannula.
- b. Rubber tubing.
- c. Scalpel handle and blade.
- d. 2 cc. syringe and needle.
- e. Sterile test tubes.
  1. a, b, c, d, e.
  2. c, d, b, e, a.
  3. d, c, a, e, b.
  4. a, e, c, b, d.

67. In preparing Mr. Kemper for the abdominal paracentesis, which of the following precautions would be of greatest importance?
1. Check his blood pressure.
2. Empty his urinary bladder.
3. Shave his abdomen.
4. Restrain his hands and feet.

68. The nurse should place Mr. Kemper in which of the following positions for paracentesis?
1. Lying supine on a stretcher.
2. Reclining on his left side.
3. Sitting upright with his back supported.
4. In the lithotomy position.

69. Throughout the paracentesis the nurse should observe Mr. Kemper especially carefully for which of the following?
1. Hiccoughs.
2. Syncope.
3. Epistaxis.
4. Incontinence.

70. Which of the following should be determined frequently while the paracentesis is being done?
1. Pulse rate and volume.
2. Oral temperature.
3. Urine specific gravity.
4. Pupillary reaction.

71. What is the preferred means of securing a dressing in place over the paracentesis puncture wound?
1. Adhesive tape.
2. Collodion.
3. Montgomery ties.
4. Abdominal binder.

72. In planning nursing care for Mr. Kemper the nurse should be aware that the physician will probably counsel Mr. Kemper in which manner concerning his future use of alcohol?
1. Instruct him to refrain from drinking any alcohol for the rest of his life.
2. Direct him to markedly and permanently reduce the volume of his alcoholic intake.
3. Suggest that he eschew whiskey and gin, limiting himself to beer and wine.
4. Advise him to drink only in conjunction with regular and well-balanced meals.

73. The nurse should weigh Mr. Kemper daily as soon as he is able to stand at the side of the bed in order to check:
1. Accumulation of edema fluid.
2. Correction of nutritional deficiencies.
3. Breakdown of tissue protein.
4. Enlargement of liver and spleen.

74. Mr. Kemper's intake of which of the following should be less than that included in a normal diet?
1. Starches.
2. Sugars.
3. Fats.
4. Minerals.

75. The sodium content of a general diet ranges between:
1. 1000 and 3000 mg.
2. 4000 and 7000 mg.
3. 8000 and 11,000 mg.
4. 12,000 and 15,000 mg.

76. As defined by the American Heart Association, a strict low sodium diet is one containing no more than:

1. 500 mg. Na per day.
2. 750 mg. Na per day.
3. 1000 mg. Na per day.
4. 1250 mg. Na per day.

77. Which of the following foods should be omitted from a strict low sodium diet?
a. Cheddar cheese.
b. Canned salmon.
c. Fresh spinach.
d. Tomato catsup.
e. Ice cream.
1. a only.
2. b and c.
3. All but e.
4. All the above.

78. Mr. Kemper's appetite could best be improved by:
a. Providing him oral hygiene before meals.
b. Providing numerous small feedings daily.
c. Serving a preponderance of highly spiced foods.
d. Serving him a cup of coffee before each meal.
e. Offering to cut up his food and feed it to him.
1. a and b.
2. b and c.
3. c and d.
4. All the above.

79. Which of the following is probably responsible for Mr. Kemper's complaint of pruritus?
1. Irritation of tissues by bilirubin.
2. Toxic inflammation of nerve fibers.
3. Alcoholic destruction of brain cortex.
4. Ischemic degeneration of end organs.

80. During his convalescence, Mr. Kemper's diet should include increased amounts of:
1. Carbohydrates.
2. Fats.
3. Proteins.
4. Water.

81. The nurse's plan for Mr. Kemper's health teaching should take into account the fact that which of the following may precipitate hepatic coma?
1. Intercurrent infection.
2. High carbohydrate intake.
3. Excessive fluid intake.
4. Lack of regular exercise.

82. Which of the following surgical procedures may be performed to relieve one of the complications of cirrhosis?
1. Cholecystectomy.
2. Gastrojejunostomy.
3. Portacaval anastomosis.
4. Temporary colostomy.

Following paracentesis Mr. Kemper's dyspnea and dyspepsia decreased markedly. With continued treatment his appetite improved and he no longer appeared to be jaundiced. Following hospital discharge Mr. Kemper went to a Salvation Army shelter. He took with him a bottle of a multivitamin preparation that he was to take daily. His physician and nurse had taught him the importance of avoiding alcoholic beverages and exposure to infection. The hospital dietitian advised the shelter director concerning preparation of the 1000 mg. sodium diet ordered for Mr. Kemper. An appointment was made for him in the hospital outpatient medical clinic so that he could receive medical follow-up care.

Hyperthyroidism and Thyroidectomy

Mrs. Nell Trimble, a 36-year-old secretary, was admitted to a large city hospital complaining of extreme nervousness, irritability and fatigue. On physical examination the doctor observed the following: height 5' 6", weight 105 pounds, temperature 99.6° F. orally. Pulse was 112 per minute, respirations 24 per minute, and blood pressure 130/65 mm. Hg. Her skin was warm and moist, she had a fine hand tremor, staring expression, exaggerated tendon reflexes, physical hyperactivity, and diffuse enlargement of the thyroid. The physician made a tentative diagnosis of toxic hyperthyroidism with exophthalmos and ordered the following tests:

1. *Protein bound iodine level of the serum.*
2. *Serum cholesterol level.*
3. *Chest x-ray.*
4. *Basal metabolism test.*
5. *Radioiodine uptake determination.*

(ANSWER BLANK ON PAGE A-85)   (CORRECT ANSWERS ON PAGE B-137)

1. It is thought that the usual cause for overproduction of thyroid hormone is:
1. Irritation of thyroid tissue by a bacterial infection.
2. Stimulation of the thyroid by a hormonotrophic serum globulin.
3. Increased stimulation of the thyroid by the vagus nerve.
4. Elevated blood pressure resulting from increased heart rate.

2. Excessive secretion of thyroid hormone over a period of time will produce:
1. Increased cellular use of adenosine triphosphate.
2. Decreased pulse pressure and pulse volume.
3. Increased conversion of glucose to glycogen.
4. Decreased stroke volume and cardiac output.

3. Mrs. Trimble's increased temperature is probably a result of:
   1. Infection.
   2. Dehydration.
   3. Hypermetabolism.
   4. Tissue necrosis.

4. Mrs. Trimble's physical examination revealed a considerably increased:
   1. Systolic pressure.
   2. Diastolic pressure.
   3. Venous pressure.
   4. Pulse pressure.

5. The variation of Mrs. Trimble's diastolic pressure from the normal value is probably the result of:
   1. Arteriosclerotic changes in the peripheral arteries.
   2. Generalized arteriolar constriction resulting from anxiety.
   3. Vasodilating effect of excessive thyroid hormone.
   4. Decreased blood flow through the renal glomerulus.

6. Mrs. Trimble's unusually moist skin was probably the result of:
   1. Increased elimination of metabolic water through perspiration.
   2. Decreased rate of evaporation of water from the body surface.
   3. Impaired ability of the renal nephron to excrete liquid waste.
   4. Reflex neurocirculatory response to feelings of acute anxiety.

7. Which of the following is a possible complication of progressive, unchecked exophthalmos:
   1. Strabismus.
   2. Cataract.
   3. Glaucoma.
   4. Blindness.

8. In addition to exophthalmos, Mrs. Trimble is apt to display which of the following eye signs?
   a. Infrequent blinking.
   b. Inequality of pupils.
   c. Inability to converge.
   d. Tortuous retinal vessels.
   e. Lid lag on downward gaze.
   1. a and b.
   2. c and d.
   3. a, c, and e.
   4. All the above.

9. Which of the following pathologic changes in Mrs. Trimble's muscles probably contributes to her feeling of extreme fatigue?

1. Atherosclerotic narrowing of small arterioles.
2. Fibrosis of motor nerve fibers and end organs.
3. Infiltration of muscle fibers with lymphocytes.
4. Replacement of muscle tissue by cysts and abscesses.

10. The enlargement of Mrs. Trimble's thyroid gland was probably a result of:
   1. Distention of the thyroid follicles with edema fluid.
   2. Presence of tumor tissue throughout the gland substance.
   3. Hyperplasia of the epithelial cells lining the follicles.
   4. Infiltration of the gland by large numbers of lymphocytes.

11. Careful history-taking might reveal that Mrs. Trimble had experienced which of the following symptoms of toxic goiter?
   a. Increased appetite.
   b. Difficulty in swallowing.
   c. Frequent outbursts of tears.
   d. Intolerance of cold.
   e. Increased number of stools.
   1. a and c.
   2. b and d.
   3. All but d.
   4. All the above.

12. In taking Mrs. Trimble's medical history, the doctor should be particularly alert to mention of which of the following as possible precipitating factors of her current episode of thyrotoxicosis?
   a. Acute infection.
   b. Surgical trauma.
   c. Psychic trauma.
   d. Reduction diet.
   e. Hay fever.
   1. a and b.
   2. a and d.
   3. a, b, and c.
   4. All the above.

13. Mrs. Trimble would be prone to which of the following gynecologic symptoms?
   1. Leukorrhea.
   2. Menorrhagia.
   3. Amenorrhea.
   4. Metrorrhagia.

Mrs. Trimble told the nurse who admitted her that she had recently been involved in a number of altercations with fellow office workers where she was employed. She explained that she had "worried a lot about the spats" and that worrying kept her from working as efficiently as usual. She confided tremulously, "I've always been a good worker and always got along with everyone. But now I'm afraid I'm going to lose my job if I can't manage to control my temper."

14. The most helpful response which the nurse could make at this time should convey which of the following thoughts?

1. Mrs. Trimble will have to trust to the innate good will and generosity of others and hope that her co-workers will forgive her outbursts of temper.
2. Friction with her co-workers could have been avoided or minimized if Mrs. Trimble had sought medical attention at an earlier stage of her illness.
3. The nurse is willing to accept Mrs. Trimble's expressions of impatience, irritability, and anger, understanding that they are a result of her illness.
4. All such temperamental outbursts will cease now that Mrs. Trimble is receiving treatment and has been relieved of the stresses of everyday life.

15. What type of hospital accommodation would be best suited to Mrs. Trimble's needs?

1. A single room at the end of a hall.
2. A double room near the ward kitchen.
3. A triple room near the nurses' station.
4. A five bed ward near the patients' lavatory.

16. In order to increase Mrs. Trimble's comfort during her hospital stay, the nurse should arrange for Mrs. Trimble's room to have:

1. Brighter than usual lighting.
2. Cooler than normal temperatures.
3. Provision for additional seating.
4. Facilities for steam humidification.

17. The basal metabolism test is based on measurement of the:

1. Level of caloric intake required to maintain constant weight for a given period of time.
2. Amount of oxygen used under resting conditions over a measured period of time.
3. Speed and degree of cardiac acceleration following specific physical exercises.
4. Ratio of respiration to pulse rate under different conditions of activity and rest.

18. In order to detect possible sources of error in Mrs. Trimble's protein bound iodine measurements, the physician should ascertain whether she has recently been subjected to which of the following?

a. Expectorant cough medicines.
b. Gallbladder x-rays.
c. Intravenous pyelogram.
d. X-ray of the bronchial tree.
e. Skin application of tincture of iodine.
   1. a only.
   2. b and c.
   3. All but e.
   4. All the above.

19. The nurse can help to ensure that the basal metabolism test will be done under standard conditions by forewarning Mrs. Trimble that the test will involve:

1. Isolating her in a soundproofed room.
2. Securing her arms and legs with restraints.
3. Obstructing her vision with a blindfold.
4. Occluding her nostrils with a clamp.

20. The nurse's responsibilities for preparing Mrs. Trimble for the basal metabolism test will include which of the following?

a. Serving only a clear liquid supper on the evening preceding the day on which the test is to be done.
b. Administering sedatives during the evening before and on the morning of the test.
c. Providing suitable surroundings for long, quiet, uninterrupted sleep before the test.
d. Withholding her breakfast on the morning of the day on which the test is to be done.
   1. a and b.
   2. b and c.
   3. c and d.
   4. All the above.

21. The nurse should understand that in order for Mrs. Trimble's test of basal metabolism to yield accurate results, her:
1. Temperature must be at the normal level.
2. Pulse rate must be less than 100 per minute.
3. Respirations must be between 18 and 22 per minute.
4. Pulse pressure must be less than 50 mm. of Hg.

22. On the morning of the metabolism test the nurse should ensure that before the test Mrs. Trimble does not:
1. Drink a glass of water.
2. Empty her bladder.
3. Smoke a cigarette.
4. Wash her face.

23. Mrs. Trimble's radioactive iodine uptake studies were ordered to enable the physician to determine the:
1. Patency of the duct through which thyroxin is secreted.
2. Ability of the thyroid gland to utilize ingested iodine.
3. Quantity of thyroxin present in the systemic circulation.
4. Causative organism responsible for the inflammatory reaction.

24. The nurse should be aware that Mrs. Trimble's radioiodine uptake studies would be invalid if Mrs. Trimble has:
1. Received an inadequate explanation of the test.
2. Previously had a greatly elevated metabolic rate.
3. Experienced a recent increase in blood pressure.
4. Recently taken a medication containing iodine.

25. Which of the following anatomic and physiologic changes are probably responsible for Mrs. Trimble's staring expression?
a. Increased retrobulbar fat.
b. Opacity of the crystalline lens.
c. Decreased blink reflex.
d. Diminished lacrimal secretion.
1. a and b.
2. a and c.
3. b and c.
4. b and d.

26. In planning care for Mrs. Trimble, the nurse should expect her to demonstrate:
a. Sudden and unexpected outbursts of tears.
b. A tendency to fumble and drop small objects.

c. Frequent requests for additional blankets.
d. Stubborn refusal to do anything for herself.
1. a and b.
2. b and c.
3. c and d.
4. All the above.

27. In caring for Mrs. Trimble, the nurse should be particularly alert to her need for:
1. Physical rest.
2. Health teaching.
3. Passive exercise.
4. Diversional therapy.

28. Which of the following occupations would be most suitable as a recreational activity for Mrs. Trimble?
1. Embroidering a tea towel.
2. Tatting edgings for handkerchiefs.
3. Hooking a rug of woolen yarn.
4. Making a petit point cushion cover.

29. The nurse noted that Mrs. Trimble was uncomfortably aware of her own heartbeat and frequently complained that her heart was "pounding" or "jumping." This symptom is known as:
1. Auricular flutter.
2. Cardiac palpitations.
3. Neurocirculatory asthenia.
4. Water hammer pulse.

30. Which of the following complications would Mrs. Trimble be most apt to develop if she were untreated or failed to respond satisfactorily to treatment for hyperthyroidism?
1. Heart failure.
2. Cerebral accident.
3. Pulmonary embolism.
4. Intestinal obstruction.

The results of Mrs. Trimble's diagnostic tests were:

1. Basal metabolic rate + 55 per cent.
2. Protein bound iodine 15 mcg. per 100 ml.
3. Radioactive iodine uptake 60 per cent.
4. Serum cholesterol 125 mg. per 100 ml.
5. Essentially normal chest x-ray.

31. The normal range for basal metabolic rate is considered to be:
1. −2 per cent to +5 per cent.
2. −15 per cent to +20 per cent.
3. −20 per cent to +35 per cent.
4. −45 per cent to +50 per cent.

32. Mrs. Trimble's blood level of protein bound iodine is:
1. Greatly decreased.

2. Slightly decreased.
3. Roughly normal.
4. Considerably increased.

33. A normal thyroid gland will accumulate or take up what percentage of a dose of radioactive iodine within twenty-four hours after administration?

1. 5 to 15 per cent.
2. 15 to 45 per cent.
3. 45 to 75 per cent.
4. 75 to 100 per cent.

34. Mrs. Trimble's blood cholesterol level was:

1. Greatly increased above normal.
2. Slightly increased above normal.
3. Within the normal range.
4. Somewhat less than normal.

The diagnosis of toxic hyperthyroidism was confirmed and the following orders were written:

1. Bedrest with bathroom privileges.
2. Propylthiouracil 100 mg. orally t.i.d.
3. Lugol's solution 10 minims orally t.i.d.
4. Phenobarbital 30 mg. orally t.i.d.
5. Pentobarbital sodium 100 mg. orally h.s.
6. Thiamine hydrochloride 50 mg. I.M. q.d.
7. Multivitamins 2 tablets daily.
8. High caloric, high carbohydrate, high protein, high vitamin diet.
9. Daily weight determination.

35. The pharmacologic action of propylthiouracil is to:

1. Interfere with the absorption of iodine by the thyroid.
2. Block the formation of thyroxin by the thyroid gland.
3. Block the biosynthesis of norepinephrine from dopamine.
4. Interfere with glucose combustion in the tissue cells.

36. Which of the following is a possible toxic effect of propylthiouracil?

1. Agranulocytosis.
2. Crystalluria.
3. Convulsions.
4. Laryngospasm.

37. Lugol's solution contains which of the following salts?

1. Potassium iodide.
2. Sodium bromide.
3. Ammonium chloride.
4. Sodium fluoride.

38. Lugol's solution was ordered for Mrs. Trimble in order to:

1. Increase the tone of myocardial and skeletal muscles.

2. Interfere with transmission of nervous impulses.
3. Accelerate glycogen storage in the liver and muscles.
4. Decrease the size and vascularity of the thyroid gland.

39. What precaution should the nurse take when administering Lugol's solution to Mrs. Trimble?

1. Pour it over ice chips.
2. Administer it on a sugar cube.
3. Dilute it with milk and give through a straw.
4. Follow it with sodium bicarbonate.

40. Which of the following are possible toxic effects of prolonged administration of Lugol's solution?

a. Excessive salivation.
b. Erythematous skin rash.
c. Temperature elevation.
d. Swollen salivary glands.
e. Ringing in the ears.

1. a and b.
2. c and d.
3. All but e.
4. All the above.

41. Phenobarbital was ordered for Mrs. Trimble for which of the following effects?

1. Sedative.
2. Anticonvulsant.
3. Spasmolytic.
4. Vasodilator.

42. Pentobarbital differs from phenobarbital in that pentobarbital:

1. Is less apt to be habituating.
2. Produces greater motor depression.
3. Relieves pain more effectively.
4. Has a shorter duration of action.

43. Pentobarbital will usually produce an effect after:

1. 10 to 15 minutes.
2. 45 to 60 minutes.
3. An hour and a half.
4. Two hours.

44. One hundred milligrams is equivalent to what dosage in the apothecary system of measurement?

1. ½ grain.
2. 1½ grains.
3. 3 grains.
4. 5 grains.

45. Another name for thiamine hydrochloride is:

1. Vitamin A.
2. Vitamin B_1.
3. Vitamin C.
4. Vitamin D.

46. Supplemental doses of thiamine hydrochloride were ordered for Mrs. Trimble in order to:

1. Facilitate carbohydrate metabolism.
2. Foster capillary proliferation.
3. Stimulate blood cell production.
4. Promote blood clot formation.

47. The nurse should warn Mrs. Trimble to expect which of the following sensations after receiving an intramuscular dose of thiamine hydrochloride?

1. A generalized feeling of warmth throughout the body.
2. Severe aching pain at the site of the injection.
3. A brief feeling of faintness, vertigo, and nausea.
4. Sudden perception of a bitter taste in the mouth.

48. A high carbohydrate diet was ordered for Mrs. Trimble in order to:

a. Facilitate a gain in weight.
b. Foster the storage of liver glycogen.
c. Prevent combustion of body protein.
d. Offset the tendency for constipation.
   1. a only.
   2. a and b.
   3. a, b, and c.
   4. All the above.

49. A high protein diet was ordered for Mrs. Trimble in order to:

1. Provide a postprandial feeling of satiety.
2. Supply raw material for tissue replacement.
3. Furnish calories in readily available form.
4. Increase the osmotic pressure of the blood.

50. Mrs. Trimble required a higher than normal intake of vitamins in order to:

1. Replace vitamins lost due to parenchymal liver cell damage.
2. Prevent deficiency diseases threatened by her long continued anorexia.
3. Manufacture the additional enzymes required for increased metabolic activities.
4. Stimulate formation of antibodies against a variety of pathogenic bacteria.

51. Which of the following adjustments might be necessary to ensure that Mrs. Trimble would eat the calories and food substances prescribed in her diet?

1. Having her husband come to visit her during mealtimes.
2. Refusing to remove the meal tray until all food is eaten.
3. Including only foods that are concentrated energy sources.
4. Serving part of the food as between-meal feedings.

52. Mrs. Trimble should be given a complete bath and several partial baths daily in order to:

1. Reduce elevated temperature by skin evaporation.
2. Stimulate arterial circulation to the periphery.
3. Remove irritating salts eliminated in perspiration.
4. Provide a relaxing effect to promote rest and sleep.

53. On making her regular patient rounds, the night nurse noticed that Mrs. Trimble's eyelids did not close completely when she slept. This observation should be recorded and reported to the physician because it:

1. Indicates that Mrs. Trimble needs a stronger dose of sedative at bedtime.
2. Suggests that measures should be instituted to protect her cornea from ulceration.
3. Invalidates the diagnosis of eye pathology previously made by the physician.
4. Contraindicates further administration of propylthiouracil in the present dosages.

54. In caring for Mrs. Trimble the nurse should adjust the usual ward nursing schedule in order to provide for Mrs. Trimble's:

1. Intolerance of close interpersonal contact over extended periods of time.
2. Need to use the bedpan at one- to two-hour intervals throughout the day.
3. Physical comfort by remaking the bed to remove wrinkles several times a day.
4. Intellectual needs by reading aloud to her during the afternoon rest hours.

55. The nurse should instruct Mrs. Trimble's visitors to:

1. Avoid bringing gifts of food and candy.
2. Refrain from discussing distressing issues with her.

3. Leave the room during mealtime and medication administration.
4. Carry the burden of conversation during the visit.

Mrs. Trimble responded well to treatment, gaining 7 pounds in the two weeks following admission to the hospital. She was then discharged to her home on continued dosage of propylthiouracil, Lugol's solution, and phenobarbital. She continued to gain weight during the next two months and was readmitted to the hospital for a thyroidectomy when her basal metabolic rate had decreased to +15 per cent.

Following readmission to the hospital Mrs. Trimble was kept at bedrest for three days during the preoperative workup. Because the workup, which included routine blood and urine tests, typing and cross-matching, and electrocardiography, yielded no contraindications to surgery, a subtotal thyroidectomy was performed under general anesthesia. Examination of the surgical specimen revealed benign hyperplasia of the acinar epithelium.

Postoperative orders included:

1. Vital signs every 15 minutes until stable, q 2 h. for 12 hours, then q 4 h.
2. Meperidine hydrochloride 25 mg. H. q 4 h. p.r.n.
3. 1000 ml. of 5 per cent dextrose in distilled water q 12 h. I.V.
4. Fluids to soft diet as tolerated.

56. Mrs. Trimble was brought to euthyroid level before surgery in order to prevent postoperative development of:
1. Incisional hemorrhage.
2. Wound dehiscence.
3. Hyperthyroid crisis.
4. Suture line infection.

57. It is especially important that Mrs. Trimble be given adequate psychological preparation for surgery because undue fear and apprehension could predispose her to:
1. Suicidal depression.
2. Cerebral accident.
3. Hysterical paralysis.
4. Thyroid crisis.

58. In preparing Mrs. Trimble for surgery, the nurse should inform her that she will experience which symptom on recovering from the anesthesia?
1. Difficulty in swallowing.
2. Decrease in visual acuity.
3. Feeling of chilliness.

4. Paroxysms of hiccoughs.

59. Preoperative instruction for Mrs. Trimble should indicate that she is apt to receive which of the following treatments during the immediate postoperative period?
a. Intravenous infusion.
b. Oxygen administration.
c. Application of an ice collar.
d. Medicated steam inhalations.
1. a only.
2. a and b.
3. b and c.
4. All the above.

60. What emergency equipment should be kept at Mrs. Trimble's bedside during her stay in the recovery room?
1. Rubber tourniquet.
2. Tracheostomy set.
3. 50 cc. syringe.
4. Large metal clamp.

61. The nurse should assemble equipment at Mrs. Trimble's bedside for which of the following treatments during her postanesthetic recovery period:
1. Gastric suctioning.
2. Nasogastric tube feeding.
3. Intravenous digitalization.
4. Oxygen administration.

62. During Mrs. Trimble's immediate postoperative period the nurse should:
1. Turn her from side to side every hour.
2. Keep her head turned to one side or the other.
3. Maintain her neck in flexed position.
4. Suction oropharyngeal secretions at frequent intervals.

63. Mrs. Trimble should be observed especially carefully postoperatively for evidence of which of the following untoward operative events?
1. Fracture of the laryngeal cartilage.
2. Laceration of the wall of the esophagus.
3. Accidental removal of parathyroid glands.
4. Perforation of the apex of the lung.

64. Mrs. Trimble's pulse and blood pressure should be monitored at frequent intervals postoperatively, since hemorrhage from the operative site could rapidly produce:
1. Shock.
2. Asphyxia.
3. Anemia.
4. Heart failure.

65. In checking Mrs. Trimble for wound hemorrhage, the recovery room nurse should:

1. Loosen one edge of the dressing and lift it to permit direct visualization of the wound.
2. Slip a hand under her neck and shoulders to check the condition of the lower bed linen.
3. Roll her to her side to permit full visualization of the sides and back of the neck.
4. Press gently on the skin surrounding the incision to express accumulated blood from the wound.

66. After awakening from anesthesia, in which position would Mrs. Trimble probably be most comfortable?

1. Prone.
2. Supine.
3. Sims'.
4. Semi-Fowler's.

67. In checking Mrs. Trimble shortly after her return to the recovery room, the nurse noted that although she was experiencing no pain or dyspnea, there was noticeable swelling of the neck tissues above the wound dressing. The nurse should:

1. Loosen and remove the neck dressing.
2. Notify the doctor of the neck swelling.
3. Lower the head of the bed completely.
4. Record the observation on the chart.

68. Mrs. Trimble should be observed during the early postoperative period for symptoms of thyroid crisis, which include:

a. Greatly increased temperature.
b. Very rapid pulse rate.
c. Irregular cardiac rate.
d. Shortness of breath.
e. Restlessness and delirium.
  1. a and b.
  2. c and d.
  3. All but e.
  4. All the above.

69. If Mrs. Trimble should develop hoarseness, that symptom should be reported immediately to the doctor because it is a possible indication of:

1. Development of a retropharyngeal or peritonsillar abscess.
2. Perforation or laceration of the trachea during intubation.
3. Toxic depression of the medulla by the anesthetic agent.
4. Injury to or edema of the recurrent laryngeal nerve.

70. Which of the following is a symptom of hypoparathyroidism?

1. Tetany.
2. Tympanites.
3. Torticollis.
4. Tinnitus.

71. During the first postoperative day the nurse should help Mrs. Trimble to sit up in bed by:

1. Grasping both her hands and pulling her forward from the hips.
2. Slipping an arm under her axilla to support and lift her shoulders.
3. Placing a hand under her head to prevent hyperextension of the neck.
4. Rolling her to one side and swinging her feet over the edge of the bed.

Mrs. Trimble recuperated rapidly following surgery. Her blood calcium and other electrolytes remained within normal limits following the operation. She was given a high caloric liquid diet on the first postoperative day, was helped to sit in a chair on the second postoperative day, and had the skin clips removed from her incision on the fourth postoperative day. She was then able to eat a soft diet, to walk to the bathroom, and to bathe herself with some assistance from the nurse. Mrs. Trimble was anxious to return to her home so her physician decided that she could be discharged from the hospital on her seventh or eighth postoperative day.

72. In giving Mrs. Trimble predischarge instructions, the nurse should explain that she should consult her doctor regularly on a long term basis in order to be checked for manifestations of:

1. Hypothyroidism.
2. Laryngitis.
3. Carcinoma.
4. Lymphadenitis.

Adenocarcinoma of the Rectum

Matthew Oakes was 68 when he was found to have adenocarcinoma of the rectum. He had consulted his family doctor because of weakness and intermittent constipation and diarrhea of several months' duration. The physician found a 4 + stool benzidine reaction and discovered a fungating mass on the posterior rectal wall on proctoscopy. Mr. Oakes was admitted to the hospital for a complete diagnostic workup and possible surgery.

(ANSWER BLANK ON PAGE A–87)   (CORRECT ANSWERS ON PAGE B–142)

1. Adenocarcinomas are malignant tumors arising from:
1. Soft fatty tissue.
2. Smooth muscle tissue.
3. Columnar epithelial tissue.
4. Fibrous connective tissue.

2. The primary cause of Mr. Oakes' weakness was probably:
1. Loss of water and electrolytes due to diarrhea.
2. Decreased oxygen carrying power of the blood.
3. Impaired intestinal absorption of nutrients.
4. Anxiety concerning the cause for his symptoms.

3. Mr. Oakes' episodes of constipation were probably caused by:
1. Obstruction of the bowel lumen by the growing tumor mass.
2. Lack of sufficient roughage because of avoidance of solid foods.
3. Physical inactivity resulting from chronic general weakness.
4. Spasm of circular smooth muscle fibers in the bowel wall.

4. Mr. Oakes' diarrhea probably resulted from:
1. Bacterial infection of the ulcerated bowel lining.
2. Accelerated peristalsis resulting from chronic anxiety.
3. Continuous ingestion of only liquid and soft foods.
4. Increased secretion of mucus as a result of mucosal irritation.

5. A 4+ reaction of Mr. Oakes' stool on testing with benzidine reagent could be interpreted as indicating the presence of:
1. Malignant cells.
2. Occult blood.
3. Excess mucus.
4. Pathogenic bacteria.

6. A fungating mass is a:
1. Soft, irregular outgrowth from a surface.
2. Hard circular swelling with an open crater.
3. Slight, flat elevation with a sharply defined edge.
4. Sharply pointed excrescence filled with pus.

7. For which of the following measures would the doctor's office nurse be responsible in preparing Mr. Oakes for a proctoscopic examination to be done in the physician's office?
a. Explaining the procedure for the examination.
b. Giving directions for necessary dietary modifications.
c. Administering a series of cleansing enemas.
d. Positioning and draping him for the examination.
   1. a and b.
   2. a, b, and d.
   3. b and c.
   4. c and d.

8. Which of the following should Mr. Oakes be advised to do in preparation for the proctoscopic examination to be done in the physician's office?
1. Administer enemas until the returns are clear on the morning of the examination.
2. Refrain from eating any food for 24 hours preceding the examination.
3. Take a strong cathartic on both the evening before and the morning of the examination.
4. Take sitz baths three times daily for three days preceding the examination.

9. The primary purpose of giving serial enemas in preparation for a proctoscopic examination is to:
1. Decrease the discomfort of instrumentation.
2. Permit optimum visualization of the bowel.
3. Prevent gas pains following the examination.
4. Increase the blood supply to the bowel wall.

10. Which of the following should the nurse assemble for the doctor's use during a proctoscopic examination?
a. Rubber gloves.
b. Lubricating jelly.
c. Sterile tongue blades.
d. Long cotton-tipped applicators.
e. Paper lined waste basket.
1. a and b.
2. c and d.
3. a, b, d, and e.
4. a, b, and e.

11. In what position would Mr. Oakes be placed for the proctoscopic examination?
1. Prone.
2. Right Sims'.
3. Lithotomy.
4. Knee-chest.

12. In preparing Mr. Oakes for the proctoscopic examination the nurse should say:
1. "You need have no anxiety concerning this procedure. You will experience no pain or discomfort at any time."
2. "You will experience a feeling of pressure and the desire to move your bowels during the brief time that the proctoscope is in place."
3. "You can reduce your discomfort

during the procedure to a minimum by bearing down as the proctoscope is introduced."
4. "You will experience no discomfort during the procedure because a topical anesthetic will be applied to the anus and rectum."

On Mr. Oakes' admission to the hospital, the following orders were written by his physician:

1. Complete blood count, hematocrit, and hemoglobin determination.
2. Barium enema and lower gastrointestinal x-ray.
3. Biopsy of rectal tumor mass.
4. Liver function tests.
5. Chest, spine, and pelvic x-rays.
6. Electrocardiogram.
7. High caloric, high protein, low residue diet.

13. Careful history-taking may reveal that Mr. Oakes had experienced which other symptoms of rectosigmoid carcinoma?
a. Loss of appetite.
b. Abdominal distention.
c. Blood in the stool.
d. Fatty food intolerance.
e. Cramping abdominal pain.
1. a and b.
2. a, c, and e.
3. All but d.
4. All the above.

14. In taking Mr. Oakes' family medical history, the physician would be particularly alert to the mention of what disease as an indication of a familial predisposition to bowel malignancy?
1. Hemorrhoids.
2. Polyposis.
3. Colitis.
4. Amebiasis.

15. In caring for Mr. Oakes after the barium enema, the nurse should realize that which of the following is a possible complication of the administration of barium to a patient with a rectal tumor?
1. Severe diarrhea.
2. Rectal fistula.
3. Anaphylactic shock.
4. Intestinal obstruction.

16. When Mr. Oakes' rectal biopsy is completed the nurse should:
a. Cleanse the anal region of excess lubricant.

b. Administer a clear tap water enema.

c. Label the biopsy specimen for the laboratory.

d. Apply a perineal pad and a T-shaped binder.

    1. a and b.

    2. a and c.

    3. b and c.

    4. b and d.

17. In caring for Mr. Oakes following biopsy of his rectal tumor, the nurse should check him for development of:

    1. Urinary retention.

    2. Rectal hemorrhage.

    3. Fecal impaction.

    4. Anal fissure.

18. The physician ordered liver function tests as part of Mr. Oakes' workup in order to:

a. Determine his ability to tolerate a general anesthetic.

b. Rule out the possibility of homologous serum hepatitis.

c. Check for indications of tumor metastases to the liver.

d. Estimate the length and severity of his nutritional deficit.

    1. a and b.

    2. a and c.

    3. b and c.

    4. b and d.

19. The physician ordered x-rays of Mr. Oakes' chest, spine, and pelvis in order to:

    1. Check for existence of osteoarthritis.

    2. Rule out gallbladder and renal stones.

    3. Look for evidence of bony metastases.

    4. Stimulate cell production by the marrow.

20. An electrocardiogram was ordered as part of the preoperative workup because Mr. Oakes would be particularly susceptible to which type of heart disease?

    1. Thyrotoxic.

    2. Rheumatic.

    3. Nutritional.

    4. Arteriosclerotic.

The result of Mr. Oakes' diagnostic tests were:

1. Red blood cell count 4,500,000 per cu. mm.

2. White blood cell count 10,000 per cu. mm.

3. Hematocrit 38 per cent.

4. Hemoglobin 10 grams per 100 ml.

5. X-ray following a barium enema revealed an irregular mass occluding the rectal lumen.

6. Liver function tests and electrocardiogram were within normal limits.

7. Biopsy of the rectal tumor mass indicated adenocarcinoma.

8. X-ray revealed a normal sized heart and some osteoarthritic changes in the bodies of the lumbar vertebrae.

21. Mr. Oakes' anemia is characterized by:

    1. Approximately equal reduction in the number of red cells and in the concentration of hemoglobin.

    2. Relative paucity of red cells and hemoglobin in comparison to the number of white blood cells.

    3. Proportionately greater decrease in number of red cells than in hemoglobin concentration.

    4. Proportionately greater decrease in hemoglobin concentration than in number of red blood cells.

22. Mr. Oakes' hematocrit and red blood cell count are suggestive of an anemia of which type?

    1. Macrocytic.

    2. Microcytic.

    3. Normocytic.

    4. Anaplastic.

23. Mr. Oakes' blood test findings are suggestive of:

    1. Acute hemorrhage.

    2. Chronic blood loss.

    3. Chronic malnutrition.

    4. Bone marrow replacement.

24. An average serving of which of the following foods contains the greatest number of calories?

    1. Soft cooked egg.

    2. Chocolate milk.

    3. Hamburger patty.

    4. Baked potato.

25. Which of the following foods is the best source of complete protein?

    1. Whole milk.

    2. Navy beans.

    3. Plain gelatin.

    4. Corn meal.

26. Which of the following foods should be eliminated from Mr. Oakes' low residue diet?

    1. Cooked farina.

    2. Hard cooked egg.

    3. Stewed prunes.

    4. Cottage cheese.

27. Which of the following foods would be permitted on a low residue diet?
- a. Poached eggs.
- b. Tomato juice.
- c. Baked chicken.
- d. White potatoes.
- e. Malted milk.
  1. a and c.
  2. b and d.
  3. All but e.
  4. All the above.

On the basis of the test findings, it was decided that Mr. Oakes' physical condition made him a suitable candidate for major surgery. The surgeon informed Mr. Oakes that he had cancer of the rectum and advised that he undergo surgery for removal of the rectum and formation of a colostomy. Mr. Oakes asked to be given a day or two to decide whether or not he wished to have the operation done. Then he sent for his wife, his two grown sons, and his parish priest. He and his family held a long and anguished consultation with the surgeon. He and his priest had several conversations. He went to Confession and to Holy Communion.

28. Which of the following factors will determine Mr. Oakes' adjustment to his illness?
- a. Understanding of his condition.
- b. Extent of metastases.
- c. Amount of family support.
- d. Basic ego strength.
- e. Attitudes of the health team.
  1. a and c.
  2. b and d.
  3. All but e.
  4. All the above.

29. Mr. Oakes' reluctance to undergo surgery may result from:
- a. Fear of undergoing a general anesthetic and a serious surgical operation.
- b. Anxiety concerning the alteration in body image effected by a colostomy.
- c. Concern about the expense of major surgery and prolonged hospitalization.
- d. Anticipation of social losses as a consequence of the colostomy.
  1. a only.
  2. a and b.
  3. a, b, and c.
  4. All the above.

30. In caring for Mr. Oakes while he is deciding whether or not to undergo surgery, it would be most helpful for the nurse to be aware of the:
1. Tenets and sacraments of the Roman Catholic church.
2. Information given to Mr. Oakes by the surgeon.
3. Attitudes of the family toward the operation.
4. Financial resources upon which Mr. Oakes can draw.

Shortly after the surgeon's conference with the entire family, Mrs. Oakes and her two sons left the hospital. An hour later, while the nurse was preparing Mr. Oakes for sleep, he said, "I've got a big decision to make and I'm not sure that I can do it."

31. What response by the nurse would be most appropriate?
1. "Isn't it possible that there really is no decision to make?"
2. "Would you like to tell me more about what concerns you?"
3. "Wouldn't it be better to let the doctor make the decision?"
4. "Do you want me to ask the priest to come visit you?"

32. In order for him to decide whether or not to undergo colostomy surgery Mr. Oakes should understand:
- a. The normal structure and function of the large bowel.
- b. The anatomic and physiologic changes brought about by colostomy.
- c. The care which he will be given postoperatively.
- d. The methods by which he will regulate colostomy functioning.
- e. The way in which his life will be modified by the colostomy.
  1. a and b.
  2. c and d.
  3. All but e.
  4. All the above.

33. In order to plan long term care for Mr. Oakes the nurse should be aware that patients with a malignancy frequently manifest which of the following responses to their disease?
- a. Dependency.
- b. Anger.
- c. Guilt.

d. Insecurity.
   1. a only.
   2. b and c.
   3. c and d.
   4. Any of the above.

The following preoperative orders were written:

1. Phthalylsulfathiazole 2 grams orally q. 6 h. for 3 days.
2. Neomycin 1 gram orally q. 1 h. × 4, then 1 gram orally q. 4 h × 1 day.
3. Cleansing enemas until returns are clear.
4. Insert a nasogastric suction tube and an indwelling catheter on the morning of surgery.
5. Meperidine hydrochloride 25 mg. H., promethazine hydrochloride 25 mg. H., and atropine sulfate 0.4 mg. H. to be given 15 minutes before going to the operating room.

34. Phthalylsulfathiazole was ordered for Mr. Oakes in order to:
   1. Prevent postoperative pneumonia.
   2. Decrease intestinal bacteria count.
   3. Remove bacteria from the blood.
   4. Eliminate urinary tract infection.

35. Phthalylsulfathiazole is better suited than sulfadiazine for the above purpose because phthalylsulfathiazole is:
   1. Effective against a greater number of bacteria.
   2. Very poorly absorbed from the intestinal tract.
   3. Less irritating to the lining of the intestine.
   4. Productive of higher blood concentrations of the drug.

36. Neomycin resembles phthalylsulfathiazole in that both drugs:
   1. Are derivatives of para-amino-benzenesulfonamide.
   2. Inhibit utilization of para-aminobenzoic acid.
   3. Are rapidly distributed to all body tissues.
   4. Are poorly absorbed from the intestinal tract.

37. Which of the following is a possible toxic effect of neomycin?
   1. Hemolytic anemia.
   2. Bronchiolar spasm.
   3. Nerve deafness.
   4. Hepatocellular necrosis.

38. Which of the following intestinal inhabitants is usually destroyed by neomycin but not by tetracycline?

1. *Escherichia coli.*
2. *Aerobacter aerogenes.*
3. *Proteus vulgaris.*
4. *Salmonella typhosa.*

39. When the nurse told Mr. Oakes that he was to receive a blood transfusion before surgery, he asked, "What for? Am I too weak to be operated on?" Which of the following responses would be most helpful?
   1. "There is nothing remarkable about your being given blood before surgery. Blood transfusions are routine in preparation for major surgery."
   2. "You have been weakened through weight loss and rectal bleeding. The doctor feels that you need a blood transfusion to build up your strength."
   3. "A transfusion now will greatly improve your strength and speed your postoperative recovery by increasing your body's defenses against stress."
   4. "The doctor ordered the transfusion as part of your preoperative preparation. He'll have to explain the purpose for giving it to you at this time."

40. The gastric suction tube was inserted before sending Mr. Oakes to surgery in order to:
   1. Facilitate administration of high caloric nutrient liquids immediately after completion of the procedure.
   2. Prevent accumulation of gas and fluid in the stomach both during and following surgical intervention.
   3. Provide a reliable means of detecting gastrointestinal hemorrhage during the operative procedure.
   4. Serve as a stimulus to restore normal peristaltic movement following recovery from anesthesia.

41. The primary purpose of inserting an indwelling catheter before taking Mr. Oakes to the operating room is to:
   1. Facilitate distention of the bladder with saline during surgery.
   2. Provide a ready check of renal function throughout surgery.
   3. Reduce the possibility of bladder injury during the procedure.
   4. Prevent contamination of the operative field due to incontinence.

42. Meperidine was ordered for Mr. Oakes preoperatively chiefly in order to:
1. Potentiate the effect of the anesthetic agent.
2. Reduce discomfort resulting from serial enemas.
3. Relieve apprehension provoked by the operation.
4. Decrease peristalsis during the surgical procedure.

43. The pharmacologic effect of promethazine hydrochloride (Phenergan) which explains its preoperative administration to Mr. Oakes is its ability to:
1. Decrease the secretions of respiratory and digestive glands.
2. Inhibit contraction of smooth muscles in the bowel wall.
3. Stimulate the cardiac and respiratory centers in the medulla.
4. Potentiate the depressant effects of narcotics and anesthetics.

44. Atropine was given to Mr. Oakes preoperatively in order to:
a. Decrease the volume of respiratory secretions.
b. Counteract the respiratory depressant effect of the anesthetic.
c. Decrease the rate and amplitude of peristalsis.
d. Produce amnesia for the immediate preoperative period.
  1. a and b.
  2. c and d.
  3. All but d.
  4. All the above.

Mr. Oakes' operation was performed under a general anesthetic. His colon was cut well above the level of the tumor and brought out through the left abdominal wall to form a colostomy. The tumor and the entire rectosigmoid segment of the bowel were then removed from below through a perineal incision. Mr. Oakes was returned to the recovery room with a nasogastric tube and an indwelling catheter in place, a clamp on the colostomy stump, and the rectal wound packed with iodoform gauze. The following orders were written:

1. 1000 cc. 5 per cent dextrose in .45 normal saline with 100 mg. ascorbic acid added.
2. Meperidine hydrochloride 50 mg. H. q. 4 h. p.r.n. for pain.

3. Intermittent positive pressure breathing for 15 minutes q. 4 h.
4. Attach nasogastric tube to intermittent suction and indwelling catheter to drainage apparatus.
5. Tetracycline 100 mg. I.M. q. 6 h.
6. Up in chair on first postoperative day.

45. Colonic tissue was removed both above and below the site of tumor tissue in order to prevent:
1. Direct extension and metastatic spread of the tumor.
2. Postoperative paralysis and distention of the bowel.
3. Accidental loosening of bowel sutures postoperatively.
4. Pressure injury to the perineal suture line.

46. The surgeon clamped off the stump of Mr. Oakes' colostomy in order to:
1. Decrease hemorrhage from vessels cut during surgery.
2. Prevent fecal contamination of the skin incision.
3. Reduce the danger of postoperative bowel distention.
4. Prevent retraction of the stoma into the abdomen.

47. In caring for Mr. Oakes immediately after his return to the recovery room, the nurse should be particularly alert to symptoms of:
a. Hemorrhage.
b. Shock.
c. Pneumonia.
d. Phlebitis.
  1. a only.
  2. a and b.
  3. b and c.
  4. All the above.

48. Which of the following factors might predispose Mr. Oakes to the development of postoperative hypotension?
a. Surgical blood loss.
b. Electrolyte imbalance.
c. Fear and apprehension.
d. Operative tissue trauma.
e. Prolonged anesthesia.
  1. a and c.
  2. b and d.
  3. c and e.
  4. All the above.

49. The side-lying position is preferred during the immediate postoperative period because it facilitates:

1. Evacuation of flatus through the colostomy.
2. Maximum expansion of the lower rib cage.
3. Ingestion of liquid and semiliquid foods.
4. Checking the rectal dressing for drainage.

50. The indwelling catheter was left in place postoperatively in order to:
   1. Avoid bacterial infection of the bladder and urethra.
   2. Facilitate healing of any trauma to the urethra during surgery.
   3. Obtain fresh serial urine specimens for analysis.
   4. Prevent soiling of the perineal dressing with urine.

51. Mr. Oakes' general condition and the nature of his surgery both predispose him to:
   a. Hypostatic pneumonia.
   b. Venous thrombosis.
   c. Wound infection.
   d. Decubitus ulcers.
      1. a only.
      2. a and b.
      3. a, b, and c.
      4. All the above.

52. Tetracycline was given to Mr. Oakes postoperatively in order to prevent:
   a. Pneumonia.
   b. Cystitis.
   c. Wound abscess.
   d. Phlebothrombosis.
      1. a only.
      2. a and b.
      3. a, b, and c.
      4. All the above.

53. Mr. Oakes asked his nurse, "I have cancer, don't I?" Which response would be most therapeutic?
   1. "When did this thought first occur to you?"
   2. "What makes you ask that question at this time?"
   3. "Has someone told you that you have cancer?"
   4. "You did have cancer, which has been cured by surgery."

54. If the nurse is unable to control her anxiety when Mr. Oakes talks to her about his malignancy, which of the following would be the most appropriate immediate response?
   1. Leave the room.
   2. Change the subject.
   3. Deny his diagnosis.
   4. Request assignment change.

On Mr. Oakes' second postoperative day the doctor removed the clamp from the colostomy stump and covered the colostomy stoma with a heavy dressing of fluff gauze.

On the third postoperative day the doctor changed Mr. Oakes' rectal dressing, which was stained with a fairly large amount of serosanguineous drainage. Over a period of five days the doctor gradually withdrew the iodoform gauze packing from the rectal wound. When the packing had been entirely removed, he instructed the nurse to irrigate the rectal wound twice daily with a weak solution of hydrogen peroxide. At the end of one week Mr. Oakes was able to have a daily sitz bath.

On Mr. Oakes' fourth postoperative day the doctor discontinued the intravenous fluid therapy, the nasogastric suction, and the intermittent positive pressure breathing device. He started Mr. Oakes on clear fluids by mouth, and tetracycline 250 mg. "I.V. piggyback" q. 8 h.

55. When the clamp was removed from the colostomy stump, Mr. Oakes should be told that:
   1. He is to ignore the colostomy entirely and let the nurse care for it.
   2. The colostomy will be nonfunctioning until he resumes normal food intake.
   3. Colostomy drainage might be semiliquid until his diet has been regulated.
   4. Defecation will always be preceded by a sensation of intra-abdominal pressure.

56. Hydrogen peroxide irrigations of Mr. Oakes' perineal wound were ordered in order to prevent the development of:
   1. Fibrous adhesions.
   2. Anal stenosis.
   3. Draining sinuses.
   4. Fecal impaction.

57. Which of the following would be most suitable for holding Mr. Oakes' perineal dressing in place?
   1. Rubber air ring.
   2. Adhesive strapping.
   3. T-shaped binder.
   4. Underwear briefs.

58. In order to ensure Mr. Oakes' maximum comfort and safety during the sitz bath, the nurse should provide him with:

    a. A rubber ring.
    b. A loin cloth.
    c. A call bell.
    d. An ice cap.
        1. a only.
        2. a and b.
        3. a, b, and c.
        4. All the above.

On the fourth postoperative day the nurse assisted Mr. Oakes to irrigate the colostomy, encountering no difficulty in either the introduction or return of the irrigating solution. A large amount of gas and a small quantity of liquid stool were expelled with the irrigating solution. Following the procedure a disposable plastic colostomy bag was applied over the stoma.

59. The nurse could best prepare Mr. Oakes for the first irrigation of his colostomy by:

    1. Telling him that the procedure will be short and painless.
    2. Giving him a pamphlet to read which outlines the procedure.
    3. Using diagrams and pictures to explain the steps in the procedure.
    4. Having him talk briefly with a well regulated colostomy patient.

60. Mr. Oakes should be instructed that the purpose for irrigating his colostomy daily is to:

    1. Stimulate return of normal peristaltic action of the surgically traumatized colon.
    2. Eliminate the possibility of fecal impaction and obstruction of the narrowing stoma.
    3. Prevent fecal drainage while he is carrying out normal daily activities.
    4. Discourage inflammation and infection of the mucosal covering of the colostomy bud.

61. What equipment should the nurse use in irrigating Mr. Oakes' colostomy for the first time?

    a. No. 16 catheter.
    b. Small funnel.
    c. Graduated pitcher.
    d. Kidney basin.
    e. Bulb syringe.
        1. a and c.

        2. b and d.
        3. All but e.
        4. All the above.

62. Which of the following would be best suited for irrigation of Mr. Oakes' colostomy?

    1. Normal saline solution.
    2. Mild soap solution.
    3. Warm tap water.
    4. Dilute hydrogen peroxide.

63. In caring for Mr. Oakes the nurse should arrange to irrigate his colostomy:

    1. Before he eats breakfast.
    2. Immediately after his breakfast.
    3. Before his bath.
    4. Just before he retires.

64. During colostomy irrigation the nurse should insert the irrigating catheter into the colon no farther than:

    1. 1 inch.
    2. 5 inches.
    3. 10 inches.
    4. 15 inches.

65. During Mr. Oakes' first colostomy irrigation the nurse should instill how much irrigating solution?

    1. 30 ml.
    2. 120 ml.
    3. 500 ml.
    4. 2000 ml.

66. Following the first irrigation procedure Mr. Oakes said bitterly, "I didn't know that I'd have to have this ugly sack strapped to me for the rest of my life!" Which response by the nurse would be most helpful?

    1. "You will have to wear a colostomy bag from now on, but you will rapidly become accustomed to it."
    2. "In time you will be able to use a much smaller colostomy bag which will not be noticeable to others."
    3. "After your colostomy has been regulated you may be able to dispense with the bag and use a simple gauze pad."
    4. "By the time you leave the hospital you will be able to occlude the stoma with a plastic cup or button."

67. During the early postoperative period, the nurse could help Mr. Oakes accept his colostomy by:

    a. Revealing her own acceptance of his colostomy through gestures and facial expression.
    b. Keeping the colostomy dressings and bed linen clean and dry at all times.

c. Encouraging him to look at the colostomy stoma during irrigations and dressing changes.

d. Inviting him to assist her in irrigating the colostomy and changing the dressings.
   1. a and b.
   2. c and d.
   3. All but d.
   4. All the above.

68. In planning care for Mr. Oakes during the postoperative period, the nurse should consider it her responsibility to instruct him concerning the:

a. Procedure for irrigation of the colostomy.

b. Care of the skin surrounding the stoma.

c. Choice and use of appliances and dressings.

d. Selection and preparation of appropriate foods.

e. Maintenance of health through hygienic measures.
   1. a and b.
   2. a, b, and c.
   3. a, b, c, and e.
   4. All the above.

69. Which of the following statements by the nurse is the most appropriate response to Mr. Oakes' comment, "Now I won't be able to go any place any more."

1. "I suppose your staying home would make you very lonely."

2. "Are you concerned about being able to control your bowel movements?"

3. "I understand what you are trying to tell me, Mr. Oakes."

4. "Initially, soiling will be a problem but you'll soon gain control."

70. Which of the following measures should the nurse employ to facilitate adherence of the disposable colostomy bag to Mr. Oakes' abdomen?

1. Cleanse the skin surrounding the stoma carefully and coat it with Karaya powder.

2. Affix the base of the bag to the skin with radiating strips of non-allergic tape.

3. Gather the plastic to the base of the colostomy stoma with a rubber band.

4. Apply a tight abdominal binder from the lower costal border to the symphysis pubis.

71. The nurse should arrange for Mr. Oakes' colostomy to be irrigated at the same time every day and choose a time:

1. About halfway between the two heaviest meals of the day.

2. That approximates his daily habit time preoperatively.

3. When his surgeon is not likely to make rounds.

4. When his family would be unable to visit.

72. Mr. Oakes should be taught that, in order to regulate the functioning of his colostomy, he should avoid eating:

a. Highly seasoned foods.

b. Fried foods.

c. Raw fruits.

d. Creamed soups.

e. Carbonated beverages.
   1. a and c.
   2. b and d.
   3. All but d.
   4. All the above.

73. In preparing him for hospital discharge the nurse should advise Mr. Oakes to budget how much time for his colostomy irrigation at home?

1. 5 to 10 minutes.

2. 20 to 30 minutes.

3. 45 minutes to 1 hour.

4. 1½ to 2 hours.

The nurse helped Mr. Oakes to order a commercially prepared irrigation set and a supply of disposable colostomy bags from a hospital supply company catalogue. Mr. Oakes selected the most expensive of several sets advertised, saying "I want the best available, so I'll have as little mess and trouble as possible after I get home." Mr. Oakes practiced irrigating his colostomy under the nurse's supervision and guidance.

74. After the colostomy had healed well to the abdominal skin, Mr. Oakes should be taught to:

1. Massage the abdomen surrounding the stoma.

2. Dilate the stoma with his forefinger.

3. Compress the colostomy bud with his palm.

4. Moisten the stomal mucosa with lubricant.

75. Mr. Oakes should be told that following hospital discharge he will be able to eat whatever foods he likes, as long as he avoids foods that:

1. Contain cellulose or fibrous connective tissue.
2. Have had seasoning added during preparation.
3. Formerly caused him flatulence or diarrhea.
4. Have been smoked, barbecued, or deep fried.

By the end of his fifth week in the hospital Mr. Oakes' colostomy was well regulated and both he and his wife had learned to irrigate the colostomy, care for the skin surrounding the bud, dilate the stoma, and apply the colostomy bag securely. His perineal wound was completely healed and nontender. Mrs. Oakes installed a hook on the bathroom wall from which to hang an irrigating bag and placed a small cabinet in the bathroom for storage of irrigating equipment and skin care supplies. Following Mr. Oakes' hospital discharge a visiting nurse made several home visits to check on his welfare and to provide instruction and support during his transition to home life and family routines.

Subdural Hematoma

When he was admitted to the hospital, 44-year-old Harvey Conklin's wife indicated that he had a three week history of generalized headache and difficulty with gait. Six weeks before admission Mr. Conklin had suffered a head injury in an automobile accident but, since x-rays revealed no skull fractures, he was released from the hospital without medical treatment. On the morning of hospital admission he had fallen and struck his head on a chair.

On physical examination Mr. Conklin was drowsy, oriented to place and person but not to time, and was complaining of severe headache. He was able to obey simple commands and responded to painful stimuli. His temperature was 99.6° F., pulse was 78 per minute, respirations were 18 per minute, and blood pressure was 140/100 mm. Hg. His right pupil was larger than the left and reacted sluggishly to light. There was slight congestion of the optic nerve heads. The left arm revealed mild weakness on extension and exaggerated deep tendon reflexes. The left leg revealed slight muscle rigidity and extensor spasms on pain stimulation. Rapid alternating movements were decreased in the left arm and leg. A positive left Babinski reflex was found. A radioactive brain scan showed increased uptake of radioactive substance on the right side. A carotid angiogram revealed the pial vessels to be widely separated from the inner table of the skull and also showed a displacement of terminal branches of the middle cerebral artery on the right.

A diagnosis was made of right chronic subdural hematoma. Mr. Conklin was taken to surgery where, under xylocaine anesthesia, right and left burr holes were made, the dura was incised, and a brown, liquefied clot under pressure was evacuated from the right side. A#8 French catheter was left in the right burr hole for 12 hours following surgery.

(ANSWER BLANK ON PAGE A-89)   (CORRECT ANSWERS ON PAGE B-148)

1. Bleeding into the subdural space usually occurs from which type of vessel?
1. Artery.
2. Arteriole.
3. Venule.
4. Capillary.

2. Mr. Conklin's headaches and locomotor difficulties were probably the result of:
1. Chemical irritation of cortical tissue by extravasated blood.
2. Ischemic necrosis of cortical tissue following hemorrhage.
3. Compression of brain tissue by a mass of clotted blood.
4. Bacterial infection of meninges following laceration.

3. In interviewing Mr. Conklin's wife concerning the history of his present illness, the nurse might learn that, in addition to headache and incoordination, he had, since his accident, displayed other symptoms of subdural hematoma, such as:
a. Slight impairment of intellectual ability.
b. Fluctuating levels of consciousness.
c. Unilateral skeletal muscle weakness.
d. Muscular twitching or convulsions.
1. a and b.
2. b and c.
3. All but d.
4. All the above.

4. It is desirable that Mr. Conklin's level of consciousness be checked immediately upon hospital admission in order to:
1. Determine whether his neurological condition is such that he can withstand a surgical procedure.
2. Provide a base line with which to compare his later levels of consciousness.
3. Familiarize him early with a procedure to which he will be subjected again and again.
4. Enable physician and nurse to simultaneously observe his responses to routine tests.

5. If Mr. Conklin's subdural bleeding were to continue and his intracranial pressure were to rise gradually, the nurse should observe the loss of the following abilities in which order?
a. Response to simple verbal commands.
b. Orientation to person.
c. Orientation to time.
d. Cough and gag reflex.
e. Response to painful stimuli.
1. a, b, c, d, e.
2. b, e, a, c, d.
3. c, b, a, e, d.
4. d, a, b, c, e.

6. Which of the following statements by the nurse would be best suited to determine Mr. Conklin's response to command?
1. "Pour a glassful of water from this pitcher."
2. "Tell me who you are and how you came here."
3. "Touch your left ear with your right hand."
4. "Extend your arms, close your eyes, and touch your nose."

7. Which of the following should be considered a purposeful response to pricking Mr. Conklin's right foot with a pin?
1. Dorsiflexion of the right foot and flexion of the right knee.
2. Tonic contraction of both arms and both legs simultaneously.
3. Frowning, grimacing, and shaking the head back and forth.
4. Rapidly alternating flexion and extension of all four limbs.

8. The nurse should note and report which of the following concerning the condition of Mr. Conklin's pupils?
a. Size.
b. Equality or inequality.
c. Response to light.
d. Speed of light response.
e. Direction of focus.
1. a and c.
2. a, b, and c.
3. All but d.
4. All the above.

9. Changes in pupillary size are regulated by which cranial nerve?
1. Second.
2. Third.
3. Fourth.
4. Fifth.

10. In the normal subject, when a bright light is directed toward the right eye, there follows:
1. Pupillary constriction of the right eye and pupillary dilation of the left.
2. Pupillary dilation of the right eye and pupillary constriction of the left.
3. Constriction of the pupil of first the right, then the left eye.
4. Dilation of the pupils of both the right and the left eye.

11. Mr. Conklin's right pupil should be checked frequently for its response to light because a fixed dilated pupil in a patient with increased intracranial pressure is a reliable indicator of:
1. Compression of the cortex.
2. Slow subdural hemorrhage.
3. Distortion of the midbrain.
4. Ischemia of the medulla.

12. The congested appearance of Mr. Conklin's optic nerve head would seem to indicate that he is suffering from:
1. Vitamin B complex deficiency.
2. Increased intracranial pressure.
3. Congestive heart failure.
4. Fluid and electrolyte imbalance.

13. Mrs. Conklin's weakness of the left arm and spasms and rigidity of the left leg are probably the result of either:
1. Intracerebral or intraventricular hemorrhage.
2. Chemical or mechanical irritation of motor cortex.
3. Cerebellar or medullary ischemia.
4. Cortical compression or brain stem distortion.

14. In spite of the fact that his subdural hematoma was over the right cerebral hemisphere, Mr. Conklin developed left sided muscle weakness because:
1. Fibers from each motor cortex cross to the opposite side in the medulla oblongata.
2. Motor fibers from anterior horn cells cross to the opposite side before leaving the cord.
3. The clot caused the right hemisphere to expand beyond the midline, compressing the opposite hemisphere.
4. Hemorrhage into one part of the brain is followed by reflex vasospasm in the opposite hemisphere.

15. When he is being tested for deep tendon reflexes, Mr. Conklin should be directed to:
1. Relax his limbs and direct his attention toward something else.
2. Steel himself against the discomfort to be generated by the test.
3. Concentrate on moving the limb as far as possible on stimulation.
4. Resist the impulse to move the limb when the tendon is struck.

16. Mr. Conklin's decreased ability to perform rapidly alternating movements (as pronation and supination) with his left arm probably indicates:
1. Increased destruction of acetylcholine at motor nerve endings.
2. Discoordinated innervation of opposing muscle groups.
3. Interruption of the reflex arc in the cervical cord.
4. Impairment of nerve transmission due to hypokalemia.

17. A positive Babinski reflex consists of:
1. Extension of the great toe when the sole of the foot is stroked.
2. Inability to maintain balance when in a standing position with eyes closed.
3. Pain on extension of the leg with the thigh flexed on the abdomen.
4. Extension of the leg on forcefully striking the patellar tendon.

18. In order to interpret the physician's notes, the nurse should know that a positive Babinski reflex indicates a lesion in the:
1. Optic chiasm.
2. Pyramidal tract.
3. Cerebral ventricles.
4. Medullary centers.

19. During a brain scan procedure more than normal amounts of radioactive material are absorbed by injured tissue as a result of:
1. Increased metabolic rate of injured tissue cells.
2. Accelerated movement of phagocytes into the tissues.
3. Breakdown of the normal blood-brain barrier.
4. Cellular starvation due to impaired blood supply.

20. Cerebral angiography should be described to Mr. Conklin as a procedure consisting of:
1. Aspiration of fluid from the subarachnoid space in order to create room for clot expansion.
2. Withdrawal of blood from the cerebral arteries in order to rapidly reduce intracranial pressure.
3. Injection of radiopaque dye into the carotid artery in order to visualize cranial vessels by x-ray.
4. Introduction of hypertonic solution into the cranial circulation in order to facilitate clot absorption.

21. During the period of observation which preceded Mr. Conklin's surgery, the single most reliable index of his neurological condition would be:

1. Eye movements.
2. Vital signs.
3. Cranial x-ray.
4. State of consciousness.

22. Mr. Conklin's temperature should be taken rectally because:

1. His susceptibility to convulsions renders oral temperature taking dangerous.
2. He is sufficiently confused that he might drop and break an oral thermometer.
3. Circulatory embarrassment following intracranial bleeding renders oral temperatures inaccurate.
4. His respiratory embarrassment would make it impossible to keep his mouth closed.

23. Which of the following findings would be most suggestive of increasing intracranial pressure?

1. Continuous rise in temperature, pulse, respirations, and blood pressure.
2. Steady decline in temperature, pulse, respirations, and blood pressure.
3. Slowing of pulse and respirations with increase in temperature and blood pressure.
4. Increase in pulse and respirations with decrease in temperature and blood pressure.

24. The blood pressure changes which are typically associated with increased intracranial pressure result from:

1. Direct application of pressure to the walls of all brain blood vessels.
2. Reflex response to increasing anoxia of cells of the vasomotor center.
3. Shunting of large volumes of cerebrospinal fluid to the circulating blood.
4. Absorption of edema fluid from brain tissue by meningeal capillaries.

25. Continuing increase in Mr. Conklin's intracranial pressure would eventually produce circulatory failure by:

1. Herniation of the medulla through the foramen magnum, followed by paralysis of vital centers.
2. Traumatic rupture of the Circle of Willis followed by sudden reduction in circulating blood volume.
3. Reducing cardiac outflow by obstructing venous return from the cranium to the heart.

4. Elevating carotid artery pressure to the point that profound reflex bradycardia occurs.

26. During the preoperative observation period Mr. Conklin should be especially protected against respiratory difficulty consequent to:

1. Shallow respirations.
2. Inadequate hydration.
3. Aspiration of vomitus.
4. Physical immobility.

27. If Mr. Conklin should have a convulsion, the nurse should observe and report the:

a. Origin and progression of the seizure.
b. Duration of convulsive movements.
c. Presence of tonic or clonic contractions.
d. Level of consciousness before, during, and after the convulsion.
e. Occurrence of urinary or fecal incontinence.
 1. a and b.
 2. a, b, and c.
 3. All but d.
 4. All the above.

28. In the event that Mr. Conklin convulses, the nurse should protect him by:

a. Remaining with him throughout the seizure.
b. Placing a small pillow under his head.
c. Placing a padded tongue blade between his teeth.
d. Loosening tight clothing about his neck and chest.
e. Applying cloth restraints to all his extremities.
 1. a and b.
 2. a, b, and c.
 3. All but e.
 4. All the above.

29. Despite the fact that Mr. Conklin complained of severe headache, his physician did not order that he be given a narcotic because:

1. It is impossible to check levels of consciousness following medication administration.
2. Such drugs tend to cause some degree of respiratory center depression.
3. He will have to be fully awake and alert during the neurosurgical procedure.
4. His pain will be sufficiently prolonged to predispose him to addiction.

30. Lumbar puncture and spinal fluid examination were not used in diagnosing Mr. Conklin's problem because:
1. Abnormal spinal fluid findings are rarely found in conjunction with subdural hematoma.
2. Sudden removal of spinal fluid might cause brain herniation through the foramen magnum.
3. Withdrawal of spinal fluid would interfere with x-ray visualization of cerebral vessels.
4. The side-lying position required for spinal puncture would increase the severity of his headache.

31. Preparation of Mr. Conklin's operative site should include:
1. Combing his hair toward the crown of his head.
2. Shaving the face and shampooing the hair.
3. Shaving the head and shampooing the scalp.
4. Cutting the hair and painting the scalp with alcohol.

32. The nurse should provide which of the following in the unit to which Mr. Conklin will be returned following surgery?
a. Bed with side rails.
b. Suction machine.
c. Tracheotomy set.
d. Canvas restraints.
e. Hypothermia machine.
    1. a and b.
    2. a, b, and c.
    3. All but d.
    4. All the above.

33. When Mr. Conklin is returned to the recovery room following surgery he should be placed in which position?
1. Trendelenburg.
2. Low Fowler's.
3. Left side-lying.
4. Supine.

34. On his arrival in the recovery room from the operating room, the nurse should check Mr. Conklin's level of consciousness every:
1. 10 minutes.
2. 30 minutes.
3. Hour.
4. 2 hours.

35. During his early postoperative period Mr. Conklin should have his position changed frequently in order to:
1. Foster drainage of blood from the cranium.
2. Prevent pooling of respiratory secretions.
3. Facilitate recovery of motor function.
4. Stimulate return to higher levels of consciousness.

36. While Mr. Conklin is stuporous and unable to take food by mouth, the nurse should provide for his oral hygiene by:
1. Giving him 50 cc. of fresh water to drink every half hour.
2. Lubricating his mouth and lips with glycerine and lemon juice.
3. Irrigating his mouth with salt and soda solution daily.
4. Brushing his teeth with 50 per cent hydrogen peroxide solution.

37. The surgeon should be notified of any decline in Mr. Conklin's level of consciousness, as that observation would indicate:
1. Failure to remove the entire clot during surgery.
2. Increase in the degree of his cerebral dysfunction.
3. Permanent damage to vital centers in the medulla.
4. Ischemic necrosis of cerebral cortical tissues.

38. Mr. Conklin's corneal reflex should be tested by:
1. Applying pressure against the supraorbital ridge.
2. Stroking the cornea lightly with a cotton wisp.
3. Brushing the eyelashes with a cotton-tipped applicator.
4. Shining a flashlight into the eye from the side.

39. If Mr. Conklin's corneal reflex were found to be absent, the nurse should:
1. Drop sterile mineral oil into the eye, close the lid, and cover the eye with a shield.
2. Instill antibiotic ointment into the eye, close the window shades, and provide indirect lighting.
3. Keep his head flat and manually rise and lower his eyelid several times each hour.
4. Cleanse his lid margins with boric acid solution and apply warm compresses to the eye.

40. The nurse should protect Mr. Conklin from postoperative respiratory complications by:
a. Turning his head to the side.

b. Frequent suctioning of his naso-pharynx.

c. Maintaining his jaw in forward position.

d. Encouraging him to sigh and cough every 15 minutes.

e. Changing his position every 15 minutes.
    1. a and c.
    2. b and d.
    3. All but e.
    4. All the above.

41. Postoperative respiratory distress would be especially threatening to Mr. Conklin because:

1. Pressure on the motor cortex would have impaired the efficiency of his respiratory muscles.

2. Coughing would tend to produce additional cranial trauma and reinstitute subdural hemorrhage.

3. Postoperative cerebral edema renders him dangerously hypersensitive to parenteral antibiotics.

4. Elevation of serum carbon dioxide dilates cranial vessels, thereby increasing intracranial pressure.

42. If, in spite of expert nursing care, Mr. Conklin should develop postoperative respiratory disturbances, he would be apt to display:

a. Tachypnea.

b. Persistent cough.

c. Chest rales.

d. Peripheral cyanosis.

e. Substernal retractions.
    1. a and b.
    2. c and d.
    3. All but e.
    4. All the above.

43. Mr. Conklin's temperature should be carefully monitored postoperatively because fever would:

1. Increase his nervous and muscular hyperirritability.

2. Decrease the coagulability of his blood.

3. Increase the oxygen need of his damaged brain.

4. Decrease the speed of cerebral blood flow.

44. Which of the following devices should be used in caring for Mr. Conklin during his postoperative period?

a. Arm sling.

b. Overhead trapeze.

c. Hand roll.

d. Footboard.

e. Bed blocks.
    1. a and b.
    2. c and d.
    3. All but d.
    4. All the above.

Carcinoma of the Tongue and Radical Neck Dissection

Claude Dyer, a 55-year-old black man, was admitted to the Mouth and Throat Surgery unit of a large hospital for treatment of carcinoma of the tongue and the floor of the mouth. As a result of anorexia and a swollen painful tongue, he had sustained a 40 pound weight loss and increasing weakness during the previous 12 months. Two months before hospital admission he developed excessive salivation and his lower teeth began to fall out. At this time, when he was able to consume only soft or liquid foods and was unable to speak clearly, he sought medical attention for his problem. ·

On hospital admission Mr. Dyer was weak, emaciated, and cachectic. His vital signs were normal, his red blood cell count was 4,500,000/mm³, hemo-

globin 12 Grams per cent, hematocrit 38 per cent, and white blood cell count 11,000/mm³. His total serum protein was 5.7 Grams per cent and his serum albumin 3 Grams per cent. Thoracic x-rays were normal. Physical examination revealed a large area of swelling and ulceration on the right floor of the mouth and right side of the tongue, enlarged right cervical lymph nodes, and an offensive odor to the breath. Biopsy of the tongue lesion revealed it to be a squamous cell carcinoma.

Following a preoperative regimen which included nasogastric tube feedings of high caloric, high protein, high vitamin liquids; irradiation of neck tissues; blood transfusions; tetracycline; trimethobenzamide (Tigan); and insertion of a tracheostomy tube, Mr. Dyer was taken to surgery for a glossectomy, right mandibulectomy, and radical neck dissection.

(ANSWER BLANK ON PAGE A–91) (CORRECT ANSWERS ON PAGE B–152)

1. In evaluating Mr. Dyer's medical history the nurse should be aware that which of the following are thought to predispose to carcinoma of the mouth?
   a. Long term use of tobacco.
   b. Chronic ingestion of alcohol.
   c. Poor dental hygiene.
   d. Poor oral hygiene.
   e. Excessive use of the voice.
      1. a and c.
      2. b and d.
      3. All but e.
      4. All the above.

2. The admitting physician learned that, several months prior to this illness, Mr. Dyer had been treated by his dentist for leukoplakia, which consists of:
   1. Deposition of tartar on the bases of the teeth just above the gum line.
   2. Collections of purulent exudate in pockets between the tooth roots and gum margins.
   3. Chalky white, thickened patches on the tongue or buccal mucosa which are removed with difficulty.
   4. Large fluid-filled vesicles covering the tongue and lips which rupture to create ulcers and fissures.

3. The long range goal for Mr. Dyer's preoperative preparation is to help him to:
   1. Face his operation without fear of diability or disfigurement.
   2. Cooperate maximally with post-operative care given by the health team.
   3. Accept the inevitable consequences of his illness and treatment.
   4. Become capable of total self-care by the time of hospital discharge.

4. Mr. Dyer's preoperative preparation should include efforts to reduce his fear of:
   a. Dependence upon others.
   b. Asphyxiation following surgery.
   c. Inability to communicate.
   d. Facial disfigurement.
   e. Rejection by others.
      1. a and c.
      2. b and d.
      3. All but d.
      4. All the above.

5. Which of the following communications by the nurse would be best suited for initiating Mr. Dyer's preoperative health teaching?
   1. "Would you like me to explain the doctor's plan for your treatment?"
   2. "Do you have any questions about your forthcoming operation?"
   3. "What reason did your doctor give you for admitting you to the hospital?"
   4. "I'm going to explain the care you will receive after surgery."

6. Mr. Dyer should be placed in which position for preoperative insertion of the nasogastric tube?
   1. Supine, with head turned toward the right.
   2. In high Fowler's position with head hyperextended.
   3. In low Fowler's position with head flexed on the chest.
   4. Lying on the left side with head slightly elevated.

7. Preoperatively, Mr. Dyer's diet should provide a daily protein intake of:
   1. 25 Grams.
   2. 50 Grams.

3. 75 Grams.

4. 100 Grams.

8. Mr. Dyer's preoperative diet should contain especially high quantities of:

1. Vitamin A.

2. Vitamin B_1.

3. Vitamin C.

4. Vitamin D.

9. Which of the following food mixtures would best meet Mr. Dyer's nutritive needs preoperatively?

1. Bouillon, strained gruel, and cranberry juice.

2. Liquid gelatin, vegetable juice, and cream.

3. Orange juice, non-fat dry milk, and eggs.

4. Tea, tomato juice, and beef broth.

10. Before administering his nasogastric tube feedings the nurse should place Mr. Dyer in which position?

1. Supine.

2. Lying on his left side.

3. Lying on his right side.

4. Semi-Fowler's.

11. Before attaching Mr. Dyer's newly inserted nasogastric tube to the gavage container holding the blenderized mixture, the end of the nasogastric tube should be inserted into a glass of water in order to:

1. Lubricate the tube in preparation for attachment to the gavage bag.

2. Ascertain whether the tube is properly positioned in the stomach.

3. Remove air from the tube before filling it with food mixture.

4. Establish a negative pressure in the tube to facilitate fluid flow.

12. In the event that Mr. Dyer should develop coughing, choking, or cyanosis during his tube feeding, the nurse should:

1. Decrease the speed of flow through the tubing.

2. Discontinue the feeding and notify the physician.

3. Withdraw the tube slightly and resume the feeding.

4. Advance the tube slowly and continue fluid flow.

13. The purpose for the preoperative irradiation therapy given Mr. Dyer was to:

1. Reverse malignant changes in tissues already infiltrated by tumor.

2. Obliterate small blood vessels in the area to be operated upon.

3. Block normal inflammatory response in structures invaded by tumor.

4. Inhibit tumor metastasis until surgery could be performed.

14. Radiation alters body tissue by:

1. Absorbing water from intra- and extracellular spaces.

2. Removing electrons from molecules of tissue protein.

3. Stimulating production of antibodies and blood cells.

4. Increasing the speed of cell maturation and division.

15. The nurse should observe Mr. Dyer for which of the following as possible symptoms of radiation sickness?

a. Itching.

b. Anorexia.

c. Nausea.

d. Tinnitus.

e. Diarrhea.

1. a and c.

2. b and d.

3. All but d.

4. All the above.

16. During the time that Mr. Dyer is receiving preoperative radiation therapy, care should be taken to protect the skin of his neck from:

a. Medicated solutions and powders.

b. Extremes of hot and cold.

c. Irritating or constrictive clothing.

d. Adhesive tape or collodion.

e. Exposure to direct sunlight.

1. a and b.

2. c and d.

3. All but e.

4. All the above.

17. The purpose for giving tetracycline preoperatively to Mr. Dyer was to:

1. Eradicate infection in the tissues to be operated upon.

2. Prevent development of postoperative bronchitis and pneumonia.

3. Destroy intestinal organisms which break down protein to ammonia.

4. Decrease the danger of thromboembolic phenomena postoperatively.

18. Which of the following is a common untoward effect of tetracycline?

1. Deafness.

2. Diplopia.

3. Diarrhea.

4. Dizziness.

19. Trimethobenzamide (Tigan) was given Mr. Dyer preoperatively for the purpose of preventing:
    1. Metastasis from the primary tumor.
    2. Nausea due to radiation sickness.
    3. Hemorrhage from the tongue lesion.
    4. Sialorrhea due to parotic stimulation.

20. In obtaining Mr. Dyer's consent for the proposed radical neck dissection, the nurse should ensure that:
    a. He understands the purpose for and the nature of the operative procedure.
    b. He appreciates the risk entailed by the procedure and the disabilities resulting from it.
    c. His consent is recorded in writing and is witnessed by a hospital employee or relative.
    d. He is not under the influence of ataraxic, sedative, or hypnotic drugs at the time of consent.
    e. The date and time of his signed consent are recorded on the operative permit.
       1. a and b.
       2. a, b, and c.
       3. All but e.
       4. All the above.

21. If Mr. Dyer's consent for the operation were fraudulently obtained, he would later have grounds for suit against the surgeon and the nurse on the charge of:
    1. Malpractice.
    2. Breach of contract.
    3. Illegal restraint.
    4. Assault and battery.

22. Mr. Dyer was tracheotomized prior to surgery in order to:
    a. Permit better visualization of the operative field.
    b. Facilitate use of resuscitative and ventilatory equipment.
    c. Prevent obstruction of airways by postoperative edema.
    d. Facilitate removal of aspirated secretions postoperatively.
    e. Inhibit production of excessive bronchopulmonary secretions.
       1. a and b.
       2. c and d.
       3. All but e.
       4. All the above.

23. Another reason for tracheotomizing Mr. Dyer preoperatively was the fact that he was apt to suffer which of the following injuries as a consequence of the surgical procedure?
    1. Paralysis of the respiratory muscles.
    2. Perforation of the apex of the lung.
    3. Fracture of the laryngeal cartilage.
    4. Severing of the superior laryngeal nerve.

24. In addition to the aforementioned effects, Mr. Dyer's tracheotomy will reduce his postoperative respiratory work load by:
    1. Decreasing the volume of his anatomical dead air space.
    2. Increasing the diameter of his upper air passages.
    3. Preventing turbulence of air flow during inspiration.
    4. Equalizing inspiratory and expiratory pressures in the alveoli.

25. Before the tracheotomy is performed Mr. Dyer should be told that immediately following the procedure:
    a. He will breathe through a hole in his trachea.
    b. He will temporarily be unable to use his voice.
    c. The air which he breathes will have to be humidified.
    d. He will communicate with the staff in writing.
    e. Secretions will frequently be aspirated from the tracheostomy.
       1. a only.
       2. a and b.
       3. All but e.
       4. All the above.

26. After the tracheostomy wound has healed, Mr. Dyer should be taught to:
    1. Swallow air and eructate in preparation for later esophageal speech.
    2. Place his finger over the tracheostomy when he wishes to speak.
    3. Remove the inner cannula of the tube to increase his speech volume.
    4. Communicate with others through means of hand and finger signals.

27. Mr. Dyer's surgeon decided to perform a radical neck dissection as well as remove the tumor tissue from the oral cavity because:
    1. Gravity drainage of secretions facilitates direct extension of oral tumors to neck structures.
    2. Enlargement of cervical nodes indicates metastatic spread of tumor to regional lymph nodes.

3. Speech difficulty indicates that tumor tissue has invaded the larynx and trachea.

4. Duration of symptoms indicates that palliation is of greater importance than tumor removal.

28. Radical neck dissection consists of the removal of which of the following types of tissue?

   a. Subcutaneous fat.

   b. Lymph nodes.

   c. Muscle.

   d. Jugular vein.

   e. Trachea.

     1. a and b.

     2. a, b, and c.

     3. All but e.

     4. All the above.

Mr. Dyer returned from the operating room to the recovery room with Hemovac suction tubes implanted in the neck wound and with a nasogastric tube and a tracheostomy tube in place. Twenty-four hours later he was returned to his unit where his postoperative care included the following:

1. Suctioning of the tracheostomy tube p.r.n.

2. 1st postoperative day: 1000 cc. 5 per cent dextrose in water q. 8 h. I.V.

3. 4th postoperative day: 200 cc. 5 per cent dextrose in water q. 4 h. by nasogastric tube and 1000 cc. 5 per cent dextrose in water q. 12 h. I.V.

4. 5th postoperative day: 3000 cc. high protein blenderized diet by nasogastric tube (20 calories per fluid ounce); 12 ounces q. 4 h. by nasogastric tube.

5. 6th postoperative day: Hemovac suction tubes removed from neck wound.

6. 14th postoperative day: Tracheostomy tube removed and tracheal opening covered with a sterile dressing.

7. 16th postoperative day: Nasogastric tube removed and a full liquid diet begun.

29. During Mr. Dyer's early postoperative period, which of the following would be an expected consequence of his surgery?

   1. Edema of the face.

   2. Cyanosis of his lips and nails.

   3. Absence of his radial pulse.

   4. Vomiting of bright red blood.

30. Which of the following should be kept at Mr. Dyer's bedside for possible emergency use during his early postoperative period?

   1. Tourniquet.

   2. Hemostat.

   3. Wire clippers.

4. Padded tongue depressor.

31. The nurse could best help Mr. Dyer to cough postoperatively by:

   1. Applying a tight binder to his abdomen.

   2. Supporting his neck with her hands.

   3. Elevating his arms over his head.

   4. Loosening the dressings over his neck wound.

32. During his immediate postoperative period Mr. Dyer will be susceptible to respiratory problems as a result of:

   a. Difficulty in swallowing pharyngeal secretions.

   b. Excessive secretion of tracheobronchial secretions.

   c. Constriction of the trachea by edema of neck tissues.

   d. Constriction of the neck by tight pressure dressings.

   e. Limitation of respiratory movement due to anxiety.

     1. a and b.

     2. a, b, and c.

     3. All but d.

     4. All the above.

33. Perforated catheters were implanted in Mr. Dyer's neck wound and attached to a portable suction device in order to prevent:

   1. Respiratory tract infection.

   2. Postsurgical shock.

   3. Delayed wound healing.

   4. Gastrointestinal obstruction.

34. For the first few days following surgery Mr. Dyer's comfort could be most increased by:

   1. Placing a gauze wick in the corner of his mouth to absorb saliva.

   2. Placing him in a side-lying position to facilitate expectoration.

   3. Encouraging him to suck ice chips to control thirst and decrease pain.

   4. Suctioning his pharyngeal cavity with a hard plastic catheter.

35. Mr. Dyer's surgeon may order that his mouth be irrigated regularly with salt and soda solution in order to:

   a. Prevent infection.

   b. Reduce odor.

   c. Promote healing.

   d. Increase appetite.

   e. Improve morale.

     1. a and c.

     2. b and d.

     3. All but d.

     4. All the above.

36. The nurse should take which of the following precautions in providing tracheostomy care for Mr. Dyer?
- a. Wear a fresh pair of sterile gloves for each suctioning procedure.
- b. Use a fresh sterile catheter each time the tube is suctioned.
- c. Flush the suction tubing with disinfectant after each use.
- d. Autoclave the inner cannula each time that it is removed.
- e. Paint the tracheostomy skin edges with disinfectant after each suctioning.
  1. a and b.
  2. c and d.
  3. All but d.
  4. All the above.

37. Before suctioning Mr. Dyer's tracheostomy tube the nurse should:
1. Instill 3 cc. of normal saline or Ringer's lactate into the tube.
2. Cleanse the tracheostomy tube opening of secretions with a dry cotton ball.
3. Untie the twill tapes which attach the outer cannula to the neck.
4. Administer I.P.P.B. treatment to increase pulmonary ventilation.

38. In aspirating secretions from Mr. Dyer's tracheostomy tube the nurse should occlude the open end of the Y-connecting tube:
1. Before turning on the electric suctioning machine.
2. Before inserting the catheter into the trachea.
3. After the catheter has been inserted into the trachea.
4. After the tube has been withdrawn from the trachea.

39. Separate catheters should be used for Mr. Dyer's oral and tracheal suctioning in order that:
1. The exact volume of both oral and tracheal secretions can be determined.
2. Neither site will be contaminated by pathogenic microorganisms inhabiting the other.
3. The tracheal catheter will not be obstructed by clotted blood and serum.
4. A multiperforate catheter be used for the mouth and a uniperforate catheter for the trachea.

40. Which of the following means would be most effective in cleansing adherent mucus from the inner cannula of the tracheostomy tube?
1. Immersing the cannula in 1:10,000 bichloride of mercury solution and rinsing it with cold water.
2. Boiling it for ten minutes and wiping it dry with a lint-free cloth.
3. Soaking it in 50 per cent hydrogen peroxide solution and cleansing it with pipe cleaners.
4. Rinsing it with normal saline and cleansing it with a test tube brush.

41. Before Mr. Dyer's tracheostomy tube is removed the physician will probably order that:
1. The tube be replaced by a series of tubes of decreasing size.
2. The cuff be released and the tube plugged for short periods of time.
3. He be given 100 per cent oxygen for several minutes through the tube.
4. The air in his room be humidified to the point of 80 per cent saturation.

42. Mr. Dyer's postoperative nasogastric tube feedings should be administered in small quantities several times a day rather than in large quantities two or three times a day in order to prevent:
1. Wide fluctuations of serum glucose levels.
2. Development of severe hunger pangs.
3. Sudden reduction in circulating blood volume.
4. Overdistention of the stomach and gut.

43. After completion of each of Mr. Dyer's nasogastric tube feedings, the nurse should:
1. Remove the tube and discard it.
2. Inject 10 cc. of air into the tube.
3. Flush the tube with clear water.
4. Immerse the end of the tube in water.

44. The nurse should begin to teach Mr. Dyer to administer fluid through his nasogastric tube:
1. On the first occasion that he is given a tube feeding.
2. When he has recovered sufficiently to sit up in a chair.
3. After his tracheostomy tube has been removed.
4. When his neck wound has completely healed.

45. Immediately following removal of Mr. Dyer's nasogastric tube he would probably have least difficulty in swallowing:
1. Hot tea.
2. Cold fruit juice.
3. Cereal gruel.
4. Plain tap water.

46. As Mr. Dyer resumes aspects of self-care following his operation he should be advised to:
1. Refrain from applying after-shave lotion over the surgical scar.
2. Seek solitude when cleansing his tracheostomy or taking tube feedings.
3. Utilize an electric razor to avoid injury to superficial neck vessels.
4. Avoid use of medicated mouthwashes, oral sprays, or gargles.

47. Mr. Dyer's physical rehabilitation should include measures to offset disabilities resulting from surgical removal of which muscle?

1. Masseter.
2. Sternocleidomastoid.
3. Trapezius.
4. Sternohyoid.

48. Which of the following exercises would be effective in protecting Mr. Dyer against postoperative deformities?
a. "Climbing" the wall with the fingers until the arms are fully extended.
b. Pulling a rope back and forth over a shower rod or curtain rod.
c. Swinging the arms pendulum-fashion while bent forward at the waist.
d. Grasping a broomstick in both hands and raising it over the head.
e. Tying a rope to a doorknob and swinging it in wide looping turns.
1. a only.
2. a and b.
3. All but e.
4. All the above.

Cataract Removal

Seventy-eight-year-old Zella Merkel was admitted to the hospital for removal of a cataract from the right eye.

Physical examination and routine diagnostic tests revealed that Zella was in good health except for a mild hypochromic anemia, for which she had been receiving iron dextran (Imferon) intramuscularly twice a week.

On the evening before surgery Mrs. Merkel was given a light diet at supper-time, chloral hydrate 500 mg. orally at bedtime, and no fluids after midnight. On the morning of surgery one drop each of atropine sulfate 1 per cent solution, neosynephrine 10 per cent solution, and cyclogyl 1 per cent solution were instilled into her right eye three times at five minute intervals. Fifty mg. of meperidine hydrochloride and 25 mg. of promethazine hydrochloride were given hypodermically. In the operating room Mrs. Merkel's right eye was massaged for three minutes, after which a peripheral iridectomy and intracapsular lens extraction were performed under 2 per cent xylocaine local anesthesia.

Mrs. Merkel was returned to her unit awake and in good condition, with a gauze dressing and a metal shield covering her right eye. Her postoperative care included:

1. Mineral oil, 1 ounce q. h.s.
2. Darvon compound 65 mg. p.r.n. for pain.
3. Gradual progression from liquid, to soft, to general diet.
4. Homatropine 5 per cent solution, one drop in right eye t.i.d.

5. *Dressing changes on the 3rd and 5th postoperative days, and dressing removal on the 7th postoperative day.*
6. *Temporary glasses after dressing removal.*
7. *Discharge from the hospital on the 10th postoperative day.*

(ANSWER BLANK ON PAGE A–93)   (CORRECT ANSWERS ON PAGE B–155)

1. A cataract can best be defined as:
   1. Ulceration of the cornea secondary to inflammation.
   2. Low-grade bacterial infection of the iris and ciliary body.
   3. Clouding or opacity of the crystalline lens.
   4. Severely increased pressure within the eye.

2. Mrs. Merkel's cataract is probably due to:
   1. Low-grade infection.
   2. Endocrine imbalance.
   3. Mechanical trauma.
   4. Degenerative change.

3. Which of the following food substances are thought to be necessary in maintaining the lens in good condition?
   a. Vitamin A.
   b. Glutathione.
   c. Vitamin B₂.
   d. Cystine.
   e. Vitamin C.
      1. a and b.
      2. a and c.
      3. a, c, and e.
      4. All the above.

4. In taking her medical history the nurse will probably learn that Mrs. Merkel has experienced:
   1. Gradual blurring of vision.
   2. Severe unilateral headaches.
   3. Itching and tearing of the eyes.
   4. Floating spots before the eyes.

5. It is typical for the patient with cataracts to indicate that bright lights produce:
   1. Enhanced visual acuity.
   2. A glaring sensation.
   3. Improved color perception.
   4. Sharp intraocular pain.

6. In evaluating Mrs. Merkel's medical history the nurse should be aware that which of the following illnesses are known to predispose to cataract development:
   a. Pernicious anemia.
   b. Diabetes mellitus.
   c. Essential hypertension.
   d. Hypothyroidism.
   e. Kidney stones.
      1. a and c.
      2. b and d.
      3. a, b, and c.
      4. All the above.

7. While admitting Mrs. Merkel to the surgical unit the nurse should take particular pains to:
   1. Show her the operating room in which her surgery will be performed.
   2. Teach her coughing, turning, and breathing routines to be used postoperatively.
   3. Introduce her to the unit personnel who will care for her postoperatively.
   4. Draw a diagram to illustrate the surgical procedure for cataract removal.

8. Mrs. Merkel's anemia is most apt to be caused by:
   1. Replacement of hematopoietic tissue in her bone marrow.
   2. Continuous loss of iron through chronic bleeding.
   3. Impaired absorption of iron from her intestines.
   4. Failure of gastric glands to produce intrinsic factor.

9. Which of the following is a common toxic effect of iron medication?
   1. Skin eruptions.
   2. Double vision.
   3. Slow pulse.
   4. High temperature.

10. Orienting Mrs. Merkel thoroughly to the physical arrangement of her room and of the nursing unit will help to protect her from postoperative:
   1. Depression.
   2. Hostility.
   3. Boredom.

4. Disorientation.

11. Preoperatively, the nurse should teach Mrs. Merkel that on the afternoon of the operative day she will be:
   a. Directed to lie quietly and hold her head still.
   b. Permitted to drink small sips of water.
   c. Fed a full liquid diet at supper time.
   d. Expected to move arms and legs through range of motion.
   e. Instructed not to cough, sneeze, or blow her nose.
      1. a and b.
      2. a, b, and c.
      3. All but d.
      4. All the above.

12. When the nurse took the operative permit to Mrs. Merkel to sign, she covered her eyes and began to cry. Which response by the nurse would be most appropriate?
   1. "You have no reason to cry. You have a fine surgeon."
   2. "It upsets you to give permission for this operation?"
   3. "The operation will almost surely restore your vision to normal."
   4. "Would you like to talk to your doctor before signing this?"

13. Preparation of Mrs. Merkel's operative site should include:
   1. Removing all facial hair and brows by shaving.
   2. Painting the right side of her face with antiseptic.
   3. Scrubbing the circumorbital skin and brows with pHisoHex.
   4. Covering the right brow, temple, and cheek with collodion.

14. In preparing equipment for the surgeon's use in removing Mrs. Merkel's eyelashes, the nurse should assemble:
   a. A pair of straight, short-blade scissors.
   b. A container of petroleum jelly.
   c. A package of gauze pledgets.
   d. A pair of sterile eyebrow tweezers.
   e. A metal eyelash curler.
      1. a only.
      2. a, b, and c.
      3. All but d.
      4. All the above.

15. One per cent atropine sulfate solution was instilled into Mrs. Merkel's eye in order to produce:

1. Capillary constriction.
2. Pupillary dilation.
3. Decreased tearing.
4. Palpebral relaxation.

16. Neosynephrine may best be classified as:
   1. An antihistaminic.
   2. A sympathomimetic.
   3. An anticholinergic.
   4. A spasmolytic.

17. Neosynephrine was instilled into Mrs. Merkel's eye in order to produce:
   1. Miosis.
   2. Ischemia.
   3. Mydriasis.
   4. Anesthesia.

18. The pharmacologic effect of tetracaine (Pontocaine) is to:
   1. Constrict capillaries and arterioles.
   2. Depress sensory cerebral cortex cells.
   3. Inactivate acetylcholine at nerve endings.
   4. Block conduction through peripheral nerves.

19. The purpose for the preoperative massage of Mrs. Merkel's eye was to:
   1. Foster absorption of anesthetic.
   2. Reduce intraocular pressure.
   3. Increase blood supply to the eye.
   4. Decrease pain sensations.

20. A local rather than a general anesthetic was used for Mrs. Merkel's operation in order to decrease the possibility of postoperative:
   1. Shock.
   2. Hemorrhage.
   3. Vomiting.
   4. Infection.

21. An iridectomy consists of:
   1. Removing a part of the iris.
   2. Creating an opening in the cornea.
   3. Perforating the capsule of the lens.
   4. Withdrawing part of the aqueous humor.

22. The purpose for Mrs. Merkel's iridectomy was to:
   1. Create an opening through which to remove the crystalline lens.
   2. Prevent formation of postoperative adhesions and scars.
   3. Improve circulation to the eye and facilitate healing.
   4. Prevent postoperative obstruction of aqueous humor flow.

23. Only the operated eye was shielded following Mrs. Merkel's surgery because covering both eyes would have produced:
   a. Greater danger of falling.
   b. More severe sensory deprivation.
   c. Less ability for self-care.
   d. Stronger feelings of isolation.
   e. Decreased communication with others.
      1. a and b.
      2. a, b, and c.
      3. All but e.
      4. All the above.

24. Postoperatively, Mrs. Merkel may develop which of the following mental manifestations as a result of sensory deprivation?
   a. Mood changes.
   b. Restlessness and irritability.
   c. Memory impairment.
   d. Thought disturbances.
   e. Disregard of instruction.
      1. a and b.
      2. c and d.
      3. All but e.
      4. All the above.

25. The nurse who cares for Mrs. Merkel postoperatively should ask the surgeon for a p.r.n. order for an:
   1. Antipyretic.
   2. Antiemetic.
   3. Anticonvulsant.
   4. Antibiotic.

26. For the first few hours following the operation Mrs. Merkel should be directed to:
   1. Turn, cough, and breathe deeply every 15 minutes.
   2. Keep her head still, avoiding sudden movement.
   3. Lie on her right side with her head slightly lowered.
   4. Remain on her stomach with her head turned to the side.

27. Which of the following safety precautions should the nurse employ in caring for Mrs. Merkel during the first few hours following her operation?
   1. Elevation of the bed side rails.
   2. Application of wrist restraints.
   3. Head immobilization with sand bags.
   4. Closing the window shades tightly.

28. In order to protect Mrs. Merkel from increase in intraocular pressure postoperatively she should be prevented from any activity which increases:
   1. Systemic arterial blood pressure.
   2. Production of lacrimal secretions.
   3. Venous pressure in the head.
   4. Tone of extraocular muscles.

29. If Mrs. Merkel should feel the urge to cough postoperatively she should be advised to:
   1. Turn her head to the right.
   2. Hold her hands over her eyes.
   3. Hang her head over the bed edge.
   4. Keep her mouth open while coughing.

30. The chief disadvantage to the use of mineral oil as a cathartic is the fact that it:
   1. Causes ulceration of the intestinal mucosa.
   2. Decreases absorption of vitamins A, D, and K.
   3. Facilitates formation of gallbladder stones.
   4. Produces severe dehydration and thirst.

31. Aspirin relieves pain by:
   1. Paralyzing sensory nerve endings peripherally.
   2. Blocking pain impulses in the thalamus.
   3. Depressing cells of the sensory cerebral cortex.
   4. Destroying cholinesterase at nerve endings.

32. Which of the following are possible complications of Mrs. Merkel's postoperative recovery?
   a. Infection.
   b. Hemorrhage.
   c. Glaucoma.
   d. Retinal detachment.
   e. Epithelial downgrowth.
      1. a and b.
      2. a, b, and c.
      3. All but e.
      4. All the above.

33. From the second to the seventh postoperative day the nurse could best protect Mrs. Merkel from postoperative complications by keeping her from:
   a. Turning her head.
   b. Falling from bed.
   c. Chewing solid food.
   d. Rubbing her eyes.
   e. Sitting upright in bed.
      1. a and c.
      2. b and d.
      3. All but d.
      4. All the above.

34. For the first week following the operation the nurse should help Mrs. Merkel to:
   a. Brush her teeth.
   b. Comb her hair.
   c. Wash her face.
   d. Tie her shoes.
   e. Eat her meals.
      1. a only.
      2. a, b, and c.
      3. All but e.
      4. All the above.

35. While Mrs. Merkel's eye is shielded, the nurse's greatest contribution toward helping her compensate for impaired reality-testing ability would be to:
   1. Foster a reliable trusting relationship between patient and nurse.
   2. Describe in detail everything and everyone in the unit.
   3. Make and explain all decisions relative to patient care.
   4. Relieve the patient of all responsibility for self-care.

36. If Mrs. Merkel's relatives should ask for suggestions in selecting a gift for her, which of the following might be therapeutic?
   a. Bottle of cologne.
   b. Transistor radio.
   c. Bouquet of roses.
   d. Box of candy.
   e. Musical powderbox.
      1. a only.
      2. a and b.
      3. All but d.
      4. All the above.

37. It is important that the nurse and the family members spend considerable time with Mrs. Merkel postoperatively in order to:
   1. Provide repeated descriptions and explanations to assist in reality orientation.
   2. Distract her from considering the complications which might follow her surgery.
   3. Relieve her of the necessity to ask questions and make decisions.
   4. Prevent her from talking to other eye patients in the same unit.

38. In addition to improving her visual acuity, Mrs. Merkel's temporary glasses serve the purpose of:
   1. Protecting her operated eye from accidental injury.
   2. Decreasing the amount of light entering her eye.

   3. Making her iridectomy less noticeable to others.
   4. Preparing her to accept the permanent cataract lenses.

39. In giving Mrs. Merkel predischarge instruction the nurse should emphasize the importance of:
   1. Irrigating her eyes daily with normal saline.
   2. Cleansing the lid margins with warm soapy water.
   3. Avoiding reading for 4 to 6 months after surgery.
   4. Wearing the metal eye shield during sleep.

40. Mrs. Merkel should be advised to obtain her doctor's permission before engaging in which of the following activities?
   1. Walking in the out-of-doors.
   2. Bending and lifting objects.
   3. Wearing dark colored glasses.
   4. Watching a television program.

41. As a consequence of her operation Mrs. Merkel will have to wear glasses for the rest of her life because lens removal causes:
   1. Increased susceptibility to infection.
   2. Loss of distance accommodation.
   3. Scarring of the corneal membrane.
   4. Loss of the corneal reflex.

42. It should be explained to Mrs. Merkel that permanent cataract lenses will not be prescribed until 3 to 4 months postoperatively because:
   1. It will take that long to determine the success of the operation.
   2. The effects of eye medications must be dissipated before refraction tests.
   3. Corneal curvature changes continually during the first few months of healing.
   4. The surgeon hopes to discourage her from reading for a long time.

43. It should be explained to Mrs. Merkel that her specially ground cataract lenses will create which of the following visual problems?
   a. Perception of double images.
   b. Magnification of objects.
   c. Inability to distinguish colors.
   d. Distortion of peripheral vision.
   e. Loss of depth perception.
      1. a and c.
      2. b and d.
      3. All but d.
      4. All the above.

Glaucoma and Iridectomy

Dominic Iago was 65 when he developed blurring of vision and pain in the eyes. He went to his oculist to have his glasses changed and the physician diagnosed his difficulty as glaucoma and hospitalized him.

Physical examination and routine diagnostic tests revealed no unusual findings except for Mr. Iago's blood pressure, which was 160/100 mm. Hg. Eye examination revealed increased intraocular pressure in both eyes and cupping of the optic disc in the right eye. A water provocative test indicated significant rise in the intraocular pressure of both eyes. Mr. Iago was diagnosed as having chronic simple glaucoma of the wide-angle type. The following orders were written:

1. *Pilocarpine hydrochloride 2 per cent, gtt. 1 t.i.d. in both eyes.*
2. *Acetazolamide (Diamox). 250 mg. Q.A.M.*

(ANSWER BLANK ON PAGE A–95) (CORRECT ANSWERS ON PAGE B–158)

1. Glaucoma can best be defined as:
   1. Chronic degenerative disease of the cornea which is characterized by severe scarring.
   2. A disorder characterized by increased intraocular pressure which damages the retina and optic nerve.
   3. A focal degeneration of the central portion of the retina which is associated with aging.
   4. Chronic infection of the vascular layer of the eye which is caused by organisms of low virulence.

2. The etiology of wide-angle glaucoma is thought to be:
   1. Infectious.
   2. Traumatic.
   3. Nutritional.
   4. Hereditary.

3. In obtaining Mr. Iago's medical history the physician would be alert for any mention of which of the following as possible symptoms of glaucoma?
   a. Loss of peripheral vision.
   b. Crusting of lid margins.
   c. Periods of foggy vision.
   d. Photophobia and excessive tearing.
   e. Rainbow halos around lights.
      1. a and b.
      2. a, c, and e.
      3. All but e.
      4. All the above.

4. In examining Mr. Iago's eyes the physician might discover which of the following symptoms of glaucoma?
   a. Clouding and insensitivity of the cornea.
   b. Dilated, sluggishly reactive pupil.
   c. Congestion of the conjunctiva.
   d. Inability to close the lids completely.
   e. Patchy exudates throughout the vitreous.
      1. a only.
      2. a, b, and c.
      3. c, d, and e.
      4. All the above.

5. Mr. Iago's medical history would probably reveal that his eye symptoms had been most severe:
   1. On arising.
   2. After meals.
   3. In midafternoon.
   4. At bedtime.

6. In evaluating Mr. Iago's medical history the nurse should be aware that transitory attacks of glaucoma are often precipitated by:
   1. Upper respiratory infection.
   2. Prolonged reading.
   3. Ingestion of alcohol.

4. Emotional upset.

7. Intraocular pressure is determined by the:

    a. Rate of aqueous humor production by the ciliary body.

    b. Pressure of cerebrospinal fluid in subarachnoid space.

    c. Resistance to outflow of aqueous humor from the eye.

    d. Width of the aperture through which the optic nerve enters the eye.

    e. Speed of blood flow through the retinal arteries and veins.

        1. a and c.

        2. b and d.

        3. All but e.

        4. All the above.

8. The pathophysiology of primary open-angle glaucoma is:

    1. Pressure of the anteriorly displaced iris against the filtration network.

    2. Clogging of the aqueous outflow tract with inflammatory debris.

    3. Thickening of the meshwork covering the Canal of Schlemm.

    4. Overproduction of aqueous humor by a hypertrophied ciliary body.

9. The instrument used to measure intraocular pressure is called a:

    1. Spirometer.

    2. Barometer.

    3. Hygrometer.

    4. Tonometer.

10. The device used to measure intraocular pressure operates by determining the:

    1. Surface tension of the fluid film covering the eye.

    2. Degree of corneal indentation produced by slight pressure.

    3. Electrical potential of the epithelial covering of the cornea.

    4. Angle at which the eye surface refracts light waves.

11. The instrument used to measure the angle between the iris and cornea is called a (an):

    1. Ophthalmoscope.

    2. Biomicroscope.

    3. Gonioscope.

    4. Stereoscope.

12. Mr. Iago should be advised to protect his eyes for an hour or two following intraocular pressure determination because:

    1. The weight of the pressure measuring device may rupture scleral vessels.

    2. Mechanical irritation of the eye produces severe temporary photophobia.

    3. Corneal anesthesia renders the eye insensitive to the presence of a foreign body.

    4. Mineral oil used as a lubricant retards normal lacrimal secretions.

13. In addition to measuring Mr. Iago's intraocular pressure, his oculist would probably also have used which of the following tests in his diagnostic workup?

    1. Transillumination of the globe.

    2. X-ray tomograms of the eye.

    3. Visual field examination.

    4. Ocular instillation of 2 per cent fluorescin.

14. Mr. Iago's loss of peripheral vision would cause him to:

    1. Bump into and stumble over furniture.

    2. Elevate his head sharply to read.

    3. Give up watching television.

    4. Avoid driving a car.

15. The cupping of Mr. Iago's optic disc is a manifestation of:

    1. Hemorrhage from an aneurysm on a retinal vessel.

    2. Degeneration due to pressure against the nerve.

    3. Inflammation of the retina by bacterial toxins.

    4. Hyperplasia of the sclera following chemical irritation.

16. For his water provocative test Mr. Iago was made to fast for 8 hours and then given a quart of water to drink, after which his intraocular pressure was measured at 15 minute intervals. In this test a significant pressure rise would be any increase over:

    1. 5 mm. Hg.

    2. 10 mm. Hg.

    3. 25 mm. Hg.

    4. 50 mm. Hg.

17. Pilocarpine is classified as a:

    1. Sympathomimetic.

    2. Secretagogue.

    3. Parasympathomimetic.

    4. Spasmolytic.

18. Pilocarpine was given to Mr. Iago for its effect as a:

    1. Miotic.

    2. Vasoconstrictor.

    3. Analeptic.

    4. Diuretic.

19. Which of the following drugs produce the same therapeutic ocular effect as pilocarpine?
   a. Physostigmine.
   b. Atropine.
   c. Carbamylcholine.
   d. Epinephrine.
   e. Pitocin.
       1. a and c.
       2. b and d.
       3. All but d.
       4. All the above.

20. Pilocarpine is effective in treating glaucoma because it:
   1. Draws the iris away from the cornea, allowing aqueous to drain from the anterior chamber.
   2. Depresses cells of the ciliary body responsible for aqueous humor production.
   3. Relaxes extraocular muscles, permitting increase in the diameter of the globe.
   4. Closes the opening between the iris and lens, preventing forward movement of vitreous.

21. In instilling medication into Mr. Iago's eyes, the most important precaution to be observed is to:
   1. Carefully check the doctor's order for medication and the label on the medicine container.
   2. Maintain the sterility of the medication solution during the procedure of instillation.
   3. Refrain from applying the medication directly to the central area of the corneal surface.
   4. Ensure prolonged contact of the drug to the eye tissues by closing the lids after instillation.

22. In administering Mr. Iago's eye drops the nurse should:
   a. Wash her hands before the instillation.
   b. Direct him to tilt his head backward.
   c. Pull down on the skin overlying the cheekbone.
   d. Steady the hand holding the dropper by placing it on his forehead.
   e. Drop medication on the everted lower eyelid.
       1. a and b.
       2. a, b, and c.
       3. All but d.
       4. All the above.

23. The pharmacologic effect of acetazolamide (Diamox) is to:
   1. Foster aqueous outflow by dilating the Canal of Schlemm.
   2. Decrease blood flow to the eye by constricting retinal vessels.
   3. Block formation of an enzyme which regulates aqueous production.
   4. Increase aqueous drainage by contraction of extraocular muscles.

24. Which of the following are possible toxic effects of acetazolamide?
   a. Paresthesias.
   b. Drowsiness.
   c. Fatigue.
   d. Dyspepsia.
   e. Tinnitus.
       1. a and b.
       2. c and d.
       3. All but e.
       4. All the above.

25. If untreated, Mr. Iago's glaucoma would probably lead to which of the following sequelae?
   1. Cerebral hemorrhage.
   2. Brain tumor.
   3. Total blindness.
   4. Corneal ulcer.

26. Mr. Iago angrily announced, "Well, it's only a matter of time until I'm blind!" In her initial response to his statement the nurse should say:
   1. "It is a possibility that you may lose your sight."
   2. "Why are you so defensive at this time?"
   3. "Most people with glaucoma retain sight for years."
   4. "What makes you think that you will become blind?"

27. After clarifying Mr. Iago's statement and recognizing his fear of possible blindness, the nurse could best help him express his feelings in the matter by saying:
   1. "I can see that blindness would be especially frightening to a man."
   2. "Can you imagine what it would be like to be completely blind?"
   3. "What is it about the possibility of blindness that frightens you?"
   4. "You feel that blindness would make it impossible for you to work?"

28. Which of the following disorders frequently develops as a complication of chronic glaucoma?
   1. Cataract.
   2. Retinal detachment.

3. Corneal ulcer.
4. Exophthalmos.

29. When walking with Mr. Iago to the men's lavatory the nurse should:
1. Wrap her arm around his waist and steer him gently in the desired direction.
2. Have him walk alongside her while holding hands with arms extended.
3. Walk behind him with her hands on his left shoulder and right elbow.
4. Allow him to follow her lead by having him place his hand on her arm.

30. Mr. Iago's medical management should include advising him to:
1. Lose weight.
2. Retire from work.
3. Avoid fatigue.
4. Exercise actively.

31. Mr. Iago would probably be directed by his physician to forgo which of the following?
1. Coffee.
2. Alcohol.
3. Tobacco.
4. Candy.

After two weeks of medical management Mr. Iago was taken to surgery where iridectomy and cyclodialysis procedures were performed on his right eye. He recovered from the surgery without incident, had an uneventful postoperative period, and was discharged to Eye Clinic ten days later.

32. In giving Mr. Iago preoperative instruction the nurse should inform him that:
a. He will be allowed to drink liquids immediately before and after the operation.
b. He will be awake during the operation but will feel no pain.
c. His vision will be completely restored following the procedure.
d. His operated eye will later be covered with an eye pad and shield.
e. He must remain flat on his back for a full week following surgery.
1. a and c.
2. b and d.
3. All but d.
4. All the above.

33. The purpose for Mr. Iago's iridectomy was to:
1. Increase flow of aqueous from the anterior to the posterior chamber and into the optic canal.

2. Increase aqueous flow from the posterior to the anterior chamber and into the chamber angle.
3. Foster movement of fluid from the anterior chamber across the cornea and into the conjunctival sac.
4. Facilitate drainage of fluid from the conjunctival sac into the lacrimal puncta and nasolacrimal duct.

34. The cyclodialysis procedure consists of:
1. Removal of a portion of the ciliary body in order to decrease aqueous humor production.
2. Creating a passage from the anterior chamber to the suprachoroid space for aqueous drainage.
3. Anastomosis of the retinal artery and vein to facilitate reduction of fluid volume in the eye.
4. Needle aspiration of the eyeball for the purpose of removing excessive aqueous humor.

35. On Mr. Iago's return from the operating room he should be placed in which position?
1. Trendelenburg position with the head turned to the right.
2. Supine with a pillow on each side of the head.
3. Right Sims' position with head flexed forward.
4. Low Fowler's position with the knees gatched.

36. During his first postoperative day Mr. Iago should be encouraged to:
1. Turn, cough, and breathe deeply several times each hour.
2. Ring the nurse's call bell whenever he needs assistance.
3. Drink large quantities of fluid at regular intervals.
4. Keep both eyes tightly closed to exclude light.

37. Following his return from the operating room Mr. Iago should be advised against which of the following as activities which increase intraocular pressure?
a. Coughing or sneezing.
b. Turning the head suddenly.
c. Rubbing the eyes.
d. Closing the lids tightly.
e. Bending over to pick up an object.
1. a and b.
2. c and d.
3. All but d.
4. All the above.

38. In order to give Mr. Iago effective health instruction the nurse should know that, as a result of his medical and surgical treatments:

1. His vision will be completely restored as soon as his incision has healed.
2. His visual loss cannot be restored but further loss can be prevented.
3. His vision will improve markedly but he will never have perfect vision.
4. His vision will continue to deteriorate but at a slower rate than before.

39. Family-centered health care for the Iagos should include:

1. Teaching Mr. Iago's wife and children how to instill eye drops.
2. Demonstrating to the entire family how to lead a partially sighted person.
3. Asking first one, then another of his children to bring Mr. Iago to the clinic.
4. Advising Mr. Iago's children to have their intraocular pressure measured.

40. Mr. Iago's 40-year-old son laughingly said to the nurse, "Like father like son. I suppose I'll get glaucoma when I'm older." Which of the following responses by the nurse would be most helpful?

1. "Tell me how you feel about the possibility of your getting glaucoma."
2. "You've made a useful observation. It would be a good idea to have your eyes examined now."
3. "Scientists haven't yet worked out all the genetic patterns involved, but glaucoma is inheritable."
4. "In this day and age there are so many diseases which have been found to be inherited."

41. In giving Mr. Iago predischarge instruction the nurse should emphasize the importance of:

a. Preventing constipation.
b. Eschewing tight fitting collars.
c. Avoiding heavy lifting.
d. Limiting television viewing.
e. Avoiding arguments and quarrels.
   1. a and c.
   2. b and d.
   3. All but e.
   4. All the above.

42. In teaching Mr. Iago how to care for himself after discharge, the nurse should advise him to:

1. Wear a gauze eye pad and metal shield during sleep.
2. Keep an extra bottle of pilocarpine at home and at work.
3. Apply warm, moist compresses to his eyes to relieve pain.
4. Avoid reading or doing close work of any kind.

43. If Mr. Iago should neglect to instill his pilocarpine drops for two days, such behavior would be most apt to signify:

1. Anger.
2. Denial.
3. Regression.
4. Acting-out.

Emphysema

Willie Hale, a 57-year-old black restaurant worker and heavy smoker, complained to his doctor of "smoker's cough," repeated respiratory infections, and dyspnea on moderate exertion. Physical examination revealed a temperature of 100.8° F., pulse 120 per minute, respirations 26 per minute, blood pressure 130/86 mm. Hg., increased anteroposterior diameter of the chest, thoracic rales, labored expiration, cyanosis of lips and nailbeds, and slight cardiomegaly. Pulmonary function tests revealed decrease in vital capacity and increased residual air volume. Arterial blood analysis revealed pO_2 of 65 mm. Hg. and pCO_2 of 50 mm. Hg.

The physician made a diagnosis of acute pulmonary emphysema and cor pulmonale. He sent Mr. Hale to the hospital and ordered the following:

1. No smoking.
2. Bedrest.
3. Tetracycline 250 mg. "O" Q.I.D.
4. Intermittent positive pressure breathing treatments of 40 per cent oxygen and air at 20 cm. of water pressure for 20 minutes t.i.d.
5. Isoproterenol (Isuprel) 1:200, gtts. V. by aerosol inhalation t.i.d. in conjunction with I.P.P.B. treatments.
6. Postural drainage with chest percussion t.i.d.
7. To Inhalation Therapy Department for breathing exercises q. A.M.
8. High protein, high vitamin, high liquid diet.

(ANSWER BLANK ON PAGE A–97)   (CORRECT ANSWERS ON PAGE B–161)

---

1. For which of the following reasons does Mr. Hale have more difficulty with expiration than with inspiration?

  a. Bronchi and bronchioles are more widely dilated during inspiration than during expiration.

  b. Elastic lung recoil is less forceful than contraction of the diaphragm and the rib levators.

  c. The carbon dioxide of expired air is heavier than the oxygen of inspired air.

  d. Respiratory cilia are more easily depressed in the caudal than in the cephalic direction.

  e. At the onset of expiration, intra-alveolar pulmonary pressure is less than atmospheric pressure.

    1. a and b.

    2. c and d.

    3. All but e.

    4. All the above.

2. Mr. Hale's elevated temperature on admission was probably due to:

  1. Dehydration resulting from inadequate fluid intake.

  2. Stimulation of hypothalamic centers by bacterial protein.

  3. Increased motor activity occasioned by persistent coughing.

  4. Emotional stress associated with admission to the hospital.

3. Mr. Hale's dyspnea on mild exertion was probably the result of:

  1. Lowered oxygen-carrying capacity of his red blood cells.

  2. Impaired diffusion between the alveolar air and blood.

  3. Thrombotic obstruction of pulmonary arterioles and capillaries.

  4. Decreased tone of the diaphragm and intercostal muscles.

4. Cyanosis is the result of:

  1. Increase in the proportion of white to red blood cells.

  2. Decreased concentration of bicarbonate ion in the serum.

  3. Decrease in the diameter of peripheral arterioles and venules.

  4. Increase in the amount of reduced hemoglobin in skin capillaries.

5. The physician could best determine whether or not Mr. Hale was cyanotic by observing the color of:

  1. The skin of his face.

  2. The palms of his hands.

  3. The lower conjunctival sac.

  4. The mucosal lining of the mouth.

6. Mr. Hale's extreme susceptibility to respiratory infections was due chiefly to:

  1. Failure of his bone marrow to produce phagocytic white blood cells.

  2. Retention of tracheobronchial secretions due to bronchospasm and mucosal edema.

  3. Decreased detoxification of body fluids by compressed liver cells.

  4. Persistent mouth breathing associated with dyspnea and coughing.

7. Which of the following results of emphysema is primarily responsible for Mr. Hale's cardiomegaly?

  1. Hypertrophy of muscles encircling the bronchi.

  2. Increased pressure in the pulmonary circulation.

  3. Decreased number of circulating red blood cells.

  4. Secretion of excessive amounts of pericardial fluid.

8. In cor pulmonale, or cardiac failure secondary to chronic obstructive pulmonary disease, which of the following symptoms tends to appear first?

1. Watery sputum.
2. Substernal pain.
3. Severe albuminuria.
4. Pedal edema.

9. The tissue change most characteristic of emphysema is:

1. Accumulation of pus in the pleural space.
2. Constriction of capillaries by fibrous tissue.
3. Filling of air passages by inflammatory coagulum.
4. Overdistention, inelasticity, and rupture of alveoli.

10. Which of the following factors commonly predisposes to emphysematous lung changes?

1. Chemical and mechanical irritation of bronchiolar and alveolar linings.
2. Sudden increase in intrapulmonary pressure coincident with hypertension.
3. Obstruction of air passages by spasms of bronchiolar muscle.
4. Senile degenerative changes in the vertebral bodies and intervertebral discs.

11. Cigarette smoking can be assumed to have contributed to Mr. Hale's pulmonary disorder by:

a. Paralyzing ciliary movement in the respiratory mucosa.
b. Decreasing the elasticity of the alveolar membrane.
c. Increasing the viscosity of tracheobronchial secretions.
d. Reducing the alveolar surface tension by altering pulmonary surfactant.
   1. a and b.
   2. b and c.
   3. c and d.
   4. All the above.

12. While waiting for the examining physician to arrive, Mr. Hale would have been most comfortable in which of the following positions?

1. Lying flat in bed.
2. Reclining on his left side.
3. Sitting on the edge of the bed.
4. Supine with his head slightly lowered.

13. It would be desirable for the admitting nurse to remain with Mr. Hale and to explain the steps of the admitting procedure because:

1. Respiratory difficulty and consequent anoxemia engender undue suspicion of strangers.
2. Anxiety provoked by strange surroundings and procedures might increase his dyspnea.
3. Instruction should begin immediately upon admission concerning the dangers of smoking.
4. Continuous observation is required to identify increasing dyspnea, cyanosis, and confusion.

14. The increased anteroposterior diameter of Mr. Hale's chest is the result of:

1. Cardiac hypertrophy secondary to obstruction of pulmonary circulation.
2. Fixation of the sternum and ribs in inspiratory position.
3. Inflammatory hyperplasia of mediastinal lymph nodes.
4. Distention of pleural and pericardial sacs by transudate.

15. The rales in Mr. Hale's chest that were heard by the examiner were produced by:

1. Blood rushing through pulmonary arteriovenous fistulas.
2. Friction between two layers of inflamed pleura.
3. Air passing through fluid in bronchi and alveoli.
4. Air being forced from the lung into the pleural sac.

16. Vital capacity is best defined as the:

1. Maximum expiration following maximum deep inspiration.
2. Volume of air which can be forcibly inhaled at the end of a normal inspiration.
3. Volume of air which can be forcibly exhaled at the end of a normal expiration.
4. Total volume of air contained in the alveoli, bronchioles, bronchi, and trachea.

17. The average tidal volume of the healthy adult is:

1. 500 cc.
2. 1500 cc.
3. 3000 cc.
4. 4500 cc.

18. Mr. Hale's reduced vital capacity is primarily the result of:

1. Reduction in lung air space.
2. Increase in residual air volume.

3. Fixed elevation of the diaphragm.
4. Flaccid paralysis of intercostal muscles.

19. In the healthy adult the partial tension of oxygen in the arterior blood (pO_2) is roughly:
1. 40 mm. Hg.
2. 60 mm. Hg.
3. 80 mm. Hg.
4. 100 mm. Hg.

20. The normal value for partial tension of carbon dioxide (pCO_2) in arterial blood is about:
1. 40 mm. Hg
2. 60 mm. Hg.
3. 80 mm. Hg.
4. 100 mm. Hg.

21. Mr. Hale's pCO_2 of 50 mm. Hg. and his pH of 7.21 indicate a physiological state of:
1. Respiratory acidosis.
2. Respiratory alkalosis.
3. Metabolic acidosis.
4. Metabolic alkalosis.

22. In healthy individuals the pH of arterial blood falls within which range?
1. 6.65 to 6.75.
2. 7.00 to 7.10.
3. 7.35 to 7.45.
4. 7.75 to 7.85.

23. Which of the following blood findings would be most compatible with Mr. Hale's diagnosis?
1. R.B.C. 6,100,000; hematocrit 55 per cent; W.B.C. 15,000; neutrophils 79 per cent; lymphocytes 15 per cent.
2. R.B.C. 5,500,000; hematocrit 47 per cent; W.B.C. 7000; neutrophils 65 per cent; lymphocytes 30 per cent.
3. R.B.C. 4,300,000; hematocrit 40 per cent; W.B.C. 30,000; neutrophils 41 per cent; lymphocytes 52 per cent.
4. R.B.C. 3,500,000; hematocrit 35 per cent; W.B.C. 5000; neutrophils 70 per cent; lymphocytes 24 per cent.

24. The physician ordered that oxygen be given to Mr. Hale in low concentration and intermittently rather than in high concentration and continuously, in order to prevent:
1. Depression of the respiratory center.
2. Decrease in red blood cell formation.
3. Rupture of emphysematous bullae.
4. Excessive drying of respiratory mucosa.

25. The administration of 100 per cent oxygen to Mr. Hale could be expected to:
1. Increase respiratory rate to the point of muscular exhaustion.
2. Precipitate cardiac failure by increasing basal metabolic rate.
3. Increase retention of CO_2 by decreasing respiratory rate and depth.
4. Induce nervous hyperirritability by sudden relief of cerebral anoxia.

26. In healthy individuals the partial pressure of oxygen (pO_2) in venous blood is:
1. 40 mm. Hg.
2. 60 mm. Hg.
3. 80 mm. Hg.
4. 100 mm. Hg.

27. Under normal conditions the partial pressure of oxygen in arterial blood is:
1. Slightly lower than the pO_2 in the alveoli.
2. Markedly higher than the pO_2 in the alveoli.
3. Somewhat lower than the pCO_2 in the alveoli.
4. Slightly higher than the total barometric pressure.

28. The normal range for partial pressure of carbon dioxide (pCO_2) in venous blood is:
1. 46 mm. Hg.
2. 56 mm. Hg.
3. 66 mm. Hg.
4. 76 mm. Hg.

29. The alterations in Mr. Hale's arterial pO_2 and pCO_2 were probably the result of:
1. Reduction in the speed of blood flow through capillaries of the pulmonary circuit.
2. Impaired exchange of inspiratory with expiratory gases in certain areas of the lung.
3. Increased numbers of red blood cells produced by hyperactive red bone marrow.
4. Faulty oxygen-carbon dioxide exchange between interstitial fluid and peripheral capillaries.

30. Mr. Hale's chronic bronchitis has contributed to his present respiratory difficulty in that:
1. Inflammatory thickening of the bronchiolar lining has tended to obstruct expiratory air flow.
2. Previous respiratory infections have sensitized him to react allergically to bacterial protein.
3. Fibrotic obliteration of pulmonary blood vessels has decreased blood flow to the alveoli.
4. Attention given him during previous respiratory illnesses encourages him to magnify present symptoms.

31. The primary goal of Mr. Hale's medical and nursing rehabilitation program should be to help him to achieve:
1. Decreased psychological dependence upon others.
2. Increased understanding of infectious disease control.
3. Decreased awareness of subjective symptoms.
4. Increased capacity for physical exertion.

32. Bedrest was ordered for Mr. Hale primarily in order to:
1. Encourage sleep as a means of alleviating fear and anxiety.
2. Facilitate the execution of diagnostic and treatment measures.
3. Decrease tissue oxygen need by decreasing basal metabolic rate.
4. Impress him with the urgency of his need to stop smoking.

33. Tetracycline has a bacteriostatic action against which of the following types of microorganisms?
   a. Gram-positive cocci.
   b. Gram-negative bacilli.
   c. Rickettsia.
   d. Viri.
   e. Fungi.
      1. a and b.
      2. b and c.
      3. All but e.
      4. All the above.

34. Mr. Hale should be observed for which of the following as a possible side effect of tetracycline?
1. Stomatitis.
2. Conjunctivitis.
3. Icterus.
4. Edema.

35. The primary purpose of Mr. Hale's intermittent positive pressure breathing treatments is to:
1. Eliminate bronchial infection.
2. Decrease bronchial irritation.
3. Increase pulmonary circulation.
4. Improve pulmonary ventilation.

36. Mr. Hale's intermittent positive pressure breathing treatments can be expected to achieve which of the following effects?
   a. Improved distribution of inhaled gases.
   b. Increased elimination of carbon dioxide.
   c. Improved removal of mucus through coughing.
   d. Increased oxygenation of arterial blood.
   e. Improved tone of respiratory muscles.
      1. a and b.
      2. a, b, and c.
      3. All but e.
      4. All the above.

37. Which of the following explanations by the nurse would best prepare Mr. Hale for the intermittent positive pressure breathing treatments?
1. "You have nothing to worry about or be fearful of. A highly trained technician, working under your doctor's order, will give you a special gas mixture through a mechanical respirator."
2. "This is a nonpainful 20 minute procedure in which you will breathe oxygen and air through a mouthpiece or mask in order to relieve your discomfort and improve your breathing."
3. "Many of your lung air sacs have been collapsed or destroyed. You will be attached to a machine which will blow pressurized air into your lungs to reexpand them."
4. "For the duration of the treatment the breathing machine will take over control of your respirations, regulating their rate and depth so as to improve oxygen delivery to your blood."

38. The nurse should give Mr. Hale which of the following directions before initiating intermittent positive pressure breathing treatments?
1. "Breathe deeply several times before the mouthpiece is applied to compensate for the machine's lag period."
2. "Once the mouthpiece is applied, hold your breath until the machine forces you to breathe."
3. "Breathe slowly and fully through the mouthpiece and the machine will be triggered by your respirations."
4. "The machine will make your breathing more difficult, but the treatment will only last 20 minutes."

39. At which of the following rates should Mr. Hale breathe in order to achieve maximum benefit from his intermittent positive pressure breathing treatments?

    1. 8 to 10 respirations per minute.
    2. 14 to 16 respirations per minute.
    3. 20 to 22 respirations per minute.
    4. 26 to 28 respirations per minute.

40. The respirator used to give Mr. Hale intermittent positive pressure breathing treatments would be of which type?

    1. Pressure controlled.
    2. Volume controlled.
    3. Temperature controlled.
    4. Density controlled.

41. It is necessary that humidification be provided with Mr. Hale's intermittent positive pressure breathing treatments in order to:

    1. Prevent thickening and crusting of tracheobronchial secretions.
    2. Seal minute air leaks between contiguous alveoli.
    3. Facilitate transport of isoproterenol across capillary membranes.
    4. Inhibit growth of microorganisms in respiratory passageways.

42. The pharmacologic effect for which isoproterenol (Isuprel) was given to Mr. Hale was which of the following?

    1. Antibiotic.
    2. Detergent.
    3. Demulcent.
    4. Bronchodilator.

43. Mr. Hale should be observed for which of the following as a possible toxic effect of isoproterenol?

    1. Headache.
    2. Tinnitus.
    3. Palpitations.
    4. Urticaria.

44. It would be best to institute postural drainage for Mr. Hale:

    1. Immediately after breakfast.
    2. Immediately before I.P.P.B. treatments.
    3. One hour before lunch.
    4. During afternoon visiting hour.

45. On the first occasion that postural drainage is carried out Mr. Hale should be maintained in postural position for how long?

    1. 2 minutes.
    2. 10 minutes.
    3. 30 minutes.
    4. 60 minutes.

46. Which of the following comfort measures should the nurse provide Mr. Hale following postural drainage?

    1. An ice cap.
    2. Oral hygiene.
    3. A partial bath.
    4. A back rub.

47. The primary purpose of the breathing improvement exercises ordered for Mr. Hale would be to:

    1. Increase the depth of inspiration by enhancing rib elevation.
    2. Improve gaseous exchange by slowing the respiratory cycle.
    3. Increase the force of exhalation by increasing diaphragmatic movement.
    4. Restore normal chest dimensions by releasing fibrous adhesions.

48. Which of the following breathing exercises would be therapeutic for Mr. Hale?

    a. Hissing through clenched teeth.
    b. Blowing a pencil across a table top.
    c. Exhaling forcefully against pursed lips.
    d. Blowing out candles at various distances.
    e. Blowing bubbles through a tube immersed in water.

        1. a and b.
        2. c, d, and e.
        3. All but a.
        4. All the above.

49. In planning long term nursing goals for Mr. Hale the nurse should be aware that he is especially apt to develop which of the following undesirable attitudes toward his prescribed treatments?

    1. Aversion to being observed during breathing exercises and treatments.
    2. Undue dependence on the intermittent positive pressure respirator.
    3. Reluctance to assume responsibility for aspects of self-care.
    4. Inability to accept instruction from younger members of the health team.

Tuberculosis

Tim Casey was graduated from nursing school in August, passed his state board examinations in September, and applied for admission to the Army Nurse Corps in October. Routine chest x-rays revealed a lesion in his right upper lobe and acid-fast bacilli were isolated from smears of his sputum. Tim indicated that he had had a negative Mantoux test on entering nursing school, had elected not to receive B.C.G. vaccine, but had had a positive Mantoux test at the end of his first year in the nursing program, at which time his chest x-ray had been negative.

Tim was admitted to a state tuberculosis hospital where, following sensitivity testing of organisms isolated from his sputum, the following treatment was ordered:

> 1. *Bedrest with bathroom privileges.*
> 2. *High protein, high vitamin diet.*
> 3. *Isoniazid 300 mg. "O" daily.*
> 4. *Rifampin 600 mg. "O" daily.*

(ANSWER BLANK ON PAGE A–99) (CORRECT ANSWERS ON PAGE B–164)

1. Tim's chest x-ray would be examined for indication of which of the following as evidence of healed primary tuberculosis?
1. Collapse of one lung or a segment of a lung.
2. A calcified peripheral nodule and a calcified hilar node.
3. Dilation and congestion of pulmonary arteries and veins.
4. Displacement of the mediastinum to the left or right.

2. Tuberculin consists of:
1. Endotoxins and exotoxins produced by the *Mycobacterium tuberculosis*.
2. Protein derived from killed cultures of tubercle bacilli.
3. Media containing the metabolic products of *Mycobacterium tuberculosis*.
4. A few tubercle bacilli suspended in normal saline solution.

3. In order to obtain reliable test results the tuberculin used for Tim's Mantoux test must have been:
a. Freshly prepared.
b. Diluted with saline.
c. Stored in a refrigerator.
d. Warmed before use.
e. Injected into two sites.
1. a and c.
2. b and d.
3. All but e.
4. All the above.

4. For the purpose of the Mantoux test tuberculin is administered:

1. Topically.
2. Intradermally.
3. Hypodermically.
4. Intramuscularly.

5. A series of different dilutions of tuberculin may be given in the Mantoux test in order to:
1. Facilitate desensitization of the host's tissues to the bacterial protein.
2. Prevent a severe local tissue reaction in a highly sensitized individual.
3. Stimulate the body's production of lymphocytes, monocytes, and plasmocytes.
4. Prevent occurrence of false positive reactions to the foreign protein.

6. The Mantoux test should be read after which interval of time?
1. 1 hour.
2. 12 hours.
3. 48 hours.
4. 1 week.

7. A positive Mantoux test consists of:
1. Formation of a vesicle followed by a pustule.
2. A sharply demarcated region of erythema.
3. A central area of induration surrounded by erythema.
4. A circle of blanched tissue surrounding the injection site.

8. A negative tuberculin reaction sometimes occurs in patients with which of the following types of tuberculosis?

1. Acute miliary tuberculosis.
2. Tuberculous meningitis.
3. Tuberculosis of the kidney.
4. Tuberculosis of the bone.

9. The Mantoux test results should be recorded as the:

1. Length of time between administration and peak reaction.
2. Distance between injection site and outermost edge of erythema.
3. Width of the largest diameter of the area of induration.
4. Degree of skin discoloration at the site of injection.

10. Tim's negative Mantoux test on entering nursing school indicated that, at that time:

1. His resistance to the tubercle bacillus had been low.
2. He had not previously been infected by the tubercle bacillus.
3. He was incapable of being infected by the tubercle bacillus.
4. He had had a tuberculous infection but had recovered from it.

11. The purpose of B.C.G. vaccination is to:

1. Render the host tissues less susceptible to infection by the *Mycobacterium tuberculosis*.
2. Destroy all tubercle bacilli then present in the host's body tissues.
3. Inject into the host antibodies against the *Mycobacterium tuberculosis*.
4. Prevent a mild initial tuberculous infection from increasing in severity.

12. B.C.G. vaccination is usually given to:

1. Asthenic persons whose ancestors or relatives have had tuberculosis.
2. Persons with a history of repeated upper and lower respiratory infection.
3. Tuberculosis-prone persons with known hypersensitivity to antibiotics.
4. Tuberculum nonreactors in whom exposure to tuberculosis is unavoidable.

13. B.C.G. vaccination is not given when the person:

1. Is less than 30 years old.
2. Is employed in a hospital or clinic.
3. Has a skin disease of any type.
4. Is allergic to penicillin or streptomycin.

14. Tim's positive Mantoux test and negative chest x-ray after one year in nursing school were indications that, at that time, he:

1. Was less susceptible to a tuberculous infection than the year before.
2. Had acquired some degree of passive immunity to tuberculosis.
3. Had sustained a tuberculous infection and had recovered from it.
4. Was harboring a mild tuberculous infection in some organ other than the lung.

15. In taking Tim's medical history the nurse should be alert for any mention of which of the following symptoms of tuberculosis?

a. Loss of weight.
b. Easy fatiguability.
c. Afternoon fever.
d. Night sweats.
e. Blood-tinged sputum.
   1. a and b.
   2. a, b, and c.
   3. All but d.
   4. All the above.

16. Through which of the following means would the physician be most apt to obtain corroborative evidence of the data obtained from Tim's chest x-ray and sputum smear?

1. Culture of concentrated fasting gastric contents.
2. Culture of serial arterial blood samples.
3. Biochemical analysis of a 24 hour sputum sample.
4. Measurement of vital capacity and residual air.

17. It may be assumed that Tim acquired the microorganisms responsible for his lung lesion by:

1. Inhalation of droplet nuclei.
2. Ingestion of contaminated food.
3. Injection with unsterile equipment.
4. Skin contact with a draining wound.

18. The *Mycobacterium tuberculosis* is not easily destroyed by exposure to ordinary disinfectants because it:

1. Forms spores during periods of quiescence.
2. Has a resistant waxy outer membrane.
3. Is composed of a carbohydrate rather than a protein.
4. Secretes an exotoxin which neutralizes antiseptics.

19. The incubation period from inoculation with tuberculosis bacilli to development of tuberculin hypersensitivity is roughly:
1. 8 to 12 hours.
2. 2 to 4 days.
3. 4 to 6 weeks.
4. 6 to 8 months.

20. The tubercle or tissue lesion produced by the *Mycobacterium tuberculosis* is characterized by:
1. Erosion of the epithelial lining of a main bronchus.
2. Dilation and sacculation of a pulmonary artery or arteriole.
3. Bacilli surrounded by inflammatory cells and fibrous tissue.
4. Hyperplasia of columnar epithelium with many immature cells.

21. Following his admission to the hospital the purpose for putting Tim on bedrest was to:
1. Reduce caloric requirements by decreasing muscular activity.
2. Foster lung healing by limiting respiratory movements.
3. Prevent disease transmission during the infectious stage.
4. Prevent nervous irritability by decreasing sensory stimuli.

22. In order to prevent the spread of tuberculosis to others the nurse should teach Tim to:
1. Cover his mouth and nose with a tissue when coughing or sneezing.
2. Wear a face mask at all times except during sleep.
3. Stifle the urge to cough by drinking a small quantity of liquid.
4. Refrain from face to face contact with relatives or hospital staff.

23. Immediately following Tim's admission to the hospital his visitors were limited to members of his immediate family in order to:
1. Decrease the possibility of transmitting tuberculosis to others.
2. Protect him from physical and emotional exhaustion.
3. Reduce bacterial contamination of his unit by outsiders.
4. Conceal from him the stigma associated with tuberculosis.

24. From Tim's standpoint, the changes which illness has wrought in his social status, occupational situation, self-view, and level of health are apt to be viewed as:
1. Sources of guilt.
2. Types of loss.
3. Punishment for sin.
4. Opportunities for learning.

25. Tim's room should be adequately ventilated with freely moving fresh air in order to:
1. Facilitate his loss of body heat by radiation and convection.
2. Dilute droplet nuclei in the air to minimum concentration.
3. Destroy tubercle bacilli by exposure to high oxygen tension.
4. Reduce unpleasant odors associated with tissue putrefaction.

26. Which of the following is a possible toxic effect of rifampin?
1. Peripheral neuritis.
2. Renal failure.
3. Bloody diarrhea.
4. Liver dysfunction.

27. Which of the following is a possible toxic effect of isoniazid?
1. Paroxysmal tachycardia.
2. Erythema multiforme.
3. Peripheral neuritis.
4. Burning on urination.

28. Which of the following is often ordered to prevent toxic effects of isoniazid?
1. Thiamine.
2. Riboflavin.
3. Cyanocobalamin.
4. Pyridoxine.

29. One day about a week after his admission to the hospital Tim coughed up a large quantity of bright red blood. In addition to calling Tim's physician the nurse should:
1. Direct him to lie on his right side, remaining as still as possible.
2. Place him in a chair with a pillow in the small of his back.
3. Have him sit upright in bed with his arms folded on an overbed table.
4. Ignore the occurrence, diverting Tim's attention through conversation.

30. The physician will probably order which of the following to relieve Tim's anxiety and dyspnea following his episode of hemoptysis?
1. Phenobarbital.
2. Aspirin.
3. Chloral hydrate.
4. Morphine.

31. Which of the following is the most frequent complication of hemorrhage in the tuberculous patient?

1. Total exsanguination and sudden death.
2. Distention of the pleural sac with blood.
3. Spread of tuberculosis to other parts of the lung.
4. Hypovolemic shock and circulatory collapse.

32. If Tim should develop paroxysms of coughing while expectorating blood, the physician would probably order which of the following drugs to control his cough?
   1. Diphenylhydramine hydrochloride.
   2. Potassium iodide.
   3. Codeine sulfate.
   4. Isoproterenol.

33. Tim's hemoptysis occurred at 3:00 P.M. Of what should his supper that evening consist?
   1. Small amounts of cold liquids.
   2. Large quantities of hot tea or cocoa.
   3. A general diet with 2 glasses of milk.
   4. A high caloric, high protein, high vitamin diet.

Because Tim developed toxic effects from rifampin, the drug was discontinued after three weeks and Tim was given ethambutol, 1 gm. orally daily.

34. Which of the following is a possible toxic effect of ethambutol?
   1. Optic neuritis.
   2. Progressive deafness.
   3. Bullous dermatitis.
   4. Muscle tremor.

35. In order to achieve the most therapeutic effect, Tim's isoniazid and ethambutol should be given:
   1. At the same time, shortly after arising.
   2. One before and one after breakfast.
   3. One after breakfast and one after lunch.
   4. One on arising and one at bedtime.

36. If Tim should develop an untoward reaction to ethambutol, which of the following drugs might be used in its stead?
   1. Ammonium nitrate.
   2. Para-amino-salicylic acid.
   3. Bismuth subsalicylate.
   4. Tetraethyl ammonium chloride.

37. Tim's failure to eat may be a manifestation of:

   a. Physical fatigue.
   b. Psychological depression.
   c. Rejection of therapy.
   d. Drug toxicity.
   e. Cultural shock.
      1. a and b.
      2. a, b, and c.
      3. All but e.
      4. All the above.

38. Which action on the nurse's part would probably be most helpful in improving Tim's nutrition at this point?
   1. Explain to him the physiologic functions of the various food groups.
   2. Ask his relatives to bring in some of his favorite dishes.
   3. Cut his food into small portions and feed it to him.
   4. Serve his trays so as to allow longer intervals between meals.

39. In order to answer Tim's questions regarding his illness and treatment, the nurse should know that he will probably be required to take medicine daily for what period of time?
   1. 6 weeks.
   2. 6 months.
   3. 2 years.
   4. For the rest of his life.

40. After he returned from his first weekend visit at home Tim said to the nurse, "Even my little sister pushes me around." In this comment he is probably expressing his:
   1. Feelings of weakness.
   2. Loss of social status.
   3. Sibling rivalry.
   4. Envy of healthy persons.

After two months of hospitalization Tim's sputum cultures were negative, he had gained 7 pounds, and he was feeling better, so he was discharged on continuing dosages of isoniazid and ethambutol. Arrangements were made for the nurse from the Municipal Tuberculosis Association to visit his home and he was directed to see his physician every month.

41. In order for Tim's treatment to be successful it is essential that he possess or develop which of the following?
   1. Self-understanding.
   2. Faith in his physician.
   3. Physical courage.
   4. Self-discipline.

42. In teaching Tim to care for himself at home, the nurse should emphasize that which of the following aspects of self care would be of greatest significance to his continuing improvement and ultimate well-being?
1. Eating a highly nutritious and well-balanced diet.
2. Adherence to a strict program of balanced rest and exercise.
3. Concurrent and terminal disinfection of articles of personal use.
4. Regular administration of medicines in prescribed amounts at specified times.

43. In preparing Tim and his family for his home care following hospital discharge, the nurse should explain that persons in which of the following categories are especially susceptible to tuberculosis?
1. Infants.
2. Teenagers.
3. Childbearing women.
4. Retirement age males.

44. In caring for Tim at home the family should arrange for him to:
1. Take his meals apart from the rest of the family.
2. Have a room of his own for sleeping and resting.
3. Have no contact with anyone but immediate family members.
4. Engage in no physical activity other than dressing and feeding himself.

45. Tim and his family should be instructed to dispose of his sputum papers by:
1. Burning them in an outdoor trash basket.
2. Double wrapping and placing them in the garbage.
3. Flushing them down the toilet.
4. Burying them in dirt or sand.

46. Tim should also be advised to:
1. Wash his hands after handling sputum papers or sputum cups.
2. Wear a mask whenever he is in direct contact with others.
3. Boil his dishes for 15 minutes after each use and before washing.
4. Burn all paper, cloth, and wooden articles when he is finished with them.

47. Which of the following complications is apt to ensue if Tim should, through feelings of discouragement or a sense of false security, fail to take his medications regularly?
1. Allergic reaction to medications.
2. Loss of tissue sensitivity to tuberculin.
3. Bacterial resistance to the drugs.
4. Calcification of hilar lymph nodes.

48. In order to ensure that Tim will receive his medications regularly after hospital discharge, the nurse should:
1. Instruct his mother to administer the ordered drugs.
2. Suggest that he record dosages on a drug calendar.
3. Phone him daily to remind him to take the medications.
4. Arrange for a public health nurse to visit him daily.

Chronic Glomerulonephritis and Hemodialysis

Walter Proxmire developed acute glomerulonephritis in childhood. Despite treatment, the disease progressed to chronic glomerulonephritis. When Walter was 25, married, the father of two children, and manager of a dime store, he was hospitalized with proteinuria, hypertension, gastritis, and anasarca. Funduscopic examination revealed narrowing of retinal arterioles and numerous exudates in both fundi. He was treated with bedrest, methyldopa (Aldomet) 250 mg. orally q. 6 h., aluminum hydroxide gel, 1 tablespoon q.i.d., and diazepam (Valium) 5 mg. t.i.d.

After 4 weeks of treatment Walter's blood pressure remained elevated, his blood urea nitrogen had risen to 80 mg. per cent, his serum creatinine was 10 mg. per cent, his serum uric acid was 8 mg. per cent, and his serum potassium was 9 mEq. per liter. A renal biopsy revealed focal obliteration of glomerular loops, hyaline degeneration of tubules, and thickening of intralobular arteries and arterioles. Walter was put on peritoneal dialysis and a 20 Gram protein diet. After three weeks on this regimen his azotemia was considerably reduced. He was discharged from the hospital and arrangements were made for him to be hemodialyzed three times a week on an outpatient basis in a nearby medical center.

(ANSWER BLANK ON PAGE A–101) (CORRECT ANSWERS ON PAGE B–167)

1. Acute glomerulonephritis is the result of:

1. Acute infection of the kidney parenchyma by gram-negative intestinal bacteria.
2. An immune response of renal tissue to the protein of the beta-hemolytic streptococcus.
3. Destruction of capillary endothelium by such heavy metals as lead, silver, and arsenic.
4. Ischemia of renal tissue resulting from atheromatous obliteration of renal vessels.

2. During his episode of acute glomerulonephritis Walter probably demonstrated which of the following symptoms?
   a. Headache.
   b. Periorbital edema.
   c. Flank pain.
   d. Oliguria.
   e. Hematuria.
      1. a and b.
      2. a, b, and c.
      3. All but e.
      4. All the above.

3. Which of the following are possible complications of chronic glomerulonephritis?
   a. Anemia.
   b. Stroke.
   c. Heart failure.
   d. Kidney stones.
   e. Uremia.
      1. a only.
      2. a and b.
      3. All but d.
      4. All the above.

4. As she takes Walter's medical history on his admission to the hospital, the nurse should be alert to any mention on his part of which of the following symptoms of chronic renal failure?

    a. Morning headaches.
    b. Visual difficulty.
    c. Nausea and vomiting.
    d. Frequent urination.
    e. Easy fatigability.
        1. a and c.
        2. b and d.
        3. All but e.
        4. All the above.

5. Walter's anasarca was primarily the result of:

    1. Increased hydrostatic capillary pressure.
    2. Increased volume of intravascular fluid.
    3. Decreased plasma colloid osmotic pressure.
    4. Inflammation of capillary endothelium.

6. The primary purpose for putting Walter on complete bedrest following hospital admission was to:

    1. Lessen the danger of his contracting infection through contact with others.
    2. Decrease the metabolic wastes to be handled by his damaged kidney.
    3. Reduce the accumulation of edema fluid in his legs and feet.
    4. Prevent falling as a consequence of sudden therapeutic reduction in blood pressure.

7. Methyldopa (Aldomet) was given to Walter in order to:

    1. Alleviate anxiety.
    2. Prevent nausea.
    3. Decrease blood pressure.
    4. Inhibit inflammation.

8. The pharmacologic effect of methyldopa is to:

    1. Increase filtration through the glomeruli.
    2. Decrease absorption of fluid from the intestine.
    3. Decrease peripheral vascular resistance.
    4. Impair absorption from the renal tubules.

9. Walter should be observed for which of the following as possible toxic effects of methyldopa?

    a. Dry mouth.
    b. Nasal congestion.
    c. Mental depression.
    d. Postural hypotension.
    e. Visual disturbances.
        1. a and b.
        2. c and d.
        3. All but e.
        4. All the above.

10. Aluminum hydroxide can best be classified as:

    1. An antacid.
    2. A cathartic.
    3. A secretagogue.
    4. A bacteriostatic.

11. Aluminum hydroxide gel was given to Walter in order to:

    1. Increase appetite.
    2. Decrease nausea.
    3. Prevent diarrhea.
    4. Eliminate edema.

12. Which of the following is a possible untoward effect of aluminum hydroxide?

    1. Gingivitis.
    2. Hiccoughs.
    3. Avitaminosis.
    4. Constipation.

13. The pharmacologic effect of diazepam (Valium) is:

    1. Diuretic.
    2. Antihistaminic.
    3. Antibiotic.
    4. Sedative.

14. The nurse should expect to observe which of the following types of effects after Walter has taken diazepam for a few days?

    1. Idiosyncratic.
    2. Paradoxic.
    3. Cumulative.
    4. Allergic.

15. Which of the following are possible toxic effects of diazepam?

    1. Nausea and vomiting.
    2. Frequency and dysuria.
    3. Erythema and pruritus.
    4. Drowsiness and lethargy.

16. Walter should be watched closely for development of uremic symptoms, which include:

    a. Lethargy.
    b. Muscle twitching.
    c. Confusion.
    d. Foul breath.
    e. Skin crystals.
        1. a and c.
        2. b and d.
        3. All but d.
        4. All the above.

17. Urea, uric acid, and creatinine constitute the:
1. Building blocks for protein synthesis.
2. Enzymes released by dying cells.
3. Molecules responsible for oncotic pressure.
4. End products of protein catabolism.

18. Which of the following is the upper limit of normal for the concentration of blood urea nitrogen?
1. 5 mg. per 100 cc.
2. 20 mg. per 100 cc.
3. 40 mg. per 100 cc.
4. 60 mg. per 100 cc.

19. Which of the following is the normal concentration of serum creatinine?
1. 1.3 mg. per 100 cc.
2. 3.5 mg. per 100 cc.
3. 5.7 mg. per 100 cc.
4. 7.9 mg. per 100 cc.

20. Which of the following is the normal concentration of serum uric acid?
1. 3.–7. mg. per 100 cc.
2. 5.–9. mg. per 100 cc.
3. 7.–11. mg. per 100 cc.
4. 9.–13. mg. per 100 cc.

21. Which of the following is the normal concentration of serum potassium?
1. 0.5–2.0 mEq. per liter.
2. 2–3.5 mEq. per liter.
3. 3.5–5.0 mEq. per liter.
4. 5–6.5 mEq. per liter.

22. Which of the following is the usual result of excessive concentrations of serum potassium?
1. Generalized edema.
2. Kidney stones.
3. Bleeding tendencies.
4. Cardiac standstill.

23. The use of peritoneal dialysis in the treatment of renal failure is based upon the principle that:
1. The peritoneum permits transfer of substances only from the interior of a vessel outward.
2. Electrolytes move across a semipermeable membrane from a higher to a lower concentration.
3. When the blood pressure is elevated, fluid passes more readily from the blood into the tissues.
4. Accumulation of toxic metabolites in uremia render tissue capillaries unusually porous.

24. The objectives for treating Walter with peritoneal dialysis were to:

a. Remove excess intra- and extracellular fluid.
b. Prevent cardiotoxic effects from rising serum potassium.
c. Decrease serum concentration of neurotoxic metabolites.
d. Stimulate urine formation by external kidney pressure.
e. Prevent fecal impaction by diluting bowel contents.
1. a and b.
2. a, b, and c.
3. All but e.
4. All the above.

25. It is the nurse's responsibility to prepare Walter for insertion of the peritoneal dialysis catheter by:
a. Placing him in side-lying position.
b. Recording his temperature, pulse, and blood pressure.
c. Administering a cleansing enema.
d. Instructing him to empty his bladder.
e. Encouraging him to push fluids.
1. a and b.
2. b and d.
3. All but d.
4. All the above.

26. The nurse's responsibility in assisting with Walter's peritoneal dialysis includes:
1. Unclamping the fluid inflow and outflow tubes simultaneously.
2. Regulating the dialysate flow rate to 60 drops per minute.
3. Encouraging him to drink large quantities of liquids.
4. Warming the dialysate to 40° C. before instillation.

27. The dialyzing solution should be allowed to remain in the peritoneal cavity for how long a period of time?
1. 3 to 5 minutes.
2. 10 to 15 minutes.
3. 30 to 45 minutes.
4. 60 to 90 minutes.

28. The physician usually takes which of the following steps to prevent obstruction of the peritoneal catheter?
1. Irrigates the catheter with normal saline solution.
2. Withdraws the catheter a few millimeters each day.
3. Adds heparin to the dialysate before instillation.
4. Insufflates the catheter with an aseptic syringe.

29. In the event that the dialysate does not drain readily from Walter's abdomen to the floor bottle, the nurse should:

1. Run more fluid into the peritoneal cavity to increase intra-abdominal pressure.
2. Apply pressure to the lower abdomen with both hands and move him from side to side.
3. Disconnect the drainage tubing and aspirate fluid through the catheter with an aseptic syringe.
4. Assist him to a standing position and direct him to cough forcefully.

30. During peritoneal dialysis Walter's temperature should be taken every 4 hours to detect development of:

1. Dehydration.
2. Shock.
3. Peritonitis.
4. Uremia.

31. Walter's pulse should be recorded every hour during dialysis in order to detect the occurrence of:

1. Intraperitoneal hemorrhage.
2. Acute anxiety.
3. Cardiac arrhythmias.
4. Intestinal perforation.

32. A sudden drop in Walter's blood pressure during dialysis would probably be the result of:

1. Congestive heart failure due to increase in circulating blood volume.
2. Reflex dilation of splanchnic vessels in response to mechanical pressure.
3. Extreme reduction in blood volume due to the osmotic effect of dialysate.
4. Traumatic rupture of mesenteric blood vessels due to overdistention.

33. Which of the following are possible complications of continuous peritoneal dialysis?

a. Decubiti.
b. Pneumonia.
c. Hemorrhage.
d. Adhesions.
e. Peritonitis.
   1. a and b.
   2. a, b, and c.
   3. All but e.
   4. All the above.

34. On the third day of peritoneal dialysis Walter complained of severe abdominal pain, which would be apt to develop as a result of:

a. Improper temperature of the dialyzing solution.
b. Incomplete removal of dialyzing solution.
c. Development of peritoneal infection.
d. Occurrence of ureteral colic.
e. Cessation of intestinal peristalsis.
   1. a or b.
   2. a, b, or c.
   3. All but e.
   4. All the above.

35. The nurse who cares for Walter during his three days of peritoneal dialysis should record the following information:

a. The amount of fluid instilled and removed at each infusion.
b. The time of beginning and ending of each infusion.
c. The exact composition of dialysate and drugs infused.
d. Vital signs obtained at intervals during the procedure.
e. His weight and blood pressure before and after dialysis.
   1. a and b.
   2. a, b, and c.
   3. All but e.
   4. All the above.

36. During his stay in the Dialysis Unit Walter should not be visited by:

1. Children under twelve.
2. Close family members.
3. Employees from his place of work.
4. Staff members with respiratory infections.

37. In evaluating Walter's response to health teaching, the nurse should make allowances for the fact that his elevated blood urea nitrogen, creatinine, and uric acid will interfere with his ability to:

a. Attend to facts presented for consideration.
b. Concentrate on details of procedures.
c. Abstract significant points in a discussion.
d. Generalize from observation of specific events.
e. Express himself accurately and succinctly.
   1. a and b.
   2. a, b, and c.

3. All but e.
4. All the above.

38. The relative unavailability of hemodialysis facilities made it necessary to screen Walter as an applicant for hemodialysis in order to determine that he:

1. Was psychologically stable and motivated to survive.
2. Had the potentiality of regaining full renal function.
3. Had one kidney which was completely free of disease.
4. Had located a kidney donor for later renal transplant.

39. In preparation for hemodialysis, a cannula was implanted in Walter's left arm to provide a semipermanent connection between:

1. Two separate points on the radial artery.
2. The radial artery and the cephalic vein.
3. The radial artery and the ulnar artery.
4. The radial vein and the median cephalic vein.

40. In some patients being prepared for hemodialysis a leg is cannulated. The chief advantage in cannulating a leg rather than an arm is the fact that the leg cannula:

1. Is less undesirable cosmetically.
2. Is less subject to trauma.
3. Enables the patient to dialyze himself.
4. Is less subject to contamination.

41. After his arm has been cannulated Walter should be instructed to:

1. Wear an arm sling to protect the cannula from injury.
2. Keep his arm elevated whenever he is lying down.
3. Carry cannula clamps on his person at all times.
4. Keep his shirt sleeve rolled to expose the cannula to view.

42. Rather than an external cannula, a surgically created subcutaneous arteriovenous fistula can be used for connection to the artificial kidney. The fistula is superior to the cannula in that it:

1. Provides greater volume of blood flow.
2. Creates less danger of hemorrhage.
3. Causes less trauma to blood vessels.
4. Eliminates the possibility of infection.

43. To which of the following complications is Walter especially subject as a result of the cannulization of his arm?

a. Hemorrhage.
b. Hypertension.
c. Infection.
d. Neuritis.
e. Contracture.
  1. a and c.
  2. b and d.
  3. All but e.
  4. All the above.

44. Dialyzing fluid differs from normal plasma in that it contains:

a. A higher concentration of glucose.
b. A higher concentration of sodium.
c. A lower concentration of urea.
d. A lower concentration of potassium.
e. A lower concentration of phosphate.
  1. a and c.
  2. a, c, and e.
  3. b and d.
  4. All the above.

45. Walter's plasma will differ from the dialyzing fluid in that it will contain:

a. A higher concentration of sodium.
b. A higher concentration of potassium.
c. A lower concentration of urea.
d. A lower concentration of bicarbonate.
e. A lower concentration of chloride.
  1. a and c.
  2. b and d.
  3. c and e.
  4. All the above.

46. During Walter's dialysis, heparin was used to:

1. Prevent clotting in the artificial kidney.
2. Retard clotting in the arm cannula.
3. Minimize intravascular clotting due to immobility.
4. Decrease embolization of clots from the cannula.

47. If Walter's blood is heparinized as it enters the dialyzer, the effect of heparin can be neutralized by the addition of which of the following to the blood being returned to Walter's arm vein?

1. Prostigmine.
2. Procainamide.
3. Pilocarpine.
4. Protamine.

48. Walter should be taught to care for his cannula at home by:

1. Cleansing the skin around the cannula daily with antiseptic solution.
2. Keeping the cannula insertion site covered with adhesive tape.
3. Irrigating the cannula daily with sterile normal saline solution.
4. "Milking" the tubing daily to prevent clot formation.

49. An antiseptic, such as 70 percent alcohol, is preferred to green soap for cleansing the cannula because the latter:

1. Irritates the wound edges, causing pain and discomfort.
2. Makes the tubing connections slippery, fostering disconnection.
3. Causes deterioration of the plastic tubing and connectors.
4. Is inactivated by the protein constituents of body fluids.

50. Walter should be instructed to do which of the following in order to offset the possibility of occlusion of his shunt by clots?

1. Apply warm compresses to the cannula q.i.d.
2. Exercise his arm at periodic intervals.
3. "Milk" the tubing with the other hand.
4. Rotate the tubing at the point of insertion.

51. In the event that Walter's cannula does become obstructed by clots, the doctor or nurse may "wash" the clots from the arterial and venous sides of the cannula by using:

1. Sterile distilled water.
2. Dilute hydrogen peroxide.
3. Warmed heparinized saline.
4. 5 per cent dextrose solution.

52. While he is being maintained on hemodialysis, Walter will probably be subjected to which of the following dietary restrictions?

1. Limitation of calories.
2. Limitation of carbohydrate.
3. Limitation of fats.
4. Limitation of protein.

53. During this same period Walter's intake of which of the following electrolytes will also be restricted?

1. Calcium and phosphorus.
2. Iron and magnesium.
3. Sodium and potassium.
4. Chlorine and sulfur.

54. Walter's intake of carbohydrate and fat is chiefly beneficial to him in:

1. Supplying the calories required to keep him slightly overweight.
2. Reducing protein catabolism, thus reducing renal work load.
3. Providing alkaline metabolic end products to combat acidosis.
4. Improving appetite by stimulating secretion of gastric juice.

55. Which of the following food servings contains the most protein?

1. One cup of cooked lima beans.
2. One tablespoon of peanut butter.
3. One boiled egg.
4. One cup of whole milk.

56. Which of the following food servings contains the least protein?

1. One cup of cooked red beans.
2. One half cup of creamed cottage cheese.
3. Two slices of whole wheat bread.
4. Three ounces of fried perch.

57. In order to evaluate the quality of Walter's self-care the nurse should know that which of the following is the usual amount of weight gain between successive dialyses?

1. 1 to 2 Kg.
2. 3 to 4 Kg.
3. 5 to 6 Kg.
4. 7 to 8 Kg.

58. In addition to hemodialysis Walter will probably occasionally need which of the following treatments to prevent symptoms of renal failure?

1. Insertion of ureteral catheters.
2. Transfusion of packed red blood cells.
3. Needle aspiration of pleural fluid.
4. Alcohol block of peripheral nerves.

59. Which of the following psychological reactions are frequently observed in patients undergoing dialysis?

a. Anxiety.
b. Denial.
c. Depression.
d. Hysteria.
e. Euphoria.

    1. a and b.
    2. a, b, and c.
    3. All but d.
    4. All the above.

60. During his thrice-weekly visits to the dialysis unit Walter made many self-deprecating remarks in his conversations with the nurse. Such diminution in his self-concept is most apt to result from:

1. The dependent position into which he has been forced by his illness.
2. The toxic effect of metabolic waste products on his nervous tissue.
3. Taunts by family and friends regarding restrictions made on his activities.
4. Fear that his illness constitutes punishment for past sins and failures.

61. As defined by Engel, psychological stress results from loss of psychic objects, injury, or frustration of drives. In Walter's case, which of the following could be considered losses?

a. Restricted use of the cannulated extremity.
b. Separation from his family during dialysis.
c. Day to day uncertainty about his state of health.
d. Uncertainty regarding his future financial status.
e. The need for Walter's wife to seek employment.
   1. a and b.
   2. b and d.
   3. All but a.
   4. All the above.

62. Which of the following threats provoked by hemodialysis would probably be most stressful to Walter?

1. Frustration created by immobilization during dialysis.
2. Reluctance to become dependent on others for survival.
3. Inability to relinquish the role of head of the household.
4. Anxiety concerning the proper functioning of his cannula.

63. During treatment for his chronic renal disease which of the following would be apt to create the greatest degree of frustration for Walter?

1. Rigid dietary restrictions.
2. Bone and joint pain.
3. Diminished sexual potency.
4. Loss of physical strength.

64. Walter's self-image will change as his chronic renal disease progresses. Which of the following adaptive mechanisms would he be most apt to use in his early adjustment to his illness?

1. Withdrawal.
2. Regression.
3. Denial.
4. Introjection.

65. Walter confided in the nurse, "I don't have as many problems as that guy being dialyzed in the next bed." His statement best illustrates the use of which defense mechanism?

1. Projection.
2. Sublimation.
3. Compensation.
4. Identification.

66. Walter said to the nuse: "Oh, once in a while I have a little pain but I just ignore it and keep on with what I'm doing." Recognizing that Walter's statement indicates use of a defense mechanism, the nurse should:

1. Respond by suggesting that he may be avoiding his problems and point out that he does have certain limitations.
2. Reflect his comment by restating his thought in similar but slightly different words and phrases.
3. Evaluate his reason for using the defense mechanism and consider its value to him at the present time.
4. Follow Walter's lead and minimize the importance of the physical limitations imposed by his illness.

67. For which of the following reasons would Walter's illness place a strain on his interactions with his family?

a. Relatives might fear that they may be asked to donate a kidney to Walter.
b. Walter's hospitalization makes it necessary for his wife to become the breadwinner.
c. Walter's discomfort makes him envious of the good health of those around him.
d. Walter's treatment regimen necessitates gross alterations in family meals and activities.
e. Relatives respond differently to Walter as they observe changes in his appearance.
   1. a only.
   2. a, b, and d.
   3. b, c, and d.
   4. All the above.

68. In talking with the nurse Mrs. Proxmire said, "Walter's illness has been a severe blow to both of us but, thank heaven, everyone has gone out of their way to help him through it all." Which statement by the nurse would be most supportive to Mrs. Proxmire?
  1. "It is at a time like this that friends can be most helpful. I hope that they continue to visit him often."
  2. "Separation from your husband, financial worries, and your concern for his welfare must be very difficult for you."
  3. "The agony of a long, drawn out illness like his is physically and emotionally stressful for everyone concerned."
  4. "We can never really understand why God allows some persons to become ill and others to enjoy good health."

69. Self-destructive behavior may appear in various forms in the chronic dialysis patient. Which of the following is a common and successful means of suicide in renal patients?
  1. Deliberate contamination of the cannula.
  2. Refusal to accept the dialysis procedure.
  3. Failure to take prescribed medicines.
  4. Overdosing with food and drink.

70. The incidence of suicide in chronic dialysis patients is how many times higher than in the general population?
  1. 2 times.
  2. 10 times.
  3. 50 times.
  4. 100 times.

71. In order to provide Walter with needed emotional support the nurse should appreciate that he is subject to economic worries deriving from:
  a. The financial demands imposed by his young family.
  b. Lack of savings to cover the expenses of illness.
  c. The long term nature of chronic renal disease.
  d. The high cost of hospitalization and dialysis.
  e. Loss of work efficiency due to his symptoms.
    1. a and b.
    2. a, b, and c.
    3. All but e.
    4. All the above.

72. The stress of chronic dialysis could be reduced for both Walter and his family by:
  a. Group therapy.
  b. Health education.
  c. Individualization of care.
  d. Financial aid.
  e. A private hospital room.
    1. a, b, and d.
    2. b, c, and d.
    3. All but e.
    4. All the above.

Ulcerative Colitis and Ileostomy

At thirty-five Edna Cavers developed flatulence and diarrhea of increasing severity. When she was passing 8 to 10 stools daily and had lost 20 pounds of weight she sought medical attention.

On hospital admission Edna appeared pale and emaciated. Her red blood cell count was 3.3 million per cubic millimeter of blood; her hemoglobin was 9.5 Grams per cent; and her hematocrit was 36 per cent. Proctoscopic examination revealed the rectal mucosa to be diffusely ulcerated, edematous, and hemorrhagic. Lower gastrointestinal x-rays revealed a narrow, rigid, pipe-like configuration of the colon consistent with a diagnosis of chronic ulcerative colitis. Stool examinations and cultures were negative.

Mrs. Cavers was treated with a low residue, high protein, high caloric diet, phenobarbital 30 mg. t.i.d., bismuth subcarbonate Gram 1 orally q. 4 h., multivitamins, iron dextran injection (Imferon) 50 mg. I.M. q.i.d., atropine sulfate 0.6 mg. H. q. 6 h., and salicylazosulfapyridine (Azulfidine) Gram 1 orally q.i.d. The physician, dietician, and floor nurses all noted that Mrs. Cavers seemed to be withdrawn and depressed concerning her condition.

After three weeks of treatment Mrs. Cavers' stools had decreased to 3 or 4 a day, so she was discharged to the Ulcerative Colitis Clinic where she was to be followed.

(ANSWER BLANK ON PAGE A–103) (CORRECT ANSWERS ON PAGE B–173)

1. The causes of ulcerative colitis are thought to be:
 a. Malignant degeneration.
 b. Auto-immune reaction.
 c. Psychosomatic response.
 d. Bacterial infection.
 e. Nutritional deficiency.
  1. a and b.
  2. b and c.
  3. c and d.
  4. d and e.

2. It has been suggested by some authorities that the patient with colitis typically reveals which of the following personality characteristics?
 a. A degree of compulsiveness about achievement and schedules.
 b. Overconcern regarding the significance of others' behavior toward him.
 c. Irritability and angry emotional outbursts at times of stress.
 d. Marked covert dependence on selected members of the health team.
  1. a and c.
  2. b and d.
  3. b, c, and d.
  4. All the above.

3. Assessment of Mrs. Cavers' relationship to her husband or mother is apt to reveal a relationship in which Mrs. Cavers:
 1. Is under strong domination but is struggling to become free.
 2. Is frightened by her desire for mature sexual experience.
 3. Placidly accepts direction but is unable to carry out commands.
 4. Aggressively controls others by manipulating important family decisions.

4. While taking Mrs. Cavers' medical history the nurse should question her specifically to determine:
 1. Which foods or food combinations have increased her diarrhea.
 2. Her evaluation of the medical care which she has received to date.
 3. Her attitudes toward assuming independence and self-direction.
 4. The immunization procedures which she has received since birth.

5. In taking Mrs. Cavers' medical history the nurse should attempt to:
 1. Determine whether her illness is anatomic or functional in nature.
 2. Identify any factor in her personal life which may have triggered the attack.
 3. Evaluate the quality of medical supervision which she has received.
 4. Obtain a detailed medical history of other family members as well.

6. In addition to diarrhea, Mrs. Cavers might be expected to have which of the following, as symptoms which are typical of ulcerative colitis?
 a. Anorexia.
 b. Nausea.
 c. Extreme thirst.
 d. Low-grade fever.
 e. Abdominal cramps.
  1. a only.
  2. a and b.
  3. a, b, and c.
  4. All the above.

7. Mrs Cavers' anemia is probably of which type?
 1. Hypochromic, microcytic.
 2. Normochromic, normocytic.
 3. Normochromic, megaloblastic.
 4. Poikilocytic, hemolytic.

8. The narrow, rigid, pipe-like appearance of Mrs. Cavers' colon was probably the result of:
1. Hypertrophy of the smooth muscle fibers encircling the bowel wall.
2. Concretization of barium salts in fissures in the bowel lining.
3. Loss of bowel elasticity and length due to fibrosis and scarring.
4. Compensatory narrowing of bowel lumen following decreased food intake.

9. Stool examinations were done as part of Mrs. Cavers' diagnostic workup primarily in order to rule out:
1. Typhoid fever.
2. Duodenal ulcer.
3. Hookworm disease.
4. Amoebic dysentery.

10. After obtaining a specimen of Mrs. Cavers' stool for examination the nurse should:
1. Deliver the specimen immediately to the laboratory in the warm and fresh state.
2. Mix the specimen with chlorinated lime solution before taking it to the laboratory.
3. Refrigerate the specimen until it is picked up by a laboratory worker or technician.
4. Store the specimen in a warm water bath until time for delivery to the laboratory.

11. Microscopic examination of Mrs. Cavers' stool would be apt to reveal the presence of:
a. Bacteria.
b. Ova.
c. Mucus.
d. Blood.
e. Pus.
   1. a, b, and c.
   2. c, d, and e.
   3. All but d.
   4. All the above.

12. Biochemical examination of Mrs. Cavers' blood serum on hospital admission would be most apt to reveal a deficiency of:
1. Chloride.
2. Sodium.
3. Potassium.
4. Nitrogen.

13. The primary purpose for giving Mrs. Cavers a high protein diet was to:
1. Prevent infection of ulcerated mucosa.

2. Facilitate healing of intestinal mucosa.
3. Decrease fermentation of intestinal contents.
4. Restore red blood cell count to normal.

14. Which of the following is the best source of protein?
1. 1 cup of whole milk.
2. 1 egg.
3. ½ cup of cottage cheese.
4. ½ cup of cooked green beans.

15. Which of the following contains the most calories?
1. 1 slice of enriched whole wheat bread.
2. ½ cup of canned corn.
3. ½ cup of creamed cottage cheese.
4. 1 egg.

16. Which of the following foods should be avoided on a low residue diet?
a. Canned green beans.
b. Fried pork chops.
c. Cooked oatmeal.
d. Orange juice.
e. Apple pie.
   1. a and c.
   2. b and d.
   3. All but d.
   4. All the above.

17. Which of the following would be the chief disadvantage of administering a low residue diet to Mrs. Cavers over an extended period of time?
1. Atrophy of muscles of the intestinal wall.
2. Gradual increase in circulating blood volume.
3. Insufficient intake of vitamins and minerals.
4. Depletion of liver glycogen stores.

18. Phenobarbital was given to Mrs. Cavers in order to:
1. Alleviate nervous tension.
2. Decrease metabolic rate.
3. Relieve abdominal cramps.
4. Retard peristaltic action.

19. Bismuth subcarbonate was given to Mrs. Cavers for which of the following effects?
a. Astringent.
b. Spasmolytic.
c. Adsorbent.
d. Vasoconstrictive.
e. Antibacterial.
   1. a and c.
   2. b and d.

3. c and e.

4. All the above.

20. A disadvantage to the use of bismuth subcarbonate is the fact that it:

1. Irritates the mucosal lining of the stomach.

2. Interferes with absorption of vitamins.

3. Causes imbalance of intestinal flora.

4. Predisposes to formation of renal stones.

21. In administering the iron-dextran injection to Mrs. Cavers the nurse should:

1. Apply a tourniquet to the extremity several minutes before inserting the intravenous needle.

2. Heat the preparation in a warm water bath to render it fluid enough for injection.

3. Rub the injection site briskly to render it hyperemic before injecting the solution subcutaneously.

4. Pull the skin aside from the subcutaneous tissue before inserting the intramuscular needle.

22. The pharmacologic effect of atropine is to:

1. Potentiate epinephrine.

2. Stimulate norepinephrine.

3. Inactivate acetylcholine.

4. Block cholinesterase.

23. Atropine was given to Mrs. Cavers in order to:

1. Decrease intestinal motility.

2. Increase anal sphincter tone.

3. Reduce intestinal secretions.

4. Improve mesenteric blood flow.

24. Which of the following are symptoms of atropine toxicity for which Mrs. Cavers should be observed?

a. Rapid pulse.

b. Flushed face.

c. Dryness of the mouth.

d. Pinpoint pupils.

e. Shallow respirations.

　　1. a only.

　　2. a and b.

　　3. All but d.

　　4. All the above.

25. Which of the following would be a pharmacologic antidote for atropine intoxication?

1. Neostigmine.

2. Epinephrine.

3. Ergot.

4. Scopolamine.

26. The purpose for giving Mrs. Cavers salicylazosulfapyridine was to:

1. Avert respiratory infections secondary to malnutrition.

2. Decrease body temperature to normal levels.

3. Prevent secondary infection of colonic ulcers.

4. Block inflammatory response in intestinal mucosa.

27. Salicylazosulfapyridine differs from sulfadiazine primarily in that the former:

1. Is more soluble in body fluids.

2. Exerts a bacteriostatic rather than a bactericidal effect.

3. Is not absorbed from the intestine.

4. Is effective against gram-negative organisms.

28. Mrs. Cavers should be informed that which of the following may occur as a side effect of her Azulfidine therapy?

1. Orange-yellow discoloration of urine.

2. Maculo-papular skin rash.

3. Muscular tremor and incoordination.

4. Marked blurring of vision.

29. Which of the following are possible toxic effects of salicylazosulfapyridine?

a. Leukocytosis.

b. Hemolysis.

c. Agranulocytosis.

d. Hemophilia.

e. Thrombosis.

　　1. a and b.

　　2. b and c.

　　3. c and d.

　　4. d and e.

30. The nurse should observe Mrs. Cavers closely for development of which of the following as symptoms of intestinal perforation?

a. Temperature elevation.

b. Rapid pulse.

c. Vomiting.

d. Abdominal pain.

e. Abdominal rigidity.

　　1. a and b.

　　2. a, b, and c.

　　3. All but e.

　　4. All the above.

31. Which of the following would be contraindicated for Mrs. Cavers?

1. Ice cold liquids.

2. Bathroom privileges.

3. Back rubs.

4. Between meal snacks.

32. Which of the following are possible complications of ulcerative colitis?
    a. Electrolyte imbalance.
    b. Intestinal hemorrhage.
    c. Polyarthritis.
    d. Anal fistulae.
    e. Colonic carcinoma.
        1. a only.
        2. a and b.
        3. All but e.
        4. All the above.

33. Which of the following devices would be especially helpful in caring for Mrs. Cavers in the hospital?
    1. An overhead frame with trapeze.
    2. Padded bedside rails.
    3. A metal bed linen cradle.
    4. An alternating air pressure mattress.

34. Which of the following would best meet Mrs. Cavers' needs for personal hygiene?
    1. A partial bed bath given by the nurse q.i.d.
    2. A complete bed bath given daily by the nurse.
    3. A daily shower taken under the nurse's supervision.
    4. A daily tub bath with the nurse's assistance.

35. How should Mrs. Cavers' physical environment be adjusted so as to increase her comfort and improve her morale?
    1. Keep the blinds down and use only indirect lighting.
    2. Provide adequate ventilation and install a room deodorizer.
    3. Decrease the room temperature to 60° F.
    4. Place a screen around her bed and a "No Visitors" sign on her door.

36. A constructive approach to Mrs. Cavers' psychological management would include:
    a. Recognition and acceptance of her need to be dependent.
    b. Reassurance regarding the accessibility of preferred health workers.
    c. Acceptance of her compulsive need to supervise care given to her.
    d. Assessment of her expressions of anger as indications of stress.
    e. Firm insistence that she rapidly accept responsibility for self-care.
        1. a only.
        2. a and b.
        3. All but e.
        4. All the above.

37. Mrs. Cavers' care should be especially designed to protect her from which of the following complications of ulcerative colitis?
    1. Pneumonia.
    2. Halitosis.
    3. Decubiti.
    4. Contractures.

38. The nurse can protect Mrs. Cavers from excoriation of the skin surrounding her anus by:
    a. Keeping a clean bedpan on the bedside chair or at the foot of the bed.
    b. Helping her to cleanse the anal area following defecation when she is too weak to do so.
    c. Washing the perianal area with warm soapy water several times a day.
    d. Applying petrolatum to the skin around the anus following each cleansing.
    e. Protecting the perineal area during sleep through use of perineal pads.
        1. a and b.
        2. a, b, and c.
        3. All but d.
        4. All the above.

39. Mrs. Cavers' mother asked the nurse whether she and other family members could bring Mrs. Cavers food from home. Which response by the nurse would be most appropriate?
    1. "I'm sorry, but you may not bring her food from home. Her doctor has put her on a special diet."
    2. "I can't answer your question. Why don't you discuss that matter with Mrs. Cavers' physician?"
    3. "That's a good idea. I'll ask the dietician to give you a list of the foods she's allowed to eat."
    4. "If you bring food in, leave it in the diet kitchen. The dietitian will decide whether she can be given it."

Mrs. Cavers was followed in the Ulcerative Colitis Clinic for five years following her discharge from the hospital. Her husband died suddenly and she shortly thereafter developed severe diarrhea, with 10 to 12 blood-tinged and mucus-flecked stools per day, weakness, and dizziness. She was hospitalized and proctoscopy revealed a severe exacerbation of acute ulcerative colitis. Because Mrs. Cavers failed to respond to medical management, her doctor decided to perform a total colectomy and ileostomy. For three days prior to surgery she was given neomycin. For 24 hours preoperatively she was given only liquids. Immediately before surgery she was catheterized, a nasogastric tube was inserted and she was given 75 mg. of meperidine hydrochloride (Demerol) and 0.4 mg. of atropine sulfate hypodermically.

Following surgery her ileostomy bud, which was elevated about 1 inch above the surrounding abdominal skin, healed slowly. She seemed markedly depressed and responded unenthusiastically to the staff's efforts to teach her self-care methods. She was finally discharged from the hospital four weeks after the operation.

40. Which of the following measures should be undertaken in preparing Mrs. Cavers for the ileostomy procedure?
  a. Explanation by the physician of the nature and results of the operation.
  b. Description by the nurse of the care which she will receive postoperatively.
  c. Discussion with a healed ileostomy patient of his experiences in rehabilitation and self-care.
  d. Demonstration by the nurse of equipment and supplies used in caring for the ileostomy.
  e. Visit to the recovery room to which she will be returned following the operation.
    1. a and b.
    2. a, b, and c.
    3. All but d.
    4. All the above.

41. Which of the following would probably be included in Mrs. Cavers' preoperative preparation?
  a. Intravenous fluids.
  b. Low residue diet.
  c. Blood transfusions.
  d. Antibiotic therapy.
  e. Nasogastric intubation.
    1. a and b.
    2. a, b, and c.
    3. All but d.
    4. All the above.

42. In preparing Mrs. Cavers for surgery the nurse should inform her that, following the ileostomy, she will:
    1. Be able to eat all foods without intestinal problems.
    2. Wear an appliance day and night for the rest of her life.
    3. Be considerably restricted in her social and recreational activities.
    4. Remain on a high liquid bland soft diet indefinitely.

43. Neomycin was given to Mrs. Cavers in order to prevent:
    1. Imbalance of intestinal flora following surgery.
    2. Inadequate absorption of fat soluble vitamins.
    3. Postoperative infection of the suture lines.
    4. Postoperative hypostatic pneumonia and thrombophlebitis.

44. What will be the condition of Mrs. Cavers' operative incision immediately following her return from the operating room?
    1. The laparatomy incision will be undressed and the two stomata will be covered with fluff gauze.
    2. Both the abdominal incision and the exteriorized loop of bowel will be covered with moistened gauze.
    3. The skin wound will be dressed and a plastic bag will be secured over the ileostomy stoma.
    4. A catheter will be inserted into the ileostomy stoma and attached to continuous suction.

45. In order to teach Mrs. Cavers how to care for her ileostomy the nurse should know that the ileostomy stoma will not shrink to its permanent size until approximately how long after the operation?
    1. 6 days.
    2. 6 weeks.
    3. 6 months.
    4. 6 years.

46. Mrs. Cavers should be taught that her primary objective in caring for her ileostomy stoma should be to:
    1. Measure the volume of fecal output accurately.
    2. Prevent skin excoriation around the stoma.
    3. Maintain medical asepsis in handling equipment.
    4. Prevent development of unpleasant body odors.

47. Which of the following times would be best suited for the nurse to change Mrs. Cavers' temporary ileostomy bag?
    1. Immediately on arising.
    2. Immediately after breakfast.
    3. During the middle of the morning.
    4. During afternoon visiting hours.

48. In addition to a clean plastic drainage bag, which of the following should the nurse assemble for use in changing Mrs. Cavers' ileostomy bag?

    a. Fluff gauze.
    b. Folded newspapers.
    c. Bandage scissors.
    d. Rubber bands.
    e. Soft rubber catheter.
        1. a and b.
        2. a, b, and c.
        3. All but e.
        4. All the above.

49. Which of the following should be applied to the skin surrounding the ileostomy to protect it from injury by digestive juices?

    1. Tincture of benzoin.
    2. Zinc oxide paste.
    3. 70 per cent alcohol.
    4. Karaya gum powder.

50. The nurse can motivate Mrs. Cavers to want to learn to change the ileostomy bag herself by:

    a. Ensuring absolute privacy on each occasion that the bag is changed.
    b. Carrying out the procedure in a calm, efficient, matter-of-fact manner.
    c. Keeping the bedside unit spotlessly clean and free of unpleasant odors.
    d. Having well-adjusted ileostomates talk with her about the procedure.
    e. Arranging for staff members to stop frequently at her bed to talk to her.

    1. a and b.
    2. a, b, and c.
    3. All but d.
    4. All the above.

51. The nurse can best help to relieve Mrs. Cavers' postoperative depression by:

    1. Respecting her wish for privacy and her right to withdraw.
    2. Encouraging her to talk about her fears and anxieties.
    3. Initiating conversations concerning her family and her home.
    4. Providing her with reading and recreational materials.

52. In preparing Mrs. Cavers to care for herself at home the nurse should teach her to wash her permanent ileostomy bag with:

    1. Cold water and mild soap.
    2. Hydrogen peroxide and salt water.
    3. Hot water and green soap.
    4. Hexachlorophene and chlorine bleach.

53. After washing and drying her permanent ileostomy appliance, Mrs. Cavers should:

    1. Cover the outside of the bag with Vaseline.
    2. Wrap it in newspaper until the next use.
    3. Dust it with talcum inside and outside.
    4. Fill the bag with tissue paper before storage.

Bladder Carcinoma and Ureterosigmoidostomy

After dysuria, hematuria, and frequency of one week, 62-year-old Mrs. Roberta Pine reported to the hospital Outpatient Clinic for care. She was admitted to the hospital where, after she had voided 300 cc. of foul-smelling urine, an additional 150 cc. of urine was obtained by catheterization. Intravenous pyelography and cystoscopy revealed contracture of the bladder neck and trabeculations of the bladder wall. Biopsy of tissue from the bladder neck revealed transitional cell carcinoma. No bowel lesion was found on rectal examination.

After a thorough preoperative workup which included the usual diagnostic tests, liquid diet, and magnesium sulfate followed by three days' administration of neomycin and phthalylsulfathiazole, Mrs. Pine was taken to surgery where a radical cystectomy, hysterectomy, bilateral oophorectomy, and bilateral ureterosigmoidostomy were performed.

Mrs. Pine returned to the recovery room following surgery with a nasogastric tube in place, intravenous fluids running, and a rectal tube attached to a gravity drainage set-up. Other aspects of her postoperative care were:

1. *Pentazocine (Talwin) 30 mg. H. p.r.n. for pain.*
2. *Leaving the rectal tube in place to drain urine for 1 week, then encouraging her to void q. 3 to 4 h.*
3. *Daily fluid intake of 3000 cc. per day.*
4. *Macrodantin 100 mg. orally t.i.d.*
5. *Sodium bicarbonate 4 Grams orally t.i.d.*
6. *Elastic stockings until out of bed.*
7. *Series of 30 radiation treatments over a period of 6 weeks.*

(ANSWER BLANK ON PAGE A–105) (CORRECT ANSWERS ON PAGE B–177)

---

1. In the normal adult the capacity of the urinary bladder is:
1. 100 to 200 cc.
2. 300 to 400 cc.
3. 500 to 600 cc.
4. 700 to 800 cc.

2. In the healthy adult residual urine in the bladder does not exceed:
1. 5 cc.
2. 15 cc.
3. 30 cc.
4. 60 cc.

3. The fact that the nurse obtained 150 cc. of urine on catheterizing Mrs. Pine immediately after she had voided indicated that Mrs. Pine's bladder was:
1. Infected.
2. Decompensated.
3. Paralyzed.
4. Perforated.

4. Analysis of urine obtained by catheterizing Mrs. Pine would be most apt to reveal:
1. Glucose and acetone.
2. Red blood cells and albumin.
3. Bacteria and pus cells.
4. Casts and crystals.

5. Before her diagnostic workup is begun the nurse should ask Mrs. Pine whether she is hypersensitive to:
1. Milk.
2. Adhesive tape.
3. Iodine.
4. Sunlight.

6. Preparation of Mrs. Pine for her intravenous pyelogram should include:
1. Pushing fluids for several hours preceding the test.
2. Withholding food and fluids for twelve hours.
3. Intravenous administration of glucose solution.
4. Insertion of a urinary catheter and a rectal tube.

7. Mrs. Pine should be told that, upon intravenous injection of the dye, she may expect to experience:
1. Muscular spasms and twitching.
2. Colicky abdominal pain.
3. A brief period of vertigo.
4. A sensation of warmth.

8. During the intravenous pyelogram the nurse who attends Mrs. Pine should observe her carefully for which of the following as a possible symptom of toxic reaction to the dye?
a. Urticaria.
b. Diaphoresis.
c. Dyspnea.
d. Cyanosis.
e. Tachycardia.
   1. a only.
   2. a and b.
   3. c and d.
   4. All the above.

9. The nurse's preparation of Mrs. Pine for cystoscopy should include:
   a. Having her sign a permit for cystoscopy.
   b. Describing the cystoscopy equipment and technique.
   c. Withholding food for several hours before the procedure.
   d. Pushing fluids for several hours before instrumentation.
   e. Dressing her in hospital gown and lithotomy boots.
      1. a and b.
      2. b and c.
      3. All but d.
      4. All the above.

10. Which of the following descriptions of the cystoscopy procedure is best suited for explaining it to Mrs. Pine?
   1. "The doctor will insert a flexible metal tube containing a light into your bladder to examine it."
   2. "While you're asleep a periscope will be used to view the inside of your bladder."
   3. "You'll be in the same position and experience the same discomfort as in a regular pelvic examination."
   4. "This is a painless procedure by which the doctor will examine your lower urinary tract."

11. In positioning Mrs. Pine on the cystoscopy table particular pains should be taken to protect her from prolonged pressure on:
   a. Hamstring muscles.
   b. Saphenous vein.
   c. Popliteal artery.
   d. Peroneal nerve.
   e. Achilles tendon.
      1. a and b.
      2. b and c.
      3. c and d.
      4. d and e.

12. What precaution should be taken in the event that Mrs. Pine must lie on the cystoscopy table for an extended period of time?
   1. She should be helped to sit erect on the edge of the table every half hour.
   2. Her legs should be removed from the stirrups at intervals and flexed and extended a few times.
   3. She should be encouraged to cough and sigh deeply from time to time.
   4. Her arms, waist, and legs should be immobilized in soft canvas restraints.

13. During Mrs. Pine's cystoscopic examination the physician will be able to observe the:
   a. Appearance of the bladder mucosa.
   b. Size of the ureteral orifices.
   c. Presence and size of tumor masses.
   d. Condition of the vesicular muscle.
   e. Evenness of bladder expansion.
      1. a and b.
      2. a, b, and c.
      3. All but d.
      4. All the above.

14. Bladder trabeculations consist of:
   1. Local areas of inflammation.
   2. Discrete growths of tumor tissue.
   3. Ridges of hypertrophied muscle.
   4. Diverticula in the bladder wall.

15. The trabeculations observed in Mrs. Pine's bladder were probably the result of:
   1. Infection.
   2. Obstruction.
   3. Perforation.
   4. Ischemia.

16. Mrs. Pine could be expected to have which of the following symptoms on her return from cystoscopy?
   1. Burning and frequency.
   2. Urinary retention.
   3. Colicky pain.
   4. Bloody urine.

17. The nurse should notify the physician if, following cystoscopy, Mrs. Pine should develop:
   a. Bloody urine with clots.
   b. Shaking chills and fever.
   c. Complete inability to void.
   d. Stiffness of the knees.
   e. Burning on urination.
      1. a only.
      2. a, b, and c.
      3. All but d.
      4. All the above.

18. If Mrs. Pine's obstruction of the bladder neck were to be left untreated, which of the following would be possible complications of her illness?
   a. Cystitis.
   b. Hydro-ureter.
   c. Hydronephrosis.
   d. Nephrolithiasis.
   e. Uremia.
      1. a and b.

2. a, b, and c.

3. All but d.

4. All the above.

19. Which of the following are the so-called "non-specific" organisms which tend to cause infection in the patient with urinary tract obstruction?

a. *Escherichia coli.*

b. *Pseudomonas aeruginosa.*

c. *Proteus vulgaris.*

d. *Staphylococcus aureus.*

e. *Mycobacterium tuberculosis.*

  1. a and b.

  2. a, b, and c.

  3. All but e.

  4. All the above.

20. The chief purpose for the liquid diet given Mrs. Pine preoperatively was to:

1. Dilute bacterial toxins in the urine.

2. Assist in preoperative cleansing of the bowel.

3. Enhance absorption of neomycin and phthalylsulfathiazole.

4. Increase blood and tissue fluid volumes.

21. The purpose for Mrs. Pine's preoperative medications was to:

1. Clear the gut of stool and bacteria.

2. Decrease the congestion of pelvic tissues.

3. Eliminate acidic end products of metabolism.

4. Re-establish optimum water and electrolyte balance.

22. Magnesium sulfate acts as:

1. A systemic alkalizer.

2. A saline cathartic.

3. An osmotic diuretic.

4. A urinary acidifier.

23. Mrs. Pine was treated with neomycin preoperatively for its effect as:

1. A urinary bacteriostatic.

2. An antifungal agent.

3. A skin disinfectant.

4. An intestinal antiseptic.

24. The nurse should be aware that Mrs. Pine may develop which of the following as a side effect of neomycin therapy?

1. Stress incontinence.

2. Loose stools.

3. Vulvar pruritus.

4. Ringing in the ears.

25. Phthalylsulfathiazole was given Mrs. Pine for its effect in:

1. Inhibiting metastases.

2. Disinfecting the gut.

3. Stimulating hematopoiesis.

4. Acidifying the urine.

26. Mrs. Pine is not apt to develop symptoms of toxicity to phthalylsulfathiazole because:

1. She is receiving much less than the usual dose of the drug.

2. Very little of the drug will be absorbed from the intestine.

3. Any symptom of sulfonamide toxicity would be masked by nitrofurantoin.

4. Her large fluid intake will dilute the drug in her circulation.

27. Mrs. Pine's preoperative recovery would be most jeopardized by the nurse's failure to provide her ample opportunity before surgery to discuss and ask questions concerning:

1. The financial cost of the operation and ensuing hospitalization.

2. The changes in body functioning which will result from her operation.

3. The alterations which she must make in food and fluid intake.

4. The personal and professional qualifications of the surgical staff.

28. The surgeon's objective in performing Mrs. Pine's surgical operation was to:

1. Relieve dysuria and prevent urinary infection.

2. Decrease urinary frequency and prevent electrolyte imbalance.

3. Decrease retention and prevent bladder rupture.

4. Relieve urinary obstruction and prevent carcinoma metastasis.

29. The complications to which Mrs. Pine will be subject following the ureterosigmoidostomy are:

a. Recurrent kidney infections.

b. Chronic atonic constipation.

c. Reabsorption of urinary electrolytes.

d. Perforation of the bowel.

e. Thrombosis of hemorrhoidal veins.

  1. a and c.

  2. b and d.

  3. All but d.

  4. All the above.

30. Postoperatively the rectal tube will probably be held in position by means of:
   1. A perineal belt.
   2. Gauze packing.
   3. Adhesive tape.
   4. An inflatable balloon.

31. The position of and drainage from Mrs. Pine's rectal tube should be checked at frequent intervals because:
   1. Liquid fecal drainage would indicate chemical irritation of the bowel wall by preoperative medications.
   2. Obstruction of the tube, with consequent back pressure, would weaken the ureterosigmoid anastomosis.
   3. Absence of urinary drainage would reveal ureteral obstruction by metastatic tumor tissue.
   4. Dark and foul-smelling drainage would suggest infection or necrosis of the suture line.

32. Pentazocine (Talwin) has an analgesic effect similar in strength to that of:
   1. Meperidine (Demerol).
   2. Codeine.
   3. Propoxyphene (Darvon).
   4. Aspirin.

33. Pentazocine differs from morphine principally in that pentazocine does not cause:
   1. Euphoria.
   2. Vomiting.
   3. Dizziness.
   4. Addiction.

34. Which of the following is the drug of choice for treatment of pentazocine toxicity?
   1. Nalorphine (Nalline).
   2. Atropine.
   3. Methylphenidate (Ritalin).
   4. Caffeine.

35. Macrodantin (a macrocrystal form of nitrofurantoin) was given to Mrs. Pine for its effect as a:
   1. Nonaddicting analgesic.
   2. Urinary bacteriocide.
   3. Smooth muscle relaxant.
   4. Systemic antacid.

36. Mrs. Pine should be observed for which of the following as a possible toxic effect of nitrofurantoin?
   1. Nausea.
   2. Pruritus.
   3. Drowsiness.
   4. Paresthesias.

37. The purpose for giving Mrs. Pine soda bicarbonate postoperatively was to:
   1. Stimulate her to drink large volumes of fluid.

2. Prevent acidosis due to urine reabsorption.
   3. Relieve gastric acidity caused by macrodantin.
   4. Compensate for inadequate respiratory gas exchange.

38. The purpose for having Mrs. Pine wear elastic stockings was to:
   1. Prevent phlebothrombosis.
   2. Eliminate pedal edema.
   3. Maintain blood pressure.
   4. Restore muscle tone.

39. During the immediate postoperative period the skin around Mrs. Pine's anus should be:
   1. Rubbed with alcohol.
   2. Covered with petrolatum.
   3. Painted with antiseptic.
   4. Dusted with talcum.

40. It may be advisable to protect Mrs. Pine from leakage of urine following removal of the rectal tube by:
   1. Applying a perineal pad and belt before preparing her for sleep.
   2. Teaching her to alternately tighten and relax her anal sphincter.
   3. Packing her rectum with Vaseline gauze after each use of the bedpan.
   4. Leaving a small padded bedpan under her hips at all times.

41. In planning rehabilitation for Mrs. Pine the nurse should operate on the assumption that Mrs. Pine will have less rectal incontinence of urine if:
   1. Her intake of food and fluid is temporarily reduced.
   2. Her requests for frequent linen change are ignored.
   3. She is successful in other activities of daily living.
   4. She is given less attention by the nursing staff.

42. Mrs. Pine should be taught to institute rectal tube drainage during sleep in order to:
   1. Decrease resorption of urinary electrolytes.
   2. Prevent soiling of bedclothes and linen.
   3. Permit accurate measurement of fluid output.
   4. Prevent reflux of urine into the ureter.

43. Mrs. Pine's preparation for self-care at home should include teaching her the importance of:
   a. Avoiding the use of harsh laxatives.
   b. Avoiding foods known to cause gas or diarrhea.

c. Emptying the rectum every 3 to 4 hours.

d. Washing the perineum daily with soap and water.

e. Washing rectal drainage equipment each morning after use.

   1. a and c.

   2. b and d.

   3. All but d.

   4. All the above.

44. Mrs. Pine should be told that, if she develops constipation at home, she should not take an enema for fear of causing:

   1. Increased resorption of urinary electrolytes from the bowel.

   2. Rupture of the anastomosis between ureter and sigmoid.

   3. Reflex smooth muscle spasm of the ureteral walls.

   4. Reflux of urine and stool into the ureter.

45. During predischarge instruction Mrs. Pine should be taught to report to her doctor which of the following symptoms, should they develop, as possible indications of electrolyte imbalance?

   a. Nausea.

   b. Diarrhea.

   c. Lethargy.

   d. Pruritus.

   e. Palpitations.

      1. a only.

      2. a, b, and c.

      3. All but d.

      4. All the above.

46. Following hospital discharge Mrs. Pine will probably be advised to eat which type of diet?

   1. Regular.

   2. Low sodium.

   3. Low fat.

   4. Low carbohydrate.

47. Following hospital discharge Mrs. Pine's daily fluid intake should be approximately:

   1. 1000 cc. per day.

   2. 2000 cc. per day.

   3. 3000 cc. per day.

   4. 4000 cc. per day.

Varicose Ulcer and Vein Stripping

Ivy Walker was 55, markedly overweight, and had been troubled with varicose veins ever since the first of her five children was born. She was admitted to the surgical unit of a small private hospital for treatment of a draining ulcer on the inner aspect of the left leg just above the medial malleolus. She commented that three months before, she had spent several days in bed with acute pain and swelling in her left calf.

The ulcer was two centimeters in diameter, covered with purulent exudate, and surrounded by an area of shiny and deeply pigmented skin. Culture of the exudate revealed staphylococci and streptococci. Mrs. Walker's physical examination revealed nothing of significance except obesity and severe varicosities of both legs. Trendelenburg test and phlebography revealed intact deep venous circulation in both legs and dilated, tortuous, superficial veins in both legs.

Mrs. Walker's leg ulcer was cleansed and debrided and the following orders were written for treatment:

   1. Complete bedrest.

   2. Tetracycline 250 mg. orally q. 6 h.

   3. Sterile cool normal saline soaks to the skin surrounding the ulcer for 30 minutes b.i.d., after which apply hydrocortisone ointment to ulcer and redress.

(ANSWER BLANK ON PAGE A–107) (CORRECT ANSWERS ON PAGE B–181)

1. Varicose veins can best be defined as:
1. Veins occluded by clots.
2. Abnormally dilated veins.
3. Inflammation of veins.
4. Fibrotic obliteration of veins.

2. Varicose veins tend to develop as a result of:
a. Incompetence of the valves.
b. Increased hydrostatic pressure in veins.
c. Inadequate support of veins by surrounding tissue.
d. Erosion of the endothelial lining of the veins.
e. Destruction of elastic fibers in venous walls.
    1. a only.
    2. a, b, and c.
    3. c, d, and e.
    4. All the above.

3. The greater and smaller saphenous veins are more subject to development of varicosities than are the deep femoral veins because the former:
1. Have thinner walls and smaller valves.
2. Are less subject to muscle pumping action.
3. Carry blood containing numerous microorganisms.
4. Are more subject to direct mechanical injury.

4. In evaluating Mrs. Walker's medical history the nurse should be aware that which of the following predispose to development of varicose veins?
a. Obesity.
b. Heredity.
c. Pregnancy.
d. Diabetes.
e. Prolonged standing.
    1. a and c.
    2. b and d.
    3. All but d.
    4. All the above.

5. Venous valves may be said to be incompetent when they:
1. Obstruct the flow of blood returning from the extremities to the heart.
2. Fail to prevent blood from flowing caudally under the influence of gravity.
3. Prevent the flow of blood between superficial and deep leg veins.

4. Fail to filter bacteria from the blood as it flows toward the heart.

6. Which of the following are common symptoms of varicose veins?
a. Easy fatigability.
b. Local heat.
c. Muscle cramps.
d. Red streaks.
e. Babinski reflex.
    1. a and c.
    2. b and d.
    3. All but e.
    4. All the above.

7. Varicose veins are most apt to develop in:
1. Postmen.
2. Dockworkers.
3. Barbers.
4. Accountants.

8. Had Mrs. Walker sought medical attention earlier, her physician would have advised her to avoid:
a. Wearing round garters.
b. Sitting with knees crossed.
c. Wearing a tight girdle.
d. Sitting for long periods of time.
e. Standing for long periods of time.
    1. a and c.
    2. b and d.
    3. All but d.
    4. All the above.

9. In giving her medical history Mrs. Walker may indicate that she has been troubled with exercise cramps in her legs, which would be the result of:
1. Irritation of sensory nerves by bacterial toxins.
2. Hypocalcemia consequent to intravascular thrombosis.
3. Pressure of edema fluid on inflamed vessel walls.
4. Decreased arterial supply secondary to venous congestion.

10. The chief cause for Mrs. Walker's leg ulcer was:
1. Pressure on overlying skin by a pulsating dilated vein.
2. Infection of skin by bacteria migrating from an underlying varix.
3. Tissue ischemia due to decreased arterial blood flow.
4. External trauma to the skin by repeated scratching.

11. Increased pigmentation of the skin surrounding Mrs. Walker's leg ulcer is probably due to:

1. Migration of numerous granulocytic white blood cells.
2. Destruction of epidermis and resultant exposure of dermis.
3. Pigmentation of tissues by extravasated red blood cells.
4. High concentration of reduced hemoglobin in skin capillaries.

12. Mrs. Walker's ulcer probably produced which of the following local symptoms?

1. Skin pallor.
2. Burning and itching.
3. Decreased skin temperature.
4. Dry gangrene.

13. The purulent exudate on the base of Mrs. Walker's leg ulcer consists of:

a. Living bacteria.
b. Dead phagocytes.
c. Blood serum.
d. Dead bacteria.
e. Devitalized tissue cells.

    1. a and b.
    2. a, b, and c.
    3. All but e.
    4. All the above.

14. Exudate from Mrs. Walker's ulcer was cultured in order to:

1. Determine the effectiveness of her physiological defenses.
2. Facilitate selection of the most effective antibiotic.
3. Discover whether the wound has been secondarily infected.
4. Obtain data for epidemiologic study of hospital infections.

15. In cleansing and dressing Mrs. Walker's leg ulcer the nurse should avoid use of:

1. pHisoHex.
2. Normal saline.
3. Cotton balls.
4. Adhesive tape.

16. In spite of the fact that Mrs. Walker's leg ulcer is infected, the nurse should use strict asepsis in treating and dressing the ulcer in order to:

1. Instruct Mrs. Walker in proper methods of wound care.
2. Prevent distortion of research data regarding hospital infections.
3. Defend herself against infection by the patient's microorganisms.
4. Protect her against secondary antibiotic resistant infection.

17. The Trendelenburg test is used to evaluate the:

1. Patency of the deep veins of the lower extremity.
2. Adequacy of arterial circulation to the feet and legs.
3. Competence of the valves of superficial and communicating veins.
4. Amount of edema in the subcutaneous tissues of the extremities.

18. In performing the Trendelenburg test the doctor had Mrs. Walker lie down with the left leg elevated to drain the veins, then applied a tourniquet around the left upper thigh and directed her to stand. The physician noted that following tourniquet application Mrs. Walker's leg veins filled rapidly from below. In the lower leg several large sacculations were visible along the course of the vein. When the tourniquet was removed the veins filled rapidly from above. These test findings indicated that:

1. Some of the superficial veins were dilated but all venous valves were competent.
2. Communicating veins of the lower leg were incompetent, those in the upper leg were competent.
3. Both the valves of the superficial veins and the valves of the communicating veins were incompetent.
4. The saphenofemoral valve, superficial veins, communicating veins, and deep veins were all incompetent.

19. Phlebography consists of:

1. Threading a catheter into the vein to record pressures.
2. Injection of air into the vein to locate local "blow-outs."
3. X-ray of the veins after injection with radiopaque material.
4. Tracing the course of a dilated vein on the overlying skin.

20. The primary purpose for placing Mrs. Walker on complete bedrest is to:

1. Reverse the negative nitrogen balance produced by infection.
2. Prevent contamination of the varicose ulcer.
3. Reduce the danger of injury to the legs.
4. Facilitate venous return flow from the legs.

21. Debridement consists of:
    1. Bringing raw wound edges into juxtaposition.
    2. Occlusion of open and bleeding vessels.
    3. Removal of infected and devitalized tissue.
    4. Reopening of an improperly healed wound.

22. The physician debrided the ulcer before initiating treatment in order to:
    1. Decrease the tissue mass to be nourished by the reduced blood supply.
    2. Eliminate foreign protein which might initiate an allergic tissue reaction.
    3. Permit better visualization of local tissue response to treatment.
    4. Remove the dead tissue which has served as a culture medium.

23. Which of the following would be best suited for cleansing Mrs. Walker's leg ulcer?
    1. Cotton balls, mild soap, and luke-warm water.
    2. Washrag, Ivory soap, and hot water.
    3. Soft brush, green soap, and cold water.
    4. Cotton-tipped applicators, iodine, and alcohol.

24. In the debridement procedure which of the following would be most helpful to flush necrotic material from the base of the ulcer?
    1. Distilled water.
    2. Normal saline.
    3. Hydrogen peroxide.
    4. Penicillin solution.

25. Staphylococci are normal inhabitants of human:
    a. Skin.
    b. Mouth.
    c. Nose.
    d. Throat.
    e. Intestine.
       1. a, b, and c.
       2. c, d, and e.
       3. All but e.
       4. All the above.

26. It is thought that tetracycline exerts a bacteriostatic effect by:
    1. Coagulation of bacterial protein.
    2. Interfering with protein synthesis.
    3. Altering pH of body fluids.
    4. Agglutination of bacteria.

27. Which of the following would be a contraindication to administration of tetracycline?
    1. Coronary heart disease.
    2. Diabetes mellitus.
    3. Chronic pyelonephritis.
    4. Hypochromic anemia.

28. It is of extreme importance that Mrs. Walker be given her tetracycline doses exactly on time in order to prevent:
    1. Irritation of gastrointestinal mucosa.
    2. Damage to liver parenchyma.
    3. Development of bacterial drug resistance.
    4. Occurrence of withdrawal symptoms.

29. For optimum effect, Mrs. Walker's tetracycline should be administered:
    1. With orange juice.
    2. In milk.
    3. One hour before meals.
    4. With meals.

30. The nurse should observe Mrs. Walker for diarrhea, which may develop during tetracycline administration due to:
    1. Overgrowth of pathological bacteria and fungi in the gut.
    2. Increase in the strength of peristaltic contractions.
    3. Chemical irritation of the lining of the intestine.
    4. Absorption of fluid from capillaries into the bowel.

31. Allergic reactions to tetracycline would probably be evidenced by:
    a. Urticaria.
    b. Excessive tearing.
    c. Angioedema.
    d. Sneezing.
    e. Convulsions.
       1. a and c.
       2. b and d.
       3. All but d.
       4. All the above.

32. Which of the following is best suited for emergency treatment of the patient with severe hives?
    1. Diphenhydramine.
    2. Chlorpheniramine.
    3. Epinephrine.
    4. Meprobamate.

33. For which of the following effects was hydrocortisone ointment ordered for Mrs. Walker's ulcer?
    1. Facilitation of protein synthesis.
    2. Interference with inflammatory response.

3. Dilation of peripheral vessels.
4. Lowering of basal metabolic rate.

34. Which of the following may be applied to the skin surrounding an ulcer to stimulate healing?
1. Silver nitrate.
2. Calamine lotion.
3. Compound tincture of benzoin.
4. Sulfamylon ointment.

After one week of treatment Mrs. Walker's leg infection had subsided so the physician discontinued the tetracycline and ordered that the ulcer be cleansed and dressed twice a week and that an Unna's paste boot be applied after each dressing.

35. Healing of the ulcer began with the appearance of granulation tissue in the base of the defect. This granulation tissue consists of:
a. Capillary buds.
b. Fibroblasts.
c. Collagen fibers.
d. Muscle fibers.
e. White blood cells.
    1. a, b, and c.
    2. c, d, and e.
    3. All but d.
    4. All the above.

36. The principal ingredients of the Unna's paste boot which was applied to Mrs. Walker's leg were:
a. Normal saline.
b. Hydrogen peroxide.
c. Gelatin.
d. Glycerine.
e. Zinc oxide.
    1. a, b, and c.
    2. c, d, and e.
    3. All but e.
    4. All the above.

37. The purposes for applying an Unna's paste boot to Mrs. Walker's leg were to:
a. Protect the ulcer from trauma.
b. Decrease contamination of the wound.
c. Provide support for superficial veins.
d. Decrease the likelihood of vasomotor collapse.
e. Prevent orthopedic deformities during bedrest.
    1. a and b.
    2. a, b, and c.
    3. All but d.
    4. All the above.

38. Preparation of Mrs. Walker for application of an Unna's paste boot should include:
a. Elevating her legs for one half hour.
b. Covering the ulcer with dry sterile gauze.
c. Wrapping the leg in sheet wadding.
d. Encasing the limb in stockinette.
e. Flexing the knee in a 15° angle.
    1. a and b.
    2. c and d.
    3. All but d.
    4. All the above.

Mrs. Walker's ulcer continued to heal under this regimen. Three weeks later she was discharged from the hospital to the vascular clinic, where she was treated with Unna's paste boot until the ulcer was completely healed. Six months later Mrs. Walker was hospitalized for a vein stripping. She had an uneventful postoperative recovery and was discharged four days after surgery.

39. Before a vein stripping can be done it must be determined that:
1. The vein to be removed has been completely obstructed by clots.
2. The deep veins are competent to return the venous blood satisfactorily.
3. The inflammation of the vein wall has completely subsided.
4. The varicosities were caused solely by incompetent valves.

40. Immediately following her return from the operating room Mrs. Walker should be placed in which position?
1. Supine with legs abducted and separated by pillows.
2. Prone with feet extended over the mattress edge.
3. Supine with legs extended and elevated at a 30° angle.
4. Sitting on the bed edge with feet on a chair.

41. Mrs. Walker was directed to ambulate on the evening of the operative day in order to:
1. Test the adequacy of venous ligatures.
2. Prevent thrombosis of deep leg veins.
3. Prevent occurrence of orthostatic hypotension.
4. Foster resorption of interstitial edema.

42. In supervising Mrs. Walker to ambulate as ordered the nurse should:
   a. Explain the therapeutic purpose for early ambulation.
   b. Assist her to stand at the side of the bed.
   c. Remain at her side during the first few walks.
   d. Plan care to alternate walks with rest periods.
   e. Remove and reapply elastic bandages when loosened.
      1. a and b.
      2. a, b, and c.
      3. All but e.
      4. All the above.

43. Mrs. Walker's predischarge instruction should include teaching her how to:
   1. Massage her legs.
   2. Apply elastic bandages.
   3. Do range of motion exercises.
   4. Cut her toenails.

Multiple Sclerosis

Beulah Hoblet, a 20-year-old office worker, told her doctor, "I stumble all the time and I drop everything I touch." Physical examination revealed nystagmus, scanning speech, intention tremor, impairment of position and vibratory sense, and ataxic gait. Beulah indicated that she had had a similar episode of incoordination and tremor during the previous year, following an acute attack of influenza. Beulah's vital signs, chest x-ray, blood and urine examinations were all normal.

The physician diagnosed Beulah's disorder as multiple sclerosis, hospitalized her, and ordered the following:

   1. Bedrest.
   2. Chlordiazepoxide hydrochloride (Librium) 10 mg. orally t.i.d.
   3. A.C.T.H. 40 units b.i.d. I.M. for 7 days, then 30 units b.i.d. for 3 days, 20 units b.i.d. for 3 days, and 10 units b.i.d. for 3 days.
   4. Potassium chloride.

(ANSWER BLANK ON PAGE A–109) (CORRECT ANSWERS ON PAGE B–184)

Beulah's tremor disappeared, her ataxia lessened, and her speech became more clear, although she still had weakness of all four extremities. After three weeks of hospitalization she was instructed in range of motion exercises and discharged to her home. Arrangements were made for a public health nurse to visit three times a week to supervise her general hygiene and to follow up on range of motion exercises.

1. Which of the following is thought to be the cause of multiple sclerosis?
   1. Heavy metal poisoning.
   2. Chronic tuberculous infection.
   3. Auto-immune reaction.
   4. Absence of an oxidative enzyme.

2. Acute attacks of multiple sclerosis are apt to be precipitated by:
   a. Excessive chilling.
   b. Acute infection.
   c. Chronic fatigue.
   d. Physical trauma.
   e. Emotional upset.
      1. a and b.
      2. b and d.
      3. All but e.
      4. All the above.

3. The pathophysiology of multiple sclerosis consists of:

1. Chronic granulomatous inflammation of the meninges covering the brain and spinal cord.
2. Patchy destruction of the myelin sheath of axons within the central nervous system.
3. Pressure upon areas of the sensory and motor cortex by circumscribed accumulations of pus.
4. Formation of a large fluid-filled cavity in the central portion of the spinal cord.

4. Examination of Beulah's spinal fluid would be most apt to reveal:

1. Increase in gamma globulin.
2. Decrease in glucose.
3. Diminution in white blood cells.
4. Presence of red blood cells.

5. In order to plan effective care for Beulah the nurse should be aware that multiple sclerosis is characterized by:

1. A steady downhill course which rapidly ends in death.
2. Gradual deterioration with progressive loss of motor ability only.
3. Recurrences and remissions extending over a period of many years.
4. Loss of motor and sensory functions in the lower extremities only.

6. According to Fox, chronic illness may be defined as any major deviation from normal health which:

a. Is permanent and has no cure.
b. Is characterized by exacerbations and remissions.
c. Necessitates training or rehabilitation.
d. Lasts longer than three months.
e. Requires lasting supervision and care.
    1. a, b, and c.
    2. a, c, and e.
    3. All but e.
    4. All the above.

7. Which of the following factors will determine how Beulah will adjust to her illness and disability?

a. Physical fitness.
b. Emotional security.
c. Occupational skills.
d. Closeness to her family.
e. Financial status.
    1. a, b, and c.
    2. a, c, and e.

3. All but e.
4. All the above.

8. Nystagmus can best be defined as:

1. Inability to close the eyelids completely.
2. Improper alignment of the two eyes.
3. Involuntary rhythmic movements of the eyes.
4. Abnormal protrusion of the eyeball.

9. In addition to nystagmus Beulah may develop which of the following eye symptoms?

a. Scotoma.
b. Blindness.
c. Diplopia.
d. Exophthalmos.
e. Strabismus.
    1. a and b.
    2. a, b, and c.
    3. All but e.
    4. All the above.

10. Intention tremor consists of:

1. Trembling of the hand on performance of a precise, willed movement.
2. Shaking of the head initiated by concentration on a fixed point.
3. Muscular trembling initiated in order to draw sympathy from others.
4. Quivering of the extremities which can be controlled by an act of will.

11. Beulah is apt to develop which of the following as additional symptoms of multiple sclerosis?

a. Weakness of extremities.
b. Tingling in extremities.
c. Vertigo and vomiting.
d. Loss of position sense.
e. Urinary frequency and urgency.
    1. a and c.
    2. b and d.
    3. All but e.
    4. All the above.

12. In planning long term care for Beulah the nurse should know that which of the following may be late complications of multiple sclerosis?

a. Urinary incontinence.
b. Difficulty in swallowing.
c. Muscle contractures.
d. Paralysis of lower extremities.
e. Convulsive seizures.
    1. a and b.
    2. c and d.
    3. All but d.
    4. All the above.

13. A.C.T.H. is an enzyme secreted by the:
    1. Anterior pituitary gland.
    2. Posterior pituitary gland.
    3. Adrenal cortex.
    4. Adrenal medulla.

14. The direct pharmacologic effect of A.C.T.H. is to:
    1. Increase secretions of all endocrine glands.
    2. Stimulate secretion of adrenal corticosteroids.
    3. Store glucose in the form of liver glycogen.
    4. Regulate the metabolic rate of tissue cells.

15. Which of the following are possible toxic effects of A.C.T.H.?
    a. Increased blood pressure.
    b. Gastrointestinal bleeding.
    c. Increase in body hair.
    d. Elevated blood glucose.
    e. Acneform skin lesions.
        1. a and b.
        2. c and d.
        3. All but e.
        4. All the above.

16. Evidence of which of the following in Beulah's past medical history would constitute a contraindication to administration of A.C.T.H.?
    1. Penicillin allergy.
    2. Healed tuberculosis.
    3. Chronic constipation.
    4. Cigarette smoking.

17. Chlordiazepoxide (Librium) was given to Beulah in order to:
    1. Relieve anxiety.
    2. Improve appetite.
    3. Decrease tremor.
    4. Prevent convulsions.

18. Chlordiazepoxide may accentuate which of the symptoms of Beulah's illness?
    1. Double vision.
    2. Slurred speech.
    3. Emotional lability.
    4. Urinary frequency.

19. Potassium chloride was given to Beulah in order to:
    1. Stimulate regeneration of myelin on motor and sensory axons.
    2. Compensate for increased potassium excretion produced by A.C.T.H.
    3. Relieve edema by fostering urinary excretion of sodium.
    4. Improve appetite by stimulating secretion of digestive juices.

20. As a consequence of her drug therapy, Beulah is apt to develop:
    1. Skin rash.
    2. Peripheral edema.
    3. Dental caries.
    4. Orthostatic hypotension.

21. The nurses on the unit noticed that Beulah seemed to be extremely euphoric. Such euphoria is common in patients with multiple sclerosis and is thought to be due to:
    1. Loss of intellectual ability to appraise reality.
    2. Attempts to conceal symptoms from family members.
    3. Demyelination of fibers in the frontal lobe.
    4. Response to the staff's expectations of symptom remission.

22. After Beulah's diagnosis of multiple sclerosis was explained to her and she had realized her loss of function, she must do which of the following in order to adjust to her illness?
    a. Go through the mourning process.
    b. Change her value system.
    c. Redeem her self-esteem.
    d. Develop defense mechanisms.
    e. Accept some dependency on others.
        1. a and b.
        2. a, c, and e.
        3. All but e.
        4. All the above.

23. The nurse noted that Beulah spilled considerable food while feeding herself and frequently failed to eat all the food on her tray. The nurse could improve Beulah's morale and nutritional state by:
    a. Providing her a half hour rest period before each meal.
    b. Positioning pillows under her elbows during each meal.
    c. Arranging for her tray to be delivered first and removed last.
    d. Arranging for her to be given a plate guard and a built up spoon.
    e. Arranging for her to eat in a dining room with other patients.
        1. a and b.
        2. b and c.
        3. All but d.
        4. All the above.

24. The nurse noticed that, though Beulah frequently asked for help in bathing and eating, she seemed to resent any help given her. This ambivalence and anger probably re-

sulted from the fact that, to her, dependency:

1. Implied inferiority.
2. Suggested indebtedness.
3. Caused regression.
4. Erased hope.

25. To which of the following postural deformities will Beulah's prolonged bedrest predispose her?

a. Radial deviation of the hand.
b. External rotation of the hip.
c. Supination of the forearm.
d. Plantar flexion of the foot.
e. Hyperextension of the neck.
   1. a and c.
   2. a and d.
   3. All but e.
   4. All the above.

26. In providing Beulah's care it would be of primary importance for the nurse to avoid:

1. Rushing her.
2. Disciplining her.
3. Protecting her.
4. Stimulating her.

27. In describing the optimum amount of physical activity for Beulah following hospital discharge, the nurse should advise her to:

1. Refrain from all but essential musculoskeletal activity.
2. Exercise daily but not to the point of provoking extreme fatigue.
3. Push herself toward maximum activity to prevent contractures.
4. Maintain activity of small rather than large skeletal muscles.

28. Beulah's family should be prepared for her to exhibit which of the following emotional responses?

1. Gradual withdrawal from interaction with others.
2. Sudden outbursts of laughing or crying.
3. Suspicion of the motives and actions of others.
4. Hostile opposition to direction from others.

29. The nurse should instruct Beulah that the reason she is to perform range of motion exercises at home is to:

1. Retard the process of nerve demyelination.
2. Maintain maximum functioning of joints.
3. Prevent increases in her symptomatology.
4. Make her less difficult to care for at home.

30. The purpose of Beulah's range of motion exercises was to:

a. Prevent joint deformity.
b. Maintain peripheral circulation.
c. Prevent muscle contracture.
d. Maintain proprioceptive reflexes.
e. Enhance her feeling of well-being.
   1. a and b.
   2. a, b, and c.
   3. All but e.
   4. All the above.

31. In passively exercising Beulah's wrist, the nurse should:

a. Hold the elbow in fixed position.
b. Support the weight of the forearm.
c. Grasp the hand in her own hand.
d. Move the wrist without Beulah's assistance.
   1. a and d.
   2. b and d.
   3. c and d.
   4. All the above.

32. During Beulah's passive exercises the degree of motion of each joint should be such so as not to produce:

1. Hyperextension.
2. Fatigue.
3. Pain.
4. Crepitus.

33. Active assistive exercises differ from active exercises in that in the former the nurse:

1. Verbally directs the action to be taken.
2. Provides physical stimulus for the desired movement.
3. Manually supports the distal part.
4. Offers physical resistance to joint movement.

34. On her first home visit the public health nurse observed that Beulah seemed despondent over the fact that she was having great difficulty dressing and undressing herself. Which action by the nurse would be most helpful to Beulah?

1. Encouraging her to persist in trying to master the activity.
2. Suggesting that she ask her mother to help her dress and undress.
3. Directing the mother to offer to help Beulah dress and undress.
4. Showing the mother how to substitute Velcro fasteners for hooks and buttons.

35. During her postdischarge clinic visits Beulah's neurologic examinations would probably include which of the following tests and observations?
    a. Ability to rise from sitting position.
    b. Typical stance and gait.
    c. Visual acuity.
    d. Strength of muscle contraction.
    e. Romberg test.
        1. a and b.
        2. c and d.
        3. All but d.
        4. All the above.

36. In dealing with her conflicts about dependency and consequent hostility, Beulah would be most likely to adopt which of the following behaviors?
    1. Verbally attacking those on whom she must rely for care.
    2. Acquiescing to all demands placed on her by others.
    3. Manipulating others to carry out her wishes through seductive behavior.
    4. Attempting to make others dependent on her in some way.

After six months at home Beulah developed stress incontinence. Cystoscopy revealed bladder atony and acute cystitis. Her physician ordered bethanechol chloride (Urecholine) 10 mg. orally t.i.d.

37. Bethanechol chloride (Urecholine) has which of the following effects?
    1. Sympathomimetic.
    2. Sympatholytic.
    3. Parasympathomimetic.
    4. Parasympatholytic.

38. Bethanechol chloride was given to Beulah in order to:
    1. Inhibit growth of bacteria in urine.
    2. Increase the tone of bladder muscle.
    3. Prevent transmission of pain impulses.
    4. Stimulate constriction of the urinary sphincter.

39. Which of the following is a possible toxic effect of Urecholine?
    1. Asthma.
    2. Epistaxis.
    3. Syncope.
    4. Tinnitus.

40. Which of the following is the pharmacologic antidote for bethanechol?
    1. Atropine.
    2. Neostigmine (Prostigmine).
    3. Epinephrine.
    4. Phentolamine (Regitine).

Beulah's urinary symptoms gradually disappeared, her strength increased, and she was eventually able to return to her job as a clerk typist.

Systemic Lupus Erythematosus

Elvira Scuggs, an 18-year-old Black girl, was admitted to the hospital with malaise, fever, chest pain, polyarthralgia, lymphadenopathy, and an erythematous butterfly-shaped rash over her nose and malar eminences. She indicated that she had experienced several similar episodes during the previous four years and had had frequent "colds" during the past year.

On admission Elvira's temperature was 102° F. orally, pulse 100 per minute, and respirations 22 per minute. Her cervical and axillary lymph nodes were enlarged. Her hematocrit was 27 per cent and her white blood cell count was 7000/mm³ with a normal differential count. Blood studies revealed hypogammaglobulinemia and the presence of numerous L. E. cells. Urinalysis revealed 3 to 5 white blood cells per high power field, 3 to 5 red blood cells per high power field, 1 + protein, and numerous casts. Nose, throat, and urine cultures were negative and the antistreptolysin-O titer was within normal limits.

Following a renal biopsy Elvira was diagnosed as having an acute exacerbation of systemic lupus erythematosus and was treated with absolute bedrest, prednisone 30 mg. orally b.i.d., propoxyphene hydrochloride (Darvon) 32 mg. orally p.r.n. for joint pain, and aspirin suppositories 0.6 Gr. rectally to decrease temperature.

(ANSWER BLANK ON PAGE A–111) (CORRECT ANSWERS ON PAGE B–187)

1. The tissue changes of lupus erythematosus are thought to be the result of:
1. Infection.
2. Auto-immunity.
3. Malnutrition.
4. Endocrine imbalance.

2. Clinical findings and laboratory data indicate that which of the following diseases may be closely related etiologically and pathologically to systemic lupus erythematosus?
a. Erysipelas.
b. Rheumatoid arthritis.
c. Pyelonephritis.
d. Scleroderma.
e. Psoriasis.
   1. a and c.
   2. b and d.
   3. All but d.
   4. All the above.

3. As well as respiratory, musculoskeletal, and urinary manifestations, systemic lupus erythematosus may produce changes in which of the following organs and tissues?
a. Retina.
b. Meninges.
c. Blood.
d. Heart valves.
e. Spleen.
   1. a and c.
   2. b and d.
   3. All but d.
   4. All the above.

4. In taking Elvira's medical history the nurse should know that which of the following symptoms frequently antedate the diagnosis of systemic lupus erythematosus by several years?
1. Episodes of severe, painless bleeding on urination.
2. Delayed healing of skin and mucosal lesions.
3. Painful ischemia of fingers on exposure to cold.
4. Occurrence of leg cramps following exercise.

5. The increased susceptibility to infection suggested by Elvira's medical history was probably due to:
a. Decreased numbers of granulocytic white blood cells.
b. Decreased integrity of skin and mucosal tissues.
c. Distortion and dysfunction of antibody molecules.
d. Inability of capillaries to dilate and constrict.
e. Infiltration of the hypothalamus by malignant cells.
   1. a and c.
   2. b and d.
   3. All but e.
   4. All the above.

6. In interpreting Elvira's medical history the nurse should be aware that which of the following often trigger acute exacerbations of systemic lupus erythematosus?
a. Exposure to sunlight.
b. Severe trauma.
c. Emotional upset.
d. Pregnancy.
e. Operative procedures.
   1. a and b.
   2. b and c.
   3. All but d.
   4. All the above.

7. Exacerbations of systemic lupus erythematosus may be triggered by which of the following drugs?
a. Potassium iodide.
b. Trimethadione.
c. Procainamide.
d. Isonicotinic acid hydrazide.
e. Hydralazine.
   1. a and b.
   2. a, b, and c.
   3. All but e.
   4. All the above.

8. In addition to the "butterfly" facial lesion, Elvira may demonstrate which of the following cutaneous symptoms elsewhere on her body?
- a. Maculopapular rash.
- b. Urticaria.
- c. Altered pigmentation.
- d. Alopecia.
- e. Purpura.
    1. a only.
    2. a, b, and c.
    3. All but d.
    4. All the above.

9. Elvira's systemic lupus erythematosus may produce which of the following symptoms of cardiovascular system involvement?
- a. Increased pulse rate.
- b. Cardiac arrhythmias.
- c. E.K.G. S-T segment changes.
- d. Pericardial friction rub.
- e. Cardiomegaly.
    1. a and b.
    2. c and d.
    3. All but e.
    4. All the above.

10. The tissue changes of systemic lupus erythematosus may produce which of the following symptoms of central nervous system dysfunction?
- a. Palsy.
- b. Convulsions.
- c. Hemiparesis.
- d. Paresthesias.
- e. Psychosis.
    1. a only.
    2. a and b.
    3. a, b, and c.
    4. All the above.

11. The L. E. cell or L. E. phenomenon, found on examination of Elvira's blood, consists of:
1. A granulocyte which has phagocytosed another leukocyte.
2. An erythrocyte of distorted or unusual shape.
3. A giant cell containing numerous peripheral nuclei.
4. A red cell from which hemoglobin has been extruded.

12. The L. E. cell phenomenon is also observed in:
- a. Dermatitis herpetiformis.
- b. Pernicious anemia.
- c. Myasthenia gravis.

- d. Penicillin hypersensitivity.
- e. Leukemia.
    1. a and b.
    2. c and d.
    3. All but d.
    4. All the above.

13. Histologic examination of Elvira's kidney tissue would be most apt to reveal:
1. Dilation of blood vessels and transudation into the tissues.
2. Replacement of normal tissue with broad bands of fibrous tissue.
3. Destruction of tissue by localized aggregations of purulent material.
4. Swelling of collagen tissue and infiltration with plasma cells.

14. Examination of Elvira's blood serum on hospital admission would probably reveal:
1. Abnormally increased concentrations of sodium, chloride, and calcium ions.
2. Numerous abnormal proteins having the characteristics of antibodies.
3. Large numbers of gram-positive cocci and gram-negative bacilli.
4. Abnormally low concentrations of glucose, cholesterol, and cholesterol esters.

15. Which of the following drugs would the physician be most apt to order to relieve Elvira's joint symptoms?
1. Aspirin.
2. Probenecid.
3. Colchicine.
4. Phenylbutazone.

16. Which of the following drugs is sometimes used to relieve the skin lesions associated with systemic lupus erythematosus?
1. Isoniazid.
2. Furadantin.
3. Chloroquine.
4. Promethazine.

17. Prednisone was given to Elvira for which of the following effects?
1. Adrenergic.
2. Anti-inflammatory.
3. Analgesic.
4. Ataractic.

18. To which of the following complications is Elvira subject as a result of her prednisone therapy?
- a. Fluid retention.
- b. Delayed healing.
- c. Peptic ulcer.

d. Intravascular thrombosis.
e. Psychotic reactions.
    1. a and b.
    2. a, b, and c.
    3. All but e.
    4. All the above.

19. Which of the following are the pharmacologic effects of propoxyphene (Darvon)?
  a. Relieves pain.
  b. Depresses cough.
  c. Decreases temperature.
  d. Blocks inflammation.
  e. Relaxes muscle spasm.
    1. a only.
    2. a and b.
    3. a, b, and c.
    4. All the above.

20. Aspirin reduces body temperature by:
  1. Decreasing the irritability of skeletal muscles.
  2. Impairing oxygen transmission to tissue cells.
  3. Inactivating oxidative enzymes in muscle cells.
  4. Resetting the hypothalamic temperature regulating center.

During the first two weeks of treatment Elvira's facial rash, joint symptoms, lymphadenopathy, and urinary findings steadily decreased. Three weeks after hospital admission Elvira became acutely disturbed, accusing the nurse of trying to kill her, refusing to eat, and pacing the floor at night. This reaction was assumed to be a drug-induced psychosis and the prednisone dosage was reduced to 20 mg. b.i.d. At this same time a guaiac test on Elvira's stool was positive and she complained of gastric distress. She was given magnesium-aluminum hydroxide suspension (Maalox), two drams in milk, p.c. and h.s.

21. Elvira was given magnesium-aluminum hydroxide suspension chiefly in order to:
  1. Improve her appetite and sense of well-being.
  2. Prevent constipation secondary to long bedrest.
  3. Correct electrolyte imbalance associated with renal dysfunction.
  4. Prevent a complication of adrenal steroid therapy.

22. Aluminum hydroxide produces which of the following untoward effects?
  1. Sialorrhea.
  2. Nausea.
  3. Diarrhea.
  4. Constipation.

23. Magnesium hydroxide exerts which of the following effects?
  a. Antihistaminic.
  b. Antacid.
  c. Choleretic.
  d. Cathartic.
  e. Depressant.
    1. a and c.
    2. b and d.
    3. All but d.
    4. All the above.

24. After four weeks of prednisone therapy Elvira presented a Cushingoid appearance, which consists of:
  a. Round face.
  b. Truncal obesity.
  c. Increased body hair.
  d. Purplish skin striae.
  e. Cervicothoracic hump.
    1. a and c.
    2. b and d.
    3. All but e.
    4. All the above.

25. Elvira's nursing care should be planned to protect her from:
  1. Tendency to undesirable weight gain.
  2. Increased susceptibility to infection.
  3. Diminution of distance and peripheral vision.
  4. Difficulty in swallowing secretions.

26. Which of the following devices should be used in providing care for Elvira in the hospital?
  1. Side rails.
  2. Footboard.
  3. Heat cradle.
  4. Balkan frame.

27. While Elvira is hospitalized, arrangements should be made to prevent her contact with:
  1. Healthy young persons of her own age.
  2. Children under the age of twelve.
  3. Relatives whom she hasn't seen for some time.
  4. Nurses with respiratory or skin infections.

28. The nurse should employ which of the following measures to keep Elvira from developing decubiti during her long period of bedrest?

    a. Keep lower sheets free of wrinkles, moisture, and foreign bodies.

    b. Turn her from back to side-lying position every two hours.

    c. Wash pressure points with mild soap and water and pat dry.

    d. Massage her back, hips, ankles, and heels with lotion daily.

    e. Protect bony prominences with sheep-skin or foam pads.

        1. a and b.

        2. a, b, and c.

        3. All but e.

        4. All the above.

29. Which of the following would be the preferred method for increasing Elvira's comfort and safety during her episode of paranoid behavior?

    1. Application of restraints to all four extremities.

    2. Attaching padded side rails to her bed.

    3. Hiring a private duty nurse to attend her.

    4. Removing all potentially harmful objects from her unit.

After three weeks' administration of 40 mg. of prednisone per day Elvira developed a temperature of 103° F. orally, sore throat, rales, and a productive cough. Her white blood cell count was 13,500/mm³, with many immature cells and her red blood cell sedimentation rate was elevated above normal. Chest x-ray revealed infiltration in the left lower lobe consistent with a diagnosis of pneumonitis. Beta-hemolytic streptococci were isolated from both sputum and blood cultures. Elvira again complained of polyarthralgia, malaise, and dyspnea. The dosage of prednisone was increased to 30 mg. orally b.i.d. and Elvira was given 4 Grams of erythromycin daily for 10 days.

Although her temperature, white blood cell count, and sedimentation rate returned to normal and her sputum and blood cultures were negative following erythromycin therapy, Elvira's joint and urinary symptoms persisted. She became progressively weaker during the ensuing four weeks and finally expired in renal failure.

30. Erythromycin is similar to which of the following antibiotics in its range of antibacterial activity?

    1. Penicillin.

    2. Streptomycin.

    3. Tetracycline.

    4. Chloramphenicol.

31. Which of the following characteristics of contemporary United States culture will make it especially difficult for Elvira to face the prospect of her impending death?

    a. The adulation of youth, vigor, and beauty expressed by advertising copy.

    b. Relative overvaluation of material and undervaluation of spiritual aspects of life.

    c. An increasing tendency for people to die in the hospital rather than at home.

    d. Widespread publication of the "miracle" cures made possible by medical science.

    e. The identification with health workers fostered by television programs portraying hospital life.

        1. a and b.

        2. a, b, and c.

        3. All but e.

        4. All the above.

32. Dying patients commonly fear:

    a. Loneliness.

    b. Regression.

    c. Loss of identity.

    d. Mutilation.

    e. Loss of control.

        1. a and c.

        2. b and d.

        3. a, b, and d.

        4. All the above.

33. Elvira will experience which of the following feelings as she goes through the process of dying?

    a. Anger.

    b. Depression.

    c. Loneliness.

    d. Anxiety.

    e. Guilt.

        1. a only.

        2. a and d.

        3. All but e.

        4. All the above.

34. The nurse can maximize her ability to meet as many as possible of Elvira's needs by recognizing that:

1. Elvira's psychosocial needs will usually take precedence over her physiological needs.
2. As death approaches, Elvira's psychosocial needs will become less significant.
3. At any one time Elvira has multiple needs at all levels of Maslow's need hierarchy.
4. Elvira herself should decide which of her needs is of primary importance.

35. When the physician told the student nurse who had worked with Elvira that Elvira's prognosis was hopeless, the student asked her clinical instructor to relieve her of responsibility for Elvira's care. The student's behavior was probably the result of her:

1. Emotional acceptance of the inevitability of Elvira's death.
2. Anger at the instructor for giving her a difficult assignment.
3. Recognition of Elvira's desire to separate herself from life.
4. Need to withdraw from a situation which was painful to her.

36. The student said to her teacher, "I've never taken care of a patient with a coronary occlusion. Tomorrow may I be assigned to Mr. Lewin instead of to Miss Scuggs?" Which response by the teacher would be most helpful to the student?

1. "No, I don't think that it would be ethical for you to change your assignment."
2. "Yes, if you like. You are more aware than I of your needs for experience."
3. "There is something about giving care to Miss Scuggs which is very difficult for you?"
4. "You should consult with your team leader before making this request to me."

37. Two weeks before her death Elvira confided to her nurse, "My doctor says there's nothing more they can do for me here. I can go home if I want to. What do you think? Should I go home to die?" Which response by the nurse would be most supportive to Elvira?

1. "Don't you think that you're best equipped to make that decision?"
2. "What do you think would make you most comfortable?"
3. "There are some advantages in your going to your own home."
4. "We should discuss this in more detail when your mother comes."

38. To assist in meeting Elvira's needs during her last days of life, nursing care should provide Elvira opportunity to:

a. Express her feelings of anger and guilt.
b. Maintain her former role in her family constellation.
c. Administer a part of her own care.
d. Keep well-informed concerning current events.
e. Assist in the planning of a definitive schedule for her nursing care.
  1. a and e.
  2. a, c, and e.
  3. All but e.
  4. All the above.

Carotid Atherosclerosis and Endarterectomy

Ray Keeler, an obese, 75-year-old retiree, consulted his doctor after three days of incapacitating vertigo. He said that while getting up at night to go to the bathroom he had lost his balance and fallen to the floor. Since then he'd had to stay in bed all day and crawl to the bathroom, since he'd become "sick" and "dizzy" every time he lifted his head from the supine position. In addition to dizziness, Mr. Keeler also complained of tinnitus, visual blurring, palpitations, exertional dyspnea, and constipation. The examining physician recorded that Mr. Keeler gave a history of transient ischemic episodes, that he had worked as an accountant before retirement, that his mother and father had both died of a stroke, that he had smoked a pack and a half of cigarettes a day for 50 years, that he drank a can of beer every night before retiring, and that he had been treated for five years for hypertension.

Physical examination revealed marked facial pallor and retinal degeneration on the left. The lungs were clear to percussion and auscultation, but there was increased antero-posterior diameter of the chest, increased thoracic resonance, decreased respiratory excursions, distant heart sounds, cardiac irregularity, a bruit over the left carotid artery, and slightly hyperactive deep tendon reflexes on the right. Mr. Keeler was referred to a vascular surgeon and, following carotid and vertebral arteriography, was diagnosed as having acute cerebral ischemia secondary to bilateral carotid atherosclerosis. Because the arteriograms revealed that the left carotid was almost completely blocked, the right was only about 50 per cent obstructed, and the vertebrals only moderately obstructed, it was decided to perform a left carotid endarterectomy immediately. Laboratory tests on admission revealed a hemoglobin concentration of 14.7 Gm.%, a hematocrit of 45%, a white blood count of 7200/mm.[3], a prothrombin time of 12.7 sec., partial thromboplastin time of 57 sec., and normal electrolytes, blood urea nitrogen, and creatinine. Chest x-ray revealed increased radiolucency of the lung fields, normal heart size, and flattening of the diaphragm. Because an electrocardiogram revealed numerous ventricular extrasystoles and evidence of an old healed infarction of the anterior wall of the left ventricle, a transvenous pacemaker was inserted prior to surgery.

(ANSWER BLANK ON PAGE A–113) (CORRECT ANSWERS ON PAGE B–190)

---

1. In investigating Mr. Keeler's chief complaint of dizziness in detail, the nurse should attempt to determine:
   a. When the dizziness occurred for the first time.
   b. Actions which appear to provoke or relieve the dizziness.
   c. Other events which seem to coincide with development of dizziness.
   d. The frequency with which attacks of dizziness occur.
   c. The duration of each attack and its usual aftermath.
      1. a only.
      2. b only.
      3. a, b, and c only.
      4. All the above.

2. Which of the following sections of Mr.

Keeler's medical history should be explored carefully as possibly yielding information useful in the differential diagnosis of his illness?

    a. Recent injury to the head.

    b. Medication currently being taken.

    c. Date and interpretation of his last eye examination.

    d. Episodes of fainting or unconsciousness.

    e. "Nervous" or seizure disorders in his immediate relatives.

        1. a only.

        2. a and b only.

        3. a, b, and c only.

        4. All the above.

3. A carefully detailed medical history may reveal that, in addition to vertigo, Mr. Keeler has experienced which of the following as a result of carotid atheromatosis?

    a. Fleeting loss of vision in the left eye.

    b. Brief inability to perform fine hand movements.

    c. Temporary weakness of muscles on the right side of the face.

    d. Temporary slurring or inability to speak.

    e. Momentary numbness of the hand or foot.

        1. a or c only.

        2. b or d only.

        3. Any but d.

        4. Any of the above.

4. The transient ischemic attacks referred to by the physican in his record of Mr. Keeler's medical history can be best described as:

    1. Periods of sudden inexplicable emotional depression.

    2. Clonic convulsions which subside quickly without treatment.

    3. Brief episodes of focal neurological impairment.

    4. Sudden brief lapses of consciousness with spontaneous recovery.

5. Customarily, a transient ischemic attack can be expected to last:

    1. 1–2 seconds.

    2. 15–30 minutes.

    3. A day or two.

    4. About a week.

6. The significance of transient ischemic attacks lies in the fact that:

    1. Repeated minor embarrassment of carotid circulation stimulates development of collateral vessels in the area.

    2. Approximately one third of patients suffering such attacks will develop cerebral infarction within a few years.

    3. Periodic recurrence of the phenomenon suggests repeated embolization from an intracardiac thrombus.

    4. Full recovery following each attack demonstrates that the carotid obstruction is functional rather than anatomic.

7. In addition to his carotid atherosclerosis, which of Mr. Keeler's other problems may have contributed to his transient ischemic attacks?

    1. Overuse of alcohol.

    2. Low hemoglobin.

    3. Cardiac arrhythmia.

    4. Thoracic immobility.

8. The pathological tissue and functional changes of atherosclerosis consist of:

    a. Deposition of lipid material subintimally.

    b. Elevation and roughening of the intima overlying lipid plaques.

    c. Protrusion or rupture of plaque into the lumen of the vessels.

    d. Formation of a clot over the roughened or ulcerated intima.

    e. Creation of abnormal eddy currents as blood flows past the obstruction.

        1. a and b only.

        2. a, b, and c only.

        3. All but e.

        4. All the above.

9. In addition to the fact that their lumens are smaller than normal, arteriosclerotic vessels tend to develop which other abnormality?

    1. Increased tortuosity.

    2. Valvular incompetence.

    3. Fistula formation.

    4. Mycotic aneurysms.

10. It may be assumed that which of the following have contributed to Mr. Keeler's development of carotid atherosclerosis?

    a. Chronic hypertension.

    b. Hereditary predisposition.

    c. Cigarette smoking.

    d. Pulmonary incompetence.

    e. Constrictive neckwear.

        1. a only.

        2. a and b only.

        3. a, b, and c only.

        4. All the above.

11. In addition to the foregoing, which other factors are thought to contribute to development of atherosclerosis?
    a. High fat intake.
    b. High caloric intake.
    c. Emotional stress.
    d. Physical inactivity.
    e. Diabetes mellitus.
        1. a and b only.
        2. a, b, and c only.
        3. All but d.
        4. All the above.

12. If Mr. Keeler's hypertension had been severe and of long duration he might be expected to display which of the following findings on funduscopic examination?
    a. Decreased arterio-venous ratio.
    b. Hemorrhages into the retina.
    c. Edema of ischemic areas of retinal tissue.
    d. Compression of retinal veins by overlying arterioles.
    e. Increased cupping of the optic disc.
        1. a and b only.
        2. c and d only.
        3. All but e.
        4. All the above.

13. On the basis of his primary diagnosis, ophthalmoscopic examination of Mr. Keeler's fundus could be expected to reveal:
    1. Opacity of the crystalline lens.
    2. Microaneurysms of the retinal arterioles.
    3. Embolic obstruction of the retinal artery.
    4. Blurring of the margin of the optic disc.

14. It is probable that Mr. Keeler's retinal degeneration was primarily the result of:
    1. Interference with circulation of aqueous humor.
    2. Inadequate blood supply to the retina.
    3. Increased intracranial pressure.
    4. Destruction of nerve cells by toxic metabolites.

15. In addition to funduscopic examination, which other eye tests might yield information to support a diagnosis of carotid atherosclerosis?
    1. Quantifying the degree of ocular tension using a tonometer.
    2. Measurement of retinal artery pressure with an ophthalmodynamometer.
    3. Measuring the angle of the anterior chamber with a gonioscope.
    4. Using a slit lamp to identify opacities within the eye.

16. Mr. Keeler's facial pallor on admission was probably the result of:
    1. Reduced volume of carotid blood flow.
    2. Subnormal hemoglobin content of the blood.
    3. Temporary decrease in the systolic blood pressure.
    4. Stress induced increase in sympathetic tone.

17. In order to interpret her findings on observing Mr. Keeler at the time of admission, the nurse should understand that, while pulsations of the carotid artery are not normally visible, they may become so in which of the following conditions?
    a. Prolonged hypertension.
    b. Severe anemia.
    c. Thyroid hypersecretion.
    d. Right heart failure.
    e. Aortic valve insufficiency.
        1. a only.
        2. a and b only.
        3. All but d.
        4. All the above.

18. Pulsations of the common carotid artery are best palpated:
    1. In the midline of the neck, just below the thyroid cartilage.
    2. Below the mandible and midway between the angle of the jaw and the chin.
    3. Medial to the sternocleidomastoid muscle and just below the angle of the jaw.
    4. Behind the clavicle in the angle formed by the origin of the sternomastoid.

19. Since Mr. Keeler's chief complaint on admission was dizziness on assuming the upright position, he should be placed in which position for palpation of his carotid pulse?
    1. Standing.
    2. Sitting.
    3. Left lateral decubitus.
    4. Supine.

20. In palpating Mr. Keeler's carotid artery the nurse should pay attention to which of the following characteristics of the pulse?
    a. Rate.
    b. Volume.

   c. Contour.

   d. Rhythm.

   e. Pattern of variability.

     1. a and b only.

     2. a, b, and c only.

     3. All but e.

     4. All the above.

21. In addition to investigating pulsations, the nurse should seek information about which of the following while palpating Mr. Keeler's carotid artery?

   1. The presence of enlarged cervical nodes.

   2. The rigidity of the arterial wall.

   3. The presence or absence of orthopnea.

   4. The strength of the sternocleidomastoid muscle.

22. Caution should be used in palpating the carotid arteries, since:

   1. Compression of the vessel may simultaneously obstruct the trachea, producing asphyxia.

   2. Compression of a rigid or friable vessel may result in sudden rupture and exsanguination.

   3. Pressure on a highly sensitive carotid sinus may produce cardiac arrhythmias and syncope.

   4. Tactile stimulation in a patient with skin hyperesthesia may provoke laryngospasm.

23. The bruit detected over Mr. Keeler's left carotid artery can best be described as:

   1. An intermittent, high-pitched crackling sound, loudest during inspiration.

   2. A continuous humming sound which is accentuated during cardiac systole.

   3. A continuous fine vibration which is best palpated with the ulnar side of the hand.

   4. A diffuse and undulating pulsation which causes the vessel to writhe beneath the skin.

24. Mr. Keeler's chest findings and his history of smoking suggest which of the following disorders?

   1. Pneumonia.

   2. Bronchiectasis.

   3. Emphysema.

   4. Empyema.

25. Mr. Keeler's greater than normal thoracic resonance was primarily the result of:

   1. Decrease in the blood volume of the pulmonary circuit.

   2. Trapping of air in permanently dilated alveoli.

   3. Disuse atrophy of the pectoral and intercostal muscles.

   4. Distention of both pleural sacs with air.

26. Which of the following findings on physical examination would support a diagnosis of left carotid artery occlusion?

   a. Decrease in caliber of the retinal artery and its branches.

   b. Hyperactive deep tendon reflexes in the right arm and leg.

   c. Impaired position and vibratory sense in the right arm and leg.

   d. Presence of the extensor plantar response.

   e. Muscle spasticity in the right arm and leg.

     1. a and c only.

     2. b and d only.

     3. All but d.

     4. All the above.

27. Which of the following portions of the physical examination might be expected to yield information helpful in diagnosing Mr. Keeler's illness?

   a. Determination of orientation to time, place, and person.

   b. Examination of the scalp for lacerations and swellings.

   c. Tests for standing balance with eyes closed and finger to nose test.

   d. Percussion of frontal sinus, maxillary sinus, and mastoid process.

   e. Inspection of the tympanic membrane.

     1. a only.

     2. b only.

     3. a, b, and c only.

     4. All the above.

28. If Mr. Keeler had not demonstrated a carotid bruit, which of the following tests might have been useful in the differential diagnosis of his illness?

   a. Differential white blood cell count.

   b. Spinal puncture.

   c. Electroencephalography.

   d. Cerebral angiogram.

   e. Radioactive brain scan.

     1. a and b only.

     2. c and d only.

     3. All but d.

     4. All the above.

29. Carotid arteriography is an x-ray procedure in which:

1. The cerebral vessels are outlined by administering an iodine dye orally, which is absorbed from the bowel and circulated systemically.
2. Dye is injected into the aortic arch by way of a catheter which is inserted into the femoral artery in the groin.
3. Serial exposures are taken of the neck in rapid sequence and at progressively greater depths from the skin surface.
4. Air is injected into a vessel blocked by a clot to provide density contrast so as to visualize the clot by x-ray.

30. The primary purpose for performing angiography as part of Mr. Keeler's diagnostic workup was to:

1. Rule out the possibility of brain tumor or abscess.
2. Identify the exact site and extent of carotid obstruction.
3. Determine whether or not cerebral hemorrhage has occurred.
4. Explore the possibility of concomitant obstruction of the jugular vein.

31. In order for Mr. Keeler to give informed consent for performance of cerebral arteriography he must be informed that in a small percentage of patients a possible untoward effect of the test is the occurrence of:

1. Stroke.
2. Heart attack.
3. Kidney failure.
4. Serum hepatitis.

32. For the first three hours following carotid arteriography Mr. Keeler's care should include:

a. Checking the puncture site for evidence of bleeding.
b. Measuring the blood pressure at hourly intervals.
c. Keeping him supine with legs in full extension.
d. Putting extremities through full range of motion every hour.
e. Fostering dye removal by gentle digital massage of the carotid.
    1. a only.
    2. a, b, and c only.
    3. All but d.
    4. All the above.

33. The primary objective in performing the carotid endarterectomy so quickly following Mr. Keeler's admission to the hospital was to prevent occurrence of:

1. Hypertensive crisis.
2. Pulmonary embolism.
3. Cerebral infarction.
4. Cardiac failure.

34. In order to give his informed consent for carotid endarterectomy, Mr. Keeler must be told that there is a small chance that the operation may increase his neurological deficit as a result of:

1. Disturbance of brain blood flow during operative manipulation of the vessel.
2. Irreversible depression of cerebral tissues by the heavy doses of anesthetic required.
3. The unavoidable sectioning of certain cranial nerve fibers in exposing the carotid artery.
4. Spinal cord trauma resulting from prolonged hyperextension of the neck during surgery.

After a three and one-half hour operative procedure Mr. Keeler's surgeon recorded: "Following occlusion of all involved vessels, arteriotomy was done, a shunt was positioned from the common carotid to the internal carotid (one and one-half minute occlusion time). Then, with circulation restored, endarterectomy was carried out and the arteriotomy was closed. Occlusion time for removal of the shunt was 1 minute and 40 seconds. During occlusion time the patient was systemically heparinized. Blood loss was 100 cc."

Mr. Keeler was returned to the Postanesthesia Recovery Room awake and alert with blood pressure of 150/90 mm. Hg., pulse of 80, respirations 24. He was receiving 40 per cent oxygen with humidity by face mask, and he had a Foley catheter in place attached to gravity drainage. Five per cent dextrose in water was running into a vein in the right forearm at a rate of 83 cc/Hr. Five per cent dextrose in water was running into a C.V.P. line at a rate of 42 cc./Hr. Intermittent positive pressure breathing treatments were ordered to be carried out every 4 hours, and a tracheotomy set was placed at the bedside.

35. Which of the following drugs would probably be given to Mr. Keeler before he leaves the Operating Room in order to counteract the effect of the heparin given during occlusion time?

1. Papaverine.
2. Physostigmine.
3. Prostigmine.
4. Protamine.

36. During the immediate postanesthetic period Mr. Keeler should be observed closely for hemorrhage from the operative site. In addition to saturation of the dressing with

blood, which of the following would be possible indications of hemorrhage?

   a. Pale, cold skin.
   b. Decreased pulse rate.
   c. Decreased systolic pressure.
   d. Increased temperature.
   e. Rapid shallow respirations.
      1. a and b only.
      2. c and d only.
      3. a, c, and e only.
      4. All the above.

37. The tracheotomy tube was kept at Mr. Keeler's bedside for emergency use in the event of respiratory embarrassment caused by:

   1. The irritant effect of the anesthetic agent.
   2. Laryngospasm due to I.P.P.B. treatments.
   3. Tracheal compression from edema due to operative tissue trauma.
   4. Laryngeal edema due to prolonged endotracheal intubation.

38. During Mr. Keeler's immediate postoperative period which of the following symptoms should be reported to the doctor immediately as a possible indication of a serious postoperative complication?

   1. Sighing.
   2. Hoarseness.
   3. Thirst.
   4. Sneezing.

39. During the first few hours postoperatively Mr. Keeler should be observed for which of the following complications?

   a. Hemorrhage.
   b. Shock.
   c. Asphyxia.
   d. Arrhythmia.
   e. Cerebral infarction.
      1. a and b only.
      2. a, b, and c only.
      3. All but d.
      4. All the above.

40. Which of the following would be the most likely cause if Mr. Keeler should demonstrate extreme restlessness during the first hour or two postoperatively?

   1. Cerebral infarction.
   2. Metabolic acidosis.
   3. Internal bleeding.
   4. Oxygen toxicity.

41. Which of the following pieces of data would be of greatest value to the nurse in evaluating Mr. Keeler's central venous pressure reading during the immediate postoperative period?

   1. The volume of parenteral fluids given during surgery.
   2. His height, body weight, and body surface area.
   3. His central venous pressure before surgery.
   4. His systolic blood pressure before surgery.

42. Appearance of which of the following during the first few hours after surgery would suggest embolization of a plaque or clot from the operative site?

   a. Sudden severe headache.
   b. Increasing confusion.
   c. Asymmetry of facial muscles.
   d. Weakness or paralysis of an extremity.
   e. Inability to speak or to comprehend spoken language.
      1. a and b only.
      2. c and d only.
      3. All but e.
      4. All the above.

43. Mr. Keeler was given oxygen during his immediate postoperative period primarily to offset the effects of which of the following intraoperative events?

   1. Interruption of cerebral blood flow.
   2. Irritation of tracheobronchial mucosa.
   3. Depression of the respiratory center.
   4. Depletion of blood volume.

44. Humidified rather than dry oxygen was administered to Mr. Keeler in order to:

   1. Correct hypovolemia.
   2. Lower body temperature.
   3. Prevent mucosal irritation.
   4. Decrease combustibility.

45. In order to protect Mr. Keeler from the risk of fire during oxygen administration the following precautions should be taken in the Recovery Room:

   a. Use three-pronged plugs on all electrical equipment.
   b. Forbid the use of extension cords and keep cords off the floor.
   c. Inspect electrical cords regularly and replace those frayed or damaged.
   d. Post and enforce "No Smoking" rules for patients, visitors, and staff.
   e. Avoid use of hair oil, mineral oil, vaseline, alcohol, and ether in patient care.
      1. a and b only.
      2. a, b, and c only.
      3. All but e.
      4. All the above.

46. In checking Mr. Keeler for skin color changes postoperatively the nurse should be aware that cyanosis would probably first be visible in the:
  1. Nailbeds.
  2. Sclera.
  3. Oral mucosa.
  4. Palms.

47. In order to interpret Mr. Keeler's postoperative blood gas readings the nurse should be aware that the normal values of partial pressure of oxygen in arterial blood are from:
  1. 35 to 40 mm. Hg.
  2. 55 to 60 mm. Hg.
  3. 95 to 100 mm. Hg.
  4. 175 to 180 mm. Hg.

48. His physician would probably try to keep Mr. Keeler's arterial pO_2 at a level slightly less than normal because of his:
  1. Previous myocardial infarction.
  2. Chronic lung disease.
  3. History of hypertension.
  4. Age and inactivity.

49. If it were suspected that Mr. Keeler had suffered a cerebral accident following surgery, it would be advisable to test his response to:
  a. Visual stimulation.
  b. Verbal commands.
  c. Pressure stimuli.
  d. Painful stimuli.
  e. Pharyngeal stimulation.
    1. a and b only.
    2. a, b, and c only.
    3. All but e.
    4. All the above.

50. The pupillary reflex should be tested by:
  1. Stroking the lateral aspect of the cornea lightly with a piece of cotton.
  2. Shining a small flashlight into the eye from the temporal side.
  3. Bringing the hand rapidly toward the face in a threatening manner.
  4. Directing the gaze into six cardinal directions while immobilizing the head.

51. Absence of the pupillary reflex would indicate impaired functioning of which cranial nerve?
  1. Optic.
  2. Oculomotor.
  3. Trigeminal.
  4. Facial.

52. In addition to testing the pupillary reflex, Mr. Keeler's eyes should be checked at intervals during the immediate postoperative period for evidence of:
  1. Inequality in pupil size.
  2. Increased intraocular pressure.
  3. Decreased scleral vascularity.
  4. Changes in iris color.

53. Response to verbal command could best be tested by directing the patient to:
  1. "Squeeze my hand."
  2. "Alternately pronate and supinate your hand."
  3. "Touch your nose with the index finger of first one hand and then the other."
  4. "Place your right heel on your left knee and run it down the shin to the foot."

54. In testing Mr. Keeler for response to painful stimuli the nurse should observe not only whether he responds to pain but also whether:
  1. His response is predominantly physical or psychological.
  2. His reaction is rapid or delayed.
  3. His response is purposeful or nonpurposeful.
  4. His pain threshold is normal or abnormal.

55. The gag reflex is mediated by which of the following?
  a. Trochlear nerve.
  b. Trigeminal nerve.
  c. Facial nerve.
  d. Glossopharyngeal nerve.
  e. Vagus nerve.
    1. a and b only.
    2. b and c only.
    3. c and d only.
    4. d and e only.

56. Mr. Keeler's gag reflex would be best tested by:
  1. Giving him water to drink while he is lying flat in bed.
  2. Touching the posterior wall of the pharynx with a tongue blade.
  3. Lifting the uvula and deflecting it to one side with a laryngeal mirror.
  4. Placing a small vial of malodorous material directly under his nostrils.

57. In observing Mr. Keeler for evidence of cerebral complications following surgery, the most reliable single indicator of neurological deterioration would be:
  1. Gradual reduction in the speed of the pupillary reflex.
  2. Progressive decrease in both pulse and blood pressure.

3. Steadily decreasing level of consciousness.
4. Decreased strength of skeletal muscle contraction.

58. Which of the following would be the best method of assessing Mr. Keeler's skeletal muscle strength during the early postoperative period?

1. Testing simultaneously his force of grip in both hands, noting equality of grip and ability to release.
2. Observing whether or not spontaneous movements of arms and legs occur at intervals during care.
3. Lifting both arms over his face and releasing them suddenly to observe the direction of fall.
4. Directing him to lift his head and shoulders from the mattress from the prone position.

59. If Mr. Keeler were to demonstrate increasing cerebral dysfunction and steadily declining level of consciousness following surgery, which of the following would indicate the greatest degree of dysfunction?

1. Grimacing in response to a strong pinch on the arm.

2. Giving a correct answer to the question, "Where are you?"
3. Lifting his arm from the bed when told to do so.
4. Giving a correct answer to the question, "What time is it?"

60. As a result of his chronic lung disease Mr. Keeler is especially susceptible to development of:

1. Hypostatic pneumonia.
2. Shock lung.
3. Pulmonary embolism.
4. Bronchopleural fistula.

61. The purpose for the I.P.P.B. treatments ordered for Mr. Keeler postoperatively was to:

1. Decrease cardiac work load.
2. Increase alveolar ventilation.
3. Restore ciliary action.
4. Release pleural adhesions.

Mr. Keeler recovered quickly and uneventfully after surgery. The stitches were removed from his neck wound on the sixth postoperative day. He was discharged on the seventh postoperative day and given an appointment to see his surgeon for a followup evaluation in one month.

Laryngeal Carcinoma and Laryngectomy

Louis Raspanti, a right-handed, fifty-seven-year-old schoolteacher, consulted an otolaryngologist with the complaint of sore throat and hoarseness of three months duration. On questioning, Mr. Raspanti indicated that he had smoked a pack and a half of cigarettes a day for 40 years, that he drank one to two beers each day, that he suffered from hay fever, and that he had recently developed a persistent cough with expectoration of thick mucus. Indirect laryngoscopy revealed a lesion of the left true vocal cord. Suspecting that the lesion was malignant, the physician admitted Mr. Raspanti to the hospital for endoscopy, biopsy, and a presurgical workup.

Endoscopy revealed, in addition to a lesion of the left cord, a 2 cm. by 2 cm. infiltrating lesion of the left pharyngeal wall. Biopsy indicated that both lesions were squamous cell carcinoma. Physical examination revealed no palpable submandibular, cervical, or subclavicular nodes and no other abnormal findings.

During his first two days in the hospital Mr. Raspanti had complete blood studies, biochemistries, chest x-rays, electrocardiography, tomogram of the larynx, and bone survey films done. On the third day after admission he was taken to the operating room for delay of a deltopectoral flap, and ten days later a radical neck dissection was performed in which the larynx was removed, the pharynx was removed from uvula to larynx, the deltopectoral flap was swung up to reconstruct the pharyngeal wall, and a split-thickness skin graft from the abdomen was used to cover the area of the left chest from which the flap was lifted.

(ANSWER BLANK ON PAGE A-115) (CORRECT ANSWERS ON PAGE B-194)

1. Mr. Raspanti's hoarseness was probably the result of:
1. Passage of air through pooled secretions in the lower pharynx and larynx.
2. Inability to completely approximate the cords because of the presence of tumor tissue.
3. Unusual eddy currents created by air passing over the pharyngeal mass.
4. Involuntary splinting of pharyngeal and tongue muscles in response to throat pain.

2. If a detailed medical history were obtained from Mr. Raspanti, it might become obvious that, in addition to hoarseness, he has experienced which other symptoms of laryngeal carcinoma?
   a. Dyspnea.
   b. Hemoptysis.
   c. Dysphagia.
   d. Wheezing.
   e. Hiccups.
      1. a only.
      2. a, b, and c only.
      3. All but d.
      4. All the above.

3. Which of the following factors in Mr. Raspanti's history is most likely to have contributed to his present problem?
   1. Respiratory allergies.
   2. Vocal strain.
   3. Prolonged smoking.
   4. Use of alcohol.

4. Which of the following are typical symptoms of pharyngeal carcinoma?
   a. Difficulty in swallowing.
   b. Sensation of a lump in the throat.
   c. Pain radiating to the ear.
   d. Eructation following meals.
   e. Regurgitation following meals.
      1. a only.
      2. a, b, and c only.
      3. All but e.
      4. All the above.

5. During indirect laryngoscopy, after the physician has pulled Mr. Raspanti's tongue forward and positioned the dental mirror in the posterior oropharynx, Mr. Raspanti should be instructed to:
   1. Take in a long deep breath and hold it.
   2. Hold his breath and bear down as if to defecate.
   3. Breathe quietly and deeply through the mouth.
   4. Remain completely immobile and breathe through the nose.

6. At some point during indirect laryngoscopy Mr. Raspanti will be directed to speak in order that the physician can determine:
   1. The motility and approximation of the vocal cords.
   2. The amount of relaxation of the pharyngeal wall.
   3. The degree of laryngeal elevation with speech.
   4. The appearance of the brachial wall below the larynx.

7. Mr. Raspanti's preparation for endoscopy should include:
   a. Withholding food and fluids for eight hours.
   b. Administering a low tap water enema.
   c. Removing his eyeglasses and dentures.
   d. Inserting an indwelling catheter.
   e. Obtaining his written consent for the procedure.
      1. a and b only.
      2. c and d only.
      3. a, c, and e only.
      4. All the above.

8. Prior to endoscopy, Mr. Raspanti should be informed that, following the procedure, he may experience a temporary:
   1. Disturbance of balance.
   2. Shortness of breath.
   3. Loss of voice.
   4. Substernal pain.

9. Mr. Raspanti's care during the first two hours following laryngoscopy should include:

1. Withholding all oral food and fluids for two to three hours.
2. Administering oxygen by face mask at four to five liters per minute.
3. Keeping him supine with a small pillow under his shoulders.
4. Encouraging him to gargle with warm saline solution.

10. For the first two to three hours following laryngoscopy, Mr. Raspanti should be checked frequently for which of the following as symptoms of possible complications?

a. Restlessness and apprehension.
b. Expectoration of bloody mucus.
c. Pain in the throat or chest.
d. Swelling of the neck.
e. Shortness of breath.
    1. a and b only.
    2. a, b, and c only.
    3. All but e.
    4. All the above.

11. For several hours following laryngoscopy Mr. Raspanti should be discouraged from coughing and talking in order to reduce the possibility of:

1. Rupture of the diseased cord.
2. Dilation of the anesthetized pharynx.
3. Bleeding from the biopsy site.
4. Mucus obstruction of the edematous larynx.

12. The nurse could most effectively discourage Mr. Raspanti from talking following laryngoscopy by:

1. Placing a plastic oxygen mask over his mouth.
2. Giving him a pad of paper and a pencil.
3. Satisfying all his needs before he can express them.
4. Talking continuously while she gives him care.

13. In order for Mr. Raspanti to give informed consent for the operation planned for him he must be told that following surgery he will:

1. Be unable to talk above a whisper.
2. Be left with a permanent tracheostomy.
3. Be fed through a permanent gastrostomy.
4. Be permanently restricted to a soft, low residue diet.

14. To prepare him for the care which he may expect to receive following surgery Mr. Raspanti should be given preoperative instruction on which of the following topics?

a. Proper methods of deep breathing and coughing.
b. The importance of scrupulous oral hygiene.
c. The appearance, placement, function, and care of a tracheostomy tube.
d. The appearance, placement, function, and care of a nasogastric feeding tube.
e. The placement, function, and care of an intravenous hyperalimentation tube.
    1. a only.
    2. a and b only.
    3. All but e.
    4. All the above.

15. As part of his preoperative preparation Mr. Raspanti should be told that, when he wakes up in the Recovery Room after surgery, he will probably find the following tubes in place:

a. A nasogastric tube.
b. A tracheotomy tube.
c. A drainage tube into the neck wound.
d. An indwelling urinary catheter.
e. A tube into a peripheral vein for fluid administration.
f. A tube into a central vein for measuring pressure.
g. A tube into a peripheral artery for measuring blood gases.
    1. a and b only.
    2. b, c, and d only.
    3. b, e, and f only.
    4. All the above.

16. In reinforcing information given to Mr. Raspanti by the surgeon, the nurse should help him to understand that, as a result of the operation, he will experience which of the following changes of function?

a. Loss of normal speech.
b. Loss of normal respiration through nose and mouth.
c. Loss of the normal sense of smell.
d. Loss of the ability to "blow" his nose.
e. Loss of the ability to lift heavy objects.
    1. a and b only.
    2. c and d only.
    3. All but e.
    4. All the above.

17. In caring for Mr. Raspanti preoperatively, it is of primary importance that the nurse provide opportunity for him to discuss at length his fear of surgery and its aftermath because:

1. Patients undergoing laryngectomy are more liable than other surgical patients to postoperative depression.
2. It gives her a chance to provide arguments to convince him of the need for surgery.
3. Lack of speech will impede communication of his feelings for several weeks following surgery.
4. Such a conversation can easily be redirected to permit instruction in deep-breathing techniques.

18. The surgeon asked a speech therapist to visit with Mr. Raspanti before surgery. The visit was scheduled to take place before the operation in order that:

1. The therapist could record his "normal" speech as a model to be followed in developing esophageal speech.
2. He be fully informed of the difficulties confronting him postoperatively before giving consent for the operation.
3. He can be taught how to swallow air and expel it slowly while he is still able to ask questions.
4. The therapist can determine whether he would be using esophageal speech or an electronic resonator following surgery.

19. In the course of Mr. Raspanti's operation the surgeon will probably remove which of the following tissues in addition to his larynx and pharynx?

a. Cervical lymph glands.
b. Sternocleidomastoid muscle.
c. Fat pad in the posterior triangle of the neck.
d. Submaxillary salivary gland.
e. Internal jugular vein.
    1. a only.
    2. a and b only.
    3. All but e.
    4. All the above.

Following the operation Mr. Raspanti was returned to the Recovery Room, with 35 per cent oxygen being delivered through a tracheostomy collar, a nasogastric tube attached to low intermittent suction, a Foley catheter attached to gravity drainage, two catheters under the neck flap attached to a Hemovac apparatus, and 1000 cc. of 5 per cent dextrose in water running into a left arm vein at 125 cc. per hour. A few hours later intravenous hyperalimentation was administered into the central venous line.

Although Mr. Raspanti developed a temperature of 100° F. and diffuse chest rales on his first postoperative day, his blood gases, pH, and serum electrolytes remained within normal limits. Chest physiotherapy and intravenous Kefzol 1 Gm. every 6 hours were ordered, and three days later his lungs were clear to percussion and auscultation and he was afebrile.

20. On his admission to the Recovery Room following surgery, Mr. Raspanti should be placed in which position?

1. Supine.
2. Trendelenberg.
3. Side lying.
4. Low Fowler's.

21. After Mr. Raspanti has regained consciousness following surgery, he should be placed in which position?

1. Supine.
2. Trendelenberg.
3. Side lying.
4. Low Fowler's.

22. During the first few hours following his operation, Mr. Raspanti must be closely observed for symptoms of respiratory embarrassment, to which complication he would be predisposed by:

a. Edema of tissues in the hypopharyngeal and tracheal region.
b. The pressure dressing applied to the cervical wound.
c. The analgesic and anesthetic medications given him.
d. Pulmonary stasis due to immobilization during surgery.
e. Excessive secretions resulting from trauma to the airway.
    1. a only.
    2. b only.
    3. a, b, and c only.
    4. All the above.

23. In the event that the nurse should observe a large amount of bleeding from Mr. Raspanti's neck wound, she should:

1. Apply a half-filled ice collar over the lower part of the neck dressing.
2. Apply additional adhesive strips to increase pressure on the dressing.
3. Apply direct manual pressure to the wound and summon help to notify the doctor.
4. Disconnect the Hemovac apparatus and replace it with a new pump.

24. Which of the following tenets of good nursing practice is even more important in caring for Mr. Raspanti than in caring for other types of postsurgical patients?

1. Promptly recording on the chart each aspect of care given and all observations made concerning significant changes in his condition.
2. Adjusting physical care routines and schedules for special procedures to fit individual needs for rest and social interaction.
3. Giving him a full explanation of the nature and purpose of each aspect of care before it is initiated.
4. Making him responsible for each aspect of self care as soon as he is physically and emotionally able to carry it out.

25. During Mr. Raspanti's first postoperative day, which of the following signs would indicate his need for tracheal suctioning?

a. Respiratory rales.
b. Motor restlessness.
c. Increased respiratory rate.
d. Increased pulse rate.
e. Mounting anxiety.
  1. a and b only.
  2. a, b, and c only.
  3. All but e.
  4. All the above.

26. The nurse should assemble which of the following equipment in preparation for tracheal suctioning?

a. Sterile catheter.
b. Sterile gloves.
c. Container of sterile water.
d. Asepto syringe.
e. 10 cc. syringe.
  1. a only.
  2. a and b only.
  3. a, b, and c only.
  4. All the above.

27. Which of the following types of catheters is best suited for tracheal suctioning?

1. A soft, rubber, closed-tip catheter.
2. A firm, plastic catheter with multiple openings along its length.
3. A transparent, plastic coudé whistle tip catheter.
4. A rigid, straight catheter with a double lumen.

28. In order to decrease the risk of transmitting infection to Mr. Raspanti in the course of tracheal suctioning, the nurse should:

a. Wear a mask while performing tracheal suctioning.
b. Wear sterile gloves while performing tracheal suctioning.
c. Maintain him in reverse isolation as long as suctioning is required.
d. Use different catheters to suction the mouth and the trachea.
e. Keep the catheter immersed in antiseptic solution between suctionings.
  1. a and c only.
  2. b and d only.
  3. All but d.
  4. All the above.

29. In aspirating Mr. Raspanti's trachea following surgery it would be advisable to apply suction intermittently for intervals no longer than:

1. 2 seconds.
2. 6 seconds.
3. 12 seconds.
4. 20 seconds.

30. It is possible for continuous tracheal suctioning for a half minute or more to cause sudden death as a result of:

a. Bradycardia and bronchospasm resulting from respiratory tract reflexes.
b. Overdistention of the heart with blood from the superior vena cava and pulmonary artery.
c. Severe cardiac arrhythmias resulting from myocardial anoxia.
d. Perforation of the trachea due to erosion by the catheter.
e. Pulmonary embolism due to pneumatic mobilization of an intracardiac thrombus.
  1. a and b only.
  2. a, b, and c only.
  3. All but e.
  4. All the above.

31. The nurse can decrease the danger of hypoxia as a complication of tracheal suctioning by:

   a. Restricting each suctioning procedure to the briefest time which will effect removal of secretions.

   b. Administering high concentrations of oxygen for several minutes before each episode of suctioning.

   c. Administering high concentrations of oxygen for several seconds at intervals throughout the procedure.

   d. Suctioning while the catheter is being introduced as well as while it is being withdrawn.

   e. Administering high concentrations of oxygen for a minute or so after suctioning has been completed.

     1. a only.
     2. a and b only.
     3. All but d.
     4. All the above.

32. In addition to or in conjunction with tracheal suctioning the respiratory therapist will probably use which of the following measures to facilitate Mr. Raspanti's respiratory functioning?

   a. Humidify the oxygen administered through the tracheostomy collar.

   b. Use chest percussion and vibration to loosen tenacious secretions.

   c. Apply postural drainage to move secretions from lung bases toward the trachea.

   d. Instill a few milliliters of sterile saline into the trachea before suctioning.

   e. Direct him to exhale forcefully and for as long as possible to stimulate coughing.

     1. a only.
     2. b only.
     3. All but c.
     4. All the above.

33. It is advisable to suction Mr. Raspanti's trachea no more frequently than necessary because:

     1. The relief he experiences from suctioning may produce psychological dependence on the machine.

     2. Tissue irritation caused during the procedure also tends to stimulate increased secretions.

     3. Artificial means of removing respiratory secretions tends to weaken the cough reflex.

     4. Repeated arousal at short intervals prevents acquisition of sufficient rapid eyeball movement phase of sleep.

34. Proper suctioning technique includes:

     1. Applying suction during insertion as well as withdrawal of the catheter.

     2. Using the widest catheter which can be inserted into the trachea without force.

     3. Moving the catheter rapidly up and down within the trachea to loosen secretion.

     4. Gently rotating the catheter and withdrawing it slowly while applying suction.

35. The derivatives of cephalosporin are generally active against which of the following?

   a. *Streptococcus pneumoniae.*
   b. *Haemophilus influenzae.*
   c. *Staphylococcus aureus.*
   d. *Escherichia coli.*
   e. *Proteus mirabilis.*

     1. a and c only.
     2. b and d only.
     3. All but e.
     4. All the above.

36. Which of the following is a typical toxic effect of the cephalosporin derivatives?

     1. Convulsions.
     2. Jaundice.
     3. Deafness.
     4. Neutropenia.

37. Since the hyperalimentation solution administered to Mr. Raspanti contained 25 per cent dextrose and 4.25 per cent amino acids, each liter of the solution contained how many calories?

     1. 293.
     2. 1170.
     3. 2420.
     4. 2633.

38. For the first few days that Mr. Raspanti is given intravenous hyperalimentation, the physician will probably check which of the following on a daily basis?

     1. Concentration of serum sodium, potassium, and chloride.

     2. Electrocardiographic tracings.

     3. Prothrombin time.

     4. Arterial blood gases.

39. For as long as Mr. Raspanti is receiving intravenous hyperalimentation the nurse should monitor which of the following parameters?

a. Daily measurement of fluid intake and output.
b. Daily determination of body weight.
c. Testing of urine for sugar and acetone Q. I. D.
d. Measurement of blood pressure every 2 hours.
e. Measurement of abdominal girth B.I.D.

    1. a only.
    2. a, b, and c only.
    3. All but e.
    4. All the above.

40. When the nurse moves Mr. Raspanti about in bed or helps him to sit up during the first few days postoperatively, she should:

1. Fold his arms over his chest.
2. Support the back of his neck.
3. Apply light pressure over his neck wound.
4. Flex his head forward sharply on his chest.

On the third postoperative day Mr. Raspanti's tracheostomy tube was replaced by a laryngectomy tube and he was moved back to the surgical unit. On his fourth postoperative day the catheters were withdrawn from his neck wound, his nasogastric tube was clamped off, and a heat lamp was applied to the chest wall donor site. Intravenous hyperalimentation was continued for another seven days, at which time nasogastric tube feedings of a high caloric, high protein, high vitamin blenderized mixture were begun.

Mr. Raspanti improved in physical strength and morale during the next five weeks, during which time he was given increasing responsibility for self care, a number of tests were performed to determine whether or not the laryngeal tumor had metastasized to distant tissues, and an electric suction machine was obtained for his use at home. Five weeks after his operation the deltopectoral flap was divided from its donor site, and the end was trimmed and sutured in final position. Mr. Raspanti recovered quickly from this second operative procedure and was discharged to his home with clinic appointments for followup care and instruction in esophageal speech.

41. Which of the following items should be kept at Mr. Raspanti's bedside during the first week or two postoperatively?

a. Tap bell.
b. Rubber tipped forceps.
c. Magic slate.
d. Tourniquet.
e. Suture scissors.

    1. a and c only.
    2. b and d only.
    3. All but e.
    4. All the above.

42. Mr. Raspanti should be taught to perform which of the following procedures as part of his self care program?

a. Suctioning of his tracheostomy tube.
b. Removal and cleaning the inner cannula of the tracheostomy tube.
c. Changing the dressing around his tracheostomy tube.
d. Administering his nasogastric tube feedings.
e. Inserting and irrigating his indwelling bladder catheter.

    1. a and b only.
    2. a and c only.
    3. All but e.
    4. All the above.

43. In order to care for him effectively, the nurse should anticipate that Mr. Raspanti's postoperative depression would be most intense about:

1. Eight hours postoperatively.
2. Three to four days following surgery.
3. Seven to ten days following surgery.
4. One month after the first operation.

44. Even though he experienced no nausea after his first postoperative day Mr. Raspanti was given nasogastric tube feedings from his third to his tenth day after surgery in order to:

a. Prevent contamination of the pharyngeal suture line.
b. Prevent fistula formation from tension on the pharyngeal suture line.
c. Ensure a precisely accurate record of fluid intake.
d. Prevent vomiting and pneumonia due to aspiration of gastric contents.
e. Provide a means by which oral medications can be administered without pain.

    1. a and b only.
    2. a, b, and c only.
    3. All but e.
    4. All the above.

45. The nurse and/or speech therapist should remain with Mr. Raspanti on the first occasion that he is given fluid to drink postoperatively, as he will be apt to:
1. Experience a feeling of choking or asphyxia.
2. Aspirate part of the fluid into the lung.
3. Expel the liquid out the tracheostomy opening.
4. Vomit a large portion of what is swallowed.

46. When Mr. Raspanti first attempts to swallow liquids postoperatively the nurse can best minimize his discomfort by:
1. Gently stroking his neck so as to assist esophageal peristalsis.
2. Pounding him on the back if he chokes while swallowing.
3. Applying pressure over the neck wound if he vomits.
4. Suctioning any tracheal secretions loosened by coughing.

47. Mr. Raspanti's first step in learning to use esophageal speech would be to practice:
1. Holding his breath for time periods of increasing length.
2. Belching air an hour or so after each oral feeding.
3. Contracting his abdominal instead of his thoracic muscles on inspiration.
4. Expiring in several short bursts rather than one continuous exhalation.

48. It is to be expected that, following his operation, Mr. Raspanti will have:
a. Pain in the shoulder.
b. Limitation of shoulder motion.
c. Loss of sensation to areas of upper chest and back.
d. Decreased motility of the lower jaw.
e. Episodes of wheezing respiration.
  1. a only.
  2. a, b, and c only.
  3. All but e.
  4. All the above.

49. It is desirable for Mr. Raspanti to progress from liquid and soft foods to a regular diet with considerable roughage as soon as it is possible for him to do so safely in order that:
1. He lose the least possible amount of weight during his illness.
2. He not become habituated to laxatives as a result of his abnormal diet.

3. His throat and abdominal muscles regain tonus needed for esophageal speech.
4. Return to normal diet will encourage resumption of other pre-morbid activities.

50. In preparing Mrs. Raspanti to be as supportive as possible to her husband during the next few weeks and months, the nurse should especially stress the importance of Mrs. Raspanti's:
1. Active encouragement of Mr. Raspanti's attempts to learn esophageal speech.
2. Insistence that Mr. Raspanti join the local laryngectomee group immediately.
3. Taking responsibility for cleansing Mr. Raspanti's tracheostomy after discharge.
4. Discouraging Mr. Raspanti's return to work until he is proficient in esophageal speech.

51. While Mr. Raspanti is beginning to learn esophageal speech he is apt to experience:
1. Severe lightheadedness.
2. Cervical swelling.
3. Substernal pain.
4. Digestive difficulty.

52. What action would the nurse take if, following surgery, Mr. Raspanti is left with areas of numbness in the neck and face due to nerve damage during the operation?
1. Advise him to massage the areas gently until normal sensation returns.
2. Caution him to avoid accidental injury to the insensitive area during shaving.
3. Instruct him to apply warm compresses to the area to hasten nerve repair.
4. Measure the extent of such numbness daily using pinprick technique.

53. Prior to his discharge from the hospital the nurse should teach Mr. Raspanti and his wife the importance of which of the following as part of his postdischarge care?
a. Air-conditioning and humidification of his home.
b. Shielding his tracheostomy against aspiration of foreign bodies.
c. Daily cleansing of crusts and secretions from the laryngectomy tube.

d. Avoidance of smoking, smokers, and smoke-laden rooms.

e. Returning to work and resuming social contacts as soon as possible.
   1. a and c only.
   2. b and d only.
   3. All but e.
   4. All the above.

54. After his discharge from the hospital Mr. Raspanti should carry an identification card which states not only that he has no vocal cords but also that:
   1. If he should need respiratory assistance, mouth to neck rather than mouth to mouth resuscitation would be required.
   2. If he develops nausea and vomiting his head should be turned to one side to prevent aspiration of vomitus.
   3. If he should require artificial respiration, the arm lift rather than the prone pressure method should be used.
   4. In the event of severe hypotension he should be given a vasopressor which will not produce bronchospasm.

Paraplegia and Skin Graft

Leonard Heller, an eighteen-year-old unemployed school dropout, was shot in the spine by an off-duty policeman as he ran to avoid capture following a gas station robbery. Leonard was taken by police ambulance to the trauma unit of the city hospital, where he complained of severe back pain and inability to move his legs and feet.

Spinal x-rays and myelograms revealed that the bullet had fractured Leonard's fourth thoracic vertebra and had severed the spinal cord, causing paraplegia. A laminectomy was performed to remove bone fragments from the spinal canal and a spinal fusion was performed to stabilize the vertebral fracture. At surgery Leonard's spinal cord was found to be completely transected. Leonard was returned to the neurosurgical unit on the day after surgery in a body cast.

(ANSWER BLANK ON PAGE A-117) (CORRECT ANSWERS ON PAGE B-198)

1. When the policeman ran up to Leonard after having shot him, Leonard was crying and complaining of pain in his back and chest. Before moving him the police should have:
   1. Summoned a physician to administer an analgesic.
   2. Asked him to move his fingers and toes.
   3. Advised him to splint his chest with his hand.
   4. Removed his shirt to determine the amount of bleeding.

2. Before the ambulance arrived the police should have cared for Leonard by:
   1. Rolling him over, log fashion, and applying direct pressure to the wound.
   2. Elevating his feet slightly above the level of his head.
   3. Keeping him supine and straight on a hard surface.
   4. Assisting his respirations by the arm lift method.

3. In order to protect Leonard from further injury while he was being moved to the hospital, what precaution should have been taken?

1. His legs should have been bound tightly together with a tie or a belt.
2. Four men should have lifted him as a unit, holding his spine straight.
3. His head should have been pulled far backward to hyperextend his neck.
4. His arms should have been folded over his chest and secured with ties.

4. Immediately following his admission to the hospital Leonard was unusually calm and quiet. When the emergency room nurse asked him how he had been injured he replied, "I don't remember." The nurse should interpret his reply as indicating:

1. Unconscious guilt.
2. Deliberate evasion.
3. Psychological shock.
4. Desire for sympathy.

5. At the time of Leonard's admission to the hospital it would be impossible to accurately predict the neurological deficit that he would ultimately be left with because:

1. With correct alignment of the severed sections of cord, some healing of fibers will occur.
2. Some of his symptoms may be the result of spinal shock rather than severance of the cord.
3. If the cord had been cut sharply it might be possible to suture the tracts together.
4. It is possible for collateral fibers to grow around the defect and permit impulse transmission.

6. For the first few weeks following Leonard's injury neurological examination of his lower extremities would probably reveal:

1. Hyperactive superficial and deep reflexes.
2. Absent superficial and deep reflexes.
3. Increasingly higher levels of motor paralysis.
4. Increasingly higher levels of sensory paralysis.

7. For the first few hours following injury Leonard's paralysis would have been of which type?

1. Flaccid.
2. Spastic.
3. Progressive.
4. Intermittent.

8. During the two days that elapsed between hospital admission and spinal fusion, Leonard could best be cared for on a:

1. Tilt table.
2. Metal stretcher-cart.
3. Stryker frame.
4. Adult-sized crib.

9. If the aforementioned device is not available, which of the following should be used in Leonard's care while he is waiting for surgery?

1. Posey belt.
2. Bedboard.
3. Foot blocks.
4. Siderails.

10. For several hours after his injury Leonard was unable to empty his bladder. Since his bladder was distended on the morning after admission, he was catheterized, resulting in the removal of 500 cc. of urine. This finding would indicate that he was suffering:

1. Bladder spasm.
2. Urinary retention.
3. Urethral stricture.
4. Unconscious withholding.

11. A few days later, immediately following an involuntary micturition of small amount, Leonard was catheterized. Two hundred cc. of residual urine was removed from his bladder. This finding would indicate development of:

1. Ureteral dilation.
2. Overflow incontinence.
3. Urinary infection.
4. Return of reflexes.

12. Even though Leonard was unable to control his bowel and bladder immediately following his injury, the doctor told his father that Leonard might later regain some control over both functions. Some control over evacuation could develop because:

1. His initial bowel and bladder problems result more from psychological than from physical injury.
2. Some of the severed motor fibers will reconnect, permitting impulse transmission.
3. Return of parasympathetic activity will permit automatic emptying of bladder and bowel.
4. With the lessening of depression,

additional energy can be mobilized for volitional control.

13. In preparing a bed to receive Leonard from the Recovery Room following his spinal fusion, the nurse should include which of the following items?
   a. Shoulder-to-hip turning sheet.
   b. Overhead frame and trapeze.
   c. Foot board or canvas foot support.
   d. Electric heat cradle.
   e. Blocks to elevate the bed foot.
      1. a only.
      2. a and b only.
      3. a, b, and c only.
      4. All the above.

14. For several days following his injury and spinal fusion, Leonard refused his meals, claiming that he wasn't hungry. His anorexia was probably the result of:
   1. Grief reaction provoked by loss of function.
   2. Inhibition of peristalsis due to spinal shock.
   3. Generalized toxicity due to urinary sepsis.
   4. Decreased energy need due to muscular inactivity.

15. Which of the following would retard Leonard's recovery from spinal shock?
   a. Premature exercise.
   b. Urinary sepsis.
   c. Psychological depression.
   d. Decubitus ulcers.
   e. Inadequate caloric intake.
      1. a and c only.
      2. b and d only.
      3. All but d.
      4. All the above.

16. Leonard would be particularly susceptible to decubitus ulcer development as a result of:
   a. Motor paralysis.
   b. Loss of sensation.
   c. Excessive perspiration.
   d. Loss of weight.
   e. Irritation from the cast.
      1. a and b only.
      2. c and d only.
      3. All but c.
      4. All the above.

17. It should be explained to Leonard that, upon recovery from spinal shock, he will experience:
   1. Uncontrolled reflex movements of the legs.

2. Reestablishment of conscious bladder control.
3. Return of sensation in the paralyzed area.
4. Resolution of grief and reversal of depression.

18. Following Leonard's recovery from spinal shock, the nurse will note which neurological change in regard to his lower extremities?
   1. Exaggeration of temperature perception.
   2. Return of deep tendon reflexes.
   3. Loss of additional motor function.
   4. Appearance of a Babinski reflex.

19. Following recovery from spinal shock Leonard will experience flexor or extensor spasms of his lower extremities, which result from:
   1. Hyperirritability of skeletal muscle fibers which are ischemic from disuse.
   2. Fibrosis and shortening of tendons and ligaments in unused joints.
   3. Release of the lower segment of the transected cord from cortical control.
   4. Erratic impulse transmission across healed motor fibers at the injury site.

20. In bathing Leonard, the nurse should be prepared for the fact that touching the skin of his lower abdomen and thighs is apt to provoke:
   a. Ejaculation of semen.
   b. Persistent penile erection.
   c. Clonic convulsions.
   d. Bladder emptying.
   e. Bowel evacuation.
      1. a and b only.
      2. c and d only.
      3. All but e.
      4. All the above.

21. Leonard's diet will probably be of which type?
   a. High vitamin.
   b. High protein.
   c. High caloric.
   d. High fat.
   e. High bulk.
      1. a only.
      2. a and b only.
      3. All but d.
      4. All the above.

22. The nurse can discourage Leonard's development of urinary infection by:
   a. Forcing intake of enough fluid to produce at least 2000 cc. of urine per day.
   b. Cleansing the external urinary meatus daily with soap and water.
   c. Irrigating the catheter three times a day through a closed drainage system.
   d. Providing early bladder training to institute automatic bladder control.
      1. a only.
      2. b only.
      3. c only.
      4. All the above.

23. Leonard should be advised to do which of the following in order to avoid development of fecal impaction?
   a. Eat three servings each day of fresh fruits and vegetables.
   b. Drink 100 cc. of prune or fig juice 30 minutes before breakfast.
   c. Attempt to move his bowels at the same time each day, after a meal.
   d. Insert a glycerine rectal suppository to initiate the evacuation reflex.
   e. Employ regular digital examination of the rectum to check for impacted feces.
      1. a and b only.
      2. a, b, and c only.
      3. All but e.
      4. All the above.

24. Leonard's susceptibility to decubitus ulcer formation can be decreased by:
   a. Changing his position every two hours.
   b. Changing his lower bed linen frequently.
   c. Placing him on an air mattress.
   d. Padding his bony prominences with lamb's wool.
   e. Applying lotion daily over his heels, sacrum, spine, and scapulae.
      1. a and b only.
      2. b and c only.
      3. All but e.
      4. All the above.

25. As a result of cord transection, Leonard will experience loss of vasomotor control in the lower extremities, the consequences of which will include:
   a. Orthostatic hypotension.
   b. Excessive sweating.
   c. Poor heat regulation.
   d. Marked pedal edema.
   e. Increased urinary output.
      1. a only.
      2. b and c only.
      3. a, b, and c only.
      4. All the above.

26. The most ambitious objective which could reasonably be set concerning treatment of Leonard's bladder dysfunction would be for him to eventually achieve:
   1. Ability to maintain catheter drainage through irrigation and receptacle emptying.
   2. Ability to regulate fluid intake and catheterize himself at 6-hour intervals.
   3. Automatic reflex emptying of his bladder at intervals of 3 to 5 hours.
   4. Complete volitional control of bladder emptying when free of infection.

27. One day Leonard complained of pain in his legs, whereupon the staff nurse asked the head nurse, "How can it be possible for Mr. Heller to feel pain in his legs? His cord is completely transected, isn't it?" Which of the following would be the most appropriate response?
   1. "He doesn't feel pain, of course. He's referring to the general discomfort which results from immobility, powerlessness, and boredom."
   2. "No, he can't feel pain. Maybe he's claiming to have pain because that's the only way he can get the staff to stop in to see him."
   3. "His pain is purely psychological. It will disappear as soon as he is able to fully accept his physical and social disability."
   4. "Some patients with cord transection experience sharp, shooting, or burning pain in the area of paralysis, which is resistant to all treatment."

After several weeks in the hospital Leonard's spinal wound healed and he managed to achieve a degree of automatic bowel and bladder control, so he was discharged to his home where he was cared for by his mother and older sister. After two visits to the Outpatient Clinic he failed to keep later appointments. Two years later he was readmitted to the hospital complaining of episodes of painful muscle spasms of the legs and a decubitus ulcer 8 cm. in diameter over the greater trochanter of the left femur.

In the admitting interview the nurse learned that Leonard had been taking Gantrisin 500 mg. "O" four times a day for two weeks. The drug had been given him by his family physician in treatment of a urinary infection. He had also been taking 50 mg. of Talwin "O" three times a day or so to relieve painful leg muscle spasms.

For five days Leonard was kept at complete bedrest, given a high-protein diet, high fluid intake, Gantrisin Q.I.D., Talwin p.r.n., and his decubitus ulcer was cleansed and dressed several times a day. On the sixth day after admission he was given 50 mg. of Demerol, 10 mg. of Valium, 0.4 mg. of Atropine, and taken to the operating room where, under nitrous oxide and halothane anesthesia, his decubitus ulcer was excised and a flap graft was mobilized from his buttock and rotated to fill in the resulting tissue defect. Two large drains were placed under the graft and attached to suction. Two strips of split-thickness skin graft from the posterior chest wall were used to cover the skin defect created by flap rotation. Pressure dressings were applied to both wounds.

28. Typically, the reflex spasms which occur in patients with cord transection consist of:

   a. Dorsiflexion of the great toe.
   b. Dorsiflexion of the ankle.
   c. Flexion of the knee on the thigh.
   d. Flexion of the thigh on the abdomen.
   e. Adduction of the thighs.
     1. a and c only.
     2. b and d only.
     3. All but e.
     4. All the above.

29. Which of the following stimuli would be apt to evoke reflex spasms in Leonard's lower extremities?

   a. Scratching the sole with a sharp object.
   b. Pricking the skin of the foot with a pin.
   c. Pinching the muscles of the thigh.
   d. Pressure of the bed linen against the leg.
   e. Passage of a draft of air across the legs.
     1. a only.
     2. a and b only.
     3. All but e.
     4. All the above.

30. Careful questioning by the nurse revealed that Leonard had been lax in taking his prescribed Gantrisin while living at home. He claimed to have had difficulty remembering to take the drug. Some doses had been omitted entirely; many had been taken late. This information is significant because:

   1. Refusal to adhere to the prescribed drug regimen indicates that he probably will not cooperate with other aspects of care.
   2. Omitted doses allow the blood concentration of the drug to fall sufficiently so that microorganisms can develop resistance to the medicine.
   3. Failure to accept prescribed treatment for an obvious physical illness indicates the existence of strong self-destructive tendencies.
   4. Memory lapses concerning an issue of such great self interest would indicate a serve degree of debility or toxicity.

31. While he was receiving Gantrisin, Leonard's daily fluid intake should have been at least:

   1. 1500 cc.
   2. 2000 cc.
   3. 2500 cc.
   4. 3000 cc.

32. The purpose for maintaining adequate fluid intake during Gantrisin administration is to prevent:

   1. Direct chemical irritation of the mucosal lining of the stomach.
   2. Blockage of kidney tubules by precipitated crystals of the drug.
   3. Constipation due to the astringent effect of the drug on the mucosa.
   4. Decreased blood volume due to the osmotic effect of the drug.

33. When Gantrisin was first prescribed for him, Leonard should have been cautioned to avoid which of the following as contributory to an untoward effect from the drug?

   1. Direct sunlight.
   2. Citrus fruits.
   3. Iced drinks.
   4. Emotional upsets.

34. Leonard should be questioned to determine whether he has experienced which of the following common and untoward side-effects of Talwin?

   1. Purpura.
   2. Tinnitus.
   3. Vertigo.
   4. Gingival hypertrophy.

35. Talwin would be preferred to morphine for relieving Leonard's pain because Talwin is less likely to cause:
  a. Constipation.
  b. Nausea.
  c. Dependency.
  d. Dizziness.
  e. Respiratory depression.
    1. a only.
    2. b and d only.
    3. a, c, and e only.
    4. All the above.

36. From the time of his spinal injury, Leonard had been unable to obtain employment of any kind, although he had sought a job as a telephone solicitor through the state employment agency. In making long-term plans for Leonard's care the nurse should consider that his inability to work during the past two years would probably have decreased his:
  1. Sense of personal worth and identity.
  2. Ability to communicate with others.
  3. Feelings of competition with age peers.
  4. Ambitions for material success.

37. Pre- and postoperatively, Leonard's diet should be especially rich in which vitamin?
  1. Vitamin A.
  2. Vitamin B_1.
  3. Vitamin C.
  4. Vitamin D.

38. Which of the following foods are especially good sources of the aforementioned vitamin?
  a. Cabbage.
  b. Lean beef.
  c. Tomatoes.
  d. Cereal grains.
  e. Milk.
    1. a and c only.
    2. b and d only.
    3. All but e.
    4. All the above.

39. In order to answer Leonard's questions concerning his surgical treatment the nurse should anticipate that preparation of his decubitus ulcer for grafting will probably require:
  1. Repeated applications of alcohol or other vasodilator to the ulcer base.
  2. Wound irrigation with antibiotic solution for several days preoperatively.
  3. Debridement of necrotic tissue from both the base and sides of the ulcer.
  4. Toughening of surrounding skin by repeated applications of tincture of benzoin.

40. Which of Leonard's preoperative laboratory values would be of greatest value in forcasting the probability of postoperative graft survival?
  1. Blood glucose level.
  2. Urine specific gravity.
  3. Serum albumin concentration.
  4. Clotting time.

41. Valium or diazepam has which of the following effects?
  a. Relieves anxiety.
  b. Relaxes skeletal muscle.
  c. Reduces restlessness.
  d. Relieves pain.
  e. Prevents convulsions.
    1. a only.
    2. a, b, and c only.
    3. All but d.
    4. All the above.

42. Which of the following are common adverse effects of diazepam?
  a. Drowsiness.
  b. Dizziness.
  c. Ataxia.
  d. Visual disturbances.
  e. Tremor.
    1. a only.
    2. a and b only.
    3. All but e.
    4. All the above.

43. The characteristic of nitrous oxide which explains its use in Leonard's anesthesia is the fact that it:
  1. Provides rapid, pleasant induction.
  2. Produces marked muscle relaxation.
  3. Fails to support combustion.
  4. Depresses salivary and mucous secretions.

44. The chief disadvantage of using nitrous oxide as an anesthetic is the danger that, during its administration, which of the following complications may occur?
  1. Anoxia.
  2. Hypotension.
  3. Explosion.
  4. Arrhythmia.

45. A flap graft, rather than a free graft, was used to cover Leonard's decubitus ulcer because, through use of the former:

a. Subcutaneous tissue as well as dermis and epidermis can be obtained to fill the defect.

b. There will be no residual defect or scar left at the site from which the tissue is taken.

c. The tissue to be transferred is never separated from its blood supply.

d. There is no need for postoperative dressing of either donor or recipient site.

e. There is no need to restrict movement during the period of graft healing.

   1. a and c only.

   2. b and d only.

   3. All but e.

   4. All the above.

46. The surgeon's primary purpose for inserting drains under the flap graft was to:

1. Prevent tension on the sutures holding the dressing in place.

2. Ensure continuous contact between the graft and the underlying tissue.

3. Aerate the dark, moist area underneath the mobilized skin flap.

4. Facilitate immediate awareness by caregivers of postoperative hemorrhage.

47. The area from which the flap was mobilized was covered by a split-thickness skin graft because:

1. The defect left by removal of a full-thickness graft is unable to heal by regeneration.

2. Coverage by a split-thickness graft yields more attractive results than does suturing skin edges together.

3. Survival of a split-thickness graft is less dependent on good blood supply than is primary wound healing.

4. The defect was covered temporarily in case additional tissue would later be needed from the site.

48. The primary purpose for the pressure dressings which were applied over the two grafts was to:

1. Prevent hemorrhage.

2. Relieve pain.

3. Minimize edema.

4. Ensure contact.

49. Which type of suction equipment should be attached to the skin catheters which were placed under the flap graft?

1. A three bottle setup in which a water seal bottle is interposed between the drainage bottle and a suction source.

2. A suction machine providing an intermittent negative pressure of fifteen centimeters of water.

3. A suction machine providing a continuous negative pressure of five centimeters of water.

4. A suction machine providing a continuous negative pressure of fifteen centimeters of water.

50. The Recovery Room nurse should observe Leonard carefully during the immediate postanesthetic period for which of the following as a common side effect of halothane anesthesia?

1. Convulsions.

2. Laryngospasm.

3. Vomiting.

4. Hypotension.

51. The dressing over the recipient site became saturated with serosanguinous drainage shortly after surgery. When the physician changed the dressing the nurse noted that the distal end of the flap was slightly darker in color than the base of the flap. The most probable cause for this phenomenon would be:

1. Venous spasm due to mechanical trauma during surgery.

2. Accumulation of clotted blood under the flap.

3. Focal inflammatory change due to bacterial invasion.

4. Necrosis of peripheral tissue due to circulatory obstruction.

52. The nurses should be especially gentle in moving Leonard after surgery because rough handling would be particularly apt to cause:

1. Displacement of the catheters which were implanted under the graft.

2. Circulatory shock through initiation of generalized systemic vasodilation.

3. Disruption of graft attachment as a result of reflex leg spasms.

4. Loss of automatic bowel control as a consequence of the startle reaction.

53. Which of the following interventions by the nurse would maximize the probability for graft survival at the recipient site?

    a. Utilizing strict aseptic technique when changing dressings over the graft.

    b. Maintaining Leonard in positions which prevent pressure on the graft.

    c. Regulating the environment so as to make mealtimes as pleasant as possible.

    d. Rolling accumulated fluid from under the graft with a cotton-tipped applicator.

    e. Applying mittens to keep Leonard from scratching the graft during sleep.

        1. a and b only.

        2. a, b, and c only.

        3. All but d.

        4. All the above.

54. Even when no drainage is visible on the dressing, it should be checked at frequent intervals during the first two to three days postoperatively because of the danger that:

    1. Openings in the suction catheter will become obstructed by clots.

    2. Local edema may cause the pressure dressings to become too tight.

    3. The graft will become displaced from its proper position.

    4. The edges of the wound will become everted and require straightening.

55. In changing Leonard's dressing postoperatively the nurse should take special pains to avoid:

    1. Movement of the catheters which were placed under the flap.

    2. Application of pressure to the central portion of the graft.

    3. Moistening the skin edges surrounding the recipient site.

    4. Disrupting contact between the graft and underlying tissue.

56. One day, while the nurse was giving him a bath, Leonard admitted that during the past two years he had not daily examined his body for pressure areas, though the clinic doctor and nurse had explained why this should be done and his mother had repeatedly reminded him to do so. His neglect of this aspect of self care was probably a manifestation of which defense mechanism?

    1. Denial.

    2. Projection.

    3. Undoing.

    4. Rationalization.

57. Several times after his surgery Leonard refused to allow the nurse to irrigate his catheter, even though it was impossible for him to carry out the procedure himself without considerable discomfort. His refusal was probably the result of:

    1. General dislike for or distrust of health care professionals.

    2. Shame concerning what he perceives as loss of manhood.

    3. Doubt that she can perform the procedure as skillfully as he can.

    4. Desire to develop some complication which would postpone hospital discharge.

58. For the first week or ten days postoperatively the nurse may expect Leonard to complain of:

    1. Pruritus of the donor and recipient graft sites.

    2. Sharp pain radiating down the posterior aspect of the left thigh.

    3. Aching pain in the region of the greater trochanter of the left femur.

    4. Burning pain in the area surrounding the site of the former ulcer.

Both the flap graft and the split-thickness graft healed slowly but without complication. The suction catheters were gradually withdrawn from the wound and the final skin sutures were removed two weeks after the operation. Leonard was again instructed concerning the need for scrupulous skin care, frequent changes in position, and high protein, high vitamin diet. In addition to giving Leonard a clinic appointment for followup regarding his plastic repair, arrangements were made for a social worker to visit him at home and help him explore educational and occupational opportunities for which he might qualify.

59. Before discharge Leonard should be provided with which of the following devices for his use at home in preventing development of additional decubitus ulcers?

    1. Back scratcher.

    2. Electric vibrator.

    3. Inflatable rubber ring.

    4. Long-handled mirror.

Arteriosclerotic Obliterative Disease and Femoral-Popliteal Bypass Graft

Willie Walker, an obese sixty-year-old watchman, sought hospital admission for relief of severe aching pain in the right calf. Mr. Walker indicated that his leg pain, which was of two years' duration, was provoked by walking the distance of a half block and was usually relieved by rest. During the past month, however, severe leg pain had several times wakened him from sleep. Mr. Walker also indicated that five years ago he had been diagnosed as having diabetes mellitus, which disorder had subsequently been well controlled on diet alone. He also had a three-year history of mild hypertension for which he had been treated with hydrochlorothiazide. He admitted to smoking a pack of cigarettes each day and to drinking three bottles of beer each week.

Physical examination revealed that Mr. Walker had normal carotid, brachial, radial, and femoral pulses, somewhat diminished popliteal pulses, and absence of the posterior tibial and dorsalis pedis pulse on the right. The posterior tibial and dorsalis pedis pulses were slightly decreased in amplitude on the left. The skin of his right foot was pale and cold. The examining physician admitted Mr. Walker to the hospital and placed him on complete bed rest while a vascular workup was performed.

Arteriography revealed severe narrowing and tortuosity of the right femoral and popliteal arteries but apparently normal arteries in the lower leg. There was also slight decrease in the caliber of the left femoral artery. Blood flow studies using Doppler ultrasound technique revealed marked decrease in blood flow through the right femoral and popliteal arteries. A diagnosis was made of arteriosclerotic obliterative disease of the extremities, most pronounced on the right.

(ANSWER BLANK ON PAGE A–119) (CORRECT ANSWERS ON PAGE B–202)

1. Which of the following factors probably predisposed Mr. Walker to obliterative vascular disease?
- a. Diabetes mellitus.
- b. Watchman's duties.
- c. Arterial hypertension.
- d. Alcoholic intake.
- e. Cigarette smoking.
    - 1. a and b only.
    - 2. c and d only.
    - 3. a, c, and e only.
    - 4. All the above.

2. Which aspect of diabetic pathophysiology contributes directly to development of atherosclerosis?
- 1. Elevation of the blood glucose level.
- 2. Decrease in serum bicarbonate level.
- 3. Increase in serum concentration of cholesterol.
- 4. Reduction in liver glycogen stores.

3. Which of the following are effects of atheromatosis which predispose to intravascular thrombus formation?

    a. Roughening of the intima.
    b. Narrowing of the lumen.
    c. Increase in serum fibrinogen.
    d. Increase in blood viscosity.
    e. Decreased speed of blood flow.
       1. a and c only.
       2. b and d only.
       3. a, b, and e only.
       4. All the above.

4. The most significant index of the degree of Mr. Walker's arterial occlusion was the:

    1. Pain on walking.
    2. Pallor of the foot.
    3. Decrease in skin temperature.
    4. Absence of peripheral pulses.

5. Mr. Walker's calf pain was principally the result of which pathological tissue change?

    1. Decrease in oxygen content.
    2. Increase in carbon dioxide content.
    3. Decrease in glucose concentration.
    4. Increase in interstitial fluid.

6. In addition to calf pain, arteriosclerotic obliterative disease of the lower extremities frequently produces which other symptoms?

    a. Thin, shiny skin.
    b. Thickening of the nails.
    c. Absence of hair on the toes.
    d. Fissuring of the heels.
    e. Dusky red discoloration of the skin.
       1. a only.
       2. a and b only.
       3. a, b, and c only.
       4. All but e.
       5. All the above.

7. Mr. Walker's recent episodes of leg pain at night indicate that:

    1. He has developed concomitant venous thrombosis.
    2. The degree of his arterial obstruction has increased.
    3. The assumption of horizontal position improves his venous return.
    4. Nervous tissue has regenerated following adaptation to oxygen lack.

8. Careful questioning would probably reveal that Mr. Walker had been able to decrease pain in his legs at night by:

    1. Elevating his leg on blankets or pillows.
    2. Hanging his foot over the edge of the bed.
    3. Applying a heating pad to his foot.
    4. Forcible flexing of his knee and ankle.

9. Femoral artery pulsations are best palpated:

    1. In the midline of the abdomen just below the umbilicus.
    2. Immediately below Poupart's ligament in the middle of the groin.
    3. On the inner aspect of the thigh, halfway between groin and knee.
    4. In the groove between the tendons at the back of the knee.

10. Pulsations of the posterior tibial artery are best detected at which point?

    1. Directly in the midline of the popliteal space.
    2. Along the shin bone, halfway between knee and ankle.
    3. Slightly distal and posterior to the medial malleolus.
    4. Between the first and second metatarsal on the dorsum of the foot.

11. While he is being kept at complete bedrest in the hospital, Mr. Walker's feet should be protected from injury by:

    a. Applying lanolin ointment to the skin daily.
    b. Wrapping the legs in elastic bandages and elevating the feet.
    c. Cushioning his feet in soft fleece-lined boots.
    d. Warming his feet with an electric blanket or pad.
    e. Supporting the upper linen with a bed cradle.
       1. a and b only.
       2. c and d only.
       3. a, c, and e only.
       4. All the above.

12. Mr. Walker could give informed consent for arteriography if the vascular surgeon and/or radiographer had explained to him that possible complications of the procedure include:

    a. Development of intravascular thrombosis.
    b. Allergic reaction to the injected dye.
    c. Embolization of a calcified plaque.
    d. Major hemorrhage from the puncture site.
    e. Perforation of the vessel by the catheter.
       1. a and b only.
       2. a, b, and c only.
       3. All but e.
       4. All the above.

13. Just before Mr. Walker was taken to the X-ray Department for arteriography of his

lower extremities, his physician started an intravenous infusion of 5 per cent dextrose in distilled water for the purpose of:

1. Overdistending his leg vessels so as to improve visualization of vascular pathology.
2. Replacing body fluids which will be lost due to the diuretic effect of the radiopaque dye.
3. Providing a reserve supply of nutrient for those tissues deprived of blood during the test.
4. Decreasing the incidence of intravascular thrombosis during the process of vascular manipulation.

14. Which of the following diagnostic tests could be used to determine more accurately the location and degree of Mr. Walker's vascular obstruction?

a. Measurement of arterial pressure in his foot, lower leg, and thigh.
b. Determination of foot temperature following application of heat to the abdomen.
c. Recording the amount of treadmill exercise required to produce claudication.
d. Timing the removal of a radioisotope which has been injected into a leg muscle.
e. Auscultation with a stethoscope along the course of the femoral artery.
   1. a only.
   2. a and b only.
   3. a, b, and c only.
   4. All the above.

Mr. Walker's routine blood, urine, serology tests, chest x-ray, and electrocardiogram were all within normal limits. Because his leg pain was severe and because it interfered with his earning a livelihood, it was decided to improve the circulation to his right leg by installing a femoral-popliteal bypass graft. However, the surgeon explained the he would delay the operation for a few months in order that Mr. Walker could lose twenty pounds and stop smoking before undergoing surgery. Accordingly, Mr. Walker was discharged on a 1200 calorie, low fat, low cholesterol diet with an appointment for follow-up in the vascular clinic.

15. Mr. Walker should be persuaded to stop smoking because nicotine produces:

1. Increase in prothrombin production by the liver.

2. Decreased sensitivity to ischemic muscle pain.
3. Spasm of small arteries providing collateral blood supply.
4. Increased restlessness and excessive motor activity.

16. Vasodilators are generally not used in treatment of chronic arteriosclerotic obliterative disease of the extremities because of their tendency to:

1. Cause capillary hemorrhage in brain and kidney tissue.
2. Produce dependent edema in the feet or lung bases.
3. Divert blood flow away from severely ischemic tissues.
4. Decrease cardiac efficiency by impairing venous return flow.

17. Which of the following points should be stressed in teaching Mr. Walker how to care for his feet at home?

a. Bathe feet daily with hot water and strong soap.
b. Prevent irritation by placing absorbent cotton between the toes.
c. Decrease callus formation by walking barefoot inside the house.
d. Wear a fresh pair of clean white wool stockings every day.
e. Wear canvas, crepe-soled shoes rather than leather oxfords.
   1. a and c only.
   2. b and d only.
   3. All but d.
   4. All the above.

18. Regarding the amount of physical activity that he should indulge in at home. Mr. Walker should be told to:

1. Remain immobile in supine or sedentary position for most of the time.
2. Limit physical activity to that absolutely necessary to self care.
3. Engage in some mild exercise daily but cease activity if pain develops.
4. Exercise the legs actively, using analgesics to control resulting pain.

19. Which of the following foods would be restricted in Mr. Walker's low cholesterol diet?

a. Egg yolk.
b. Olive oil.
c. Cheddar cheese.
d. Muscle meats.
e. Shellfish.
   1. a and b only.
   2. c and d only.
   3. a, c, and e only.
   4. All the above.

20. In preparing Mr. Walker for discharge the nurse should instruct him concerning the dangers of self medication, especially warning him against using any of the commercially available:

    1. Headache anodynes.
    2. Sinus remedies.
    3. Gastric antacids.
    4. Bulk-producing laxatives.

21. Mr. Walker should be instructed to avoid which of the following as hazards to foot health?

    a. Cold exposure.
    b. Corn remedies.
    c. Hot water bottles.
    d. Loose-fitting shoes.
    e. Sitting with crossed knees.
        1. a and c only.
        2. b and d only.
        3. All but e.
        4. All the above.

22. Mr. Walker should be taught that, as a result of his diabetes, any foot lesion which he might develop would be especially subject to:

    1. Swelling.
    2. Hemorrhage.
    3. Infection.
    4. Scarring.

23. Before leaving the hospital, Mr. Walker should be told to contact his physician immediately if he should develop:

    a. Sudden sharp pain in the leg.
    b. Discoloration of the toe or foot.
    c. Numbness of the foot or leg.
    d. Fissuring of the skin between the toes.
    e. Pallor and coldness of the limb.
        1. a only.
        2. a and b only.
        3. a, b, and c only.
        4. Any of the above.

24. During the interval between diagnosis of Mr. Walker's arterial disease and installation of a bypass graft, his treatment would be principally aimed at preventing:

    1. Pain.
    2. Paralysis.
    3. Hemorrhage.
    4. Gangrene.

25. Both the hospital nurse and the clinic nurse should encourage Mr. Walker to examine his legs and feet daily for injury because:

    1. His alcoholic drinking habit renders him prone to physical trauma.
    2. Diabetic neuropathy may have decreased his perception of pain.
    3. A low fat diet will predispose him to capillary weakness.
    4. Ulcers resulting from arterial insufficiency are typically painless.

Four months after hospital discharge Mr. Walker had lost 25 pounds and had stopped smoking. However, the rest pain in his right leg had increased in frequency and severity, so he was readmitted to the hospital and an autogenous saphenous vein graft was applied to circumvent his occluded right femoral and popliteal arteries. Preoperatively Mr. Walker's legs were measured for below-the-knee elastic stockings to be applied postoperatively, and his right groin and leg scrubbed in preparation for surgery. The operative area was scrubbed again and shaved in the operating room immediately before Mr. Walker was anesthetized.

26. Mr. Walker should be in which position while he is being measured for his below the knee elastic stockings?

    1. Standing upright with his weight evenly distributed on both legs.
    2. Sitting in a straight chair with his feet planted firmly on the floor.
    3. Sitting on a bed with his legs dangling over the side of the mattress.
    4. Lying supine with his legs slightly elevated and feet in relaxed position.

27. As part of Mr. Walker's preparation for surgery the nurse should teach him how to perform which of the following activities?

    1. Simple wound dressing.
    2. Three-point crutch walking.
    3. Quadriceps setting exercises.
    4. Measuring of arterial blood pressure.

28. Which of the following antiseptics would be best suited for use in Mr. Walker's preoperative skin preparation?

    1. 70 per cent ethyl alcohol.
    2. 0.5 per cent sodium hypochlorite.
    3. 50 per cent hydrogen peroxide.
    4. 0.5 per cent providone-iodine.

29. In preoperative skin preparation a disposable rather than a reusable razor should be employed because use of the former minimizes:

    1. Discomfort.
    2. Infection.

3. Time expenditure.

4. Expenses.

30. Mr. Walker should be handled gently when he is moved from the operating table to the recovery bed, as rapid, rough movement during transfer would be apt to cause:

   a. Too rapid recovery from anesthesia.

   b. Weakening of the suture line.

   c. Sudden lowering of blood pressure.

   d. Rebellious or combative behavior.

     1. a and b only.

     2. b and c only.

     3. c and d only.

     4. All the above.

31. Mr. Walker was transported from the operating room with an oropharyngeal airway in place. The airway should be removed:

   1. Immediately on admission to the recovery room.

   2. When he begins to recover consciousness.

   3. When he is fully conscious and oriented.

   4. When his vital signs have been stabilized.

32. Mr. Walker was semi-comatose on admission to the recovery room. He should be placed in which position?

   1. Fowler's position, with the knee gatch elevated slightly.

   2. Supine, with his head turned to one side.

   3. On his left side, with his right leg supported full length on pillows.

   4. Prone, with his toes extended over the end of the mattress.

33. Immediately after positioning Mr. Walker in bed, the recovery room nurse should ascertain his general condition and immediate needs. To do this she should first:

   1. Ask the accompanying anesthetist for an evaluation of Mr. Walker's condition.

   2. Check Mr. Walker's vital signs, wound dressing, and level of consciousness.

   3. Review the description of anesthesia and surgical procedure on the Operative Record.

   4. Read the surgeon's written orders for Mr. Walker's postoperative care.

34. Immediately upon Mr. Walker's admission to the Recovery Room, the nurse should check his femoral, popliteal, posterior tibial, and dorsalis pedis pulses in order to:

   1. Ascertain the effectiveness of the operation in restoring circulation.

   2. Obtain baseline information against which to evaluate subsequent findings.

   3. Detect evidence of occult bleeding from the site of vascular anastamosis.

   4. Determine his state of general hydration and need for intravenous fluid therapy.

35. Mr. Walker's bed position should be changed frequently during the first few hours following the operation in order to prevent:

   a. Pooling and infection of respiratory secretions.

   b. Collapse of peripheral pulmonary alveoli.

   c. Shunting of blood in the pulmonary circuit.

   d. Edema of tissues traumatized during surgery.

   e. Formation of postoperative adhesions.

     1. a only.

     2. a and b only.

     3. a, b, and c only.

     4. All the above.

36. After his oropharyngeal airway was removed, Mr. Walker seemed somewhat drowsy, but he complained of nausea. The position of choice for Mr. Walker at this time would be:

   1. High Fowler's.

   2. Trendelenburg.

   3. Side-lying.

   4. Prone.

37. In addition to checking his femoral, popliteal, posterior tibial, and dorsalis pedis pulses, the Recovery Room nurse should ascertain the adequacy of circulation in Mr. Walker's right leg postoperatively by determining the:

   1. Circumference of the right thigh at half-hour intervals.

   2. Femoral artery pressure difference between the left and right legs.

   3. Interval between leg elevation and occurrence of calf pain.

   4. Time required for capillary filling following release of toenail compression.

38. The nurse can best determine when Mr. Walker has regained full consciousness by:
1. Checking his pupillary reaction to light.
2. Asking him to identify where he is.
3. Giving him sips of water to drink.
4. Pinching the skin of his arms or legs.

39. As soon as Mr. Walker regains consciousness the nurse should:
1. Give him ice chips or sips of water.
2. Direct him to breathe deeply and cough.
3. Encourage active exercise of both legs.
4. Elevate the head of the bed slightly.

40. For the first two to three hours following Mr. Walker's operation, which of the following physical findings would be expected?
a. Higher skin temperature in the right foot than the left.
b. Swelling and tension along the skin suture line.
c. Absence of the dorsalis pedis pulse on the right.
d. Oozing of dark blood at upper and lower poles of the incision.
e. Pallor and mottling of the right foot and leg.
  1. a and c only.
  2. b and d only.
  3. All but d.
  4. All the above.

41. While searching for the dorsalis pedis pulse in Mr. Walker's right foot, the nurse was able to detect only a faint pulsation. To determine whether it was her own or Mr. Walker's pulse that she had perceived, the nurse should:
1. Count her own radial pulse to see if it is the same rate and rhythm as that she has just counted.
2. Palpate his radial and dorsalis pedis pulses simultaneously to see if a radial beat slightly precedes each pedal beat.
3. Palpate his femoral pulse to see if it is the same rate as that she has just counted.
4. Increase her own pulse rate through brief exercise and then recount his pedal pulse to see if the rate remains constant.

42. Which characteristics of Mr. Walker's pulse should be noted by the nurse?

a. Rate.
b. Rhythm.
c. Volume.
d. Contour.
e. Variability.
  1. a only.
  2. a and b only.
  3. a, b, and c only.
  4. All the above.

43. The purpose for applying below-the-knee elastic stockings to Mr. Walker's legs postoperatively was to prevent development of:
1. Hypotension.
2. Hemorrhage.
3. Edema.
4. Varicosities.

44. The Recovery Room nurse should measure Mr. Walker's blood pressure frequently during the immediate postanesthetic period, as a hypotensive episode would considerably increase his risk of postoperative:
1. Hemorrhage.
2. Pneumonia.
3. Thrombosis.
4. Convulsions.

45. Which of the following would be the most likely cause of a fall in Mr. Walker's blood pressure during the first eight hours following surgery?
1. Vasodilation produced by the anesthetic agent.
2. Hemorrhage from the site of vascular anastomosis.
3. Blockade of vasomotor reflexes by analgesic drugs.
4. Myocardial inefficiency due to impaired venous return.

46. In addition to observing Mr. Walker's wound dressings for drainage, the Recovery Room nurse should also check for postoperative hemorrhage by:
1. Serial measurements of the circumference of his leg.
2. Palpating the incision for swelling and tension.
3. Observing capillary flush after compression of the nail.
4. Comparing the skin temperature of the two legs.

47. Four hours postoperatively the Recovery Room nurse detected both the posterior tibial and dorsalis pedis pulses in Mr. Walker's right leg. If at a later time she should be unable to palpate a pulse at either site she should interpret such pulse lack as probably the result of:

1. Transient hypotension.
2. Vascular spasm.
3. Graft thrombosis.
4. Dependent edema.

48. In dressing Mr. Walker's leg postoperatively the nurse should:

1. Apply pressure along the suture line to express accumulated blood or serum.
2. Keep the inner layer of gauze well moistened with normal saline solution.
3. Apply the outer roller gauze tightly, rolling from the groin toward the toe.
4. Avoid attaching adhesive tape directly to the skin of the leg.

Mr. Walker's leg wound healed quickly and without complication. His skin sutures were removed on the eleventh postoperative day, and he was discharged with a referral to the Vascular Clinic for long-term follow-up.

49. Readying Mr. Walker for hospital discharge should include counseling him to:

a. Refrain from smoking.
b. Avoid gaining weight.
c. Remove corns carefully.
d. Massage his feet daily.
e. Elevate his legs frequently.
 1. a and b only.
 2. c and d only.
 3. All but d.
 4. All the above.

50. Mr. Walker should be told that if, following surgery, he should again experience intermittent claudication he can decrease his leg pain or delay its occurrence by:

1. Adopting a more high-stepping, free-swinging stride.

2. Stamping his feet occasionally to improve blood flow.
3. Shortening his steps and slowing his gait somewhat.
4. Wearing socks and shoes a size larger than his regular size.

51. Mr. Walker should be taught to avoid cold injury to his feet in winter by:

1. Wearing battery heated shoes or boots.
2. Sprinkling pepper inside his stockings.
3. Bathing his feet in liniment daily.
4. Staying indoors in extremely cold weather.

52. If, in spite of the foregoing precaution, Mr. Walker is unable to sleep because of cold feet, it would be safest for him to relieve this discomfort by:

1. Rubbing his feet briskly with a soft woolen cloth.
2. Applying an electric heating pad to the soles of his feet.
3. Applying oil to his feet and soaking them briefly in hot water.
4. Placing an insulated hot water bottle on his abdomen before retiring.

53. As part of Mr. Walker's preparation for self care at home he should be persuaded to buy and to use:

1. A pumice stone.
2. A bath thermometer.
3. Stainless steel toe nail clippers.
4. Rubber shower thongs.

54. Proper foot care for Mr. Walker would include application of which of the following to his feet after bathing them each day?

1. Rubbing alcohol compound.
2. Lanolin containing ointment.
3. Anti-fungal powder.
4. Mild boric acid solution.

Viral Hepatitis

Kerry Mottram had worked as a clinical specialist in renal nursing for several years prior to becoming ill one morning at work. She was examined on the unit by the attending physician, who knew that she had a positive hepatitis B surface antigen (HB_sAg). He obtained a blood sample and ordered liver function studies.

Ten months ago Kerry had told the attending physician and her nurse co-workers that she had pricked her thumb with a needle from a jaundiced patient that had been dialyzed in the unit. Kerry had then had monthly blood studies done and one month before had developed a positive HB$_s$Ag but no other symptoms. Early in the morning of the day she became ill she had had symptoms which she attributed to a mild cold and reasoned that she would feel better after she ate breakfast and got busy at work.

The laboratory technician reported the following results from Kerry's blood tests:

Serum glutamic oxaloacetic transaminase (SGOT)	*810 U/ml.*
Serum glutamic pyruvate transaminase (SGPT)	*750 U/ml.*
Gamma glutamyl transpeptidase (GGT)	*80 U/ml.*
Alkaline phosphatase	*260 U/ml.*
Bilirubin, direct (conjugated)	*5.8 mg/100 ml.*
Bilirubin, indirect (unconjugated)	*2.0 mg/100 ml.*
Prothrombin time	*20 Sec.*
Elevated globulin (IgG, IgM, IgA)	
Decreased albumin 2.5 Gm/100 ml. (about 33 per cent total protein)	

Kerry was hospitalized and placed in isolation on bed rest. She had a fever and vomited periodically. The nurses caring for her encouraged her to drink many liquids and to eat the food served to her. Intravenous infusions of 5 per cent dextrose in water were administered for two days until she stopped vomiting.

Several days later Kerry's urine darkened, she became jaundiced and complained of pruritus. Then the fever subsided and, with the exception of her profound fatigue, her general condition improved.

(ANSWER BLANK ON PAGE A–121) (CORRECT ANSWERS ON PAGE B–206)

---

1. The liver normally weighs:
   1. 0.5–1.0 kg.
   2. 1.0–1.5 kg.
   3. 1.5–2.0 kg.
   4. 2.0–2.5 kg.

2. The hepatic artery of the liver receives arterial blood from which of the following arteries?
   1. Celiac.
   2. Superior mesenteric.
   3. Inferior mesenteric.
   4. Splenic.

3. Blood from which of the following veins flows directly into the portal vein?
   a. Splenic.
   b. Left gastric.
   c. Prepyloric.
   d. Superior mesenteric.
   e. Inferior mesenteric.
      1. a only.
      2. a, b, and d.
      3. All but d.
      4. All the above.

4. In contrasting the hepatic artery with the portal vein the nurse should know that the hepatic artery has:
   1. Higher oxygen content, more blood, lower blood pressure.
   2. Higher oxygen content, less blood, higher blood pressure.
   3. Lower oxygen content, less blood, higher blood pressure.
   4. Higher oxygen content, more blood, higher blood pressure.

5. Blood flowing out of the liver follows which of the following routes?
   1. Sinusoid – central vein – hepatic vein – inferior vena cava.
   2. Sinusoid – hepatic vein – inferior mesenteric vein – inferior vena cava.
   3. Sinusoid – sublobular vein – superior mesenteric vein – inferior vena cava.
   4. Sinusoid – splenic vein – hepatic vein – inferior vena cava.

6. Pathophysiology of the liver can lead to which of the following alterations in normal functioning of the body?
   a. Decreased immunocompetence.
   b. Electrolyte imbalance.
   c. Metabolic disruptions.
   d. Inadequate oxygenation of cells.
   e. Distortion of perception.
       1. a and c.
       2. a, c, and d.
       3. All but e.
       4. All the above.

7. Damage to the parenchymal cells and obstruction to blood flow in the sinusoids could cause increased portal vein pressure and venous engorgement of which of the following organs?
   a. Spleen.
   b. Esophagus.
   c. Rectum.
   d. Colon.
   e. Stomach.
       1. a and b only.
       2. a, b, and c.
       3. All but d.
       4. All the above.

8. The liver sinusoids act most like which of the following vessels?
       1. Arteries.
       2. Capillaries.
       3. Veins.
       4. Lymphatics.

9. The liver sinusoids normally contain which of the following types of fluids?
       1. Arterial blood only.
       2. Venous blood only.
       3. Mixed arterial-venous blood.
       4. Lymph and bile combined.

10. Which of the following most accurately describes the function of the Kupffer cells in the liver sinusoids?
       1. Gluconeogenesis.
       2. Phagocytosis.
       3. Detoxification.
       4. Glycogenolysis.

11. The function of bile is best described by which of the following statements?
       1. A pigment responsible for the breakdown of hemoglobin from fragile erythrocytes.
       2. A green pigment produced in the intestines to split fat into free fatty acids.
       3. A brownish substance which oxidizes urobilinogen into stercobilin in the intestine.
       4. A substance required for the emulsification of fats during digestion.

12. Another name for Type B-viral hepatitis is:
       1. Short incubation hepatitis.
       2. Epidemic hepatitis.
       3. Infectious hepatitis.
       4. Serum hepatitis.

13. Type B-viral hepatitis is transmitted most frequently by which of the following substances?
       1. Feces.
       2. Blood.
       3. Semen.
       4. Shellfish.

14. What is the usual length of incubation for the virus causing Type B-viral hepatitis?
       1. 1–15 days.
       2. 15–50 days.
       3. 50–150 days.
       4. 150–300 days.

15. Kerry's doctor ordered a dye clearance study to estimate the amount of liver cell damage. Which of the following dyes are typically used for this study?
   a. Para-amino hippuric acid (PAH).
   b. Bromsulphalein (BSP).
   c. Para-aminobenzoic acid (PAB).
   d. Indocyanine green (ICG).
   e. Inulin.
       1. a and b.
       2. b and d.
       3. All but d.
       4. All the above.

16. Kerry's liver biopsy would be apt to reveal which of the following pathologic changes?
       1. Inflammation of biliary ducts.
       2. Necrosis of liver parenchymal cells.
       3. Disruption of lobular architecture.
       4. Fatty hyaline membrane deposits.

17. SGPT is usually elevated 10–20 times normal in Type B-viral hepatitis. What is the significance of the elevation of this enzyme in Kerry's serum?
       1. The SGPT elevation is directly proportional to the amount of liver cell damage.
       2. Liver cells are damaged, but enzyme elevation may not reflect the amount of pathology.
       3. SGPT analysis is insignificant without directly correlating SGPT and SGOT elevation.
       4. SGPT is elevated because the enzyme responsible for its inhibition is not metabolized in hepatitis.

18. Which of the following best describes gamma glutamyl transpeptidase (GGT)?
1. An enzyme found in the biliary tract but not in cardiac or skeletal muscle.
2. An enzyme found predominantly in liver, and cardiac and skeletal muscle.
3. A hormone synthesized in the body and degraded by the liver cells.
4. An enzyme responsible for the production of bilirubin in the liver.

19. Kerry's alkaline phosphatase was elevated for which of the following reasons?
1. Damage to liver parenchyma.
2. Damage to bone tissue.
3. Renal obstruction.
4. Biliary obstruction.

20. Total bilirubin is elevated in hepatitis for which of the following reasons?
a. Direct (conjugated) bilirubin is increased due to obstruction of biliary ducts.
b. Indirect (unconjugated) bilirubin is increased due to obstruction of biliary ducts.
c. Impaired excretion of conjugated bilirubin through damaged kidneys.
d. Excessive excretion of unconjugated bilirubin from lysed red cells.
e. Indirect bilirubin is elevated because of damaged liver cells.
   1. a only.
   2. a and d.
   3. a, c, and e.
   4. b and c.

21. Deficiency of which of the following enzymes would result in increased indirect (unconjugated) bilirubin?
1. Glycolytic transferase.
2. Carbonic anhydrase.
3. Lipolytic transaminase.
4. Glucuronyl transferase.

22. The Dane particle, a virus-like particle found in the serum of patients with Type B hepatitis, has a core antibody (HB_cA_b) and a surface coat which contains the antigen (HB_sA_g). Which of the following best describes an antigen?
1. A foreign substance which, when introduced into the body, stimulates the production of antibodies.
2. A protein that is produced in the body in response to invasion by a foreign agent.

3. An agent that enhances immunocompetence by destroying foreign proteins.
4. Any substance which inhibits the thymus T cell production of immunologic particles.

23. Which of the following best describes an antibody?
1. A foreign substance which when introduced into the body stimulates the production of antibodies.
2. A protein that is produced in the body in response to invasion by a foreign agent.
3. An agent that enhances immunocompetence by destroying foreign proteins.
4. Any substance which inhibits the thymus T cell production of immunologic particles.

24. Which of the following quantities of blood is thought to be sufficient to transmit Type B-viral hepatitis?
1. 0.0005 ml.
2. 0.005 ml.
3. 0.05 ml.
4. 0.5 ml.

25. On physical examination Kerry would be most apt to show which of the following symptoms?
a. Urticarial rash.
b. Arthralgia.
c. Pharyngitis.
d. Enlarged lymph nodes.
e. Right upper quadrant pain.
   1. c only.
   2. a, c, and d.
   3. All but d.
   4. All the above.

26. Isolation precautions for Kerry should include which of the following?
a. Private room with a shower and toilet facilities.
b. Wearing a mask and gown when giving her care.
c. Careful handling and disposal of Kerry's needles and syringes.
d. Scrupulous handwashing before and after giving her nursing care.
e. Saving each stool specimen in a paper cup.
   1. a and c.
   2. a, c, and d.
   3. All but e.
   4. All the above.

27. To avoid some of the complications of prolonged inactivity and/or bedrest, Kerry should be encouraged to:
1. Have a high intake of fluids.
2. Eat a high fat, low protein diet.
3. Engage in an hour of isometric exercise daily.
4. Increase her intake of ionized calcium.

28. The diet most likely to be ordered for Kerry would be one:
1. High in fat and protein.
2. Low in fat and carbohydrate.
3. High in carbohydrate and protein.
4. Low in carbohydrate and protein.

29. Which of the following foods should not be served to Kerry?
1. Broiled fillet of white fish.
2. Deep fried liver croquettes.
3. Orange or pineapple sherbet.
4. Uncooked fruit or vegetables.

30. How many liters per day of fluid should the nurse ensure that Kerry drink or receive by intravenous infusion?
1. 0.5–1 liter.
2. 1–2 liters.
3. 2–3 liters.
4. 3–5 liters.

31. In which of the phases of Type B-viral hepatitis would Kerry's total bilirubin probably be most elevated above normal?
1. Incubation.
2. Prodromal.
3. Icteric.
4. Convalescence.

32. Jaundice does not become apparent until the serum bilirubin concentration is the same as or greater than:
1. 0.5–1.4 mg per 100 ml.
2. 1.5–2.4 mg per 100 ml.
3. 2.5–3.4 mg per 100 ml.
4. 3.5–4.4 mg per 100 ml.

33. Jaundice in persons with Type B-viral hepatitis usually occurs:
1. One week prior to other prodromal symptoms.
2. At the same time as other prodromal symptoms.
3. One week after appearance of prodromal symptoms.
4. At the same the HB_sAg becomes positive.

34. Which of the following contribute to pruritus?

a. Tissue anoxia.
b. Perfuse perspiration.
c. Emotional stress.
d. Dry skin.
e. Electrolyte imbalance.
1. a only.
2. b, c, and d.
3. All but e.
4. All the above.

35. Which of the following nursing interventions would reduce pruritus?
a. Frequent bathing.
b. Nail cutting.
c. Room ventilation.
d. Enjoyable distractions.
e. Fluid restriction.
1. a, b, and d.
2. b, c, and d.
3. All but e.
4. All the above.

36. Which of the following drugs is thought to be most effective in reducing pruritus?
1. Cholestyramine (Cuemid).
2. Chlorphenesin (Maolate).
3. Carisoprodol (Soma).
4. Deslanoside (Cedilanid).

37. A nursing intervention which would be helpful during the acute phase of her illness is to remind Kerry and her family that the jaundice is:
1. Noticeable.
2. Pruritic.
3. Diagnostic.
4. Transient.

38. Human immune serum globulin (ISG) is thought to be useful in prevention of Type A-viral hepatitis but not Type B-viral hepatitis, unless which of the following can be established?
1. A high titer of HB_sAg.
2. A high titer of HB_cAb.
3. Negative HB_sAg in the serum.
4. Negative HB_cAb in the serum.

39. If possible, Kerry should not be given which of the following hepatotoxic drugs?
a. Chlorpromazine (Thorazine).
b. Chlordiazepoxide (Librium).
c. Tetracyclines.
d. Phenobarbital.
e. Methyldopa (Aldomet).
1. a and b.
2. a, b, and e.
3. All but e.
4. All the above.

40. If Kerry had developed a fulminating case of Type B-viral hepatitis which resulted in permanent parenchymal cell damage, administration of vitamin K would result in which of the following?

    1. Prothrombin time would return to normal.

    2. Prothrombin time would remain elevated.

    3. Prothrombin time would remain decreased.

    4. No change at all in prothrombin time.

41. Since stress would prolong the length of time that Kerry will experience symptoms, the nurse should help Kerry assess which factors would be most stressful. Which of the following are apt to be most stress producing for her?

    a. Prolonged confinement.

    b. Watching others work.

    c. Having jaundice.

    d. Boredom and guilt.

    e. Receiving intravenous fluids.

        1. a only.

        2. a, c, and d.

        3. All but d.

        4. All the above.

42. Complete recovery is possible for Kerry if she does which of the following?

    a. Obtains adequate rest.

    b. Eats a nutritious diet.

    c. Drinks enough fluids.

    d. Reduces stress and boredom.

    e. Receives immunoserum globulin.

        1. a and b.

        2. a, b, and c.

        3. All but e.

        4. All the above.

43. Spread of Type B-viral hepatitis has been most significantly prevented by which of the following procedures?

    1. Cold storage of blood for four weeks.

    2. Screening of blood donors for Hb_sAg.

    3. Administration of immune serum globulin.

    4. Voluntary donation of blood.

44. How can nurses minimize spread of Type B-viral hepatitis to themselves and other patients?

    a. Identification of carriers of Type B-virus through blood screening for Hb_sAg.

    b. Donation of own blood prior to surgery and avoidance of unnecessary transfusions.

    c. Testing of blood for Hb_sAg during pregnancy and hemodialysis and prior to surgery.

    d. Use of disposable equipment and sterilization by autoclaving of non-disposable items.

    e. Wearing of gloves when directed to avoid direct contact with patients' blood, feces, and secretions.

        1. a and d.

        2. a, b, and d.

        3. All but e.

        4. All the above.

45. Kerry needs to be reminded that as a result of her hepatitis and treatment she would be prone to which of the following for several weeks post-hospital discharge?

    1. Infection.

    2. Fainting.

    3. Dehydration.

    4. Hypoglycemia.

46. After Kerry recovers from her Type B-viral hepatitis she will be immune to which of the following diseases?

    1. Type A-viral hepatitis.

    2. Type B-viral hepatitis.

    3. Both Type A and B-viral hepatitis.

    4. None of the above.

Kerry was discharged after 10 days of hospitalization and told that during convalescence at home she could eat any food she could tolerate. She was cautioned to gradually increase her activities and to avoid new intimate contacts until her Hb_sAg assay was normal on two subsequent analyses.

The nurse caring for Kerry reminded her that she probably would fatigue easily for months and that her enzymes might remain abnormal for six months.

Polycystic Kidney and Renal Failure

Ben Toczek, a twenty-five-year-old trucker in chronic renal failure, was referred from a small rural community to a large university hospital for hemodialysis.

His letter of referral indicated that Ben had apparently been in good health until three months before, when, following an attack of the "flu," he had suddenly developed generalized edema. A medical workup consisting of a flat plate of the abdomen, cystoscopy, intravenous urogram, and various renal function tests yielded a diagnosis of renal failure secondary to polycystic kidney disease. He was treated briefly with a low-protein, low-sodium, and potassium-free diet, fluid restriction, Aldomet, and Amphojel. When dietary, fluid, and electrolyte management failed to relieve his edema and biochemical abnormalities, his physician decided that hemodialysis was indicated.

On admission to the university hospital Ben was experiencing headache, dizziness, anorexia, and weakness. The nurse noted an ammoniacal odor to his breath, erosions on the buccal mucosa, and ecchymoses on the extensor surfaces of his arms and legs. His temperature was 98.8 orally, his pulse 96, his respirations 28, and his blood pressure 190/110 mm. Hg. His serum pH was 7.29, his blood urea nitrogen 61 mg.%, his serum creatinine 8 mg.%, his serum potassium 5.8 mEq./L. and his serum bicarbonate 20.9 mEq./L. His urine pH was 6.5, specific gravity 1.008, albumin ++, and negative for sugar and acetone.

The admitting physician wrote the following orders for Ben's care:
1. *Bedrest.*
2. *Record daily weight and intake and output.*
3. *Take vital signs Q.4H.*
4. *Lasix 40 mg. P.O. Stat.*
5. *Aldomet 250 mg. P.O. B.I.D.*
6. *Amphojel 2 Tbsp. T.I.D.*
7. *Low protein (30 G.) protein, high carbohydrate, 1 Gram sodium, no potassium diet*
8. *Limit fluid intake to 1000 c.c./day*

(ANSWER BLANK ON PAGE A–123) (CORRECT ANSWERS ON PAGE B–210)

1. It may be assumed that Ben's bout of influenza precipitated his development of edema by:
1. Destroying large numbers of renal parenchymal cells.
2. Depressing impulse transmission through cardiac conductive tissue.
3. Upsetting his already precarious fluid-electrolyte balance.
4. Interfering with production of serum albumin by the liver.

2. A flat plate film of Ben's abdomen could be expected to reveal:
1. The general size, shape, and location of the kidney.
2. Dilation or constriction of the pelvis of the kidney.
3. The outline of the ureters, bladder, and urethra.
4. The patency of the abdominal aorta and renal arteries.

3. The nurse could decrease Ben's discomfort during cystoscopy by:
1. Placing him in a warm sitz bath for half an hour before the procedure.
2. Directing him to bear down forcefully as the cystoscope is introduced.
3. Teaching him how to use deep breathing exercises during the procedure.
4. Withholding fluids for several hours prior to the procedure.

4. As part of Ben's preparation for cystoscopy he should be told that when the cystoscope is passed through the urethra he may expect to experience:
1. A strong desire to void.
2. Burning pain in the penis.
3. Cramping or gripping pelvic pain.
4. A feeling of rectal fullness.

5. Ben should not be allowed to stand or walk immediately following cystoscopy, as, for some time following the procedure, he will be particularly susceptible to:
1. Anaphylactic shock.
2. Bladder hemorrhage.
3. Pulmonary embolism.
4. Orthostatic hypotension.

6. Ben's preparation for the intravenous urogram should include:
a. Withholding fluids for eight hours.
b. Withholding food for eight hours.
c. Administration of cleansing enemas.
d. Insertion of an indwelling catheter.
e. Investigating possible iodine sensitivity.
   1. a and b only.
   2. c and d only.
   3. All but d.
   4. All the above.

7. Which of the following are expected side effects of iodine-containing intravenous dyes which Ben should be warned about before his intravenous urogram?
a. A generalized feeling of warmth.
b. Crushing pain in the precordium.
c. A salty taste in the mouth.
d. A sharp stabbing pain in the flank.
e. Seeing flashes of light or spots before the eyes.
   1. a and c only.
   2. b and d only.
   3. All but e.
   4. All the above.

8. The sudden development of which of the following during intravenous urography would suggest that Ben was experiencing a sensitivity reaction to the dye used?
a. Dyspnea.
b. Cyanosis.
c. Diaphoresis.
d. Urticaria.
e. Hypotension.
   1. a and b only.
   2. c and d only.
   3. All but e.
   4. All the above.

9. The urine concentration test is used chiefly to determine:
1. The volume of renal blood flow.
2. The permeability of the glomerular membrane.
3. The functional efficiency of tubular cells.
4. The adequacy of cellular hydration.

10. The standard urine concentration test consists of:
1. Measuring the kidney's ability to vary urine concentration following administration of different amounts of fluid.
2. Comparing urine specific gravity with the type of solute found in a given urine specimen.
3. Determining the osmolality of three urine specimens obtained at hourly intervals following a twelve-hour fast.
4. Determining the speed with which the kidney can clear the blood of an intravenously administered dye.

11. Under the circumstances which characterize the standard urine concentration test, the normal range of urine specific gravity would be:
1. 1.000 to 1.005.
2. 1.005 to 1.010.
3. 1.010 to 1.020.
4. 1.020 to 1.035.

12. The phenolsulfonphthalein excretion test is chiefly used to determine:
1. The caliber of the renal arteries.
2. The contour of the renal pelvis.
3. The efficiency of renal tubular secretion.
4. The presence or absence of kidney infection.

13. In order to ensure accuracy of Ben's phenolsulfonphthalein excretion test the nurse should instruct Ben to:
1. Drink no liquid after the previous midnight.
2. Empty his bladder completely at each test voiding.

3. Save only a midstream specimen for testing purposes.
4. Collect his urine specimens in sterile containers.

14. Which of the following is the pathological process which is responsible for Ben's renal failure?
1. Obstruction of arterial blood flow to the kidney.
2. Progressive destruction of nephrons by compression.
3. Invasion of renal parenchyma by pus-producing organisms.
4. Obliteration of renal tubules by fibrous scar tissue.

15. Ben's headache and dizziness are most likely the result of:
1. Generalized tissue dehydration.
2. Persistent elevation of blood pressure.
3. Obstruction of retinal arteries.
4. Infarction of cerebral tissue.

16. Which of the following are consequences of impaired renal functioning which may have contributed to Ben's anorexia?
a. Metallic taste in the mouth.
b. Decreased flow of saliva.
c. Inflammation of oral mucosa.
d. Ulceration of gastric mucosa.
e. Decreased secretion of bile.
  1. a and b only.
  2. c and d only.
  3. All but e.
  4. All the above.

17. Ben's edema would differ from that of a patient with congestive heart failure in that Ben's abnormal fluid accumulation is:
1. Less liable to pit on pressure.
2. Generalized rather than gravity dependent.
3. More readily relieved by bed rest.
4. Less likely to lead to skin breakdown.

18. Ben's anemia is predominately the result of:
1. Decreased production of erythropoietin by the kidney.
2. Escape of red blood cells through damaged glomeruli.
3. Interference with transportation of iron to bone marrow.
4. Decreased absorption of vitamin B_{12} and folic acid.

19. The ecchymoses noted on the extensor surfaces of Ben's arms and legs were probably the result of:

1. Repeated minor trauma due to muscular incoordination.
2. A clotting disturbance due to abnormal platelet function.
3. Spontaneous hemorrhage due to increased capillary fragility.
4. Minute infarctions due to embolization of renal abscesses.

20. The ammoniacal odor of Ben's breath may best be countered by:
1. Urging him to use chlorophyll breath mints.
2. Having him use a mouthwash containing sodium acid phosphate.
3. Administering frequent small doses of an antacid.
4. Brushing the teeth and gums vigorously after meals.

21. Which of the following biochemical abnormalities is most commonly associated with renal failure?
1. Elevation of serum albumin.
2. Elevation of serum potassium.
3. Elevation of serum calcium.
4. Elevation of serum bicarbonate.

22. The level of Ben's serum bicarbonate is indicative of:
1. Malnutrition.
2. Dehydration.
3. Acidosis.
4. Sepsis.

23. Ben should be closely observed for development of which of the following as possible neurological manifestations of uremia?
a. Impaired concentration.
b. Emotional depression.
c. Muscle twitching.
d. Clonic convulsions.
e. Deepening stupor.
  1. a and b only.
  2. c and d only.
  3. All but e.
  4. All the above.

24. Ben's long-term care should be planned with consideration that he will have increasing susceptibility to which of the following cardiovascular complications?
a. Cerebral hemorrhage.
b. Pericardial effusion.
c. Congestive heart failure.
d. Coronary occlusion.
e. Mitral stenosis.
  1. a and b only.
  2. a, b, and c only.
  3. All but d.
  4. All the above.

25. By taking a detailed medical history the nurse may discover that, in addition to anorexia, ecchymoses, and ammoniacal breath odor, Ben has experienced which other symptoms of uremia?
    a. Easy fatigability.
    b. Marked irritability.
    c. Mental confusion.
    d. Numbness and tingling of the toes.
    e. Nausea and vomiting.
        1. a and c only.
        2. b and d only.
        3. All but e.
        4. All the above.

26. When the pH of his serum was 7.29 and his serum bicarbonate level was 20.9 mEq./L, Ben was in a state of:
    1. Respiratory acidosis.
    2. Respiratory alkalosis.
    3. Metabolic acidosis.
    4. Metabolic alkalosis.

27. The principal effect of Ben's rapid deep respirations at the time of his hospital admission would be to:
    1. Eliminate increased amounts of water and decrease the pH of his body fluids.
    2. Eliminate increased amounts of carbon dioxide and increase the pH of the serum.
    3. Take up increased amounts of oxygen and bind excess hydrogen ions as water.
    4. Reduce blood urea by eliminating volatile nitrogenous compounds through the alveoli.

28. The ulcerations of Ben's oral mucosa are most likely the result of:
    1. Inadequate intake of vitamin C and protein.
    2. Vasoconstriction due to emotional stress.
    3. High ammonia content of body fluids.
    4. Generalized dehydration of body tissues.

29. Which of the following are typical symptoms of hyperkalemia?
    a. Paresthesias.
    b. Tetany.
    c. Muscle weakness.
    d. Tachypnea.
    e. Cardiac arrhythmia.
        1. a and b only.
        2. c and d only.
        3. a, c, and e only.
        4. All the above.

30. Each day, while giving Ben his bath, the nurse should examine his skin carefully for:
    1. Pigmentation changes.
    2. Pulsatile angiomas.
    3. Urate crystals.
    4. Fungus infection.

31. Each day as the nurse gives Ben morning care, her physical assessment of his condition should include particularly investigation for evidence of:
    1. Carotid artery thrills and bruits.
    2. Hepatic and splenic enlargement.
    3. Pleural and pericardial friction rubs.
    4. Extensor plantar reflexes.

32. The principal action of furosemide or Lasix is to:
    1. Block the action of carbonic anhydrase in tubular cells.
    2. Dilate the glomerulus, making it more permeable.
    3. Inhibit resorption of sodium in the renal tubule.
    4. Increase osmotic pressure in the efferent arteriole.

33. The nurse should expect the onset of diuretic action within what interval of time following administration of Lasix?
    1. 2 to 5 minutes.
    2. 30 to 60 minutes.
    3. 3 to 4 hours.
    4. 6 to 8 hours.

34. Which of the following are common toxic effects of Lasix?
    a. Weakness.
    b. Muscle cramps.
    c. Paresthesias.
    d. Dermatitis.
    e. Stomatitis.
        1. a only.
        2. a, b, and c only.
        3. All but c.
        4. All the above.

35. The pharmacological effect of Aldomet is to:
    1. Block impulse transmission through sympathetic ganglia.
    2. Depress smooth muscle fibers in the arterial wall.
    3. Inhibit an enzyme involved in epinephrine synthesis.
    4. Block impulse transmission from the vasomotor center.

36. Ben may complain of which of the following as a side effect of Aldomet?
    1. Blurring of vision.
    2. Joint pain.

3. Nasal stuffiness.

4. Bizarre dreams.

37. The primary objective in administering Amphojel to Ben was to:

1. Offset the hyperchlorhydria associated with metabolic acidosis.

2. Constrict vessels in the inflamed gastric mucosa.

3. Prevent the diarrhea associated with uremia.

4. Facilitate phosphate excretion through the bowel.

38. The physician ordered that Ben's protein intake be reduced below the amount usually ingested by a man of his age in order to:

1. Decrease the amount of nitrogenous wastes to be handled by his kidney.

2. Discourage edema formation by limiting production of serum albumin.

3. Facilitate weight reduction as a first step in decreasing cardiac load.

4. Eliminate the chief dietary source of potassium, sulfates, phosphates, and acids.

39. On a 30 Gram protein diet the following foods would be eliminated:

a. Meat.

b. Eggs.

c. Fish.

d. Beans.

e. Cheese.

1. a and b only.

2. a, c, and e only.

3. All but e.

4. All the above.

40. A high-carbohydrate diet was ordered for Ben at this time in order to:

1. Replace weight lost as a result of treatment-induced diuresis.

2. Provide sufficient calories that body protein will not be catalyzed.

3. Foster an increase in perirenal fat as protection against renal injury.

4. Offset the feeling of psychological deprivation caused by sodium restriction.

41. Ben and his wife should be instructed that on a one Gram sodium diet:

1. Salt may be used as usual during food preparation, but only limited amounts of salt may be added at table.

2. A limited amount of salt is allowed in cooking and a limited amount of salt may be added at the table.

3. Only a limited amount of salt is allowed in cooking and no salt may be added at the table.

4. No salt is added during cooking and only one slice of buttered bakery bread may be eaten each day.

42. Ben should be taught that in following a sodium-restricted diet he will have to avoid which of the following foods?

a. Fresh strawberries.

b. Smoked meats.

c. Condiments and relishes.

d. Frozen peas and lima beans.

e. Orange marmalade.

1. a and b only.

2. b, c, and d only.

3. All but d.

4. All the above.

43. In addition to being taught the sodium content of various naturally occurring foods, Ben and his wife need to know about some less obvious sources of sodium. These include:

a. Baking powder.

b. Food preservatives.

c. Flavor enhancers.

d. Cough medicines.

e. Water softening compounds.

1. a only.

2. a and b only.

3. All but d.

4. All the above.

44. In order to achieve zero potassium intake Ben will have to avoid which of the following:

a. Orange juice.

b. Instant coffee.

c. Fresh spinach.

d. Peanut butter.

e. Vegetable oil.

1. a only.

2. a and b only.

3. All but e.

4. All the above.

After his laboratory test results were reviewed, Ben's physician created an external shunt in his left forearm and arranged for hemodialysis to be done for 6 hours twice weekly. Following his first dialysis Ben's blood pressure fell to 130/90 mm. Hg. and his serum potassium decreased to 5 mEq./L. On the day after his second dialysis he was taken to the Operating Room and an arteriovenous fistula was created in his left forearm. Following his third dialysis his blood pressure was 132/86 mm. Hg., his serum potassium was 4.8 mEq./L., and his serum creatinine was 2 mg.%. At that point he was discharged with an appointment to return to the renal unit for hemodialysis twice a week.

45. The chief advantage of hemodialysis over peritoneal dialysis is the fact that with hemodialysis:
  1. The serum concentration of toxic substances is lowered more gradually.
  2. There is no need to monitor vital signs during the procedure.
  3. Serum albumin is not lost into the dialysate during the procedure.
  4. There is less danger of infection from use of faulty technique.

46. The biophysical principle upon which hemodialysis operates is the fact that:
  1. The pressure of a gas dissolved in a liquid is greater than the pressure of the same gas in a gaseous mixture.
  2. Substances of low molecular weight will pass across a semipermeable membrane from an area of greater to an area of lesser concentration.
  3. Molecules which are too large to be transferred through a living membrane can be forced through an inert membrane with centrifugal force.
  4. Toxic substances adsorbed to red and white blood cells can be removed from the cells by diluting the blood with a hypotonic solution.

47. In talking with the nurse on the day of hospital admission, Ben confided, "I didn't want to come to the hospital, 'cause I didn't want dialysis. I'm afraid that once I get tied to that machine it'll be downhill from then on." After she has encouraged Ben to vent his feelings on this subject, the nurse could best decrease his anxiety about his upcoming dialysis by:
  1. Describing in detail and in proper sequence each step in the hemodialysis procedure.
  2. Allowing him to read an article about the proven effectiveness of hemodialysis.
  3. Allowing him to observe and to talk with other patients as they undergo dialysis.
  4. Showing him a movie explaining the rationale for hemodialysis in treating renal failure.

48. Ben's preparation for hemodialysis should include:

  1. Signifying in writing his consent for the procedure and his knowledge of possible complications.
  2. Taking no solid food for eight hours prior to the dialysis procedure.
  3. Drinking no liquids for eight hours prior to the dialysis procedure.
  4. Catheterization of the urinary bladder and administration of a cleansing enema.

49. Before Ben's hemodialysis is begun the nurse should measure and record the following parameters:
  a. Body weight.
  b. Blood pressure.
  c. Pulse rate.
  d. Urine specific gravity.
  e. Abdominal girth.
    1. a only.
    2. a, b, and c only.
    3. All but d.
    4. All the above.

50. During the time that the arteriovenous shunt was being used, daily care of the shunt should include:
  a. Washing the tubing and surrounding skin with hexachlorophene and rinsing with saline.
  b. Applying antibiotic ointment to the skin around the cannula exit sites.
  c. Covering all but the distal loop of the shunt with a sterile dressing.
  d. Occluding the shunt with clamps between dialysis treatments.
  e. "Milking" the tubing between treatments to remove clotted blood.
    1. a only.
    2. b only.
    3. a, b, and c only.
    4. All but e.

51. As a safety precaution during the time that the external shunt is being used, which of the following items should be attached to Ben's arm dressing?
  1. A safety pin.
  2. Two cannula clamps.
  3. Suture scissors.
  4. A 2 cc. syringe and needle.

52. Which of the following would be the preferred means of testing the external arteriovenous shunt for patency?
  1. Pinching the shunt and noting the speed of filling on release.
  2. Palpating the cannula throughout its length to perceive pulsations.

3. Palpating the cannulized vein to discern the presence of a thrill.
4. Using a needle and syringe to aspirate blood from the cannula.

53. The nurse should expect that Ben may experience which of the following symptoms during the course of hemodialysis?
  a. Headache.
  b. Nausea.
  c. Palpitations.
  d. Precordial pain.
  e. Muscular tremor.
    1. a and b only.
    2. b and c only.
    3. c and d only.
    4. d and e only.

54. Ben should be observed closely during hemodialysis, as the effects of the procedure predispose him to:
  1. Hypochloremic alkalosis.
  2. Hypovolemic shock.
  3. Pulmonary embolism.
  4. Increased intracranial pressure.

55. Throughout hemodialysis the nurse should monitor Ben's response to the procedure by checking his:
  1. Rectal or axillary temperature every hour.
  2. Blood pressure and pulse every 30 minutes.
  3. Urine specific gravity every hour.
  4. Heart and lung sounds every thirty minutes.

56. During hemodialysis Ben's care should include:
  a. Changing his position frequently to relieve fatigue and pressure areas.
  b. Checking the cannulas, the coil, and the dialysate for hemorrhage.
  c. Informing him of the reasons for each step in the procedure.
  d. Reinforcing the instruction given him about dietary and fluid restrictions.
  e. Questioning him at intervals to determine his comfort and mental acuity.
    1. a and c only.
    2. b and d only.
    3. All but c.
    4. All the above.

57. Appearance of which of the following symptoms during dialysis should alert the nurse to the possibility that osmotic disequilibrium induced by the treatment has produced hypovolemia?
  a. Anxiety.
  b. Restlessness.
  c. Diaphoresis.
  d. Dizziness.
  e. Tachycardia.
    1. a and b only.
    2. c and d only.
    3. a, b, and e only.
    4. All the above.

58. In the event that hypovolemia develops during dialysis, the nurse should:
  1. Lower the head of the bed and notify the physician.
  2. Persuade Ben to drink a cup of hot tea or coffee.
  3. Occlude both the arterial and venous cannulas with clamps.
  4. Increase the pressure of blood in the coil through machine adjustment.

59. Near the end of dialysis excess electrolytes and nitrogenous wastes may be removed from the blood more rapidly than they can be cleared from the tissues of the central nervous tissue, resulting in an osmotic disequilibrium between nervous tissues and the blood. Which of the following symptoms would indicate that such an osmotic disequilibrium had developed?
  a. Headache.
  b. Restlessness.
  c. Mental confusion.
  d. Vomiting.
  e. Convulsions.
    1. a and b only.
    2. c and d only.
    3. All but e.
    4. All the above.

60. When the dialysis has been completed, what care should be given Ben?
  a. Application of a pressure dressing over the needle puncture sites in his arm.
  b. Measure his weight, compare it with pre-treatment weight, and record the loss.
  c. Draw a blood sample for measurement of electrolytes, urea, and creatinine.
  d. Wash his back and massage the pressure points with lotion.
  e. Rinse out his mouth with mouthwash and serve any meal that was omitted.
    1. a and b.
    2. c and d.
    3. All but e.
    4. All the above.

61. The nurse who cares for Ben should be aware that which of the following would predispose hin to thrombotic obstruction of his arteriovenous fistula?
- a. Measuring blood pressure in his left arm.
- b. Applying circumferential bandages over the fistula.
- c. Using improper technique in inserting needles into the fistula.
- d. Wearing garments with constrictive sleeves or cuffs.
- e. Rolling over on his left arm during sleep.
    1. a and b only.
    2. a, b, and c only.
    3. All but d.
    4. All the above.

62. It should be expected that Ben will use which of the following defense mechanisms in order to cope with the stresses of his illness and treatment?
    1. Conversion.
    2. Denial.
    3. Projection.
    4. Sublimation.

63. In planning for Ben's long-term care, the clinic nurse should be aware that Ben's relationship with his wife is apt to be altered by development of which of the following as a complication of chronic renal failure?
    1. Amnesia.
    2. Aphasia.
    3. Impotence.
    4. Deafness.

64. As a result of his illness and treatment Ben will probably require professional assistance in handling such problems as:
- a. Loss of his job and recreational outlets.
- b. Inability to pay for needed drugs and treatments.
- c. Difficulty in accepting his new role in the family.
- d. Grief provoked by loss of strength and health.
- e. Resistance to modifying dietary and drinking habits.
    1. a and b only.
    2. c and d only.
    3. All but e.
    4. All the above.

65. In order to provide needed psychological support to Ben and his family during clinic followup after his discharge from the hospital, the clinic nurse should determine:
    1. Whether or not Ben is to be a candidate for renal transplant.
    2. The total family income and the cost of his present treatment.
    3. The percentage of his renal parenchyma which is capable of functioning.
    4. His activities and feelings from hour to hour throughout a typical day.

Pancreatitis and Pancreatic Pseudocyst

Judson Teeple, a 38-year-old black garage mechanic, came to the examining room of University Hospital complaining of sharp abdominal pain and vomiting of three days' duration. The pain, which was most severe in his left upper quadrant, was somewhat relieved by flexing his left thigh on his abdomen. When he vomited on entering the examining room, the nurse noted that his vomitus was watery, greenish-yellow in color, and contained no food particles. On questioning, Mr. Teeple indicated that he was married and had two sons. He said that he had smoked one pack of cigarettes per day since adolescence and admitted having drunk from a pint to a pint and a half of whisky a day for 15 years. He indicated too that he had been drinking heavily the night before his abdominal pain and vomiting had developed.

Mr. Teeple's physical examination was negative except for abdominal distention, abdominal muscle guarding, epigastric and right upper quadrant tenderness, rebound tenderness in the left upper quadrant, and absent bowel sounds. His vital signs on admission were blood pressure of 130/72, oral temperature 101°F., pulse 110, and respirations 24. Initial laboratory test results were as follows: red blood cell count 4.17 million per mm.³, hemoglobin 12.1 Gm.%, hematocrit 36%, white blood cell count 18,500/mm.³, with 85 per cent polymorphonuclears, 9 per cent lymphocytes, 4 per cent monocytes, and 2 per cent band cells. Blood chemistries were within normal limits. Serum amylase concentration was 420 Somogyi units/100 ml. Blood gases were within normal limits. Chest x-ray on admission showed linear densities in the bases of both lungs and elevation of the left hemidiaphragm.

The physician made a tentative diagnosis of acute pancreatitis, inserted a Foley catheter and a nasogastric tube, and wrote the following orders:

(ANSWER BLANK ON PAGE A–125) (CORRECT ANSWERS ON PAGE B–215)

1. Start I.V. infusion 5 per cent Dextrose in Ringer's Lactate, 100 cc. to run in 8 hours.
2. Monitor arterial blood gas values daily.
3. Measure serum amylase concentration every day.
4. Measure 2 hour urine amylase concentration every day.
5. Measure serum enzymes, SGOT, SGPT, LDH, and CPK.
6. Take flat plate of the abdomen.

1. Which of the following are known to contribute to development of chronic pancreatitis?
   a. Excessive alcohol intake.
   b. Inadequate intake of vitamins.
   c. Stones in the common bile duct.
   d. Prolonged psychological stress.
   e. Chronic diabetes mellitus.
      1. a and c only.
      2. b and d only.
      3. All but d.
      4. All the above.

2. Which of the following nutritional imbalances is thought to play a role in the etiology of pancreatitis?
   1. Vitamin B deficiency.
   2. Protein deficiency.
   3. Excess of animal fat.
   4. Sodium excess.

3. Which of the following drugs has been known to cause pancreatitis in certain subjects?
   a. Dilantin.
   b. Digitalis.
   c. Chlorothiazide.
   d. Cortisone.
   e. Tetracycline.
      1. a and b only.
      2. b and c only.
      3. c and d only.
      4. d and e only.

4. The symptoms of pancreatitis result primarily from injury to pancreatic parenchymal cells by:
   1. Toxic metabolites elaborated by intestinal bacteria.
   2. External pressure by enlarged spleen, stomach, or liver.
   3. Auto-digestion of pancreatic tissue by activated trypsinogen.
   4. Intestinal microorganisms which ascend the pancreatic duct.

5. In questioning Mr. Teeple concerning the history of his present illness, the nurse should be aware that it is not uncommon for the pain of pancreatitis to radiate to the:
   a. Shoulder.
   b. Hand.
   c. Back.
   d. Hip.
   e. Leg.
      1. a and c only.
      2. b and d only.
      3. All but d.
      4. All the above.

6. In attempting to rule out possible causes for Mr. Teeple's pain other than pancreatitis, which of the following would be "significant negatives" to the nurse or physician who investigates the history of his present illness?

    a. No history of melena.
    b. No history of fatty food intolerance.
    c. No history of hematemesis.
    d. No history of jaundice.
    e. No history of belching.

        1. a and c only.
        2. b and d only.
        3. All but e.
        4. All the above.

7. In a patient with chronic pancreatitis, ingestion of a large amount of alcohol tends to precipitate acute exacerbations of illness by:

    a. Increasing gastric secretion of hydrochloric acid.
    b. Increasing the tone of the sphincter of Oddi.
    c. Overstimulating pancreatic islet cells to secrete.
    d. Producing fatty infiltration of pancreatic parenchyma.
    e. Dulling the appetite for vitamin rich foods.

        1. a and b only.
        2. c and d only.
        3. All but e.
        4. All the above.

8. Persistent severe vomiting would be apt to accentuate Mr. Teeple's problems by producing:

    1. Rupture of distended veins at the base of the esophagus.
    2. Reflux of duodenal content into the pancreatic duct.
    3. Telescoping of a length of bowel into an adjoining segment.
    4. Weakening and separation of muscles of the abdominal wall.

9. Mr. Teeple's higher than normal temperature on hospital admission was probably primarily the result of:

    1. General increase in metabolic rate produced by the exertion of vomiting.
    2. Severe loss of body water due to vomiting and gastric suctioning.
    3. Resetting of the hypothalamic thermostat by pyrogens released in tissue breakdown.

    4. Sympathetic nervous system hyperactivity produced by fear and anxiety.

10. Rebound tenderness is defined as:

    1. Abdominal discomfort which increases in severity as the effect of an analgesic wears off.
    2. Abdominal distress which is felt when the body is rocked vigorously from side to side.
    3. Abdominal pain experienced when, after application of steady manual pressure, the hand is suddenly removed.
    4. Abdominal tenderness which is felt when percussion is used to outline the liver, spleen, kidney, or bladder.

11. The finding of rebound tenderness signifies the presence of:

    1. Peritonitis.
    2. Ascites.
    3. Pancreatolithiasis.
    4. Intestinal distention.

12. The absence of bowel sounds at the time of Mr. Teeple's admission was probably the result of:

    1. Muffling of sounds by distended segments of bowel.
    2. Removal of fluid from the bowel by reverse peristalsis.
    3. Paralytic ileus secondary to chemical peritonitis.
    4. Lack of food intake during the recent drinking bout.

13. If the abdominal x-ray taken on Mr. Teeple's admission to the hospital had shown multiple small calcifications in the region of the pancreas, such finding would probably have been interpreted as evidence of:

    1. Chronic, recurrent pancreatitis.
    2. Healed· miliary tuberculosis.
    3. Primary or metastatic tumor tissue.
    4. Migration of gallstones into the pancreatic duct.

14. Mr. Teeple's blood test values can best be interpreted as indicating:

    1. Leukemia.
    2. Leukemoid reaction.
    3. Leukopenia.
    4. Leukocytosis.

15. The foregoing finding is probably representative of:

    1. The expected response to inflammatory tissue change.

2. One aspect of a systemically disseminated malignancy.

3. The result of toxic depression of bone marrow.

4. Hemoconcentration secondary to rapid body fluid loss.

16. In order to interpret Mr. Teeple's laboratory findings, the nurse should know that the upper limit of normal serum amylase concentration (in Somogyi units per 100 ml.) is:

   1. 50.

   2. 150.

   3. 250.

   4. 350.

17. The upper limit of normal urine amylase concentration (in Somogyi units per hour) is:

   1. 50.

   2. 150.

   3. 250.

   4. 350.

18. Elevation of serum amylase is not, in itself, diagnostic of pancreatitis, as serum levels of the enzyme are frequently higher than normal in which other conditions?

   a. Perforated ulcer.

   b. Acute cholecystitis.

   c. Intestinal strangulation.

   d. Splenic infarction.

   e. Colon carcinoma.

     1. a only.

     2. a, b, and c only.

     3. All but e.

     4. All the above.

19. The physician ordered that the levels of both serum and urine amylase be measured as part of Mr. Teeple's diagnostic workup because, generally:

   1. Serum amylase alone is elevated in pancreatitis, urine amylase alone is elevated in gall bladder disease.

   2. The amount of pancreatic damage is directly proportional to the total of serum and urinary amylase.

   3. Elevation of serum amylase alone indicates the disease is reversible; elevation of both indicates poor prognosis.

   4. Serum amylase is elevated during the first few days of illness, but urine amylase remains elevated longer.

20. In addition to elevation of serum amylase levels, Mr. Teeple's laboratory tests would probably reveal which other abnormal finding?

   1. Decreased urinary urobilinogen.

   2. Elevated serum protein bound iodine.

   3. Decreased urinary 17 ketosteroids.

   4. Elevated serum lipase concentration.

21. A nasogastric tube was inserted during Mr. Teeple's treatment primarily in order to:

   1. Obtain serial samples of duodenal content for enzyme analysis.

   2. Prevent digestion of blood and absorption of urea from the bowel.

   3. Empty the bowel in preparation for possible emergency surgery.

   4. Prevent pancreatic stimulation by gastric content in the duodenum.

22. After bringing the intravenous fluid, tubing, and angiocath to Mr. Teeple's bedside and informing him about the purpose and procedure for intravenous fluid administration, the nurse should do which of the following before starting the infusion?

   1. Wash her hands.

   2. Take his pulse.

   3. Auscultate his lung bases.

   4. Place him flat in bed.

23. Which of the following sites would be best for the nurse to use in starting Mr. Teeple's intravenous infusion?

   1. Dorsum of the hand.

   2. Lower forearm.

   3. Antecubital fossa.

   4. Slightly above the ankle.

24. If, after applying the tourniquet, the nurse should not be able to find a vein large enough to start the infusion, which of the following measures should be undertaken to further distend the selected vein?

   a. Allow the extremity to hang over the side of the bed for a short time.

   b. Apply a warm moist pack over the selected site for 10 to 15 minutes.

   c. Apply counter pressure while Mr. Teeple flexes and extends the extremity.

   d. Apply a cold compress over the desired site for a minute or two.

   e. Remove the tourniquet, elevate the limb briefly, then reapply the tourniquet.

     1. a and b only.

     2. b and c only.

     3. c and d only.

     4. All but e.

25. Before inserting the venipuncture needle through the skin, the nurse should:
1. Release the tourniquet from the extremity.
2. Place a rolled piece of gauze under the needle hub.
3. Remove air from the fluid tubing.
4. Adjust the clamp to regulate the drip rate.

26. The physician should specify the rate at which intravenous fluid should be infused. If he does not, and it is necessary that the infusion be started immediately, the nurse should adjust the fluid flow at what rate until she can obtain an order concerning the flow rate?
1. 5 cc./hour.
2. 50 cc./hour.
3. 100 cc./hour.
4. 150 cc./hour.

27. Too rapid rate of intravenous infusion is especially hazardous in persons with which of the following types of problems?
a. Severe anemia.
b. Arteriosclerotic heart disease.
c. Chronic obstructive lung disease.
d. Degenerative liver disease.
e. Chronic renal failure.
   1. a and c only.
   2. b and d only.
   3. e only.
   4. All the above.

28. In order to prevent microbial contamination of the intravenous fluid line, the nurse must refrain from:
1. Pinching the tubing to check for proper positioning of the needle or angiocath.
2. Applying ointment or solution to the venipuncture site.
3. Pushing a dislodged needle or angiocath back into a vein.
4. Changing needle, catheter, or tubing on an infusion which is running properly.

29. When discontinuing an intravenous infusion the nurse should examine the needle or catheter to determine whether it is intact. If she should find a piece of the tip to be missing, she should first:
1. Hang the extremity over the edge of the bed.
2. Place the patient in high Fowler's position with pillows under his arms.
3. Fully extend the extremity and lower the head of the bed.

4. Place a tourniquet around the upper part of the extremity.

30. If Mr. Teeple should later require an intravenous admixture solution, it should be prepared by a pharmacist or a pharmacist-directed nurse in a specially constructed area within the hospital pharmacy in order to decrease the possibility of which of the following complications of intravenous fluid therapy?
a. Fluid overload.
b. Drug incompatibility.
c. Chemical incompatibility.
d. Microbial contamination.
e. Anaphylactic shock.
   1. a, b, and c.
   2. b, c, and d.
   3. c, d, and e.
   4. All the above.

On his fifth hospital day Mr. Teeple's serum enzyme levels were as follows: SGOT, 831; SGPT, 521; LDH, 851; CPK, 135. A flat plate of the abdomen on that same date revealed an area of increased density in the left hypochondrium which was read as suggestive of a mass displacing the stomach anteriorly and the kidney and the splenic flexure of the colon inferiorly. On the basis of this finding a sonogram was ordered, revealing a large cystic mass in the left upper abdomen. The mass was diagnosed as a pseudocyst of the pancreas.

31. During Mr. Teeple's first few days in the hospital he would be at greatest risk for which of the following possible complications?
1. Shock.
2. Peritonitis.
3. Uremia.
4. Septicemia.

32. While Mr. Teeple's pain is most severe he would be most comfortable in which position?
1. Supine.
2. Prone.
3. Fowler's.
4. Left Sims.

33. Which of the following analgesics would be best suited for relieving Mr. Teeple's abdominal pain?
1. Aspirin.
2. Codeine.
3. Morphine.
4. Meperidine.

34. While caring for Mr. Teeple the nurse

should observe him carefully for symptoms of shock, to which complication he is predisposed as a result of which aspects of his disease process?

   a. Loss of fluid by vomiting and nasogastric suctioning.

   b. Direct depression of the myocardium by a toxic metabolite.

   c. Exudation of fluid into the peritoneal and retroperitoneal cavities.

   d. Sequestration of fluid in loops of paralyzed bowel.

   e. Depression of medullary vasomotor center by excess hydrogen ions.

     1. a and b.
     2. c and d.
     3. All but e.
     4. All the above.

35. During Mr. Teeple's bout of acute pancreatitis he is in danger of hemorrhage from the pancreas or other abdominal viscera, as a result of:

   1. Dissolving of elastic fibers in blood vessel walls by an enzyme activated by trypsin.

   2. Traumatic rupture of vessels due to blood pressure elevation secondary to psychological stress.

   3. Decrease in prothrombin production by liver cells damaged by biliary obstruction and stasis.

   4. Loss of capillary integrity due to lack of vitamin C intake during vomiting and gastric suctioning.

36. If Mr. Teeple's pancreatitis were so severe that little or no pancreatic lipase were to reach his bowel, his stools would tend to be:

   1. Black and gummy in consistency.
   2. Rock hard and pellet shaped.
   3. Streaked with blood and mucus.
   4. Bulky, oily, and malodorous.

37. Mr. Teeple might develop subnormal serum concentration of calcium as a result of:

   1. Increased binding of calcium ions in disseminated intravascular clotting reactions.

   2. Decreased calcium absorption due to lack of oral feedings for several days.

   3. Combination of calcium ions with fatty acids freed during peritoneal fat necrosis.

   4. Excretion of excessive amounts of calcium by damaged renal tubular cells.

38. The normal range for serum calcium concentration is:

   1. 9–11 mg. %.
   2. 15–30 mg. %.
   3. 40–60 mg. %.
   4. 80–120 mg. %.

39. Which of the following is a test that a nurse or physician can use to elicit a neurological symptom of low serum calcium concentration?

   1. Applying a vibrating tuning fork to the external malleolus.

   2. Having Mr. Teeple rapidly pronate and supinate his hands.

   3. Tapping the facial nerve against the facial bone just in front of his ear.

   4. Striking his patellar tendon with a percussion hammer.

40. The nurse should observe Mr. Teeple for which of the following symptoms of low serum calcium concentration?

   1. Hiccoughs.
   2. Tetany.
   3. Diarrhea.
   4. Pruritus.

41. While giving Mr. Teeple daily care the nurse should observe him for bluish discoloration around the umbilicus or in the flank, which finding should be suggestive of:

   1. Biliary cirrhosis.
   2. Congestive heart failure.
   3. Intraperitoneal hemorrhage.
   4. Renal failure.

42. A pancreatic pseudocyst is a saclike structure which usually contains a mixture of:

   a. Pancreatic juice.
   b. Gastric juice.
   c. Necrotic tissue.
   d. Bile.
   e. Purulent material.

     1. a and b only.
     2. c and d only.
     3. a, c, and e only.
     4. All the above.

43. In addition to pseudocyst formation, which of the following are possible complications of acute pancreatitis?

   a. Diabetes mellitus.
   b. Duodenal perforation.
   c. Paralytic ileus.
   d. Mesenteric vein thrombosis.
   e. Abdominal abscesses.

     1. a and b only.
     2. a, b, and c only.
     3. All but d.
     4. All the above.

44. During his preoperative period Mr. Teeple should be observed for symptoms of which of the following, as possible complications of the pseudocyst?

   a. Rupture of esophageal varices.
   b. Obstruction of the common bile duct.
   c. Ascites.
   d. Peritonitis.
   e. Septicemia.
      1. a and c only.
      2. b and d only.
      3. All but d.
      4. All the above.

Ten days after hospital admission Mr. Teeple's condition had stabilized sufficiently that he could be taken to the Operating Room for drainage of his pancreatic pseudocyst. Following surgery he recovered rapidly, with discontinuation of intravenous fluids and nasogastric suctioning on his second postoperative day and progression to a bland, low fat diet on his third postoperative day. He was discharged a few days later, with referrals for outpatient treatment in the Alcoholism Clinic and the Surgical Clinic.

BIBLIOGRAPHY   MEDICAL-SURGICAL NURSING

Aagaard, George: Treatment of hypertension. American Journal of Nursing, *73*:620–623, April, 1970.

Abram, H. S.: The psychiatrist, the treatment of chronic renal failure, and the prolongation of life. I. American Journal of Psychiatry, *124*:1351–1358, 1968.

Abram, H. S.: The psychiatrist, the treatment of chronic renal failure, and the prolongation of life. II. American Journal of Psychiatry, *126*:157–167, 1969.

Abram, H. S., Moore, G., and Westervelt, F.: Suicidal behavior in chronic dialysis patients. American Journal of Psychiatry, *127*:1194–1198, March, 1971.

Adler, Sol: Speech after laryngectomy. American Journal of Nursing, *69*:2138–2141, October, 1969.

Alba, A., and Papeika, J.: The nurse's role in preventing circulatory complications in the patient with a fractured hip. Nursing Clinics of North America, *1*:57–61, March, 1961.

Albers, J.: Evaluation of blood volume in patients on hemodialysis. American Journal of Nursing, *68*:1677–1679, August 1968.

Andreoli, K. G.: The cardiac monitor. American Journal of Nursing, *69*:1238–1243, June 1969.

Arden, G., Harrison, S., and Ansell, B.: Rheumatoid arthritis: surgical treatment. British Medical Journal, *4*:604–609, December 5, 1970.

Artz, C., Cohn, I., and Davis, J.: Brief Textbook of Surgery. Philadelphia, W. B. Saunders Company, 1976.

Asperheim, M., and Eisenhauer, L.: The Pharmacological Basis of Patient Care, 3rd ed. Philadelphia, W. B. Saunders Company, 1976.

Bacon, H.: Cancer of the Colon, Rectum, and Anal Canal. Philadelphia, J. B. Lippincott Co., 1969.

Bailey, W., Shinedling, M., and Payne, I.: Obese individuals' perception of body image. Perceptual and Motor Skills, *31*:617–618, October 1970.

Bargen, J. A.: Chronic Ulcerative Colitis. Springfield, Illinois, Charles C Thomas, 1969.

Bates, D., Macklem, P., and Christie, R.: Respiratory Function in Disease: An Introduction to the Integrated Study of the Lung. 2nd ed. Philadelphia, W. B. Saunders Co., 1971.

Beeson, P. B., and McDermott, W., eds.: Cecil-Loeb Textbook of Medicine. 14th ed. Philadelphia, W. B. Saunders Co., 1975.

Beland, I. C.: Clinical Nursing: Pathophysiological and Psychosocial Approaches. 3rd ed. New York, The Macmillan Co., 1975.

Bergersen, B., ed.: Current Concepts in Clinical Nursing. Vol. I and II. St. Louis, C. V. Mosby Co., 1967, 1969.

Bergersen, B., and Goth, A.: Pharmacology in Nursing, 13th ed. St. Louis, C. V. Mosby Co., 1976.

Betson, C., and Ude, L.: Central venous pressure. American Journal of Nursing, *69*:1466–1468, July 1969.

Bluestone, R.: Rheumatoid arthritis: medical management. British Medical Journal, *4*:602–604, December 5, 1970.

Bockus, H.: Gastroenterology. Vol. 3. 3rd ed. Philadelphia, W. B. Saunders Co., 1976.

Bondy, P. K., and Rosenberg, L. E.: Duncan's Diseases of Metabolism. 7th ed. Philadelphia, W. B. Saunders Co., 1974.

Bordicks, K.: Patterns of Shock: Implications for Nursing Care. New York, The Macmillan Co., 1965.

Bouchard, R., and Owens, N.: Nursing Care of the Cancer Patient, 2nd ed. St. Louis, C. V. Mosby Co., 1972.

Bouzarth, W. F.: Neurosurgical watch sheet for craniocerebral trauma. Journal of Trauma, 8:29–31, February 1968.

Bray, A. P., and Thomas, J. R.: Severe fat embolism syndrome following multiple fractures. Nursing Times, 65:109–110, January 23, 1969.

Brennan, K. S.: Epilepsy. Nursing Times, 67:435–438, April 15, 1971.

Breslau, R. C.: Intensive care following vascular surgery. American Journal of Nursing, 68:1670–1676, August 1968.

Brunner, L. S., Emerson, C. P., Ferguson, L. K., and Suddarth, D.: Textbook of Medical-Surgical Nursing. 3rd ed. Philadelphia, J. B. Lippincott Co., 1975.

Buchan, D. J.: Mind-body relationships in gastrointestinal disease. Canadian Nurse, 67:35–37, March 1971.

Buckingham, W., et al.: A Primer of Clinical Diagnosis. New York, Harper and Row, 1971.

Busse, E.: Geriatrics today: an overview. American Journal of Psychiatry, 123:1226–1233, April 1967.

Caldwell, J. R., Cobb, S., Dowling, M. D., and DeJongh, D.: The dropout problem in antihypertensive treatment. Journal of Chronic Diseases, 22:579–592, February 1970.

Carini, E., and Owens, G.: Neurological and Neurosurgical Nursing. 5th ed. St. Louis, C. V. Mosby Co., 1970.

Carnevali, D. L.: Preoperative anxiety. American Journal of Nursing, 66:1536–1538, July 1966.

Cassel, J. C., ed.: Symposium Issue: Evans County cardiovascular and cerebrovascular epidemiologic study. Archives of Internal Medicine, 128:883–986, December 1971.

Catt, K. J.: VI. The thyroid gland. Lancet, 1 (7661):1383–1389, June 27, 1970.

Chodil, J., and Williams, B.: The concept of sensory deprivation. Nursing Clinics of North America, 5:453–465, September 1970.

Chrisman, M.: Dyspnea. American Journal of Nursing, 74:643–646, April, 1974.

Christian, Charles L., ed.: Rheumatoid arthritis. Arthritis and Rheumatism, 13:472–498, 1970.

Condl, E. D.: Ophthalmic nursing: the gentle touch. Nursing Clinics of North America, 5:467–476, September 1970.

Condon, R., and Nyhus, L. (eds.): Manual of Surgical Therapeutics, 3rd ed. Boston, Little, Brown and Company, 1975.

Conn, H., ed.: Current Therapy, 1977. Philadelphia, W. B. Saunders Company, 1977.

Connor, G. H., Hughes, D., Mills, M. J., Rittmanic, B., and Sigg, L. V.: Tracheostomy: when it is done; how it is done; details of care. American Journal of Nursing, 72:68–74, January 1972.

Coopersmith, S.: Studies in self esteem. Scientific American, 218:96–106. February 1968.

Corbeil, M.: Nursing process for the patient with a body image disturbance. Nursing Clinics of North America, 6:155–163, March 1971.

Crawley, M.: The care of a patient with a myocardial infarction. American Journal of Nursing, 61:68–70, February 1961.

Cummings, J. W.: Hemodialysis: feelings, facts, fantasies. American Journal of Nursing, 70:70–76, January 1970.

Daly, J., Zeigler, B., and Dudrick, S.: Central venous catheterization. American Journal of Nursing, 75:820–824, May, 1975.

Davis, W.: Psychologic aspects of geriatric nursing. American Journal of Nursing, 68:802–804, April 1968.

Degroot, J.: Indwelling catheters. American Journal of Nursing, 75:448–449, March 1975.

DeJong, R.: The Neurological Examination. 3rd ed. New York, Harper and Row, 1967.

Delp, M., and Manning, R.: Major's Physical Diagnosis. Philadelphia, W. B. Saunders Company, 1975.

Deluca, J.: The ulcerative colitis personality. Nursing Clinics of North America, 5:23–33, 1970.

Denman, A. M.: Rheumatoid arthritis: aetiology. British Medical Journal, 4:601–602, December 5, 1970.

Ditunno, J., and Ehrlich, G. E.: Care and training of elderly patients with rheumatoid arthritis. Geriatrics, 25:164–172, March 1970.

Dolan, P., and Greene, H.: Renal failure and peritoneal dialysis. Nursing '75, 5:40–49, July, 1975.

Downing, S. R.: Nursing support in early renal failure. American Journal of Nursing, 69:1212–1216, June 1969.

Downs, F.: Bedrest and sensory disturbances. American Journal of Nursing, 74:434–438, March, 1974.

Druss, R. G., O'Conner, J. F., and Stern, L. O.: Psychologic response to colostomy. Archives of General Psychiatry, 20:419, April 1969.

Elliott, C.: Radiation therapy: how you can help. Nursing '76, 6:34–41, September, 1976.

Engel, G.: Grief and grieving. American Journal of Nursing, 64:93–98, September 1964.

Fagin, C.: Psychotherapeutic Nursing. American Journal of Nursing, 67:298–304, February 1967.

Falconer, M., Norman, M., Patterson, R., and Gustafson, E.: The Drug, The Nurse, and The Patient. 5th ed. Philadelphia, W. B. Saunders Co., 1974.

Fass, G.: Sleep, drugs, and dreams. American Journal of Nursing, 71:2316–2320, December 1971.

Ferebee, S. H.: Controlled chemoprophylaxis trials in tuberculosis. A general review. Advances in Tuberculosis Research, 17:29–106, 1969.

Feustel, D.: Autonomic hyperreflexia. American Journal of Nursing, 76:228–230, February 1976.

Flatter, P. A.: Hazards of oxygen therapy. American Journal of Nursing. 68:80–84, January 1968.

Flynn, W. E.: Managing the emotional aspects of peptic ulcer and ulcerative colitis. Postgraduate Medicine, 47:119–122, May 1970.

Fort, J.: Comparison chart of major substances used for mind alteration. American Journal of Nursing, 71:1950, September 1971.

Foss, G.: Postural drainage. American Journal of Nursing, 73:666–669, April, 1973.

Foulk, W., ed.: Diseases of the Liver. New York, McGraw Hill Book Co., 1968.

Francis, G. M.: Cancer: the emotional component. American Journal of Nursing, 69:1677–1681, August 1969.

Gehrink, A.: Changing trends in appendicitis. American Journal of Nursing, 63:88–89, October 1963.

Gerdes, L.: The confused or delirious patient. American Journal of Nursing, 68:1228–1233, June 1968.

Germain, C.: Exercise makes the heart grow stronger. American Journal of Nursing, 72:2169–2173, December 1972.

Given, B., and Simmons, S.: Care of a patient with a gastric ulcer. American Journal of Nursing, 70:1472–1475, July 1970.

Glaser, B., and Strauss, A.: Awareness of Dying. Chicago, Aldine Publishing Co., 1965.

Glaser, B., and Strauss, A.: The social loss of dying patients. American Journal of Nursing, 64:119–121, June 1964.

Goffman, E.: Stigma. Englewood Cliffs, N. J., Prentice Hall Inc., 1963.

Goodman, L., and Gilman, A., eds.: The Pharmacological Basis of Therapeutics. 4th ed. New York, The Macmillan Co., 1970.

Goss, C. M., ed.: Gray's Anatomy of the Human Body. 29th ed. Philadelphia, Lea and Febiger, 1973.

Grant, J. A., Moir, E., and Fago, M.: Parenteral hyperalimentation. American Journal of Nursing, 69:2392–2395, November 1969.

Greisheimer, E., and Wiedeman, M.: Physiology and Anatomy, 9th ed. Philadelphia, J. B. Lippincott, 1972.

Guyton, A.: Textbook of Medical Physiology. 5th ed. Philadelphia, W. B. Saunders Co., 1976.

Harvey, A., and Bordley, J., III: Differential Diagnosis: The Interpretation of Clinical Evidence. Philadelphia, W. B. Saunders Co., 1972.

Hayten, J.: Impaired liver function and related nursing care. American Journal of Nursing, 68:2374–2379, November 1968.

Healy, K. M.: Does preoperative instruction make a difference. American Journal of Nursing, 68:62–67, January 1968.

Heinemann, E., and Estes, N.: Assessing alcoholic patients. American Journal of Nursing, 76:785–789, May 1976.

Javid, H., et al.: Surgical treatment of cerebral ischemia. Surgical Clinics of North America, 54:239–255, February 1974.

Jensen, V.: Better techniques for bagging stomas. Part 3: Ileostomies. Nursing '74, 4:60–63, September 1974.

Kahn, D. R., Strang, R. H., and Wilson, W. S.: Clinical Aspects of Operable Heart Disease. New York, Appleton-Century-Crofts, 1968.

Katona, E.: Learning colostomy control. American Journal of Nursing, *67*:534–541, March 1967.

Kegney, F.: Psychosomatic gastrointestinal disturbances: a multifactor interactional concept. Postgraduate Medicine, *47*:109–113, May 1970.

Kerr, J. A.: Appendicitis: The Seven Anomalies. New York, Appleton-Century-Crofts, 1970.

Keuhnelian, J. G., and Sanders, V. E.: Urologic Nursing. New York, The Macmillan Co., 1970.

King, I., ed.: Symposium on Neurologic and Neurosurgical Nursing. Nursing Clinics of North America, *4*:199–300, June 1969.

King, J.: Denial. The American Journal of Nursing, *66*:1010–1013, May 1966.

Kintzel, K. D., ed.: Advanced Concepts in Clinical Nursing. Philadelphia, J. B. Lippincott Co., 1971.

Kirsner, J. B.: The challenges of ulcerative colitis. Postgraduate Medicine, *49*:109–112, March 1971.

Krause, M., and Hunscher, M.: Food, Nutrition and Diet Therapy. 5th ed. Philadelphia, W. B. Saunders Co., 1972.

Kubler-Ross, E.: On Death and Dying. New York, The Macmillan Co., 1969.

Lee, C., Stroot, V., and Schaper, C.: What to do when acid-base problems hang in the balance. Nursing '75, *5*:32–37, August 1975.

Lehninger, A.: Biochemistry: The Molecular Basis of Cell Structure and Function. New York, Worth, 1970.

LeMaitre, R., and Finnegan, J.: The Patient in Surgery: A Guide for Nurses, 3rd ed. Philadelphia, W. B. Saunders Company, 1975.

Lesse, S.: Hypochondriasis and psychosomatic disorders masking depression. American Journal of Psychotherapy, *21*:607–620, July 1967.

Lewis, E. P.: Nursing in Cardiovascular Diseases. New York, American Journal of Nursing Company, 1971.

Libman, R., and Keithley, J.: Relieving airway obstruction in the recovery room. American Journal of Nursing, *75*:603–605, April 1975.

Lilijefors, I., and Rahe, R.: An identical twin study of psychosocial factors in coronary heart disease in Sweden. Psychosomatic Medicine, *32*:523–542, 1970.

Lindemann, E.: Symptomatology and management of acute grief. American Journal of Psychiatry, *101*:141–148, September 1944.

Lindh, K., and Rickerson, G.: Spinal cord injury: you can make a difference. Nursing '74, *4*:41–45, February, 1974.

Lockie, L. M.: Current evaluation of drugs for treating arthritis. Postgraduate Medicine, *49*:100–104, April 1971.

Long, B.: Sleep. American Journal of Nursing, *69*:1896–1899, September 1969.

Long, M., et al.: Hypertension: what patients need to know. American Journal of Nursing. *76*:765–770, May 1976.

Luce, G. G., ed.: Biological Rhythms in Psychiatry and Medicine. U. S. Department of Health, Education, and Welfare, Public Health Service Publication No. 2088. Washington, D. C., U.S. Government Printing Office, 1970.

Luckman, J., and Sorenson, K.: Medical-Surgical Nursing: A Psychophysiologic Approach. Philadelphia, W. B. Saunders Company, 1974.

MacBryde, C., ed.: Signs and Symptoms: Applied Pathologic Physiology and Clinical Interpretation. 5th ed. Philadelphia, J. B. Lippincott Co., 1970.

MacRae, I.: Some aspects of nursing care of rheumatic diseases. Nursing Times, *65*: 327–329, March 13, 1969.

McFarland, H. R.: The management of multiple sclerosis. II. Serial neurological examination and use of corticotropin and glucocorticoids. Missouri Medicine, *66*:113–116, February 1969.

Mei-Tal, V., Meyerowitz, S., and Engel, G. L.: The role of psychological process in a somatic disorder: multiple sclerosis. Psychosomatic Medicine, *32*:67–86, January-February 1970.

Mehtzer, L. E., Abdellah, F. G., and Kitchell, J. M., eds.: Concepts and Practices of Intensive Care. Philadelphia, Charles Press, 1969.

Mehtzer, L. E., Pinneo, R., and Kitchell, J. R.: Intensive Coronary Care: A Manual for Nurses. Philadelphia, Presbyterian Hospital Coronary Care Unit Fund, 1965.

Merritt, H. H.: A Textbook of Neurology. 4th ed. Philadelphia, Lea and Febiger, 1967.

Minckley, B. B.: Physiologic hazards of position changes on the anesthetized patient. American Journal of Nursing, *69*:2606–2611, December 1969.

Moidel, H., Sorenson, G., Gilbin, E., and Kaufman, M. eds.: Nursing Care of Patients With Medical and Surgical Disorders. New York, McGraw-Hill Book Co., 1971.

Moldofsky, H., and Chester, W.: Pain and mood patterns in patients with rheumatoid arthritis. Psychosomatic Medicine, *32*:309–318, May-June 1970.

Moody, L.: Primer for pulmonary hygiene. American Journal of Nursing, 77:104–106, January 1977.

Morgan, W., and Engel, G.: The Clinical Approach to the Patient. Philadelphia, W. B. Saunders Company, 1969.

Morony, J.: Surgery for Nurses. Edinburgh, Churchill Livingstone, 1971.

Mountjoy, P., and Wythe, B.: Nursing Care of the Unconscious Patient. London, Bailliere Tindall and Cassell, 1970.

Muslin, H. C.: On acquiring a kidney. American Journal of Psychiatry, 129:1185–1188, March 1971.

Nelson, J., and Hall, J.: Detection, diagnostic evaluation, and treatment of dysplasia and early carcinoma of the cervix. CA: Cancer Journal for the Clinician, 20:150–163, 1970.

Newcombe, B.: Care of the patient with head and neck cancer. Nursing Clinics of North America, 2:599–607, December 1967.

Norris, C. M.: The work of getting well. American Journal of Nursing, 69:2118–2121, October 1969.

Oakes, A., and Morrow, H.: Understanding blood gases. Nursing '73, 3:15–21, September 1973.

Oberhelman, H.: Physiological Principles of Gastric Surgery. Springfield, Illinois, Charles C Thomas, 1968.

O'Brien, M. J.: The Care of the Aged. St. Louis, C. V. Mosby Co., 1971.

Parsa, M., Thornton, B., and Ferrer, J.: Central venous alimentation. American Journal of Nursing, 72:2042–2047, November 1972.

Parsons, M. C., et al.: Difficult patients do exist. Nursing Clinics of North America, 6:173–187, March 1971.

Pattison, E. M.: The experience of dying. American Journal of Psychotherapy, 21:32–43, January 1967.

Peoples-Veiga, C.: Get into hypertension to improve patient compliance. Nursing '76, 6:32–35, October, 1976.

Peplau, H.: Interpersonal Relations in Nursing. New York, G. P. Putnam's Sons, 1952.

Picconi, J.: Human sexuality—a nursing challenge. Nursing '77, 7:72D–72M, February 1977.

Pinneo, R.: Nursing in a coronary care unit. American Journal of Nursing, 65:76–79, February 1965.

Pitorak, E. F.: Laryngectomy. American Journal of Nursing, 68:780–786, April 1968.

Plummer, E. M.: The MS patient. American Journal of Nursing, 68:2161–2167, October 1968.

Prior, J., and Silberstein, J.: Physical Diagnosis. St. Louis, C. V. Mosby Company, 1973.

Purintun, L. R., and Nelson, L. I.: Ulcer patient: emotional emergency. American Journal of Nursing, 68:1930–1933, September 1968.

Quarrell, E. J.: Pulmonary tuberculosis. 4. Signs and symptoms of pulmonary tuberculosis. Nursing Times, 65:242–245, February 20, 1969.

Quarrell, E. J.: Pulmonary tuberculosis. 7. Community aspects of tuberculosis. Nursing Times, 65:338–340, March 13, 1969.

Quint, J.: The Nurse and Dying Patient. New York, The Macmillan Co., 1967.

Rawlings, M. S.: Inside the coronary care unit: trends in therapeutic management. American Journal of Nursing, 67:2321–2328, November 1967.

Reed, J.: Lead poisoning—silent epidemic and social crime. American Journal of Nursing, 72:2181–2184, December 1972.

Regina, Sr.: Sensory stimulation techniques. American Journal of Nursing, 66:281, 1968.

Robinson, L.: Psychological Aspects of the Care of Hospitalized Patients. Philadelphia, F. A. Davis, 1968.

Rodman, M., and Smith, D.: Pharmacology and Drug Therapy in Nursing. Philadelphia, J. B. Lippincott Company, 1968.

Rodman, T., Myerson, R. M., Lawrence, L. T., Gallagher, A. P., and Kasper, A.: The Physiologic and Pharmacologic Basis of Coronary Care Nursing. St. Louis, C. V. Mosby Co., 1971.

Roy, R., Sauer, W., et al.: Experience with ileostomies. American Journal of Surgery, 70:77–86, January 1970.

Rusk, H.: Rehabilitation Medicine, 3rd ed. St. Louis, C. V. Mosby Company, 1971.

Ryan, R.: Thrombophlebitis: assessment and prevention. American Journal of Nursing, 76:1634–1636, October 1976.

Sabiston, D. C.: Davis-Christopher Textbook of Surgery, 10th ed. Philadelphia, W. B. Saunders Company, 1972.

Santopietro, M.: Meeting the emotional needs of hemodialysis patients and their spouses. American Journal of Nursing, 75:629–632, April 1975.

Schulman, H., and Thetford, W.: A comparison of personality traits in ulcerative colitis and migraine patients. Journal of Abnormal Psychology, 76:443–452, 1970.

Schwaid, M. C.: The impact of emphysema. American Journal of Nursing, 70:1247–1250, June 1970.

Schwartz, S., et al.: Principles of Surgery, 2nd ed. New York, McGraw Hill, 1974.

Scott, B. H.: Tensions linked with emphysema. American Journal of Nursing, 69:538–540, March 1969.

Secor, J.: Patient Care in Respiratory Problems. Philadelphia, W. B. Saunders Co., 1969.

Selye, H.: The stress syndrome. American Journal of Nursing, 65:97–99, March 1965.

Shafer, K., et al.: Medical-Surgical Nursing. 6th ed. St. Louis, C. V. Mosby Co., 1975.

Sherlock, S.: Diseases of the Liver and Biliary System. 4th ed. Philadelphia, F. A. Davis, 1968.

Simborg, D. W.: The status of risk factors and coronary heart disease. Journal of Chronic Disease, 22:515–552, 1970.

Smith, B.: Congestive heart failure. American Journal of Nursing, 69:278–282, February 1969.

Smith, D., Conant, N., and Overman, J.: Zinsser Microbiology, 13th ed. New York, Appleton Century-Crofts, 1964.

Smith, J.: Essentials of Gastroenterology. St. Louis, C. V. Mosby Co., 1969.

Smith, J., and Bullough, B.: Sexuality and the severely disabled person. American Journal of Nursing, 75:2194–2197, December 1975.

Smith, P. H.: Benign enlargement of the prostate. Nursing Times, 66:524–527, April 23, 1970.

Sobel, D.: Personalization on the coronary care unit. American Journal of Nursing, 69:1439–1442, July 1969.

Sodeman, W., and Sodeman, W., Jr.: Pathologic Physiology. 5th ed. Philadelphia, W. B. Saunders Co., 1974.

Spellburg, M.: The treatment of ascites and esophageal varices. American Journal of Gastroenterology, 51:208–226, 1969.

Standards for tuberculosis treatment in the 1970's. Bulletin of the National Tuberculosis Respiratory Disease Association, 57:9–11, March 1971.

Sweetwood, H.: Nursing in the Intensive Respiratory Care Unit. New York, Springer, 1971.

Taif, B.: Diet therapy in renal failure. Journal of Practical Nursing, 26:23–25, February 1976.

Thomas, S.: Fat embolism: a hazard of trauma. Nursing Times, 65:105–108, January 23, 1969.

Trowbridge, J.: Caring for patients with facial or intraoral reconstruction. American Journal of Nursing, 73:1930–1934, November 1973.

Ujhely, G.: What is realistic emotional support? American Journal of Nursing, 68:758–762, April 1968.

Van Meter, M., and Lavine, P.: What every nurse should know about EKGs. Part I. Nursing '75, 5:19–27, April 1975.

Veber, D.: Fluid and electrolyte problems in the postoperative period. Nursing Clinics of North America, 1:275, 1966.

Watkins, F.: The patient who has peritoneal dialysis. American Journal of Nursing, 66:1572–1577, July 1966.

Watson, J.: Medical-Surgical Nursing and Related Physiology. Philadelphia, W. B. Saunders Company, 1972.

Weg, John: Tuberculosis and the generation gap. American Journal of Nursing, 71:495–500, March 1971.

Wenckert, A., and Hallgren, T.: Evaluation of conservative treatment of acute cholecystitis. Acta Chirurgica Scandinavica, 135:701–706, 1969.

Westfall, V.: Electrical and mechanical events in the cardiac cycle. American Journal of Nursing, 76:231–235, February 1976.

Whitehead, S.: Nursing Care of the Adult Urology Patient. New York, Appleton-Century-Crofts, 1970.

Whiteley, H., Stevens, M., et al.: Radiation therapy in the palliative management of patients with recurrent cancer of the rectum and colon. Surgical Clinics of North America, 49 (2):381–387, 1969.

Whittington, T.: Forty years of looking at diabetics' eyes. Postgraduate Medical Journal, 47:62–65, January Supplement, 1971.

Williams, D.: Sleep and disease. American Journal of Nursing, 71:2321–2324, December 1971.

Wintrobe, M. M., et al.: Harrison's Principles of Internal Medicine. 6th ed. New York, McGraw-Hill Book Co., 1970.

Wolff, K.: The Biological, Sociological, Psychological Aspects of Aging. Springfield, Illinois, Charles C Thomas, 1959.

Zyzanski, S. J., and Jenkins, C. D.: Basic dimensions within the coronary prone behavior pattern. Journal of Chronic Disease, 22:781–795, 1970.

4
PSYCHIATRIC— MENTAL HEALTH NURSING

Anxiety Reaction

Eva Kowalski was 28 years old when her father left home to escape the nagging of his extremely religious and demanding wife. Eva, her father's favorite, grieved over his departure, but her sense of duty to her mother kept her from following him. Shortly thereafter, on her way to work in a large business machines corporation, Eva suffered an acute attack of palpitations, dizziness, and shortness of breath, which subsided spontaneously within a few minutes. Fearing serious heart disease, Eva consulted an internist who was unable to find evidence of any anatomic or physiologic disorder in a complete diagnostic workup.

Eva returned to work but continued to suffer occasional attacks of palpitations and shortness of breath and to worry about having heart disease. She gradually became unable to enjoy any of her usual activities. During the next six months Eva's mother urged Eva to marry the young office co-worker whom she had been dating. Somewhat unenthusiastically Eva set the date for the marriage, but three days before the wedding she suffered a severe attack of palpitations and shortness of breath. Remembering the internist's assurances that there was nothing wrong with her heart and lungs, she decided that she must be losing her mind and went for help to a nearby community mental health center.

Eva told the community mental health nurse who interviewed her that she was afraid that she was losing control and that she must have help to keep from acting irrationally. Eva also told the nurse that she had almost died of pneumonia during infancy and had suffered repeated attacks of asthma throughout childhood, during which her overly protective mother had become even more solicitous concerning her welfare. Eva described herself as having been a superior student in both high school and business school. She had held a responsible position in the business machines company for eight years, had had several promotions, earned a substantial salary, and was well-liked by her co-workers, but she now felt inadequate in her work and did not, she said, "really enjoy life."

(ANSWER BLANK ON PAGE A–127) (CORRECT ANSWERS ON PAGE B–220)

1. In 1926, Freud reformulated his theory concerning the normal anxiety which most persons experience in every day life. Which of the following statements best describes his new theory?

1. Anxiety develops as a result of an overwhelming influx of stimuli or from anticipation of a situation which is potentially harmful.
2. An abnormal accumulation of libidinous energy within the psyche stimulates production of a counterforce which takes the form of anxiety.
3. When the individual feels threatened by overwhelming sexual impulses, the superego restricts overt response through the production of anxiety.
4. The individual suffers feelings of anxiety when confronted with a conflict between internalized and external social values.

2. The capacity for reacting with anxiety to a potentially dangerous situation has survival value for the individual in that it serves as a:

1. Power source.
2. Fictive force.
3. Action deterrent.
4. Protective signal.

3. Since according to Freudian theory it is part of the ego's function both to master incoming stimuli and to discharge them effectively, it would be expected that anxiety is most easily provoked during the:
  1. First year of life.
  2. Oedipal period.
  3. Adolescent period.
  4. Postclimacteric period.

4. Which of the following statements best describes normal or signal anxiety as defined by Freud in 1926?
  a. Signal anxiety is elicited by the danger situations which typically occur in childhood.
  b. Signal anxiety stimulates the ego to check or inhibit id impulses in a dangerous situation.
  c. The strength of a noxious stimulus and the amount of signal anxiety produced by it are proportional.
  d. Signal anxiety is an attenuated form of anxiety which is characteristically protective to the ego.
      1. a only.
      2. b and d.
      3. All but d.
      4. All the above.

5. Freud stated that all neurotic processes are developed in an attempt to avoid:
  1. Reality.
  2. Anxiety.
  3. Responsibility.
  4. Aggression.

6. An anxiety reaction is basically a response to:
  1. Change in libidinal energy.
  2. Loss of ego control.
  3. Increased repressive forces.
  4. Shift in object cathexis.

7. Normal anxiety differs from fear in that the stimulus for anxiety is:
  1. An easily observable external threat to security.
  2. Not immediately available to the conscious mind.
  3. A more serious threat to one's social welfare.
  4. Completely unrelated to one's life situation.

8. Which of the following are typical somatic symptoms of an anxiety reaction?
  a. Tachycardia and palpitations.
  b. Dyspnea and air hunger.
  c. Nausea and diarrhea.
  d. Dizziness and weakness.
  e. Haziness of vision.
      1. a, b, and c.

  2. b, c, and d.
  3. All but e.
  4. All the above.

9. Eva's palpitations and shortness of breath could most accurately be interpreted as expressions of her:
  1. Grief.
  2. Anger.
  3. Suspicion.
  4. Fear.

10. Differential diagnosis of Eva's problem requires that the nurse therapist rule out which of the following disorders?
  a. Hyperventilation syndrome.
  b. Conversion hysteria.
  c. Bronchial asthma.
  d. Impending psychosis.
  e. Paroxysmal tachycardia.
      1. a and b.
      2. c and d.
      3. All but e.
      4. All the above.

11. The community mental health nurse who interviews Eva should assess whether or not she:
  a. Needs hospitalization.
  b. Can care for herself.
  c. Has an adequate support system.
  d. Is able to pay for therapy.
  e. Requires a physical examination.
      1. a only.
      2. a, b, and c.
      3. All but d.
      4. All the above.

12. In determining whether Eva's reaction to anxiety is neurotic or psychotic, the nurse will be guided by the fact that neurotic anxiety is:
  1. Based on realistic fears.
  2. Disproportionate to its cause.
  3. Accompanied by delusions.
  4. Incapable of reduction.

13. Sullivan defined anxiety as:
  1. A sign that self-esteem had been endangered.
  2. An inevitable part of every interpersonal relationship.
  3. A phenomenon evoked by a situation of autonomy.
  4. Disguised guilt arising from the use of security operations.

14. According to Sullivanian theory, anxiety develops as a result of:
  1. Innate biological drives which create overwhelming demands for action.
  2. Persistent asynchrony between personal and social moral values.

3. Inability to avoid those social situations which bring punishment.
4. Distorted perception of others' evaluation of one's worth.

15. According to Sullivan's concept of an anxiety continuum, complete absence of anxiety would be known as:
1. Euphoria.
2. Mirth.
3. Detachment.
4. Ecstasy.

16. According to Sullivan's concept of an anxiety continuum, an extremely high level of anxiety is known as:
1. Fear.
2. Panic.
3. Agitation.
4. Tremor.

17. In the past Eva probably controlled conflicting forces and minimized anxiety chiefly through the use of:
a. Memory.
b. Identification.
c. Fantasy.
d. Repression.
e. Sublimation.
  1. a and b.
  2. b, c, and e.
  3. a, c, and d.
  4. All the above.

18. Sublimation can most accurately be defined as:
1. Substitution of a similar goal for one that is being blocked.
2. Adopting the ideas, feelings, and behavior of another idealized person.
3. Finding a socially acceptable expression for one's id impulses.
4. Escaping painful situations through recourse to daydreams and fantasies.

19. Repression can be best understood as:
1. The barring of unacceptable id impulses from consciousness.
2. The resumption of behavior typical of an earlier developmental level.
3. The conscious forgetting of one's acts, impulses, or desires.
4. Maintenance of a trait in the unconscious by expression of its opposite.

20. Fantasy consists of:
1. A sensual experience for which no external stimulus exists.
2. Imaginary construction of scenes and events through memory manipulation.
3. Misinterpretation of a sensual stimulus through inattention.
4. Providing varied and inconsistent accounts of past events.

21. Identification is achieved through the use of which of the following defense mechanisms?
1. Fixation.
2. Projection.
3. Sublimation.
4. Introjection.

22. Anxiety results when the security of the ego is threatened by:
1. Failure of significant others to fulfill one's expectations concerning their behavior.
2. Danger that repressed desires and feelings will break through to consciousness.
3. Confrontation with an object or problem that one has been unable to master.
4. A gradual and steady elevation in one's moral percepts or ideal aspirations.

23. Eva's terror, confusion, and sense of helplessness were related to her subjective fears of:
a. Fear.
b. Irrationality.
c. Disease.
d. Psychosis.
e. Death.
  1. a and c.
  2. b and d.
  3. All but e.
  4. All the above.

24. The nurse should be aware that, after Eva's acute anxiety reaction subsides, her conflicts could be resolved by:
a. A return to normal functioning with sublimation of her conflict through socializing or work.
b. Encapsulation and insulation of the conflict, which renders it totally inaccessible to conscious thought.
c. Channeling the anxiety to an organ system with the production of a psychosomatic illness.
d. Adoption of a pattern of thought that ignores the factors of time, condition, or logic.
e. Focusing the anxiety on an object or idea, with the development of a phobia.
  1. a or b.
  2. c or d.
  3. a, c, or e.
  4. All the above.

25. Eva's conflict can best be understood as:
    1. Vacillation, from a positive to a negative feeling toward an object.
    2. The tendency to rapidly alter her attitudes toward a situation.
    3. The existence of two opposing goals of approximately equal strength.
    4. Transfer of feelings from one situation to another situation or object.

26. The symptoms of an anxiety reaction differ from those of the other classic psychoneuroses in that the symptoms of an anxiety reaction:
    1. Give no indication of the nature of the underlying conflict.
    2. Are less apt to produce a severe degree of conscious discomfort.
    3. Are so sufficiently entrenched as to be inaccessible to treatment.
    4. Tend to be less closely related to one's view of himself.

27. Eva's prognosis for recovery from her anxiety reaction is good because she has:
    1. Expressed dissatisfaction with her present life situation.
    2. Presented herself voluntarily for diagnosis and treatment.
    3. Experienced little secondary gain from her symptoms.
    4. Readily accepted the evidence refuting an organic illness.

Following a screening interview with Eva, the nurse consulted with a psychiatrist, who agreed with the nurse's opinion that Eva was experiencing an anxiety reaction and ordered that Eva be given chlordiazepoxide hydrochloride (Librium) 10 mg. q.i.d. orally. It was decided that Eva would be given out-patient crisis intervention therapy with the community mental health nurse as the primary therapist. When Eva's mother and father were contacted, they indicated that they both felt considerable guilt concerning what they believed to be their own responsibility for Eva's problem and stated that they were willing to re-examine their relationship with Eva and modify it if necessary.

During her interview with the nurse therapist Eva was able to identify her anxiety and said that she thought she should make some change in her life but didn't know what that change should be. Initially, she blamed her somatic symptoms for her anxiety, but as the interviews progressed she began to see that she had strongly identified with her father and blamed her mother for having driven him away from home. Eva also blamed her mother for having pushed her toward an unwanted marriage, which she saw as an effort to drive her from home too. Guilt concerning her wish to be like her father made Eva feel unworthy of success and satisfaction. The nurse helped her to see the relationship between her feelings and her symptoms and supported Eva in her decision to call off the marriage and return to the job she enjoyed.

28. The chief pharmacologic effect of chlordiazepoxide hydrochloride (Librium) is to:
    1. Produce amnesia for recent events.
    2. Relieve moderate anxiety and tension.
    3. Depress the sympathetic nervous system.
    4. Induce deep, dreamless, natural sleep.

29. From the standpoint of psychiatric theory, a crisis is a situation that:
    a. Produces a sudden alteration in one's expectations of himself and others.
    b. Provokes discomfort that lingers beyond the duration of the event.
    c. Cannot be handled by one's usual mechanisms for coping with problems.
    d. Evokes extreme fear and anxiety that are relieved by the use of defense mechanisms.
    e. Prevents one from accepting support from persons in his environment.
       1. a, b, and c.
       2. b, c, and d.
       3. c, d, and e.
       4. All the above.

30. Crises differ from more usual stress situations in that following a crisis, one is more apt to demonstrate:
    1. A change in the level of psychological functioning.
    2. A decrease in the number of defense mechanisms used.
    3. An improvement in the ability to face adversity.
    4. A severe decline in self-confidence and trust in others.

31. Crisis intervention therapy can be categorized in Caplan's theory of levels of disease prevention as:
    1. Primary prevention.
    2. Secondary prevention.
    3. Tertiary prevention.
    4. Quaternary prevention.

32. Which of the following statements best describes Caplan's concept of tertiary level of disease prevention?
1. Reducing the incidence of affective disorders in the community.
2. Reducing the duration of psychotic illnesses in the community.
3. Understanding treatment philosophies and related therapeutic interventions.
4. Reducing impairment resulting from mental illness in the community.

33. Eva would seem to be a good candidate for crisis intervention therapy because:
a. The event precipitating her reaction was readily identifiable.
b. Her previous level of adjustment had been fairly stable.
c. The coping patterns used to reduce anxiety were not yet fixed.
d. She presented herself for treatment during the early stage of the reaction.
e. Her family and close friends evidenced willingness to modify their behavior.
1. a and c.
2. b and d.
3. All but d.
4. All the above.

34. Eva's father returned home in an effort to improve his interpersonal relationships with his wife, but the nagging and conflicts continued. Which of the following actions would be most therapeutic for Eva at this time?
1. Move to her own apartment.
2. Immediately marry the office co-worker.
3. Identify more strongly with her mother.
4. Ponder her problems in silence.

35. The success of Eva's crisis therapy would be influenced by:
a. The quality of her previous life experiences.
b. The relative strengths of her id, ego, and superego.
c. The coping mechanisms used to resolve the conflict.
d. The responses elicited currently from significant others.
e. The current availability and use of helping resources.
1. a and c.
2. b and d.
3. All but e.
4. All the above.

36. Eva would be most apt to profit from therapy during the early stage of her anxiety reaction because:
1. Her acute discomfort would render her especially receptive to guidance.
2. The therapist would be more optimistic about the outcome of treatment.
3. She would clearly remember the symptoms of the acute reaction.
4. She would welcome therapy as a legitimate excuse to avoid marriage.

37. Eva's crisis intervention therapy would include:
a. Identifying and focusing her anxiety.
b. Relating her anxiety to its cause.
c. Ventilation of her feelings about her conflict.
d. Communication of dormant feelings among family members.
e. The therapist's introjection of corrective observations.
1. a and b.
2. a, b, and c.
3. All but e.
4. All the above.

38. The factor that precipitated Eva's current crisis was:
1. The fear of death produced by her palpitations and dyspnea.
2. Tension created by her fears concerning the impending marriage.
3. Her feeling of guilt relative to her success in her job.
4. Her unresolved grief concerning her father's leaving home.

39. In describing her mother to the nurse Eva said, "She's really a very good woman... You know what I mean?" What response by the nurse would be most helpful?
1. "No, I'm not sure that I follow what you're trying to tell me."
2. "You say that your mother is really a very good woman?"
3. "It's apparently important to you to have a very good mother."
4. "What makes you think that your mother is a very good person?"

40. In explaining her reaction to her father's having left home, Eva said, "I was just lost when I found out he had left." Which response would be most therapeutic?
1. "What did you do then?"
2. "How did your mother react?"
3. "Tell me more about that."
4. "I understand how you felt."

41. In another interview Eva told the nurse, "You don't know what it's like to feel that you're suffocating." What response should the nurse make?
1. "When were you suffocating?"
2. "No, I guess I don't."
3. "Tell me how you feel."
4. "Suffocating? What do you mean?"

42. In one of her interviews with the nurse Eva said, "When I had that attack I thought I was dying." What response by the nurse would be most appropriate?
1. "You thought you were dying?"
2. "What made you think that?"
3. "Then what did you do?"
4. "Describe how you felt."

43. During therapy Eva was presented with the idea that her physical symptoms were an expression of her feelings. Eva replied, "I have to express myself that way." Which response would be most helpful?
1. "Why must you express yourself through physical symptoms?"
2. "I see that you feel strongly about this."
3. "What feelings do you need to express."
4. "Is that the best way of expressing yourself?"

44. In talking about her forthcoming wedding, Eva said, "Maybe I'm not ready to get married." The nurse could best respond with:
1. "You'll know when you're ready."
2. "Do you want to get married?"
3. "Do you think you'd be happy?"
4. "There's something you must do first?"

45. In attempting to formulate plans for her future, Eva said, "I don't know. I liked my job. But I can't go back there now, can I?" Which response would be most appropriate?
1. "What do you think?"
2. "What have you done?"
3. "You liked working there?"
4. "You have to do something."

The aims of Eva's treatment were realized after 10 interviews with the therapist. During the process of treatment Eva's most pressing fears and conflicts were brought out into the open and dealt with in a logical manner. As a result of treatment, Eva's ego was strengthened and she acquired greater freedom in communicating with her parents and friends. After she made the decision to continue working and postpone marriage, her anxiety seemed to abate.

At a followup contact one year later the nurse-therapist learned that Eva had been free of anxiety attacks during the year, continued to be successful at work, and had married a few weeks earlier.

Obsessive-Compulsive Reaction

The rural community in which Dolly Handmacher grew up was 15 miles from the small town in which she completed high school, worked as a secretary for four years, and met and married her husband. Dolly had been the oldest of three children but had felt distant from her parents and siblings. She had been a lonely, naïve child. Although her controlling mother frequently warned Dolly about the dangers of close contact with boys and with public toilet fixtures, she had given her no sex instruction. Dolly's father, grandfather, and uncle, it was rumored, had all been guilty of marital infidelity. Dolly entered marriage feeling that sex was dirty, that men were untrustworthy, and that she had been soiled by her awkward experimentation with premarital sexual experiences.

Early in their marriage Dolly's husband Fred, a factory foreman, noted his wife's extreme personal fastidiousness. One day he came home from work to find that the water in the toilet had backed up, flooding the bathroom floor and soaking through to the kitchen ceiling. After Dolly had thoroughly cleaned the bathroom and kitchen, she had spent hours scrubbing her body and clothing, feeling that she had been contaminated by the contents of the toilet. Following this event Dolly developed a number of compulsive washing rituals, with which her husband sometimes cooperated in an effort to reduce her persistent fear of contamination.

By means of these rituals Dolly managed to control her anxiety and to maintain the appearance of a conventional, efficient housewife for nine years. One year after the birth of their first child, Dolly's husband was promoted to the position of plant supervisor, which required that he become more socially active than formerly. The demands of child rearing and increased socializing left Dolly less time for her compulsive cleaning routines, and she developed insomnia, irritability, and even more time-consuming rituals. Finally her husband persuaded her to see a psychoanalyst, whose therapy helped reduce her anxiety for a period of one year. Then Dolly became confused, had difficulty remembering the proper sequence of her routines, and began to experience suicidal thoughts. Shortly thereafter her psychiatrist hospitalized her for psychological testing and more intensive treatment.

The results of Dolly's Rorschach, Draw-a-Person, and Thematic Apperception Tests gave no evidence of an underlying schizophrenic process. The psychiatrist therefore reaffirmed his earlier diagnosis of obsessive-compulsive neurosis.

(ANSWER BLANK ON PAGE A–129) (CORRECT ANSWERS ON PAGE B–222)

---

1. Neurotic symptoms develop in response to unconscious:
1. Anxiety.
2. Guilt.
3. Hostility.
4. Conflict.

2. Fleeting obsessions or compulsions that do not interfere with the individual's activities of daily living are considered:
1. Normal.
2. Neurotic.
3. Psychotic.
4. Dissociative.

3. An obsessive-compulsive neurosis is characterized by:
1. The expression of unconscious conflict through physiologic disturbances.
2. The absence of voluntary activity and a tendency to extreme negativism.
3. The presence of fixed, systematized, and well-concealed delusions.
4. Compelling, repetitive, and stylized patterns of behavior and ideation.

4. An obsession is:
1. A pathologically persistent, repetitive, and unwelcome thought.
2. A clouding of consciousness with the production of illusions.
3. An exaggerated concern over one's physical health and well-being.
4. Interpretation of all events as being significantly related to oneself.

5. Compulsion is best defined as:
1. A group of repressed, emotionally charged ideas that influence behavior.
2. The development of a desirable trait to disguise its undesirable opposite.
3. The morbid and irresistible urge to repeat a defensive act again and again.
4. The automatic tendency to oppose and resist what is suggested by others.

6. Dolly's behavioral rituals served the purpose of:
1. Blocking delusions and hallucinations from awareness.
2. Providing temporary and partial relief from her anxiety.
3. Drawing attention and approval from significant others.
4. Increasing the inhibitory powers of her superego.

7. Which of the following most accurately describes Dolly's attitude toward her own behavior?

    1. She viewed her behavior as reasonable, productive, and protective of her family.

    2. She was able to relate her behavior to the underlying feelings precipitating it.

    3. She recognized her behavior as unrealistic but was unable to control it.

    4. She found her greatest enjoyment in performing the highly structured rituals.

8. Unconsciously, Dolly viewed her rituals as:

    1. Trivial time passers.

    2. Dramatic declamations.

    3. Secret signals.

    4. Magical manipulations.

9. Dolly's presentation of herself as an upright, conventional, self-disciplined housewife was an attempt to control her thoughts of:

    1. Love and romance.

    2. Doubt and suspicion.

    3. Weakness and inferiority.

    4. Guilt and hostility.

10. According to Sullivanian theory, the individual is apt to develop an obsessive-compulsive neurosis who utilizes which of the following devices in an effort to achieve security in childhood?

    1. Clinging to the expression of certain word combinations, then doubting their effectiveness in reducing anxiety.

    2. Developing disguised reaction formations to combat or nullify unconscious impulses or wishes.

    3. Diverting the energies of repressed sexual impulses into stereotyped behavior.

    4. Employing patterned motor behavior in order to discharge excess nervous energy.

11. Sullivan stated that the type of home situation which predisposes to development of an obsessive-compulsive neurosis is one in which:

    1. Open expression of hostility is replaced by platitudes and moralizing.

    2. The child regressed to avoid the threat of seductive behavior by one parent.

    3. There is a total lack of respect and affection between parents and child.

    4. Verbal communication between parent and child has been largely supplanted by physical contact.

12. According to Erikson's theory of psychosocial development the obsessive-compulsive person is one who struggles with the alternating attitudes of:

    1. Trust versus mistrust.

    2. Autonomy versus shame and doubt.

    3. Initiative versus guilt.

    4. Industry versus inferiority.

13. Freud designated the obsessive-compulsive individual as being fixated at or regressed to which developmental level?

    1. Oral dependent.

    2. Muscle training.

    3. Oedipal.

    4. Latent.

14. Nurses who interact with Dolly should know that which of the following are typical behaviors of a person with an obsessive-compulsive neurosis?

    a. Frugality.

    b. Stubbornness.

    c. Obedience.

    d. Hoarding.

    e. Cleanliness.

        1. a, b, and e.

        2. b, c, and d.

        3. All but e.

        4. All the above.

15. Nursing assessment of Dolly's needs shortly after admission should include determination of which of the following?

    a. Whether she continues to have suicidal thoughts and the likelihood that she might act on these thoughts.

    b. How much structuring of time and activities Dolly would need in order to decrease her anxiety.

    c. What approach in dealing with Dolly would force her to see that her rituals are not solutions to problems.

    d. What adjustments could be made in unit routine or room assignments to accommodate Dolly's needs.

    e. Whether Dolly's compulsive behavior needs to be discussed with other patients on the unit.

        1. a, b, and c.

        2. a, b, d, and e.

        3. All but e.

        4. All the above.

16. The most therapeutic nursing intervention for Dolly after admission would be to:

1. Assure Dolly of a united approach from the nurses.
2. Provide a portable timer with a long ringing bell.
3. Discuss the schedule of her activities for the day.
4. Type out a list of her compulsive rituals for reference purposes.

17. The nurses discussed the differences between regression and fixation and accurately defined fixation as:
1. Returning to an earlier level of development for gratification.
2. Fearing an object that carries no realistic threat to welfare.
3. Persistence of pregenital interests into later psychosexual development.
4. Loving oneself excessively, to the exclusion of heterosexuality.

18. Dolly's behavior differs from that of a neurotic individual with a phobic reaction in that Dolly:
1. Attempts to avoid those objects which frighten her.
2. Converts her fears into various physical symptoms.
3. Actively protects herself from what she fears.
4. Effectively represses her conflicts and experiences no fear.

19. Reaction formation can best be understood as:
1. Emphasizing a strong point to cover up a feeling of inadequacy or failure.
2. Keeping one of a pair of ambivalent attitudes unconscious by expressing the opposite.
3. The barring from conscious awareness of unwanted emotions, memories, or impulses.
4. The shifting of an emotion to a less dangerous object than that causing the emotion.

20. Dolly used the unconscious ego defense mechanism of isolation, which is:
1. Determination of consciously acceptable reasons for one's actions, wishes, or shortcomings.
2. Withdrawal into extreme passivity in order to protect oneself from painful emotions.
3. A regressive thought process in which problems are solved by the use of fantasy.
4. Defensive separation of feelings and impulses from the reality of an event.

21. Undoing can best be understood as:
1. Opposition to direction by using contrary behavior.
2. Avoidance of an anxiety-provoking situation or thought.
3. Neutralization of and atonement for anxiety-ridden acts.
4. Reversal of feelings by turning interests inward.

22. Nurses interacting with Dolly should recognize that her use of reaction formation, isolation, and undoing are all expressions of:
1. Hostility.
2. Ambivalence.
3. Confusion.
4. Sexuality.

23. Dolly used reaction formation, isolation, and undoing chiefly as defenses against the wish to:
1. Eat.
2. Smear.
3. Masturbate.
4. Make love.

24. In psychoneuroses other than obsessive-compulsive neurosis, which of the following defense mechanisms is most frequently used to protect the ego against unacceptable impulses?
1. Regression.
2. Repression.
3. Sublimation.
4. Denial.

25. Dolly's recurrent idea of being contaminated was formed by the process of:
a. Displacement.
b. Identification.
c. Symbolization.
d. Conversion.
e. Condensation.
    1. a and b.
    2. c and d.
    3. a, c, and e.
    4. All the above.

26. Dolly's fears of dirt and contamination were probably displaced and symbolized fears of:
1. Impulses.
2. Infection.
3. Humiliation.
4. Closeness.

27. Dolly's superego could best be described as:
1. Demanding and punitive.
2. Fragmented and inconsistent.
3. Adequate but incomplete.
4. Mature and realistic.

28. Which of the following are among the important concepts of psychoanalysis?
- a. Free association.
- b. Transference.
- c. Resistance.
- d. Repression.
- e. Libido.
    1. a and b.
    2. a, b, and d.
    3. All but e.
    4. All the above.

29. Resistance in psychoanalysis may best be defined as:
1. Inability of the client to verbally express the emotions which he feels.
2. Intentional or unintentional attempts by family members to sabotage the therapy.
3. Reluctance on the part of the client to enter upon the process of psychoanalysis.
4. Strong opposition to bringing repressed material from unconsciousness into awareness.

30. Which of the following are considered to be forms of resistance?
- a. Becoming silent during an analytic session.
- b. Clinging to discussion of superficial material.
- c. Forgetting material previously discussed in analysis.
- d. Speaking exclusively about the analyst.
- e. Misunderstanding most remarks and questions of the analyst.
    1. b and d.
    2. a, c, and e.
    3. All but e.
    4. All the above.

31. Freud described a sexual energy or drive which has specific but changing aims and objects. He called this energy:
1. Instinct.
2. Cathexis.
3. Libido.
4. Narcissism.

32. In psychoanalysis, insight may best be defined as the:
1. Extent of the patient's genuine understanding of the origins and unconscious dynamisms of his behavior.
2. Phenomenon of sudden awareness when a thought is first linked with its related strong emotion.
3. Awareness of those thought processes which are determined by genetic control mechanisms.
4. Therapist's ability to distinguish factual from fantasized content in the client's free association.

33. Any acting out which Dolly would display during psychoanalysis would be an attempt to express herself through action rather than through verbal communication. Such acting out is always relative to:
1. Failure in therapy.
2. The therapist's anxiety level.
3. An unresolved anger.
4. The transference situation.

34. The first objective for Dolly's psychoanalysis would probably be to:
1. Offer interpretations of the content of material in Dolly's stream of consciousness talk.
2. Emphasize the reality of her regression and assist her to adjust to a dependent existence.
3. Encourage her to relate in detail the progressive development of her ritualistic symptoms.
4. Help her to free blocked emotions by dynamic interpretation of the ego defense of isolation.

35. In order to contribute maximally to Dolly's therapy, her nurse should know that which of the following are true of the interpretations made to Dolly by her analyst?
- a. An interpretation is a working hypothesis that Dolly may test, work through, or ignore.
- b. The accuracy of interpretations is necessarily uncertain and seldom precisely correct.
- c. Interpretations will not provide Dolly with insight, but may stimulate disclosure of repressed material.
- d. Interpretations will help Dolly to correlate her behavior, past history, and future aims.
- e. A decreased need for rituals on Dolly's part would confirm the accuracy of interpretations.
    1. a and c.
    2. a, c, and d.
    3. All but e.
    4. All the above.

36. At the time she was hospitalized Dolly probably managed her feelings of anger by:
1. Externalizing hostility in her interactions with others.

2. Turning her hostile feelings inward, against herself.
3. Talking out her aggressive feelings with other persons.
4. Converting rage to symptoms of psychosomatic illness.

In the hospital interviews with her psychiatrist Dolly expressed a desire to be cured, but she continued to deny her hostility and to rationalize her behavior. She seldom expressed her feelings openly but rather filled her treatment hours with superficial intellectualizations concerning her life situation and attitudes.

Dolly was accepted by the patients on the unit even though she tended to be controlling in her interactions with them. Near the end of her stay they began to taunt her concerning her routines. Dolly interacted frequently and communicated openly with the nurses. At times, she took independent actions, but on other occasions she was dependent upon the nurses to tell her what she should do. Either Dolly's husband or her neighbor came to visit her every day.

37. A primary difficulty the psychiatrist would encounter in treating Dolly is the fact that:
1. She would be strongly suspicious and distrustful of the psychiatrist.
2. She would easily become discouraged and would miss many appointments.
3. She would be prone to discuss her thoughts rather than to express her feelings.
4. She would be unable to agree with his goals for her treatment.

38. Dolly's extensive use of reaction formation could give rise to secondary narcissistic gain which might, in turn, increase her:
1. Resistance to psychoanalysis.
2. Thoughts of suicide.
3. Panicky anxiety attacks.
4. Adherence to rituals.

39. Dolly said angrily, "My psychiatrist said that I only see things from my own point of view. Is that true?" Which response by the nurse would be most appropriate?
1. "Since that upsets you, don't think about it."
2. "Well, after all, isn't that true of everyone?"
3. "Do you think that describes your viewpoint accurately?"

4. "It doesn't seem to me that you're that selfish."

40. In order to construct a therapeutic plan of nursing care for Dolly the nurse should be aware of Dolly's:
a. Intellectual ability and level of educational achievement.
b. Degree of social and sexual adjustment in her marriage.
c. Former experiences in living and working with groups.
d. Underlying conflict and the meaning of her symptoms.
    1. a and c.
    2. a and d.
    3. All but d.
    4. All the above.

41. The nurse who worked most closely with Dolly observed that many of Dolly's characteristics were much like her own. Which of the following characteristics would the nurse and Dolly be most apt to have in common?
a. Rigidity.
b. Orderliness.
c. Cautiousness.
d. Conscientiousness.
e. Dependability.
    1. a and b.
    2. a, b, and d.
    3. All but d.
    4. All the above.

42. In order to plan Dolly's care the nurse must accept the fact that Dolly does not recognize:
1. That she is a human being separate and independent from other persons.
2. Either the cause for her symptoms or the concomitant secondary gains.
3. The therapeutic abilities of the various members of the treatment team.
4. The degree to which her rituals interfere with the activities of living.

43. Which methods other than psychoanalysis have been successful in treatment of obsessive-compulsive neurosis?
a. Behavior therapy.
b. Milieu or systems therapy.
c. Electroconvulsive therapy.
d. Role playing.
e. Supportive psychotherapy.
    1. a only.
    2. a, b, and e.
    3. All but c.
    4. All the above.

44. The nurse should aim at helping Dolly toward increasing:
1. Self-esteem.
2. Self-control.
3. Self-examination.
4. Self-denial.

45. In order to understand the meaning of the cleaning rituals the nurse should appreciate that to Dolly:
1. Pleasure is felt in opposing the wishes of others.
2. Power is obtained by counteracting hostile fate.
3. Acceptance is assured by doing the socially approved thing.
4. Safety is achieved by following prescribed formulas.

46. Shortly after she entered the hospital Dolly began to increase her ritualistic washing at bedtime, to the point that she was losing several hours of sleep. Which action by the nurse would be most helpful?
   a. Talk with her to determine the cause of her bedtime anxiety.
   b. Modify her retirement routine so as to diminish her bedtime anxiety.
   c. Remind Dolly daily to begin to perform her rituals early in the evening.
   d. Limit the amount of time which Dolly may spend on her washing rituals.
   e. Ignore her washing activities and make no comments about them.
      1. a and b.
      2. a, b, and d.
      3. All but e.
      4. All the above.

47. The psychiatrist insisted that Dolly participate in recreational and occupational therapy in the hospital so that she might have:
1. A means to release tension and to develop interests outside herself.
2. An opportunity to produce an object expressing her aspirations and fears.
3. Regular and enforced change of physical and social environment.
4. Stimulation for the acquisition of new and non-ritualistic motor skills.

48. In order to avoid increasing Dolly's anxiety, what attitude should the nurse take toward the cleansing rituals?
1. Encourage the cleansing routines by performing them with or for Dolly.
2. Ignore the rituals, making no allowances for consideration of Dolly's habits.

3. Work with Dolly to develop compromises and to set limits on her behavior.
4. Assume responsibility for forcibly restraining her from the rituals.

49. It would be inadvisable for the nurse to use logic and reason in an attempt to discredit Dolly's need for compulsive routines because:
1. Dolly's hysterical temperament causes her to be distrustful of logic.
2. Pressure to relinquish the rituals would produce increased anxiety.
3. Compulsive routines can be abandoned only in response to personal pleas.
4. Dolly's lack of contact with reality renders her immune to logic.

50. In order to handle the interaction problem among Dolly and other patients on the unit, the nurse who has established the best relationship with Dolly should first:
1. Inform the other nurses that a problem exists and outline the reasons for its occurrence.
2. Tell the psychoanalyst that Dolly is creating problems on the unit.
3. Point out to Dolly that her controlling behavior is contributing to the problem.
4. Instruct the other patients on the unit to stop teasing and taunting Dolly.

51. Dolly will not be able to relinquish her compulsive washing routines until she:
1. Acquires sufficient increase in superego strength to break well-entrenched habits.
2. Recognizes the unrealistic and undesirable nature of her ritualistic behavior.
3. No longer needs them to manage her feelings of guilt and aggression.
4. Regains sufficient contact with reality to relate comfortably with others.

52. One morning Dolly said to the nurse "I started to menstruate just now. Should I give up my trip to occupational therapy?" Initially, how should the nurse respond?
1. "Do as you like. Go or stay as you see fit."
2. "You know you're expected to keep appointments."
3. "What are you trying to tell me?"
4. "You have a lot of pain with menstruation?"

53. Dolly's prognosis for total recovery is not especially favorable because of her inability to:

1. Restrain herself from her well-entrenched rituals long enough to form new habits.
2. Experience the depth of emotion that would be apt to lead to a change in behavior.
3. Communicate her troublesome thoughts clearly enough to be understood by others.
4. Develop sufficient motivation to continue with the proposed program of therapy.

After only two weeks of hospitalization, Dolly's confusion and suicidal ideas had disappeared. Her rituals continued, but in greatly attenuated form. She was discharged from the hospital and decided to continue therapy with her psychiatrist on a weekly basis for the next year, after which her anxiety was well controlled by minimal use of routines and she had had no further episodes of confusion.

Psychotic Depressive Reaction

Thirty-five-year-old Gertrude Cowert was brought to the admission center of a large state mental hospital by her husband, Kenneth, who gave the social worker a résumé of his wife's health history. Mrs. Cowert had previously been hospitalized for treatment of psychotic depressive reactions at the age of 24, after the birth of her second child, and again at the age of 31. During her second hospitalization Mrs. Cowert had been given electroconvulsive therapy. During the six weeks preceding the present hospital admission Mrs. Cowert had demonstrated behavior similar to that which had necessitated her previous hospitalizations. She had become progressively unable to sleep, eat, talk, or perform any of her routine housework. She had sat silently for long periods of time, smoking one cigarette after another, apparently oblivious to her family's activities.

During the admission interview with the psychiatrist Mrs. Cowert was oriented to time, place, and person, but appeared to be preoccupied, withdrawn, and frightened. Sitting slumped forward, with her head in her hands, she responded to a few of the psychiatrist's questions in a mumbled monotone. She said that she was unable to decide what to say and didn't know why she felt so bad. The psychiatrist's diagnosis of psychotic depressive reaction was confirmed by psychological testing.

Mr. Cowert told the admitting nurse that his wife's relationship with her psychotic mother had been very poor and that Mrs. Cowert had been brutally treated by her mother until the latter's death five years earlier. Mrs. Cowert's father had spent little time in the home.

Mr. Cowert described his own childhood as also having been unhappy. He said that life with his wife had been filled with crises, arguments, and periods of silence between the two of them. He said that while his wife was extraordinarily dependent upon him, he could depend only upon himself. He had recently begun to sell insurance in his spare time in order to earn money to send his children to college.

Mrs. Cowert was admitted to a locked unit and placed in a room with a quiet patient of about the same age. The doctor wrote the following orders for Mrs. Cowert:

1. *Imipramine hydrochloride (Tofranil) 25 mg. orally, q.i.d.*
2. *Multi-vitamin with iron, 1 tablet, q.a.m.*
3. *To leave unit only to attend occupational therapy.*
4. *Must be accompanied to occupational therapy by a staff member.*
5. *Close supervision on the unit.*
6. *May have visitors without restriction.*

(ANSWER BLANK ON PAGE A–131) (CORRECT ANSWERS ON PAGE B–225)

---

1. The birth of Mrs. Cowert's second child probably contributed to her initial episode of an affective disorder by:

1. Increasing the demands of others upon her at a time when her own dependency needs were especially acute.
2. Depleting her reserves of physical strength during the periods of pregnancy, labor, and delivery.
3. Threatening the family economy through the additional expense associated with hospitalization and delivery.
4. Emphasizing her feeling of social isolation with the increase in size and complexity of her family.

2. It is thought that electroshock therapy relieves the symptoms of psychotic depression in part by:

1. Interrupting long established invalid thought patterns and realigning them constructively.
2. Satisfying the patient's felt needs for punishment to expiate strong guilt feelings.
3. Interrupting impulse transmission from the prefrontal to the central cerebral cortex.
4. Providing strong sensory stimuli to distract attention from self-deprecating delusions.

3. There is indirect evidence that underproduction of which of the following chemical substances may cause psychotic depression?

1. Aminobutyric acid and vitamin B_6.
2. Acetyl coenzyme A and pyruvic acid.
3. Dexamethasone and ACTH.
4. Norepinephrine and serotonin.

4. Which of the following is the most plausible explanation for Mr. Cowert's delay in bringing his wife for treatment during her current illness?

1. His inability to recognize a qualitative behavioral change in someone with whom he has had continuous contact.
2. His reluctance to acknowledge the fact that Mrs. Cowert's previous affective disorder had recurred.
3. His inattention to complaints and behavior to which he had become accustomed through previous exposure.
4. A lack of attention to his wife deriving from her decreased attractiveness and responsiveness to him.

5. The nurse should appreciate that Mrs. Cowert's recent insomnia, anorexia and inactivity would tend to accentuate her depression primarily by:

1. Disrupting family routines.
2. Decreasing her ego strength.
3. Exhausting her physical energy.
4. Reducing her interpersonal contacts.

6. In addition to insomnia and anorexia, Mrs. Cowert would be apt to develop which of the following physical complaints?

1. Menorrhagia.
2. Sordes.
3. Melena.
4. Constipation.

7. The nurse who receives Mrs. Cowert on the unit should assess which of the following?

a. Mrs. Cowert's general health and nutritional status.
b. Mrs. Cowert's verbal and nonverbal behavior.
c. Her own reactions to Mr. and Mrs. Cowert.
d. Mrs. Cowert's interaction ability at this time.
e. Amount of observation that Mrs. Cowert needs.

1. b and d.
2. a, c, d, and e.
3. All but c.
4. All the above.

8. Special structuring of unit activities and furniture were required as an initial effort to meet Mrs. Cowert's physical and emotional needs. Which of the following changes would be therapeutic for Mrs. Cowert early in her hospitalization?

a. Monitor Mrs. Cowert's activity in her room by closed circuit television.

b. Permit only those unit and occupational therapy activities in which Mrs. Cowert can participate without increasing her anxiety.

c. Arrange all furniture in the television room and lounge in a circle so Mrs. Cowert can interact with ease.

d. After an explanation is given, remove all forks and knives from the dining area and instruct patients to eat with teaspoons.

e. Assign other patients in the unit to help watch Mrs. Cowert during the evening and night hours.

    1. a only.
    2. a and e.
    3. b and d.
    4. All but d.
    5. All the above.

9. Mr. Cowert asked, "What made my wife sick this time?" Which of the following responses by the nurse would be most instructive?

1. "Your question indicates an unreasonable feeling of guilt on your part."

2. "No single person or event is responsible for your wife's health or illness."

3. "I know you're worried about the cause of her illness, but that's no longer important."

4. "The psychiatrist will be able to answer that question only after several interviews."

10. Then Mr. Cowert began to cry and said, "It's all my fault. I should never have taken that extra job." Which reply by the nurse would be most supportive to Mr. Cowert?

1. "You mean it was difficult to decide to take the job and it's hard to know now whether the decision was wise?"

2. "We all do things we regret later, but I see no need for you to blame yourself."

3. "You may be partially responsible for her illness, but she is somewhat responsible, too."

4. "You are too upset to talk about that now. I'll come back later to discuss it with you."

11. In saying, "I can depend only on myself," Mr. Cowert revealed that:

1. He is unusually independent and stable.

2. He holds the usual view of a man's role.

3. Mrs. Cowert infrequently supported his views.

4. He has never learned to trust other people.

12. It is probable that which of the following contributed significantly to the development of Mrs. Cowert's depression?

a. A predominantly oral personality.

b. A wholly instinctual id.

c. An extremely punitive superego.

d. An unresolved Oedipal conflict.

    1. a only.
    2. a and c.
    3. b and d.
    4. All the above.

13. Psychoanalytically, libido is the term used to describe the:

1. Energy associated with the instincts of the id.

2. Instability of one's affect or unconscious feelings.

3. Investment of an object with special significance.

4. Censor of dangerous impulses from consciousness.

14. Healthy ego functioning contributes to mastery of the environment through mediation of:

a. Motor control.
b. Sensory perception.
c. Memory storage.
d. Affective response.
e. Thinking processes.

    1. a and b.
    2. c and d.
    3. All but e.
    4. All the above.

15. The chief function of the ego is to:

1. Harbor instincts.
2. Censor behavior.
3. Test reality.
4. Project ideals.

16. According to current psychoanalytic theory, ego development begins:
1. At the moment of birth.
2. About six months of age.
3. About three years of age.
4. About seven years of age.

17. Which of the following is the best example of the reality testing function of the ego?
1. The ability to evaluate the quality of one's own behavior.
2. The ability to distinguish between external and internal stimuli.
3. The tendency to like or dislike certain activities or people.
4. The ability to weigh the validity of certain ideas and concepts.

18. The psychodynamics of depression are such that the nurse may assume that during the early stage of Mrs. Cowert's illness, she used which of the following defense mechanisms to protect herself from extreme anxiety?
   a. Regression.
   b. Projection.
   c. Introjection.
   d. Reaction formation.
   e. Identification.
      1. a and c.
      2. b and d.
      3. a, c, and e.
      4. All the above.

19. Introjection is best defined as an unconscious process whereby one:
1. Symbolically incorporates a loved or hated object.
2. Attributes one's own feelings to significant others.
3. Fails to respond to the overtures and pleas of another.
4. Adopts a pessimistic attitude toward one's life situation.

20. The superego develops from:
1. Analysis of experience in terms of cause and effect relationships.
2. Spontaneous maturation of a cognitive ability dormant at birth.
3. Successful resolution of the struggle between the id and the ego.
4. Internalization of values presented to the child by significant adults.

21. Psychological guilt is best defined as:
1. Intellectual acceptance of responsibility for an unethical or illegal action.

2. A feeling of blameworthiness for thoughts or behavior unacceptable to the superego.
3. A sense of weakness or inability to withstand prolonged external temptation.
4. A defensive maneuver by which the ego protects itself against anxiety.

22. Freud regarded which of the following factors as necessary to the development of psychotic depression?
   a. Strong fixation on the love object.
   b. Narcissistic choice of love object.
   c. Ambivalent relationship with the love object.
   d. Strict and rigid superego.
   e. Equating of ego and love object.
      1. a only.
      2. c and d.
      3. All but e.
      4. All the above.

23. In addition to environmental influences, which other factors determined the intensity of Mrs. Cowert's present depressive reaction?
   a. The manner in which she had resolved previous losses.
   b. Her relationship with the real or imagined loss object.
   c. The degree of her ambivalence toward the lost love object.
   d. The characteristics of her superego, id, and ego.
      1. a and b.
      2. c and d.
      3. All but d.
      4. All the above.

24. Freud thought that, in contradistinction to mourning, melancholia is characterized by:
1. Realizing what has been lost and effectively separating oneself from the lost object.
2. Having difficulty in identifying the lost love object and its significance.
3. Failing to recognize any loss while becoming depressed due to diminution of positive reinforcement.
4. Misinterpretation of events in the environment, and despondence over lack of insight.

25. Ambivalence is best defined as:
1. Unusual strength or persistence of an unpleasant feeling or impression.
2. The ability to change one's attitude when confronted with meaningful evidence.

3. The tendency for a feeling to remain below the level of consciousness.
4. The coexistence of conflicting emotions toward an object or person.

26. Mrs. Cowert's depression is probably a manifestation of:
1. Paralyzing fear.
2. Conflicting responsibilities.
3. Physical exhaustion.
4. Internalized aggression.

27. The feeling Mrs. Cowert is most apt to demonstrate during her psychotic depression is:
1. Agitation.
2. Loneliness.
3. Suspicion of others.
4. Disillusionment with self.

28. A nursing problem arose from Mrs. Cowert's withdrawal behavior, since the other patients ignored her, both on the unit and during team meetings. If the nurse should allow this pattern of behavior to continue, Mrs. Cowert's initial response would probably be to:
1. Increase the externalization of anger.
2. Decrease her ability to relate with others.
3. Re-evaluate her need for hospitalization.
4. Increase her feelings of unworthiness.

29. The chief reason why Mrs. Cowert feels worthless is the fact that she:
1. Feels that she has accomplished little of importance during her life.
2. Concludes that she is responsible for the loss of the love object.
3. Has received little positive reinforcement of her worth from her husband.
4. Realizes that she has regressed and regrets having done so.

30. The Rorschach test administered to Mrs. Cowert consists of:
1. Having her draw a house, a tree, and a person, and then having her tell a story about them.
2. Presenting her with unstructured stimuli in order to call forth subjective responses.
3. Presenting her with problem situations for which she is to select a solution.
4. Having her write a descriptive exposition of her evaluation of a current social problem.

31. Which of the following is the same type of test as the Rorschach?
1. Downey Will-Temperament Test.
2. Stanford-Binet Test.
3. Minnesota Multiphasic Personality Inventory.
4. Thematic Apperception Test.

32. The chief action of imipramine hydrochloride (Tofranil), which explains its having been given to Mrs. Cowert, is its ability to:
1. Induce a state of euphoria.
2. Stimulate the central nervous system.
3. Lessen fatigue, anorexia, and delusions.
4. Potentiate the barbiturate hypnotics.

33. Side effects of imipramine hydrochloride (Tofranil) which the nurse may observe in Mrs. Cowert are:
1. Hot flashes, flushing, and fainting.
2. Hypertrophy and tenderness of lymph nodes.
3. Gingival hypertrophy and bleeding.
4. Dryness of the mouth, tachycardia, and constipation.

34. Which of the following attitudes of the nurse would be most helpful in overcoming Mrs. Cowert's reluctance to take her medication?
1. Firm kindness.
2. Rigid insistence.
3. Humble entreaty.
4. Gentle bantering.

35. Which of the following occupational therapy activities would be most directly related to Mrs. Cowert's treatment goals?
1. Writing poetry.
2. Baking cookies.
3. Interpretive dancing.
4. Sanding furniture.

36. The chief therapeutic objective in having Mrs. Cowert participate in occupational therapy activities is to enable her to:
1. Develop an interest in the appearance of her surroundings.
2. Express aggression externally through motor activity.
3. Acquire a skill that may later have economic value.
4. Relieve boredom through participation in a new activity.

Mrs. Cowert remained withdrawn during the first three weeks of her hospitalization and failed to respond significantly to individual psychotherapy with the psychiatrist.

She was aloof, suicidal, and unable to achieve any insight into her own behavior. On one occasion when the nurse was sitting beside her, Mrs. Cowert mumbled, "I think the children are burning." On several occasions the nurse found Mrs. Cowert alone, hunched in the corner of the dayroom and shivering.

37. Mrs. Cowert's withdrawal served a defensive function by:
1. Giving her sufficient time to think out solutions to her problems.
2. Reducing the number and complexity of her interactions with others.
3. Decreasing the number of ideas with which she must deal intellectually.
4. Decreasing the demands for her to formulate her thoughts into words.

38. General nursing approaches to Mrs. Cowert during her deep depression should include:
   a. Offering nourishment and facilitating elimination.
   b. Protecting her from physical and emotional trauma.
   c. Sitting silently by when she is unable to talk.
   d. Staying with her constantly throughout the day.
   e. Encouraging her to pursue her interests and exercise her abilities.
      1. a, b, and c.
      2. b, c, and e.
      3. All but e.
      4. All the above.

39. Which of the following could the nurse profitably use as indications of the depth of Mrs. Cowert's depression at any given point in time?
   a. Her eating, eliminating, and sleeping patterns.
   b. Her interactions with patients and staff.
   c. Her facial expressions, posture and gestures.
   d. Her choice of words and the content of her drawings.
   e. The degree of her participation in planned and spontaneous activities.
      1. a, b, and c.
      2. a, c, and d.
      3. All but e.
      4. All the above.

40. In order to protect Mrs. Cowert from suicide the nurse should recognize which of the following as clues of suicidal thought?
   a. A tendency to hoard sleeping pills.
   b. The collection of sharp objects.
   c. A preference to remain alone.
   d. The expression of somatic complaints.
   e. Demonstration of marked mood change.
      1. a, b, and c.
      2. b, c, and e.
      3. All but e.
      4. All the above.

41. Mrs. Cowert is most apt to attempt to commit suicide during which of the following phases of her hospitalization?
1. Immediately after hospital admission.
2. At the point of her deepest depression.
3. When her depression begins to abate.
4. Shortly before hospital discharge.

42. Which of the following best explains what was implied when Mrs. Cowert was described as being a dependent person?
1. She tends to exaggerate the importance of her sensual needs.
2. She employs cunning in persuading others to her viewpoint.
3. She continuously seeks support and protection from others.
4. She is unable to verbalize her needs clearly and directly.

43. In responding to Mrs. Cowert's expression of delusional thought, "I think my children are burning," the nurse must understand that she should *not*:
1. Explore the delusional content.
2. Try to reason away the delusion.
3. Show her disbelief in the delusion.
4. Convey the idea that delusions are temporary.

44. Following Mrs. Cowert's refusal to eat several meals the nurse should:
   a. Provide frequent small feedings and between-meal nourishment.
   b. Deliver the meal tray, cut the meat, and butter the bread.
   c. Suggest to Mrs. Cowert that she begin by eating her bread.
   d. Place a glass of milk in her hand and guide it to her mouth.

e. Omit several scheduled meals, to increase her desire for food.
    1. a only.
    2. a, b, and c.
    3. b, c, and d.
    4. All but e.

45. The nurse should do which of the following when she observes Mrs. Cowert shivering in the corner of the dayroom?
    1. Ignore her shivering in order to force Mrs. Cowert either to get a sweater or request one.
    2. Get a sweater from Mrs. Cowert's locker and, without comment, drape it over her shoulders.
    3. Direct Mrs. Cowert to go to her locker, get her sweater, and put it on before she returns to the dayroom.
    4. Comment to Mrs. Cowert that she observes her shivering and go with Mrs. Cowert to get a sweater for her.

46. Mrs. Cowert's complaints, self-deprecation, inactivity, and withdrawal are apt to provoke which of the following feelings in the nurse?
  a. Inadequacy.
  b. Helplessness.
  c. Fear.
  d. Anger.
  e. Guilt.
    1. a and b.
    2. a, c, and e.
    3. All but e.
    4. All the above.

47. In order to maintain the therapeutic relationship which she has established with her patient, the nurse must accept the fact that Mrs. Cowert:
  a. May express considerable hostility toward her.
  b. Will portray ambivalent feelings toward the nurse.
  c. Will have much difficulty in making decisions.
  d. Will need to test out new responses to old problems.
  e. Will be acutely sensitive to veiled criticism.
    1. b and d.
    2. a, c, and d.
    3. All but e.
    4. All the above.

By her sixth week of hospitalization Mrs. Cowert's mood had improved. She slept, ate, talked, and participated in ward activities. However, when she began to talk she expressed self-deprecatory ideas and made many critical comments about the staff and hospital.

48. Mrs. Cowert said to the nurse, "I'm terrible. I don't deserve to live." Which of the following responses by the nurse would be most appropriate?
    1. "Yes, it has occured to us that you had that opinion of yourself."
    2. "If you continue to talk this way, I can't listen to you anymore."
    3. "What has led you to think that you don't deserve to live?"
    4. "I don't think you're terrible. You seem to be well-liked here."

49. In criticizing her psychiatrist one day Mrs. Cowert said, "He doesn't understand me. He's just making me worse." How should the nurse reply?
    1. "It sounds like you feel very angry toward your psychiatrist."
    2. "Give him a chance. It takes time for treatment to take effect."
    3. "Do you hold him wholly responsible for your return to health?"
    4. "Today you feel that you are worse. Tomorrow may be different."

50. Mrs. Cowert's criticism of her psychiatrist can most accurately be interpreted as indicating that she has:
    1. Achieved a degree of identification with him.
    2. Become more regressed and unable to manage aggression.
    3. Recognized that he is especially intolerant of criticism.
    4. Discovered the natural human shortcomings of the staff.

51. One of the psychiatric team's treatment goals for Mrs. Cowert was to help her achieve a positive, realistic self-concept. Which of the following would be included in such a self-concept?
  a. A degree of self-esteem.
  b. A feeling of acceptance by others.
  c. A feeling of self-respect.
  d. A feeling of belonging.
  e. A feeling of humility.
    1. a and c.
    2. b and d.
    3. All but e.
    4. All the above.

52. After a week of looking unkempt and disheveled, Mrs. Cowert arose one morning, took a tub bath, put on an attractive pink dress, and combed her hair before going to breakfast. How should the nurse respond to this change in Mrs. Cowert's behavior?

1. "Why Mrs. Cowert, how you've changed! I see you've got a pretty new dress. You must be getting better."
2. "Now that you've demonstrated that you can bathe and dress yourself, we hope you'll maintain a good appearance."
3. "As long as you were getting yourself dressed up this morning, why didn't you put on some lipstick and powder?"
4. "I see that you got up early, took a bath, combed your hair and put on a fresh dress before coming to breakfast."

Mrs. Cowert continued in individual psychotherapy while participating in 10 family therapy sessions. At the end of 12 weeks of hospitalization she appeared to be symptom free but still did not have significant insight into her behavior. Following two successful weekend visits to her home she was discharged as improved and was counseled to adopt a day by day attitude toward her problems and not to expect to feel perfectly well for a while.

53. The family is an example of which of the following types of groups?

1. Primary.
2. Secondary.
3. Artificial.
4. Intimate.

54. Which of the following statements is an accurate description of family interactions?

1. Roles within the family are explicitly defined and relatively unchanging.
2. The behavior of each family member is affected by that of every other.
3. Family life protects its members against conflict and anxiety.
4. The emotional climate of the family remains relatively the same through time.

55. The Cowert's family therapy would be directed chiefly toward understanding and improving:

1. Aggressive and hostile expressions by Mrs. Cowert.
2. Mr. Cowert's understanding of his wife's behavior.
3. Anxiety provoking situations inherent in family life.
4. Disturbed psychosocial relationships within the family.

56. Which of the following would the Cowerts' family therapist probably wish to accomplish in his initial contacts with the family members?

a. Explain the nature of family therapy to each family member.
b. Explore each family member's expectations of group therapy.
c. Clarify the fact that Mrs. Cowert is the family's main problem.
d. Identify any symptoms of disharmony within the family's interactions.
e. Determine which member is principally responsible for the family's pain.

1. a and b.
2. a, b, and d.
3. All but e.
4. All the above.

57. Virginia Satir teaches that, in any family therapy situation, the group treatments should not be terminated until:

a. Parents view themselves as a pair of individuals with identical feelings and motives.
b. All family members have freed themselves from the need to emulate unhealthy models.
c. Individual members have learned to effectively suppress their hostilities.
d. The members can tell each other what they hope, fear, and expect from each other.
e. The member can find faults in each other and still feel warmth toward each other.

1. a and c.
2. b and d.
3. All but e.
4. All the above.

58. After his wife was discharged, Mr. Cowert refused to continue family therapy, saying "I don't have time for chatting." What was probably the main motive behind his decision?

1. He valued earning money for his children's education more than his wife's health.
2. He wanted to expose the family therapist who wasn't meeting his wife's needs.
3. He was trying to protect the children from the effects of family therapy.
4. He desired to escape a situation which was making him recognize his own needs and defenses.

59. Mrs. Cowert's children were 11 and 12 years old. Their responses to their mother's illness and to family therapy would probably be:

a. Anger.
b. Regression.
c. Shame.
d. Guilt.
e. Fear.

    1. a only.
    2. a and b.

3. All but d.
4. All the above.

60. As the nurse evaluated the care given Mrs. Cowert, she observed that insufficient discharge planning had been done. Which of the following is the most important assessment for the nurse to make in discharge planning for Mrs. Cowert?

1. Whether she has all her personal belongings collected and how and when she will be leaving for home.
2. Whether she has anyone to help care for her children and whether she can obtain and remember to take her medicines.
3. Whether she knows when her next appointment is and whether she can see her therapist on that day at that time.
4. Whether her husband has sufficient love for his wife to re-evaluate his need for a second job.

Manic Reaction

Victoria Clapper was 48 years old when her husband brought her to a state mental hospital in an acute manic state. Victoria's history, as conveyed to the psychiatrist by her husband, was as follows. When she was four years old her mother died. Soon afterward her father married a younger woman, who had five children in the next seven years. Victoria's stepmother relegated to Victoria much of the responsibility for the care of her stepbrothers and stepsisters but, at the same time, somehow managed to keep Victoria at the periphery of family life and activity.

A college scholarship enabled Victoria to leave home immediately after she was graduated from high school to study music. On being graduated from college she married Henry Clapper, a college chemistry professor, and took a position as a high school music teacher in the small community in which her husband taught.

During the six months preceding her hospitalization Victoria first complained of a variety of somatic symptoms, then became exceedingly jealous of what she considered to be her husband's excessive attentions toward his young, female laboratory assistant. Finally, after three days of severe depression, Victoria made a vituperative verbal attack on the judges who had failed to award her favorite pupil the first prize in a state music contest.

On admission to the hospital Victoria moved about restlessly, waving her arms in a threatening manner while loudly berating her husband, the hospital personnel, and the state music judges. She demanded to be released from "this jail" and cursed the nurse and psychiatrist who interviewed her. The psychiatrist described Victoria as a possessive and dependent person who feared rejection and abandonment and was in an acute manic state. He wrote the following orders:

1. *Chlorpromazine (Thorazine) 50 mg. orally q.i.d.*
2. *Chlorpromazine (Thorazine) 50 mg. I.M. p.r.n.*
3. *Lithium carbonate 600 mg. orally t.i.d.*
4. *Restrict to the unit.*

(ANSWER BLANK ON PAGE A–133) (CORRECT ANSWERS ON PAGE B–229)

---

1. Assessment of Victoria Clapper by the nurse who admits her to the unit should include determining:
  a. Which of her physical needs require attention.
  b. When she should be isolated from other patients.
  c. Her ability to control her own behavior.
  d. In what ways she needs physical protection.
  e. What made her feel loved in the past.
    1. c only.
    2. a, c, and d.
    3. All but d.
    4. All the above.

2. In orienting Victoria to the unit the nurse should do which of the following:
  a. Direct Victoria to the isolation room and restrain her.
  b. Introduce her to each patient and nurse individually.
  c. Orient her to the patient areas of the unit.
  d. Show her her room and the ladies' bathroom.
  e. Determine whether she is hungry, thirsty, or has any questions.
    1. a only.
    2. c, d, and e.
    3. All but a.
    4. All the above.

3. Which of the following best describes the most suitable environment for Victoria during her acute mania?
    1. A seclusion room with a large window.
    2. A spacious room with few people in it.
    3. A dayroom filled with other patients.
    4. A well-lighted, four bed room.

4. Which of the following traumas precipitated Victoria's manic episode?
  a. Ego threats precipitated by the menopause.
  b. Sudden impairment of physical health.
  c. Suspicion of her husband's infidelity.
  d. Loss of freedom upon hospitalization.
  e. Presumed failure of her protégé.
    1. a and b.
    2. c and d.
    3. a, c, and e.
    4. All the above.

5. The nurse should understand that the events precipitating Victoria's manic episode were incidents which she could perceive as a:
    1. Threat to life.
    2. Loss of love.
    3. Increase in freedom.
    4. Decrease of restraint.

6. During the acute stage of mania, Victoria's predominant feeling would appear to be that of:
    1. Freedom.
    2. Elation.
    3. Joviality.
    4. Ecstasy.

7. Dynamically, Victoria's manic behavior was an attempt on her part to avoid consciously recognizing and experiencing feelings of:
    1. Depression.
    2. Hostility.
    3. Euphoria.
    4. Acceptance.

8. Mrs. Clapper's fear of being abandoned derives from the fact that in her relationships with others she has been:
    1. Guarded and suspicious.
    2. Distant and reserved.
    3. Dependent and possessive.
    4. Empathic and considerate.

9. In order to gratify her needs, Mrs. Clapper unconsciously attempted to manipulate and exploit others. Frustrations of such efforts probably gave rise to:
    1. Guilt.
    2. Hostility.

3. Resignation.
4. Relief.

10. Mrs. Clapper's fear of being abandoned by significant others would have led to:
1. An increase in her anxiety.
2. Physical withdrawal from others.
3. An accentuation of self-reliance.
4. An absence of reality testing.

11. Which of the following nursing interventions would be most helpful to Victoria immediately following admission?
1. Providing a calm and safe environment.
2. Staying with her and talking to her.
3. Helping her to set limits on her behavior.
4. Administering medications as ordered.

12. What is the probable initial reaction of the other patients on the unit to Victoria immediately after her admission?
1. Fear.
2. Amusement.
3. Disgust.
4. Anger.

13. Mrs. Clapper's excessive demands, hostility, and meddling in the affairs of her husband and school music personnel accentuated her problems chiefly by:
1. Exhausting her physical energy.
2. Distracting her from work.
3. Giving her a sense of power.
4. Precipitating rejection by others.

14. The psychodynamic basis for Victoria's acute manic episode can be assumed to have been a:
1. Weak ego, powerful id, and strong superego.
2. Strong ego, powerful id, and strong superego.
3. Weak ego, weak id, and weak superego.
4. Strong ego, weak id, and weak superego.

15. Contributing to her mania is the fact that Victoria has chiefly employed which of the following defense mechanisms in protecting her ego from disintegration?
1. Suppression.
2. Sublimation.
3. Denial.
4. Identification.

16. The nurse should expect Victoria to display which of the following types of behavior during her manic phase?
a. Exhibitionistic.

b. Domineering.
c. Boastful.
d. Meddlesome.
e. Intolerant.
   1. a and c.
   2. b and d.
   3. All but e.
   4. All the above.

17. Victoria's speech during the manic episode would probably be characterized as:
1. Slow, deliberate, and threatening.
2. Bizarre, unconnected, and unintelligible.
3. Light, humorous, and fanciful.
4. Rapid, rhyming, and circumstantial.

18. The content of Victoria's speech constitutes a response to:
1. Ideas originating in her disordered thought processes.
2. Stimuli received from her external environment.
3. Stimuli below the threshold of awareness of others.
4. Others' expectations regarding her behavior.

19. During her first few days in the hospital Victoria frequently addressed the nurse with "You Bitch!" At this point the nurse should deal with Victoria's inappropriate language by:
1. Ignoring it.
2. Interpreting it.
3. Forbidding it.
4. Returning it.

20. One day the nurse overheard Victoria say to a patient whose physician had refused his request for a home visit, "Forget about it. He doesn't control the passes, anyway. I have the last word in these matters." Victoria's statement should be interpreted as being indicative of her.
1. Disregard for the truth.
2. Inability to recognize authority.
3. Delusion of grandeur.
4. Sympathy for the underdog.

21. Chlorpromazine was ordered for Victoria for the purpose of:
1. Inducing a deep, dreamless, persistent sleep.
2. Minimizing agitation, anxiety, tension, and confusion.
3. Decreasing the force of skeletal muscle contraction.
4. Preventing the occurrence of grand mal convulsions.

22. Victoria should be observed carefully for which of the following as undesirable side effects of chlorpromazine?
   a. Drowsiness.
   b. Dry mouth.
   c. Hypotension.
   d. Dermatitis.
   e. Ataxia.
      1. a and b.
      2. c and d.
      3. All but e.
      4. All the above.

23. Frequent side effects of the lithium carbonate ordered to control Victoria's mania are:
   a. Tremor.
   b. Anorexia.
   c. Nephrotoxicity.
   d. Diarrhea.
   e. Ataxia.
      1. a and c.
      2. b, c, and d.
      3. All but e.
      4. All the above.

24. The toxic effects of lithium carbonate would be most apt to appear if the blood level of the drug were to exceed:
      1. 0.08–.12 mEq. per liter.
      2. 0.8–1.2 mEq. per liter.
      3. 8.0–12.0 mEq. per liter.
      4. 80–120 mEq. per liter.

The delirious stage of Victoria's mania subsided after three days in the hospital. The physician reduced the lithium carbonate to 300 mg. t.i.d. and discontinued the Thorazine 50 mg. orally q.i.d. Shortly thereafter the psychiatrist initiated brief psychotherapeutic interviews in an effort to establish rapport and emotional involvement. Victoria responded by becoming extremely dependent on the psychiatrist, to the point that she attempted to manipulate him into making even the smallest decisions for her.

When Victoria was permitted to associate with other patients she showed an inclination to supervise their activities and to establish her superiority by promising them gifts and privileges which she was not able to confer. The other patients were both amused and irritated by Victoria and occasionally entertained themselves by encouraging her to engage in mischievous and inappropriate behavior. The principal problems in Victoria's nursing care continued to be protecting her from irritating others and from being irritated by them, and dealing with her voracious appetite for food and drink.

25. Rapport can be most accurately defined as:
   1. Mutually advantageous give and take between participants in a meaningful relationship.
   2. Unqualified acceptance of the ideas and attitudes of an unfamiliar person.
   3. Willing submergence of one's own needs to the preferences of another person.
   4. Loss of one's own individuality through conscious identification with another.

26. It would be helpful for the nurse to have knowledge of Victoria's premorbid personality in order to:
   1. Anticipate her probable reaction to various hospital events and experiences.
   2. Predict the degree of recovery she can be expected to make.
   3. Regulate the hospital situation so as to frustrate her undesirable behavior.
   4. Structure her hospital environment to ensure maximal permissiveness.

27. In general, Victoria's nursing care during her manic phase should be directed toward:
   a. Protecting her from injury from her environment.
   b. Controlling and directing her excess energy.
   c. Providing for satisfaction of her physical needs.
   d. Decreasing the number of stimuli impinging upon her.
   e. Manifesting reliability, acceptance, and firmness.
      1. a and c.
      2. b and d.
      3. All but e.
      4. All the above.

28. During her acute manic phase Victoria would require protection against:
   a. Inflicting physical injury on herself.
   b. Performing socially indiscreet acts.
   c. Giving away all her possessions.
   d. Eliciting the wrath of other patients.
      1. a and b.
      2. c and d.

3. All but d.

4. All the above.

29. As Victoria's acute manic phase subsided, she began to give away her furniture, car, and other property. Would a bill of sale or deed signed by Victoria while she was hospitalized be considered a legal document?

    1. No, because she is a woman and can't sell property.

    2. No, because she is being treated in a mental hospital.

    3. Yes, because she still has all her civil rights.

    4. Yes, because no one can be stopped from selling property.

30. According to the law in some countries, patients can be committed to a hospital if:

    a. They have been proven to be dangerous to self or others.

    b. They are unable to care for themselves at home.

    c. Inpatient treatment is more beneficial than outpatient treatment.

    d. They are unable to differentiate time, person and place.

    e. They consistently perform antisocial acts in public.

        1. a only.

        2. a and d.

        3. a, b, and c.

        4. All the above.

31. In order to convince Victoria that she will not be able to manipulate the hospital personnel as she has others, the psychiatrist and the nurse should:

    1. Carefully explain how their relationship with her will differ from her superficial interactions of the past.

    2. Give her a short clear definition of the limits that will be set on her behavior.

    3. Outline the consequences of any attempt on her part to manipulate or exploit them.

    4. Acquaint her with the complete health history they have obtained from her husband.

32. At 1:00 A.M. one night during her second week of hospitalization Victoria rushed up to the nurses' station and demanded that her therapist come to the ward immediately to write an order giving her a pass. Which should be the first response by the nurse?

    1. "Okay, Victoria, go to the dayroom and wait. I'll call him immediately."

    2. "Victoria, you are just being difficult. You know that I cannot do that.

    3. "Your request is unreasonable and I will not call your doctor now."

    4. "You must be very upset to want a pass immediately."

33. Which of the following would be ways in which Victoria's acting out and manipulative behavior could be managed by the nurses on the unit?

    a. Increasing both the thorazine and lithium carbonate dosages.

    b. Responding positively to any mood shift toward depression.

    c. Rejecting her when she disobeys or is loud in public.

    d. Spending extra time with her regardless of her behavior.

    e. Writing out and enforcing limits set on her behavior.

        1. a and b.

        2. a, b, and c.

        3. a, c, and e.

        4. a, d, and e.

34. The chief aim of Victoria's occupational therapy would be to:

    1. Force her to confront and accept reality.

    2. Provide a constructive outlet for her excessive energy.

    3. Teach her social skills required for group living.

    4. Stimulate interest in her physical surroundings.

35. Which of the following activities would be suitable for Victoria's occupational therapy?

    a. Fingerpainting and drawing.

    b. Writing letters and stories.

    c. Tearing rags for rugs.

    d. Playing table tennis.

    e. Engaging in group singing.

        1. a and c.

        2. b and d.

        3. All but e.

        4. All the above.

36. The chief difficulty to be encountered in providing Victoria with occupational therapy will probably be her:

    1. Physical weakness.

    2. Easy distractibility.

    3. Fear of others.

    4. Lack of coordination.

37. Victoria had difficulty in sleeping, rarely sleeping longer than two or three hours at a time. In attempting to alleviate Victoria's insomnia, the nurse might:
  a. Give her a hot drink at bedtime.
  b. Encourage her to take a warm bath.
  c. Administer a sedative for sleep.
  d. Provide an evening of quiet activity.
  e. Avoid rewarding awakening with special attention.
    1. a, b, and c.
    2. a, b, and d.
    3. All but e.
    4. All the above.

38. In order to be most therapeutic to Victoria the nurse should attempt to convey which of the following attitudes?
    1. You can depend on me to meet all your needs.
    2. You are both meaningful and important to me.
    3. You can trust me to accept your behavior.
    4. You will not be able to provoke me to anger.

39. In talking to Victoria during her acute phase of mania the nurse should:
    1. Raise her voice pitch and intensity in order to claim Victoria's wandering attention.
    2. Refer chiefly to the feelings conveyed rather than to the verbal content expressed.
    3. Refute or modify any erroneous statements as soon as Victoria expresses them.
    4. Attempt to explore the motivations for behavior by direct questioning.

40. Victoria learned that she could irritate the head nurse by describing her as tomboyish and frequently referred to her in that fashion. What approach to the problem should the head nurse adopt?
    1. Tell Victoria that she is sensitive to reflections concerning her femininity.
    2. Promise to provide extra privileges when Victoria learns to curb her comments.
    3. Recognize that Victoria is mentally ill and that her opinions are not valid.
    4. Remain nonjudgmental and respond without anger or retaliation.

41. In planning her interactions with Victoria the nurse should remember that:

    1. It is not acceptable to have feelings of anger toward dependents.
    2. It is not advisable to express one's feelings of anger.
    3. It is therapeutic to recognize and deal with one's anger.
    4. It is usually impossible to curtail direct expressions of anger.

Although Victoria was able to acquire only limited insight into her feelings and behavior, there was a decrease in her physical activity, speed of talk, and demanding attitude toward others in her environment. Because Victoria had functioned on a high level of efficiency for many years before her acute psychotic episode, the psychiatrist felt that her prognosis for future adjustment was good. Therefore, he discharged her after five weeks of hospitalization, arranged for Victoria and her husband, Henry (age 50), to participate in family therapy on an outpatient basis, and prescribed a maintenance dose of lithium carbonate for Victoria.

During family therapy with the psychiatrist and nurse, the Clappers said that they had had what could be called a companionate marriage. By design, they had no children of their own. Victoria devoted an inordinate amount of time and energy to certain of her public school pupils whom she considered her protégés and to whom she gave special piano and voice lessons. Recently, Henry spent extra time preparing his lectures and setting up the laboratory for the students' experiments.

42. Erikson identified eight stages in the human life cycle. Chronologically, the Clappers are in which one of the following stages?
    1. Identity vs. role confusion.
    2. Intimacy vs. isolation.
    3. Generativity vs. ego stagnation.
    4. Integrity vs. despair.

43. Which of the following are basic emotional tasks for the young adult?
  a. Achieving independence from parental controls.
  b. Establishing intimate relationships outside the family.
  c. Establishing a personal set of values.
  d. Developing a sense of personal identity.
  e. Identifying with a peer group of one's own sex.
    1. a only.

2. a, b, and d.

3. All but e.

4. All the above.

44. Which of the following should be dimensions of Victoria's (age 48) and Henry's (age 50) life in their current phase of psychosocial development?

a. Planning for the future together.

b. Sustaining application of abilities.

c. Investing energy in future generations.

d. Accomplishing routine work of daily life.

e. Engaging in self interests and ideas.

   1. a only.

   2. a, b, and c.

   3. All but e.

   4. All the above.

45. Sheehy identified the prevalent life patterns for men in the middle years. Which of the following would most accurately describe Henry?

1. Transient.

2. Wunderkind.

3. Locked in.

4. Paranurturer.

46. Sheehy identified the prevalent life patterns for women in the middle years. Which of the following would most accurately describe Victoria?

1. Caregiver.

2. Nurturer who defers achievement.

3. Achiever who defers nurturing.

4. Integrator.

47. Which of the following will be the primary determiner of the richness or paucity of Henry Clapper's middle years?

1. His ability to make changes.

2. Victoria's health or illness.

3. Degree of his physical decline.

4. His own view of himself.

48. Problems which the middle-aged Clappers should discuss and work out in family therapy would include their:

a. Reacting to Victoria's hospitalization.

b. Evaluation of a childless marriage.

c. Facing the stigma of mental illness.

d. Growing older without grandchildren.

e. Adjusting to declining physical stamina.

1. a and c.

2. b, c, and d.

3. All but e.

4. All the above.

49. Henry Clapper's response to his wife's illness probably would be influenced most strongly by:

1. His understanding of the nature of his wife's illness.

2. His personal philosophy toward mental illness.

3. His wife's response to her recent mental illness.

4. The type of feelings he has toward his wife.

50. If Victoria is to achieve and maintain mental health, the family therapists will need to assess and help Victoria confront which of the following?

a. Her feelings toward menopause.

b. Her excessive dependency needs.

c. Her manipulative behavior.

d. Her ability to take medications.

e. Henry's reaction to her illness.

   1. a, c, and d.

   2. b, c, and e.

   3. All but d.

   4. All the above.

51. Aguilera and Messick have developed a paradigm for crisis intervention which, if applied in the Clappers' family therapy, might be therapeutic for them. Which of the following techniques are included in this model?

a. Helping the Clappers to gain an intellectual understanding of their problems.

b. Finding and using any situational supports available to Henry and Victoria.

c. Assisting Henry and Victoria to bring feelings out in the open.

d. Exploring Henry's and Victoria's past and present coping patterns.

e. Anticipatory planning for physical, economic, and sexual adjustments of aging.

   1. a, b, and c.

   2. b, c, and e.

   3. All but d.

   4. All the above.

Schizophrenic Reaction

During his early childhood years, Irving Gold's parents had described him as a timid, sensitive boy who had frequent nightmares. Following each bad dream his mother would comfort him, but his father was disappointed by his son's unmanly fearfulness. During adolescence, Irving had been shy in the company of women and had experienced numerous somatic symptoms and acute attacks of guilt as a consequence of his masturbation.

During medical school, Irving was aloof toward his classmates. His mother discouraged him from socializing with other young people by carefully screening his phone calls and by insisting that he study at home rather than at the university library. In spite of his mother's open objections, he married at 30, after a very short courtship.

After he had completed his medical education, his residency, and had undertaken private practice with an older, well-known cardiologist, Dr. Gold accepted an appointment as director of the cardiac physiology laboratory of a private hospital. His research in cardiac physiology was reported widely in the professional literature and won him the admiration of his medical colleagues.

When he was 38 years old, and following the birth of his second child, increasing fear of financial responsibilities caused Dr. Gold to leave his position as a full time hospital medical staff member to enter private practice. At the same time he accepted an appointment as an associate professor of internal medicine at the state university in order to satisfy his teaching interests.

During his first months in private practice Dr. Gold became increasingly agitated and worried about his work. He confided to his wife that he was afraid of being sued for malpractice and doubted his ability to earn enough money to support his growing family. Although he had been an interested and affectionate father toward his older son, he demonstrated marked antipathy toward his newborn son, claiming that the birth of this child had precipitated his present financial problems. At about the same time he expressed fear that his fellow physicians at the university had instigated a plot to discredit his research and deprive him of his faculty position. At his wife's suggestion he consulted a private psychiatrist, to whom he divulged his fear of making a serious diagnostic error and his guilt concerning his inability to be perfectly honest in telling his patients the true nature and significance of their illnesses. He expressed concern, too, about his increasing consumption of alcohol, his insomnia, and his growing discomfort in face-to-face conversations with people.

Finally, Dr. Gold cancelled the appointments of his private patients, failed to appear for his scheduled lectures in the medical school, and spent his time in bed at home, refusing to see anyone but his wife. When he was told that his older son had undergone emergency surgery for acute appendicitis, he evidenced no concern for the child's welfare. His wife called her husband's psychiatrist, who convinced Dr. Gold to enter a private psychiatric hospital for treatment.

On admission to the hospital Dr. Gold was ataxic, uncommunicative, and suspicious. He refused to eat, avoided contact with other patients, and displayed an arrogant, contemptuous, and hostile attitude toward patients and personnel. The psychiatrist made a diagnosis of schizophrenic reaction, paranoid type, and decided to treat Dr. Gold with psychotherapy, family therapy, and trifluoperazine (Stelazine).

(ANSWER BLANK ON PAGE A–135) (CORRECT ANSWERS ON PAGE B–231)

1. According to a widely accepted theory, schizophrenia is caused by:
1. Metabolic imbalances produced by genetic influences of a recessive type.
2. Interaction of a variety of diverse social and biologic factors.
3. Failure of a constitutionally weak personality to mature completely.
4. Establishment of poor habits of thinking and interacting with others.

2. There is some experimental evidence that which of the following hereditary biochemical aberrations predisposes to development of schizophrenia?
1. Inadequate production of messenger RNA.
2. Impaired transmission of glucose across the cell membrane.
3. Episodic overproduction of cholinesterase.
4. Impairment of the noradrenergic reward system.

3. Bateson postulated a theory concerning the etiology of schizophrenia which he called the double-bind theory. Which of the following are terms used by him in relation to this theory?
a. Context – metacontext.
b. Autointoxication syndrome.
c. Disharmonious splitting.
d. Dyssocial patterning.
e. Collective unconscious.
   1. a only.
   2. b and c.
   3. All but e.
   4. All the above.

4. According to Bateson, which of the following causes schizophrenia to develop?
1. Conflict between self-love and other-love in relationships.
2. Discordance between the primary context and metacontext.

3. Dyssocial patterning prominence during late adolescence.
4. Reaction to a severe, universal state of anxiety.

5. Which of the following disturbances in interpersonal relationships most often predisposes to the development of schizophrenia?
1. Faulty family atmosphere and interaction.
2. Absence of a parent of the opposite sex.
3. Extreme competition with authority figures.
4. Lack of participation in peer groups.

6. The communication pattern in Dr. Gold's original family was probably one in which he was frequently:
1. A witness to obscure intellectual debates between his erudite elders.
2. The recipient of much confusing information with multiple or contradictory meanings.
3. The target of much sensual language which engendered sexual fantasies.
4. An observer of confrontations between an aggressive mother and a passive father.

7. Since schizophrenia is a name for a group of reactions and a single etiology has not been found, the nurse in her assessment of schizophrenic patients will observe variety in the:
a. Type of symptoms.
b. Severity of symptoms.
c. Amount of regression.
d. Degree of dependency.
e. Level of intellectual functioning.
   1. a and b.
   2. c, d, and e.
   3. All but e.
   4. All the above.

8. After completion of the nursing assessment of Dr. Gold's needs, the nurses outlined a plan for interacting with him on the unit. Their plan should include which of the following?
  a. Assigning one nurse to develop a therapeutic interpersonal relationship with Dr. Gold.
  b. Structuring the milieu so that Dr. Gold has only minimal interaction with other patients.
  c. Restricting him to the unit for several days until initial assessments are confirmed.
  d. Requesting that Dr. Gold instruct other patients on the unit to address him as "Irv."
  e. Administering his medication with caution, being careful not to overmedicate.
    1. a only.
    2. a, c, and e.
    3. All but d.
    4. All the above.

9. The psychopathology of schizophrenia typically includes:
  a. Regressive withdrawal to infantile behavior of omnipotence and rage.
  b. Loss of ego strength with consequent inability to perceive reality.
  c. Impaired sense of identity together with confusion of the sexual role.
  d. Lack of ability to discriminate between fantasy and reality.
  e. Progressive deterioration of the processes of interpersonal communication.
    1. a and b.
    2. c and d.
    3. All but e.
    4. All the above.

10. Which of the following best summarizes the functions of the ego?
  1. Supplementation.
  2. Compromise.
  3. Analysis.
  4. Synthesis.

11. In order for the child to develop a healthy ego, he must:
  a. Relinquish his early infantile expectations of magical wish fulfillment.
  b. Establish firm boundaries between his mother and his "self."
  c. Interrelate with warmly affectionate parental and sibling figures.
  d. Find free expression of his physical and emotional drives.
  e. Express only the positive aspect of conflicting instincts.
    1. a and b.
    2. a, b, and c.
    3. All but e.
    4. All the above.

12. In order for Dr. Gold to respond to family therapy, his ego must be strong enough to:
  a. Postpone gratification.
  b. Identify with the therapists.
  c. Integrate interpretations.
  d. Control regression.
  e. Verbalize feelings.
    1. b and d.
    2. a, b, and c.
    3. All but e.
    4. All the above.

13. Which of the following is most apt to induce regression of the ego to a fantasied union between the self and the mother.
  1. Wish frustration.
  2. Overgratification.
  3. Harsh discipline.
  4. Rigid control.

14. In modifying Freud's theories concerning ego functioning, Hartmann suggested that:
  1. The ego is continuously redefined through successful interpersonal relationships.
  2. The ego arises through internalization of parental and social standards.
  3. Not all areas of ego functioning develop through resolution of conflict.
  4. The ego consists of a perceptive distillate of instinctual experiences.

15. According to Erikson, the child's first social achievement should be to:
  1. Smile when his mother and father talk to him or stroke his face and lips.
  2. Trust his mother to meet his needs for nutrition, affection, and protection.
  3. Deposit his urinary and fecal excretions in an appropriate container.
  4. Utter vocal sounds to express sensations of physical and emotional pleasure and pain.

16. Which of the following were responsible for Dr. Gold's schizophrenic behavior?
  a. His inability to avoid or cope with conflict and anxiety.
  b. A defensive regression to the narcissistic level of functioning.

c. Disruption of his relationships with persons in his environment.
d. Flooding of his repressed instinctual impulse into consciousness.
e. Attempts to minimize anxiety through wish-fulfilling fantasies.
   1. a only.
   2. b and d.
   3. All but e.
   4. All the above.

In a family therapy session Dr. Gold's wife said that, prior to the birth of their second child, she was indulgent of her husband's moods and devoted much of her time to meeting his needs. Recently she hadn't had the energy or interest to be indulgent toward him. Also, she had begun to think that her husband hadn't achieved the financial or social level that she had expected him to.

Dr. Gold explained that his need to be more productive conflicted with his feeling that he should spend more time at home. Finally, he didn't know what to do.

17. The stresses which caused the breakdown of Dr. Gold's defenses and led to his schizophrenic reaction were produced by:
a. Birth of his second child.
b. Establishing a private medical practice.
c. Relinquishing his research position.
d. Assuming a university teaching post.
e. Increasing dependence upon his wife.
   1. a, b, and d.
   2. a, c, and e.
   3. All but e.
   4. All the above.

18. Goals of family therapy for Dr. Gold and his family should include which of the following?
1. Finding a different family scapegoat.
2. Reinforcing the family's double bind.
3. Correcting distorted perceptions of needs.
4. Role playing deviant behavior patterns.

19. Dr. Gold's withdrawal from reality was an attempt to:
1. Avoid stimulation of his exaggerated sexual and aggressive impulses.
2. Relieve discomfort by seeking security in a subjective world.
3. Provide uninterrupted periods of time for critical thinking.

4. Protect himself from continuous competitive striving for superiority.

20. Dr. Gold's withdrawal probably resulted from his:
1. Overconcern with his physical and psychological discomforts.
2. Excessively demanding professional and family responsibilities.
3. Inability to invest in enduring emotional attachments.
4. Lack of attractive personality and character traits.

21. Regression can be most accurately defined as:
1. Resumption of behavior typical of an earlier level of development.
2. Banishment of unacceptable wishes or ideas from conscious awareness.
3. Unconscious symbolic efforts to eradicate a previous painful experience.
4. Turning of interests inward to total preoccupation with the self.

22. Dr. Gold displayed which of the following typical features of schizophrenia?
a. Denial of external reality.
b. Overinvestment of interest in himself.
c. Substitution of fantasy for reality.
d. Blunting and distortion of affect.
e. Disturbances in thinking processes.
   1. a and c.
   2. b and d.
   3. All but e.
   4. All the above.

23. Denial can best be understood as:
1. Unconscious refusal to recognize unwelcome thoughts and wishes.
2. Keeping one trait unconscious by conscious expression of its opposite.
3. An action designed to atone for an unacceptable act or impulse.
4. Offering justification for one's undesirable or unacceptable behavior.

24. The defense mechanism of projection consists of:
1. Shifting one's emotion to a less dangerous object than that engendering it.
2. Transferring one's unacceptable impulses and thoughts to others in the environment.
3. Remembering a painful incident without recognition of the feelings provoked by it.
4. Making up for inadequacy in one personality area by overemphasis on another.

25. In order for Dr. Gold to attribute his hostilities and fears to his medical colleagues, he must first employ:
1. Denial.
2. Suppression.
3. Sublimation.
4. Identification.

26. Dr. Gold's tendency to distort personal experience can be expected to result in:
a. Flatness of affective tone.
b. Decrease of repressed instincts.
c. Disharmony in thought and feeling.
d. Ease in social interaction.
    1. a and c.
    2. b and d.
    3. All but d.
    4. All the above.

27. Dr. Gold's retreat to his bed and his lack of concern for his son's illness can be interpreted as resulting from his increasing:
1. Masochism.
2. Rationalization.
3. Hypochondriasis.
4. Narcissism.

28. Dr. Gold's delusions and hallucinations serve the functions of:
a. Fulfilling unacceptable wishes.
b. Preventing overt depression.
c. Externalizing overwhelming guilt.
d. Reducing anxiety and fear.
e. Simulating interpersonal contacts.
    1. a and b.
    2. c and d.
    3. a, c, and d.
    4. All the above.

29. Dr. Gold's use of delusional thinking signifies that he is:
1. Eager to excuse his behavior to friends and relatives.
2. Aware of his unusual vulnerability to external attack.
3. Unable to differentiate between thoughts and external reality.
4. Unusually perceptive of the feelings and intentions of others.

30. Dr. Gold's delusions of persecution constituted:
1. Satisfaction of his conscious needs for humiliation and punishment.
2. Compensatory efforts to reduce internal threats to personal integrity.
3. Unconscious identification with the martyred others of his ethnic group.
4. Thinly disguised jealousy of the work of his medical colleagues.

31. The phenothiazine tranquilizers are extremely effective psychotropic agents which influence the central and autonomic nervous systems and the endocrine system. These effects are thought to occur by:
a. Blockade of adrenergic (epinephrine) synapses.
b. Stimulation of extrapyramidal nerve tracts.
c. Direct action of the hypothalamic nuclei.
d. Weak blockade of peripheral cholinergic nerves.
e. Stimulation of the chemoemetic center in the medulla.
    1. a and b.
    2. a, b, and d.
    3. All but e.
    4. All the above.

32. The nurse should give Dr. Gold and his wife precautionary information about the effects of Stelazine. Which of the following statements reflects accurate teaching for a person receiving phenothiazines?
1. "You may experience increased libido."
2. "Your blood pressure will increase."
3. "You should not drive an automobile."
4. "Your drug is an experimental drug."

33. Benztropine mesylate (Cogentin) might be administered to Dr. Gold to treat a specific side effect of trifluoperazine (Stelazine). If used for such purpose, Cogentin would be given to:
1. Stimulate cerebral cortical, glial cells.
2. Counteract extrapyramidal, pseudo-parkinsonism symptoms.
3. Stimulate smooth muscle of blood vessels.
4. Counteract muscle weakness of the extremities.

34. Dr. Gold's auditory hallucinations result from:
1. A tendency to distrust visual, tactile, and olfactory perceptions.
2. Overinvestment of libidinal energy in the hearing apparatus.
3. Increased hearing acuity developed during medical practice.
4. Inability to distinguish memory traces from current sensory stimuli.

35. Dr. Gold told the nurse that the editorial in the daily newspaper contained a coded message telling him that his cardiac research findings had been discredited by

Russian scientists. This behavior indicates that he was experiencing:

1. Distortion of sensation.
2. Delusions of grandeur.
3. Ideas of reference.
4. Ideas of transference.

36. The nurse should observe Dr. Gold for the expression of feelings of depersonalization, which tend to develop from:

1. Focusing all libidinal energies on objects and persons external to the self.
2. Increasing investment of interest in the self and withdrawal from the world.
3. Decreased acuity of visual, auditory, olfactory, and tactile perception.
4. Retardation of impulse transmission between the voluntary and autonomic nervous systems.

37. The nurse's chief goal in her care of Dr. Gold should be:

1. Interpreting his speech and behavior.
2. Directing his activity on the ward.
3. Anticipating and satisfying his needs.
4. Providing a warm human experience.

38. In order to provide maximal therapeutic advantage for Dr. Gold, the nurse's relationship with him should be one in which:

1. She spends a specified amount of time with him according to a pre-arranged schedule.
2. They meet frequently and spontaneously at different times of day in different types of situations.
3. He can feel free to request her presence in any situation that arouses his anxiety.
4. She initiates conversations with him when she believes that he needs immediate behavioral control.

39. A therapeutic relationship between nurse and patient differs from a social relationship in that the former is characterized by:

1. Reciprocity of need expression and gratification.
2. Satisfaction of the emergent needs of the client.
3. Major personality reconstruction of one participant.
4. Concern with the latent meanings of behavior.

40. Which of the following are characteristics of a therapeutic relationship?

a. One person is responsible for goal direction of the communication.
b. Interaction between the participants is guided by a plan.
c. The counselor recognizes her own needs but concentrates on the patient's needs.
d. Communication results in improvement of the patient's problem-solving ability.
c. The counselor and client examine and modify their behavior as indicated.

   1. a and c.
   2. b and d.
   3. All but e.
   4. All the above.

41. An interview can most accurately be described as:

1. A face-to-face meeting of persons having the object of accomplishing some purpose.
2. An exchange of information between persons for the purpose of establishing or increasing trust.
3. A conversation in which a professional servant accumulates needed information from a client.
4. A communication between non-friends in which the method and content are formally structured.

42. The nurse should understand that her communication with Dr. Gold may be considered successful when:

1. He begins to describe his hallucinations to her.
2. She develops empathy for his thoughts and feelings.
3. He experiences the feeling of being understood.
4. She becomes able to decipher his symbolic speech.

43. Communication can best be understood as:

1. The transmission of ideas from sender to receiver with little or no distortion.
2. Involvement of two or more persons in a reciprocal exchange of information.
3. Establishment of rapport and sympathy between persons through oral or written language.
4. Mutual interchange of ideas in which the opinions of all participants are modified.

44. Involving Dr. Gold in an activity program may be expected to increase his communication abilities through:
1. Improving his action language.
2. Establishing consistent daily routines.
3. Creating insight into his problems.
4. Increasing his contacts with people.

45. During one of the nurse's conversations with him, Dr. Gold lapsed into a lengthy silence, crossed his legs, and swung his foot rapidly back and forth. In order to be most therapeutic at this point the nurse should:
1. Comment that she observes that he seems anxious.
2. Direct his attention to the activities of nearby patients.
3. Switch to a completely different topic of conversation.
4. Touch his knee in a gently restraining fashion.

46. Which of the following actions by the nurse could be expected to prevent effective communication between Dr. Gold and herself?
a. Offering reassurance freely.
b. Initiating changes of subject.
c. Giving her opinion of his situation.
d. Suggesting solutions for his problems.
e. Emphasizing medical or psychiatric terminology.
    1. a and c.
    2. b and d.
    3. All but e.
    4. All the above.

47. In her interactions with Dr. Gold, which of the following actions by the nurse would have therapeutic value for him?
a. Recognizing that his behavior is meaningful.
b. Helping him become more aware of his feelings.
c. Encouraging him to describe significant events in detail.
d. Leading him to clarify and reorganize his experiences.
e. Assisting him to derive sounder conclusions from his observations.
    1. a and b.
    2. c and d.
    3. All but e.
    4. All the above.

48. According to Sullivan, Dr. Gold's anxiety would be:
1. Interpersonally created and interpersonally reduced.
2. Precipitated by identifiable current stressors.
3. Short-lived and completely self-limited.
4. Evoked only by analytic techniques.

49. In describing the pathogenesis of schizophrenia Sullivan theorized that:
1. The individual avoids assumption of unwanted adult responsibilities by adopting irrational, irresponsible behavior.
2. The individual forfeits his independence and forms a symbiotic union with his mother in order to avoid anxiety.
3. The individual labors under such a burden of intrapsychically generated stimuli that his poorly developed ego is overwhelmed.
4. The individual is confronted with psychosocial development tasks which he cannot master and he protectively retreats to fantasy.

50. An increase in the level of Dr. Gold's anxiety during his first few days of hospitalization would render him:
1. More receptive to the hospital staff's direction and control.
2. Intractable to treatment and incapable of communication.
3. Less able to focus attention on the reality of his situation.
4. More insightful concerning his illness and need for care.

51. As the nurse approached Dr. Gold he said, "I don't want to talk today." What response by the nurse would be most appropriate?
1. "You say you don't want to talk?"
2. "Why are you so reluctant to talk?"
3. "There is no need for you to talk."
4. "I'll sit here with you for a while."

52. Which of the following would be the most effective broad question for the nurse to use in initiating conversation with Dr. Gold?
1. "Have you any family here in the city?"
2. "What would you like to talk about today?"

3. "Have you become accustomed to the hospital?"

4. "Are you beginning to feel any better?"

53. During one conversation Dr. Gold said to the nurse, "I'm not going to talk to you about that. How do I know you're not reading a part, too?" Which response by the nurse would be most helpful in clarifying his meaning?

1. "I'm not involved in any plan designed to harm you."

2. "You're wondering whether or not I'm reading a part, too?"

3. "I can't understand you at all when you talk that way."

4. "I'm not sure that I follow what you're trying to tell me."

54. Dr. Gold said to the nurse, "I offended a lot of patients during my last week at the office. Do you think I should try to resume my practice when I get out of here?" Which of the following responses by the nurse would be most helpful?

1. "Do you think that you should resume your practice?"

2. "Tell me more about how you offended your patients."

3. "What might you do other than reenter private practice?"

4. "Yes, I think you will be able to do that."

55. On his 21st day in the hospital Dr. Gold greeted the nurse by announcing loudly, "I just found out that my wife has rented my office!" Which response by the nurse would be most appropriate?

1. "I wonder what reason she might have had for doing that?"

2. "How did you find out that she has rented your office?"

3. "Don't think about that now. It's out of your control."

4. "I see that you are very angry about her doing that."

56. During one of her conversations with Dr. Gold the nurse became acutely uncomfortable and found it necessary to abruptly excuse herself and leave the room. Her behavior probably was motivated by:

1. Intolerance.

2. Anxiety.

3. Identification.

4. Regression.

57. After working with Doctor Gold for two months, the nurse began to think that although she had initially been helpful, her relationship with him had not yielded the fullest possible therapeutic result. Upon recognizing this possibility she should:

a. Review the process recordings of her verbal and nonverbal communications with Dr. Gold.

b. Determine her own and Dr. Gold's patterns of behavior during their contacts.

c. Identify her own feelings toward Dr. Gold as a consequence of their interaction.

d. Seek guidance from a nurse specialist or psychiatrist regarding the relationship.

e. Formulate a new or reaffirm her original approach to Dr. Gold as indicated.

1. a and b.

2. c and d.

3. All but d.

4. All the above.

58. The nurse recognized that Dr. Gold's prognosis was more favorable than that of many patients diagnosed as having schizophrenia because:

a. His illness had a sudden onset with obvious precipitating factors.

b. He had no previous history of schizophrenic attacks.

c. His symptoms had been present for a short period of time.

d. He had a job to return to after discharge.

e. He had a family that was willing to help him.

1. a and c.

2. b and d.

3. All but d.

4. All the above.

59. The usual "institutionalized" schizophrenic patients differ from Dr. Gold in that they typically:

a. Have a history of previous hospitalization.

b. Are of a lower socioeconomic class.

c. Have a family history of mental illness.

d. Have symptoms obvious for years.

e. Have a lower intelligence quotient.

1. a and c.

2. a, c, and d.

3. All but e.

4. All the above.

60. In preparing Dr. Gold for hospital discharge it would be particularly important that the nurse structure her interactions with him to provide:

1. Advice concerning typical postdischarge problems and their solution.
2. Instruction regarding proper dosage of his prescribed medications.
3. Opportunity for gradual termination of their relationship.
4. Approbation of his efforts to achieve health and maturity.

61. The nurse should anticipate that during the termination of her relationship with Doctor Gold, he will manifest:

1. Euphoria.
2. Relief.
3. Indifference.
4. Anger.

62. The nurse should begin the process of terminating her relationship with Dr. Gold when:

1. She initiates her treatment relationship with him.
2. Dr. Gold begins to arouse negative feelings in her.
3. She determines that Dr. Gold thinks of her as a mother.

4. Dr. Gold asks to terminate the relationship.

63. Ideally, Dr. Gold's outpatient psychotherapy should be terminated when:

a. His major conflicts have been identified, interpreted, and worked through.
b. His nonadaptive ego defenses have been explored and abandoned.
c. His capacity for love and work operate under healthy ego control.
d. His transferences have been therapeutically utilized and their intensities attenuated.
e. He feels he is no longer deriving benefit from psychotherapy.

   1. a, b, and c.
   2. a, c, and d.
   3. All but e.
   4. All the above.

After 10 weeks of hospitalization Dr. Gold was discharged as improved. He was no longer delusional but still experienced difficulty in communicating with others. Plans were made for him to continue supportive psychotherapy on an out-patient basis.

Adolescent Adjustment Reaction

Ben Sturmer, a 17-year-old high school senior, became so preoccupied, confused, and unkempt when his parents left town for a month's vacation that his uncle hastily admitted him to a private psychiatric hospital. The uncle told the psychiatrist that Ben, the oldest of three boys, had been a model son and a good student until the beginning of his senior year, when he began to cut classes, fail courses, and openly defy his father's rules against smoking, drinking, swearing, and drug abuse. Ben admitted to his father that he frequently used marijuana and occasionally took amphetamines.

In his initial interviews with the psychiatrist Ben revealed extreme antagonism toward his father's impossibly high expectations for his sons' behavior and achievement. Ben also indicated that for a short time he had enjoyed being a part of a neighborhood gang, occasionally engaging in minor delinquent acts, but close contact with these boys had provoked frightening sexual thoughts which made him feel sinful. He had, therefore, fled the company of boys and had become fanatically religious, denying him-

self physical pleasure and devoting his time to charitable activities. He began to date a minister's daughter, a college senior, and they talked of preparing themselves to become missionaries.

The psychiatrist diagnosed Ben's illness as an adolescent adjustment reaction and believed that it had been precipitated when his parents left town with their two younger sons, producing a marked increase in Ben's anxiety.

Ben was given a series of projective personality tests, which ruled out an underlying schizophrenic process. Ben was placed on a psychiatric ward with other adolescents and adults. The psychiatrist ordered that Ben participate in the hospital's adolescent program, which included structured time for school, recreational activity, therapeutic interviews, and free time for the pursuit of his own interests.

Ben's parents and two brothers were asked to participate in several family conferences. During these sessions the therapists attempted to assess the family interaction patterns and to increase interactions between Ben and members of his family.

(ANSWER BLANK ON PAGE A–137) (CORRECT ANSWERS ON PAGE B–235)

---

1. Adolescence can best be understood as that stage of life characterized by:
1. The highest possible development of the individual's physical, mental, and spiritual capabilities.
2. Personality reorganization that affords constructive adult resolution of the conflicts precipitated by puberty.
3. Final relinquishing of feelings, interests, and defenses experienced during childhood.
4. The adoption of a totally new and socially oriented system of interests and values.

2. Puberty can most accurately be defined as that period of life which is characterized by:
1. Occurrence of sexual maturity and appearance of secondary sex characteristics.
2. Substitution of adult interests and value systems for childhood interests.

3. The most rapid rate of physical and mental growth and development.
4. The awakening of sexual feelings and the initiation of sexual experience.

3. The several rapid physical changes occurring at puberty produce significant changes in the individual's:
a. Body image.
b. Self-concept.
c. Sexual role.
d. Social status.
   1. a and c.
   2. b and d.
   3. All but d.
   4. All the above.

4. During puberty, rapid physical changes and consequent psychological and social discomfort tend to produce:
1. Conscious death wishes.
2. Relaxed superego control.
3. Increased reality testing.
4. Decreased ego strength.

5. The tasks that Ben should complete during the adolescent or young adulthood period include:

  a. Emancipation from domination by his parents.

  b. Achievement of personal individuality and independence.

  c. Development of interest in the opposite sex.

  d. Attainment of defenses adequate to control his impulses.

  e. Selection of an occupation suited to his interests and abilities.

    1. a and c.
    2. b and d.
    3. a, c, and e.
    4. All the above.

6. According to Freudian theory, one of the major tasks in the adolescent period is to:

    1. Establish oneself as a member of a peer group outside the home.
    2. Compete successfully for the affections of the parent of the opposite sex.
    3. Direct one's sexual drives toward a love object outside of the family.
    4. Build up libidinal energy and focus it on the erotogenic zones.

7. According to Freud's theory of psychosexual development, there is in adolescence a reactivation of conflicts carried over from which of the following periods of development?

    1. Oral.
    2. Anal.
    3. Oedipal.
    4. Latency.

8. The emotionally healthy individual demonstrates the:

  a. Ability to translate insight into action.

  b. Ability to cope with frustration and anxiety.

  c. Capacity for facing conflicts in life.

  d. Feeling of inner coherence and continuity.

  e. Ability to maintain and to lose control.

    1. a, b, and c.
    2. a, b, and d.
    3. All but e.
    4. All the above.

9. Which of the following would be considered abnormal behavior for an adolescent boy?

    1. Inconsistent attitudes.
    2. Emotional equilibrium.
    3. Extreme anger.
    4. Intense involvements.

10. In an adolescent it is difficult to differentiate between a temporary upset and a frank neurosis or psychosis, because the adolescent:

    1. Normally manifests behavior which resembles that seen in major forms of mental illness.
    2. Tends to conceal his feelings behind a facade of superficiality and superiority.
    3. Lacks the ability and the inclination to communicate his problems to others.
    4. Has not achieved sufficient personality differentiation to permit analysis.

11. Which defense mechanisms did Ben use to protect himself against frightening sexual impulses?

  a. Withdrawal.

  b. Denial.

  c. Intellectualization.

  d. Conversion.

  e. Regression.

    1. a and c.
    2. b and d.
    3. All but d.
    4. All the above.

12. Ben utilized the aforementioned defenses chiefly to protect himself from:

    1. Overwhelming dependency needs.
    2. Unmanageable hostile urges.
    3. Frightening sexual impulses.
    4. Subconscious death wishes.

13. Which of Ben's actions best exemplifies denial?

    1. Devoting a great deal of energy to church activities.
    2. Cultivation of friendship with the minister's daughter.
    3. Directing himself toward a missionary career.
    4. Decreasing his efforts toward scholastic goals.

14. Intellectualization can best be understood as:

    1. Concentration of psychic energy in scholarly rather than physical pursuits.
    2. Avoidance of affective experiences through superficial talk about how one might feel.

3. The conscious justification for thoughts and behavior having unconscious motivation.
4. Transference of emotion to a less dangerous object than that engendering it.

15. Which of Ben's actions best exemplifies his regression?
1. His failure to dress and groom himself appropriately.
2. His inability to maintain satisfactory scholastic achievement.
3. His homosexual thoughts concerning boys of his own age.
4. His exaggerated interest in religion and altruistic activities.

16. Ben's efforts to deny himself pleasurable experiences is referred to as:
1. Sublimation.
2. Undoing.
3. Reaction formation.
4. Asceticism.

17. Ben's flight into religion represented:
1. Adoption of the value system of his parents.
2. An attempt to control his sexual impulses.
3. The idealism characteristic of the adolescent.
4. A need for companionship with morally strong people.

18. Some degree of which of the following could be considered normal behavior in a boy of Ben's age?
a. Homosexuality.
b. Hypochondriasis.
c. Exhibitionism.
d. Aggression.
e. Masturbation.
   1. a, b, and e.
   2. b, c, and d.
   3. All but e.
   4. All the above.

19. Ben's feelings of ambivalence are apt to be most pronounced in reference to:
1. Love and hate.
2. Goodness and badness.
3. Dependence and independence.
4. Truth and falsehood.

20. According to Erikson the major task to be accomplished during adolescence is the:
1. Formation of heterosexual interests.
2. Establishment of ego identity.
3. Selection of an adult occupation.
4. Final refinement of the superego.

21. The sense of ego identity to which Erikson refers can most accurately be described as:
1. The adoption of ideas, ideals, and values held by one's parents and peers.
2. Confidence that one's inner self-definition matches the meaning one has to others.
3. The ability to pursue goals to which the majority of one's group does not subscribe.
4. The acceptance of one's feelings, thoughts, and way of life as being right and inevitable.

22. Erikson believes that there is some danger during adolescence of "identity diffusion," which is:
1. The tendency to follow the example of others rather than to make one's own decisions.
2. The attempt to efface one's individuality and to become as unobtrusive as possible.
3. The feeling that one has not firmly established the kind of person one is.
4. The development of interest and skill in a wide variety of different activities.

23. Ben's rebellion against his father's ban on smoking, drinking, profanity and drug abuse can best be understood as:
1. A test of his father's conviction that the rules had real importance.
2. An effort to devalue his father's strength and masculinity in his mother's eyes.
3. An attempt to overthrow his infantile superego and submission to peer pressure.
4. An attempt to punish his parents for the suffering he is experiencing.

24. Ben's smoking, drinking, swearing, drug abuse, delinquency, and later extreme self-denial were all efforts to:
1. Establish independence from his parents.
2. Manage his heightened aggressive drives.
3. Demonstrate his completely adult status.
4. Identify with strong parent surrogates.

25. Ben's anger derived both from the normal adolescent increase in aggressive drives and from:

1. Weakening of his infantile superego.
2. Rejection by both his parents.
3. Inability to express his new feelings.
4. Insecurity regarding his future.

26. By turning his back on his peer group of adolescent boys, Ben denied himself a valuable opportunity for:

1. Safe experimentation with a variety of social roles.
2. Sharing vicariously in the experiences of others.
3. The selection and refinement of social skills.
4. Developing facility in verbal and nonverbal communication.

27. Membership in a gang can be advantageous to an adolescent boy by giving him opportunity for:

a. Playing a leadership role in relation to his peers.
b. Experience in following the leadership of various age-mates.
c. Re-enactment of the nuclear family struggle outside of the family.
d. Talking out wishes, fears, and problems with an understanding audience.
e. Relating to others as part of a group rather than on a one-to-one basis.
   1. a and b.
   2. c and d.
   3. All but e.
   4. All the above.

28. Membership in a gang is apt to be disadvantageous to an adolescent boy in that he may be encouraged to:

a. Regress to behavior of an earlier level of development.
b. Emulate the antisocial behavior of another group member.
c. Accept a dependent role that prevents emotional growth.
d. Limit his interests to those common only to adolescents.
e. Perpetuate his problems by talking too openly about them.
   1. a and b.
   2. c and d.
   3. a, b, and c.
   4. All the above.

29. The basic plan for Ben's hospital care should include:

a. Consistency in the behavior of all treatment team members.
b. The setting of specific limits for Ben's behavior.
c. Provision of appropriate punishment for infraction of rules.
d. Structuring of activities to include work, study, and play.
   1. a and b.
   2. c and d.
   3. All but d.
   4. All the above.

30. Ideally, Ben's hospital treatment program should for the most part be planned by:

1. Ben himself.
2. Ben's psychiatrist.
3. The nursing personnel.
4. The entire treatment team.

31. It would be particularly helpful for a nursing student or a young graduate to care for Ben because such a person would:

1. Be more inclined than an older person to comprehend and use adolescent slang.
2. Serve as a model of someone who has recently achieved adult identity and status.
3. Be better equipped to understand and to sympathize with his problems.
4. Be less intolerant and judgmental concerning his acting-out or antisocial behavior.

32. Which of the following games would be best suited for Ben during his hospitalization?

1. Bridge.
2. Football.
3. Scrabble.
4. Post office.

33. Which of the following rules should guide the nurse in her conversations with Ben?

a. Discuss subjects in which Ben has demonstrated some interest.
b. Offer examples of effective problem solving from her own adolescent experience.
c. Avoid commenting to him concerning probable meanings of his behavior.
d. Forbid him to use profanity or to discuss his sexual feelings.
e. Prevent him from revealing too much personal information too quickly.
   1. a and c.
   2. b and d.

3. a, c, and e.

4. All the above.

34. One morning during Ben's first week in the hospital the nurse directed him to dress and go to the dining room for breakfast. He spat in her face. Which initial response by the nurse would be most appropriate?

1. "That makes me very angry and I will not tolerate such behavior."

2. "The next time you do that I'm going to put you in seclusion."

3. "Surely you can find a more appropriate way to express yourself."

4. "You must be very angry. I'll sit here while you tell me about it."

35. In order to be most therapeutic the nurse should encourage Ben to manage his anger by:

1. Acting it out.

2. Talking it out.

3. Displacing it.

4. Turning it inward.

36. It is important that Ben perceive the nurse's attitude toward him as being one of:

1. Genuine interest.

2. Selfless devotion.

3. Penetrating curiosity.

4. Spiritual attachment.

37. The nurse's accurate interpretation of Ben's clothing, personal possessions, and room arrangement would constitute her perception of his:

1. Unconscious motivation.

2. Object language.

3. Personality type.

4. Superego strength.

38. The nurse's unique contribution to Ben's care, as compared with the contributions of other team members, would be her ability to:

1. Provide a safe, accepting mother figure whom he can trust and from whom he can expect continuing support.

2. Stimulate him to frequent examination of his behavior and feelings in a variety of daily situations.

3. Elicit his expression of disturbing sexual fantasies engendered by his contacts with patients on the unit.

4. Coordinate, integrate, and evaluate the plans and efforts of the several members of the treatment team.

39. Ben's adjustment to life outside the hospital will be facilitated if:

1. His activities are continuously supervised by authority figures.

2. His community guides rather than labels his behavior.

3. Others make major decisions concerning his welfare.

4. He is steered toward companionships with well-adjusted persons.

40. In discharge planning for Ben the nurse should include which of the following in her assessments?

a. Ben may be the identified patient in a troubled family.

b. Ben will need continual psychotherapy throughout adolescence.

c. The Sturmers would benefit from attendance at community parents' meetings.

d. Ben's problems in adjusting to adolescence were unique.

e. Ben may be devalued by his brothers, who would be apt to view him as weak.

1. a only.

2. a and c.

3. All but e.

4. All the above.

At the end of three weeks of hospitalization, during which he was given supportive psychotherapy, Ben was no longer confused and disorganized. He was therefore discharged. Psychotherapy had been helpful to Ben because he had been able to tolerate a close relationship with an adult male therapist, he had been reassured that his fears of sexuality were typical, and he had experienced a strengthening of his ego.

In the family conferences Ben had been able to ventilate much of his anger toward himself and his father. His parents had been able to re-evaluate dependence-independence in their own marital relationship and to establish reasonable limits and expectations for their son's behavior.

Drug Addiction

Five days prior to hospital admission, 22-year-old Wade Hyskell developed swelling and pain of the inner aspect of the left elbow. Four days later he developed fever, chills, malaise, headache, and diarrhea. Even though he feared police arrest, he allowed his wife to take him to a general hospital.

On admission Mr. Hyskell stated that he had been a heroin addict for the past two years and had supported his increasingly expensive habit (currently $120.00 per day) by playing in a dance band and by stealing. The examining physician noted an enlarged liver, fever, and tender, thickened veins on the dorsum of the left hand and forearm. Mr. Hyskell told the nurse that he was in the habit of taking three "fixes" of heroin a day and that he occasionally smoked a "joint," but that he no longer took amphetamines, to which he had been habituated some years before. He indicated that he had injected his last dose of heroin five hours before admission. The doctor restricted him to the unit and ordered blood, stool, urine, and throat cultures, a complete blood count, bedrest, chest x-rays, and an electrocardiogram.

Six hours after admission Mr. Hyskell complained of rhinorrhea and abdominal cramps and threatened to leave the hospital, saying that the methadone (10 mg. orally q. 12 h.) which the admitting physician had ordered to relieve heroin withdrawal symptoms wouldn't be effective. The following morning he refused breakfast but talked the aide into preparing a snack for him at 10:30 A.M. That same afternoon Mr. Hyskell requested a pass for "personal business reasons." His request was refused and he was advised to remain in the hospital to be treated for possible Type B-viral hepatitis and to talk with the counselor from the local therapeutic community for the treatment of drug addiction. On the following day Mr. Hyskell signed out of the hospital against medical advice saying, "This is something I just have to do."

Six months later, following a severe episode of Type B-viral hepatitis, Mr. Hyskell presented himself to a therapeutic community for treatment of heroin addiction.

(ANSWER BLANK ON PAGE A–139) (CORRECT ANSWERS ON PAGE B–237)

---

1. Which of the following is the best estimate of the number of heroin users in the United States?
1. 20,000.
2. 50,000.
3. 200,000.
4. 500,000.

2. Drug abuse has replaced accidents as the leading cause of death in which of the following age groups?
1. 1 to 14 years.
2. 15 to 34 years.
3. 35 to 54 years.
4. 55 to 74 years.

3. Which of the following is the most common reason underlying drug self-administration?
1. A desire to evade problems and to ease stress.
2. A need to relieve physical pain and discomfort.
3. An attempt to improve performance in motor skills.
4. A wish to be included in one's social group.

4. The danger of drug addiction is greatest among which of the following?
1. Lawyers.
2. Writers.

3. Athletes.

4. Physicians.

5. If Wade had not informed the examining physician of his drug habit, the physician could probably have suspected his addiction on the basis of which physical finding?

1. Lateral nystagmus.

2. Enlarged liver.

3. Venous tattooing.

4. Scleral icterus.

6. Wade's original motives for self-administration of drugs probably included the wish to:

a. Have a new, pleasurable experience.

b. Achieve increased insight.

c. Achieve a sense of belonging.

d. Escape from a threatening situation.

e. Express independence and hostility.

1. a and c.

2. b and d.

3. All but e.

4. All the above.

7. The chief pharmacologic effect of the amphetamines is:

1. Stimulation of the cerebral cortical cells.

2. Potentiation of cholinesterase at the myoneural junction.

3. Depression of the reticular activating system.

4. Neutralization of acetylcholine at nerve endings.

8. Indiscriminate use of amphetamines often develops in an individual who ingests the drug in an effort to:

a. Relieve physical discomfort and pain.

b. Improve performance through prevention of fatigue.

c. Distort visual and auditory sense perceptions.

d. Engender a temporary sense of euphoria.

e. Relieve nervousness, irritability, and insomnia.

1. a and c.

2. b and d.

3. All but d.

4. All the above.

9. In which of the following occupational groups is habituation to amphetamines most common?

1. Obese housewives.

2. Aging secretaries.

3. Reserved teachers.

4. Aggressive salesmen.

10. Which of the following is a slang term frequently applied to methamphetamine hydrochloride (Methedrine) by illegal drug users?

1. "Snow."

2. "Speed."

3. "Hash."

4. "Tea."

11. Marijuana use differs from heroin addiction in that:

1. Marijuana use is accompanied by increasing tolerance to the drug.

2. Marijuana abuse develops in neurotic rather than in psychotic individuals.

3. Dependency on marijuana is psychological rather than physical.

4. Addiction to marijuana can only be broken by gradual withdrawal.

12. Heroin is a member of which of the following drug groups?

1. Barbiturates.

2. Ataractics.

3. Antidepressants.

4. Opiates.

13. Which of the following is a slang term frequently applied to heroin by illegal drug users?

1. "Coke."

2. "Bonita."

3. "Smack."

4. "Hemp."

14. Which of the following addictive drugs exert a depressant effect on the central nervous system?

a. Dilaudid.

b. Meperidine.

c. Pentobarbital.

d. Cocaine.

e. Mescaline.

1. a and b.

2. a, b, and c.

3. c, d, and e.

4. All but e.

5. All the above.

15. Which of the following drugs can produce an hallucinogenic effect?

a. Amphetamine.

b. Phenobarbital.

c. Marijuana.

d. Lysergic acid diethylamide.

e. Heroin.

1. a and b.

2. a, c, and d.

3. All but e.

4. All the above.

16. During his two years of addiction Wade had increased his daily dosage of heroin as a result of:

1. The tendency for a "pusher" to sell increasingly dilute heroin to a customer.
2. Inability of the body to excrete heroin as rapidly as it is absorbed.
3. The tendency to develop increasing tolerance to heroin with continued usage.
4. An exhibitionistic tendency to exceed the drug dosage of addict peers.

17. Which of the following are frequent sequelae of indiscriminate use of opiates?

a. Acute toxic overdosage.
b. Loss of perceptive acuity.
c. Occurrence of withdrawal symptoms.
d. Diminution of productivity.
e. Reduction of intellectual capacity.
    1. a and c.
    2. b and d.
    3. All but e.
    4. All the above.

18. It can be assumed that Wade's heroin addiction has interfered with his welfare by engendering:

a. Preoccupation with drug taking.
b. Personal neglect.
c. Malnutrition.
d. Infections.
e. Economic distress.
    1. a and b.
    2. b and c.
    3. c and d.
    4. All the above.

19. The heroin addict is especially subject to external threat as a result of his vulnerability to:

a. Drug overdosage.
b. Criminal action.
c. Economic exploitation.
d. Social ostracism.
e. Medical neglect.
    1. a and b.
    2. c and d.
    3. a, b, and c.
    4. All the above.

20. Wade is particularly subject to which of the following medical sequelae as a result of his heroin addiction?

a. Skin abscess.
b. Thrombophlebitis.
c. Septicemia.
d. Bacterial endocarditis.
e. Tetanus.
    1. a and b.
    2. a, b, and c.
    3. All but d.
    4. All the above.

21. In addition to rhinorrhea and abdominal cramps, Wade might also have demonstrated which other symptoms of heroin withdrawal?

a. Yawning.
b. Sneezing.
c. Pupillary dilation.
d. Weight loss.
e. Profuse perspiration.
    1. a and b.
    2. c and d.
    3. All but e.
    4. All the above.

22. Wade's withdrawal or abstinence symptoms will probably reach their peak in how many hours after his last dose of heroin?

1. 3 to 6 hours.
2. 6 to 12 hours.
3. 12 to 24 hours.
4. 24 to 48 hours.

23. Methadone is useful in treatment of heroin addiction as a result of its tendency to:

1. Increase the electric potential across the myoneural junction.
2. Stimulate repair of the myelin sheath of the central nerve fibers.
3. Correct fluid and electrolyte imbalance in brain tissue.
4. Eliminate drug hunger and block the physiologic effects of heroin.

24. Which of the following is a disadvantage of methadone treatment for chronic heroin dependence?

1. Methadone causes blunting of intellectual functions.
2. Methadone produces many dangerous side effects.
3. Methadone is addicting and addicts dislike its effect on them.
4. Continually increasing doses of methadone are required for control.

25. Methadone treatment for Wade's heroin addiction would be apt to be successful only if:

1. He entered the treatment program voluntarily.
2. His dosage of methadone exceeded that of heroin.
3. His dependence on heroin was psychological rather than physical.
4. He remains under the close personal supervision of an ex-addict.

26. In caring for Wade during treatment for heroin withdrawal the nurse should know that which of the following are possible side effects of methadone?
- a. Nausea.
- b. Gingivitis.
- c. Constipation.
- d. Jaundice.
- e. Pruritus.
    1. a and b.
    2. b and c.
    3. a, b, and c.
    4. All the above.

27. In addition to methadone, which of the following drugs has been successful in treating some heroin addicts?
1. Naloxone.
2. Antabuse.
3. Paraldehyde.
4. Reserpine.

28. Which single factor would have the greatest influence on the success or failure of Wade's treatment program?
1. His nurse's attitudes toward drug addicts.
2. The drugs prescribed by his physician.
3. Wade's wife's understanding of his problems.
4. Wade's desire to change his habits.

29. The chief aim for Wade's psychotherapeutic program would be to:
1. Prevent his injection of heroin.
2. Increase his economic productivity.
3. Alter his response to stress.
4. Reshape and strengthen his super-ego.

30. Which of the following aspects of his rehabilitation program would be apt to be most difficult for Wade?
1. Alleviating his symptoms of drug withdrawal.
2. Finding an economically satisfying job.
3. Eliminating his psychic dependence on heroin.
4. Re-establishing his family and community relationships.

31. Major aspects of Wade's physical care as provided by the nurse should include:
- a. Nutritious food and fluid intake.
- b. Restriction to the unit.
- c. No telephone calls.
- d. Warm moist arm packs.
- e. Continuing observation.
    1. a and b.
    2. a, b, and c.
    3. All but d.
    4. All the above.

32. The nurse may assume that Wade will have experienced which of the following feelings in conjunction with his role as an addict?
- a. Anxiety.
- b. Loneliness.
- c. Hopelessness.
- d. Depression.
- e. Anger.
    1. a and c.
    2. b and d.
    3. All but d.
    4. All the above.

33. The nurse may expect that, as a result of his underlying personality characteristics, Wade will establish with her a relationship characterized on his part by:
1. Clinging dependence.
2. Approach-avoidance.
3. Concealed manipulation.
4. Passive aggression.

34. A nursing approach which would be most therapeutic in dealing with Wade would be one in which Wade could perceive the nurse as:
1. Permissive.
2. Protective.
3. Controlling.
4. Straightforward.

35. Since he is apt to have difficulty with male-female relationships, therapeutic nursing interventions for Wade might be hampered, since he would tend to view the nurse as which of the following?
- a. Sexual object.
- b. Seductive peer.
- c. Mother figure.
- d. Father figure.
- e. Intellectual superior.
    1. a only.
    2. a and c.
    3. All but e.
    4. All the above.

36. As the nurse makes her assessment of Wade, she should recognize that Wade, as a drug abuser, differs from a typical teenage drug user in which of the following ways?
1. Physiologically he can no longer increase his heroin tolerance.
2. He can never recover his extreme socioeconomic loss.
3. His addiction has severely isolated him from his peer group.
4. His self-identity is secure in that he no longer is an adolescent.

37. From what is known of the psychodynamics of addiction the nurse should reason that Wade would probably derive greatest psychic satisfaction from which of the following activities?
  1. Discussing theater.
  2. Playing chess.
  3. Collecting coins.
  4. Smoking a pipe.

38. The initial objective of a therapeutic community in rehabilitating the drug addict is to provide:
  1. Stimulation for the addict to examine the developmental causes for his abuse of drugs.
  2. Occupational, educational, and recreational activities to consume his waking hours.
  3. Steady, direct confrontation of the addict with the nature and consequences of his current behavior.
  4. Alteration of the addict's self-image through changes in his social contacts and activities of daily living.

39. In order to fulfill her role in the primary prevention of drug abuse, the nurse should realize that:
  a. In settings where a particular drug is socially acceptable, moderate use tends to be widespread.
  b. When large numbers of persons use a drug, a significant increase in drug dependence occurs.
  c. The sensational manner in which news of drug users is publicized stimulates drug experimentation.
  d. Deviant use of drugs tends to be associated with conditions of rapid socioeconomic change.
  e. Deviant use of drugs may reflect a weakening of cultural controls and changing mores.
      1. a and b.
      2. a, b, and c.
      3. All but e.
      4. All the above.

40. The community mental health nurse can help to reduce the incidence of drug dependence by taking which of the following actions?
  a. Establishing and justifying the credibility of her own opinions concerning the dangers of drug abuse.
  b. Helping to deglamorize drugs and to nullify the status given addicts in some communities.
  c. Supporting academic organizations addressing themselves to the dangers of frequently abused drugs.
  d. Legislating and educating for improved distribution control of potentially addicting drugs.
  e. Promoting development and viability of groups which provide alternatives to preoccupation with drugs.
      1. a and c.
      2. b and d.
      3. All but d.
      4. All the above.

Alcoholism

William Peabody was 42 years old but everyone called him "Billy." The only son and youngest child of a wealthy small town lumberman, he had studied business administration in college and had returned to his home town, married the banker's daughter, and taken a job as agent in a real estate firm. Mr. Peabody was tall, slender, and good looking. He talked a lot, and engagingly, of his philosophy, feelings, and plans to anyone who would listen.

Mr. Peabody first drank alcohol in his parents' home and continued to drink both in college and during his army service in Europe. Following the war his consumption of alcohol increased as he struggled to support his growing family. Although his wife objected to his drinking, she made excuses for him when drunkenness kept him from business appointments. Finally Mr. Peabody disgraced himself and his firm with a display of intoxication, profanity, and belligerence in a contract closure meeting and was fired. His humiliation and remorse led to a week-long bout of heavy and continuous drinking in a nearby town. At the end of this spree he wrecked his car and was arrested for drunken driving, vagrancy, and creating a public disturbance.

During hospitalization for possible head injuries following his accident, Mr. Peabody developed delirium tremens, for which he was treated with sedatives, tranquilizers, and vitamins. When he returned to his home his wife and teen-age children urged him to join Alcoholics Anonymous. A member of that organization came to the home to explain their program to Mr. Peabody, but he refused to participate. A year later, after a series of short term jobs and long term binges, Mr. Peabody recognized his inability to manage his problems alone and sought help from a community mental health center.

In his initial screening interview with the psychiatrist Mr. Peabody revealed strong feelings of guilt and remorse concerning his drinking, resentment toward his strong and capable wife on whom he was dependent, ambivalence toward his domineering mother on whom he was still emotionally dependent, and fear of his successful and distant father. It was decided that Mr. Peabody would be accepted into the center's alcoholic treatment program and be treated in group psychotherapy. The psychiatrist ordered that Mr. Peabody take chlordiazepoxide hydrochloride (Librium), vitamin B complex, and a high caloric diet at home.

(ANSWER BLANK ON PAGE A–141) (CORRECT ANSWERS ON PAGE B–240)

---

1. Addiction is best defined as:
1. The formation of a habit which strengthens through time.
2. The overinvestment of emotion in a pleasurable pursuit.
3. An intense and prolonged desire for something forbidden.
4. A harmful dependence on one or more chemical substances.

2. The principal pharmacologic effect of ethyl alcohol is to:
1. Stimulate the peripheral nervous system.
2. Depress central nervous system functioning.
3. Increase the irritability of muscle fibers.
4. Decrease the motility of the digestive tract.

3. It is likely that Mr. Peabody developed alcoholism while many of his drinking companions did not because he:
1. Experienced drinking as highly pleasurable and his friends did not.
2. Was born with a high tolerance for alcohol and his friends were not.
3. Was unable to metabolize alcohol quickly and his friends were.
4. Was extremely sensitive to others' pain and his friends were not.

4. Tolerance to alcohol consists of:
1. The production of antibodies to combine with and render it inactive.
2. Elimination of alcohol unchanged, without subjecting it to catabolism.
3. A developed ability to endure or resist its more harmful effects.
4. The acquisition of a mental state resistive to depressant effects.

5. Underlying the loneliness and anxiety that led to Mr. Peabody's drinking was excessive:
1. Suspicion.
2. Fear.
3. Indulgence.
4. Frustration.

6. Prodromal symptoms of delirium tremens are:
   a. Apprehensiveness.
   b. Anorexia.
   c. Sweating.
   d. Insomnia.
   e. Tremor.
      1. a and c.
      2. b and e.
      3. All but d.
      4. All the above.

7. Mr. Peabody's delirium tremens could best be described as:
1. A rhythmic tremor of the hands which increases with intentional movement.
2. A fearful, excited state accompanied by thought and perceptual disorders.
3. A generalized shaking of the body most noticeable in the resting state.
4. Gross incoordination and disorganization of body speech and muscle activity.

8. Hallucinations which occur in the alcoholic patient with delirium tremens are typically:
1. Olfactory.
2. Visual.
3. Gustatory.
4. Tactile.

9. The alcoholic individual usually perceives his hallucinations as:
1. Pleasurable.
2. Unreal.
3. Frightening.
4. Ridiculous.

10. The Alcoholics Anonymous organization offers relief from alcoholism through a stepwise program consisting of:
a. Accepting one's powerlessness to manage the use of alcohol.
b. Recognizing the existence of a supernatural power greater than oneself.
c. Making restitution to those one has harmed as a result of drinking.
d. Taking regular inventory of one's motives and actions through meditation.
e. Providing instruction and support for others needing release from alcoholism.
    1. a and b.
    2. c and d.
    3. All but d.
    4. All the above.

11. The consequences of Mr. Peabody's excessive drinking affected the activities of:
a. His family.
b. His employer.
c. His friends.
d. The police.
e. The court.
    1. a, b, and c.
    2. b, c, and e.
    3. All but e.
    4. All the above.

12. Physical changes which typically occur in the chronic alcoholic are:
a. Brain deterioration.
b. Malnutrition.
c. Cirrhosis.
d. Gastritis.
e. Pancreatitis.
    1. a and b.
    2. c and d.
    3. All but e.
    4. All the above.

13. Chronic alcoholism leads in some cases to Korsakoff's psychosis, which is characterized by:
a. Marked irritability.
b. Memory defects.
c. Frequent confabulation.
d. Peripheral neuritis.
    1. a and c.
    2. b and d.
    3. All but d.
    4. All the above.

14. Confabulation can be most accurately defined as:
1. A deliberate attempt to deceive a listener concerning one's feelings, motives, and actions.
2. Filling in memory gaps with detailed but inaccurate accounts of fantasized activities.
3. The unconscious refusal to recognize or accept unwelcome thoughts, wishes, and deeds.
4. The conscious subjugation and control of dangerous impulses, ideas, and feelings.

15. By the time he lost his job, Mr. Peabody had probably developed which of the following behaviors in reference to his alcoholism?
a. Worrying about his drinking problem.
b. Concealing the amount of his drinking.
c. Showing resentment of his wife's criticism.
d. Defending his need to drink excessively.
e. Thinking continuously of drinking.
    1. a and b.
    2. c and d.
    3. All but e.
    4. All the above.

16. Psychodynamically, Mr. Peabody is apt to have a:
1. Strong ego and punitive superego.

2. Weak ego and weak superego.

3. Strong ego and weak superego.

4. Weak ego and harsh superego.

17. Mr. Peabody's sprees were cyclical phenomena produced and perpetuated by:

   a. His scarcity of pleasant memories.

   b. His low tolerance for frustration.

   c. Asocial behavior provoked by drinking.

   d. Remorse felt for his drinking and behavior.

   e. Ability of alcohol to relieve his tensions.

     1. a and c.

     2. b and d.

     3. All but e.

     4. All the above.

18. The community mental health center staff should expect Mr. Peabody to display:

   a. Inability to postpone need gratification.

   b. A charming but superficial sociability.

   c. Feelings of inferiority and unworthiness.

   d. Strong needs for dependence on others.

     1. a and b.

     2. c and d.

     3. All but d.

     4. All the above.

19. The most serious effect of Mr. Peabody's alcoholism was that his:

   1. Wife and children were deprived of the financial support they needed.

   2. Time was largely spent with socially undesirable individuals.

   3. Antisocial behavior when drinking caused embarrassment to his family.

   4. Energies were devoted to drinking rather than to his family and community.

20. The townspeople considered Mr. Peabody's alcoholism to be more disgraceful than his sister's psychomotor epilepsy because:

   1. Alcoholism produces more antisocial behavior.

   2. Alcoholism is more apt to be inherited.

   3. Alcoholism is obviously self-inflicted.

   4. Alcoholism is more destructive of intelligence.

21. Probably alcoholism is a major problem in the United States because:

   a. Most persons are exposed to drinking and can afford to purchase alcohol.

   b. Competitive, highly mobile societies create extreme psychological stress.

   c. Cultural patterns encourage excessive dependence on the maternal figure.

   d. Broad scale advertising programs feature alcohol consumption as being sophisticated.

     1. a only.

     2. b and d.

     3. a, b, and d.

     4. All the above.

22. Rather than a criminal act, alcoholism is currently considered to be:

   1. An ineffectual attempt to adjust to tension created by underlying problems.

   2. A conscious attempt to avoid acceptance of one's social responsibilities.

   3. A mental disease characterized by genetically determined metabolic imbalances.

   4. An acute individual manifestation of a disturbed or imbalanced social order.

23. In constructing a treatment plan for Mr. Peabody the community health center staff would operate on the principle that:

   1. All alcoholics have the same underlying personality structure but differ in their physical response to alcohol.

   2. All alcoholics have similar personality patterns but differ markedly in intelligence, potential, and drive.

   3. All alcoholics have a common problem but differ considerably in their underlying personality patterns.

   4. Alcoholics differ in so many respects that no single treatment method is widely applicable to them.

24. The chief aim of Mr. Peabody's treatment should be to help him to:

   1. Feel completely independent and self-sufficient.

   2. Become dependent on people rather than alcohol.

   3. Give up all alcohol and association with drinkers.

   4. Appreciate the grief he has caused others.

25. It would be unwise for any of the center's staff to adopt an attitude of dictatorial authority toward Mr. Peabody because:

 1. He would interpret such an approach as a slur against his masculinity.

 2. He would be apt to have had experiences rendering him suspicious of authority.

 3. He would then be reluctant to confide his shortcomings to them.

 4. He would then expect cold impartiality rather than support from the staff.

26. In order to be therapeutic in relating to Mr. Peabody the nurse should operate on which of the following premises?

 1. All alcoholics can be cured.

 2. No one drinks without a reason.

 3. Breaking habits requires time.

 4. Alcoholics never keep promises.

27. Mr. Peabody was probably not treated with either sedative or antidepressant drugs because:

 1. Long term malnutrition would render him overreactive to both.

 2. Both would be potentiated by the alcohol remaining in his system.

 3. Transfer of addictions is easily accomplished in the vulnerable person.

 4. Administration of either would jeopardize his impaired motor abilities.

28. In the nurse's first meeting with Mr. Peabody in the center he offered her a cigarette. If the nurse smokes, how should she respond to his gesture?

 1. "No thank you."

 2. "Thanks, I'd like one, but I don't smoke on duty."

 3. "Yes, thank you. Won't you sit down and have one with me?"

 4. "Yes, I'll take one and smoke it later at my desk."

29. Mr. Peabody said to the nurse therapist, "You can't make me stop drinking!" Which response of the nurse reflects the most helpful attitude?

 1. "I know I can't. You have to do it by yourself."

 2. "That's true, but with help you will, won't you?"

 3. "With such an attitude you will never stop drinking."

 4. "What makes you think I want to control your behavior?"

30. Mr. Peabody is more apt to profit from group therapy than from individual therapy because of:

 1. His inability to identify the group with his controlling mother.

 2. The lesser tendency to develop crippling dependence on a group.

 3. The greater challenge in having to relate to a number of people.

 4. The pressure provided by the expression of his current feelings and the counter-feeling of other group members.

31. The basic requirements which must be met in order for a group to function are:

 a. Similar backgrounds.

 b. A common goal.

 c. Small size.

 d. Effective leadership.

 e. Continuous contact.

  1. a and c.

  2. b and d.

  3. All but d.

  4. All the above.

32. The primary goals of group psychotherapy for Mr. Peabody were to improve his:

 a. Level of morale.

 b. Problem solving.

 c. Social poise.

 d. Communication skills.

 e. Frustration tolerance.

  1. a and c.

  2. b, d, and e.

  3. All but e.

  4. All the above.

33. The task of the group is to:

 1. Adapt to the changing needs of its members.

 2. Organize individuals for efficient working.

 3. Conform to the leader's ideals and goals.

 4. Provide for effective transmission of ideas.

34. In group psychotherapy the functions of the therapist include:

 a. Receiving transference from a number of group members.

 b. Absorbing or interpreting the affectionate and hostile expressions of participants.

 c. Entering actively into give and take

discussions between group members.

   d. Monitoring the analysis of members' behavior made by other participants.

   e. Limiting or channeling acting-out behavior of participants.

     1. b and c.

     2. a, d, and e.

     3. All but e.

     4. All the above.

35. In respect to the transference situation, group psychotherapy differs from individual psychotherapy in that, in the group:

   1. Transferences are made only to the primary therapist.

   2. Dependence upon the primary therapist is more pronounced.

   3. The therapist represents an externalized and strict superego.

   4. Transferences are less intense and derive from less early repressions.

36. In contradistinction to individual psychotherapy, group therapy is apt to engender in the participant more feelings of:

   1. Anxiety.

   2. Aggression.

   3. Love.

   4. Guilt.

37. When Mr. Peabody arrived for the second group meeting the nurse therapist noted that he was meticulously dressed and groomed. Her comment to him conveying this observation would be:

   1. Threateningly seductive.

   2. Inappropriate socialization.

   3. Beside the point.

   4. Ego building.

38. In order to be effective leaders in the alcoholic treatment group, the psychologist and the nurse therapist should be able to:

   a. Perceive what the group needs or wants.

   b. Contribute stimuli to move the group toward its goal.

   c. Present ideas in a fashion acceptable to the group.

   d. Evaluate the group's progress and respond accordingly.

   e. Strengthen the group through sensitivity to their needs.

     1. a and c.

     2. b and d.

     3. All but d.

     4. All the above.

39. Leadership responsibilities in the alcoholic treatment group:

   1. Remain at all times with the designated leaders.

   2. Are taken over by the most hostile member.

   3. May shift back and forth among the members.

   4. Need not be fulfilled for successful functioning.

40. In one of the group meetings another member remarked that he had been cured of alcoholism through treatment with tetraethylthiuram disulfiram (Antabuse), the effect of which is to:

   1. Compete with the alcohol molecule for its attachment sites on the nerve cell membrane.

   2. Interfere with the normal metabolic breakdown of alcohol, with accumulation of acetaldehyde.

   3. Counteract the depressant effects of alcohol by directly stimulating nervous tissue.

   4. Destroy the cerebral area in which memories of pleasurable alcoholic experiences are stored.

41. Members of the alcoholic treatment group should come to understand that:

   1. The role of each member should be carefully outlined and closely adhered to.

   2. Each individual has both a right and a responsibility to contribute to the group.

   3. The treatment team will select both problems needing solution and methods of attack.

   4. Each member should concentrate on the realization of his own long term goals.

42. Group cohesiveness is:

   1. The degree to which members resemble each other in experience and ability.

   2. The strength of the external forces which separate the group from society.

   3. The amount of identification which has taken place between the members.

   4. The willingness of members to abandon their individuality and lose their identity.

43. In the working-through phase of the group process it is hoped that the members can see a relationship between their:
1. Unpleasant experiences in early childhood, in late adolescence, and in early adulthood.
2. Deficiency of constructive interactions in the past and their current need for psychotherapy.
3. Behavior within the group and their behavior with significant others outside the group.
4. Attitudes toward giving and taking and their attitudes toward eating and drinking.

44. Communication within groups is impeded by:
a. Excessive levels of anxiety.
b. Feelings of rejection.
c. Feelings of inadequacy.
d. Conforming-submissive members.
e. Hostile-resistive members.
1. a and b.
2. a, b, and c.
3. All but e.
4. All the above.

45. The work of the alcoholic treatment group will be furthered by assumption of which of the following roles by group members?
a. Antagonist.
b. Instrumentalist.
c. Conciliator.
d. Expressivist.
1. a and c.
2. b and c.
3. b and d.
4. All the above.

46. The community mental health nurse would assist patients in the Alcoholic Treatment Program by:
a. Giving instruction in proper nutrition.
b. Assisting in the structuring of leisure activities.
c. Assuring provision of medical care when needed.
d. Participating in individual or group therapy.
e. Working with family, friends, and employer.
1. a and c.
2. b and d.
3. All but e.
4. All the above.

47. The functions of the nurse as a co-therapist in Mr. Peabody's psychotherapy group were probably altered as the:
1. Phases in the group process changed.
2. Mood of the patient group altered.
3. Topics discussed by the group shifted.
4. Membership in the group varied.

48. In working with Mr. Peabody's family the nurse therapist should urge them to:
a. Plan weekends in the country as a departure from former activities.
b. Establish friendships with new people to stimulate additional interests.
c. Request his help in performance of home-centered projects and chores.
d. Involve him in increased interaction with the children.
e. Remove alcohol from the home and avoid any mention of alcohol.
1. a and b.
2. c and d.
3. All but e.
4. All the above.

49. The nurse therapist could be most helpful to Mr. Peabody by:
1. Supporting him in his plans for working out his problems.
2. Advising him concerning methods for avoiding the temptation to drink.
3. Protecting him from disappointment by his family and coworkers.
4. Deterring him from the tendency to indulge in unhealthy thinking.

50. In working with Mr. Peabody's employer, the nurse therapist should urge him to provide Mr. Peabody with:
1. Close and continuous supervision of all of his job functions.
2. Special consideration in regard to work deadlines and hours of duty.
3. A clear job description and regular evaluation of his performance.
4. Payment for services in the form of direct deposits in a bank account.

Mr. Peabody met daily with his treatment group for three weeks, then weekly for a year. During this time his wife and children participated in related family groups. As group cohesiveness and communication skills increased in Mr. Peabody's group, the individual members developed facility in examining their own and others' behavior and motivation. Mr. Peabody felt accepted by the group even though he managed to ventilate considerable anger during group psychotherapy sessions. Throughout the year he maintained sobriety, good physical health, and an acceptable work record. During the following year the nurse therapist maintained contact with Mr. Peabody, his family, and his employer, and he was allowed to return to the community mental health center for assistance and encouragement as needed. It was considered that his alcoholism was well controlled.

Chronic Arteriosclerotic Brain Syndrome

Lydia Lightfoot had been widowed for ten years and lived alone in a small house on the corner of her son's farm. A wiry, energetic 75-year-old lady who enjoyed reading, sewing, entertaining, and housework, Lydia lived comfortably on income from her well chosen investments. Her only complaints were loneliness and occasional morning headache and dizziness.

Knowing that Lydia had had influenza, her granddaughter stopped by to visit one morning. Lydia was wandering aimlessly about the kitchen in her nightgown and greeted her visitor with, "Is that you, George? Is it time to go?" Lydia's granddaughter put her to bed, called the doctor, and stayed with her for the next few days. After a week of bedrest Lydia recovered from her respiratory infection and became oriented to her surroundings, but had difficulty in remembering names, dates, and recent events, and had to grope for once familiar words. She began to disregard her appearance, failing to wash her body and clothing as often as she had been accustomed to doing. She stopped cleaning house, and preferred snacking on cookies, candy, canned milk and cereal to cooking regular meals. Her worried family took her to the doctor, who determined that Lydia's blood pressure was elevated and ordered antihypertensive medications. Lydia forgot to take the drugs, just as she frequently forgot to eat.

Lydia fell while getting out of bed one morning and was left with temporary aphasia, confusion, and weakness of her right arm and leg. She was hospitalized briefly, was found to have suffered a cerebrovascular thrombosis, and with her son's consent was transferred to a nursing home for care. Upon arrival in the institution Lydia demonstrated only slight loss of physical strength, but marked fatigue, irritability, confusion, and obstinacy. During her first few months in the home Lydia had several outbursts of temper in response to the staff's efforts to restrain her from walking about at night, entering other patients' rooms, and running away from the institution.

(ANSWER BLANK ON PAGE A–143) (CORRECT ANSWERS ON PAGE B–243)

1. An organic psychosis is a mental disorder:
   1. Produced by exposure to harmful chemicals.
   2. Occurring in psychologically healthy persons.
   3. In which neuropathology can be demonstrated.
   4. Which is secondary to an infectious process.

2. Possible causes of organic psychoses are:
   a. Arteriosclerosis.
   b. Alcoholism.
   c. Syphilis.
   d. Epilepsy.
   e. Trauma.
      1. a, b, and c.
      2. a, b, and e.
      3. All but d.
      4. All the above.

3. The relatively permanent impairment of cerebral function which occurs in chronic organic brain damage typically produces defects in:
   a. Memory.
   b. Orientation.
   c. Judgment.
   d. Comprehension.
   e. Affect.
      1. a and b.
      2. a, b, and c.
      3. All but e.
      4. All the above.

4. Orientation can best be understood as:
   1. A realistic awareness of place, time, circumstances, and interpersonal relationships.
   2. Tendency to behave at a fairly concrete level of perception of one's environment.
   3. Recognition of one's situation, its probable causes and its logical consequences.
   4. The ability to correctly interpret facts and their logical interrelationships.

5. Lydia's impairment of orientation is apt to be most marked in regard to:
   1. Her physical surroundings.
   2. Identity of other persons.
   3. Time of day, week, or year.
   4. Her own identity.

6. The nurse could most effectively minimize Lydia's disorientation by:
   a. Keeping a night light burning throughout the hours of darkness.
   b. Posting at her bedside a written schedule of her daily activities.
   c. Providing a Big Ben alarm clock and a large print calendar.
   d. Directing her daily to recite the names of her relatives and caretakers.
   e. Restricting her visitors to members of her own immediate family.
      1. a and c.
      2. a, c, and d.
      3. All but e.
      4. All the above.

7. Lydia's memory defect is apt to be of which type?
   1. Greatest difficulty in retrieving material stored first.
   2. Greatest impairment for recall of recent events.
   3. Most pronounced loss for person and place names.
   4. Daily variation in acuity of total memory function.

8. On their visits with her in the nursing home, Lydia's family members noted that, while she responded to their conversational overtures courteously, she rarely initiated a topic of conversation. This reduction in spontaneous conversation on her part was probably the result of:
   1. Physical fatigue.
   2. Hidden resentment.
   3. Separation anxiety.
   4. Impoverished ideation.

9. Lydia's chronic brain syndrome differs from an acute organic brain disorder in that her illness:
   1. Tends to be progressive and irreversible.
   2. Produces a greater degree of incapacity.
   3. Derives from more specific pathology.
   4. Responds more favorably to treatment.

10. The psychopathologic manifestations which typically accompany arteriosclerotic brain damage are:
   1. Paranoid.
   2. Schizophrenic.
   3. Affective.
   4. Nonspecific.

11. A fundamental requirement of therapeutic care for Lydia would be:
   1. Removal of all externally induced irritation.

2. Providing a well-regulated mode of life.
3. Reconstruction of her personality patterns.
4. Substitutions of new interests for old.

12. The plan for Lydia's care in the nursing home should take into consideration the fact that her disorientation would tend to produce:

1. Inability to dress herself.
2. Reversal of her sleeping patterns.
3. Loss of basic social skills.
4. Diminished knowledge of current events.

13. Lydia's physician would be most apt to order that she be given supplementary doses of which of the following vitamins, as having a therapeutic effect on nervous tissue?

1. Vitamin A.
2. Vitamin B.
3. Vitamin C.
4. Vitamin D.

14. The nurse should inform Lydia's family that immediately following her admission to the nursing home Lydia would be apt to:

  a. Display increased irritability, confusion, depression, and insomnia.
  b. Criticize the care given her as being inadequate for her needs.
  c. Make frequent threats or attempts to run away from the home.
  d. Express irritation concerning lack of privacy and independence.
    1. a and c.
    2. b and d.
    3. All but d.
    4. All the above.

15. In telling her family of her dissatisfactions with life in the nursing home Lydia said, "They're always telling me what to do! Who gave these people authority over me?" What would be the best response?

1. "What do you mean, telling you what to do? Is someone here treating you badly?"
2. "We haven't given anyone here complete authority over you. They just carry out the doctor's orders."
3. "We gave them authority to care for you, so as to relieve you of responsibilities you can no longer manage."
4. "We know you're unhappy, but this is the right place for you. Try to make the best of it."

16. An important part of Lydia's care would be efforts to:

1. Correct her memory defect.
2. Make her function independently.
3. Weaken her family attachments.
4. Keep her regression to a minimum.

17. In addition to regression, aged persons with arteriosclerotic brain damage tend to use which of the following defense mechanisms?

1. Denial and projection.
2. Isolation and undoing.
3. Suppression and sublimation.
4. Condensation and symbolization.

18. Lydia is apt to display which of the following emotional responses to the nursing home personnel?

1. Strongly affectionate ties.
2. Continuous hostile accusations.
3. Wide fluctuations in mood.
4. Cold and silent withdrawal.

19. Those aspects of Lydia's behavior which are not directly the result of cerebral ischemia can best be understood as arising from her underlying feelings of:

1. Independence.
2. Depersonalization.
3. Martyrdom.
4. Insecurity.

20. One afternoon two of Lydia's lady friends called on her. She greeted them enthusiastically, sat visiting with them for a few minutes in the reception room, then excused herself, saying, "Just a minute, I'm going to get you some candy." She walked down the hall, entered her room, sat down in her chair, and began to read a magazine. Her behavior probably resulted from:

1. Embarrassment at having her friends see her in a nursing home.
2. Resentment of her friends' better health and more fortunate circumstances.
3. Forgetting her visitors as soon as they were out of her sight.
4. Withdrawal from persons with whom she felt she had nothing in common.

21. After Lydia had abandoned her guests in the reception room, the nurse could be most helpful to all concerned by:

1. Explaining to the guests that Lydia was quickly tired by visitors.
2. Reminding Lydia that her friends were waiting in the reception room.
3. Escorting the ladies to Lydia's room and providing them with chairs.
4. Asking the ladies to leave and return to visit on another day.

22. Important considerations in treating a person with organic brain syndrome are to determine his:
   a. Actual degree of cerebrovascular damage.
   b. Attitude and reaction to his physical changes.
   c. Previous level of intellectual productiveness.
   d. Life experiences during infancy and early childhood.
      1. a only.
      2. a, b, and d.
      3. All but d.
      4. All the above.

23. In order to understand Lydia's behavior in the nursing home the nurse should understand that her illness would tend to result in:
   1. Total reversal of personality and character traits.
   2. Marked exaggeration of premorbid personality characteristics.
   3. Complete regression to the level of infantile development.
   4. Severe psychological disorganization and loss of control.

24. One morning Lydia greeted the nurse with, "I'm going to take my driver's test today." Which response would be most therapeutic?
   1. "What makes you think that you want to take a driver's test today?"
   2. "I find that hard to believe. You've sold your car and don't drive now."
   3. "Why don't you spend the day watching television in the reception room?"
   4. "Don't you remember that you lost your driver's license for poor eyesight?"

25. Lydia hoarded useless odds and ends in her bedside stand. It is thought that this tendency in aged persons represents:
   1. An attempt to achieve security by surrounding themselves with a large number of material possessions.
   2. A return to the pattern of indiscriminate incorporation characteristic of the oral stage of development.
   3. An effort to antagonize their caretakers by making their housekeeping duties needlessly complex.
   4. An inability to give of themselves or their belongings to those with whom they associate.

26. One evening Lydia told her nurse, "My former minister called on me this afternoon." The nurse replied, "How nice. What did you talk about?" After a pause Lydia mumbled, "I don't know . . . God, I guess." Lydia's primary reason for initiating this conversation was probably:
   1. Worry about the state of her immortal soul.
   2. Chagrin that she had forgotten the content of the conversation.
   3. Pleasure at having an old friend call on her.
   4. A desire to convince the nurse of her respectability.

27. On one of her granddaughter's visits, Lydia greeted her by asking, "Did Mother come with you?" Which response would be most appropriate?
   1. "No, she wasn't able to come with me today."
   2. "Hello, Grandma, don't you recognize me? It's Julia."
   3. "No, your mother isn't here. She died ten years ago."
   4. "Have you forgotten that your mother died long ago?"

28. One day Lydia's aged lady friend came to visit her at the nursing home. On her friend's departure Lydia said, "Now I want you to come to my house for Thanksgiving." Which response would be most supporting?
   1. "You don't live in your house any more. I'll visit you here in the nursing home."
   2. "You know that's not possible. You're in no condition to entertain company."
   3. "Oh, let's talk about that later on. No need to rush the holiday season."
   4. "All right, I'll plan on that. Is there anything you'd like me to bring?"

29. After Lydia had been in the home for some time, the nurse should prepare Lydia's family for the possibility that Lydia might develop:
   1. Progression of brain damage and additional strokes.
   2. Sufficiently improved health to return to her home.
   3. Pressure sores, urinary infections, and constipation.
   4. Accident proneness resulting from motor incoordination.

30. In one conversation with her son, Lydia asked bluntly, "What will they say about me when I'm gone?" Which would be the best response?

1. "They will say that you were a good Christian and never did anyone any harm."
2. "Why do you care what other people are going to say about you after you're gone?"
3. "Are you trying to tell me that you have been thinking about dying?"
4. "When you go home the people here will probably want you to come back again."

31. Nurses who work with geriatric patients may be more aware than other persons of the advisability of preparing for old age by:

1. Accumulating sufficient financial savings throughout life to be able to afford custodial care in a total care institution.
2. Beginning in young adulthood to acquire diverse interests and habits contributing to mental and physical health.
3. Marrying a man younger than oneself to decrease the chances of living through a long, lonely widowhood.
4. Buying a home of the size, type, and location that will provide safe and comfortable retirement living.

32. In planning nursing care for Lydia the nurse should recognize that which of the following are psychological tasks of old age?

a. Maintaining old interests and developing new ones.
b. Becoming as self-supporting as one's health permits.
c. Transferring to others wisdom accumulated through experience.
d. Avoiding social withdrawal, inflexibility, and despair.
e. Planning for the future years of life.
   1. a and b.
   2. b, c, and d.
   3. All but e.
   4. All the above.

33. Which of the following are typical needs of aged persons?

a. Security.
b. Sexual activity.
c. Novelty.
d. Esteem.
e. Self-actualization.
   1. a and d.
   2. a, c, and d.
   3. All but e.
   4. All the above.

After she had been in the nursing home for two years, she talked less and less about her home, her former friends, her relatives, and her distant past. She was pleasant, but detached, and in spite of participation in an orientation group, her memory continued to fail. It seemed possible that she might continue to live on in this condition for some time.

Obesity and Behavior Modification

Maggie Anthony, who had been obese most of her life, wrote the following letter to the state university hospital:

Dear Sir:

I'm writing concerning the bypass intestinal operation. I was told by an ex-patient of your hospital of your work. I would like to obtain this operation but no one will help me. I have been in the hospital 4 times in the last 1 year simply because of my obesity hurting my legs and nerves. I can't cope with my weight any more. I am 29, 5' 11" tall, and more than 150 pounds overweight. I've tried everything for the past 21 years I've been heavy. Please help me if you can. My nerves are shot for the depression of my weight. I can't control it at all. Would you please tell me all you can on the procedure and price of it for my medical insurance wouldn't pay for this. I haven't been able to work for over a year because of my weight. So, you see it really is a problem to me. I'm divorced and have two daughters. Thanks.

Mrs. Margaret Anthony

Maggie's letter was referred to the Chief of Surgery, who invited Maggie to the Surgery Clinic the following month. Maggie traveled from the small town where she lived to the University Hospital, 100 miles away. After a brief examination in Surgery Clinic she was referred to the Metabolic Clinic for evaluation and prescription of a diet program. The endocrinologist made the assessment that Maggie had neither endocrinopathy nor life-threatening obesity. He prescribed a diet and referred her to the clinic's psychologist who, in collaboration with the nurse practitioner, elicited a more detailed history and started Maggie on a program of behavior modification.

Maggie said that her parents had obtained a divorce shortly after she was born. Her mother was not overweight but her father was a pleasant, 5' 3", 300 pound man. Maggie lived with her dominating mother, who remarried, and her two older siblings. When they were very young Maggie's brother and sister began to work outside the home, so Maggie was assigned the task of cleaning house, for which work she was rewarded with candy. Maggie recalled that she had been heavy at eight years. The family doctor told her she weighed 42 pounds at 15 months of age. At 14 years she jogged, starved herself, and lost weight until she weighed 132 pounds.

She married at 18 and had two children, then divorced her alcoholic husband, enrolled in beautician's school, and worked as a beautician until her "legs and nerves got bad." Finally, she "settled in at home, ate, and worried." She tried to lose weight through dieting, Weight Watchers and TOPS, achieving a degree of success with each endeavor. During the three years before she contacted University Hospital, Maggie said, "I just went crazy and gained 70 pounds. I hate myself when I overeat."

(ANSWER BLANK ON PAGE A–145) (CORRECT ANSWERS ON PAGE B–245)

---

1. Most health science workers would accept which of the following as an accurate definition of obesity?

1. Body weight is 7 kg. in excess of ideal body weight, and the triceps skin fold is in excess of 15–30 mm.
2. Body weight is 12 kg. in excess of ideal body weight and the triceps skin fold is in excess of 15–30 mm.
3. Body weight is 15 kg. in excess of ideal body weight and the triceps skin fold is in excess of 30–40 mm.
4. Body weight is 21 kg. in excess of ideal body weight and the triceps skin fold is in excess of 30–40 mm.

2. The majority of health professionals would agree to which of the following as the most common etiology of obesity?

1. Amounts of food consumed are in excess of that needed for energy.
2. Metabolic enzymes required for fat degradation are deficient.
3. Adrenergic synthetic pathways in the brain are over-stimulated.
4. Hormones secreted by the hypothalamus over-stimulate the adrenal cortex.

3. Rather than being viewed as a symptom of some kind of disease, obesity is viewed by proponents of the behavior modification theory as:

1. A dynamic process which demon-

strates that we are what we eat in spite of environmental demands.

2. A manifestation of psychoendocrinology which results in an abundance of internal stimuli.

3. A way that the individual has learned to cope with environmental and self imposed demands.

4. An individualized adjustment of the body's metabolic processes to constantly changing social stimuli.

4. Which two of the following probably had the strongest influence on Maggie's energy intake?

a. Habitual diet.
b. Satiety.
c. Hunger.
d. Social pressures.
e. Metabolic work.
    1. a and d.
    2. b and c.
    3. c and a.
    4. d and e.

5. Hunger and satiety are thought to be controlled by which of the following organs?

1. Thalamus.
2. Hypothalamus.
3. Amygdala.
4. Pituitary.

6. In order to determine whether Maggie's obesity was due to Cushing syndrome, the endocrinologist would order which of the following measurements?

1. Serum cortisol.
2. Glucose tolerance.
3. 24 hour urine calcium.
4. Serum aldosterone.

7. One's repertoire of eating behaviors is influenced by biological, psychological, cultural and familial forces. In addition to these factors, which of the following determines when food ingestion is initiated or terminated?

a. Tolerance of hunger.
b. Time of day and place.
c. Rate of ingestion.
d. Cost and palatability of food.
e. Physical position during eating.
    1. a and c.
    2. a, c, and d.
    3. All but e.
    4. All the above.

8. A biological factor which may have influenced Maggie's inability to maintain normal body weight is the fact that a person who has been fat as an infant experiences which of the following changes in metabolism of fat?

1. Fat cells increase in size.
2. Fat cells increase in number.
3. Fat cells increase the metabolic rate.
4. Fat cells contain more cyclic AMP.

9. Maggie's obesity predisposes her to which of the following diseases?

a. Thrombophlebitis.
b. Hypertension.
c. Arthritis.
d. Diabetes mellitus.
e. Malignancy.
    1. a and c.
    2. b, c, and d.
    3. All but e.
    4. All the above.

10. Even though she is obese now, Maggie could possibly hold a body image of herself as a normal weight person. What is the best explanation of how this phenomenon might occur?

1. Because her mother who rewarded her was of normal weight.
2. Because she was of normal weight during many of her adolescent years.
3. Because fantasy plays an important role in the process of becoming obese.
4. Because her obesity developed after her marriage and pregnancies.

11. Hilde Bruch proposed that obesity is caused by which of the following?

1. Inability of the body to differentiate between physiological hunger and an emotional state.
2. The initiation and termination of eating behavior by external rather than internal cues.
3. The initiation and termination of eating behavior by internal cues unrelated to external environment.
4. Inability of the individual to differentiate between hunger and satiety as a function of caloric value.

12. Behavior modification treatment can best be described as:

1. Role re-patterning.
2. Medical intervention.
3. Social learning.
4. Somatic conditioning.

13. The desired outcome of Maggie's behavior modification therapy for her obesity would be:

1. A weight reduction of 30 kg.
2. An elimination of fat from her diet.
3. An increase in social interactions.
4. An alteration of her eating behavior.

14. Behavior modification in a noninstitutional setting differs from that which can be initiated in a hospital because at home one's behavior is primarily self controlled. Self control, from a behavioral point of view, is derived principally from:
1. Adaptive mechanism regulated by the superego.
2. Fear of the social consequences of acting out.
3. Limbic system's modification of aggression.
4. Responses received for behavior demonstrated.

15. Before helping Maggie to shape new eating behaviors, which of the following should be done?
a. Complete a health assessment.
b. Assess her pattern of eating behavior.
c. Describe behavior modification techniques.
d. Identify reinforcers which would be effective for her.
e. Evaluate whether or not she will lose weight.
  1. a and b.
  2. a, b, and d.
  3. b, c, and e.
  4. All the above.

16. To be successful, the first step in behavior modification treatment of overeating should be based on a functional analysis of which of the following?
a. Oral aggressive behavior.
b. Topography of eating responses.
c. Situations which provoke overeating.
d. Consequent conditions.
e. Anal-fictive patterns.
  1. a and c.
  2. b, c, and d.
  3. All but e.
  4. All the above.

17. The nurse asked Maggie to monitor her own food intake patterns in order to evaluate her eating behavior and its determinants. Which of the following should the nurse ask Maggie to record accurately and in detail?
a. When and where eating occurs.
b. Description of how she eats.
c. The specific foods selected.
d. Behavior which typically precedes eating.
e. Feeling and mood consequent to eating.

  1. a and c.
  2. a, c, and e.
  3. All but d.
  4. All the above.

18. Analysis of Maggie's records of her eating behaviors revealed that her behavior generally resembled that of most obese individuals. Which of the following eating behaviors did she probably record?
a. Consumed large bites of food too fast.
b. Ate in rooms other than kitchen or diningroom.
c. Consumed quantities of high caloric density food.
d. Ate snacks lying, standing, or walking.
e. Ate until she consumed all food on her plate.
  1. a and c.
  2. a, c, and e.
  3. All but d.
  4. All the above.

19. In order to help Maggie in weight reduction, the nurse should assess which of the following?
a. Which eating activities occur with high frequency?
b. Which responses to eating occur with high frequency?
c. Whether losing weight is a positive reinforcer?
d. Whether gaining weight is a negative reinforcer?
e. What types of activities are rarely engaged in?
  1. a and b.
  2. c and d.
  3. All but e.
  4. All the above.

20. Which of the following are characteristics of a positive reinforcer?
a. Acts by increasing the desired behavior.
b. Its delivery can be uniformly controlled.
c. Can be delivered immediately and consistently.
d. Following its withdrawal, antecedent behavior is increased.
e. Its schedule of delivery can be carefully planned.
  1. a and b.
  2. a, c, and d.

3. a, b, c, and e.

4. All the above.

21. In attempting to modify Maggie's eating behavior, it would be especially important for the nurse to evaluate which of the following?

1. Whether Maggie uses eating as a reward to herself.

2. Whether Maggie usually eats alone in the evenings.

3. Areas of Maggie's body that contain large fat deposits.

4. The degree to which Maggie's genes resemble her father's.

22. In order to help Maggie lose weight, the nurse should reinforce Maggie for which of the following?

a. Consuming large amounts of protein early in each meal.

b. Eating her food and drinking liquids more slowly.

c. Discriminating between acceptable food and nonacceptable food.

d. Buying for snacks only those foods which have nutritional value.

e. Leaving food on her plate for a couple of meals each day.

1. a and b.

2. b, c, and e.

3. All but d.

4. All the above.

23. Attempts to extinguish Maggie's overeating behavior would be unsuccessful if, inadvertently, which of the following conditions should obtain?

1. Rapid eating was reinforced.

2. Eating with others occurred.

3. Eating while sitting was reinforced.

4. Stimuli for eating were narrowed.

24. For Maggie the strongest reinforcer of weight reduction was the decreasing frequency of her leg and back pain. Which of the following would be another positive reinforcer for Maggie's dieting?

1. Desire for employment.

2. Low fat diet.

3. Medication.

4. A hobby.

25. The behavior therapist helping Maggie requested that she weigh herself and record her weight four times a day. Why was this request made?

1. Because the average of four weights taken on the same scale is more accurate than a single recording.

2. Because, in most situations, behavior is not likely to change unless the im-

mediate consequences of that behavior also change.

3. Because requesting that Maggie record her weight on a sheet is one way to train her to participate in activities other than eating.

4. Because the control that Maggie learns through properly recording her weight will introduce her to the concept of self control.

26. The nurse gave Maggie some helpful tips regarding grocery shopping. Which of the following would encourage weight loss?

a. "Shop only after meals."

b. "Never buy snack foods."

c. "Ignore food sale items."

d. "Buy foods which require preparation."

e. "Do your own grocery shopping."

1. a and d.

2. a, b, and c.

3. All but e.

4. All the above.

Maggie lost several pounds and proceeded through several steps of the program outlined by her and the therapists for eliminating her compulsive overeating. She seemed pleased with her progress and told the nurse that she had resumed her crocheting and was learning to do needlepoint.

Maggie made dietary changes and was ingenious in devising ways to prevent overeating. Unfortunately, she persisted in overindulging in high caloric–low nutrient value snacks each evening after she put her children to bed.

27. How much weight should Maggie be advised to lose per week?

1. 1 kg.

2. 2 kg.

3. 3 kg.

4. 4 kg.

28. Initially, Maggie was told to stop eating and place her utensils on her plate for about 2 minutes in the middle of each meal in order to:

1. Allow her hot foods to get cold and greasy.

2. Lengthen the meal time and decrease snacking time.

3. Give her a conscious experience in controlling her eating.

4. Allow her to attend to sounds and other stimuli in the room.

29. Maggie was instructed to do nothing but eat during mealtime because:

1. Maggie needs to concentrate on chewing her food and looking at her large, bulging body.
2. Activities associated with eating become identified with and, therefore, stimuli for eating.
3. Associated experiences to any activity tend to lessen the impact of each individual event.
4. Early in the behavior modification program for Maggie, there is danger of overloading her with stimuli.

30. Maggie felt compelled to eat in the evening after her children are in bed. She might try which of the following to break herself of the habit?

1. Go to bed when the children do.
2. Practice a new needlepoint pattern.
3. Crochet a vest for herself.
4. Keep the children up late.

31. Too severe restriction of calories in an obese patient may provoke which of the following results?
   a. Irritability.
   b. Depression.
   c. Decreased libido.
   d. Bradycardia.
   e. Decreased metabolic rate.
      1. a and b.
      2. b, c, and d.
      3. All but d.
      4. All the above.

32. Since behavior which is not reinforced becomes extinct, Maggie is in danger of not maintaining her early weight loss because:

1. She doesn't have adult family members nearby to reward her for weight reduction.
2. In the past, Maggie lost weight and regained it several times but never could maintain normal weight.
3. She is apt to return to work when she feels better, and her leg and back pain will recur.
4. She will reach a plateau in weight loss and become discouraged by the lack of progress reflected in her own weight record.

33. Researchers have explained why losing weight and maintaining decreased body weight are very difficult in an industrialized society. Which of the following summarizes their thinking?
   a. Obesity is a way to control the behavior of others and to feel powerful.
   b. Consequences for overeating are not closely associated in time with eating behavior.
   c. Normal caloric intake during adulthood can cause weight gain in a person with childhood onset obesity.
   d. Stigma attached to obesity is not as great as that attached to anorexia.
   e. Obesity represents a metabolic balance and caloric restriction provokes a starvation-like syndrome.
      1. a and b.
      2. a, b, and c.
      3. All but d.
      4. All the above.

Maggie lost about 15 kg. in 9 months, and then weight loss became minimal each month for 6 months. Finally, she told the doctors in the surgery clinic that what she had really wanted all along was bypass surgery. They explained the procedure to her and informed her that side effects (diarrhea, vitamin deficiency, electrolyte imbalances) might occur. After consultation with the psychologist, anesthesiologist, endocrinologist and psychiatrist, a jejunoileal bypass operation was performed. Her only complaint during hospitalization was that she had back pain due to the poor mattress on her hospital bed.

Six months after the jejunoileal bypass, Maggie wrote to her doctor at the University Hospital:

Because of financial problems I am not able at this time to return for a checkup. My family physician would like to know which tests he should run and where he should send the results. Two questions he wanted me to ask you are: (1) How much intestine was bypassed; and (2) should I stay on a diet and what can I eat. I am feeling much better, have lost 40 pounds, and have only minimal trouble with my back now. I'll call you and make an appointment for a checkup as soon as I can afford the trip. Thank you.

Maggie Anthony

Suicide and Suicide Prevention

Bonnie Sue, a well-qualified and highly successful nursing instructor, committed suicide when she was thirty-five. Her grief-stricken friends and colleagues conducted a "psychological autopsy" in order to determine why she had taken her own life.

They recalled that, when her mother had died shortly after Bonnie's birth, her father, a Baptist missionary, had arranged for Bonnie to be reared by his wife's sister, who had a young daughter of the same age. Bonnie's aunt was kind to her, and the two children got along well until it became obvious that Bonnie was more intelligent and socially apt than her cousin, LaVerne. After that time Bonnie was often ignored in order that LaVerne could be accorded the central position in family activities.

After Bonnie Sue completed high school, she was able to enroll in a nursing program at the state university as a result of a scholarship grant which she had been awarded for academic excellence. Although her college years were fraught with conflict and dissatisfaction, she graduated from nursing school with high honors and took a job at the local hospital. After a few stormy years of employment as a staff nurse, Bonnie enrolled in a Master's Degree nursing program. When the stresses of studying, severe financial worries, and dissatisfaction with her teachers caused her to withdraw from school, she took a teaching position in a diploma nursing school. Her students, who delighted in her enthusiasm for nursing and her devotion to excellent patient care, never criticized her for carelessness in grooming or for a tendency to drink more heavily than any of her wide circle of friends.

As time passed, Bonnie's deep concern for the rights of patients and her inability to rectify the social injustices that she saw all around her made her increasingly critical of what she called "Establishment Medicine." Because she was extremely articulate, she talked loudly and persuasively about needed changes in patient care and hospital administration to anyone who would listen. She and her boy friend spent a week of Bonnie's vacation making a photographic study of "conditions" in the hospital where she worked. Her supervisors advised Bonnie to be less aggressive in seeking reforms in the health care establishment.

One evening, after the housemother in the Nurses' Residence criticized Bonnie for the untidiness of her room, Bonnie impulsively gathered up her belongings and moved into a nearby commune. Her argument with the housemother so enraged Bonnie that she sought employment in another hospital. As she deliberated about this change of job, her concern for patients in the City Hospital where she worked seemed to increase, and she became more and more critical of her colleagues for their seeming lack of commitment to excellence in patient care.

A few days later Bonnie gave her new coat and her treasured sewing machine to a friend who stopped by to visit. Then she made several telephone calls to other friends and talked excitedly about her new job, her menstrual difficulties, and her plans to campaign for an improved Patients' Bill of Rights. Her friends attributed her agitation to the fact that she had been drinking. One *person to whom she talked invited her out for a cup of coffee, but Bonnie declined the offer. After she hung up the telephone, Bonnie smashed several dishes, wrote a suicide note, drove into the garage, closed the door, and killed herself by inhaling carbon monoxide gas from the car exhaust.*

In her lengthy suicide note Bonnie railed against her colleagues' insensitivity to her own and the patients' needs for care and attention. The letter concluded by saying: "I hope that by my death I may become the sacrificial lamb for all future patients in City Hospital in the same way that Jesus Christ died to save sinners from the threat of Hell."

Although her death seemed to have no immediate effect on hospital operation, several hospital policies which she had criticized publicly were changed during the year following her suicide. Bonnie's colleagues still talk about her affectionately, describing her to hospital newcomers as a sensitive eccentric who suffered excessively because she appointed herself the conscience for the entire local medical community.

(ANSWER BLANK ON PAGE A–147) (CORRECT ANSWERS ON PAGE B–247)

1. Attempts have been made by sociologists and psychologists to classify suicide as which of the following?

    a. Communication.
    b. Revenge.
    c. Rebirth.
    d. Unconscious flight.
    e. Magical reunion.

      1. a and b.
      2. a, b, and d.
      3. All but d.
      4. All of the above.

2. Which of the following are factors commonly cited as a cause for suicide?

    a. Problems with family.
    b. Financial problems.
    c. Problems with the opposite sex.
    d. Academic and social pressures.
    e. Identity crisis.

      1. a and b.
      2. a, c, and e.
      3. All but e.
      4. All the above.

3. Bonnie Sue was atypical of women suicides in that they commit suicide most frequently by:
    1. Jumping off a bridge.
    2. Shooting self with a gun.
    3. Driving a car recklessly.
    4. Taking overdose of drugs.

4. Women account for what per cent of the unsuccessful suicide attempts?
    1. 25 per cent.
    2. 33 per cent.
    3. 50 per cent.
    4. 66 per cent.

5. Men comprise what per cent of the completed suicide population?
    1. 25 per cent.
    2. 33 per cent.
    3. 50 per cent.
    4. 66 per cent.

6. Which of the following are *not* true about suicide and suicidal persons?
    a. Suicide is usually inherited.
    b. Suicide happens without warning.
    c. Most people just talk about suicide.
    d. Once suicidal, always suicidal.
    e. Suicide is a rich man's disease.

      1. a, b, and c.
      2. a, b, c, and e.
      3. All but e.
      4. All the above.

7. Which of the following is a fact about suicide?
    1. Suicidal people are intent on dying and habitually gamble with death.
    2. Suicides occur at the height of the individual's morbid feelings.
    3. Suicidal individuals are mentally ill and most are psychotic.

4. Suicidal people are frequently undecided about living or dying.

8. Suicidal deaths occur most frequently during which times of day?

1. 6 A.M.–12 noon.
2. 1 P.M.–5 P.M.
3. 6 P.M.–12 midnight.
4. 1 A.M.–5 A.M.

9. Bonnie Sue's nurse friends probably knew that suicidal intentions are strongest during life crisis situations which appear:

1. Undesirable, but tolerable.
2. Detrimental to the person.
3. Capable of releasing growth energy.
4. Insoluble to the person.

10. Bonnie Sue's abuse of alcohol may have contributed to her suicide in which of the following ways?

1. Increased ingestion of alcohol resulted in increased rejection.
2. Alcohol made obstacles smaller and wish fulfillments nearer.
3. Alcohol disrupted nerve pathways which controlled impulse repression.
4. Feelings of guilt over her drinking increased anxiety and frustration.

11. Following her suicide, Bonnie's friends and family would be most apt to ask which of the following questions?

1. "What was her problem?"
2. "Why did she do it?"
3. "Where was her common sense?"
4. "Who caused this to happen?"

12. Suicide is a behavioral attempt to communicate. What was Bonnie Sue probably trying to communicate?

1. Supernatural ability and feelings of superiority.
2. Persistent rebellion and feelings of ambivalence.
3. Hidden immorality and feelings of sinfulness.
4. Extreme frustration and feelings of unworthiness.

13. Which of the following emotions was probably strongest in Bonnie Sue's colleagues after they were told of her suicide?

1. Anger.
2. Guilt.
3. Depression.
4. Indifference.

14. In addition to recognizing a "suicidal threat" as an individual's expressed intent to kill himself, Bonnie Sue's nurse friends probably knew that which of the following is also true of such threats?

1. Any mentally ill person should be considered suicidal.
2. Suicidal threats are often attempts to get attention.
3. Families usually ignore verbal suicide threats.
4. Another's talk of suicide awakens fears within an individual.

15. Which of the following was an indication of Bonnie's suicidal intentions which her friends could probably recognize only in retrospect?

1. Seeking a new job in the university.
2. Moving out of the nurses' residence.
3. Calling her friends late in the evening.
4. Giving away her coat and sewing machine.

16. Bonnie Sue's composition of a lengthy suicide note to her friends may best be interpreted as which of the following?

a. A wish to explain why she committed suicide.
b. An expression of her ambivalence toward committing suicide.
c. A lasting written record of her beliefs and ideals.
d. An irrelevant essay of a disturbed, confused mind.
e. A calculated effort to make her colleagues feel guilty.

1. a only.
2. a, b, and e.
3. All but e.
4. All the above.

17. Some theorists believe that the risk of suicide in alcoholic persons increases immediately following the loss of an external object. Which of the following might Bonnie have interpreted as significant losses?

a. Being ridiculed by the resident director.
b. Sudden move from the nurses' residence.
c. Seeking and being offered a new teaching job.
d. Inability to effect changes in patient care.
e. Giving away her coat and sewing machine.

1. a only.
2. a, b, and c.
3. All but e.
4. All the above.

18. An individual who experiences the impact of his mother's death during the first 10 years of his life tends to attempt suicide more often than members of the general population. Which of the following factors would most strongly condition such a person to later suicidal inclinations?
1. Age of the surviving parents and whether or not they remarry.
2. Number of community organizations available to give economic and emotional guidance.
3. Quality of physical and emotional care the grieving child subsequently receives.
4. Sex of the parent who committed suicide and the sex of the surviving child.

19. Community responses to the marital partner or other close relative of the suicide victim frequently heighten the guilt and shame of the survivors. Which of the following events is probably *most* destructive to the surviving spouse, family, and/or significant others?
1. Clergymen who refuse to conduct traditional burial services.
2. In-laws and friends who thrust blame for the suicide on the survivors.
3. Coroner's office and insurance representatives who show insensitivity.
4. Police officers who suggest homicide as a possible cause of the death.

20. A child whose parent has committed suicide must deal not only with resolution of his own grief but also with stresses resulting from problems encountered by the surviving parent, such as:
a. Surviving parent's preoccupied withdrawal.
b. Changes made in basic living arrangements.
c. Surviving parent's shock, guilt, and blaming.
d. Intertwining of their own and parent's grieving.
e. Realignment of family dynamics due to the loss.
   1. a and c.
   2. b and d.
   3. All but d.
   4. All the above.

21. The psychological impact of suicide on the children of a suicide victim can lead to ambivalent feelings of:
a. Resentment.
b. Guilt.
c. Shame.
d. Abandonment.
e. Depression.
   1. a and d.
   2. a, c, and d.
   3. All but b.
   4. All the above.

22. Which of the following are thought to be forms of chronic suicide?
a. Reckless driving.
b. Drug addiction.
c. Alcohol addiction.
d. Chronic overeating.
e. Persistent risk taking.
   1. a and c.
   2. a, b, and c.
   3. All but d.
   4. All the above.

23. Following his study of suicide etiology, Emile Durkheim concluded that:
1. The risk of suicide varies inversely with the degree of the individual's integration within the social group of which he is a part.
2. The risk of suicide varies inversely with the number of persons within the social group of which the individual is a member.
3. The risk of suicide exists when an individual learns oral dependent patterns of interaction which are unfulfilled in adulthood.
4. Suicide occurs in persons who have been highly industrious before their creativity is suddenly thwarted.

24. Durkheim theorized that men are most protected from suicide by which of the following:
1. Marital relationship.
2. Physical health.
3. Financial success.
4. Aggressive traits.

25. A major problem in suicide prevention is the suicidal person's lack of easy entry into a service facility which is equipped to give needed help. Which of the following are obstacles to suicide prevention?

a. Most persons in crisis fear police officers.
b. Admitting psychiatrists do not work 24 hours a day.
c. Welfare cases are not admitted to many hospitals.
d. Lack of empathy for suicidal persons from emergency personnel.
e. Mental health centers are usually available only in large cities.
    1. a and b.
    2. a, b, and c.
    3. All but d.
    4. All the above.

26. What percentage of persons who commit suicide communicate their intent in advance?
    1. 25 per cent.
    2. 50 per cent.
    3. 66 per cent.
    4. 80 per cent.

27. Within the white population the suicide rate among those who have made previous unsuccessful suicide attempts is how many times greater than for those with no previous suicide attempts?
    1. 4.
    2. 16.
    3. 32.
    4. 64.

28. Nationally, the black and white males' suicide rate (about 34 per 100,000) is highest in which age range?
    1. 20–25.
    2. 30–35.
    3. 40–45.
    4. 50–55.

29. The suicide rate for blacks who have previously attempted suicide differs from that of blacks who have made no previous suicide attempts in that:
    1. The suicide rate is 10 times greater than that of blacks with no previous attempts.
    2. Suicide attempts are negatively related to further self-destructive behavior.
    3. Suicide attempts are predictive of future successful suicides.
    4. The suicide rate is 100 times greater than that of blacks in the general population.

30. In San Francisco, California, approximately how many calls does the suicide prevention center receive monthly from persons who identify themselves as suicidal?
    1. 250.
    2. 750.
    3. 1200.
    4. 1600.

31. In telephone conversation with a person who is potentially suicidal, the listener at a Suicide Prevention Center should ask the caller directly for which of the following information?
a. The caller's name, address, and phone number.
b. Prior attempts at suicide and when they occurred.
c. Whether or not he is presently planning an attempt.
d. If he has the means available to carry out his plans.
e. Why he wishes to kill himself at this time.
    1. a only.
    2. a, b, and c.
    3. All but e.
    4. All the above.

32. Which of the following tasks can be handled effectively by a telephone volunteer in a Suicide Prevention Center?
a. Listening to obtain information.
b. Recording information obtained.
c. Evaluating suicidal potential.
d. Diagnosing the precipitating factors.
e. Recommending a course of help.
    1. a and b.
    2. a, b, and c.
    3. All but d.
    4. All the above.

33. Volunteers offer valuable assistance at Suicide Prevention Centers. Which of the following would be desired qualities in such a volunteer?
a. Willingly accepts responsibility for own feelings and actions.
b. Normal hearing and clear verbal expression.
c. Accepting of manners and mores unlike his own.
d. Tends to keep personal information confidential.
e. Recognizes his own limitations as a counselor.
    1. a and b.
    2. a, b, and d.
    3. All but c.
    4. All the above.

34. Nurses can help prevent suicide in persons of suicidal intent by doing which of the following?
   a. Reassuring the person of his ability to tolerate the stress experienced in his present situation.
   b. Offering continual support through numerous personal and telephone interviews.
   c. Assessing the client's strengths and past experience in coping with stress.
   d. Tolerating the ambiguity of whether or not the client will commit suicide when unattended.
   e. Mobilizing resources to relieve the client of personal responsibilities.
      1. a only.
      2. a, b, and c.
      3. All but e.
      4. All the above.

35. When a family hospitalizes a member in order to prevent his suicide, the nurse should help the family to accept the fact that:
   1. Only rarely does a hospitalized patient commit suicide.
   2. Suicide can and does occur in hospitalized patients.
   3. Danger of suicide increases directly with increasing length of hospitalization.
   4. Reintegration into the family may be impossible following hospitalization.

36. In conversations with the suicidal person's family the nurse should reinforce which of the following concepts?
   1. The most effective way to help the suicidal member is to avoid him until his stress is relieved.
   2. Family and friends should not discuss suicide with the patient because it stimulates his suicidal ideation.
   3. Family members cannot behave objectively toward a suicidal relative, so should leave him to the care of health professionals.
   4. Family members can best help by decreasing the degree of social isolation felt by the suicidal member.

37. In a telephone conversation with a person who is suicidal, the nurse should follow which of the following principles?
   a. Encourage the caller to do most of the talking.
   b. Write down all important facts related by the caller.
   c. Be optimistic and reassure the caller that problems will abate.
   d. Use the words "hope" and "hopeful" in realistic contexts.
   e. Mobilize help for the caller, if indicated.
      1. a and b.
      2. a, b, d, and e.
      3. All but d.
      4. All the above.

BIBLIOGRAPHY

PSYCHIATRIC—MENTAL HEALTH NURSING

Ackerman, N.: The Psychodynamics of Family Life. New York, Basic Books, Inc., 1958.

Agoston, T.: Insight Therapy. Columbus, Ohio. Columbus Blank Book Co., 1969.

Aguilera, D. C., and Messick, J. M.: Crisis Intervention, 2nd ed. St. Louis, C. V. Mosby Company, 1974.

Alexander, F.: Fundamentals of Psychoanalysis. New York, W. W. Norton Co., 1948.

Armstrong, J.: Alcoholism as a disease. The Canadian Nurse, 61:614–617, August 1965.

Armstrong, S., and Rouslin, S.: Group Psychotherapy in Nursing Practice. New York, The Macmillan Co., 1963.

Aronson, M.: Resistance in individual and group psychotherapy. American Journal of Psychotherapy, 21:86–94, January 1967.

Astrup, C.: Functional Psychoses: Diagnostic and Prognostic Models. Springfield, Illinois, Charles C Thomas, 1966.

Axelrod, J.: Noradrenaline: Fate and control of its biosynthesis. Science, 173:598–606, August 13, 1971.

Banton, A. L., ed.: Behavioral Change in Cerebrovascular Disease. New York, Harper and Row, 1968.

Bateson, G.: Minimal requirements for a theory of schizophrenia. Archives of General Psychiatry, 2:477–491, 1960.

Bellak, L., and Small, L.: Emergency Psychotherapy and Brief Psychotherapy. New York, Grune and Stratton, 1965.

Bergersen, B., and Krug, E.: Pharmacology in Nursing. 13th ed. St. Louis, C. V. Mosby Co., 1976.

Berni, R., and Fordyce, W. E.: Behavior Modification and the Nursing Process. St. Louis, C. V. Mosby, 1973.

Betts, V.: Psychotherapeutic intervention with the addict-client. Nursing Clinics of North America, 11:551–558, 1976.

Bibring, G., and Kahana, R.: Lectures in Medical Psychology. New York, International Universities Press, 1968.

Bindman, A. M.: Perspectives in Community Mental Health. Chicago, Aldine, 1969.

Bloom, V.: An analysis of suicide at a training center. American Journal of Psychiatry, 123:918–925, February 1967.

Blos, P.: On Adolescence. Glencoe, Illinois, The Free Press, 1962.

Bosselman, B.: Neurosis and Psychosis. 3rd ed. Springfield, Illinois, Charles C Thomas, 1964.

Brenner, C.: An Elementary Textbook of Psychoanalysis. Garden City, New York, Doubleday and Co., 1957.

Brickner, P. W., ed.: Care of the Nursing Home Patient. New York, The Macmillan Co., 1971.

Brown, M., and Fowler, G.: Psychodynamic Nursing: A Biosocial Orientation. 4th ed. Philadelphia, W. B. Saunders Co., 1971.

Bruch, H.: Eating Disorders: Obesity, Anorexia Nervosa, and the Person Within. New York, Basic Books, 1973.

Burd, S., and Marshall, M., eds.: Some Clinical Approaches to Psychiatric Nursing. New York, The Macmillan Co., 1963.

Busse, E.: Geriatrics today: an overview. American Journal of Psychiatry, 123:1226–1233, April 1967.

Cameron, D. C.: Facts about drugs. World Health, pp. 4–11, April 1971.

Caplan, C.: Support Systems and Community Mental Health: Lectures on Concept Development. New York, Behavioral Publications, 1974.

Caplan, G.: Principles of Preventive Psychiatry. New York, Basic Books, Inc., 1964.

Cartwright, D., and Zander, A.: Group Dynamics: Research and Theory. 3rd ed. New York, Harper and Row, 1968.

Chodoff, P., Friedman, S. B., and Hamburg, D. A.: Stress, defenses, and coping behavior. American Journal of Psychiatry, 120:743–749, 1964.

Clare, A.: Psychiatry in Dissent: Controversial Issues in Thought and Practice. London, Tavistock, 1976.

Davis, A.: A comparative analysis of Laing and Arieti on schizophrenia. Perspectives in Psychiatric Care, 14:78–88, 1976.

Dembicki, E. L.: Selected bibliography for students and teachers in drug dependency and drug abuse. Journal of Psychiatric Nursing, 9:37–38, May-June, 1971.

Detre, R. P., and Jarecki, H. G.: Modern Psychiatric Treatment. Philadelphia, J. B. Lippincott Co., 1971.

Deutsch, H.: Neuroses and Character Types. New York, International University Press, 1965.

Deutsch, H.: The Psychology of Women. Vols. I and II. New York, Grune and Stratton, 1944.

DeYoung, C., and Tower, M.: The Nurse's Role in Community Health Centers. Out of Uniform and Into Trouble. St. Louis, C. V. Mosby Co., 1971.

Draper, E.: Developmental theory of suicide. Comprehensive Psychiatry, 17:63–80, 1976.

Erikson, E.: Childhood and Society. 2nd ed. New York, W. W. Norton Co., 1963.

Erikson, E.: Identity and the life cycle. Psychological issues. Monograph Series No. 1, New York, International Universities Press, Inc., 1959.

Fagin, C.: Family Centered Nursing in Community Psychiatry. Philadelphia, F. A. Davis, 1970.

Feldman, L.: Strategies and techniques of family therapy. American Journal of Psychotherapy, 30:14–28, 1976.

Fenichel, O.: The Psychoanalytical Theory of Neurosis. New York, W. W. Norton Co., 1945.

Fox, R.: Alcoholism and reliance upon drugs as depressive equivalents. American Journal of Psychotherapy, 21:585–596, July 1967.

Fox, R.: Aspects of Alcoholism. Vol. 2. Philadelphia, J. B. Lippincott Co., 1966.

Francis, G., and Munjas, B.: Manual of Social Psychologic Assessment. New York, Appleton-Century-Crofts, 1976.

Freedman, A., and Kaplan, H., eds.: Comprehensive Textbook of Psychiatry. 2nd ed. Baltimore, Williams and Wilkins, 1975.

Freud, A.: Psychotherapy seen against the background of normal development. The British Journal of Psychiatry, 129:401–406.

Freud, A.: Adolescence. Psychoanalytic Study of the Child, 13:255–278, 1958.

Freud, S.: The Ego and the Mechanisms of Defense. London, Hogarth Press, 1937.

Freud, S.: The Complete Psychological Works of Sigmund Freud. The Standard Edition. Translated by J. Strachey. 24 Vols. London, Hogarth Press, 1953–1966.

Freud, S.: Introductory Lectures on Psychoanalysis. The Standard Edition. Vols. 15–16. London, Hogarth Press, 1963.

Freud, S.: Group Psychology and the Analysis of the Ego. The Standard Edition. 18: 67–143, London, Hogarth Press, 1955.

Freud, S.: Neurosis and Psychosis. The Standard Edition. 19:149–153, London, Hogarth Press, 1961.

Fromm, E.: The Crisis of Psychoanalysis. New York, Holt, Rinehart, and Winston, 1970.

Fromm-Reichmann, F.: Psychoanalysis and Psychotherapy. Chicago, University of Chicago Press, 1959.

Furberow, N. L., and Shneidman, E. S. (eds.): The Cry for Help. New York, McGraw-Hill, 1961.

Gardner, G. E.: Aggression and violence: the enemies of precision learning in children. American Journal of Psychiatry, 128:445–450, October 1971.

Goffman, E.: Asylums. New York, Doubleday and Co., 1961.

Goldstein, A.: Heroin addiction: Sequential treatment employing pharmacologic supports. Archives of General Psychiatry, 33:353–358, 1976.

Goodman, L., and Gilman, A., eds.: The Pharmacological Basis of Therapeutics, 5th ed. New York, The Macmillan Co., 1975.

Gorton, J. V.: Behavioral Components of Patient Care. New York, The Macmillan Co., 1970.

Gray, W., Duhl, F., and Rizzo, N., eds.: General Systems Theory and Psychiatry. Boston, Little, Brown and Co., 1969.

Greenacre, P., ed.: Affective Disorders. New York, International Universities Press, 1953.

Grossman, S. P.: A Textbook of Physiological Psychology. New York, Wiley, 1967.

Group for the Advancement of Psychiatry: Psychiatry and the Aged: An Introductory Approach. Vol. 5, Report 59. New York, Group for the Advancement of Psychiatry, 1965.

Hartmann, H.: Ego Psychology and the Problem of Adaptation. New York, International Universities Press, Inc., 1958.

Hirsch, E. A.: The Troubled Adolescent. New York, International Universities Press, 1970.

Hoffman, F.: Handbook on Drug and Alcohol Abuse. New York, Oxford University Press, 1975.

Horman, R. E., and Fox, Allan, eds.: Drug Awareness. New York, Avon Books, 1970.

Horney, K.: The Neurotic Personality of Our Time. New York, W. W. Norton Co., 1937.

Huey, F. L.: In a therapeutic community. American Journal of Nursing, 71:926–933, May 1971.

Jacobson, E.: Psychotic Conflict and Reality. New York, International Universities Press, 1967.

Johnson, A. M.: Experience, Affect and Behavior. Chicago, University of Chicago Press, 1969.

Johnson, J. A.: Group Therapy: A Practical Approach. New York, McGraw-Hill Book Co., 1963.

Johnson, M. K.: Mental Health and Mental Illness. Philadelphia, J. B. Lippincott, 1971.

Jordan, H. A., and Levitz, L. S.: A behavioral approach to the problem of obesity. In Silverstone, T.: Obesity: Its Pathogenesis and Management. Acton, Massachusetts, Publishing Sciences Group Inc., 1975.

Kalkman, M., and Davis, A.: New Dimensions in Mental Health—Psychiatric Nursing. 4th ed. New York, McGraw-Hill Book Co., 1974.

Kyes, J., and Hofling, C.: Basic Concepts in Psychiatric Nursing. 3rd ed. Philadelphia, J. B. Lippincott Company, 1974.

Lederer, W.: Dragons, delinquent and destiny: an essay on positive super ego function. Psychological Issues, Vol. 4: No. 3, Monograph 15, 1964.

Leininger, M. (ed.): Contemporary Issues in Mental Health Nursing. Boston, Little, Brown and Company, 1973.

Leitenberg, H. (ed.): Handbook of Behavioral Modification. New York, Appleton-Century-Crofts, 1974.

Lidz, T.: The Person: His Development Throughout the Life Cycle. New York, Basic Books, 1968.

Lorand, S., and Schneer, H., eds.: Adolescents: Psychoanalytic Approach to Problems and Therapy. New York, Harper and Row, 1964.

Lynch, V.: Narcissistic loss and depression in late adolescence. Perspectives in Psychiatric Care, *14*:133–135, 1976.

MacGregor, R., et al.: Multiple Impact Therapy with Families. New York, McGraw-Hill Book Co., 1964.

Marais, P.: Community psychiatric nursing: An alternative to hospitalization. Nursing Times, *72*:1708–1710, 1976.

Masserman, J. (ed.): Current Psychiatric Therapies. Vol. 16. New York, Grune and Stratton, 1976.

May, R.: The Meaning of Anxiety. New York, Ronald Press, 1950.

McDermott, R. Sr.: Maintaining the methadone patient. Nursing Outlook, *18*:22–26, December 1970.

Mellow, J.: Nursing therapy. American Journal of Nursing, *68*:2365–2369, November 1968.

Mereness, D.: Essentials of Psychiatric Nursing. 9th ed. St. Louis, C. V. Mosby Co., 1974.

Moulton, R.: Some effects of the new feminism. The American Journal of Psychiatry, *134*:1–6, 1977.

Mullahy, P.: A Study of Interpersonal Relations. New York, Hermitage House, 1950.

Mullahy, P.: Oedipus: Myth and Complex. New York, Heritage House, 1952.

Mullahy, P.: Psychoanalysis and Interpersonal Psychiatry. New York, Science House, 1970.

Noyes, A., and Kolb, L.: Modern Clinical Psychiatry. 8th ed. Philadelphia, W. B. Saunders Co., 1973.

Panzetta, W. F.: Community Mental Health. Myth and Reality. Philadelphia, Lea and Febiger, 1971.

Parad, H. J., and Caplan, G.: A framework for studying families in crisis. Social Work, *5*:3–16, July 1960.

Parens, H., and Saul, L.: Dependence in Man: A Psychoanalytic Study. New York, International Universities Press, 1971.

Peplau, H.: Interpersonal Relations in Nursing. New York, G. P. Putnam's Sons, 1952.

Peplau, H.: Interpersonal techniques, the crux of psychiatric nursing. American Journal of Nursing, *62*:50–54, June 1962.

Rainwater, L.: American underclass: red, white, black. Transaction, *6*:9, February 1969.

Redl, F., and Wineman, D.: Children Who Hate. Glencoe, Illinois, The Free Press, 1951.

Richardson, S. A., and Guttmacher, A. F., eds.: Childbearing, Its Social and Psychological Aspects. Baltimore, Williams and Wilkins, 1967.

Richter, C.: Biological Clocks in Medicine and Psychiatry. Springfield, Illinois, Charles C Thomas, 1965.

Riessman, F., Cohen, J., and Pearl, A., eds.: Mental Health of the Poor. Glencoe, Illinois, Glencoe Free Press, 1964.

Rogers, C.: Carl Rogers on Encounter Groups. New York, Harper and Row, 1971.

Rothenberg, A.: On anger. American Journal of Psychiatry, *128*:454–460, October 1971.

Rowe, C. J.: An Outline of Psychiatry, 6th ed. Dubuque, Iowa, Wm. C. Brown Company, 1975.

Ruesch, J.: Disturbed Communication. New York, W. W. Norton Co., 1957.

Ruesch, J.: Therapeutic Communication. New York, W. W. Norton Co., 1961.

Ruesch, J., and Bateson, G.: Communication: The Social Matrix of Psychiatry. New York, W. W. Norton Co., 1951.

Sabshin, M., and Miller, A. A.: Psychotherapy in psychiatric hospitals. Archives of General Psychiatry, *9*:71–81, July 1963.

Satir, V.: Conjoint Family Therapy. Palo Alto, California, Science and Behavior Books, 1967.

Sheehy, G.: Passages: Predictable Crises of Adult Life. New York, E. P. Dutton and Company, 1976.

Shneidman, E. (ed.): Suicodology: Contemporary Development. New York, Grune and Stratton, 1976.

Smythies, J. R.: Brain Mechanisms and Behavior: An Outline of the Mechanisms of Emotion, Memory, Learning, and Origins of Behavior. New York, Academic Press, 1970.

Snyder, J., and Wilson, M.: Elements of a psychological assessment. American Journal of Nursing, *77*:235–239, 1977.

Spiegel, R.: Anger and acting out: masks of depression. American Journal of Psychotherapy, *21*:597–606, July 1967.

Stein, L., and Wise, C. D.: Possible etiology of schizophrenia: progressive damage to the noradrenergic reward system by 6-hydroxydopamine. Science, *177*:1032–1036, March 12, 1971.

Steiner, C.: Games Alcoholics Play. New York, Grove Press, Inc., 1971.

Stuart, R. B.: Behavior control of overeating. Behavior Research and Therapy, *5*:357–365, 1967.

Stunkard, A., and Burt, V.: Obesity and the body image. II. Age at onset of disturbances in the body image. American Journal of Psychiatry, *123*:1443–1447, May 1967.

Sullivan, H. S.: Collected Works. New York, W. W. Norton Co., 1965.

Sullivan, H. S.: Schizophrenia as a Human Process. New York, W. W. Norton Co., 1962.

Sullivan, H. S.: The Interpersonal Theory of Psychiatry. Perry, H. S. and Gawel, M. L., eds. New York, W. W. Norton Co., 1953.

Susser, M. W.: Community Psychiatry: Epidemiologic and Social Themes. New York, Random House, 1968.

Tallman, I.: The family as a small problem solving group. Journal of Marriage and the Family, *32*:94, February 1970.

Thompson, C.: The different schools of psychoanalysis. American Journal of Nursing, *57*:1304–1307, October 1957.

Walker, L.: Crisis of change: A case study of a heroin-dependent patient. Perspectives in Psychiatric Care, *12*:20–25, 1974.

Weiner, Irving B.: Psychological Disturbances in Adolescence. New York, Wiley Interscience, 1970.

Whitaker, D., and Lieberman, M.: Psychotherapy through the Group Process. New York, Atherton Press, 1964.

Yowell, S., and Brose, C.: Working with drug abuse patients in the ER. American Journal of Nursing, *77*:82–85, 1977.

Zalss, A., et al.: Treatment of opiate dependence with high dose oral naloxone. Journal of the American Medical Association, *215*:2108–2110, March 24, 1971.

Zinberg, N. E., ed.: Psychiatry and Medical Practice in a General Hospital. New York, International Universities Press, 1964.

Index

NAME _____ LAST _____ FIRST _____ MIDDLE _____ DATE OF BIRTH _____ AGE _____ SEX _____ M OR F

SCHOOL _____ CITY _____ GRADE OR CLASS _____ INSTRUCTOR _____

NAME OF TEST _____ PART _____

SCORES

1	5
2	6
3	7
4	8

DIRECTIONS: Read each question and its numbered answers. When you have decided which answer is correct, blacken the corresponding space on this sheet with the special pencil. Make your mark as long as the pair of lines, and move the pencil point up and down firmly to make a heavy black line. If you change your mind, erase your first mark completely. Make no stray marks; they may count against you.

SAMPLE:

1—1 a country
1—2 a mountain
1—3 an island
1—4 a city
1—5 a state

1. Chicago is

BE SURE YOUR MARKS ARE HEAVY AND BLACK.
ERASE COMPLETELY ANY ANSWER YOU WISH TO CHANGE.

(Answer grid: items 1–90, each with choices 1 2 3 4, arranged in three columns: 1–30, 31–60, 61–90)

IBM FORM I.T.S. 1000 B 108

	1	2	3	4		1	2	3	4		1	2	3	4		1	2	3	4		1	2	3	4
91					117					143					169					195				
92					118					144					170					196				
93					119					145					171					197				
94					120					146					172					198				
95					121					147					173					199				
96					122					148					174					200				
97					123					149					175					201				
98					124					150					176					202				
99					125					151					177					203				
100					126					152					178					204				
101					127					153					179					205				
102					128					154					180					206				
103					129					155					181					207				
104					130					156					182					208				
105					131					157					183					209				
106					132					158					184					210				
107					133					159					185					211				
108					134					160					186					212				
109					135					161					187					213				
110					136					162					188					214				
111					137					163					189					215				
112					138					164					190					216				
113					139					165					191					217				
114					140					166					192									
115					141					167					193									
116					142					168					194									

NAME _____ DATE _____

     LAST   FIRST   MIDDLE

SCHOOL _____ CITY _____

1 _____ 2 _____

DATE OF BIRTH _____ AGE _____ SEX _____

                                       M OR F

GRADE OR CLASS _____ INSTRUCTOR _____ PART _____

NAME OF TEST _____

SCORES

1	_____	5	_____
2	_____	6	_____
3	_____	7	_____
4	_____	8	_____

DIRECTIONS: Read each question and its numbered answers. When you have decided which answer is correct, blacken the corresponding space on this sheet with the special pencil. Make your mark as long as the pair of lines, and move the pencil point up and down firmly to make a heavy black line. If you change your mind, erase your first mark completely. Make no stray marks; they may count against you.

SAMPLE:

1—1 a country
1—2 a mountain
1—3 an island
1—4 a city
1—5 a state

1. Chicago is

1 ::::
1 2 3 4 5 :::: ▌ ::::

BE SURE YOUR MARKS ARE HEAVY AND BLACK.
ERASE COMPLETELY ANY ANSWER YOU WISH TO CHANGE.

#	1	2	3	4
1				
2				
3				
4				
5				
6				
7				
8				
9				
10				
11				
12				
13				
14				
15				
16				
17				
18				
19				
20				
21				
22				
23				
24				
25				
26				
27				
28				
29				
30				

#	1	2	3	4
31				
32				
33				
34				
35				
36				
37				
38				
39				
40				
41				
42				
43				
44				
45				
46				
47				
48				
49				
50				
51				
52				
53				
54				
55				
56				
57				
58				
59				
60				

#	1	2	3	4
61				
62				
63			▬	
64				
65				
66				
67				
68				
69				
70				
71				
72				
73				
74				
75				
76				
77				
78				
79				
80				
81				
82				
83				
84				
85				
86				
87				
88				
89				
90				

IBM FORM I.T.S. 1000 B 108

NAME _____
LAST   FIRST   MIDDLE   DATE _____

SCHOOL _____ CITY _____

DATE OF BIRTH _____ AGE _____ SEX _____ M OR F

GRADE OR CLASS _____ INSTRUCTOR _____

NAME OF TEST _____ PART _____

SCORES

1	5
2	6
3	7
4	8

DIRECTIONS: Read each question and its numbered answers. When you have decided which answer is correct, blacken the corresponding space on this sheet with the special pencil. Make your mark as long as the pair of lines, and move the pencil point up and down firmly to make a heavy black line. If you change your mind, erase your first mark completely. Make no stray marks; they may count against you.

SAMPLE:

1—1 a country
1—2 a mountain
1—3 an island
1—4 a city
1—5 a state

1. Chicago is

1   2   3   4   5

1 ▦

BE SURE YOUR MARKS ARE HEAVY AND BLACK.
ERASE COMPLETELY ANY ANSWER YOU WISH TO CHANGE.

Questions 1–30 (columns 1 2 3 4)
Questions 31–60 (columns 1 2 3 4)
Questions 61–90 (columns 1 2 3 4)

1 2 3 4 ... 31 ... 61
(answer grid 1 through 90)

IBM FORM I.T.S. 1000 B 108

A-5

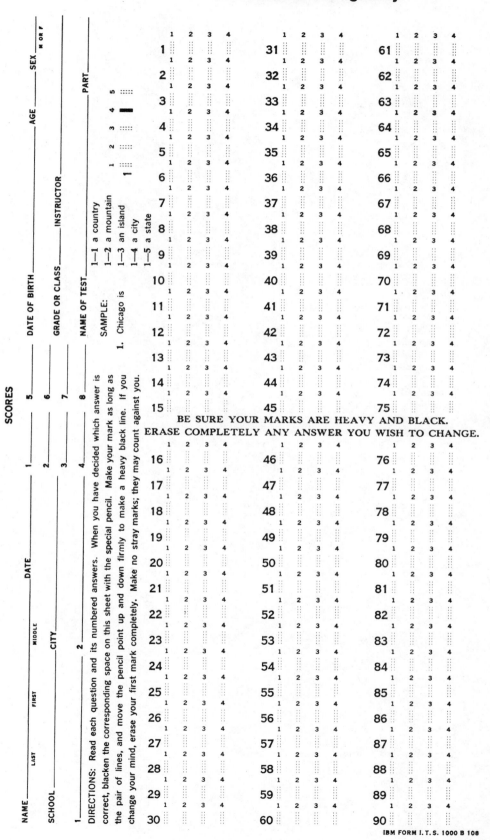

NAME _____
LAST   FIRST   MIDDLE

SCHOOL _____
CITY

DATE _____

DATE OF BIRTH _____

AGE _____ SEX _____ M OR F

GRADE OR CLASS _____ INSTRUCTOR _____

NAME OF TEST _____ PART _____

SCORES

1	5
2	6
3	7
4	8

DIRECTIONS: Read each question and its numbered answers. When you have decided which answer is correct, blacken the corresponding space on this sheet with the special pencil. Make your mark as long as the pair of lines, and move the pencil point up and down firmly to make a heavy black line. If you change your mind, erase your first mark completely. Make no stray marks; they may count against you.

SAMPLE:
1—1 a country
1—2 a mountain
1—3 an island
1—4 a city
1—5 a state

1. Chicago is

BE SURE YOUR MARKS ARE HEAVY AND BLACK.
ERASE COMPLETELY ANY ANSWER YOU WISH TO CHANGE.

IBM FORM I. T. S. 1000 B 108

NAME _____

LAST   FIRST   MIDDLE   DATE _____

SCHOOL _____

CITY _____

DATE OF BIRTH _____   AGE _____   SEX M OR F

GRADE OR CLASS _____   INSTRUCTOR _____

NAME OF TEST _____   PART _____

SCORES

1 _____ 5 _____
2 _____ 6 _____
3 _____ 7 _____
4 _____ 8 _____

DIRECTIONS: Read each question and its numbered answers. When you have decided which answer is correct, blacken the corresponding space on this sheet with the special pencil. Make your mark as long as the pair of lines, and move the pencil point up and down firmly to make a heavy black line. If you change your mind, erase your first mark completely. Make no stray marks; they may count against you.

SAMPLE:

1. Chicago is

1—1 a country
1—2 a mountain
1—3 an island
1—4 a city
1—5 a state

1 1 ═══ 2 ┊┊ 3 ┊┊ 4 ┊┊ 5 ┊┊

BE SURE YOUR MARKS ARE HEAVY AND BLACK.
ERASE COMPLETELY ANY ANSWER YOU WISH TO CHANGE.

1–30	31–60	61–90
1	31	61
2	32	62
3	33	63
4	34	64
5	35	65
6	36	66
7	37	67
8	38	68
9	39	69
10	40	70
11	41	71
12	42	72
13	43	73
14	44	74
15	45	75
16	46	76
17	47	77
18	48	78
19	49	79
20	50	80
21	51	81
22	52	82
23	53	83
24	54	84
25	55	85
26	56	86
27	57	87
28	58	88
29	59	89
30	60	90

(Each item provides answer choices 1, 2, 3, 4)

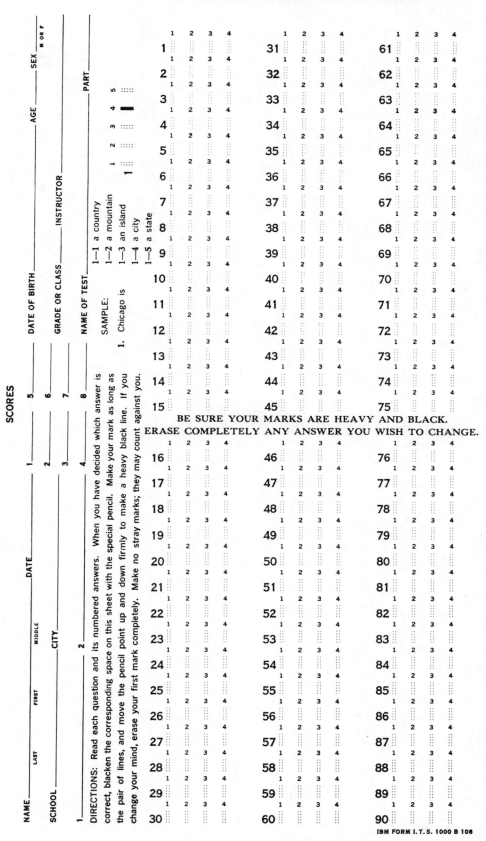

NAME _____
LAST   FIRST   MIDDLE

SCHOOL _____

DATE _____

CITY _____

DATE OF BIRTH _____

GRADE OR CLASS _____ INSTRUCTOR _____

NAME OF TEST _____

AGE _____ SEX   M OR F

PART _____

SCORES

1	5
2	6
3	7
4	8

DIRECTIONS: Read each question and its numbered answers. When you have decided which answer is correct, blacken the corresponding space on this sheet with the special pencil. Make your mark as long as the pair of lines, and move the pencil point up and down firmly to make a heavy black line. If you change your mind, erase your first mark completely. Make no stray marks; they may count against you.

SAMPLE:

1. Chicago is

1—1 a country
1—2 a mountain
1—3 an island
1—4 a city
1—5 a state

BE SURE YOUR MARKS ARE HEAVY AND BLACK.
ERASE COMPLETELY ANY ANSWER YOU WISH TO CHANGE.

IBM FORM I.T.S. 1000 B 108

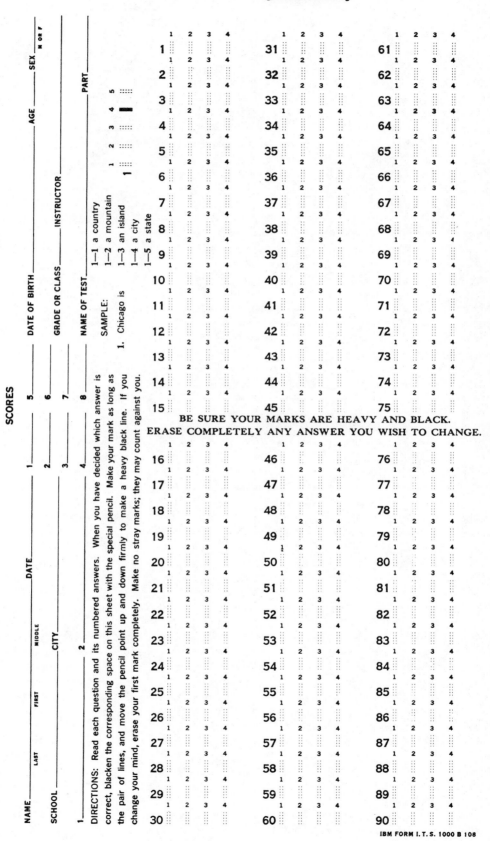

SCORES

1	5
2	6
3	7
4	8

NAME ___ LAST ___ FIRST ___ MIDDLE ___ DATE ___

SCHOOL ___ CITY ___

DATE OF BIRTH ___ AGE ___ SEX ___ M OR F

GRADE OR CLASS ___ INSTRUCTOR ___

NAME OF TEST ___ PART ___

DIRECTIONS: Read each question and its numbered answers. When you have decided which answer is correct, blacken the corresponding space on this sheet with the special pencil. Make your mark as long as the pair of lines, and move the pencil point up and down firmly to make a heavy black line. If you change your mind, erase your first mark completely. Make no stray marks; they may count against you.

SAMPLE:

1—1 a country
1—2 a mountain
1—3 an island
1—4 a city
1—5 a state

1. Chicago is

BE SURE YOUR MARKS ARE HEAVY AND BLACK.
ERASE COMPLETELY ANY ANSWER YOU WISH TO CHANGE.

IBM FORM I.T.S. 1000 B 108

A-13

NAME _____ LAST _____ FIRST _____ MIDDLE _____ DATE _____

SCHOOL _____ CITY _____

DATE OF BIRTH _____ AGE _____ SEX M OR F

GRADE OR CLASS _____ INSTRUCTOR _____

NAME OF TEST _____ PART _____

SCORES

1 ___ 5 ___
2 ___ 6 ___
3 ___ 7 ___
4 ___ 8 ___

DIRECTIONS: Read each question and its numbered answers. When you have decided which answer is correct, blacken the corresponding space on this sheet with the special pencil. Make your mark as long as the pair of lines, and move the pencil point up and down firmly to make a heavy black line. If you change your mind, erase your first mark completely. Make no stray marks; they may count against you.

SAMPLE:

1—1 a country
1—2 a mountain
1—3 an island
1—4 a city
1—5 a state

1. Chicago is

1 2 3 4 5

1 ::::

BE SURE YOUR MARKS ARE HEAVY AND BLACK.
ERASE COMPLETELY ANY ANSWER YOU WISH TO CHANGE.

	1	2	3	4		1	2	3	4		1	2	3	4
1					31					61				
2					32					62				
3					33					63				
4					34					64				
5					35					65				
6					36					66				
7					37					67				
8					38					68				
9					39					69				
10					40					70				
11					41					71				
12					42					72				
13					43					73				
14					44					74				
15					45					75				
16					46					76				
17					47					77				
18					48					78				
19					49					79				
20					50					80				
21					51					81				
22					52					82				
23					53					83				
24					54					84				
25					55					85				
26					56					86				
27					57					87				
28					58					88				
29					59					89				
30					60					90				

IBM FORM I.T.S. 1000 B 108

1 Postpartum Adjustment

SCORES

NAME ______ (LAST) ______ (FIRST) ______ (MIDDLE) ______ DATE ______ 1 ______ 5 ______ DATE OF BIRTH ______ AGE ______ SEX ______ (M OR F)

SCHOOL ______ CITY ______ 2 ______ 6 ______ GRADE OR CLASS ______ INSTRUCTOR ______

3 ______ 7 ______

1 ______ 2 ______ 4 ______ 8 ______ NAME OF TEST ______ PART ______

DIRECTIONS: Read each question and its numbered answers. When you have decided which answer is correct, blacken the corresponding space on this sheet with the special pencil. Make your mark as long as the pair of lines, and move the pencil point up and down firmly to make a heavy black line. If you change your mind, erase your first mark completely. Make no stray marks; they may count against you.

SAMPLE:

1. Chicago is
1—1 a country
1—2 a mountain
1—3 an island
1—4 a city
1—5 a state

1 2 3 4 5 (answer 4 marked)

Item	Choices	Item	Choices	Item	Choices
1	1 2 3 4	31	1 2 3 4	61	1 2 3 4
2	1 2 3 4	32	1 2 3 4	62	1 2 3 4
3	1 2 3 4	33	1 2 3 4	63	1 2 3 4
4	1 2 3 4	34	1 2 3 4	64	1 2 3 4
5	1 2 3 4	35	1 2 3 4	65	1 2 3 4
6	1 2 3 4	36	1 2 3 4	66	1 2 3 4
7	1 2 3 4	37	1 2 3 4	67	1 2 3 4
8	1 2 3 4	38	1 2 3 4	68	1 2 3 4
9	1 2 3 4	39	1 2 3 4	69	1 2 3 4
10	1 2 3 4	40	1 2 3 4	70	1 2 3 4
11	1 2 3 4	41	1 2 3 4	71	1 2 3 4
12	1 2 3 4	42	1 2 3 4	72	1 2 3 4
13	1 2 3 4	43	1 2 3 4	73	1 2 3 4
14	1 2 3 4	44	1 2 3 4	74	1 2 3 4
15	1 2 3 4	45	1 2 3 4	75	1 2 3 4

BE SURE YOUR MARKS ARE HEAVY AND BLACK.
ERASE COMPLETELY ANY ANSWER YOU WISH TO CHANGE.

Item	Choices	Item	Choices	Item	Choices
16	1 2 3 4	46	1 2 3 4	76	1 2 3 4
17	1 2 3 4	47	1 2 3 4	77	1 2 3 4
18	1 2 3 4	48	1 2 3 4	78	1 2 3 4
19	1 2 3 4	49	1 2 3 4	79	1 2 3 4
20	1 2 3 4	50	1 2 3 4	80	1 2 3 4
21	1 2 3 4	51	1 2 3 4	81	1 2 3 4
22	1 2 3 4	52	1 2 3 4	82	1 2 3 4
23	1 2 3 4	53	1 2 3 4	83	1 2 3 4
24	1 2 3 4	54	1 2 3 4	84	1 2 3 4
25	1 2 3 4	55	1 2 3 4	85	1 2 3 4
26	1 2 3 4	56	1 2 3 4	86	1 2 3 4
27	1 2 3 4	57	1 2 3 4	87	1 2 3 4
28	1 2 3 4	58	1 2 3 4	88	1 2 3 4
29	1 2 3 4	59	1 2 3 4	89	1 2 3 4
30	1 2 3 4	60	1 2 3 4	90	1 2 3 4

IBM FORM I.T.S. 1000 B 108

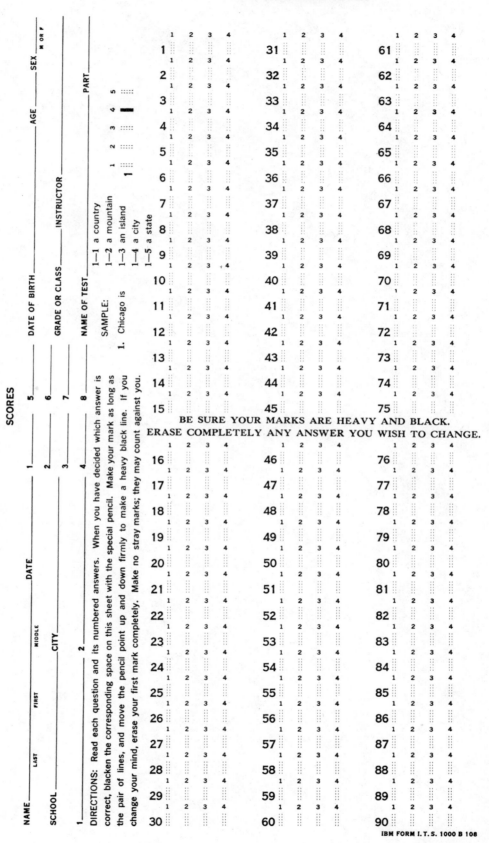

NAME _____ LAST _____ FIRST _____ MIDDLE _____ DATE _____

SCHOOL _____ CITY _____ GRADE OR CLASS _____ INSTRUCTOR _____ DATE OF BIRTH _____ AGE _____ SEX _____ M OR F

NAME OF TEST _____ PART _____

SCORES

1	5
2	6
3	7
4	8

DIRECTIONS: Read each question and its numbered answers. When you have decided which answer is correct, blacken the corresponding space on this sheet with the special pencil. Make your mark as long as the pair of lines, and move the pencil point up and down firmly to make a heavy black line. If you change your mind, erase your first mark completely. Make no stray marks; they may count against you.

SAMPLE:
1—1 a country
1—2 a mountain
1—3 an island
1—4 a city
1—5 a state

1. Chicago is

BE SURE YOUR MARKS ARE HEAVY AND BLACK.
ERASE COMPLETELY ANY ANSWER YOU WISH TO CHANGE.

IBM FORM I. T. S. 1000 B 108

A-19

NAME _____ DATE _____

LAST   FIRST   MIDDLE

SCHOOL _____ DATE OF BIRTH _____ AGE _____ SEX _____

CITY   GRADE OR CLASS _____ INSTRUCTOR _____ M OR F

SCORES

1 _____ 5 _____
2 _____ 6 _____
3 _____ 7 _____
4 _____ 8 _____

1 _____ 2 _____

DIRECTIONS: Read each question and its numbered answers. When you have decided which answer is correct, blacken the corresponding space on this sheet with the special pencil. Make your mark as long as the pair of lines, and move the pencil point up and down firmly to make a heavy black line. If you change your mind, erase your first mark completely. Make no stray marks; they may count against you.

NAME OF TEST _____ PART _____

SAMPLE:

1—1 a country
1—2 a mountain
1—3 an island
1—4 a city
1—5 a state

1. Chicago is

1 ┊:::┊
2 ┊:::┊
3 ▬▬
4 ┊:::┊
5 ┊:::┊

	1	2	3	4		1	2	3	4		1	2	3	4
1					31					61				
2					32					62				
3					33					63				
4					34					64				
5					35					65				
6					36					66				
7					37					67				
8					38					68				
9					39					69				
10					40					70				
11					41					71				
12					42					72				
13					43					73				
14					44					74				
15					45					75				

BE SURE YOUR MARKS ARE HEAVY AND BLACK.
ERASE COMPLETELY ANY ANSWER YOU WISH TO CHANGE.

	1	2	3	4		1	2	3	4		1	2	3	4
16					46					76				
17					47					77				
18					48					78				
19					49					79				
20					50					80				
21					51					81				
22					52					82				
23					53					83				
24					54					84				
25					55					85				
26					56					86				
27					57					87				
28					58					88				
29					59					89				
30					60					90				

IBM FORM I.T.S. 1000 B 108

NAME _____ DATE _____

LAST   FIRST   MIDDLE

SCHOOL _____ CITY _____

DATE OF BIRTH _____ AGE _____ SEX __ OR F

GRADE OR CLASS _____ INSTRUCTOR _____

NAME OF TEST _____ PART _____

SCORES

1	5
2	6
3	7
4	8

DIRECTIONS: Read each question and its numbered answers. When you have decided which answer is correct, blacken the corresponding space on this sheet with the special pencil. Make your mark as long as the pair of lines, and move the pencil point up and down firmly to make a heavy black line. If you change your mind, erase your first mark completely. Make no stray marks; they may count against you.

SAMPLE:
1—1 a country
1—2 a mountain
1—3 an island
1—4 a city
1—5 a state

1. Chicago is

BE SURE YOUR MARKS ARE HEAVY AND BLACK.
ERASE COMPLETELY ANY ANSWER YOU WISH TO CHANGE.

(Answer grid, columns 1–4 for items 1 through 90)

1 2 3 4 ... 31 ... 61
2 ... 32 ... 62
3 ... 33 ... 63
4 ... 34 ... 64
5 ... 35 ... 65
6 ... 36 ... 66
7 ... 37 ... 67
8 ... 38 ... 68
9 ... 39 ... 69
10 ... 40 ... 70
11 ... 41 ... 71
12 ... 42 ... 72
13 ... 43 ... 73
14 ... 44 ... 74
15 ... 45 ... 75
16 ... 46 ... 76
17 ... 47 ... 77
18 ... 48 ... 78
19 ... 49 ... 79
20 ... 50 ... 80
21 ... 51 ... 81
22 ... 52 ... 82
23 ... 53 ... 83
24 ... 54 ... 84
25 ... 55 ... 85
26 ... 56 ... 86
27 ... 57 ... 87
28 ... 58 ... 88
29 ... 59 ... 89
30 ... 60 ... 90

IBM FORM I.T.S. 1000 B 108

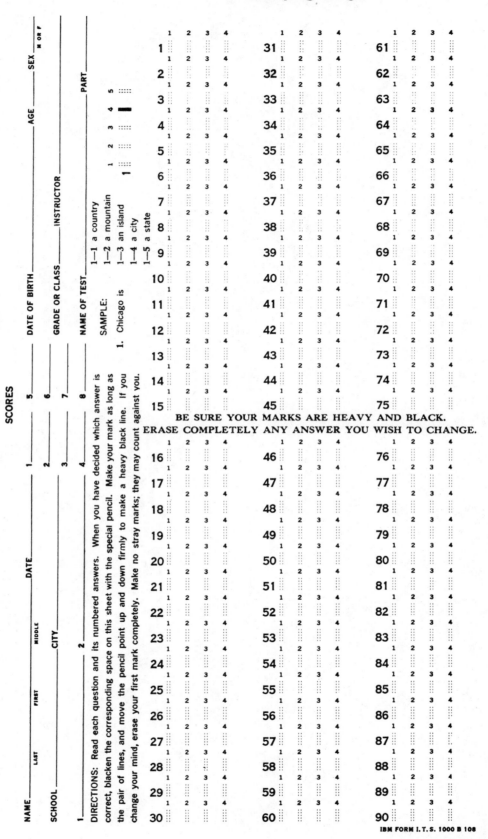

SCORES

1	5
2	6
3	7
4	8

NAME _____ LAST ___ FIRST ___ MIDDLE ___ DATE _____

SCHOOL _____ CITY _____

DATE OF BIRTH _____ AGE ___ SEX M OR F

GRADE OR CLASS _____ INSTRUCTOR _____

NAME OF TEST _____ PART _____

DIRECTIONS: Read each question and its numbered answers. When you have decided which answer is correct, blacken the corresponding space on this sheet with the special pencil. Make your mark as long as the pair of lines, and move the pencil point up and down firmly to make a heavy black line. If you change your mind, erase your first mark completely. Make no stray marks; they may count against you.

SAMPLE:

1—1 a country
1—2 a mountain
1—3 an island
1—4 a city
1—5 a state

1. Chicago is

BE SURE YOUR MARKS ARE HEAVY AND BLACK.
ERASE COMPLETELY ANY ANSWER YOU WISH TO CHANGE.

IBM FORM I.T.S. 1000 B 108

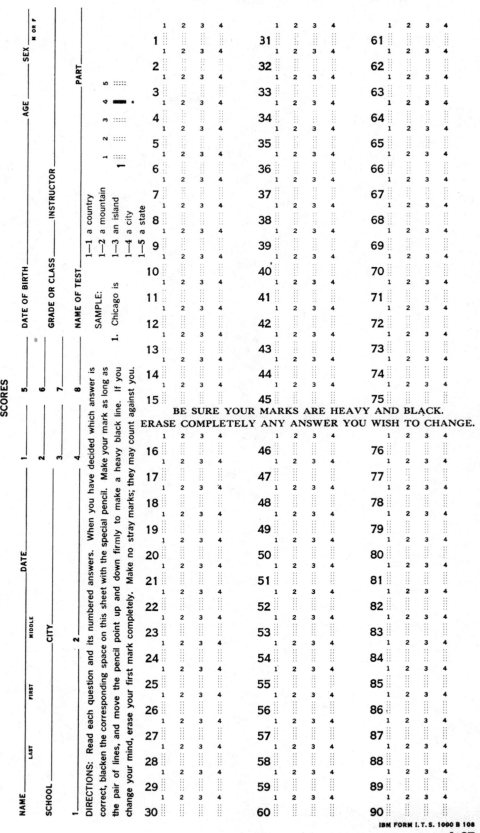

SCORES

	1	5
	2	6
	3	7
	4	8

NAME _____ LAST _____ FIRST _____ MIDDLE _____ DATE _____

SCHOOL _____ CITY _____

DATE OF BIRTH _____ AGE _____ SEX M OR F

GRADE OR CLASS _____ INSTRUCTOR _____

NAME OF TEST _____ PART _____

DIRECTIONS: Read each question and its numbered answers. When you have decided which answer is correct, blacken the corresponding space on this sheet with the special pencil. Make your mark as long as the pair of lines, and move the pencil point up and down firmly to make a heavy black line. If you change your mind, erase your first mark completely. Make no stray marks; they may count against you.

SAMPLE:

1. Chicago is

1—1 a country
1—2 a mountain
1—3 an island
1—4 a city
1—5 a state

BE SURE YOUR MARKS ARE HEAVY AND BLACK.
ERASE COMPLETELY ANY ANSWER YOU WISH TO CHANGE.

IBM FORM I. T. S. 1000 B 108

A-27

SCORES

1	5
2	6
3	7
4	8

NAME _____
LAST   FIRST   MIDDLE

DATE _____

SCHOOL _____
CITY _____

DATE OF BIRTH _____   AGE _____   SEX _____ M OR F

GRADE OR CLASS _____   INSTRUCTOR _____

NAME OF TEST _____   PART _____

DIRECTIONS: Read each question and its numbered answers. When you have decided which answer is correct, blacken the corresponding space on this sheet with the special pencil. Make your mark as long as the pair of lines, and move the pencil point up and down firmly to make a heavy black line. If you change your mind, erase your first mark completely. Make no stray marks; they may count against you.

SAMPLE:

1—1 a country
1—2 a mountain
1—3 an island
1—4 a city
1—5 a state

1. Chicago is

1 :::::
    1   2   3   4   5
         :::::   ▨   :::::

BE SURE YOUR MARKS ARE HEAVY AND BLACK.
ERASE COMPLETELY ANY ANSWER YOU WISH TO CHANGE.

Answer grid columns (1 2 3 4):

1–15, 31–45, 61–75 (first block)

16–30, 46–60, 76–90 (second block)

IBM FORM I. T. S. 1000 B 108

SCORES

1	5
2	6
3	7
4	8

NAME _____ DATE _____

    LAST   FIRST   MIDDLE

SCHOOL _____ CITY _____

DATE OF BIRTH _____ AGE _____ SEX ___ M OR F

GRADE OR CLASS _____ INSTRUCTOR _____

NAME OF TEST _____ PART _____

DIRECTIONS: Read each question and its numbered answers. When you have decided which answer is correct, blacken the corresponding space on this sheet with the special pencil. Make your mark as long as the pair of lines, and move the pencil point up and down firmly to make a heavy black line. If you change your mind, erase your first mark completely. Make no stray marks; they may count against you.

SAMPLE:

1—1 a country
1—2 a mountain
1—3 an island
1—4 a city
1—5 a state

1. Chicago is

    1   2   3   4   5

BE SURE YOUR MARKS ARE HEAVY AND BLACK.
ERASE COMPLETELY ANY ANSWER YOU WISH TO CHANGE.

Questions 1–90, each with answer columns 1 2 3 4.

#					#					#			
1	1 2 3 4				31	1 2 3 4				61	1 2 3 4		
2	1 2 3 4				32	1 2 3 4				62	1 2 3 4		
3	1 2 3 4				33	1 2 3 4				63	1 2 3 4		
4	1 2 3 4				34	1 2 3 4				64	1 2 3 4		
5	1 2 3 4				35	1 2 3 4				65	1 2 3 4		
6	1 2 3 4				36	1 2 3 4				66	1 2 3 4		
7	1 2 3 4				37	1 2 3 4				67	1 2 3 4		
8	1 2 3 4				38	1 2 3 4				68	1 2 3 4		
9	1 2 3 4				39	1 2 3 4				69	1 2 3 4		
10	1 2 3 4				40	1 2 3 4				70	1 2 3 4		
11	1 2 3 4				41	1 2 3 4				71	1 2 3 4		
12	1 2 3 4				42	1 2 3 4				72	1 2 3 4		
13	1 2 3 4				43	1 2 3 4				73	1 2 3 4		
14	1 2 3 4				44	1 2 3 4				74	1 2 3 4		
15	1 2 3 4				45	1 2 3 4				75	1 2 3 4		
16	1 2 3 4				46	1 2 3 4				76	1 2 3 4		
17	1 2 3 4				47	1 2 3 4				77	1 2 3 4		
18	1 2 3 4				48	1 2 3 4				78	1 2 3 4		
19	1 2 3 4				49	1 2 3 4				79	1 2 3 4		
20	1 2 3 4				50	1 2 3 4				80	1 2 3 4		
21	1 2 3 4				51	1 2 3 4				81	1 2 3 4		
22	1 2 3 4				52	1 2 3 4				82	1 2 3 4		
23	1 2 3 4				53	1 2 3 4				83	1 2 3 4		
24	1 2 3 4				54	1 2 3 4				84	1 2 3 4		
25	1 2 3 4				55	1 2 3 4				85	1 2 3 4		
26	1 2 3 4				56	1 2 3 4				86	1 2 3 4		
27	1 2 3 4				57	1 2 3 4				87	1 2 3 4		
28	1 2 3 4				58	1 2 3 4				88	1 2 3 4		
29	1 2 3 4				59	1 2 3 4				89	1 2 3 4		
30	1 2 3 4				60	1 2 3 4				90	1 2 3 4		

IBM FORM I. T. S. 1000 B 108

SCORES

1	5
2	6
3	7
4	8

NAME _____ LAST _____ FIRST _____ MIDDLE _____ DATE _____

SCHOOL _____ CITY _____

DATE OF BIRTH _____ AGE _____ SEX M OR F

GRADE OR CLASS _____ INSTRUCTOR _____

NAME OF TEST _____ PART _____

DIRECTIONS: Read each question and its numbered answers. When you have decided which answer is correct, blacken the corresponding space on this sheet with the special pencil. Make your mark as long as the pair of lines, and move the pencil point up and down firmly to make a heavy black line. If you change your mind, erase your first mark completely. Make no stray marks; they may count against you.

SAMPLE:

1. Chicago is

1—1 a country
1—2 a mountain
1—3 an island
1—4 a city
1—5 a state

BE SURE YOUR MARKS ARE HEAVY AND BLACK.
ERASE COMPLETELY ANY ANSWER YOU WISH TO CHANGE.

(Answer grid, questions 1–90, columns labeled 1 2 3 4)

IBM FORM I.T.S. 1000 B 108

A-33

NAME _____
LAST   FIRST   MIDDLE   DATE _____

SCHOOL _____ CITY _____

SCORES

1 ___ 5 ___
2 ___ 6 ___
3 ___ 7 ___
4 ___ 8 ___

DATE OF BIRTH _____ AGE _____ SEX M OR F

GRADE OR CLASS _____ INSTRUCTOR _____

NAME OF TEST _____ PART _____

DIRECTIONS: Read each question and its numbered answers. When you have decided which answer is correct, blacken the corresponding space on this sheet with the special pencil. Make your mark as long as the pair of lines, and move the pencil point up and down firmly to make a heavy black line. If you change your mind, erase your first mark completely. Make no stray marks; they may count against you.

SAMPLE:

1—1 a country
1—2 a mountain
1—3 an island
1—4 a city
1—5 a state

1. Chicago is

	1	2	3	4	5
1	┊	┊	┊	▅	┊

BE SURE YOUR MARKS ARE HEAVY AND BLACK.
ERASE COMPLETELY ANY ANSWER YOU WISH TO CHANGE.

Items 1–90, each with answer choices 1 2 3 4:

1–30, 31–60, 61–90

IBM FORM I.T.S. 1000 B 108

A-35

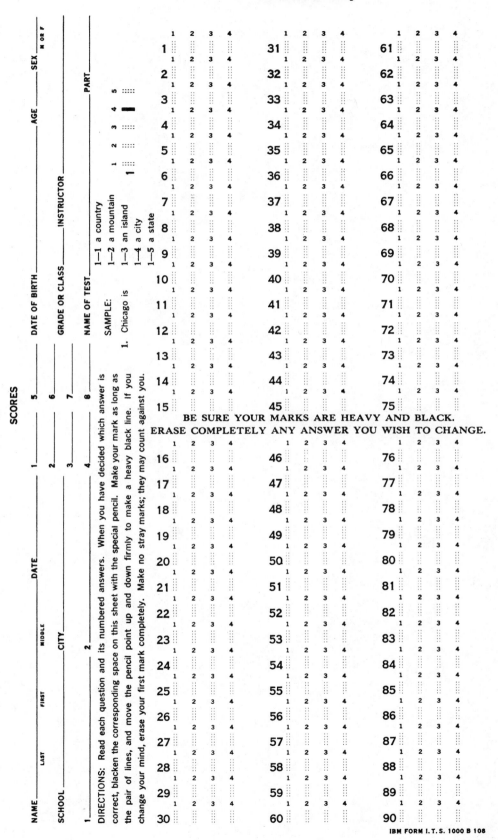

SCORES

NAME _____ LAST _____ FIRST _____ MIDDLE _____ DATE _____

SCHOOL _____ CITY _____

DATE OF BIRTH _____ AGE _____ SEX _____ M OR F

GRADE OR CLASS _____ INSTRUCTOR _____

NAME OF TEST _____ PART _____

DIRECTIONS: Read each question and its numbered answers. When you have decided which answer is correct, blacken the corresponding space on this sheet with the special pencil. Make your mark as long as the pair of lines, and move the pencil point up and down firmly to make a heavy black line. If you change your mind, erase your first mark completely. Make no stray marks; they may count against you.

SAMPLE:

1—1 a country
1—2 a mountain
1—3 an island
1—4 a city
1—5 a state

1. Chicago is

BE SURE YOUR MARKS ARE HEAVY AND BLACK.
ERASE COMPLETELY ANY ANSWER YOU WISH TO CHANGE.

IBM FORM I.T.S. 1000 B 108

NAME _____ DATE _____ AGE _____ SEX ___ M OR F

LAST   FIRST   MIDDLE

SCHOOL _____ CITY _____ DATE OF BIRTH _____

GRADE OR CLASS _____ INSTRUCTOR _____

1 _____   2 _____   NAME OF TEST _____ PART _____

SCORES

1 ___ 5 ___
2 ___ 6 ___
3 ___ 7 ___
4 ___ 8 ___

DIRECTIONS: Read each question and its numbered answers. When you have decided which answer is correct, blacken the corresponding space on this sheet with the special pencil. Make your mark as long as the pair of lines, and move the pencil point up and down firmly to make a heavy black line. If you change your mind, erase your first mark completely. Make no stray marks; they may count against you.

SAMPLE:

1—1 a country
1—2 a mountain
1—3 an island
1—4 a city
1—5 a state

1. Chicago is   1 |::::| 2 |::::| 3 |▮| 4 |::::| 5 |::::|

	1	2	3	4		1	2	3	4		1	2	3	4
1					31					61				
2					32					62				
3					33					63				
4					34					64				
5					35					65				
6					36					66				
7					37					67				
8					38					68				
9					39					69				
10					40					70				
11					41					71				
12					42					72				
13					43					73				
14					44					74				
15					45					75				

BE SURE YOUR MARKS ARE HEAVY AND BLACK.
ERASE COMPLETELY ANY ANSWER YOU WISH TO CHANGE.

	1	2	3	4		1	2	3	4		1	2	3	4
16					46					76				
17					47					77				
18					48					78				
19					49					79				
20					50					80				
21					51					81				
22					52					82				
23					53					83				
24					54					84				
25					55					85				
26					56					86				
27					57					87				
28					58					88				
29					59					89				
30					60					90				

IBM FORM I. T. S. 1000 B 108

A-39

NAME _____ LAST ___ FIRST. ___ MIDDLE ___ DATE _____

SCHOOL _____ CITY _____

DATE OF BIRTH _____ AGE ___ SEX ___ M OR F

GRADE OR CLASS _____ INSTRUCTOR _____

NAME OF TEST _____ PART _____

SCORES

1	5
2	6
3	7
4	8

DIRECTIONS: Read each question and its numbered answers. When you have decided which answer is correct, blacken the corresponding space on this sheet with the special pencil. Make your mark as long as the pair of lines, and move the pencil point up and down firmly to make a heavy black line. If you change your mind, erase your first mark completely. Make no stray marks; they may count against you.

SAMPLE:

1. Chicago is

1—1 a country
1—2 a mountain
1—3 an island
1—4 a city
1—5 a state

```
          1  2  3  4  5
       1  ⋮  ⋮  ⋮  ⋮  ⋮
```

BE SURE YOUR MARKS ARE HEAVY AND BLACK.
ERASE COMPLETELY ANY ANSWER YOU WISH TO CHANGE.

Questions 1–90, each with answer columns 1 2 3 4

1, 2, 3, 4, 5, 6, 7, 8, 9, 10, 11, 12, 13, 14, 15, 16, 17, 18, 19, 20, 21, 22, 23, 24, 25, 26, 27, 28, 29, 30

31, 32, 33, 34, 35, 36, 37, 38, 39, 40, 41, 42, 43, 44, 45, 46, 47, 48, 49, 50, 51, 52, 53, 54, 55, 56, 57, 58, 59, 60

61, 62, 63, 64, 65, 66, 67, 68, 69, 70, 71, 72, 73, 74, 75, 76, 77, 78, 79, 80, 81, 82, 83, 84, 85, 86, 87, 88, 89, 90

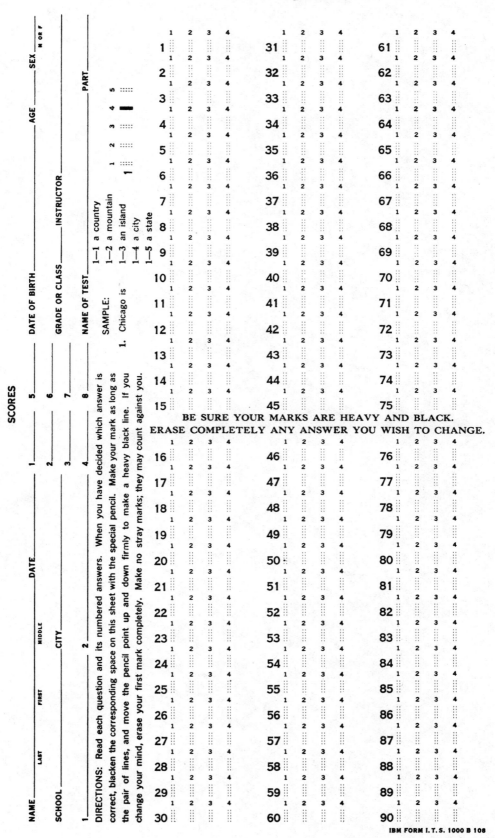

NAME _____ LAST _____ FIRST _____ MIDDLE _____ DATE _____

SCHOOL _____ CITY _____

1 _____ 2 _____

DATE OF BIRTH _____ AGE _____ SEX _____ M OR F

GRADE OR CLASS _____ INSTRUCTOR _____

NAME OF TEST _____ PART _____

SCORES

1	5
2	6
3	7
4	8

DIRECTIONS: Read each question and its numbered answers. When you have decided which answer is correct, blacken the corresponding space on this sheet with the special pencil. Make your mark as long as the pair of lines, and move the pencil point up and down firmly to make a heavy black line. If you change your mind, erase your first mark completely. Make no stray marks; they may count against you.

SAMPLE:

1—1   a country
1—2   a mountain
1—3   an island
1—4   a city
1—5   a state

1.   Chicago is

**BE SURE YOUR MARKS ARE HEAVY AND BLACK.
ERASE COMPLETELY ANY ANSWER YOU WISH TO CHANGE.**

IBM FORM I.T.S. 1000 B 108

NAME _____ DATE _____
LAST   FIRST   MIDDLE

SCHOOL _____ CITY _____

DATE OF BIRTH _____ AGE _____ SEX _____ M OR F

GRADE OR CLASS _____ INSTRUCTOR _____

NAME OF TEST _____ PART _____

SCORES

1 _____ 5 _____
2 _____ 6 _____
3 _____ 7 _____
4 _____ 8 _____

DIRECTIONS: Read each question and its numbered answers. When you have decided which answer is correct, blacken the corresponding space on this sheet with the special pencil. Make your mark as long as the pair of lines, and move the pencil point up and down firmly to make a heavy black line. If you change your mind, erase your first mark completely. Make no stray marks; they may count against you.

SAMPLE:

1—1 a country
1—2 a mountain
1—3 an island
1—4 a city
1—5 a state

1. Chicago is

1 :::: 2 :::: 3 :::: 4 :::: 5 ::::

BE SURE YOUR MARKS ARE HEAVY AND BLACK.
ERASE COMPLETELY ANY ANSWER YOU WISH TO CHANGE.

IBM FORM I.T.S. 1000 B 108

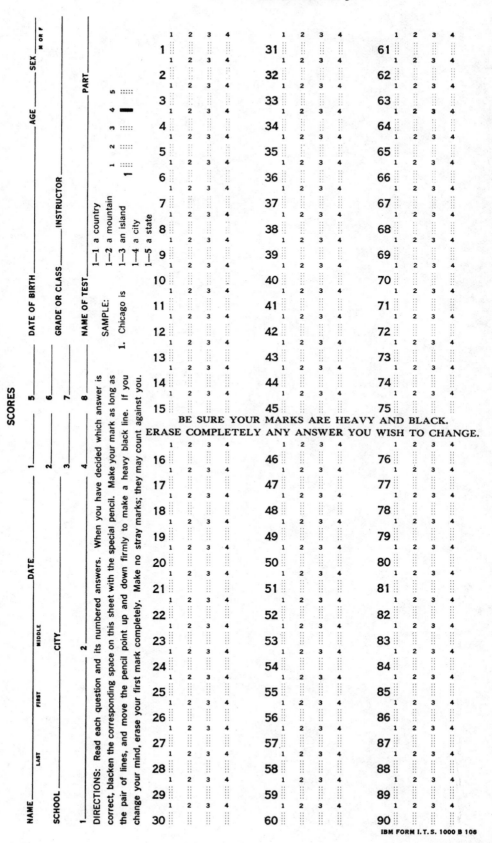

NAME _____ LAST _____ FIRST _____ MIDDLE _____ DATE _____

SCHOOL _____ CITY _____

DATE OF BIRTH _____ AGE _____ SEX M OR F

GRADE OR CLASS _____ INSTRUCTOR _____

NAME OF TEST _____ PART _____

SCORES

1	5
2	6
3	7
4	8

1 _____ 2 _____

DIRECTIONS: Read each question and its numbered answers. When you have decided which answer is correct, blacken the corresponding space on this sheet with the special pencil. Make your mark as long as the pair of lines, and move the pencil point up and down firmly to make a heavy black line. If you change your mind, erase your first mark completely. Make no stray marks; they may count against you.

SAMPLE:

1—1 a country
1—2 a mountain
1—3 an island
1—4 a city
1—5 a state

1. Chicago is

1   2   3   4   5

BE SURE YOUR MARKS ARE HEAVY AND BLACK.
ERASE COMPLETELY ANY ANSWER YOU WISH TO CHANGE.

(Answer grid items numbered 1–90, each with columns 1, 2, 3, 4)

1 2 3 4 5 6 7 8 9 10 11 12 13 14 15
16 17 18 19 20 21 22 23 24 25 26 27 28 29 30
31 32 33 34 35 36 37 38 39 40 41 42 43 44 45
46 47 48 49 50 51 52 53 54 55 56 57 58 59 60
61 62 63 64 65 66 67 68 69 70 71 72 73 74 75
76 77 78 79 80 81 82 83 84 85 86 87 88 89 90

IBM FORM I.T.S. 1000 B 108

NAME _____ DATE _____
     LAST   FIRST   MIDDLE

SCHOOL _____
                        CITY

SCORES

1 ___ 5
2 ___ 6
3 ___ 7
4 ___ 8

DATE OF BIRTH _____ AGE _____ SEX _____ M OR F

GRADE OR CLASS _____ INSTRUCTOR _____

NAME OF TEST _____ PART _____

SAMPLE:

1. Chicago is

1—1 a country
1—2 a mountain
1—3 an island
1—4 a city
1—5 a state

DIRECTIONS: Read each question and its numbered answers. When you have decided which answer is correct, blacken the corresponding space on this sheet with the special pencil. Make your mark as long as the pair of lines, and move the pencil point up and down firmly to make a heavy black line. If you change your mind, erase your first mark completely. Make no stray marks; they may count against you.

BE SURE YOUR MARKS ARE HEAVY AND BLACK.
ERASE COMPLETELY ANY ANSWER YOU WISH TO CHANGE.

Answer columns, numbered 1–90, each with options 1 2 3 4.

1–30 (first column), 31–60 (second column), 61–90 (third column).

IBM FORM I. T. S. 1000 B 108

A-49

NAME ___ LAST ___ FIRST ___ MIDDLE ___ DATE ___

SCHOOL ___ CITY ___

DATE OF BIRTH ___ AGE ___ SEX ___ M OR F

GRADE OR CLASS ___ INSTRUCTOR ___

NAME OF TEST ___ PART ___

SCORES

1	5
2	6
3	7
4	8

DIRECTIONS: Read each question and its numbered answers. When you have decided which answer is correct, blacken the corresponding space on this sheet with the special pencil. Make your mark as long as the pair of lines, and move the pencil point up and down firmly to make a heavy black line. If you change your mind, erase your first mark completely. Make no stray marks; they may count against you.

SAMPLE:

1. Chicago is

1—1 a country
1—2 a mountain
1—3 an island
1—4 a city
1—5 a state

Questions 1–90, each with answer columns 1 2 3 4.

Columns: 1–30, 31–60, 61–90.

BE SURE YOUR MARKS ARE HEAVY AND BLACK.
ERASE COMPLETELY ANY ANSWER YOU WISH TO CHANGE.

IBM FORM I. T. S. 1000 B 108

A-51

NAME _____ LAST _____ FIRST _____ MIDDLE _____ DATE _____

SCHOOL _____ CITY _____

DATE OF BIRTH _____ AGE _____ SEX _____ M OR F

GRADE OR CLASS _____ INSTRUCTOR _____

NAME OF TEST _____ PART _____

SCORES

1	5
2	6
3	7
4	8

DIRECTIONS: Read each question and its numbered answers. When you have decided which answer is correct, blacken the corresponding space on this sheet with the special pencil. Make your mark as long as the pair of lines, and move the pencil point up and down firmly to make a heavy black line. If you change your mind, erase your first mark completely. Make no stray marks; they may count against you.

SAMPLE:

1—1 a country
1—2 a mountain
1—3 an island
1—4 a city
1—5 a state

1. Chicago is

1 2 3 4 5

BE SURE YOUR MARKS ARE HEAVY AND BLACK.
ERASE COMPLETELY ANY ANSWER YOU WISH TO CHANGE.

(Answer grid: items 1–90 each with response columns 1, 2, 3, 4)

IBM FORM I.T.S. 1000 B 108

NAME _____ LAST _____ FIRST _____ MIDDLE _____ DATE _____

SCHOOL _____ CITY _____

DATE OF BIRTH _____ AGE _____ SEX _____ M OR F

GRADE OR CLASS _____ INSTRUCTOR _____

NAME OF TEST _____ PART _____

SCORES

1	5
2	6
3	7
4	8

SAMPLE:

1—1 a country
1—2 a mountain
1—3 an island
1—4 a city
1—5 a state

1. Chicago is

DIRECTIONS: Read each question and its numbered answers. When you have decided which answer is correct, blacken the corresponding space on this sheet with the special pencil. Make your mark as long as the pair of lines, and move the pencil point up and down firmly to make a heavy black line. If you change your mind, erase your first mark completely. Make no stray marks; they may count against you.

BE SURE YOUR MARKS ARE HEAVY AND BLACK.
ERASE COMPLETELY ANY ANSWER YOU WISH TO CHANGE.

IBM FORM I.T.S. 1000 B 108

SCORES

NAME _____
LAST   FIRST   MIDDLE

SCHOOL _____
CITY

DATE _____

DATE OF BIRTH _____   AGE ___   SEX ___
M OR F

GRADE OR CLASS _____   INSTRUCTOR _____

NAME OF TEST _____   PART ___

1	5
2	6
3	7
4	8

SAMPLE:

1—1 a country
1—2 a mountain
1—3 an island
1—4 a city
1—5 a state

1. Chicago is

1   2   3   4   5
1 :::: :::: ::::: ▬▬

DIRECTIONS: Read each question and its numbered answers. When you have decided which answer is correct, blacken the corresponding space on this sheet with the special pencil. Make your mark as long as the pair of lines, and move the pencil point up and down firmly to make a heavy black line. If you change your mind, erase your first mark completely. Make no stray marks; they may count against you.

1   2   3   4
1
2
3
4
5
6
7
8
9
10
11
12
13
14
15

1   2   3   4
31
32
33
34
35
36
37
38
39
40
41
42
43
44
45

1   2   3   4
61
62
63
64
65
66
67
68
69
70
71
72
73
74
75

BE SURE YOUR MARKS ARE HEAVY AND BLACK.
ERASE COMPLETELY ANY ANSWER YOU WISH TO CHANGE.

1   2   3   4
16
17
18
19
20
21
22
23
24
25
26
27
28
29
30

1   2   3   4
46
47
48
49
50
51
52
53
54
55
56
57
58
59
60

1   2   3   4
76
77
78
79
80
81
82
83
84
85
86
87
88
89
90

IBM FORM I.T.S. 1000 B 108

NAME _____
     LAST   FIRST   MIDDLE   DATE _____

SCHOOL _____   CITY _____

SCORES

1	5
2	6
3	7
4	8

1. _____

2. _____

DATE OF BIRTH _____   AGE _____   SEX _____ M OR F

GRADE OR CLASS _____   INSTRUCTOR _____

NAME OF TEST _____   PART _____

SAMPLE:

1. Chicago is

1—1 a country
1—2 a mountain
1—3 an island
1—4 a city
1—5 a state

DIRECTIONS: Read each question and its numbered answers. When you have decided which answer is correct, blacken the corresponding space on this sheet with the special pencil. Make your mark as long as the pair of lines, and move the pencil point up and down firmly to make a heavy black line. If you change your mind, erase your first mark completely. Make no stray marks; they may count against you.

BE SURE YOUR MARKS ARE HEAVY AND BLACK.
ERASE COMPLETELY ANY ANSWER YOU WISH TO CHANGE.

1	31	61
2	32	62
3	33	63
4	34	64
5	35	65
6	36	66
7	37	67
8	38	68
9	39	69
10	40	70
11	41	71
12	42	72
13	43	73
14	44	74
15	45	75
16	46	76
17	47	77
18	48	78
19	49	79
20	50	80
21	51	81
22	52	82
23	53	83
24	54	84
25	55	85
26	56	86
27	57	87
28	58	88
29	59	89
30	60	90

IBM FORM I. T. S. 1000 B 108

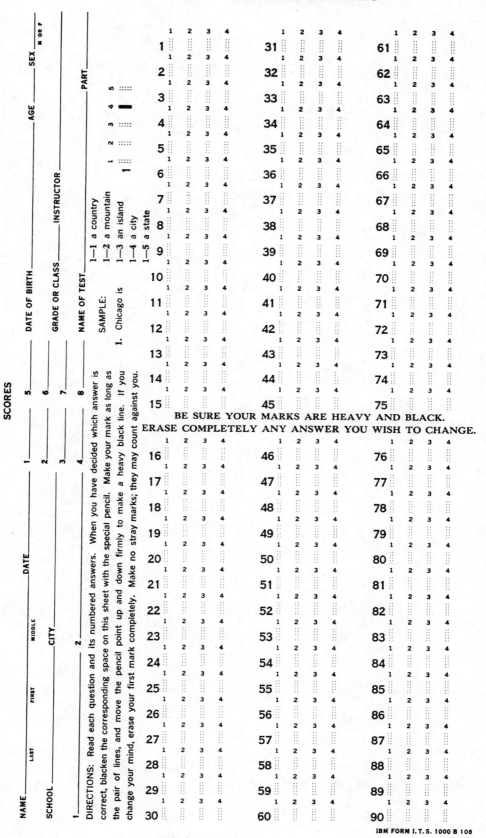

BE SURE YOUR MARKS ARE HEAVY AND BLACK.
ERASE COMPLETELY ANY ANSWER YOU WISH TO CHANGE.

IBM FORM I.T.S. 1000 B 108

A-61

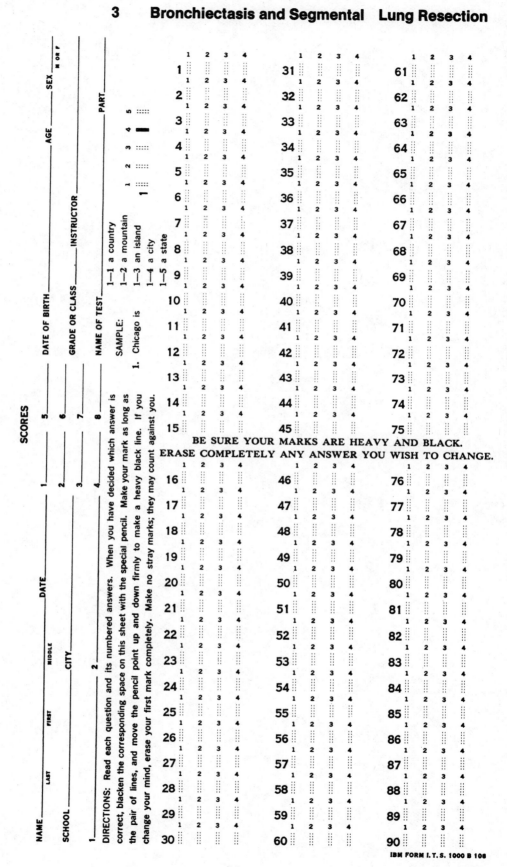

SCORES

NAME ___ LAST ___ FIRST ___ MIDDLE ___ DATE ___

SCHOOL ___ CITY ___

DATE OF BIRTH ___ AGE ___ SEX ___ M OR F

GRADE OR CLASS ___ INSTRUCTOR ___

NAME OF TEST ___ PART ___

SAMPLE:

1—1 a country
1—2 a mountain
1—3 an island
1—4 a city
1—5 a state

1. Chicago is

DIRECTIONS: Read each question and its numbered answers. When you have decided which answer is correct, blacken the corresponding space on this sheet with the special pencil. Make your mark as long as the pair of lines, and move the pencil point up and down firmly to make a heavy black line. If you change your mind, erase your first mark completely. Make no stray marks; they may count against you.

BE SURE YOUR MARKS ARE HEAVY AND BLACK.
ERASE COMPLETELY ANY ANSWER YOU WISH TO CHANGE.

IBM FORM I.T.S. 1000 B 106

A-63

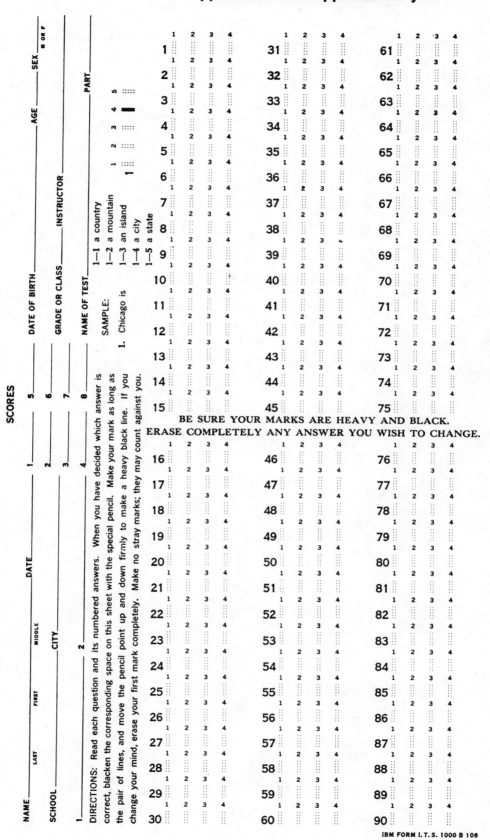

NAME _____ LAST _____ FIRST _____ MIDDLE _____ DATE _____

SCHOOL _____ CITY _____

SCORES

1	5
2	6
3	7
4	8

DATE OF BIRTH _____ AGE _____ SEX _____ M OR F

GRADE OR CLASS _____ INSTRUCTOR _____

NAME OF TEST _____ PART _____

DIRECTIONS: Read each question and its numbered answers. When you have decided which answer is correct, blacken the corresponding space on this sheet with the special pencil. Make your mark as long as the pair of lines, and move the pencil point up and down firmly to make a heavy black line. If you change your mind, erase your first mark completely. Make no stray marks; they may count against you.

SAMPLE:

1. Chicago is

1—1 a country
1—2 a mountain
1—3 an island
1—4 a city
1—5 a state

BE SURE YOUR MARKS ARE HEAVY AND BLACK.
ERASE COMPLETELY ANY ANSWER YOU WISH TO CHANGE.

IBM FORM I. T. S. 1000 B 108

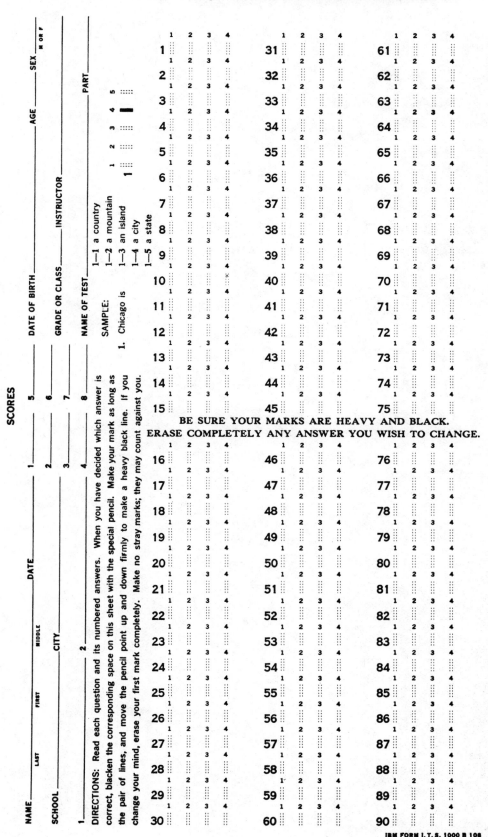

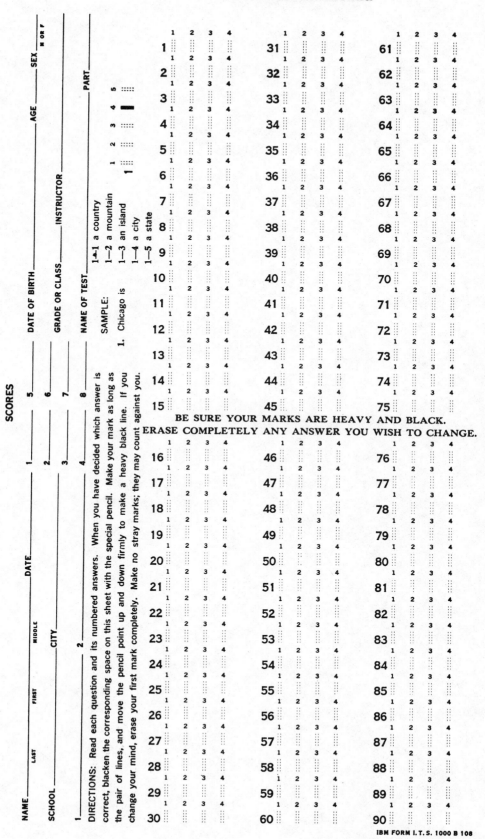

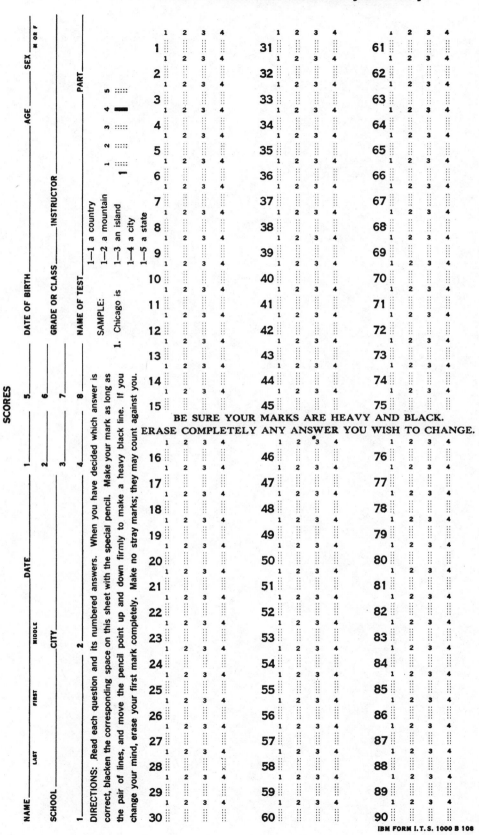

NAME _____
LAST   FIRST   MIDDLE

SCHOOL _____
CITY

SCORES

1	5
2	6
3	7
4	8

DATE OF BIRTH _____

GRADE OR CLASS _____ INSTRUCTOR _____

NAME OF TEST _____

DATE _____   AGE _____ SEX _____ M OR F

PART _____

SAMPLE:

1—1 a country
1—2 a mountain
1—3 an island
1—4 a city
1—5 a state

1. Chicago is

DIRECTIONS: Read each question and its numbered answers. When you have decided which answer is correct, blacken the corresponding space on this sheet with the special pencil. Make your mark as long as the pair of lines, and move the pencil point up and down firmly to make a heavy black line. If you change your mind, erase your first mark completely. Make no stray marks; they may count against you.

BE SURE YOUR MARKS ARE HEAVY AND BLACK.
ERASE COMPLETELY ANY ANSWER YOU WISH TO CHANGE.

IBM FORM I.T.S. 1000 B 108

A-71

NAME _____ LAST _____ FIRST _____ MIDDLE _____ DATE _____

SCHOOL _____ CITY _____

1 _____ 2 _____

DIRECTIONS: Read each question and its numbered answers. When you have decided which answer is correct, blacken the corresponding space on this sheet with the special pencil. Make your mark as long as the pair of lines, and move the pencil point up and down firmly to make a heavy black line. If you change your mind, erase your first mark completely. Make no stray marks; they may count against you.

DATE OF BIRTH _____ AGE _____ SEX M OR F _____

GRADE OR CLASS _____ INSTRUCTOR _____

NAME OF TEST _____ PART _____

SAMPLE:

1—1 a country
1—2 a mountain
1—3 an island
1—4 a city
1—5 a state

1. Chicago is

SCORES

1 _____ 5 _____
2 _____ 6 _____
3 _____ 7 _____
4 _____ 8 _____

BE SURE YOUR MARKS ARE HEAVY AND BLACK.
ERASE COMPLETELY ANY ANSWER YOU WISH TO CHANGE.

(Answer grid: items 1–90, each with answer columns 1 2 3 4)

NAME _____ LAST _____ FIRST _____ MIDDLE _____ DATE _____

SCHOOL _____ CITY _____

DATE OF BIRTH _____

GRADE OR CLASS _____ INSTRUCTOR _____

NAME OF TEST _____

AGE _____ SEX M OR F _____

PART _____

SCORES

1	5
2	6
3	7
4	8

DIRECTIONS: Read each question and its numbered answers. When you have decided which answer is correct, blacken the corresponding space on this sheet with the special pencil. Make your mark as long as the pair of lines, and move the pencil point up and down firmly to make a heavy black line. If you change your mind, erase your first mark completely. Make no stray marks; they may count against you.

SAMPLE:

1. Chicago is

   1—1 a country
   1—2 a mountain
   1—3 an island
   1—4 a city
   1—5 a state

BE SURE YOUR MARKS ARE HEAVY AND BLACK.
ERASE COMPLETELY ANY ANSWER YOU WISH TO CHANGE.

1 2 3 4	1 2 3 4	1 2 3 4
1	31	61
2	32	62
3	33	63
4	34	64
5	35	65
6	36	66
7	37	67
8	38	68
9	39	69
10	40	70
11	41	71
12	42	72
13	43	73
14	44	74
15	45	75
16	46	76
17	47	77
18	48	78
19	49	79
20	50	80
21	51	81
22	52	82
23	53	83
24	54	84
25	55	85
26	56	86
27	57	87
28	58	88
29	59	89
30	60	90

IBM FORM I.T.S. 1000 B 108

A-75

SCORES

1	5
2	6
3	7
4	8

NAME _____ DATE _____
    LAST   FIRST   MIDDLE

SCHOOL _____ CITY _____

DATE OF BIRTH _____ AGE _____ SEX _____
                                          M OR F

GRADE OR CLASS _____ INSTRUCTOR _____

NAME OF TEST _____ PART _____

DIRECTIONS: Read each question and its numbered answers. When you have decided which answer is correct, blacken the corresponding space on this sheet with the special pencil. Make your mark as long as the pair of lines, and move the pencil point up and down firmly to make a heavy black line. If you change your mind, erase your first mark completely. Make no stray marks; they may count against you.

SAMPLE:

1—1 a country
1—2 a mountain
1—3 an island
1—4 a city
1—5 a state

1. Chicago is

   1   2   3   4   5
1   ⋮   ⋮   ⋮   ▮   ⋮

BE SURE YOUR MARKS ARE HEAVY AND BLACK.
ERASE COMPLETELY ANY ANSWER YOU WISH TO CHANGE.

Answer grid, questions 1–90, each with columns 1 2 3 4:

1	31	61
2	32	62
3	33	63
4	34	64
5	35	65
6	36	66
7	37	67
8	38	68
9	39	69
10	40	70
11	41	71
12	42	72
13	43	73
14	44	74
15	45	75
16	46	76
17	47	77
18	48	78
19	49	79
20	50	80
21	51	81
22	52	82
23	53	83
24	54	84
25	55	85
26	56	86
27	57	87
28	58	88
29	59	89
30	60	90

IBM FORM I. T. S. 1000 B 106

NAME _____

LAST   FIRST   MIDDLE   DATE _____

SCHOOL _____ CITY _____

DATE OF BIRTH _____ AGE _____ SEX __ OR F

GRADE OR CLASS _____ INSTRUCTOR _____

NAME OF TEST _____ PART _____

SCORES

1	5
2	6
3	7
4	8
1	2

DIRECTIONS: Read each question and its numbered answers. When you have decided which answer is correct, blacken the corresponding space on this sheet with the special pencil. Make your mark as long as the pair of lines, and move the pencil point up and down firmly to make a heavy black line. If you change your mind, erase your first mark completely. Make no stray marks; they may count against you.

SAMPLE:

1—1 a country
1—2 a mountain
1—3 an island
1—4 a city
1—5 a state

1. Chicago is

	1	2	3	4	5
1					

BE SURE YOUR MARKS ARE HEAVY AND BLACK.
ERASE COMPLETELY ANY ANSWER YOU WISH TO CHANGE.

Questions 1–90, each with answer columns 1 2 3 4:

1–30, 31–60, 61–90 (columns)

IBM FORM I.T.S. 1000 B 108

NAME _____

LAST   FIRST   MIDDLE   DATE _____

SCHOOL _____   CITY _____

DATE OF BIRTH _____

GRADE OR CLASS _____   INSTRUCTOR _____

NAME OF TEST _____   PART _____

AGE _____   SEX _____ M OR F

SCORES

1 _____ 5 _____
2 _____ 6 _____
3 _____ 7 _____
4 _____ 8 _____

DIRECTIONS: Read each question and its numbered answers. When you have decided which answer is correct, blacken the corresponding space on this sheet with the special pencil. Make your mark as long as the pair of lines, and move the pencil point up and down firmly to make a heavy black line. If you change your mind, erase your first mark completely. Make no stray marks; they may count against you.

SAMPLE:

1—1 a country
1—2 a mountain
1—3 an island
1—4 a city
1—5 a state

1. Chicago is   1 ⦚ 2 ⦚ 3 ⦚ 4 ▮ 5 ⦚

	1	2	3	4		1	2	3	4		1	2	3	4
1					31					61				
2					32					62				
3					33				x	63				
4					34					64				
5					35					65				
6					36					66				
7					37					67				
8					38					68				
9					39					69				
10					40					70				
11					41					71				
12					42					72				
13					43					73				
14					44					74				
15					45					75				

BE SURE YOUR MARKS ARE HEAVY AND BLACK.
ERASE COMPLETELY ANY ANSWER YOU WISH TO CHANGE.

	1	2	3	4		1	2	3	4		1	2	3	4
16					46					76				
17					47					77				
18					48					78				
19					49					79				
20					50					80				
21					51					81				
22					52					82				
23					53					83				
24					54					84				
25					55					85				
26					56					86				
27					57					87				
28					58					88				
29					59					89				
30					60					90				

IBM FORM I. T. S. 1000 B 108

A-81

NAME

LAST   FIRST   MIDDLE   DATE

SCHOOL   CITY

SCORES

1	5
2	6
3	7
4	8

DIRECTIONS: Read each question and its numbered answers. When you have decided which answer is correct, blacken the corresponding space on this sheet with the special pencil. Make your mark as long as the pair of lines, and move the pencil point up and down firmly to make a heavy black line. If you change your mind, erase your first mark completely. Make no stray marks; they may count against you.

DATE OF BIRTH   AGE   SEX   M OR F

GRADE OR CLASS   INSTRUCTOR

NAME OF TEST   PART

SAMPLE:

1—1 a country
1—2 a mountain
1—3 an island
1—4 a city
1—5 a state

1. Chicago is

1 :::::
2 :::::
3 :::::
4 ▉
5 :::::

1 2 3 4   31 ... 1 2 3 4   61 ... 1 2 3 4
2   32   62
3   33   63
4   34   64
5   35   65
6   36   66
7   37   67
8   38   68
9   39   69
10   40   70
11   41   71
12   42   72
13   43   73
14   44   74
15   45   75

BE SURE YOUR MARKS ARE HEAVY AND BLACK.
ERASE COMPLETELY ANY ANSWER YOU WISH TO CHANGE.

16   1 2 3 4   46   1 2 3 4   76   1 2 3 4
17   47   77
18   48   78
19   49   79
20   50   80
21   51   81
22   52   82
23   53   83
24   54   84
25   55   85
26   56   86
27   57   87
28   58   88
29   59   89
30   60   90

IBM FORM I. T. S. 1000 B 108

NAME _____ LAST _____ FIRST _____ MIDDLE _____ DATE _____

SCHOOL _____ CITY _____

DATE OF BIRTH _____ AGE _____ SEX _____ M OR F

GRADE OR CLASS _____ INSTRUCTOR _____

NAME OF TEST _____ PART _____

SCORES

1 _____ 5 _____
2 _____ 6 _____
3 _____ 7 _____
4 _____ 8 _____

DIRECTIONS: Read each question and its numbered answers. When you have decided which answer is correct, blacken the corresponding space on this sheet with the special pencil. Make your mark as long as the pair of lines, and move the pencil point up and down firmly to make a heavy black line. If you change your mind, erase your first mark completely. Make no stray marks; they may count against you.

SAMPLE:

1—1 a country
1—2 a mountain
1—3 an island
1—4 a city
1—5 a state

1. Chicago is

1   2   3   4   5

BE SURE YOUR MARKS ARE HEAVY AND BLACK.
ERASE COMPLETELY ANY ANSWER YOU WISH TO CHANGE.

Questions 1–90, each with answer options 1 2 3 4:

1, 2, 3, 4, 5, 6, 7, 8, 9, 10, 11, 12, 13, 14, 15, 16, 17, 18, 19, 20, 21, 22, 23, 24, 25, 26, 27, 28, 29, 30

31, 32, 33, 34, 35, 36, 37, 38, 39, 40, 41, 42, 43, 44, 45, 46, 47, 48, 49, 50, 51, 52, 53, 54, 55, 56, 57, 58, 59, 60

61, 62, 63, 64, 65, 66, 67, 68, 69, 70, 71, 72, 73, 74, 75, 76, 77, 78, 79, 80, 81, 82, 83, 84, 85, 86, 87, 88, 89, 90

IBM FORM I. T. S. 1000 B 108

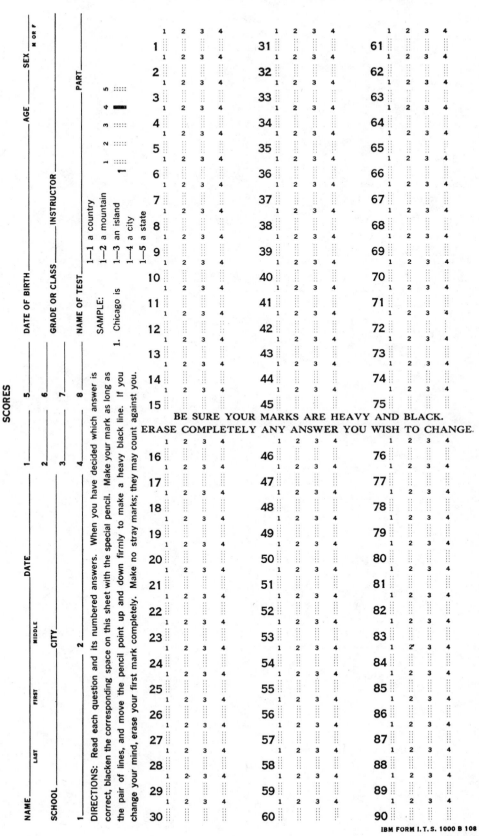

NAME _____ LAST ___ FIRST ___ MIDDLE ___ DATE _____

SCHOOL _____ CITY _____

SCORES

1	5	
2	6	
3	7	
4	8	

1 _____ 2 _____

DATE OF BIRTH _____ AGE ___ SEX ___ M OR F

GRADE OR CLASS _____ INSTRUCTOR _____

NAME OF TEST _____ PART _____

DIRECTIONS: Read each question and its numbered answers. When you have decided which answer is correct, blacken the corresponding space on this sheet with the special pencil. Make your mark as long as the pair of lines, and move the pencil point up and down firmly to make a heavy black line. If you change your mind, erase your first mark completely. Make no stray marks; they may count against you.

SAMPLE:

1—1 a country
1—2 a mountain
1—3 an island
1—4 a city
1—5 a state

1. Chicago is

BE SURE YOUR MARKS ARE HEAVY AND BLACK.
ERASE COMPLETELY ANY ANSWER YOU WISH TO CHANGE.

IBM FORM I.T.S. 1000 B 108

SCORES

1	5
2	6
3	7
4	8

NAME _____ LAST _____ FIRST _____ MIDDLE _____ DATE _____

SCHOOL _____ CITY _____

DATE OF BIRTH _____ AGE _____ SEX _____ M OR F

GRADE OR CLASS _____ INSTRUCTOR _____

NAME OF TEST _____ PART _____

DIRECTIONS: Read each question and its numbered answers. When you have decided which answer is correct, blacken the corresponding space on this sheet with the special pencil. Make your mark as long as the pair of lines, and move the pencil point up and down firmly to make a heavy black line. If you change your mind, erase your first mark completely. Make no stray marks; they may count against you.

SAMPLE:

1—1 a country
1—2 a mountain
1—3 an island
1—4 a city
1—5 a state

1. Chicago is

BE SURE YOUR MARKS ARE HEAVY AND BLACK.
ERASE COMPLETELY ANY ANSWER YOU WISH TO CHANGE.

(Answer grid, questions 1–90, each with choices 1 2 3 4)

IBM FORM I. T. S. 1000 B 108

A-89

NAME _____ DATE _____

_____ LAST _____ FIRST _____ MIDDLE

SCHOOL _____

_____ CITY

DATE OF BIRTH _____ AGE _____ SEX _____ M OR F

GRADE OR CLASS _____ INSTRUCTOR _____

NAME OF TEST _____ PART _____

SCORES

1		5	
2		6	
3		7	
4		8	

DIRECTIONS: Read each question and its numbered answers. When you have decided which answer is correct, blacken the corresponding space on this sheet with the special pencil. Make your mark as long as the pair of lines, and move the pencil point up and down firmly to make a heavy black line. If you change your mind, erase your first mark completely. Make no stray marks; they may count against you.

SAMPLE:

1—1 a country
1—2 a mountain
1—3 an island
1—4 a city
1—5 a state

1. Chicago is

1 ::::   2 ::::   3 ::::   4 ▓▓▓▓   5 ::::

Questions 1–90, each with answer choices 1 2 3 4:

1, 2, 3, 4, 5, 6, 7, 8, 9, 10, 11, 12, 13, 14, 15

31, 32, 33, 34, 35, 36, 37, 38, 39, 40, 41, 42, 43, 44, 45

61, 62, 63, 64, 65, 66, 67, 68, 69, 70, 71, 72, 73, 74, 75

BE SURE YOUR MARKS ARE HEAVY AND BLACK.
ERASE COMPLETELY ANY ANSWER YOU WISH TO CHANGE.

16, 17, 18, 19, 20, 21, 22, 23, 24, 25, 26, 27, 28, 29, 30

46, 47, 48, 49, 50, 51, 52, 53, 54, 55, 56, 57, 58, 59, 60

76, 77, 78, 79, 80, 81, 82, 83, 84, 85, 86, 87, 88, 89, 90

IBM FORM I. T. S. 1000 B 108

3   Cataract Removal

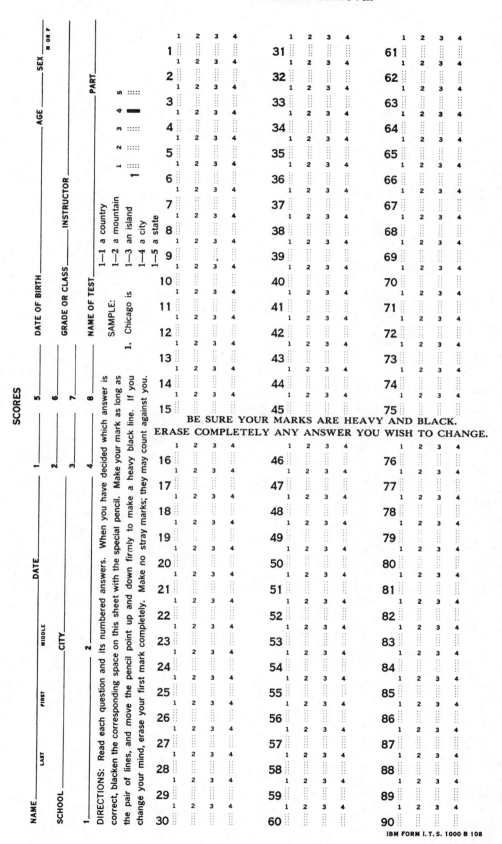

NAME

LAST   FIRST   MIDDLE   DATE

SCHOOL   CITY

DATE OF BIRTH   AGE   SEX   M OR F

GRADE OR CLASS   INSTRUCTOR   PART

NAME OF TEST

SCORES

1   5
2   6
3   7
4   8

SAMPLE:

1—1 a country
1—2 a mountain
1—3 an island
1—4 a city
1—5 a state

1. Chicago is

DIRECTIONS: Read each question and its numbered answers. When you have decided which answer is correct, blacken the corresponding space on this sheet with the special pencil. Make your mark as long as the pair of lines, and move the pencil point up and down firmly to make a heavy black line. If you change your mind, erase your first mark completely. Make no stray marks; they may count against you.

BE SURE YOUR MARKS ARE HEAVY AND BLACK.
ERASE COMPLETELY ANY ANSWER YOU WISH TO CHANGE.

IBM FORM I. T. S. 1000 B 108

A-93

SCORES

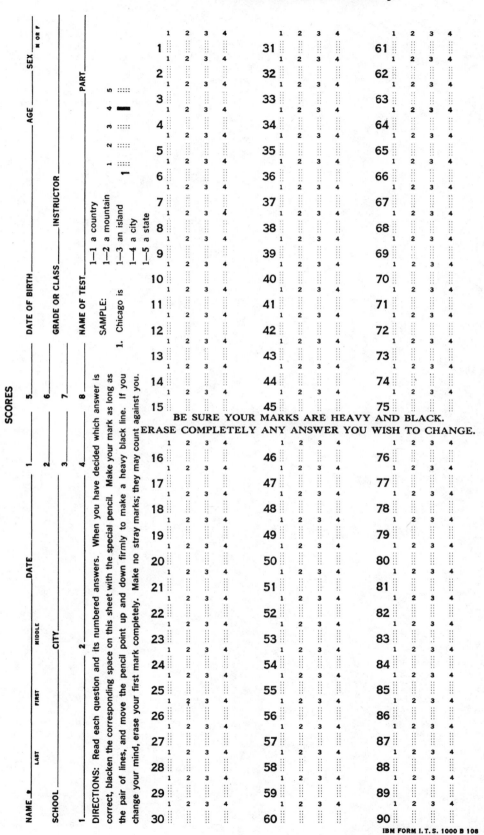

NAME ___ LAST FIRST MIDDLE ___ DATE ___ 1 ___ 5 ___ DATE OF BIRTH ___ AGE ___ SEX ___ M OR F

SCHOOL ___ CITY ___ 2 ___ 6 ___ GRADE OR CLASS ___ INSTRUCTOR ___

3 ___ 7 ___

1 ___ 2 ___ 4 ___ 8 ___ NAME OF TEST ___ PART ___

DIRECTIONS: Read each question and its numbered answers. When you have decided which answer is correct, blacken the corresponding space on this sheet with the special pencil. Make your mark as long as the pair of lines, and move the pencil point up and down firmly to make a heavy black line. If you change your mind, erase your first mark completely. Make no stray marks; they may count against you.

SAMPLE:

1. Chicago is
1—1 a country
1—2 a mountain
1—3 an island
1—4 a city
1—5 a state

1 ⁞ 1 ⁞ 2 ⁞ 3 ▮ 4 ⁞ 5

1	1 2 3 4	31	1 2 3 4	61	1 2 3 4
2	1 2 3 4	32	1 2 3 4	62	1 2 3 4
3	1 2 3 4	33	1 2 3 4	63	1 2 3 4
4	1 2 3 4	34	1 2 3 4	64	1 2 3 4
5	1 2 3 4	35	1 2 3 4	65	1 2 3 4
6	1 2 3 4	36	1 2 3 4	66	1 2 3 4
7	1 2 3 4	37	1 2 3 4	67	1 2 3 4
8	1 2 3 4	38	1 2 3 4	68	1 2 3 4
9	1 2 3 4	39	1 2 3 4	69	1 2 3 4
10	1 2 3 4	40	1 2 3 4	70	1 2 3 4
11	1 2 3 4	41	1 2 3 4	71	1 2 3 4
12	1 2 3 4	42	1 2 3 4	72	1 2 3 4
13	1 2 3 4	43	1 2 3 4	73	1 2 3 4
14	1 2 3 4	44	1 2 3 4	74	1 2 3 4
15	1 2 3 4	45	1 2 3 4	75	1 2 3 4

BE SURE YOUR MARKS ARE HEAVY AND BLACK.
ERASE COMPLETELY ANY ANSWER YOU WISH TO CHANGE.

16	1 2 3 4	46	1 2 3 4	76	1 2 3 4
17	1 2 3 4	47	1 2 3 4	77	1 2 3 4
18	1 2 3 4	48	1 2 3 4	78	1 2 3 4
19	1 2 3 4	49	1 2 3 4	79	1 2 3 4
20	1 2 3 4	50	1 2 3 4	80	1 2 3 4
21	1 2 3 4	51	1 2 3 4	81	1 2 3 4
22	1 2 3 4	52	1 2 3 4	82	1 2 3 4
23	1 2 3 4	53	1 2 3 4	83	1 2 3 4
24	1 2 3 4	54	1 2 3 4	84	1 2 3 4
25	1 2 3 4	55	1 2 3 4	85	1 2 3 4
26	1 2 3 4	56	1 2 3 4	86	1 2 3 4
27	1 2 3 4	57	1 2 3 4	87	1 2 3 4
28	1 2 3 4	58	1 2 3 4	88	1 2 3 4
29	1 2 3 4	59	1 2 3 4	89	1 2 3 4
30	1 2 3 4	60	1 2 3 4	90	1 2 3 4

IBM FORM I.T.S. 1000 B 106

NAME _____ DATE _____

     LAST   FIRST   MIDDLE

SCHOOL _____ CITY _____

DATE OF BIRTH _____ AGE _____ SEX _____

                                             M OR F

GRADE OR CLASS _____ INSTRUCTOR _____

NAME OF TEST _____ PART _____

SCORES

1	5
2	6
3	7
4	8
1	2

DIRECTIONS: Read each question and its numbered answers. When you have decided which answer is correct, blacken the corresponding space on this sheet with the special pencil. Make your mark as long as the pair of lines, and move the pencil point up and down firmly to make a heavy black line. If you change your mind, erase your first mark completely. Make no stray marks; they may count against you.

SAMPLE:

1—1 a country
1—2 a mountain
1—3 an island
1—4 a city
1—5 a state

1. Chicago is

     1   2   3   4   5

1   2   3   4   5

BE SURE YOUR MARKS ARE HEAVY AND BLACK.
ERASE COMPLETELY ANY ANSWER YOU WISH TO CHANGE.

Items 1–90, each with answer options 1 2 3 4:

1	31	61
2	32	62
3	33	63
4	34	64
5	35	65
6	36	66
7	37	67
8	38	68
9	39	69
10	40	70
11	41	71
12	42	72
13	43	73
14	44	74
15	45	75
16	46	76
17	47	77
18	48	78
19	49	79
20	50	80
21	51	81
22	52	82
23	53	83
24	54	84
25	55	85
26	56	86
27	57	87
28	58	88
29	59	89
30	60	90

IBM FORM I.T.S. 1000 B 108

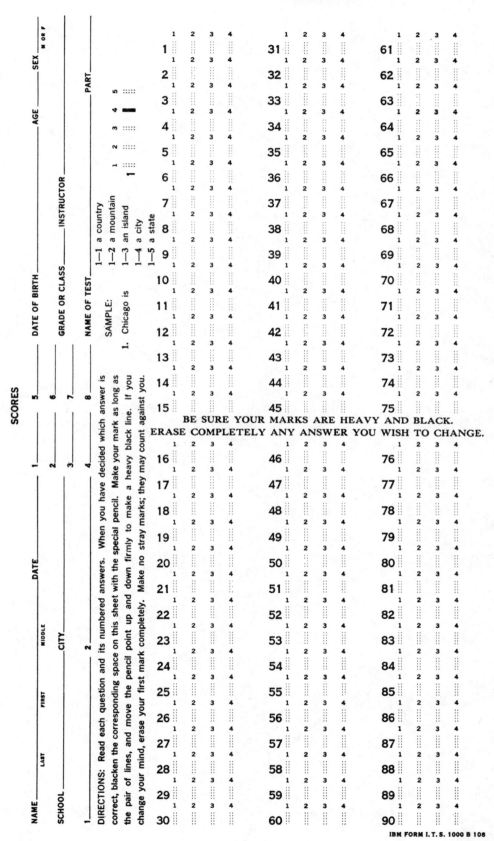

NAME _____ DATE _____ DATE OF BIRTH _____ AGE _____ SEX M OR F

LAST   FIRST   MIDDLE

SCHOOL _____ CITY _____ GRADE OR CLASS _____ INSTRUCTOR _____

1 _____ 2 _____ NAME OF TEST _____ PART _____

SCORES

1	5
2	6
3	7
4	8

DIRECTIONS: Read each question and its numbered answers. When you have decided which answer is correct, blacken the corresponding space on this sheet with the special pencil. Make your mark as long as the pair of lines, and move the pencil point up and down firmly to make a heavy black line. If you change your mind, erase your first mark completely. Make no stray marks; they may count against you.

SAMPLE:

1—1 a country
1—2 a mountain
1—3 an island
1—4 a city
1—5 a state

1. Chicago is

BE SURE YOUR MARKS ARE HEAVY AND BLACK.
ERASE COMPLETELY ANY ANSWER YOU WISH TO CHANGE.

IBM FORM I. T. S. 1000 B 108

NAME _____ LAST ___ FIRST ___ MIDDLE ___ DATE _____

SCHOOL _____ CITY _____

SCORES

	1		5
	2		6
	3		7
	4		8

1 _____ 2 _____

DATE OF BIRTH _____ AGE ___ SEX M OR F

GRADE OR CLASS _____ INSTRUCTOR _____

NAME OF TEST _____ PART ___

SAMPLE:

1—1 a country
1—2 a mountain
1—3 an island
1—4 a city
1—5 a state

1. Chicago is

```
        1   2   3   4   5
        1 ::::: :::::
        1   2   3   4   5
        1 ::::: :::::
        1 ▆▆▆
```

DIRECTIONS: Read each question and its numbered answers. When you have decided which answer is correct, blacken the corresponding space on this sheet with the special pencil. Make your mark as long as the pair of lines, and move the pencil point up and down firmly to make a heavy black line. If you change your mind, erase your first mark completely. Make no stray marks; they may count against you.

BE SURE YOUR MARKS ARE HEAVY AND BLACK.
ERASE COMPLETELY ANY ANSWER YOU WISH TO CHANGE.

	1	2	3	4		1	2	3	4		1	2	3	4
1					31					61				
2					32					62				
3					33					63				
4					34					64				
5					35					65				
6					36					66				
7					37					67				
8					38					68				
9					39					69				
10					40					70				
11					41					71				
12					42					72				
13					43					73				
14					44					74				
15					45					75				
16					46					76				
17					47					77				
18					48					78				
19					49					79				
20					50					80				
21					51					81				
22					52					82				
23					53					83				
24					54					84				
25					55					85				
26					56					86				
27					57					87				
28					58					88				
29					59					89				
30					60					90				

IBM FORM I. T. S. 1000 B 108

SCORES

1	5
2	6
3	7
4	8

NAME _____ LAST _____ FIRST _____ MIDDLE _____ DATE _____

SCHOOL _____ CITY _____

DATE OF BIRTH _____

GRADE OR CLASS _____ INSTRUCTOR _____

AGE _____ SEX _____ M OR F

NAME OF TEST _____ PART _____

SAMPLE:

1. Chicago is
   1—1 a country
   1—2 a mountain
   1—3 an island
   1—4 a city
   1—5 a state

DIRECTIONS: Read each question and its numbered answers. When you have decided which answer is correct, blacken the corresponding space on this sheet with the special pencil. Make your mark as long as the pair of lines, and move the pencil point up and down firmly to make a heavy black line. If you change your mind, erase your first mark completely. Make no stray marks; they may count against you.

1   2   3   4

1
2
3
4
5
6
7
8
9
10
11
12
13
14
15

31
32
33
34
35
36
37
38
39
40
41
42
43
44
45

61
62
63
64
65
66
67
68
69
70
71
72
73
74
75

BE SURE YOUR MARKS ARE HEAVY AND BLACK.
ERASE COMPLETELY ANY ANSWER YOU WISH TO CHANGE.

16
17
18
19
20
21
22
23
24
25
26
27
28
29
30

46
47
48
49
50
51
52
53
54
55
56
57
58
59
60

76
77
78
79
80
81
82
83
84
85
86
87
88
89
90

IBM FORM I. T. S. 1000 B 108

NAME _____ LAST _____ FIRST _____ MIDDLE _____ DATE _____

SCHOOL _____ CITY _____

SCORES

1	5
2	6
3	7
4	8

DATE OF BIRTH _____ AGE _____ SEX ___ M OR F

GRADE OR CLASS _____ INSTRUCTOR _____

NAME OF TEST _____ PART _____

SAMPLE:

1—1 a country
1—2 a mountain
1—3 an island
1—4 a city
1—5 a state

1. Chicago is

DIRECTIONS: Read each question and its numbered answers. When you have decided which answer is correct, blacken the corresponding space on this sheet with the special pencil. Make your mark as long as the pair of lines, and move the pencil point up and down firmly to make a heavy black line. If you change your mind, erase your first mark completely. Make no stray marks; they may count against you.

BE SURE YOUR MARKS ARE HEAVY AND BLACK.
ERASE COMPLETELY ANY ANSWER YOU WISH TO CHANGE.

Answer grid, questions 1–90, each with columns 1 2 3 4.

IBM FORM I.T.S. 1000 B 108

A-105

NAME _____ LAST _____ FIRST _____ MIDDLE _____ DATE _____

SCHOOL _____ CITY _____

DATE OF BIRTH _____

GRADE OR CLASS _____ INSTRUCTOR _____

NAME OF TEST _____

AGE _____ SEX _____ M OR F

PART _____

SCORES

1	5
2	6
3	7
4	8

DIRECTIONS: Read each question and its numbered answers. When you have decided which answer is correct, blacken the corresponding space on this sheet with the special pencil. Make your mark as long as the pair of lines, and move the pencil point up and down firmly to make a heavy black line. If you change your mind, erase your first mark completely. Make no stray marks; they may count against you.

SAMPLE:

1—1 a country
1—2 a mountain
1—3 an island
1—4 a city
1—5 a state

1. Chicago is

1 ::::
1 2 ::::
1 2 3 ::::
1 2 3 4 █████
1 2 3 4 5 ::::

Columns (each item has answer choices 1 2 3 4):

1, 2, 3, 4, 5, 6, 7, 8, 9, 10, 11, 12, 13, 14, 15

31, 32, 33, 34, 35, 36, 37, 38, 39, 40, 41, 42, 43, 44, 45

61, 62, 63, 64, 65, 66, 67, 68, 69, 70, 71, 72, 73, 74, 75

BE SURE YOUR MARKS ARE HEAVY AND BLACK.
ERASE COMPLETELY ANY ANSWER YOU WISH TO CHANGE.

16, 17, 18, 19, 20, 21, 22, 23, 24, 25, 26, 27, 28, 29, 30

46, 47, 48, 49, 50, 51, 52, 53, 54, 55, 56, 57, 58, 59, 60

76, 77, 78, 79, 80, 81, 82, 83, 84, 85, 86, 87, 88, 89, 90

IBM FORM I.T.S. 1000 P 108

A-107

NAME _____ _____ _____ DATE _____

LAST   FIRST   MIDDLE

SCHOOL _____ CITY _____

SEX ___ M OR F

AGE _____

DATE OF BIRTH _____

GRADE OR CLASS _____ INSTRUCTOR _____

NAME OF TEST _____

PART _____

SCORES

1 _____ 5

2 _____ 6

3 _____ 7

4 _____ 8

1 _____ 2 _____

DIRECTIONS: Read each question and its numbered answers. When you have decided which answer is correct, blacken the corresponding space on this sheet with the special pencil. Make your mark as long as the pair of lines, and move the pencil point up and down firmly to make a heavy black line. If you change your mind, erase your first mark completely. Make no stray marks; they may count against you.

SAMPLE:

1—1 a country
1—2 a mountain
1—3 an island
1—4 a city
1—5 a state

1. Chicago is

BE SURE YOUR MARKS ARE HEAVY AND BLACK.
ERASE COMPLETELY ANY ANSWER YOU WISH TO CHANGE.

(Answer grid, columns numbered 1 2 3 4 for each item)

1–30, 31–60, 61–90

IBM FORM I. T. S. 1000 B 108

A-109

SCORES

1 ———	5 ———
2 ———	6 ———
3 ———	7 ———
4 ———	8 ———

NAME ——— LAST — FIRST — MIDDLE — DATE ———

SCHOOL ——— CITY ———

DATE OF BIRTH ——— AGE ——— SEX M OR F

GRADE OR CLASS ——— INSTRUCTOR ———

NAME OF TEST ——— PART ———

DIRECTIONS: Read each question and its numbered answers. When you have decided which answer is correct, blacken the corresponding space on this sheet with the special pencil. Make your mark as long as the pair of lines, and move the pencil point up and down firmly to make a heavy black line. If you change your mind, erase your first mark completely. Make no stray marks; they may count against you.

SAMPLE:

1—1 a country
1—2 a mountain
1—3 an island
1—4 a city
1—5 a state

1. Chicago is

         1   2   3   4   5
         1 ::: 2 ::: 3 ::: 4 ■■ 5 :::

BE SURE YOUR MARKS ARE HEAVY AND BLACK.
ERASE COMPLETELY ANY ANSWER YOU WISH TO CHANGE

(Answer grid: items 1–90, each with bubbles 1 2 3 4, arranged in three columns: 1–30, 31–60, 61–90.)

IBM FORM I. T. S. 1000 B 108

NAME_____
LAST   FIRST   MIDDLE

SCHOOL_____

DATE OF BIRTH_____   AGE_____ SEX_____ M OR F

GRADE OR CLASS_____ INSTRUCTOR_____

NAME OF TEST_____ DATE_____ PART_____

CITY_____

SCORES

1	5
2	6
3	7
4	8

SAMPLE:

1—1 a country
1—2 a mountain
1—3 an island
1—4 a city
1—5 a state

1. Chicago is

DIRECTIONS: Read each question and its numbered answers. When you have decided which answer is correct, blacken the corresponding space on this sheet with the special pencil. Make your mark as long as the pair of lines, and move the pencil point up and down firmly to make a heavy black line. If you change your mind, erase your first mark completely. Make no stray marks; they may count against you.

BE SURE YOUR MARKS ARE HEAVY AND BLACK.
ERASE COMPLETELY ANY ANSWER YOU WISH TO CHANGE.

(Answer grid, items 1–90, columns 1 2 3 4)

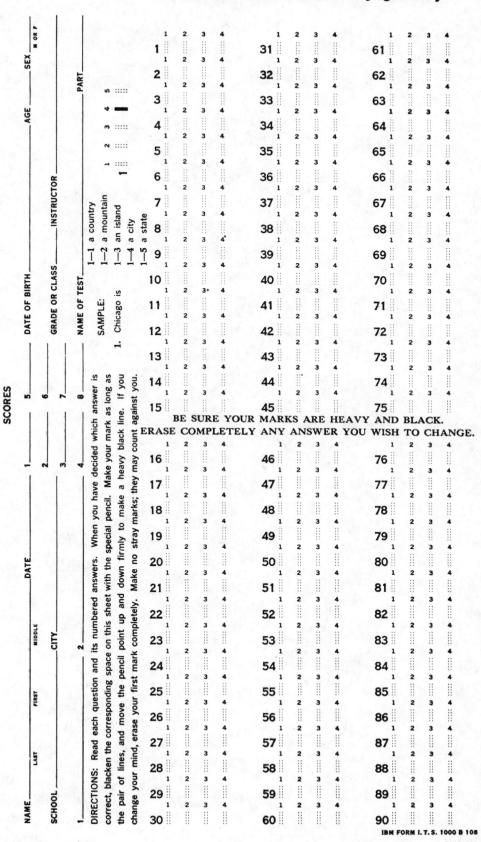

NAME _____
LAST   FIRST   MIDDLE

SCHOOL _____ CITY

SCORES

	5
1	
2	6
3	7
4	8

DATE OF BIRTH _____ AGE ____ SEX __ M OR F

GRADE OR CLASS _____ INSTRUCTOR _____

NAME OF TEST _____ DATE _____ PART ____

DIRECTIONS: Read each question and its numbered answers. When you have decided which answer is correct, blacken the corresponding space on this sheet with the special pencil. Make your mark as long as the pair of lines, and move the pencil point up and down firmly to make a heavy black line. If you change your mind, erase your first mark completely. Make no stray marks; they may count against you.

SAMPLE:

1—1 a country
1—2 a mountain
1—3 an island
1—4 a city
1—5 a state

1. Chicago is

BE SURE YOUR MARKS ARE HEAVY AND BLACK.
ERASE COMPLETELY ANY ANSWER YOU WISH TO CHANGE.

IBM FORM I. T. S. 1000 B 108

A-115

NAME _____

SCHOOL _____ CITY _____

LAST   FIRST   MIDDLE   DATE _____

DATE OF BIRTH _____   AGE _____   SEX M OR F

GRADE OR CLASS _____   INSTRUCTOR _____

NAME OF TEST _____   PART _____

SCORES

1	5
2	6
3	7
4	8

DIRECTIONS: Read each question and its numbered answers. When you have decided which answer is correct, blacken the corresponding space on this sheet with the special pencil. Make your mark as long as the pair of lines, and move the pencil point up and down firmly to make a heavy black line. If you change your mind, erase your first mark completely. Make no stray marks; they may count against you.

SAMPLE:

1—1 a country
1—2 a mountain
1—3 an island
1—4 a city
1—5 a state

1. Chicago is

BE SURE YOUR MARKS ARE HEAVY AND BLACK.
ERASE COMPLETELY ANY ANSWER YOU WISH TO CHANGE.

IBM FORM I. T. S. 1000 B 108

A-117

3 Arteriosclerotic Obliterative Disease and Femoro-Popliteal Bypass Graft

NAME _____
LAST   FIRST   MIDDLE   DATE _____

SCHOOL _____ CITY _____

DATE OF BIRTH _____ AGE _____ SEX M OR F

GRADE OR CLASS _____ INSTRUCTOR _____

NAME OF TEST _____ PART _____

SCORES

1	5
2	6
3	7
4	8

1 _____ 2 _____

DIRECTIONS: Read each question and its numbered answers. When you have decided which answer is correct, blacken the corresponding space on this sheet with the special pencil. Make your mark as long as the pair of lines, and move the pencil point up and down firmly to make a heavy black line. If you change your mind, erase your first mark completely. Make no stray marks; they may count against you.

SAMPLE:

1. Chicago is
1—1 a country
1—2 a mountain
1—3 an island
1—4 a city
1—5 a state

BE SURE YOUR MARKS ARE HEAVY AND BLACK.
ERASE COMPLETELY ANY ANSWER YOU WISH TO CHANGE.

(Answer grid columns numbered 1–90, each with response options 1 2 3 4)

Columns: 1–30, 31–60, 61–90

IBM FORM I. T. S. 1000 B 105

A-119

NAME _____ LAST _____ FIRST _____ MIDDLE _____ DATE _____

SCHOOL _____ CITY _____

SCORES

1	5
2	6
3	7
4	8

DATE OF BIRTH _____ AGE _____ SEX _____ M OR F

GRADE OR CLASS _____ INSTRUCTOR _____

NAME OF TEST _____ PART _____

DIRECTIONS: Read each question and its numbered answers. When you have decided which answer is correct, blacken the corresponding space on this sheet with the special pencil. Make your mark as long as the pair of lines, and move the pencil point up and down firmly to make a heavy black line. If you change your mind, erase your first mark completely. Make no stray marks; they may count against you.

SAMPLE:

1. Chicago is
   1—1 a country
   1—2 a mountain
   1—3 an island
   1—4 a city
   1—5 a state

BE SURE YOUR MARKS ARE HEAVY AND BLACK.
ERASE COMPLETELY ANY ANSWER YOU WISH TO CHANGE.

Questions 1 through 90 with answer columns 1 2 3 4 for each.

Items 1–15, 31–45, 61–75 (top section)
Items 16–30, 46–60, 76–90 (bottom section)

IBM FORM I. T. S. 1000 B 108

A-121

NAME _____ DATE _____

LAST   FIRST   MIDDLE

SCHOOL _____ CITY _____

DATE OF BIRTH _____ AGE _____ SEX ___ M OR F

GRADE OR CLASS _____ INSTRUCTOR _____

NAME OF TEST _____ PART _____

SCORES

1	5
2	6
3	7
4	8

DIRECTIONS: Read each question and its numbered answers. When you have decided which answer is correct, blacken the corresponding space on this sheet with the special pencil. Make your mark as long as the pair of lines, and move the pencil point up and down firmly to make a heavy black line. If you change your mind, erase your first mark completely. Make no stray marks; they may count against you.

SAMPLE:

1—1 a country
1—2 a mountain
1—3 an island
1—4 a city
1—5 a state

1. Chicago is

	1	2	3	4	5
1				�In	

	1	2	3	4			1	2	3	4			1	2	3	4
1						31						61				
2						32						62				
3						33						63				
4						34						64				
5						35						65				
6						36						66				
7						37						67				
8						38						68				
9						39						69				
10						40						70				
11						41						71				
12						42						72				
13						43						73				
14						44						74				
15						45						75				

BE SURE YOUR MARKS ARE HEAVY AND BLACK.
ERASE COMPLETELY ANY ANSWER YOU WISH TO CHANGE.

	1	2	3	4			1	2	3	4			1	2	3	4
16						46						76				
17						47						77				
18						48						78				
19						49						79				
20						50						80				
21						51						81				
22						52						82				
23						53						83				
24						54						84				
25						55						85				
26						56						86				
27						57						87				
28						58						88				
29						59						89				
30						60						90				

IBM FORM I.T.S. 1000 B 108

A-123

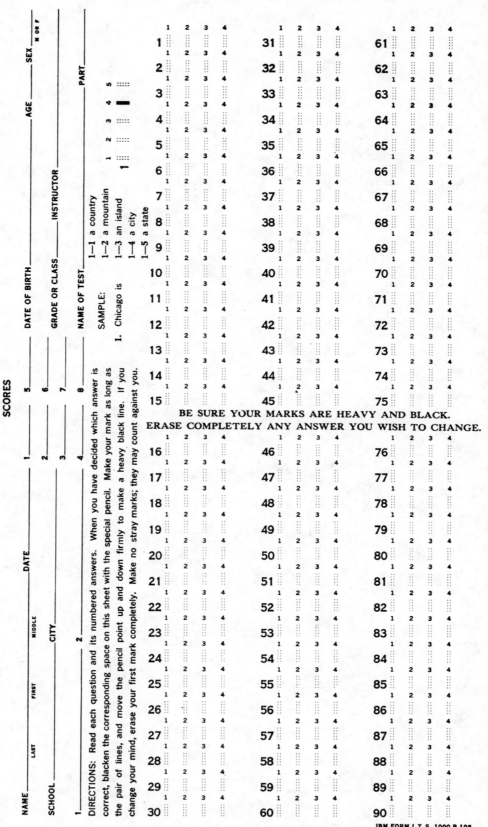

NAME _____ _____ _____ DATE _____
LAST   FIRST   MIDDLE

SCHOOL _____ CITY _____

SCORES

1	5
2	6
3	7
4	8

DATE OF BIRTH _____ AGE _____ SEX _____ M OR F

GRADE OR CLASS _____ INSTRUCTOR _____

NAME OF TEST _____ PART _____

DIRECTIONS: Read each question and its numbered answers. When you have decided which answer is correct, blacken the corresponding space on this sheet with the special pencil. Make your mark as long as the pair of lines, and move the pencil point up and down firmly to make a heavy black line. If you change your mind, erase your first mark completely. Make no stray marks; they may count against you.

SAMPLE:
1—1 a country
1—2 a mountain
1—3 an island
1—4 a city
1—5 a state

1. Chicago is

BE SURE YOUR MARKS ARE HEAVY AND BLACK.
ERASE COMPLETELY ANY ANSWER YOU WISH TO CHANGE.

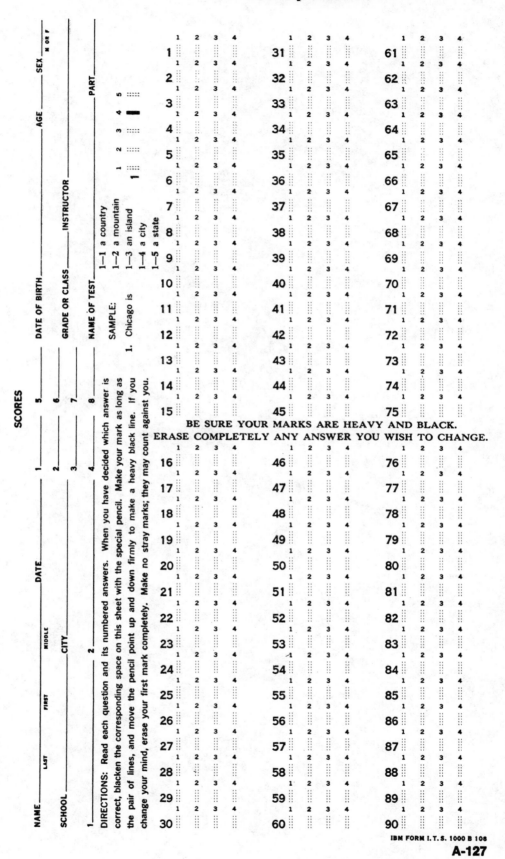

NAME _____ LAST _____ FIRST _____ MIDDLE _____ DATE _____

SCHOOL _____ CITY _____

DATE OF BIRTH _____

GRADE OR CLASS _____ INSTRUCTOR _____

NAME OF TEST _____

AGE _____ SEX _____ M OR F

PART _____

SCORES

1	5
2	6
3	7
4	8

DIRECTIONS: Read each question and its numbered answers. When you have decided which answer is correct, blacken the corresponding space on this sheet with the special pencil. Make your mark as long as the pair of lines, and move the pencil point up and down firmly to make a heavy black line. If you change your mind, erase your first mark completely. Make no stray marks; they may count against you.

SAMPLE:

1—1 a country
1—2 a mountain
1—3 an island
1—4 a city
1—5 a state

1. Chicago is

BE SURE YOUR MARKS ARE HEAVY AND BLACK.
ERASE COMPLETELY ANY ANSWER YOU WISH TO CHANGE.

IBM FORM I. T. S. 1000 B 108

A-127

SCORES

1	5
2	6
3	7
4	8

NAME _____ LAST _____ FIRST _____ MIDDLE _____ DATE _____

SCHOOL _____ CITY _____

DATE OF BIRTH _____ AGE _____ SEX _____ M or F

GRADE OR CLASS _____ INSTRUCTOR _____

NAME OF TEST _____ PART _____

DIRECTIONS: Read each question and its numbered answers. When you have decided which answer is correct, blacken the corresponding space on this sheet with the special pencil. Make your mark as long as the pair of lines, and move the pencil point up and down firmly to make a heavy black line. If you change your mind, erase your first mark completely. Make no stray marks; they may count against you.

SAMPLE:

1—1 a country
1—2 a mountain
1—3 an island
1—4 a city
1—5 a state

1. Chicago is

1 2 3 4 5

BE SURE YOUR MARKS ARE HEAVY AND BLACK.
ERASE COMPLETELY ANY ANSWER YOU WISH TO CHANGE.

1 2 3 4   31 ... 61 ...
2 ...   32 ... 62 ...
3 ...   33 ... 63 ...
4 ...   34 ... 64 ...
5 ...   35 ... 65 ...
6 ...   36 ... 66 ...
7 ...   37 ... 67 ...
8 ...   38 ... 68 ...
9 ...   39 ... 69 ...
10 ...   40 ... 70 ...
11 ...   41 ... 71 ...
12 ...   42 ... 72 ...
13 ...   43 ... 73 ...
14 ...   44 ... 74 ...
15 ...   45 ... 75 ...
16 ...   46 ... 76 ...
17 ...   47 ... 77 ...
18 ...   48 ... 78 ...
19 ...   49 ... 79 ...
20 ...   50 ... 80 ...
21 ...   51 ... 81 ...
22 ...   52 ... 82 ...
23 ...   53 ... 83 ...
24 ...   54 ... 84 ...
25 ...   55 ... 85 ...
26 ...   56 ... 86 ...
27 ...   57 ... 87 ...
28 ...   58 ... 88 ...
29 ...   59 ... 89 ...
30 ...   60 ... 90 ...

IBM FORM I. T. S. 1000 B 108

A-129

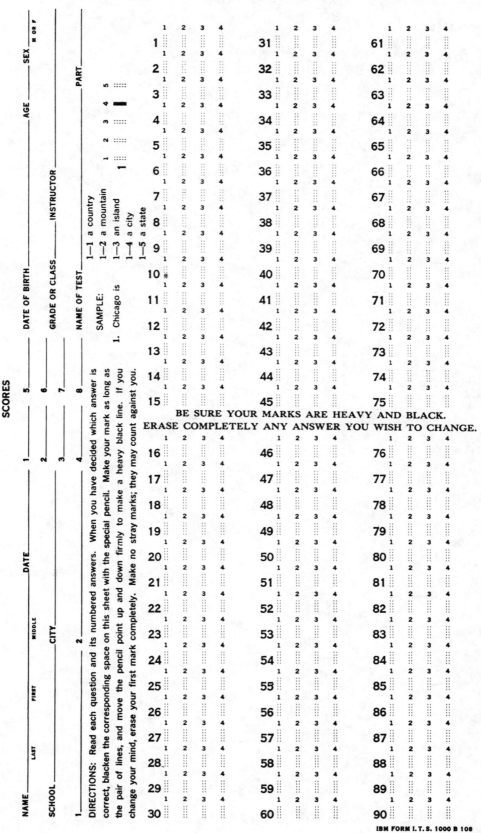

NAME _____ LAST ___ FIRST ___ MIDDLE ___ DATE _____

SCHOOL _____ CITY _____

DATE OF BIRTH _____

GRADE OR CLASS _____ INSTRUCTOR _____

NAME OF TEST _____ PART _____

AGE ___ SEX ___ M OR F

SCORES

1	5
2	6
3	7
4	8

DIRECTIONS: Read each question and its numbered answers. When you have decided which answer is correct, blacken the corresponding space on this sheet with the special pencil. Make your mark as long as the pair of lines, and move the pencil point up and down firmly to make a heavy black line. If you change your mind, erase your first mark completely. Make no stray marks; they may count against you.

SAMPLE:

1—1 a country
1—2 a mountain
1—3 an island
1—4 a city
1—5 a state

1. Chicago is

BE SURE YOUR MARKS ARE HEAVY AND BLACK.
ERASE COMPLETELY ANY ANSWER YOU WISH TO CHANGE.

NAME _____ LAST _____ FIRST _____ MIDDLE _____ DATE _____

SCHOOL _____ CITY _____

1 _____ 2 _____

DATE OF BIRTH _____ AGE _____ SEX M OR F _____

GRADE OR CLASS _____ INSTRUCTOR _____

NAME OF TEST _____ PART _____

SCORES

1 _____ 5 _____
2 _____ 6 _____
3 _____ 7 _____
4 _____ 8 _____

DIRECTIONS: Read each question and its numbered answers. When you have decided which answer is correct, blacken the corresponding space on this sheet with the special pencil. Make your mark as long as the pair of lines, and move the pencil point up and down firmly to make a heavy black line. If you change your mind, erase your first mark completely. Make no stray marks; they may count against you.

SAMPLE:

1—1 a country
1—2 a mountain
1—3 an island
1—4 a city
1—5 a state

1. Chicago is

1   2   3   4   5

BE SURE YOUR MARKS ARE HEAVY AND BLACK.
ERASE COMPLETELY ANY ANSWER YOU WISH TO CHANGE.

(Answer grid, columns numbered 1–4 for each item)

1–30, 31–60, 61–90

Items 1 through 90 arranged in three columns with answer positions 1 2 3 4.

IBM FORM I. T. S. 1000 B 108

A-133

NAME

LAST   FIRST   MIDDLE   DATE

SCHOOL

CITY

DATE OF BIRTH   AGE   SEX   M OR F

GRADE OR CLASS   INSTRUCTOR

NAME OF TEST   PART

SCORES

1   5

2   6

3   7

4   8

1   2

DIRECTIONS: Read each question and its numbered answers. When you have decided which answer is correct, blacken the corresponding space on this sheet with the special pencil. Make your mark as long as the pair of lines, and move the pencil point up and down firmly to make a heavy black line. If you change your mind, erase your first mark completely. Make no stray marks; they may count against you.

SAMPLE:

1—1 a country
1—2 a mountain
1—3 an island
1—4 a city
1—5 a state

1. Chicago is

1   2   3   4   5

BE SURE YOUR MARKS ARE HEAVY AND BLACK.
ERASE COMPLETELY ANY ANSWER YOU WISH TO CHANGE.

(Answer grid, questions 1–90, each with columns 1 2 3 4)

1 2 3 4 5 6 7 8 9 10 11 12 13 14 15 16 17 18 19 20 21 22 23 24 25 26 27 28 29 30

31 32 33 34 35 36 37 38 39 40 41 42 43 44 45 46 47 48 49 50 51 52 53 54 55 56 57 58 59 60

61 62 63 64 65 66 67 68 69 70 71 72 73 74 75 76 77 78 79 80 81 82 83 84 85 86 87 88 89 90

IBM FORM I. T. S. 1000 B 108

A-135

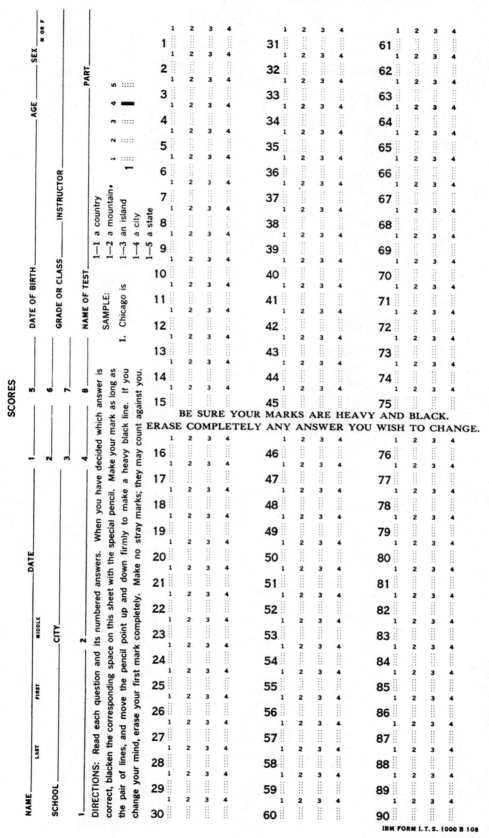

NAME

LAST   FIRST   MIDDLE   DATE

SCHOOL   CITY

DATE OF BIRTH   AGE   SEX M OR F

GRADE OR CLASS   INSTRUCTOR

NAME OF TEST   PART

SCORES

1—5   2—6   3—7   4—8

1   2   3   4

DIRECTIONS: Read each question and its numbered answers. When you have decided which answer is correct, blacken the corresponding space on this sheet with the special pencil. Make your mark as long as the pair of lines, and move the pencil point up and down firmly to make a heavy black line. If you change your mind, erase your first mark completely. Make no stray marks; they may count against you.

SAMPLE:

1—1 a country
1—2 a mountain
1—3 an island
1—4 a city
1—5 a state

1. Chicago is   1   2   3   4   5

BE SURE YOUR MARKS ARE HEAVY AND BLACK.
ERASE COMPLETELY ANY ANSWER YOU WISH TO CHANGE.

IBM FORM I.T.S. 1000 B 108

A-137

NAME _____ _____ _____ _____ DATE _____ AGE _____ SEX _____
   LAST   FIRST   MIDDLE   M OR F

SCHOOL _____ CITY _____ DATE OF BIRTH _____

SCORES

1	5
2	6
3	7
4	8

GRADE OR CLASS _____ INSTRUCTOR _____

NAME OF TEST _____ PART _____

1 _____ 2 _____

DIRECTIONS: Read each question and its numbered answers. When you have decided which answer is correct, blacken the corresponding space on this sheet with the special pencil. Make your mark as long as the pair of lines, and move the pencil point up and down firmly to make a heavy black line. If you change your mind, erase your first mark completely. Make no stray marks; they may count against you.

SAMPLE:

1—1 a country
1—2 a mountain
1—3 an island
1—4 a city
1—5 a state

1. Chicago is

BE SURE YOUR MARKS ARE HEAVY AND BLACK.
ERASE COMPLETELY ANY ANSWER YOU WISH TO CHANGE.

(answer grid, items 1–90, each with options 1 2 3 4)

IBM FORM I. T. S. 1000 B 108

A-139

SCORES

1		5	
2		6	
3		7	
4		8	

1

2

NAME _____
LAST   FIRST   MIDDLE   DATE _____

SCHOOL _____   CITY _____

DATE OF BIRTH _____   AGE _____   SEX _____ M OR F

GRADE OR CLASS _____   INSTRUCTOR _____

NAME OF TEST _____   PART _____

SAMPLE:

1—1 a country
1—2 a mountain
1—3 an island
1—4 a city
1—5 a state

1. Chicago is

DIRECTIONS: Read each question and its numbered answers. When you have decided which answer is correct, blacken the corresponding space on this sheet with the special pencil. Make your mark as long as the pair of lines, and move the pencil point up and down firmly to make a heavy black line. If you change your mind, erase your first mark completely. Make no stray marks; they may count against you.

BE SURE YOUR MARKS ARE HEAVY AND BLACK.
ERASE COMPLETELY ANY ANSWER YOU WISH TO CHANGE.

(Answer grid, items 1–90, each with choices 1 2 3 4)

IBM FORM I.T.S. 1000 B 108

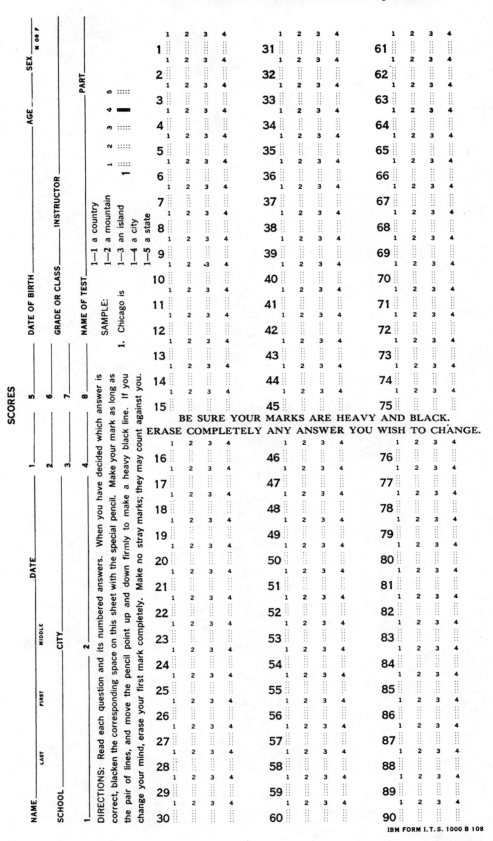

NAME _____
LAST   FIRST   MIDDLE

SCHOOL _____
CITY

DATE _____

DATE OF BIRTH _____

GRADE OR CLASS _____ INSTRUCTOR _____

AGE _____ SEX _____ M OR F

PART _____

NAME OF TEST _____

SCORES

1	5
2	6
3	7
4	8

SAMPLE:

1—1 a country
1—2 a mountain
1—3 an island
1—4 a city
1—5 a state

1. Chicago is

DIRECTIONS: Read each question and its numbered answers. When you have decided which answer is correct, blacken the corresponding space on this sheet with the special pencil. Make your mark as long as the pair of lines, and move the pencil point up and down firmly to make a heavy black line. If you change your mind, erase your first mark completely. Make no stray marks; they may count against you.

BE SURE YOUR MARKS ARE HEAVY AND BLACK.
ERASE COMPLETELY ANY ANSWER YOU WISH TO CHANGE.

IBM FORM I. T. S. 1000 B 108

A-143

NAME _____
LAST   FIRST   MIDDLE

SCHOOL _____ CITY _____

DATE _____

DATE OF BIRTH _____

GRADE OR CLASS _____ INSTRUCTOR _____

NAME OF TEST _____

AGE _____ SEX ___ M OR F

PART _____

SCORES

1	5
2	6
3	7
4	8

SAMPLE:

1—1 a country
1—2 a mountain
1—3 an island
1—4 a city
1—5 a state

1. Chicago is

1 [1] [2] [3] [4] [●] 5

DIRECTIONS: Read each question and its numbered answers. When you have decided which answer is correct, blacken the corresponding space on this sheet with the special pencil. Make your mark as long as the pair of lines, and move the pencil point up and down firmly to make a heavy black line. If you change your mind, erase your first mark completely. Make no stray marks; they may count against you.

BE SURE YOUR MARKS ARE HEAVY AND BLACK.
ERASE COMPLETELY ANY ANSWER YOU WISH TO CHANGE.

Items 1–90, each with answer choices 1 2 3 4:

1, 2, 3, 4, 5, 6, 7, 8, 9, 10, 11, 12, 13, 14, 15, 16, 17, 18, 19, 20, 21, 22, 23, 24, 25, 26, 27, 28, 29, 30

31, 32, 33, 34, 35, 36, 37, 38, 39, 40, 41, 42, 43, 44, 45, 46, 47, 48, 49, 50, 51, 52, 53, 54, 55, 56, 57, 58, 59, 60

61, 62, 63, 64, 65, 66, 67, 68, 69, 70, 71, 72, 73, 74, 75, 76, 77, 78, 79, 80, 81, 82, 83, 84, 85, 86, 87, 88, 89, 90

IBM FORM I.T.S. 1000 B 108

A-145

4 Suicide and Suicide Prevention

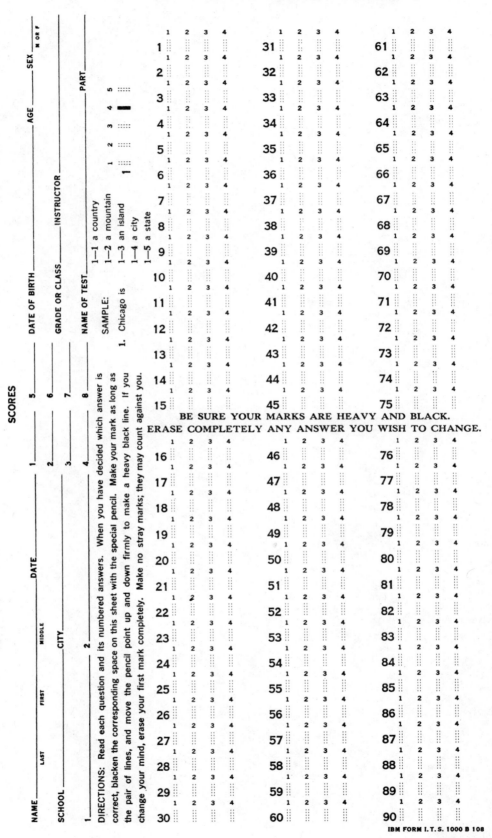

NAME ___ LAST ___ FIRST ___ MIDDLE ___ DATE ___

SCHOOL ___ CITY ___

DATE OF BIRTH ___ AGE ___ SEX M OR F

GRADE OR CLASS ___ INSTRUCTOR ___

NAME OF TEST ___ PART ___

SCORES

1 ___ 5 ___
2 ___ 6 ___
3 ___ 7 ___
4 ___ 8 ___

DIRECTIONS: Read each question and its numbered answers. When you have decided which answer is correct, blacken the corresponding space on this sheet with the special pencil. Make your mark as long as the pair of lines, and move the pencil point up and down firmly to make a heavy black line. If you change your mind, erase your first mark completely. Make no stray marks; they may count against you.

SAMPLE:
1—1 a country
1—2 a mountain
1—3 an island
1—4 a city
1—5 a state

1. Chicago is

BE SURE YOUR MARKS ARE HEAVY AND BLACK.
ERASE COMPLETELY ANY ANSWER YOU WISH TO CHANGE.

IBM FORM I.T.S. 1000 B 108

A-147

ANSWERS
AND
RATIONALES

1 MATERNITY AND GYNECOLOGIC NURSING

Normal Pregnancy

1. (2) Under the influence of follicle-stimulating hormone (FSH) and luteinizing hormone (LH), endometrium changes and ovarian development occur. The source of FSH and LH is the anterior pituitary gland. It receives messages regarding the secretion rate of FSH and LH from the hypothalamus. Thus, the anterior pituitary and the hypothalamus are responsible for uterine and ovarian development.

2. (2) Release of FSH acts on the ovaries to develop an ovum from the surrounding follicular cells. As the follicular cells develop, more estrogen is secreted; thus, plasma estrogen increases and circulates back to the hypothalamus.

3. (2) An ovary is composed of cell clusters called "follicles," which contain an ovum surrounded by the theca folliculi. The theca consists of an inner circle of secretory cells and an outer ring of connective tissue. It is mainly the theca interna cells that secrete the hormone estrogen during the first half of pregnancy.

4. (3) The follicular and ovulatory phase of ovarian function is approximately the first 14 days of the menstrual cycle.

5. (3) Meiosis is the process of reduction of chromosomes to their haploid number.

6. (3) The mature human ovum contains 23 chromosomes.

7. (1) Of the 23 chromosomes found in the human ovum, one is an X chromosome.

8. (4) Chromosomes are made up of molecules of deoxyribonucleic acid (DNA). They carry the genetic information that determines the characteristics of an individual.

9. (3) DNA is composed of repeating units of a five carbon sugar, purine-pyrimidine base pairs, and phosphoric acid.

10. (2) The gene is the basic unit of heredity. The genetic character is determined by the sequence of purine and pyrimidine bases.

11. (3) Midcycle or ovulatory pain is also known as mittelschmerz.

12. (3) Estrogen secretion is highest during the preovulatory or follicular phase. Its maximal secretion occurs at about day 13.

13. (1) Serum estrogen levels are lowest at the beginning of the menstrual cycle.

14. (4) Effects of estrogen influence are most seen in the uterine myometrium, the lactiferous ducts of the breasts, and the alteration of cervical mucus. High levels of serum estrogen act to inhibit FSH and LH release.

15. (3) During the last half of the menstrual cycle, LH is released from the anterior pituitary. Anterior pituitary hormones are transported via the circulatory system to their target organs.

16. (3) During the luteal phase of ovarian function, progesterone is secreted in substantial amounts by the corpus luteum.

17. (4) Progesterone acts to increase basal body temperature, promotes smooth muscle relaxation, and continues to facilitate implantation by enhancing the uterine endometrium.

18. (4) If fertilization has not occurred the corpus luteum degenerates. The resultant decrease of both progesterone and estrogen leads to the sloughing of the endometrial lining (menstruation).

19. (3) The decline in estrogen and progesterone levels results in the constriction of uterine blood vessels and the subsequent sloughing of the endometrium.

20. (3) The average blood loss per menstrual period measures 50–150 ml. over a three- to five-day period.

21. (4) The side effects of oral contraceptives can be attributed to the estrogen increase and include nausea, dizziness, headache, weight gain, and breast discomfort.

22. (3) Conception is most likely to occur within 24 hours of ovulation.
23. (2) Fertilization usually occurs in the distal portion of the fallopian tube.
24. (2) Implantation occurs at the blastocyst stage, or at six to seven days after fertilization. This would be approximately 20–21 days since the last menstrual period.
25. (3) The corpus luteum secretes levels of estrogen and progesterone sufficient to maintain the pregnancy until the placenta is able to function as an endocrine gland.
26. (4) Presumptive signs of pregnancy are subjective and recognized by the woman. They include: amenorrhea, nausea/vomiting, breast changes (tenderness and pigmentation), urinary frequency, quickening, pigmentation of the skin, and fatigue.
27. (2) Nausea and vomiting during pregnancy have been attributed to hormonal changes, gastrointestinal alterations, and hypoglycemia. Small, frequent carbohydrate-rich meals have been found to be effective in combating morning sickness.
28. (2) By the end of the third month the maternal system has adapted to the body changes evoked by pregnancy, and nausea and vomiting have disappeared.
29. (4) Under the influence of progesterone, estrogen, and prolactin the breasts undergo changes during pregnancy. Breast size, with prominence of nipples and areolar sweat glands, increases as a result of the growth of the secretory ductile system. Nipple pigmentation is more pronounced secondary to melanocyte-stimulating hormone (MSH) influence.
30. (3) Chadwick's sign (purplish discoloration of vaginal mucosa), Goodell's sign (softening of the cervix), and Hegar's sign (softening of the lower uterine segment) can be observed by the second month of pregnancy. Increase in uterine size can be determined by pelvic examination early in pregnancy.
31. (1) Chadwick's sign is attributed to the intense congestion of the pelvic vessels.
32. (2) EDC is calculated using Nägele's rule: take the first day of the last menstrual period, add seven days, and then subtract three months, changing to the appropriate year.

$$
\begin{array}{llll}
\text{LMP} = & 12 \text{ (December)} & & 15 \\
& \underline{-\quad 3} & & \underline{+\quad 7} \\
\text{EDC} = & 9 \text{ (September)} & & 22
\end{array}
$$

33. (4) Laboratory tests performed in the initial prenatal visit include: pelvic; Pap smear; hemoglobin and hematrocrit; Rh factor and blood type. Serology test for syphilis is usually mandated by the state law. Blood pressure, clean-catch urine specimen, and weight are obtained as baseline data.
34. (4) H.C.G. (human chorionic gonadotropin) is produced by the placental trophoblasts. Its presence in the maternal urine provides the basis for many bioassay and immunoassay tests for pregnancy.
35. (2) The chorionic cells of the developing placenta almost immediately secrete H.C.G., a glycoprotein hormone with properties similar to LH. H.C.G. strongly stimulates the corpus luteum to secrete estrogen and progesterone until placental functioning is established.
36. (2) Immunoassay tests can give positive results in pregnancy about 10 days after a missed menstrual period. This would approximate 4 weeks' gestation.
37. (3) The size of the pelvic inlet can be estimated by deducting 1.5 to 2 cm. from the diagonal conjugate. The diagonal conjugate can be used to estimate the anterior posterior diameter of the pelvis from the symphysis pubis in front to the sacral promontory in back.
38. (1) The distance between the sacral promontory and the lower margin of the symphysis pubis would approximate the diagonal conjugate — the most significant pelvic measurement. It normally is 12.5 to 13 cm.
39. (1) V.D.R.L. is a serologic test used to detect the presence of syphilis.
40. (1) A class 1 Pap smear is negative for the presence of malignant cells.

41. (4) Hemoglobin may be lower because of the physiologic hemodilution that accompanies pregnancy. Total blood volume increases 35–50 per cent; however, the proportion of plasma increase is greater than that of red cells, thus accounting for lower-than-normal values of hemoglobin.

42. (3) Slight bleeding episodes during pregnancy, although not uncommon, need to be evaluated by the health professional before treatment is recommended.

43. (3) Garters or stretch bands that restrict the venous circulation of the lower extremities, and predispose to or aggravate varicose veins, are to be avoided.

44. (3) Usually the pregnant patient is seen every month until the seventh month of pregnancy, every two weeks during the eighth month, and weekly during the ninth month.

45. (3) Ongoing physical evaluation of the pregnant patient includes growth of the uterus and assessment of estimation of fetal size, auscultation of fetal heart tones, weight gain, blood pressure, urinalysis for glucose and protein, and checking for edema.

46. (3) Minimal weight gain should be 24 lbs., with no defined maximum.

47. (4) Factors contributing to poor pregnancy outcomes include: low pre-pregnancy weight, low weight gain during pregnancy, and poor nutritional status.

48. (4) The foods listed are considered minimal requirement by the USDA for well-balanced human nutrition. Pregnancy requirements are based on these nutritional needs.

49. (4) Dark green and yellow vegetables provide high sources of vitamin A. Spinach per ½-cup serving provides 6000 IUs of vitamin A.

50. (1) Thiamine functions in the release of energy from the metabolism of carbohydrate. Lean pork is especially high in its thiamine concentration.

51. (4) Riboflavin aids in the metabolism of amino acids and carbohydrates. Particularly good sources are organ meats and milk.

52. (2) Good sources of ascorbic acid include citrus fruits, greens, broccoli, and Brussels sprouts.

53. (3) Since the usual diet is not likely to provide sufficient quantities of iron, the Committee on Maternal Nutrition recommends that all women receive 30–60 mg. of iron as a daily supplement during the second and third trimester of pregnancy.

54. (1) Good sources of calcium include cheese, spinach, greens, and oysters.

55. (2) Iron is necessary for maternal and fetal well-being. Good sources are liver, beans, raisins, lean pork, and beef.

56. (1) The natural sodium content of animal foods is relatively high. Shellfish and greens also contain high levels of sodium. Since bouillon has a meat base, its sodium content is significant.

57. (4) Foods to avoid on a sodium-restricted diet include all salted foods, canned fish, meat, vegetables, pickles, relish, salted butter, bread, and nuts. Foods containing regular baking powder or soda should also be limited.

58. (2) Varicosities occur in about 20 per cent of all pregnant women, and tend to become more prominent with each successive pregnancy. The gravid uterus causes pressure on the vessels of the vulva and lower extremities, thus obstructing venous return.

59. (2) Douching is not recommended during pregnancy. Should vaginal infection occur, use of appropriate medications and good perineal hygiene is usually sufficient.

60. (2) Heartburn is probably due to relaxation of the cardiac sphincter (at the junction of the esophagus and the stomach) and relaxation of the lower end of the esophagus. Pressure of the gravid uterus on the stomach and decreased gastric motility facilitate regurgitation of the stomach contents into the esophagus.

61. (4) Pregnancy need not be an indication for curtailing most forms of exercise that the pregnant patient enjoys. Activities can be continued as long as she feels able and well.

62. (2) The integumentary system is more active during pregnancy. Daily bathing is encouraged, both as a hygienic practice and because the skin assumes an

added role in the elimination of waste products produced by the growing fetus.

63. (4) Sexual relations can continue throughout pregnancy without restriction. Contraindications are usually limited to ruptured membranes, incompetent cervix, and spotting/bleeding.

64. (4) Bowel function can often be maintained by ensuring a liberal water intake, by exercise, by an intake of generous amounts of fruits and vegetables, and by avoiding unnecessary tensions.

65. (2) Sensation of fetal movements may be experienced as early as 16 weeks by most women. This is viewed as a presumptive sign of pregnancy, since it can be confused with intestinal peristalsis.

66. (4) Successful adaptation to pregnancy can be facilitated if personal, social, and cultural supports are available. The relationship between the parents, their ability to adjust to new situations and the acceptance of the pregnancy all foster adaptation.

67. (2) After 2–3 weeks' gestation, fetal red blood cells and vascular changes develop within the projecting villi. Thus, differentiation between placenta and fetal and maternal membranes become possible.

68. (4) Oxygen and nutrients must cross from the maternal intervillous spaces into the fetal capillary vessels within the villi. Waste products and carbon dioxide must pass in the reverse direction. Bacteria normally do not cross the placenta, and large molecule transfer is inhibited. The placenta also functions as an endocrine gland responsible for the needs of the developing fetus and for maintenance of the pregnancy.

69. (3) The principal known hormones produced by the placenta are estrogen, progesterone, human chorionic gonadotropin (H.C.G.), and human placental lactogen (H.P.L.).

70. (2) Substances of small molecular size can pass across the placenta by diffusion. The passage of other molecules is selectively enhanced by either facilitated diffusion, active transfer, or pinocytosis.

71. (1) The chorion mediates the exchange of nutrients and metabolic wastes between maternal and fetal circulation.

72. (1) The amnion and chorion compose the fetal membranes.

73. (1) The umbilical cord consists of three vessels: an umbilical vein that carries oxygenated blood from placenta to fetus, and two umbilical arteries that carry deoxygenated blood from fetus to placenta. The vessels are enclosed in a gelatinous substance.

74. (2) At term the placenta is about 15–20 cm. in diameter, is 2–3 cm. thick at the center, and weighs approximately 500 grams.

75. (1) The ambivalence of early pregnancy is well documented. Initial unhappiness with pregnancy has been reported in 25–80 per cent of women studied.

76. (4) Provision of the pregnant couple with knowledge and "tools" to cope with labor and delivery can interrupt the fear-tension-pain cycle. Ways to facilitate the exchange of information include classes, counseling, tours, and the learning of relaxation and breathing techniques.

77. (2) Breathing deeply and regularly and relaxing the pelvic muscles decrease the discomfort of the pelvic examination.

78. (3) *Candida albicans*, which is the causative organism of monilial vaginitis, can cause thrush (monilial infection of oral mucosa) in the neonate.

79. (1) Gentian violet when applied locally has an antiseptic action.

80. (4) Gentian violet causes permanent staining on clothing and linen.

81. (3) Nystatin is an antibiotic effective against fungi. Vaginal tablets of 100,000 Units are usually prescribed twice daily for two weeks.

82. (3) Rh incompatibility is not a problem with the first pregnancy.

83. (3) During fetal development any agent (environmental or ingested) that can have a deformity-producing effect on the fetus should be avoided.

84. (2) Pap smears are used in the diagnosis of cervical cancer.

85. (1) Many pregnant women experience a deficiency in iron. In microcytic anemia, erythrocytes are decreased in size. In hypochromic anemia, decrease in hemoglobin is greater than the decrease in the number of erythrocytes.

86. (3) Ferrous sulfate can produce side-effects of gastrointestinal upset, with possible nausea and/or vomiting. These can be minimized if the drug is taken on a full stomach, and therefore ingestion after meals is most appropriate.

87. (2) By 13 weeks of pregnancy the fundus of the uterus rises out of the pelvis and can be palpated just above the symphysis pubis. The fundus reaches the lower border of the umbilicus at 20 weeks and the xiphoid process at 36 weeks.

88. (3) Fetal heart tones can be auscultated with a fetoscope by 20 weeks of gestation. If an ultrasonic Doppler is used, they can be heard as early as 16 weeks.

89. (2) The rhythm of the fetal heart rate is regular at 120–160 beats per minute. Very slow or acclerated heart rates are usually indicative of fetal distress.

90. (3) In addition to fetal heart sounds, abdominal auscultation can reveal funic souffle (placental vessels), uterine souffle (secondary to increased blood flow), and maternal pulse.

91. (3) The funic souffle is heard as a sharp, whistling sound. It has the same rate per minute as the fetal heart.

92. (3) Actually, both 2 and 3 could be considered correct options. Although the mother has identified with her "real" baby, ambivalence *may* continue with regard to wanting the baby and yet rejecting the restrictions of parenthood.

93. (3) Since the focus of the woman's concern in labor is not the monitoring of her possessions, it is best to leave all valuables at home.

94. (3) Lightening refers to the settling of the presenting part of the fetus into the maternal pelvis. It is a subjective sensation accompanied by ease in breathing due to lack of pressure of the uterus on the diaphragm.

95. (3) In spite of the increase in their intensity, frequency, and duration, contractions are not a constant occurrence. An interval between contractions is necessary for the fetus and uterine cells to accommodate the vasoconstriction or compression caused by contractions.

96. (1) The concentration of myometrial cells is greatest at the fundus, as contrasted with the lower portion, which has less concentration of myometrium. This explains "fundal dominance," in that contractions initiate at the fundus (top) and radiate down.

97. (2) The muscle layer (myometrium) of the fundus is unique. The fibers run longitudinally, circularly, and spirally, and crisscross in every direction.

98. (2) The isthmus is located below the uterine fundus and above the cervix.

99. (3) The uterosacral ligaments are located on each side of the uterus. They extend from the cervix, and insert on the posterior wall of the pelvis. By exerting traction on the cervix, the uterus is held in position.

100. (3) The ridge between the upper and lower uterine segments has been described as the contraction ring.

101. (4) The exact physiologic mechanisms leading to the initiation of labor are unknown. Theories regarding its onset include: the uterine-distention stretch theory; increased levels of oxytocin (secondary to fetal production); changes in ratio between estrogen and progesterone, with estrogen becoming dominant; aging of the placenta, resulting in altered vasculature.

102. (1) Abdominal examination of a fetus in the left occiput anterior (LOA) position would reveal: breech in the uterine fundus, the back of the fetus on the left side, with small parts palpated on the right, and the head fixed in the pelvis.

103. (3) During labor the motility of the gastrointestinal system decreases considerably, predisposing the patient to nausea and vomiting.

104. (3) Frequency and duration of contractions can be ascertained only after several have been timed to determine if a pattern exists.

105. (4) By placing the fingertips gently on the fundus of the uterus, the nurse can approximately evaluate the strength and duration of the contraction.

106. (3) The duration pattern is measured in seconds, and tells how long the contraction lasted from its onset to its end.

107. (4) The frequency pattern is measured in minutes, and reflects the interval between the beginning of one contraction and the beginning of the next.

108. (4) An enema can stimulate uterine contractions, and serves to remove fecal

material from the rectum that may interfere with fetal descent and adequate examination. It can also prevent postpartum discomfort.

109. (3) The presenting part descends and engages into the midpelvis. This movement occurs first and continues throughout the labor.

110. (2) The fetal head enters the maternal midpelvis transversely, to accommodate to the largest diameter of the pelvis.

111. (2) Flexion of the fetal head allows presentation of the smallest diameter of the skull into the pelvis.

112. (2) Internal rotation follows flexion. This occurs when the head reaches the pelvic floor, and involves alignment of the head with the anteroposterior diameter of the pelvic outlet.

113. (3) With each contraction the uterine muscle fibers become progressively shorter and thicker. This results in the thickening and shortening of the fundus and the thinning and widening of the lower, less muscular portion of the uterus.

114. (1) Since absorption of stomach contents and gastric motility is considerably slower during labor, solid foods should be avoided. Liquids can be ingested.

115. (1) Specific breathing exercises during contractions promote oxygenation and provide distraction from the pain of the contraction.

116. (3) The transition phase is the most physically and emotionally exhaustive for most women. Physical occurrences during this time include nausea and vomiting, chills, leg tremors, the urge to push, and lower back pain. Counterpressure to the small of the back can alleviate the pressure caused by the presenting part.

117. (1) Assessments of the fetal heart rate pattern should increase proportionately with the progress of labor in the first stage. Suggested minimal intervals in the various phases are: latent — minimum every hour; active — minimum every half-hour; transitional — minimum every 15 minutes.

118. (2) Early deceleration of the fetal heart rate produces a uniform pattern, the shape of which reflects the uterine pressure curve. The pattern is thought to be due to application of mechanical forces of uterine contractions to the fetal head by the dilating cervix. This pattern is not associated with fetal distress.

119. (2) During transition the woman needs to be reminded that this is the hardest *but also* the shortest period of labor. It is time-limited, and relief occurs with complete dilatation.

120. (2) Cervical effacement is the process whereby the cervix becomes soft and thin. The contractions of the uterine myometrium pull the cervix upward, resulting in the thinning of its dense fibrous connective tissue.

121. (3) Cervical effacement and dilatation occur primarily as the result of uterine contractions. Additionally, the pressure of the fetal presenting part or the bag of waters serves to act as a "dilating wedge," and thus influences the process of dilatation.

122. (2) The removal of amniotic fluid, which served as an equalizing force, can allow the presenting part to descend more completely on the cervix and become a more efficient dilating wedge.

123. (2) Engagement of the fetal head eliminates a space fo the umbilical cord to slip downward.

124. (3) The first stage of labor, the stage of dilatation, begins with the onset of regular uterine contractions and ends with the complete dilatation of the cervix.

125. (2) Cervical dilatation is measured in centimeters, from 0–10. The completely dilated cervix is 10 cm. in width.

126. (4) Contractions cause stretching of the cervix, traction upon the peritoneum and supporting ligaments, pressure on the urethra and bladder, distention of soft tissues, ischemia of the uterine cells, and pressure on nerve ganglia adjacent to the cervix and vagina. The pain experience for the patient in labor does not have physiologic validity.

127. (4) Vaginal or rectal examinations during labor provide information as to the status of the cervix, the level of the presenting part, and the presentation and position of the fetus.

128. (4) With the numerous stimuli from cervical dilatation, descent of the fetus, and stretching of the perineum, the urge to urinate may be decreased. A distended bladder impedes the progress of labor. Thus, all women during labor need to be assessed for bladder distention and offered the bedpan at regular intervals.

129. (2) The second stage of labor is more intense than the first. Contractions became more expulsive in nature and have a duration of about 1 minute.

130. (1) The contractions of the second stage occur at frequent intervals, generally 1–3 minutes.

131. (2) Contractions of prolonged duration (over 90 seconds), constant with no interval or relaxation phase or of extreme tonus, are abnormal and should be reported to the physician.

132. (2) During the second stage the woman bears down with uterine contractions to provide intra-abdominal pressure to aid in the expulsion process.

133. (3) Station refers to the level of the presenting part in the pelvic midplane. When the presenting part is at the level of the ischial spines, the station is referred to as "zero" and indicates engagement. Levels above the ischial spines refer to a "minus" (−1, −2, −3) station. Levels below the ischial spines refer to a "plus" (+1, +2, +3) station, and indicate passage onto the perineal floor.

134. (2) Engagement indicates that the fetal presenting part has traversed the pelvic inlet and has settled into the midpelvis.

135. (2) Position refers to the more specific relationship of the presenting part to the maternal pelvis. This relationship is the point on the presenting part that is being directed to either the front, back, or left-right sides of the maternal passage.

136. (2) In addition to an increase in blood pressure, respiratory rate is altered and usually increased between contractions.

137. (2) Fetal heart rate must be carefully monitored during the second stage. During the early second stage, auscultation should occur at least every 5 minutes. As the second stage advances, fetal heart rate should be assessed after every contraction.

138. (1) Molding is the overlapping of the bones of the skull and the narrowing of sutures caused by normal compression during delivery to accommodate passage through the birth canal.

139. (3) Asepsis should be the rule for any procedure that involves the penetration of the skin or entrance into a body cavity of the woman in labor.

140. (2) As the head begins to crown, have the mother pant. Support the perineum and allow the head to be delivered between contractions. This action will protect the infant's intracranial structure and minimize the danger of perineal laceration.

141. (3) The mother should not be left unattended if delivery is near. The nurse should call for help, instruct the patient not to push, and slowly deliver the head between contractions.

142. (2) The occiput anterior position occurs most often, since 97 per cent of presentations are vertex, and the left occiput anterior position is more common than the right.

143. (3) The main purposes of an episiotomy are to alleviate pressure of the fetal head on the perineum, prevent laceration of perineal tissue and muscle, and facilitate delivery by enlarging the vaginal orifice.

144. (2) As soon as the head is delivered, feel about the neck for the cord. If it is present and is loose, the cord is slipped over head. If it is too tight to remove, it will be necessary to clamp the cord in two places and cut between the ties.

145. (3) Once the neck has been checked for the cord, the head is supported with one hand, and the mucus and fluid are wiped from the nose and mouth.

146. (3) The stage of expulsion or delivery begins with the complete dilatation of the cervix, and ends with the birth of the baby.

147. (2) Transfusion from placenta to infant can occur if the infant is placed below the level of the perineum.

148. (3) The cord must be double-clamped before it is cut to prevent hemorrhage

from either the maternal or the infant system. The cord is cut between the clamps.

149. (2) Mild tactile stimulation can assist the infant to initiate respirations.

150. (4) The Apgar score is a tool to assess the neonate's cardiopulmonary functions. It consists of five criteria, with an optimal score of 10 points. Heart rate is scored 0 — absent, 1 — below 100, and 2 — over 100. Since the maximal score was achieved, the baby was given a 2 — over 100 for heart rate.

151. (4) Respiratory effort is scored 0 — absent, 1 — slow and irregular, and 2 — good with a strong cry. Since the maximal score was achieved, respiratory efforts are at the 2 level.

152. (4) Color is scored 0 — blue or pale, 1 — acrocyanosis, and 2 — completely pink. Since the maximal score was achieved, the color is at the 2 level.

153. (4) Infants with scores of 10 usually do not need extra therapy beyond the routines to ensure patent airway, heat, and continued observation.

154. (2) The first few contractions following delivery of the baby shear the placenta from the myometrium.

155. (2) As the placenta separates and descends into the lower uterine segment, the fundus rises and becomes globular.

156. (1) In addition to the change in the uterine fundus, the amount of umbilical cord visible increases, and vaginal blood flow is more evident, thus indicating placental separation.

157. (2) The third stage, the placental stage, begins after the complete birth of the baby and ends with the delivery of the placenta. The goal is the separation and expulsion of the placenta.

158. (3) The fourth stage of labor, the "immediate recovery period," begins after the expulsion of the placenta and lasts for at least one hour.

159. (2) Methylergonovine stimulates uterine contractions, and thus helps prevent postpartum hemorrhage.

160. (2) Methylergonovine acts to stimulate uterine contractions. Its use is limited to the postpartum period.

161. (3) During the fourth stage of labor the position and tonus of the uterus, amount and character of lochia, pulse, and blood pressure should be monitored every 15 minutes.

162. (4) In addition to observation of the lochial flow, monitoring of maternal vital signs is used to assess the patient for symptoms of postpartum hemorrhage.

163. (2) Uterine atony is the most frequent cause of postpartum hemorrhage. Immediate action involves massage of the fundus until it becomes firm.

164. (2) Average blood loss during the immediate postpartal period indicates that a perineal pad is soaked within 30 minutes.

165. (4) Silver nitrate is effective against the gonorrhea bacillus that may have been present in the maternal tissues and passed on to the baby.

166. (3) Use of an identification band that verifies the mother, date and time of birth, and sex of the child is the identification method of choice.

167. (2) Identification of the infant should occur in the delivery room in the presence of the mother, as soon as possible after birth.

168. (3) Namebands with corresponding numbers and dates are attached to the mother's wrist and to two of the infant's extremities.

169. (4) Goals of postpartum care include promotion of health, facilitation of maternal-infant adaptation, assumption of maternal role, and prevention of complications.

170. (1) A full bladder will displace the fundus upward and to the right of the midline.

171. (2) The patient's recovery from anesthesia, physical condition and hemoglobin count are evaluated prior to ambulation. She generally is up within a few hours after delivery, and usually within 24 hours.

172. (4) The fundus during the period of involution is palpated as smooth and hard, secondary to the contracted myometrium.

173. (2) The "taking-in" period of the early postpartal period includes a therapeutic sleep, increased interest in food, desire to be cared for, and a need to recount the labor/delivery process.

174. (1) The behavior of the early postpartal period is characterized by dependency and the new mother's attempts to have her own needs met.

175. (4) The position of the fundus is generally at the umbilicus on the first postpartum day. It descends one to two fingerbreadths per day during the process of involution.

176. (2) Relaxation and contraction of the uterine myometrium are responsible for "afterpains."

177. (4) Various treatments can be utilized to alleviate perineal pain: heat (either by lamp or sitz bath) will increase vasodilatation; local anesthetics penetrate the sensory nerve endings and reduce the responsiveness of sensory stimuli; and analgesics may be necessary to relieve the pain.

178. (2) The transitory depression of the postpartal period is believed to be precipitated by environmental pressures, role changes, and endocrine changes.

179. (2) Lochia serosa is present during days 3–8. It is pink or dark brown in color, and consists of erythrocytes, leukocytes, shreds of decidua, mucus from the cervix, and microorganisms.

180. (4) Good perineal hygiene procedures are essential in reducing the possibility of puerperal infection. The new mother should refrain from sexual intercourse until the episiotomy is healed (usually 2–3 weeks).

181. (4) Factors that predispose women to infections during the puerperal period include trauma and/or excessive blood loss during labor, prolonged rupture of membranes, and any deviation from maternal health.

182. (3) Infections in the puerperal period originate from two primary sources: endogenous — bacteria in the normal flora, which become virulent when tissues are traumatized; and exogenous — pathogens introduced via excessive obstetric manipulations or a break in aseptic technique.

183. (4) In addition to positive lochial cultures, foul-smelling and excessive lochia, and persistent pain, a temperature elevation of 100.4° F. (38° C.) after the first 24 hours following delivery, and which remains elevated on two or more assessments, is diagnostic of puerperal infection.

184. (2) The most common causative organism of puerperal infection is anaerobic streptococcus.

185. (2) Endometritis is the main manifestation of puerperal infection because the endometrium acts as a particularly good medium for bacterial growth.

186. (1) Appropriate antibiotic therapy is the usual treatment for puerperal sepsis.

187. (4) The infectious process can extend into the surrounding pelvic tissues, travel via the blood or lymphatics, and establish new infection sites in heart, lungs, and kidneys.

188. (2) Retention of tissue fluid adds to the weight gain in the last weeks of pregnancy. The loss of this fluid accounts for a portion of the weight loss during the postpartal period.

189. (4) About 76 grams of protein per day is recommended during pregnancy. A 20-gram increase in protein during lactation beings the requirement to 96 grams per day during lactation.

190. (4) The high levels of estrogen and progesterone secreted by the placenta inhibit the release of prolactin by the anterior pituitary.

191. (3) Colostrum contains more protein materials and salt, but less fat and slightly less sugar than human milk.

192. (4) Prolactin stimulates synthesis of a large quantity of fat lactose and casein by the mammary glands. It takes about 3 days for this to occur and for sufficient milk to be produced.

193. (4) Nipples should be cleansed with clear, warm water. Since soap removes protective skin oils, it should not be used on the nipples.

194. (1) Engorgement is due to an exaggeration of the normal venous and lymphatic circulation to the breasts. It is not an overaccumulation of milk.

195. (2) Pain due to breast engorgement can be relieved by breast support, ice packs, and analgesia.

196. (1) Wearing a brassiere can help alleviate the discomfort of engorgement and provide a measure of protection for the nipples.

197. (3) Drinking this quantity of milk will replace the protein being given to the infant.

198. (1) Sucking time is limited to prevent soreness and cracking of the nipples. However, current practice in many hospitals is not to limit nursing time since sucking promotes milk secretion.

199. (2) Nursing care of the woman who is breast-feeding includes education and support. The infant should be sucking and well-positioned. Constant supervision is unnecessary and may inhibit the mother.

200. (3) Handwashing is the most effective method of preventing contamination of the infant.

201. (3) If nipples become sore and cracked, the feeding time can be shortened. Exposure of the sore nipple to a heat lamp will promote vasodilatation, and thereby facilitate healing. The use of a nipple shield is recommended but controversial.

202. (1) Poor handwashing technique and contamination between infants has been proved to be the greatest source of infection in the neonatal nursery.

203. (3) Normal range for vital signs in the newborn are respirations 30–40/minute, heart rate 120–140/minute, and temperature 36.5–37°C. These values are applicable within 4–6 hours after birth.

204. (4) In order to maintain an adequate respiratory pattern, careful attention must be given to mucus secretion and drainage. Positioning the infant to facilitate drainage, gentle suctioning with bulb syringe, and careful observation are essential. Accurate recording and reporting are also important.

205. (4) The normal newborn exhibits the rooting, sucking, swallowing, and gag reflexes. There may be uncoordinated suck/swallow responses during the first attempts at feeding; "retrusive" reflex refers to the infant's regurgitation of food before swallowing it.

206. (3) The Moro reflex consists of two phases: first, quick flexion of the forearm, followed by abduction of the arm at the shoulder, and extension of the forearm and fingers; second, adduction of the arm at the shoulder. This is also referred to as the "startle response."

207. (4) Prophylactic treatment with 1 per cent silver nitrate is mandated by law in most states. Since chemical conjunctivitis is not an uncommon response to its instillation, daily cleansing and irrigation are appropriate, utilizing the correct scientific principles.

208. (3) Water is usually given as the first feeding to ascertain if feeding problems exist. Attention is given to suck/swallow coordination. Also, sterile water, if aspirated, is less irritating to the lungs than formula.

209. (3) Stool patterns change in consistency, color, amount, and frequency depending on the food intake. Transitional stools are best described as greenish-brown and of a somewhat watery consistency.

210. (2) Absence of the passage of meconium may indicate an imperforate anus or obstruction in the ileum.

211. (4) Jaundice appearing after 72 hours of life has been defined as "physiologic," and occurs in approximately 80 per cent of all infants.

212. (2) The umbilical cord stump usually separates between 10 and 14 days after birth. There may be some slight bleeding at the time of separation.

213. (1) Care of the umbilical stump includes cleansing, application of alcohol to the base, and air-drying.

214. (4) Successful adaptation of the maternal role requires that the new mother feel confident and secure in each "task" that she attempts. Multiple tasks may be simultaneously undertaken, although success may occur at varying rates.

215. (2) Douching should be avoided until the process of involution is complete. Good perineal hygiene will help to remove the odor from lochial flow.

216. (2) Lactating mothers usually experience anovulation and amenorrhea for varying degress of time — some for as long as they lactate, others for only 2 months. The average menstruation delay is 4 months.

217. (4) By six weeks the process of involution should be complete. All of the procedures listed would re-establish baseline values and assure proper postdelivery healing.

Preeclampsia

1. (4) Toxemia of pregnancy is a general category that includes preeclampsia and eclampsia.
2. (4) Predisposing causes for toxemia include: hypertension, renal disease, diabetes, polyhydramnios, multiple pregnancy, hydatidiform mole, anemia, and poor nutritional status.
3. (3) The classic symptoms of toxemia include hypertension, edema, and proteinuria. Convulsions and/or coma occur in eclampsia.
4. (3) In general, an elevation of 30 mm. Hg systolic pressure or more and/or 15 mm. Hg diastolic pressure or more over baseline are abnormal, and considered characteristic of toxemia.
5. (1) The exact cause of toxemia is unknown, although several theories have been proposed. Uterine ischemia is currently thought to be a probable cause of toxemia of pregnancy.
6. (3) Eclamptic toxemia is a disease state that occurs only in pregnancy.
7. (3) Since toxemia is dependent on a functioning pregnancy in order to continue, termination of the pregnancy will result in termination of the disease.
8. (3) Hemoconcentration, generalized vasospasm, and edema are the pathophysiologic changes evidenced with toxemia.
9. (2) Vasoconstriction of the afferent glomerular arterioles alters the permeability of the glomerular membrane, thus predisposing to proteinuria.
10. (1) The etiology of all of the signs of toxemia are related to generalized vasospasm. Arteriolar vasoconstriction and peripheral vascular spasms are reflected in elevation of blood pressure.
11. (3) The major organs affected are the cerebrum, kidney, and uterus. Decreased blood flow to the cerebrum can result in headaches, blurred vision, convulsions and/or coma. Proteinuria results from vasoconstriction of the glomerular arterioles, and uteroplacental insufficiency can be attributed to vasospasms.
12. (2) Many symptoms of preeclampsia (blood pressure elevation, proteinuria, edema) require an examination by a health professional to determine their severity.
13. (4) Energy conservation is important in decreasing the metabolic rate to minimize the demand for oxygen. Lowered oxygen tension in toxemia is the result of vasoconstriction and decreased blood flow that diminishes the amount of nutrients and oxygen in the cells.
14. (4) Uterine oxygen supply is compromised with vasoconstriction, thereby predisposing the fetus to hypoxia. If the disease state endangers the mother or the fetus, early termination of the pregnancy may be required.
15. (4) All the complications listed are possible if the toxemia does not respond to therapy. They are the result of continued vasoconstriction and an imbalance between intra- and extra-cellular fluid.
16. (4) Eclampsia differs from preeclampsia in that the eclamptic patient exhibits convulsions and/or coma.
17. (4) Fluid accumulation in the tissue results in a shift of fluid from the intravascular to the extravascular compartment. This produces hemoconcentration, as reflected by an increased hematocrit.
18. (3) Edema of the ankles and fingers occur in about 60 per cent of women whose pregnancy is considered normal. Facial edema reflects increased fluid retention (considered 3+) and cannot be classified as a normal occurrence.
19. (4) Progression of the disease is indicated by blurred vision, headaches, dizziness, nausea and vomiting, epigastric pain, and oliguria.
20. (3) Warning signs that a convulsion is imminent include severe epigastric pain, chest tightness, increased restlessness, and decreased pulse and respirations.
21. (1) Examination of the eyegrounds will reveal arteriolar vasospasm, and possibly retinal hemorrhages.
22. (4) All the listed blood chemistry changes would be evident, secondary to vasoconstriction, fluid shifts, and compensation.
23. (2) Toxemia of pregnancy predisposes patients to abruptio placenta. Women with toxemia complicated by underlying hypertensive vascular disease are at even greater risk.

24. (2) Monitoring of intake and output will indicate the degree of renal impairment due to decreased circulation, and can assist in ascertaining the amount of fluid being retained.
25. (1) The normal pregnant woman should not exceed 300 mg./day excretion of protein. Levels greater than this are indicative of preeclampsia.
26. (3) Urine protein levels, weight determination to check fluid retention, serum sodium levels, and deep tendon reflexes to determine central nervous system excitability are evaluated on a daily basis.
27. (3) Phenobarbital is administered for its sedative effect. The aim of this therapy is to encourage relaxation and thus decrease metabolic oxygen demands.
28. (1) In hypnotic doses sodium secobarbital produces sedation and rest, with minimal side effects for both mother and fetus.
29. (4) Phenobarbital is a long-acting barbiturate with a duration of action of 8–16 hours. Secobarbital is a short-acting barbiturate with a duration of action of 3–6 hours and an onset of action of 10–15 minutes.
30. (3) Moderate sodium-restricted diet would prohibit the addition of any salt prior to or following cooking.
31. (4) All foods listed have a high sodium content.
32. (1) Animal proteins, such as meat, poultry, fish, milk, cheese, and eggs, which provide essential amino acids, are also relatively high in sodium. These foods, however, are essential for good nutrition.
33. (3) The side-lying position will promote renal blood flow and encourage diuresis.
34. (2) Examination of the eyegrounds would be performed on a daily basis to assess arteriolar spasms and retinal hemorrhage.
35. (4) All the visual disturbances listed might be experienced as vasoconstriction increases, creating edema and spasm in the retinal area.
36. (1) Sudden sensory stimulation can precipitate a convulsion. A quiet, darkened environment is helpful in preventing this complication.
37. (4) Nursing response should not increase anxiety or create fear. Option 4 provides the patient with a supportive and understandable explanation.
38. (3) Energy conservation is a primary goal of therapy. Care is needed to minimize sensory stimulation and promote relaxation.
39. (4) As the disease progresses, all the symptoms listed may indicate that a convulsion is imminent.
40. (3) Both tonic and clonic convulsions occur in eclampsia. At first all muscles are in a state of tonic contraction, and then muscles alternately contract and relax.
41. (2) Precautions that can protect the patient from injuries during a convulsion include: use of an airway, no restraints on limbs, padding the siderails of the bed, and constant attendance by the nurse.
42. (3) Nursing care is directed toward patient comfort. All actions are appropriate except those that might be too stimulating and would not facilitate energy conservation.
43. (3) Contractions during early labor are infrequent and of mild intensity. Heavy sedation may interfere with the patient's perception of contractions.
44. (4) Labor was induced because the toxemia was progressing and all the listed complications might develop.
45. (1) Oxytocin increases the permeability of the cell membrane to sodium ion. This augments the numbers of contracting myofibrils, thus promoting rhythmic contractions of uterine muscle fibers.
46. (3) Hypotonic uterine dysfunction and/or uterine inertia can be effectively treated with oxytocin infusion.
47. (3) The patient receiving oxytocin therapy must be continuously monitored. Optimal management includes constant attendance by a physician or nurse, and use of electronic fetal monitoring.
48. (3) In addition to monitoring the rate of infusion, blood pressure and fetal heart rate are checked every 15 minutes.
49. (1) The contraction pattern established by oxytocin infusion should have a duration of 60 seconds or less and a frequency of at least every 2–3 minutes.
50. (2) Fetal bradycardia, uterine hypertonicity, or tetanic contractions indicate a reaction to the oxytocin infusion, and require it to be discontinued.

51. (2) Fetal heart rate should be monitored every 5 minutes to assess tolerance of the effects of oxytocin.
52. (1) Although a decrease in fetal heart tone is a frequent occurrence late in pregnancy, this phenomenon is an abnormal but benign pattern.
53. (1) Valium is used for its sedative and relaxing effects.
54. (3) Magnesium sulfate causes central nervous system depression, thus preventing convulsions, promoting vasodilatation, and enhancing diuresis.
55. (4) Magnesium toxicity is characterized by loss of the patellar deep tendon reflex, quickly followed by depression of respiration and lowered pulse.
56. (1) Calcium gluconate is the antidote for magnesium toxicity.
57. (3) Deladumone is an androgen-estrogen preparation that inhibits the release of lactogenic hormone from the pituitary, thus preventing lactation and breast engorgement.
58. (2) There is a danger of an eclamptic convulsion for approximately 48 hours after delivery.
59. (2) After delivery there usually is rapid improvement of toxemia. The most favorable response is that of increased urinary output.
60. (2) Maintenance of self-respect and ego strength are essential to turn the crisis of single parenthood into a growth-producing experience.
61. (1) Acceptance of the present in relation to the future will facilitate the maintenance of self-respect.
62. (4) Generally, the effects of toxemia are limited to the disease process and leave no residual effects.
63. (4) Agencies generally consider all the factors listed when interviewing prospective adoptive parents.
64. (3) The unwed mother generally is viewed as having erred and being undeserving of any understanding.
65. (2) The concerns of the unwed father are usually ignored and generally discounted by society.

Placenta Praevia

1. (3) In placenta praevia the placenta is implanted low in the uterus, either on the lower uterine segment or over the internal os.
2. (1) Although the exact cause of placental praevia is unknown, it is more common in multiparas, and its incidence increases with advancing maternal age.
3. (4) Placenta praevia may be related to spontaneous abortion in that lower segment implantations have a lower probability of continuing to term.
4. (3) As the lower uterine segment retracts and dilates during the last weeks of pregnancy, the villi are torn from the uterus. The placental site is thus denuded and hemorrhage occurs.
5. (3) Cervical dilatation causes the placental villi to be torn, thus opening the uterine sinuses and resulting in hemorrhage.
6. (3) Abnormal fetal presentation usually accompanies placenta praevia.
7. (4) Since the bleeding that accompanies placenta praevia can occur as early as the sixth month of gestation, the risk of prematurity is great for the neonate.
8. (1) The management of placenta praevia depends on the length of gestation and the amount of bleeding. In all cases, bedrest and observation are indicated.
9. (4) Vaginal examination to diagnose placenta praevia is carried out only when fetal gestation is at least 37 weeks, or when repeated hemorrhages pose a threat to the mother's life. The examination is referred to as a "double set-up" and is performed only in the operating room.
10. (3) The "double set-up" vaginal examination requires that everything be available to perform a cesarean section should a hemorrhage be provoked. Abdominal skin preparation is required should surgery prove to be necessary.
11. (4) Since the vaginal examination is done as a sterile procedure with surgery as a possible outcome, all the equipment listed should be assembled.
12. (2) Laboratory tests that can diagnose placenta praevia include placental localization by radioisotopes and ultrasound scan.

13. (3) Constant observation is important so that complications can be identified quickly.
14. (1) As soon as the patient is able to understand what has occurred, an explanation should be provided. This will provide a framework for future supportive discussions.
15. (1) The husband should be advised on the status of mother and infant as soon as the surgery is completed.
16. (1) The initial stage of the grief process is shock and disbelief. If the death was unexpected, this stage may be prolonged.
17. (4) It is inadvisable for the nurse to remind the mother that she is "blessed" with other children. The mother needs to work through this loss, and cannot focus on other aspects of her life until this crisis has begun to resolve. This response gives the mother the opportunity to verbalize and begin to deal with the crisis.
18. (2) Mothers may blame themselves for any abnormalities in the fetus. The nurse's question allows Alice to explore, with help, the cause of placenta praevia and its relationship to the death of the fetus.
19. (1) Although the chance of having another normal child is good, the nurse is cautioned against being unduly optimistic. Inquiry about the patient's wishes is appropriate because it continues to help her with the crisis resolution.
20. (3) The actions of the nurse depend on her assessment of the individual. The request may be appropriate and may reflect the patient's attempt to resolve the grief process.

Diabetes and Pregnancy

1. (4) Obesity, history of diabetes, stillbirth or spontaneous abortion, and delivery of a large infant place the pregnant woman at risk for the development or exacerbation of diabetes. Diabetes in pregnancy is a major cause of maternal and perinatal morbidity and mortality.
2. (4) All the physiologic changes listed can be attributed to either fetal drain of maternal glucose and amino acids and/or the antagonistic effects of the placental hormones on maternal insulin.
3. (3) Adrenal corticosteroids, anterior pituitary hormones, and thyroxine are increased during pregnancy and are thought to explain the diabetogenic effect of pregnancy. These hormones, directly or indirectly, increase the concentration of glucose in the serum.
4. (4) All the complications listed can occur with a history of long-standing diabetes compounded by vascular changes. The variety of hormones produced by the placenta, and increased maternal levels of corticosteroids during gestation, diminish the effectiveness of insulin.
5. (4) The diabetic patient is at risk for all the complications listed. They can be attributed to altered carbohydrate metabolism and vascular compromise.
6. (2) The normal fasting serum glucose level ranges from 80 to 120 mg. per 100 ml. of blood.
7. (2) In the nonpregnant patient, two-hour postprandial glucose levels should not exceed 110 mg. per 100 ml.
8. (3) Arteriosclerotic heart disease is a complication that can occur as a result of diabetes. The basement membrane of the capillary beds thickens primarily in the retina, kidney, and skeletal muscle.
9. (2) Tolbutamide acts on the islet cells of the pancreas to stimulate the release of endogenous insulin.
10. (1) Oral agents are contraindicated during pregnancy. They have been associated with congenital abnormalities, and rarely provide sufficient control of diabetes. Oral thiazides are thought to have a diabetogenic effect.
11. (1) Postprandial serum glucose is determined by venous blood drawn at hourly intervals following a glucose meal.
12. (2) The renal threshold for glucose decreases during pregnancy, producing a lower tubular capacity to reabsorb glucose, and thus resulting in glycosuria.

13. (3) Obese persons have less body water per kg. than normal-weight persons. High concentration of glucose filters into the renal tubules and acts as an osmotic diuretic, resulting in dehydration.

14. (3) One gram of pure carbohydrate will yield 4 calories. Therefore, 150 grams of carbohydrate represents 600 calories.

15. (4) One gram of pure fat will yield 9 calories. Therefore, 70 grams of fat represents 630 calories.

16. (3) Fruit exchanges represent 10 grams of carbohydrate; protein and fat are negligible. The fruits may be used fresh, cooked, canned, frozen, or unsweetened. Included as one fruit exchange are: one grapefruit half, one orange, and one cup of strawberries. These fruits are also excellent sources of ascorbic acid.

17. (4) One fruit exchange contains 10 grams of carbohydrate and 40 kcal. The fruits may be used fresh, cooked, canned, or unsweetened.

18. (2) Group A vegetables provide major sources of vitamin A and iron and are a good source of B-complex vitamins. Included in group A vegetables are broccoli, tomatoes, and spinach.

19. (4) Class A vegetables can be eaten as desired. Their protein, carbohydrate, and fat value are negligible.

20. (3) Butter and margarine contain higher proportions of saturated fatty acids than do the vegetable oils.

21. (2) The classes of beta-lipoproteins greatly increase after age 30. The increase has been associated with a high incidence of coronary artery disease and atherosclerosis. Type IV abnormality of hyperlipoproteinemia is common in diabetes.

22. (3) Chicken is the meat that is lowest in saturated fats.

23. (4) The symptoms describe a hypoglycemic reaction, and therefore ingestion of a concentrated carbohydrate is indicated.

24. (4) When blood sugar levels are abnormally high, the excess glucose eventually spills into the urine. Fractional urine tests assist in assessing the degree of control. The usual time to test urine is one half-hour before meals and at bedtime. The results of the tests are used to determine insulin dosage.

25. (2) Insulin reactions can be the result of insulin overdose, omission of food, or overexertion without caloric compensation. The time of the reaction depends on the type of insulin. Since Lente insulin is intermediate-acting, the most likely time for a reaction would be 8–10 hours after administration.

26. (2) Since an insulin reaction can result from the omission of meals or from eating less food than prescribed, the appropriate action is to compensate for the carbohydrate loss.

27. (3) Light exercise would be appropriate for all purposes shown except d. Renal damage secondary to vascular disease has no relationship to activity level.

28. (4) a, b, and d are routinely performed on all pregnant women. Eyegrounds are visualized to assess vascular status of the retina, which is important in persons with diabetes.

29. (3) Insulin requirements during pregnancy reflect the availability of circulating carbohydrate and the antagonistic effects of the placental hormones toward insulin. Since the effects of the hormones are more pronounced during the second half of pregnancy, the insulin requirements at that time are greater than during the first half of pregnancy.

30. (4) Hospitalization of the diabetic patient is intended to assess maternal and fetal status and insure diabetic control.

31. (2) The biparietal diameter is checked to assess gestational age, thus providing an indication of the expected date of confinement.

32. (4) The lecithin-sphingomyelin ratio is used to assess fetal lung maturity. Adequate pulmonary development is reflected by a ratio of at least 2:1.

33. (3) Respiratory distress syndrome does not occur usually when the L/S ratio is greater than 2:1. The ratio may become as great as 5:1 at 40 weeks' gestation.

34. (2) Urinary estriol represents the metabolic activity of th fetoplacental unit. Since estriol values increase as pregnancy advances, they can be used to assess gestational age.

35. (3) The oxytocin challenge test is used to assess placental reserve and fetal response to fairly mild uterine contractions.
36. (3) The FHR pattern described is that of late deceleration. The physiologic basis for this pattern is uteroplacental insufficiency.
37. (1) Preoperative skin cleansing is intended primarily to remove bacteria mechanically.
38. (3) Insertion of an indwelling urinary catheter is considered part of routine preparation for surgery.
39. (2) Labor represents a severe exercise state; as such, it uses all available glucose and may deplete glycogen stores.
40. (4) Low transverse incision is preferred for all the reasons stated and because it is associated with low maternal morbidity and complications.
41. (2) The infant of a diabetic mother is easily identified. In addition to the baby's being large for gestational age, the heart, spleen and liver are enlarged. The increased size and abundant fat tissue stores can be attributed to the effects of excessive insulin.
42. (3) Increased size of an infant is primarily a result of excessive fat tissue, glycogen storage, and increased organ size. Retention of excessive interstitial fluids is also a factor, but is less contributory to size increase.
43. (4) Metabolic and growth abnormalities observed in the infants of diabetic mothers are secondary to excessive maternal hormones and fetal hyperglycemia, with its resultant hyperinsulinemia.
44. (4) The generic name for Demerol is meperidine.
45. (2) Demerol is intended to relieve moderate-to-severe pain. The drug acts on those areas of the brain involved in the perception of pain.
46. (3) Promethazine is the generic name for Phenergan.
47. (3) Phenergan was originally introduced for its antihistamine properties. It is also useful as a sedative, antiemetic, and tranquilizer.
48. (3) Recovery room care of the patient who has undergone a cesarean section involves the same precautions as for the patient whose infant is vaginally delivered, plus the monitoring of abdominal dressings.
49. (1) Hemorrhage poses the greatest risk during the immediate postpartum period. Bleeding may be evident, as in excess vaginal flow, or concealed, as evidenced by alterations in vital signs.
50. (3) Shock is manifested by alterations in vital signs and appearance as the body attempts to compensate for decreased blood volume. Respiratory rate is rapid, as is pulse rate. Blood pressure initially is normotensive and then begins to fall. The patient is cool and pale, and exhibits behavior characteristic of anxiety and apprehension.
51. (3) Pelvic thrombosis is a complication of cesarean delivery. Most frequently, the ovarian vein is the site of involvement.
52. (2) Conversion of serum glucose to lactose occurs in all postpartum patients. It will, however, be more evident in the diabetic patient, for whom closer monitoring of glucose levels is done.
53. (4) Early ambulation following abdominal surgery has been associated with increased peristalsis and lower incidence of maternal complications.
54. (1) Hypocalcemia is a frequent complication in infants of diabetic mothers. It can be associated with a higher incidence of prematurity, birth asphyxia, and tissue damage, which adds to the phosphate "load."
55. (1) Birth injury is not uncommon in infants of diabetic mothers because of their large body size. The injury occurs most frequently in the head and neck area, and can also be associated with prematurity.
56. (2) Immediate care of the infant of a diabetic mother includes provision and maintenance of a patent airway, respiratory stimulation, and prevention of heat loss.
57. (3) Hypoglycemia occurs frequently in the infant of a diabetic mother because the supply of maternal glucose is terminated at delivery. However, fetal insulin levels are high. The decrease in circulating carbohydrate and the continued high level of insulin predispose the newborn to hypoglycemia.
58. (3) Respiratory distress syndrome is a frequent complication. Symptoms appear within hours after birth, and are secondary to prematurity of the pulmonary system.

59. (2) Early and frequent feedings are appropriate in the management of the infant of a diabetic mother. The initial feeding of glucose water would provide calories and be less irritating to the lungs if aspiration should occur.

60. (3) Neonatal death rate is higher for infants of diabetic mothers. The events associated with prematurity, birth injury, and other congenital anomalies have been implicated as the leading causes.

Heart Disease and Pregnancy

1. (1) Rheumatic fever is an acute or chronic inflammatory process that affects connective tissue in organs throughout the body. Rheumatic carditis involves one or all three of the layers of the heart.

2. (3) During pregnancy the heart enlarges, presumably because of greater diastolic filling secondary to an increased stroke volume. The heart sounds are louder on auscultation, with evidence of a split second sound and faint systolic murmur. Dependent or mechanical edema occurs in a high percentage of normal pregnancies.

3. (2) Organic heart disease involves underlying vascular, valve, or tissue damage. Since the patient did have confirmed mitral stenosis, the disease was classified as organic.

4. (1) During pregnancy, polycythemia tends to occur near term and influences the sedimentation rate.

5. (2) Mitral stenosis is the most common lesion of the mitral valve. As the valve calcifies and becomes immobile, the flow of blood from the left atrium to the left ventricle becomes turbulent instead of flowing in the normal laminar, noiseless manner.

6. (2) Any situation that would further stress the heart poses a risk for the pregnant patient with heart disease. Factors that predispose to the development of complications include: excessive weight gain, anemia, hypertension, anxiety, fatigue, and infectious processes.

7. (1) Promotion of rest is the major component in the care of the patient with heart disease. Rest helps prevent fatigue in cardiac functioning.

8. (3) Sleep and rest patterns should include a minimum of 8–10 hours per night, with frequent rest periods throughout the day.

9. (3) Physical activity should be encouraged as long as it does not lead to shortness of breath and fatigue. If these symptoms occur, the most strenuous activities should be limited.

10. (1) A diet high in iron is essential to meet the increased needs for oxygen and plasma volume. Should anemia occur, cardiac output would increase as a compensatory mechanism for oxygen deficit.

11. (4) Any infectious process predisposes the patient with heart disease to cardiac failure. The woman should be well-nourished and well-rested, and should avoid possible sources of infection.

12. (4) If the patient shows signs of cardiac failure, fluid may also be restricted to decrease the circulating volume and reduce cardiac work.

13. (3) Blood volume increases approximately 35 per cent during pregnancy. This additional load can produce symptoms of cardiac failure in the patient with pre-existing heart disease.

14. (1) Cardiac output increases in response to physiologic anemia and the demands of the fetus for oxygen. Mitral stenosis inhibits flow of blood from the left atrium to the left ventricle, thus preventing an adequate increase in cardiac output. Congestion of blood may occur in the lungs and venous system.

15. (2) As congestive heart failure progresses, an increased amount of fluid may be evident in the lungs, compromising gas exchange.

16. (3) Although edema is not uncommon during pregnancy, and can be attributed to the pressure of the gravid uterus, venous congestion due to heart failure compounds this edema.

17. (3) Cough is a common symptom of left-sided heart failure. The cough is usually moist and productive as a result of the fluid which moves from pulmonary capillaries into alveolar spaces.

18. (4) Since white cell count is not elevated, it can be assumed that there is no current infectious process. The damage is attributed to a previous inflammatory process.

19. (2) Class II heart disease places slight limitation on physical activities, since fatigue, dyspnea, and angina occur with normal activity.

20. (3) Rales and cough are indicative of pulmonary edema. Since venous congestion reduces peripheral blood flow, cyanosis occurs. Rapid pulse is indicative of the compensatory efforts of the myocardium.

21. (2) Rest will decrease the energy demands of the body, and thus reduce the oxygen and nutrient requirements of the tissues and organs.

22. (4) Complete bedrest indicates that the patient is not to exert any energy. This requires that even routine activities of daily living are severely restricted.

23. (1) The sitting position allows for maximal expansion of the thoracic cavity, thus providing optimal ventilation.

24. (3) The most important action of digitalis is its direct effect on myocardial contraction. Completeness of ventricular emptying and force of systolic contraction are increased.

25. (3) Chlorothiazide (Diuril) increases renal excretion of sodium, chloride, and water. It is administered orally; the onset of action is after 4 hours, but the duration of action is 6–12 hours.

26. (3) Hypokalemia is a side of chlorothiazide therapy. This can be offset by administering a K^+ supplement or providing a diet high in potassium.

27. (4) All the foods listed should be avoided. Table salt should not be added to the sodium-restricted diet, and salted foods and those with high sodium content, including those with preservatives, should also be avoided.

28. (4) Pregnancy is a stressor to heart disease in that it creates an increased workload for an already burdened heart. The patient should be made aware of this so that she may be spared unnecessary guilt feelings.

29. (4) Major symptoms of digitalis toxicity are: gastrointestinal (anorexia, nausea, vomiting, diarrhea); CNS-related (headache, lethargy, irritability); ocular ("colored" vision, diplopia); and cardiovascular (arrhythmias, cardiac failure).

30. (2) Although withholding oral food and fluid is not as popular currently as it once was, the theory behind this is to decrease oxygen demand resulting from metabolism of foods, and to decrease blood volume.

31. (2) Pulse rate is the most sensitive indicator of impending cardiac failure during the first stage of labor. Although pulse rate may increase with contractions, the baseline pulse is not elevated during labor.

32. (2) The ideal position for labor is semirecumbent, with head and shoulders elevated and supported. This allows for maximal expansion of the thoracic cage.

33. (2) Lumbar epidural anesthesia involves the injection of local anesthesia at the lumbar level outside of the dura mater. Epidural anesthesia blocks the nerves that transmit the pain of the first stage of labor.

34. (3) In addition to the normal assessment activities used to monitor the laboring patient, pulse and respiratory rate should be checked at least every 15 minutes, and more often as labor progresses.

35. (1) Care of the cardiac patient during the second stage of labor involves efforts to decrease its length and minimize bearing-down efforts. This will reduce the strain on the heart.

36. (1) Prophylactic procaine penicillin is used to prevent a recurrence of a streptococcal infection.

37. (3) Risks of cardiac failure are great during the postpartum period. Following delivery there is a remobilization of extravascular fluid into the blood stream, and a significant rise in cardiac output. These changes increase cardiac workload and predispose the patient to cardiac failure.

38. (2) The heart's capacity to tolerate the stress imposed by pregnancy must be evaluated, and future planning based on a realistic prognosis.

39. (1) Oral contraceptives are contraindicated in women with a history of heart disease. Side effects of estrogen excess include fluid retention, hypertension, and thromboembolytic disease.

40. (4) Vasectomy is a permanent sterilization procedure that involves severing the vas deferens, thus preventing the sperm from traveling from the testes.

Hemolytic Disease of the Newborn

1. (3) A determinant that will influence whether this couple's children will inherit Paul's Rh positive factor is dependent on whether Paul's trait is heterozygous or homozygous. If he is homozygous Rh positive (genotype DD) and the mother is negative, all the children will be Rh positive.

Father	Mother	
	d	d
D	Dd	Dd
D	Dd	Dd

   If he is heterozygous Rh positive (genotype Dd), the chances are that only half the children will be Rh positive.

Father	Mother	
	d	d
D	Dd	Dd
d	dd	dd

2. (2) Corrine's blood could contain both AA and AO antigens as a result of her ABO genotype.

3. (1) If both parents are type AA, Corrine's genotype for ABO type blood would have to be homozygous.

4. (2) Corrine's blood serum contains anti B antibodies, which are normal constituents of her blood type. If she received types B or AB blood transfusions, agglutination would occur because of the anti B present in the transfusion. If she received O blood, agglutination would not occur because type O blood does not react with anti B.

5. (1) Paul's blood serum contains anti A antibodies, which are normal constituents of his blood type. If this was transfused with types A or AB, agglutination would occur because of the anti A present. If he received O blood, agglutination would not occur because type O blood does not react with anti A.

6. (1) For example, anti Rh antibodies could develop in Corrine (Rh negative) in response to the Rh positive erythrocytes (antigens) of the fetus crossing the placenta into Corrine's body.

7. (2) Examples of antigens are bacteria, toxins, and foreign blood cells.

8. (1) Specific antibodies develop in response to specific antigens. A newer term for antibodies is immunoglobulins, e.g., IgG, IgA, IgM, IgE, IgD.

9. (4) Type AB blood contains no antibodies against A or B antigens; therefore, persons with type AB can receive A, B, or O transfusions. However, a type AB transfusion is preferred.

10. (1) During her first pregnancy Corrine, who is Rh negative, developed anti Rh antibodies only after the Rh positive blood passed through the placenta from the baby to her. During the second pregnancy, the anti Rh antibody level was sufficiently high to cause mild hemolytic disease in the infant.

11. (2) See rationale #10.

12. (4) Rh immunoglobulin inactivates antigens on the RBC membrane, thus blocking the development of maternal anti Rh antibodies.

13. (2) Fetal neonatal hemoglobin is typically higher than that of adults, most likely because of the increased metabolic needs of the fetus.

14. (3) In the direct Coombs' test, a sample of the infant's RBCs are washed and added to Coombs' serum (anti-human IgG). If the RBCs agglutinate the test is positive, demonstrating maternal antibodies on the infant's RBCs and the possibility of the development of hemolytic disease.

15. (1) See rationale #14.

16. (2) Bilirubin is an orange-brown pigment produced by the breakdown of heme. Heme is the iron-containing component of the hemoglobin molecule.

17. (3) a, Rapid or increased destruction of RBCs producing increased degradation of hemoglobin, results in excess bilirubin in the blood. c, Bilirubin is transported to the liver and conjugated to bilirubin glucuronide. This combination is facilitated by the enzyme, glucuronyl transferase. If an adequate amount is not

available owing to prematurity or liver disease, hyperbilirubinemia can occur. e, With the other components of bile, bilirubin enters the bowel, where it is converted by bacteria to urobilinogen. Any intestinal obstruction may interfere with excretion of bilirubin; thus, large amounts may be reabsorbed into the portal and general circulatory systems.

18. (2) Albumin/bilirubin binding is pH-dependent. When acidosis occurs accompanied by increased fatty acid levels in the blood, the binding process may be inhibited. Sulfonamides and sodium benzoate also compete for albumin-binding sites. These factors can result in decreased bonding of bilirubin with albumin.

19. (1) a, It is believed that, through a process of photodegradation, unconjugated bilirubin is reduced to biliverdin after which it is excreted. b, The exchange transfusion replaces most of the infant's Rh positive blood with Rh negative blood, thus slowing the hemolytic process. The exchange also replaces blood high in unconjugated bilirubin with blood free of unconjugated bilirubin, and high in albumin.

20. (1) See rationale #19.

21. (1) The range of normal bilirubin of an adult is 0.3–1.1 mg. per 100 ml. of blood. The higher bilirubin level in the infant is probably due to immature liver functioning. This state is referred to as physiologic jaundice.

22. (2) The isoimmunization process results in maternal anti Rh antibodies causing hemolysis of fetal RBC's. In this process, large amounts of heme are released. When heme is broken down, bilirubin is one of the end products that will enter the blood stream, causing hyperbilirubinemia.

23. (3) Although this rationale is controversial, some people believe that this level of hyperbilirubinemia causes deposition of bilirubin in the brain tissue because of the immature blood barrier in the premature infant.

24. (3) The genotype for ABO blood has the potential for developing a number of different antigens. If the mother and child possess certain combinations of antigens and antibodies, ABO incompatability occurs, and hemolytic disease could result.

25. (3) In erythroblastosis there is a rapid destruction of RBC's. In an attempt to replace the destroyed cells, the bone marrow accelerates RBC production and release. The RBC's, however, are not mature.

26. (4) The lecithin-sphingomyelin (L/S) ratio determined through amniocentesis is a mode for assessing fetal maturity. Ratios 2:1 indicate that the fetus has lung maturity and is at least at 36 weeks' gestation. Chromosome and enzyme studies can be readily performed on the amniotic fluid sample. Tay-Sachs disease is an example of a genetic disease that can be diagnosed through enzyme studies.

27. (2) Both light and heat can alter amniotic fluid. If immediate analysis is not possible, the specimen should be refrigerated in an opaque container to prevent the bilirubinoid pigments from breaking down into other components, thus causing alternations of the analysis findings.

28. (2) Initially, most fluid is derived from the maternal blood. Later, the fetus makes a contribution by excreting urine into the amniotic fluid. The fluid resembles a transudate of maternal plasma. It is isotonic, but has a reduced protein concentration.

29. (2) Isotope studies used to check the rate of amniotic fluid formation in infants of 40 weeks' gestation reveal that the water in amniotic fluid is normally replaced every 3 hours; electrolytes, sodium, and potassium are replaced approximately every 15 hours.

30. (3) See rationale #26 for discussion of the L/S ratio. Creatinine production is evidence of muscle development and kidney maturation. Levels of 1.8 or greater indicate that a fetus is at least at 36 weeks' gestation. Oxytocinase is the enzyme that splits the oxytocin molecule. It is detected in the pregnant mammary gland, uterus (placenta), and maternal blood stream after 36 weeks, or during labor and delivery, when there may be increased RBC degradation. It is *not* an estimate of fetal age, but more of maternal hormone state.

31. (4) It is imperative to institute all the nursing responsibilities listed because of the instability of the infant's adaptive mechanisms and the immaturity of organ development.

32. (2) Fetal morbidity and mortality rates relative to the safety of amniocentesis vary, depending on the number of subjects in the study and the nature of the complication. Overall, however, the risk rates are about 0.8 per cent mortality and morbidity in studies of 1000 subjects. The complications that could develop include maternal hemorrhage, infection, fetal puncture wounds, pneumothorax, laceration of the fetal spleen, damage to placental and umbilical vessels, and sudden death from fetal exsanguination.

33. (2) An intraperitoneal transfusion of O-negative packed cells into the fetus would be indicated because type O blood would not cause any further detrimental AB antibody formation against the fetal RBCs. Packed red cells would provide sufficient mature RBCs to ensure adequate oxygenation.

34. (1) Corrine's infant inherited the Rh positive trait from her father. Corrine has Rh negative blood. Corrine became immunized against the fetus' Rh positive trait and developed anti Rh antibodies (agglutinins), which crossed the placenta and coated and destroyed the infant's RBCs, releasing large quantities of bilirubin into the plasma.

35. (3) The physician's decision limited the extent of the hemolytic disease and prevented severe anemia and potential death of the infant.

36. (2) Prompt clamping will prevent further transfer of maternal antibodies to the infant. Leaving a four-inch umbilical stump will allow for umbilical vessel cannulization if exchange transfusions are warranted.

37. (3) After blanching of the skin, yellowing of the skin can easily be seen.

38. (1) Early jaundice is always an indication of pathophysiology, and requires prompt and close investigation.

39. (4) Destruction of RBC's at a rate faster than production can cause anemia. Hypoproteinemia and decreased intravascular colloidal pressure can arise and cause a fluid shift from the blood stream to the intercellular spaces. As a result, massive edema and atelectasis can occur. The anemia also requires the heart to pump more vigorously in an attempt to circulate the decreased number of RBC's more rapidly so that the oxygenation needs of body cells are met. Pump overwork can eventually result in cardiac failure.

40. (2) The deposition of bilirubin in brain tissue occurs when there is no more available blood plasma albumin to which it can bind. Other factors that affect this problem are the predilection of bilirubin to deposit in soft tissue, and the underdevelopment of the blood-brain barrier of the newborn infant.

41. (3) Unconjugated bilirubin is water-insoluble and has an affinity for lipids. If the blood-brain barrier is underdeveloped, the bilirubin may bind to lipids and be deposited in the brain, producing serious neurologic damage. It is hypothesized that existing systemic hypoxia, caused by extreme hemolysis or acidosis, may play a role in rendering the barrier abnormally permeable.

42. (4) All the symptoms listed occur as a result of the deposition of bilirubin in the brain, which interferes with cerebral oxygenation and creates electrolyte imbalances.

43. (4) Depending on the area of the brain most severely affected, the result of the damage will vary. Muscle spasticity, however, is almost the universal outcome, coupled with one or more of the other problems listed.

44. (1) The hemopoietic tissues of the baby attempt to replace the hemolyzing red blood cells, thus the liver and the spleen become greatly enlarged from overactivity.

45. (2) Bilirubin conjugation depends on an adequate supply of binding protein, albumin, an adequate supply of hepatic acceptor proteins Y and Z, and adequate amounts of hepatic enzyme, glucuronyl transferase, which may be at low levels in the premature infant.

46. (4) In the exchange, the new infant's blood is replaced with type O, Rh negative blood. This prevents further antibody destruction, RBC hemolysis, and kernicterus.

47. (2) a, The infant's stomach should be emptied to prevent aspiration. c, Central venous pressure is monitored because it may demonstrate hypervolemic congestive heart failure, necessitating withdrawal of blood to decrease the pressure, or hypovolemia, which would require expansion of the vascular space and correction of the acidosis.

48. (3) ACD contains sugar, which can stimulate the neonatal insulin output, result-

ing in rebound hypoglycemia. ACD lowers the blood pH, which in turn lowers the PaO$_2$. In acidosis, hydrogen ions move into the RBC's and potassium ions are liberated from the cell. This exchange alters the electrical potential of the cell membrane, which is reflected in a prolonged P-R interval, depressed ST segment, and a depressed T wave.

49. (4) a, As a result of the exchange, intravascular oncotic pressure may rise, causing fluid shifts from the intercellular spaces to the intravascular space, resulting in circulatory overload. b and c, The preservative in the blood can cause hypoglycemia and electrolyte imbalances. d, Because of the instability of the temperature-regulating center in the premature infant, hypothermia may occur. e, Air may imperceptibly be introduced through the catheter during the exchange procedure, and this could cause an air embolus.

50. (3) This infant would probably have a circulatory volume of about 200 ml. Most exchange infusions are double volume exchanges, i.e., an amount equal to twice the assumed blood volume is used, since it is believed that this quantity will assure 85–90 per cent effective replacement of circulating erythrocytes. Fifteen to 20 aliquots are removed and replaced at each exchange, since this represents up to 10 per cent of the infant's circulating volume.

51. (4) If the blood is not warmed to body temperature, hypothermia can result and cause vascular constriction, hypoxia, cardiac arrhythmia, and eventual cardiac arrest.

52. (3) The citrate in the blood preservative binds with the circulating calcium, causing a calcium depletion. Hypocalcemia can cause seizures, cardiac fibrillation, tetany, and arrest.

53. (4) See rationale #52.

54. (2) The calcium ion is important in the process of muscle contraction. Hypocalcemia can result in muscle irritability and muscle spasms.

55. (3) Venous pressure is measured after each 100 ml. of exchange because, as the blood level of RBCs increases, with a resultant rise in intravascular oncotic pressure, fluid shifts from the intercellular space to the blood. Monitoring the venous pressure facilitates detection of circulatory overload and the progress of the exchange.

56. (4) a and b, Dyspnea and cyanosis can be caused by hypo- or hypervolemia, or hypothermia. c, Bleeding can occur from the site where the umbilical artery catheter was inserted. d, Hypoglycemia can result from the blood preservative causing rebound hypoglycemia. e, Listlessness occurs from electrolyte imbalances.

57. (3) Corrine has type A, Rh negative blood, and should be given the same type in order to prevent an antigen-antibody reaction.

58. (3) Because of the differences in Rh factors in mother and infant, the remaining antibodies in the baby will cause some continuing destruction of RBC's.

59. (3) a, The amount of warmth the baby needs depends on his size and age. The goal is to maintain the infant at a neutral temperature, i.e., the temperature at which oxygen consumption will be kept at a minimum. c, The exact mechanisms causing low resistance to infection in the infant are very complex. d, Overfeeding may result in regurgitation, with the associated danger of aspiration.

Hysterectomy

1. (3) Early diagnosis is an important factor influencing the prospects for cure in treatable malignant tumors. Screening tests that detect cervical cancer in its initial growth are highly valid.

2. (2) Approximately 10,000 women die annually from carcinoma of the cervix, and it is suggested that this disease of the reproductive tract develops in roughly 2 per cent of all women. Deaths each year from breast cancer are even higher, about 33,000.

3. (1) The quantity of menstrual bleeding varies in individual women, so the best way to determine whether flow is excessive, average, or scanty is to compare each woman's change in flow with her usual amount of bleeding.

4. (4) The list of reasons why women neglect to obtain regular screening is long, and includes those listed. Apparently the recognition of vulnerability is weighed against the perception of future liability.

5. (1) A full bladder not only interferes with the examination procedure, but increases the physical discomfort experienced during it. Additionally, the urine specimen obtained is analyzed.

6. (2) Breathing deeply and regularly helps to relax the pelvic muscles and decrease the discomfort of the pelvic examination.

7. (3) The office nurse can be instrumental in decreasing the potential physical and psychologic discomfort of the pelvic examination by reminding Mrs. Grayling about what she should do.

8. (3) The purpose of the pelvic examination is to permit visual and digital examination of the external and internal genitals and pelvic contours; a rectal examination is not part of the procedure.

9. (3) In the Pap test, secretory cells are obtained to detect abnormalities of cell growth in the squamocolumnar junction, cervix, or vagina.

10. (3) Leiomyomas are true benign tumors of smooth muscle cell origin, and fibrosis becomes evident only after atrophic and degenerative changes.

11. (1) Estrogen promotes growth of leiomyoma (fibroids) when these are present during pregnancy, and also in postmenopausal women to whom this hormone is given. Uterine fibroids invariably cease enlarging following menopause.

12. (4) Fatigue is caused by blood loss, anemia, or iron deficiency. All of these contribute to a decreased oxygen supply to the body cells.

13. (2) "Hypochromic" is a word used to refer to lack of (hypo) color intensity (chromic). In this patient's anemia, the hypochromia is due to lack of hemoglobin content inside the erythrocyte.

14. (4) The pressure on structures adjoining the uterus enlarged by fibroids causes urinary retention and constipation. Fatigue is due to blood and iron loss. Cramping pain is associated with menstruation, and less often occurs intermenstrually.

15. (3) The acute pain is associated with infarction due to sudden degeneration of a pedunculated fibroid.

16. (2) Hysterectomy as a form of contraception is 100 per cent effective. Following hysterectomy, sexual activity can be normal.

17. (4) Proteins, carbohydrates, and fats all contain carbon, hydrogen, and oxygen. In addition, proteins contain sulfur, phosphorus, and nitrogen.

18. (4) Protein substances in the body are essential for structure and function because cell walls, various membranes, connective tissue, and muscles are primarily protein. Albumin is a key protein of the plasma and serves as a transport vehicle. It also helps to maintain water balance through its osmotic action in the capillaries.

19. (2) Complete proteins provide amino acids necessary for the body's metabolism, and contain amino acids that the body cannot synthesize independent of protein intake.

20. (4) Major sources of protein are animal products such as eggs, meat, fish, and milk. Normal concentration of protein in the plasma is 6–8 grams per 100 ml. blood.

21. (4) Vitamins are instrumental in enzyme production and thus help transform other food substances into bone, skin, nerves, brain, and blood. For example, vitamin A is essential for normal maintenance of epithelial, skeletal, and soft tissue.

22. (3) Vitamin C is essential for normal vascular function, the production of osteoid tissue, tissue respiration, and wound healing. A deficiency of vitamin C can cause hemorrhages and loose teeth, both of which are symptoms of scurvy.

23. (4) Optimal wound healing can only occur if Vitamin C is adequate in the body. Normal daily requirement for vitamin C is 70 mg. for an adult and 30–80 mg. for a child.

24. (1) Citrus and some other fruits are a main source of vitamin C. Other sources include tomatoes, cabbage, and green pepper. Cottage cheese, cereal, and lima beans are poor sources of vitamin C.

25. (2) Fish, liver, milk, eggs, and green or yellow vegetables are the principal sources of vitamin A. Deficiency of vitamin A causes night blindness.

26. (4) Vitamin B_2 (riboflavin) promotes growth or general health, and is essential for cellular oxidation.

27. (3) Oxidation refers to the combining of substances with oxygen. Riboflavin seems to play a role in the oxidative processes that occurs in cells. Thiamine enhances glucose metabolism.

28. (2) The best sources of B complex vitamins are yeast, legumes (a pod or fruit such as peas or beans), and organ meats (liver, kidney, heart).

29. (4) The purpose of the douche preoperatively is to reduce the number of potential contaminants in the vagina or cervix. This cleansing can be best accomplished by using sterile equipment and solution.

30. (3) The preoperative skin preparation for a hysterectomy includes scrubbing and shaving the abdominal wall and pubic and perineal areas, and cleansing the umbilicus. The purpose is to reduce the number of potential contaminants.

31. (2) The surgical procedure of hysterectomy includes removal of the uterine fundus, body, and cervix. A *radical* hysterectomy refers to removal of ovaries, fallopian tubes, uterus with the cervix, and parametrial tissue.

32. (3) Morphine and anesthetics depress ventilation. Patients in shock may experience oxygen deficit, and exhibit labored and difficult breathing.

33. (4) In addition to the monitoring activities listed, the nurse should assess urinary output and central venous pressure.

34. (3) The microorganisms that cause pneumonia are always present in the upper respiratory tract. When resistance is seriously lowered, pneumococci may invade the lungs.

35. (1) The side-lying position is indicated in the recovery phase of anesthesia until the patient is alert, can cough, and is able to move about in the bed.

36. (2) Thiamine (B_1) functions specifically to enhance glucose metabolism. It is essential for normal metabolism of pyruvic acid (a compound formed in glycolysis).

37. (1) During the performance of a hysterectomy, dissection of the ureter may occur. This can be prevented by good surgical technique, which includes the insertion of a catheter.

38. (1) "Gas pains" following surgery are painful, and can be relieved in part by insertion of a rectal tube.

39. (4) Thrombophlebitis occurs following trauma to the veins that allows an inflammatory process to develop. The pelvic area is a highly vascular area, so that a vein can easily be occluded or damaged during surgical intervention.

40. (3) Mobility decreases susceptibility to venous stasis. Movement or exercise of the legs will increase venous return by pulsatile flow (rhythmic contraction of leg muscles forces blood through the veins toward the heart).

41. (1) Intestinal distention is a frequent sequela to abdominal hysterectomy. Early reestablishment of normal peristalsis and bowel function is essential.

42. (2) Sliding first to the left side of the bed allows for safe rolling to the right side and for positioning in good alignment.

43. (4) Support of the arms and legs on pillows following abdominal surgery is a comfort measure.

44. (3) Bowel sounds should resume approximately one day following surgery. These signs are an indirect indication that motility has resumed in the gastrointestinal tract and that paralytic ileus is not present.

45. (3) Loss of the uterus is perceived differently by different women. The patient's age, hormonal status, desire to have children, and emotional support influence the intensity of the postoperative depression.

46. (3) The husband's support and expressions of love are more important and helpful at this time than are comments by nurses, physicians, or children.

47. (1) Protein supports wound healing and blood formation. Recall the earlier discussion of the vital role of good protein intake.

48. (3) Any activity that causes pressure on the abdominal viscera or muscles and vaginal "stump" will be contraindicated early in the postoperative rehabilitation period.

49. (3) Not only will a girdle relieve tension on the incision area, but it will decrease general discomfort due to the "strain" of abdominal muscles.

Carcinoma of the Cervix

1. (2) Metrorrhogia, the most common early symptom, refers to uterine bleeding that occurs at completely irregular intervals. Menorrhogia and watery vaginal discharge are other early signs of cervical carcinoma.

2. (3) The health history of an individual with carcinoma of the cervix often includes bleeding following sexual intercourse. The bleeding may also occur after douching, defecating, or heavy lifting. Pelvic pain is a symptom of advanced disease.

3. (2) "Indurated" refers to abnormally hardened tissue resulting from hyperemia, inflammation, or infiltration by neoplasm.

4. (4) The parametrium is connective tissue surrounding the uterus. The endometrium is the mucous membrane lining the uterus.

5. (2) As noted in the rationale for #1, a watery vaginal discharge may be present in early stages of cervical cancer. If infection occurs the drainage changes to a thicker, discolored discharge.

6. (3) Blood loss and low iron intake are two common causes of low hemoglobin concentration. The most likely cause in this case is blood loss.

7. (3) Inflammation is a tissue response to injury or destruction of cells. Infection refers to the invasion of body tissues by pathogenic organisms. In this case, the change in normal cells allowed organisms ordinarily present in the vagina and cervix to cause an infection. Common signs of an infection are fever, elevated sedimentation rate, and elevated leukocyte count.

8. (2) Chronic local irritation (i.e., veneral disease), frequent sexual intercourse with multiple partners over a number of years, and inadequate medical care (poor pre- and postnatal care, no annual Pap smear) predispose to cervical cancer.

9. (4) In performing a vaginal Pap test, a vaginal spectrum is inserted; secretions are removed with wooden spatulas or long, cotton-tipped applicators. The secretions removed are smeared on glass plates that are "fixed" by immersing them into mixtures of alcohol and ether. The plates are then studied microscopically for abnormal or cancerous cells.

10. (1) Malignant tumors slough off cells into surrounding fluids. Cervical and vaginal secretions are studied to ascertain if malignant cells are present. The areas scraped to obtain secretions for this study are the squamous-columnar cell junction in the cervix and the posterior fornix (vaultlike space) of the vagina.

11. (1) In cervical carcinoma, also known as epidermoid or squamous-cell cancer, there is a loss of normal stratification of the normal squamous epithelial pattern.

12. (1) The reasons for failure to have a Pap smear are numerous, and to various degrees could include all of those listed. Modesty has been thought to be a chief reason for not having an annual Pap test.

13. (2) Class III Pap test indicates suspicious cellular abnormalities suggestive of, but not definitive for, malignant cells. A Class I test means only normal cells; Class II smear contains cells with atypical features but not suggestive of malignant cells (i.e., inconclusive).

14. (2) Glycogen is present in normal cervical and vaginal mucosa, and these cells will stain with iodine. Abnormal areas will have lighter stain and can be localized as the biopsy site.

15. (3) Colposcopy is examination of cervical and vaginal tissue by means of brightly illuminated optical instruments after the cervix has been treated with acetic acid. Biopsy is obtained from the most extreme abnormality visualized.

16. (2) Squamous cells (scaly or platelike) cover the vaginal portion of the cervix. The vagina is lined with mucous membrane.

17. (2) In addition to the Pap smear Classes (I–IV), tumor cells of the cervix are assigned clinical stages to reflect either localization or spread of the malignant changes. International Stage 2 means that the carcinoma extends beyond the cervix into the vagina, but not into the pelvic wall or into the lower one third of the vagina. Stage 1 means that the cancer is confined to the cervix. In Stage 3 there is metastasis to the pelvic wall, and in Stage 4 metastasis is beyond the pelvic wall into the bladder and rectum.

18. (4) Anemia (due to blood loss), weight loss, anorexia, and fatigue are the symptoms most apt to occur. Note that pain is *not* one of those symptoms.

19. (4) Review of the distractors (a–d), which are all correct, certainly shows why early detection is crucial for recovery. The cure rate for early diagnosed cervical carcinoma (Classes I–III, Stages 0–1) is usually 100 per cent.

20. (4) Although malignant cells can spread from their site of origin in all the ways listed, metastasis in cervical carcinoma is by direct extension into adjoining cells.

21. (2) Since carcinoma of the cervix, Stage 4, involves metastasis to the bladder, the physician is evaluating whether malignant changes have occurred in the bladder.

22. (3) Radiation is a major method for treatment of cervical carcinoma because it kills cells undergoing early malignant changes, and it can retard malignant spread while the feasibility of surgical intervention is being evaluated.

23. (2) External radiation is used to reduce the tumor mass in order to make it more amenable to radium implant or surgery. The effect of radium on cells is degeneration and necrosis, and this effect is greater on malignant cells than on normal cells.

24. (4) Radiologists consider the ray type, length of time for radiation, and distance from radioactive source. Protection of adjoining areas is accomplished by careful shielding.

25. (4) Undergoing radiation therapy is at best a formidable experience. Any instruction of the patient (such as that listed) that helps to reduce the unpleasantness or stress of the treatment is recommended.

26. (4) Patients should be informed about the side effects of radiation exposure and told what symptoms to report.

27. (3) Chlorpromazine (Thorazine) has an antiemetic effect, as do the antihistamines (e.g., Dramamine, Tigan). Chlordiazepoxide (Librium) and chloral hydrate (which is hypnotic) do not have major antiemetic effects.

28. (4) Vaginal douching prior to insertion of the radium applicator removes secretions that may interfere with radium placement, and reduces, to some extent, the foul-smelling vaginal discharge that develops as cells are destroyed. Good perineal care is essential.

29. (3) Before radium insertion, a cleansing enema and low-residue diet are given to prevent distention of the bowel.

30. (3) The vaginal packing holds the radium applicator in the desired position. If the stem of the radium applicator is inserted through the cervix into the uterus, severe uterine contractions will arise as a result of cervical dilation. A narcotic may be given to counteract the pain that accompanies these contractions.

31. (4) Since proximity to the source of radiation is one factor that determines the amount of radioactive ray exposure, the distance from the source should be maximized for the health team and visitors to the unit.

32. (3) The catheter prevents distention of the bladder and lessens its exposure to radiation.

33. (4) Nursing care during radium treatment includes attending to physical needs and providing sufficient emotional support to reduce the stress of the treatment. It is very important that patients know when the therapy will end.

34. (2) "Iatrogenic" refers to any disorder that is inadvertently produced as a result of treatment efforts. Destruction of the bladder muscle cells during treatment is decreased if the bladder remains empty during the radium insertion. Drinking at least 3 liters of fluid per day helps relieve irritation of the urinary system.

35. (1) Patients with a radium applicator in the uterus are restricted to a recumbent position in bed, and only allowed to move from side to side. Maintaining this position helps prevent any displacement of the radioactive substance.

36. (1) Beta rays can be blocked by the patient's body or heavy plastic, but gamma ray emissions (such as used in this patient) must be shielded by lead. The nurse will limit her exposure to this patient to a maximum of 30 minutes at a time. Radiation exposure is accumulative, and if treatment were to be prolonged it would be advisable (although not maximally therapeutic) for nurses to rotate the person who gives a bed bath and perineal care each day.

37. (2) Patients do not wish to cause harm to those attending to their needs, so they need to be reassured that you are taking precautions to protect yourself and

them. Nurses should discuss with family members what constitutes safe exposure, and help them monitor their length of contact.

38. (2) Since patients with radium insertion must remain on bedrest, nursing care is directed toward maintaining urinary system competence, electrolyte balance, skin integrity, and muscle strength. Frequent back care will relieve discomfort and prevent skin breakdown.

39. (3) Radioactivity does not remain after the radium source has been removed and placed in a lead container.

40. (1) A solid radium source was used instead of a liquid radioactive substance, so there was no contamination of linens, and no special handling is required.

41. (1) Radium implantation in the cervix can cause temporary radiation sickness (nausea, vomiting, diarrhea, malaise, fever) or more permanent symptoms (vaginal stenosis, fistula, vagina bleeding for 1–3 months, rectal irritation). Sexual functioning is *not* usually impaired.

42. (3) The skin should not be cleaned or covered with anything that will be irritating or that will remove the radiologist's markings. Strong sunlight and extremes in temperature should be avoided.

43. (2) There is no need for scissors or suture. Safe practice with sealed internal radium includes the factors of time, distance, and shielding. Gloves should be worn since the radium should never come into direct contact with the skin. Distance is provided by the use of long-bladed forceps. The radium is placed in a lead container so that it is safe from accidental handling or loss. It also prevents spread of radioactivity since the radioactive particles and rays are absorbed by the lead.

44. (1) Radiologists insert the radium and determine the duration of the treatment. Nurses' responsibility to the patient includes assuring, in any way possible, that radiation overdose does not occur.

Postpartum Adjustment

1. (1) About 0.2 per cent of maternity patients experience serious psychiatric illness. Of this percentage, over half the episodes occur in the early puerperium. Most mothers experience only mild postpartum "blues."

2. (3) Temporary moments of crying, outbursts of anger, or slight depression are due to hormonal imbalances and are typical events of the early puerperium. All these symptoms are usually transitory, and last from 1–2 hours to several days.

3. (2) When mothers don't behave as they "always do," insensitive or thoughtless family members may mislabel a normal phenomenon.

4. (4) A mother of any age and from any race, socioeconomic class, or educational group is vulnerable to postpartum depression. The person deemed "least likely" to have emotional distress following delivery not uncommonly does so.

5. (3) "Mental illness" seems a harsh description for the reactions to the hormonal imbalances, changes in body image, increasing responsibilities, and decreasing freedom that often accompanying pregnancy and mothering. These reactions, however, do occur within three months following birth of the infant.

6. (1) An anxiety reaction indicates the threat to the self-esteem that occurs in the postpartum period.

7. (4) Rubin described the stages of the puerperal periods as the "taking-in" and the "taking-hold" phases. During the taking-in phase, the first 1–3 days following delivery, the nurse may observe that the mother's expressed needs center on her own requirements for food, sleep, and rest. The mother also needs to discuss the labor and delivery events. As these demands are met, the mother's interaction with the infant is facilitated. Nurses can assess the nature of this interaction by observing how the mother holds, explores, looks at, and talks to her baby.

8. (4) This maternal behavior indicates that the infant is becoming a more central focus in her life.

9. (4) The type and rate of maternal attachment to her infant is influenced by previ-

ous life experiences of the mother, and the baby's behavior during initial contacts.

10. (3) Although new mothers interviewed in this study scored as significantly more submissive than did women in general, they were not found to be neurotic.

11. (1) According to Paschall and Newton, "tendermindedness" refers to the tendency to be overprotected and cultured, with protected emotional sensitivity. "Depressiveness" refers to a tendency to be inhibited, sober, and serious.

12. (3) As defined by Paschall and Newton, "submissiveness" includes tendencies to be suggestible and dependent. "Anxiety" means worry, guilt-proneness, high tension from frustration, ego weakness, or emotional immaturity and or instability.

13. (4) Having Karla attend classes and talk with a person experienced in mothering would increase her knowledge, skill, and confidence in caring for herself and her infant.

14. (4) Although research shows that dysmenorrhea contributes to maladjustment in the puerperium, it is not known whether this influence is hormonal or psychologic.

15. (4) Knowledge of a woman's physical health, her reaction to pregnancy, and her attitudes toward sex, child rearing, her own femininity, and her mother's child-rearing abilities all help the nurse to identify any special needs that the individual pregnant women or mother may manifest.

16. (1) Change usually produces some level of stress. The intensity of the stressful event depends on the individual's perception of that event.

17. (2) The habit of always doing things well may have set a precedent that Karla wasn't sure she could carry over into mothering. Those persons most likely to help her "do good" either did too much (her mother took over mothering while Karla rested) or not enough (her husband focused his efforts on studying in graduate school). Karla wasn't able at that time either to ask for more support or to manage without it.

18. (3) Anxiety frequently produces physical signs, including hyperventilation and tachycardia.

19. (1) A threat to the self-esteem produces anxiety that causes a narrowing of interests. If the anxiety level is high, individuals tend to focus on themselves.

20. (4) Any person or event that is perceived as a threat to the self, or disrupts established equilibria, will contribute to stress.

21. (2) Typically, the early signs of impending postpartum illness are insomnia and mood change during the first few days following delivery. Karla's complaint of "excessive" lochia most likely was an attempt to draw attention to her need.

22. (2) Caring for the baby was the area in which Karla had the least experience and confidence.

23. (3) Almost traditionally, the significance of the fathering role has been given secondary importance. In recent years fathers have been involved actively in every phase of pregnancy, labor, delivery, and child care. It is just as important to ascertain Lennie's perceptions as it is to assess Karla's feelings and attitudes.

24. (1) Pregnancy probably brings out the best and worst in the persons involved. The overall or predominant response is shaped chiefly by the strength of the ego, the variety of experiences, and how these persons would have handled the crisis prior to pregnancy.

25. (2) Research data are not conclusive, but mothers of children who fail to thrive or who have congenital anomalies seem to be more vulnerable to emotional problems following childbirth. Such mothers are thought to experience guilt or to blame themselves for contributing to the infant's physical problems.

26. (2) Pregnancy can be considered a crisis. A typical definition of crisis is "an event that threatens the life style," i.e., a person or event that forces individuals to alter their usual routine: a turning point for better or worse. Everyone experiences a developmental crisis, identity crisis, or situational crisis at some juncture in life.

27. (4) The forms of behavior listed are all techniques used in crisis intervention to facilitate a positive outcome.

2 PEDIATRIC NURSING

Premature Infant

1. (3) Pulse rate cannot be used as a criterion for the diagnosis of prematurity because, even though main pulse rates for various gestational ages have been ascertained, the pulse itself is contingent on many variables.

2. (4) All of those listed are considered to be risk factors: the more factors present, the greater the risk that the mother will give birth to a premature or high risk infant.

3. (4) 2.2 lbs. = 1 kg.; 1000 gm. = 1 kg.; 1170 gm. = 1.170 kg.; 1.17 kg. × 2.2 lbs. = 2.6 lbs., or 2 lbs. 9 oz.

4. (4) The Apgar score is a reliable method of assessing the need for resuscitation within the first minute of life. The 5-minute Apgar is felt to be an indicator of morbidity/mortality in the first year of life. A score of 0–3 at 1 minute indicates the need for cardiopulmonary resuscitation; 4–6, oxygen per mask; 7–10, normal. Of the items scored, heart rate is the most sensitive indicator; below 100 means that life support assistance is required.

5. (1) Acidosis is a potent pulmonary vasoconstrictor. Constriction of pulmonic vessels in the premature can lead to cellular death and decreased surfactant synthesis, resulting in hyaline membrane disease.

6. (3) Assessment of airway patency is a universal first step, since oxygen is a primary need.

7. (2) The premature infant is incapable of independently maintaining adequate ventilation in the extrauterine environment because of functional and structural immaturity. At 35 weeks, gestation is beginning to peak.

8. (1) Absent or scant sole skin creases and little or no cartilage in the ear are typical of structural immaturity. These are two of the physical criteria used to determine gestational age.

9. (3) Neural structures are poorly developed in premature infants; thus, the Babinski reflex, an abnormal neural reflex, would not occur even if underlying pathology existed.

10. (3) The first three reasons cited for inefficient temperature regulation are due to prematurity.

11. (2) Breakdown of brown fat is an effective means of producing heat. Brown fat is deposited in areas of high vascularity besides being vascular itself. When chilling occurs, brown fat breaks down to triglycerides and gives off heat, warming the circulating blood.

12. (4) Hypothermia results in bodily efforts to raise the temperature, producing increased circulation and respiration. However, these efforts are also exhausting. All options represent objective manifestations of the body's attempt to maintain an efficient temperature.

13. (3) The normal infant's response to chilling is reflected in an increased metabolic rate, causing increased O_2 consumption and increased respiratory rate. The premature infant cannot sustain the hyperpnea; thus, apnea develops and leads to hypoxic acidosis and hypoglycemia. The resulting azotemia and hyperkalemia are due to the excessive breakdown of protein for energy or heat production.

14. (4) The premature infant has structural and functional immaturity of the respiratory system; therefore, all the options listed are correct.

15. (4) The reserves or compensatory abilities of the premature infant are limited; thus, any of the complications listed can occur.

16. (3) The combination of capillary fragility, small fat deposits, and decreased clotting make premature infants more susceptible to hemorrhage and less able to reverse it.

17. (4) Respiratory and pulse rates fluctuate owing to many variables. The PaO_2 (partial pressure of oxygen in arterial blood) is most reliable because it measures the amount of O_2 that diffuses across the alveolar membrane and is in solution in the plasma.

18. (3) Immature retinal vessels are susceptible to vasoconstriction when increased arterial oxygen tension occurs during breathing of high O_2 concentrations.

The vasoconstriction causes hypoxia to the areas of retina supplied by these vessels. New vessels are formed as a result of the hypoxia, but their fragility causes breakage and hemorrhage. This results in scar tissue formation behind the lens (retrolental fibroplasia), which may produce retinal detachment and possibly blindness.

19. (1) Oxygen cannot diffuse readily across dry mucosal membranes. This can result in drying of bronchial secretions. High-risk neonates are prone to insensible water loss through the skin and lungs. Humidification helps to deter these problems.

20. (4) Immunoglobulin G (IgG), the only antibody that crosses the placenta, is transferred maximally during the last trimester. Premature infants do not have full benefit of this IgG transfer. They can manufacture IgM but only in limited amounts. They also are plagued with structural and functional immaturity.

21. (1) Increased metabolic rate increases oxygen need and consumption.

22. (4) In addition to all the factors listed, a significant reduction of nursery spread infection is effected through good handwashing technique.

23. (4) Structural and functional immaturity causes the premature infant to have a high percentage of immature red blood cells, decreased vitamins and iron stored in the liver, and fragile capillaries. It also causes low hemoglobin concentration due to inadequacy in hemoglobin concentration in relation to the relatively rapid rate of growth and increased blood volume.

24. (3) Infection, trauma, and exhaustion can occur because of immaturity. Kernicterus, the deposition of bile pigments in the brain, has no known relationship to the amount of handling of the child.

25. (4) Growth is critical to the premature's survival. Calories should be expended toward promoting growth and not toward unnecessary energy expenditure.

26. (1) The neonate's jaundice is probably due to a combination of factors including shorter life span and greater destruction of RBCs, higher level of nonerythrocyte bilirubin (obtained from breakdown of cellular elements), and the low ability of the kidneys to clear hemoglobin.

27. (2) The central nervous system of the premature infant is extremely vulnerable to damage due to immaturity of the blood-brain barrier. Thus, fat-soluble, unconjugated bilirubin can be deposited in brain tissues. Untreated excessive blood concentration of bilirubin may cause severe brain damage.

28. (3) Although its action is not fully understood, it is thought that blue or ultraviolet light breaks down bilirubin trapped in the subcutaneous tissue by a photooxidative process to water-soluble compounds that can be excreted from the body.

29. (1) The premature baby may not be fed during the initial hours of the first day for a variety of reasons relating to gastrointestinal and pulmonary functioning. These include poorly developed gag, cough, and swallowing reflexes; delayed stomach emptying; reduced intestinal mobility; and reduced secretions of digestive and hepatic enzymes.

30. (1) The daily nutritional requirements for a premature infant are: calories, 110–140 kcal./kg./day; water, 120–150 ml./kg./day; protein, 3–4 gm./kg./day; fat, 5–7 gm./kg./day; carbohydrates, 10–15 gm./kg./day. The caloric requirements are influenced by the metabolic rate, growth rate, and large body surface area relative to body weight. The major consideration in choosing a formula is that it be low in saturated fats, because these are not metabolized well by the premature infant.

31. (2) Whole milk contains a high percentage of saturated fats not readily digested by the premature infant owing to insufficient production of enzymes for fat degradation.

32. (4) The premature is prone to muscular fatigue resulting in weakness in sucking, and has a small stomach capacity (about 4 ml.). Respiratory work and growth consume calories, and therefore energy requirements are not met easily. Respiratory embarrassment may be an early sign of nutritional failure.

33. (4) The four functions listed are common practice, designed to conserve energy while providing the required nutrients.

34. (1) The premature infant is prone to functional intestinal obstructions as well as

necrotizing enterocolitis (NEC), which is thought to be due to anoxic ischemia of the bowel and bacterial overgrowth. Death of part of the bowel can impair peristalsis and cause rupture of the gut. Measurements of abdominal circumferences and stool tests are ways of assessing whether or not bowel impairment is occurring.

35. (3) The number is variable, but four to five is an approximation of normal stool frequency.

36. (2) Prematures do not readily break down fats because of their low levels of enzymes.

37. (3) Premature infants do not digest and absorb fats well, and therefore have insufficient storage of fat-soluble vitamins (A, D, and K).

38. (4) Vitamin K is necessary for the synthesis of prothrombin in the liver. Deficiency of vitamin K therefore impairs blood coagulation and clotting.

39. (4) Premature infants have insufficient stores of immunoglobulins (antibodies), and relatively little protection against gram-negative organisms. Broad-spectrum antibodies are frequently given for prophylaxis.

40. (3) These organisms are all gram-negative.

41. (3) Penicillin is ineffective against *E. coli* and *P. vulgaris*.

42. (1) Although it is controversial, some physicians order ferrous sulfate for premature infants to prevent iron deficiency.

43. (4) Prolonged separation of a mother and infant can seriously affect the bonding process started in the early hours after birth when the mother can touch and "explore" her infant. Disruption of the process can lead to feelings of incompetence in the mother, and has been known to contribute to child neglect or abuse.

44. (3) The central nervous system develops at a steady, predictable rate in normal infants. Premature birth does not result in acceleration of this growth. Because Francis was born at 35 weeks' gestation, his maturity at 1 month will parallel that of 39–40 weeks' gestation. In time he will "catch up," but prediction of mental status at this point is not well defined. The 5 min. (0–4) Apgar score has been correlated with poor mental development.

Cleft Lip and Palate

1. (4) The etiology of cleft lip and cleft palate is the result of many teratogenic, genetic, and developmental factors. Parents frequently are focused on a genetic etiology.

2. (2) Most parents envison having a perfect baby. A congenital defect, especially of the face, can provoke an acute crisis response and self-deprecating feelings.

3. (2) Data from twin studies suggests that genetic factors may be of greater significance in the etiology of cleft lip and palate than in etiology of cleft palate alone.

4. (2) The grief process as outlined by Kübler-Ross includes: shock and denial, anger, bargaining, depression, acceptance.

5. (2) Shock and denial are often manifested by unrealistic goals and expectations.

6. (1) Nurses probably would ask her not to touch the defect owing to the danger of infection. If Mrs. Griffin is holding her infant, looking at his face, cuddling him, and speaking to him, she is showing signs of acceptance.

7. (4) See the rationale for item 2.

8. (3) Although early surgery may increase acceptance of the child by the parents, many surgeons prefer to achieve steady weight gain and stable hemoglobin in the infant prior to the repair. It is felt that delaying the surgery increases the parent's eventual satisfaction because the cosmetic repair appears so much better than the original defect.

9. (4) Either a large, soft nipple with large holes or a long lamb's nipple are used to feed the infant with cleft lip and palate. The infant should be held in such a position as to encourage the use of muscles for sucking, which is important for speech development (see item 10).

10. (3) The upright position allows excess milk to drain out of the side of the

mouth rather than accumulating in the anterior pharynx, as it would if the head were held in the normal bottle-feeding position. Upright positioning helps prevent aspiration pneumonia.

11. (3) Because Homer cannot form a seal around a nipple (owing to the cleft palate), he will tend to swallow more air with his feedings than normal infants.

12. (4) The benefit of nose-breathing is to filter, warm, and humidify the air. Breathing through the mouth allows the sensitive mucosa of the pharynx and trachea to become dry and cracked, creating an excellent focus for entry of bacteria.

13. (3) The newborn has characteristic hand-to-mouth activity. Because of the nature of Homer's defect, this must be prevented. The nurse should be aware of both the physiologic and the psychologic stress of limb immobilization.

14. (1) The Logan bar is used to prevent the infant from rubbing the incision.

15. (1) The newborn infant with cleft lip and palate is prone to respiratory difficulty postoperatively as a result of anesthesia. The lip and palate defects are also excellent portals of entry for bacteria (see rationale 12).

16. (3) Elbow restraints allow arm movement while preventing the elbow's being bent and the hand's being brought to the mouth.

17. (1) Many practitioners now leave the suture line dry. If the physician orders moistening, saline solution is generally used.

18. (4) Irritation and crusting cause increased scarring.

19. (4) Crying creates tension along the suture line and may result in improper healing and scarring.

20. (1) Keeping Homer quiet and immobilized will enhance stasis of pulmonary secretions.

21. (2) The trachea of the newborn measures 6 mm. in diameter compared with the adult's, which measures 20 mm. Even though a small endotracheal tube is inserted, the small diameter of the infant trachea makes edema a relatively common side effect.

22. (3) There are two schools of thought on this issue. Humidity is used to keep the irritated airway moist and prevent cracking and subsequent infection. Humidity probably has no effect on edema reduction, and so it is used infrequently at present.

23. (4) Since the cleft palate is not yet repaired, there is still a danger of aspiration. Slow feedings in an upright position will facilitate swallowing. The nurse should avoid touching the suture line to prevent injury and infection.

24. (2) Sustaining a vacuum during bottle-feeding is necessary for normal sucking and swallowing.

25. (2) Because of the palate defect there is an increased portal of entry for bacteria.

26. (4) Care of cleft lip and palate requires a multidisciplinary approach for the rehabilitative aspects of child care and to provide emotional support for the family.

27. (2) Often the presence of one congenital defect is a clue that others may be present. Cleft lip and palate frequently are accompanied by hearing disorders.

28. (1) Parents of infants with congenital defects often feel guilty. Their response to this feeling is often to "protect" the child from further "trauma" or injury.

29. (3) An intact palate is necessary for correct word formation. Loss of the vacuum needed to enunciate can cause improper speech development, which will not be ameliorated once the palate is repaired.

Pyloric Stenosis

1. (3) Vomiting leads to loss of fluid and electrolytes. Particularly significant are the loss of H^+ and Cl^- ions (HCl) from the stomach, and resulting metabolic alkalosis. Persistent vomiting prevents gastric absorption of ingested food and fluids, thus causing progressive dehydration and weight loss.

2. (4) The pyloric obstruction prevents gastric emptying, so that gastric contents increase with each feeding. The increased intra-abdominal pressure causes projectile vomiting; emesis is characterized by undigested formula. There is no stimulus for nausea.

3. (3) Little, if any, formula is able to pass through the pyloric obstruction, and fecal material is not formed.

4. (3) The etiology of pyloric stenosis is not fully understood, but involves thickening of the circular musculature of the pylorus.

5. (1) Food will be unable to pass the thickened pylorus, so that the epigastric area is distended. Epigastric peristalsis is visible owing to the emaciated appearance of the infant and the hyperactivity of the pylorus in its attempt to pass the formula through the obstruction.

6. (4) Loss of fluids due to vomiting will alter the solute/solvent ratio. All of the options are noted, and reflect a loss of fluid from the extracellular fluid compartments.

7. (1) Prior to the initiation of intravenous fluids Rexford was apt to have the following serum changes: a low calcium (lack of intake and retention of formula); a low potassium, low chloride, low hydrogen ion, and high pH (vomiting); and a high bicarbonate. The administration of intravenous fluids should help correct these abnormalities.

8. (1) The body attempts to compensate for excessive fluid loss and resultant dehydration by shifting fluid from one compartment to another. Rexford's fluid transport was from the plasma (ECF) to intracellular fluid volume. The loss of fluid from the intravascular space might cause circulating volume deficit and shock.

9. (1) Vitamin K is necessary for the formation of prothrombin and factor VIII by the liver. It is given to infants prior to surgery to prevent a delayed prothrombin time, which might result in hemorrhage.

10. (1) The rationale for item 9 applies here.

11. (1) Infant feedings should not be deficient, and practitioners are aiming to prevent this by increased attention to nutrition. The vitamin deficiency is not caused by inadequate liver stores of vitamin K, but by the inability of the liver to secrete bile, which is necessary for the absorption of vitamin K, a fat-soluble vitamin. In Rexford's case, his inability to retain feedings might reduce the amount of normal bacterial flora and contribute to vitamin deficiencies.

12. (3) Vitamin C aids in the stimulation of fibroblasts and the proliferation of capillaries that enhances oxygenation, necessary for postoperative tissue growth and wound healing.

13. (1) Vitamin B enhances the glycolysis and glucose utilization that is needed during the stress of surgery, particularly while the infant is taking nothing by mouth.

14. (3) Additional B-complex vitamins include options a, b, and d. Ascorbic acid is vitamin C; viosterol is the same as calciferol.

15. (2) Delaying the emptying time of the stomach increases satiety and makes vomiting less likely than does ingestion of a dilute liquid.

16. (2) The lack of oral stimulation during the gavage feeding increases the importance of holding and cradling during feedings.

17. (1) While the catheter is being passed it may be displaced into the trachea rather than the esophagus. Lubricants other than normal saline could have serious adverse effects (e.g., pneumonia).

18. (2) This measurement accounts for the distance from the nose to the posterior oropharynx, and from the oropharynx to the cardiac sphincter outlet.

19. (3) As the tip of the catheter touches the posterior pharynx it stimulates cranial nerves IX and XII, and causes gagging and coughing. This in turn stimulates a Valsalva response, inducing flushing.

20. (2) To confirm that the tube is in the stomach, the nurse can inject 3–5 ml. of air while listening over the stomach with a stethoscope. Hearing the air entering the stomach confirms correct placement. An earlier method to determine correct tube placement was to immerse the free end of the tube into water and watch for bubbles: rapid bubbling at the site of the immersed free end of the catheter would indicate passage of the catheter into the lung.

21. (1) Pinching the tube will prevent any "dripping" of formula from the catheter tip that could be aspirated and lead to a lipid pneumonia. Option 2 might lead to gastric distention.

22. (1) This form of restraint, called "mummying," safely and securely immobilizes the infant during the procedure.
23. (3) This surgical procedure, called the Rashkind or pylorotomy, allows release of the pyloric muscle in order to enlarge the pyloric outlet.
24. (4) All options are correct and reflect the adrenergic response of atropine.
25. (2) This position facilitates a patent airway and allows for drainage of oral secretions.
26. (2) Usually the microdrops are equal to 60 drops per 1 ml.

$$\frac{100 \text{ ml.}}{6 \text{ hrs.}} \times \frac{1 \text{ hr}}{60 \text{ min.}} \times \frac{60 \text{ microdrops}}{\text{ml.}} = \frac{100}{6} = 16\text{–}17 \text{ microdrops/min.}$$

27. (3) The infant's kidneys do not mature fully until 1 year of age. If Rexford is given too much I.V. fluid, he will be unable to excrete the excess, and increased intravascular volume and cardiac work will be caused.
28. (2) Rexford should be restrained to prevent him from pulling the tube out.
29. (1) This is to ensure that Rexford obtains only a small amount of formula, thereby reducing stress at the pylorus, the surgical site. Remember that he also was receiving I.V. fluids
30. (4) An upright position promotes downward flow of formula and a rise of gastric air. If vomiting occurs, the possibility of aspiration is minimized.
31. (1) Usually a collodion seal rather than a gauze dressing is applied to the incision after pylorotomy. Applying the diaper low prevents irritation and contamination of the site.
32. (4) The literature supports clinical evidence that pylorotomy relieves the obstruction caused by a hypertrophied pylorus. Therefore, it would be appropriate to reassure the mother that recurrence is highly unlikely. Her use of the word "tumor" shows that she has some misunderstanding of Rexford's pyloric stenosis.

Whooping Cough

1. (2) Pertussis is a member of the *Hemophilus* group of bacilli. It is a small, gram-negative, nonmotile coccoid bacillus.
2. (3) The pertussis bacillus incubates in the secretions of the upper airway.
3. (1) This is the definition of incubation.
4. (3) The incubation period for pertussis may vary from 5 to 10 days.
5. (2) Actually, there *is* passive transference of the pertussis antibody from immunized mothers to their infants. The concern is that women vaccinated as infants have low levels of antibodies. During pregnancy there is an insufficient transfer of antibodies to infants to protect them before immunization.
6. (4) Sidney is too young to begin a vaccination program. He needs to be protected from exposure to the bacillus. Fortunately, the incidence of whooping cough has been greatly reduced.
7. (2) A diphtheria, pertussis, and tetanus vaccine in combination is given to the infant at the appropriate age.
8. (2) Practitioners prefer the child to be approximately 2–3 months of age when active immunization is initiated.
9. (1) The pertussis bacillus invades the tracheal mucosa, eroding the tissue and causing an increase of mucus production. The mucus, thick and tenacious, obstructs the bronchial airways.
10. (4) The pertussis bacillus is encapsulated and remains virulent for a long time.
11. (2) Obstruction by mucous plugs stimulates paroxysms of coughing, which propel the plugs outward.
12. (4) When Sidney sleeps he is not drinking fluids and the mucus becomes thickened. Also, the decrease in activity and a recumbent position facilitate pooling of secretions.
13. (2) Frequent paroxysms of coughing increase caloric utilization and prevent sufficient oral caloric intake.

14. (4) These actions would improve oral intake and assist in monitoring nutritional status.
15. (4) The infant has frequent paroxysms of coughing that may cause vomiting. If vomiting occurs during feeding, the formula should be offered again after the coughing episode, as Sidney will still be hungry.
16. (1) The paroxysms are frightening, and staying with the child will ease his apprehension. Supporting the abdomen reduces abdominal strain during coughing.
17. (1) The paroxysms of coughing increase pressure in the vessels of conjunctiva, which causes them to rupture.
18. (3) The current antibiotic of choice for pertussis is erythromycin, which is similar in effect to penicillin G procaine. However, compared to penicillin, erythromycin produces fewer allergic reactions and has greater effectiveness in attacking gram-negative bacteria.
19. (1) The thick mucus "coats" the cilia and prevents propulsion of foreign material and secretions out of the respiratory tract.
20. (4) Pneumonia, bronchitis, and bronchiectasis are caused by the pooling of mucous secretions in the respiratory tract, which provides an excellent medium for infection, inflammation, and tissue breakdown. The mucous secretions and plugs obstruct the bronchioles and prevent air entry into alveoli, which results in atelectasis. If the obstruction allows air entry into alveoli but minimal air exit, alveoli may rupture and emphysema may develop.
21. (4) All these measures will help to keep the airway free of mucous obstruction and will loosen secretions in the lower airway. Chilling, leading to pulmonary complications, is rare in a child of this age.
22. (2) These complications result from increased intra-abdominal pressure created by coughing.
23. (2) Since Sidney is only 8 weeks old, options d and e are unnecessary.
24. (4) All these actions are appropriate.
25. (2) The paroxysms of coughing will continue as long as there is formation of mucus.

Meningomyelocele and Hydrocephalus

1. (1) A meningomyelocele is a hernial protrusion of the meninges and spinal cord through a defect in the vertebral column.
2. (3) Spina bifida is the loss of continuity of the vertebral column due to imperfect union of the paired vertebral arches at the midline.
3. (1) This position allows for application of sterile, moist dressings and provides maximal protection of the meningomyelocele.
4. (2) The spinal defect obstructs the normal flow of CSF, resulting in cerebral accumulation of spinal fluid and cranial enlargement.
5. (1) Normally, cerebral spinal fluid, found in the subarachnoid spaces surrounding the brain and spinal cord, is continuously produced by the choroid plexus of the lateral ventricles, and reabsorbed through the arachnoid villi at approximately the same rate. Besides meningomyelocele, hydrocephalus may also result from overproduction of CSF from the choroid plexus (as in tumor), or from impaired absorption from the arachnoid villi (as in meningitis).
6. (1) The child with lumbosacral meningomyelocele often develops concomitant bladder problems owing to the involvement of those nerves that control bladder tone.
7. (3) See the rationale for item 5.
8. (3) See the rationale for item 5.
9. (2) Cerebrospinal fluid continuously bathes the brain, spinal cord, and meninges, and provides a protective cushion to absorb mechanical shocks. The major constituents of CSF include water, glucose, sodium chloride, and protein.
10. (3) All but d may potentially obstruct normal flow of CSF.

11. (4) All of these may result from the accumulation of CSF under pressure. The infant's head circumference increases abnormally, sutures separate, and fontanels become tense and bulging. The excessive CSF also exerts pressure on the orbital plate, resulting in the "sunset eyes" phenomenon; increased compression of cerebral tissue causes irritability, anorexia, and vomiting.

12. (3) These ducts, which exit from the third ventricle, are narrow and easily obstructed.

13. (4) All these conditions can be mistaken for hydrocephalus. Prematurity and dwarfism are characterized by a larger-than-normal head-to-body ratio. Subdural hematoma and intracranial tumor may also elicit symptoms similar to those of hydrocephalus.

14. (1) See the rationale for items 5 and 11.

15. (2) This explains the mechanism by which hydrocephalus causes mental retardation.

16. (1) The increased intracranial pressure results in anorexia and vomiting. This accounts for Dolores' malnourished appearance.

17. (4) These are appropriate measures to reduce vomiting after feeding. The nurse may also try thickened feedings.

18. (1) This facilitates access to the meningomyelocele and prevents contamination.

19. (1) Some practitioners intially perform a CAT scan, and then utilize a ventriculogram as necessary to provide additional information.

20. (1) Possible side effects of a ventriculogram include headache, nausea, vomiting, diaphoresis, changes in intracranial pressure, and changes in vital signs.

21. (3) Following the ventriculogram Dolores should be kept supine for 12 to 15 hours and any side effects should be treated symptomatically. Response to the procedure is documented through observation of vital signs and possible changes in intracranial pressure (see the rationale for item 11). In an appropriate manner, hydration is encouraged to assist in the production of CSF, and oxygen may be utilized prophylactically for prevention of hyperpyrexia.

22. (4) Phenolsulfonphthalein is the dye used in tracer studies.

23. (3) Failure of the dye to appear in the lumbar spinal fluid indicates obstruction to normal flow of CSF.

24. (4) The one-way valve allows CSF, when under pressure, to enter the peritoneal cavity, but prevents backflow into the ventricles.

25. (4) All of these are potential complications.

26. (1) Elevating the head facilitates flow of CSF by gravity, but combined with the action of the Pudenz valve it may cause hypotension from the large and sudden decrease of intracranial pressure.

27. (1) Intake and output, urine specific gravities, and daily weights are necessary to calculate fluid requirements. In the early postoperative period a high urine output indicates functioning of the ventriculoperitoneal shunt and removal of excessive CSF.

28. (2) Assessment of shunt function includes palpation of the anterior fontanel. Tenseness of the fontanel indicates that intracranial pressure remains high and may signify shunt failure. A reduction in head circumference and decreased irritability are also desirable.

29. (1) The surgical procedure carries the risk of infection that may develop after insertion of a foreign body. Prophylaxis is important since antibiotic therapy after the development of infection in the shunt invariably fails.

30. (4) These are all side effects of ampicillin.

31. (1) Dolores needs normal nurturing interventions such as holding and cuddling. During feedings the lesion is covered with a sterile dressing, and the infant held so as to prevent pressure or contamination of the site.

32. (1) Prior to repair of the lesion, feeding is usually a problem for an infant such as Dolores. Mrs. Sommersett needs to be assisted in helping her deal with this problem (see the rationale for item 31).

33. (4) All these are appropriate in providing good skin care.

34. (1) To preserve as much neurologic functioning as possible, it is now thought that repair of the defect should be done within the first few hours of life. At this time, there are fewer adhesions between the nervous tissue and the sac, and the risk of infection is decreased.

35. (4) See the rationale for item 34.
36. (1) Should the shunt fail to function again it would be reflected in increasing head size.
37. (4) All of these reflect CSF accumulation and increased intracranial pressure.
38. (3) If pressure is kept off the surgical repair the infant can be held while being fed.
39. (4) These are all important for the parents' understanding and successful management of Dolores' condition.
40. (1) This is the range of mild retardation.
41. (2) This requires cognitive abilities that Dolores may not possess.

Cystic Fibrosis

1. (4) Because the pulmonary secretions are thick and block small airways, cystic fibrosis was at one time called "mucoviscidosis." This term is now considered archaic.
2. (3) Cystic fibrosis is an autosomal recessive disease, and thus both parents must carry the gene for this disease to be transmitted to their offspring. There is a high incidence of subsequent children also having the disease.
3. (3) Carriers do not have the disease. Since the disease is recessive, the only way it can be expressed is for both parents to transmit the gene for the disease.
4. (1) In any given pregnancy in which both parents carry the gene for cystic fibrosis, the offspring has a 1 in 4 chance of inheriting the disease. This percentage remains constant with each pregnancy.
5. (3) The secretions are altered in consistency and increased in amount.
6. (2) The increased amount and tenacity of the secretions obstruct glands and ducts, especially those in the pancreas, and prohibit the secretion of the pancreatic enzymes needed for digesting of nutrients.
7. (1) The increased viscosity of the mucus leads to bronchial obstruction. Ciliary action is also impaired, reducing expectoration.
8. (3) Bronchiole obstruction allows air to enter on inspiration but prevents air exit on expiration. This leads to terminal air trapping, eventually causing emphysema.
9. (4) The increased, viscoid respiratory secretions enhance bacterial growth, which affects the temperature regulating center.
10. (2) Neutrophilia frequently is associated with a bacterial infection.
11. (4) This is a common complication of cystic fibrosis whereby the pulmonary changes increase pulmonary vascular pressure and increase the workload of the right ventricle. This eventually causes right ventricular failure.
12. (3) Pancreatic obstruction and atrophy prevent secretion of enzymes that normally assist in the absorption of fats. Thus, most of the ingested food is excreted as unabsorbed fats and proteins.
13. (3) This complication is due to obstruction of the bile ducts by thick or viscoid mucus.
14. (1) Owing to pancreatic obstruction, enzymes are absent in the duodenum. The absence of trypsin on stool analysis is indicative of cystic fibrosis.
15. (2) Pilocarpine, a cholinergic drug, enhances nerve impulse transmission to the exocrine glands and stimulates sweat production. The sweat is then analyzed for sodium and chloride concentrations.
16. (2) Usually a 4-by-4-inch area is needed to conduct the test. The forearm and extensor surface of the thigh are ideal sites.
17. (3) It is important to cleanse the skin thoroughly before testing. Distilled water is preferable because it does not add elements to the skin surface.
18. (4) This is a common complication in infancy and childhood due to straining, emaciation of the buttocks, and weak musculature in the rectal area.
19. (2) Elevated sweat electrolyte levels are diagnostic of cystic fibrosis, although high levels may also occur in siblings and their relatives who have no clinical manifestation of the disease. The reason for the elevated levels is not completely known.
20. (3) Gentamicin is selective for gram-negative organisms.

21. (4) Gentamicin is potentially toxic to renal, auditory, and vestibular functions. Additional untoward effects include headache and skin eruptions.
22. (1) Methicillin is a semisynthetic penicillin unaffected by penicillinase.
23. (1) Propylene glycol was added to the mucolytic agent administered in aerosol form to lower the surface tension, making treatment more effective than normal saline solution or water. The goal of this therapy is to assure that the droplets are inhaled into the terminal airways to help liquefy thickened sputum.
24. (4) Fat-soluble vitamins are poorly absorbed and need to be supplemented.
25. (2) Vitamin K is necessary for the synthesis of prothrombin or plasma protein essential for normal coagulation.
26. (2) Owing to the thick mucoid secretions, children with cystic fibrosis are especially prone to respiratory infections.
27. (4) All these factors contribute to skin breakdown.
28. (1) This position best utilizes and mobilizes lower airway secretions to be coughed up or suctioned out.
29. (3) Methicillin injections are painful and irritating to subcutaneous tissue. Children under 2 years of age should receive I.M. injections deep into the vastus lateralis or rectus femoris since gluteal muscles are underdeveloped. Correct I.M. injection technique does include options 2 and 4.
30. (4) These are all examples of respiratory infections.
31. (3) Heat prostration results from a high environmental temperature and excessive loss of electrolytes in perspiration.
32. (1) These measures assist in preventing excessive insensible water loss through sweating.
33. (4) A mist tent assists in liquefying the tenacious mucus of the respiratory tract.
34. (2) Both of these methods facilitate removal of the pulmonary secretions.
35. (3) It is important to provide a balanced diet high in protein and low in fat.
36. (3) Cystic fibrosis and its management often interfere with normal growth and development. The unrelenting treatments such as daily postural drainage can lead to resentment and frustration. Encouragement of normal physical activity is physiologically and psychologically beneficial.

Eczema

1. (4) This is the average weight of a male fetus of 40 weeks' gestation following a normal pregnancy.
2. (2) The usual age for weaning is between 5 and 6 months.
3. (2) Weaning should be done gradually over several weeks to allow for physiologic and emotional transition. In addition, upon hospitalization of his mother, Victor probably experienced a separation reaction that complicated the weaning process.
4. (4) Eczema, the most frequent allergic state seen in infancy, is considered to be an atopic manifestation of a specific allergen.
5. (4) The chronicity of the disease and strict dietary and treatment regimens may lead to overprotective and controlling tendencies in the mother.
6. (4) Any of these, whether ingested or in contact with the skin, may be responsible for infantile eczema. The specific cause for the sensitivity is not fully understood.
7. (3) The anti-inflammatory effect of adrenocorticosteroids is not fully understood, but may be due to stabilization of the lysosome membranes, decreased formation of bradykinin, and decreased capillary membrane permeability.
8. (3) Diphenhydramine, by competing for histamine receptor sites, blocks histamine action that promotes capillary permeability and edema formation.
9. (2) Most immunization sera are made from chick embryos, and children with eczema usually are highly allergic to eggs and egg albumin. Therefore, eczematous lesions may flare up if prophylactic immunization is carried out.
10. (2) Smallpox vaccine is no longer routinely given, but if an eczematous child comes in contact with a vaccinated individual caution must be exercised to prevent a generalized vaccinia.

11. (4) All these are important in identifying and removing causative allergens and initiating a therapeutic regimen.
12. (1) Acetaminophen acts directly on hypothalamic heat-regulating centers, facilitating peripheral vasodilation and heat loss.
13. (3) This method is mechanically and chemically the least traumatic to the skin.
14. (4) Zinc oxide, a water-insoluble topical protectant, has astringent, antipruritic, and antiseptic properties.
15. (3) See the rationale for item 14.
16. (3) A face mask facilitates close contact between medication and skin, and discourages Victor from rubbing the paste off the lesions.
17. (2) The normal response to increased body temperature includes capillary dilation and diaphoresis. The accompanying warmth and moisture at the skin surface intensifies itching of the lesions.
18. (1) The eczematous lesions may cause intense itching, and secondary bacterial infection may result if the infant is allowed to scratch afflicted areas. Extensive lesions may heal poorly and result in scarring.
19. (2) The alkaline solution neutralizes the pH of the exudate of the lesions and relieves itching.
20. (2) Diversion and judicious use of restraints both help to prevent Victor from scratching during the bath procedure. Options a, c, and e are inappropriate.
21. (1) Although selected authorities recommend the use of plastic over the bed sheets, this procedure must be weighed against the discomfort caused the child by sleeping on plastic rather than the sheet.
22. (1) Mineral oil is less irritating to the skin. Options 2, 3, and 4 are irritating and painful if used with open lesions.
23. (4) This cleanses the skin without causing increased irritation of the existing lesions.
24. (1) S. aureus, commonly found on the skin, is the most likely organism to cause secondary infection.
25. (1) These restraints best prevent scratching while allowing some physical mobility.
26. (2) Scratching becomes a manipulative, attention-seeking device.
27. (3) These activities meet both physiologic (prevention of hypostatic pneumonia) and psychologic (love and attention) needs.
28. (2) Most immunization sera are developed in chick embryos. Eczematous children usually are highly allergic, and thus are particularly prone to allergic reactions following immunization.
29. (1) This ensures that Victor receives the recommended daily allowance of vitamins.
30. (3) These concepts are important if the parents are to achieve realistic and successful treatment of their infant.
31. (3) These actions alleviate any concerns Mrs. Skinner may have relative to Victor's skin care, and allow her to demonstrate her ability to follow skin care procedures correctly.
32. (3) These measures reduce allergens, promote good skin care, and prevent exacerbation of existing lesions.
33. (2) Children with eczema frequently develop asthma as the eczematous condition subsides. Both conditions are associated with specific allergens that initiate the clinical manifestations.

Laryngotracheobronchitis

1. (1) Inspiratory stridor and clear breath sounds are also observed in a child with upper airway obstruction. This is most frequently due to foreign body aspiration.
2. (4) Although not commonly seen, diphtheria is an infection of the upper airway also accompanied by stridor, hyperpyrexia, tachycardia, and dyspnea.
3. (3) In the clinical progression of laryngotracheobronchitis (LTB), the laryngeal mucosa becomes inflamed, edematous, and covered with exudate. Airway obstruction and respiratory arrest may result.

4. (4) All of these have been implicated.

5. (2) See the rationale for item 3.

6. (1) Stridor is a high-pitched sound made as air attempts to pass through the laryngeal openings, which are narrowed as a result of inflammation and edema.

7. (2) See the rationales for items 3 and 6.

8. (4) The thick tracheobronchial secretions cover the cilia and prevent the outward propulsion of mucus.

9. (2) As a 2-year-old, Lena will demonstrate heightened anxiety due to separation from her parents. Attempts to make her hospitalization as normal as possible promote feelings of security.

10. (4) These responses may be demonstrated by the toddler experiencing parental separation. They reflect anxiety, regression, and depression.

11. (1) See the rationales for items 3 and 9.

12. (1) Frequent inspection of the chest is necessary to assess respiratory rate and depth, chest excursion, and use of accessory muscles.

13. (3) Phonation normally results from vibration of the larynx. Increasing inflammation and edema affects the vibratory action of the larynx and may produce hoarseness or aphonia.

14. (4) This position prevents pooling of secretions in the upper airway.

15. (3) Children between the ages of 6 months and 6 years may develop seizures when the body temperature exceeds 103° F. rectally. It is thought that hyperpyrexia may trigger seizure activity.

16. (4) There is a significant correlation between increased fluids, less tenacious mucus, prevention of dehydration, and dilution of bacterial toxins.

17. (2) Ampicillin is a broad-spectrum antibiotic. Penicillin is primarily effective only against gram-positive organisms. Muscular absorption is approximately the same; both may provoke allergic reactions; and both may be inactivated by penicillinase.

18. (3) Cool humidity constricts the vessels and reduces edema.

19. (1) Airway obstruction may result in "air hunger," or a feeling of being unable to take in adequate amounts of air.

20. (4) Atelectasis may result from mucous plugs (causing complete obstruction of small airways) and alveoli secretions. The anatomic uniqueness of the eustachian tube in the young facilitates accumulation of upper airway secretions in the tube. This may result in otitis media. Hyperpyrexia may lower the seizure threshold. Changes in the lungs may lead to cardiac drainage and complications.

21. (2) See the rationale for item 20 concerning atelectasis. Unequal chest expansion reflects aeration of the unaffected side but lack of air entry on the affected side.

22. (3) Extreme quiet may reflect hypoxia (Pa_{O_2} 50 mm. Hg), with decreased cellular oxygenation and immense fatigue.

23. (4) These are all symptoms of laryngeal obstruction leading to increased ventilatory effort and cyanosis.

24. (4) Ampicillin is a semisynthetic, broad-spectrum penicillin effective against all these organisms.

25. (3) Humidification moistens and thins secretions, facilitating their removal.

26. (4) These are all correct. Constant nursing attention is necessary to ensure patency of the airway.

27. (4) Options a and b are necessary so that the second tracheostomy tube may be inserted should the original tube be accidentally withdrawn. Option c is needed to remove secretions. Option d is necessary to moisten the airway and prevent localized swelling at the tracheostomy site.

28. (1) Initial placement may cause excess accumulation of secretions, since the tube is foreign to the airway.

29. (2) It is important to prevent introduction of bacteria into the respiratory tract. Suctioning is always performed with aseptic technique.

30. (1) Applying suction during insertion of the catheter traumatizes the tracheal mucosa.

31. (2) Saline liquefies secretions and facilitates their removal.

32. (1) Cleaning the inner cannula removes mucus accumulation and dried secre-

tions, and ensures patency of the airway. It should be noted that many pediatric tracheostomy tubes do not contain inner cannulas owing to their already small diameter.

33. (3) Pipe cleaners are flexible and conform to the tube. Hydrogen peroxide removes mucoid concretions adhering to the cannula. Some institutions use roller gauze instead of pipe cleaners.

34. (1) Immediate action must be taken by the nurse to ensure a patent airway. The duplicate tracheostomy tube should be opened and reinserted as quickly and gently as possible, using the obturator as a guide.

35. (3) These are normal developmental, gross motor skills characteristic of a 2-year-old.

36. (1) Parallel play is typical of the toddler. Interaction with people has gained importance but not to the point of sharing.

37. (4) The toddler is striving for autonomy through bowel and bladder control, and control of others.

38. (3) These conditions would be the result of bacterial invasion of the lower airway resulting in significant parenchymal damage.

39. (2) It would be best for Mrs. Barcus to have a cool steam or room humidifier. The measures are substitutes. She would need to be alert to the highly investigative nature of the 2-year-old in order to prevent an accident (e.g., burn).

Bronchial Asthma

1. (2) These pathologic changes, due to a hyperresponsiveness of the airway, account for the obstructive nature of asthma.

2. (4) The many theories advanced to explain the etiology of bronchial asthma include immunologic, infectious, metabolic, chemical, and psychologic causes.

3. (4) In sensitive individuals any of these may act as irritants or allergens, and trigger an asthmatic attack.

4. (2) In asthma the bronchi and bronchioles are obstructed with thick, tenacious mucous plugs that contain portions of the respiratory epithelium.

5. (3) The contracted and edematous bronchial musculature and increased mucus production prevent the passage of air. Air in the alveoli distal to the occlusion cannot escape, and becomes overdistended.

6. (3) This is a compensatory mechanism to facilitate expiration of air.

7. (2) This indicates increased ventilatory effort.

8. (2) To prevent toxicity, oxygen should be used only in hypoxemia, which would be manifested by cyanosis.

9. (2) A cold for three days prior to admission would have interfered with sleep and nutrition.

10. (2) This position facilitates lung expansion and prevents pooling of secretions.

11. (1) Asthma may precipitate paroxysms of coughing, which can cause vomiting.

12. (4) An increased number of eosinophils occurs in allergic diseases, although their exact role has not yet been defined. It is thought that they may suppress the inflammatory response by neutralizing histamine.

13. (1) Respiratory failure is indicated by a pCO_2 greater than 50 mm. Hg and a pH less than 7.35.

14. (1) The aunt has been her caretaker since her mother's death.

15. (4) Epinephrine is a hormone produced by the adrenal medulla.

16. (1) Epinephrine, a sympathomimetic, stimulates adrenergic receptors and relaxes the smooth muscles of the bronchioles.

17. (1) Aminophylline, a xanthine, relaxes smooth muscle of bronchi and pulmonary vessels by direct action. Unlike the situation with sympathomimetic agents, tolerance to the bronchodilator effects of aminophylline rarely develops, but it should be used cautiously in children.

18. (1) Ephedrine, an indirect-acting sympathomimetic amine, is pharmacologically similar to epinephrine but less potent, with slower onset and more prolonged action.

19. (2) See rationales for items 16 and 18.
20. (3) Adverse effects of ephedrine (usually with large doses) include headache, insomnia, nervousness, tachycardia, sweating, nausea, and vomiting.
21. (1) The sedative effects of phenobarbital are due primarily to inhibition of the reticular activating system and interference with impulse transmission to the cerebral cortex.
22. (4) By direct action on bronchial tissue, potassium iodide increases secretion of respiratory fluids, thereby decreasing mucous viscosity. Thus, it is used to facilitate bronchial drainage and ease cough.
23. (1) The liquefaction of the secretions by the potassium iodide can increase nasal discharge.
24. (2) These measures loosen and mobilize bronchial secretions, and improve oxygenation.
25. (2) Increased fluids maintain hydration and liquefy bronchial secretions.
26. (4) Maria is already apprehensive about not being able to breathe and being hospitalized. She will be very sensitive to the attitudes of others. A nurse displaying irritation would increase Maria's anxiety.
27. (2) Nonallergenic factors such as these may precipitate an asthma attack. Intense cold and strenuous exercise can decrease oxygen, whereas sudden emotion can decrease adenylcyclase and cause bronchial constriction.
28. (4) These are all potential allergens that may precipitate an asthma attack.
29. (3) See the rationale for item 17.
30. (2) See the rationale for item 17.
31. (2) Adverse effects of aminophylline include nausea, vomiting, irritability, headache, hyperexcitability, tachycardia, flushing, and rectal irritation.
32. (2) Isoproterenol, a synthetic sympathomimetic amine, is pharmacologically similar to epinephrine, but acts almost exclusively on beta adrenergic receptors and produces relaxation of the bronchial tree.
33. (3) See the rationales for items 15 and 32.
34. (4) Again, the purpose is to identify both allergenic and nonallergenic factors that may be precipitating the asthma attacks.
35. (1) Of these areas in the home, Maria probably spends most of the time in her bedroom.
36. (4) Skin testing may be performed by any of these methods. The intracutaneous method is also known as intradermal.
37. (4) It is important to observe Maria's reaction to the control scratch, which may appear to be a skin test reaction (false-positive) and make the allergen identification inaccurate.
38. (1) Skin testing is performed to identify specific allergens. Patients are often unaware of the sensitivities they possess, and the nurse must always be prepared for the possibility of systemic anaphylaxis. In this event, epinephrine, 0.5 ml 1:1000 strength, S.Q. or I.V., is the drug of choice.
39. (4) These are all appropriate measures to reduce allergens and minimize the severity and number of asthma attacks.

Cerebral Palsy

1. (4) Cerebral palsy (CP) is a nonprogressive disease of the pyramidal motor system characterized by abnormal muscle tone and coordination.
2. (3) In diplegia all extremities are involved, but generally the spasticity is greater in the legs than in the arms.
3. (4) These answers reflect the variety of etiologic factors thought to cause CP. In determining the cause, prenatal, perinatal, and postnatal factors are ruled out. Cerebral anoxia is considered the leading cause in prenatal and perinatal complications.
4. (1) Erythroblastosis fetalis is associated with increased RBC hemolysis. The hemolysis contributes to anemia, which can cause cerebral hypoxia.
5. (3) The pyramidal tract consists of the motor cortex, basal ganglia, and cerebellum.
6. (2) This information is important in order to determine Buddy's current capa-

bilities as compared to normal growth and developmental milestones, and to predict his potential.

7. (4) These are all correct and reflect the multiplicity of problems associated with CP. Of the associated problems, mental retardation is probably the most serious.

8. (1) Spastic CP, the most common form, is due to upper motor neuron involvement and is characterized by increased muscle tone, increased extension, and muscle weakness. The hypertonic muscles are continuously contracted, whereas other muscles are overstretched, resulting in the characteristic scissor and toe-pointing position.

9. (2) See the rationale for item 8.

10. (1) This is due to disruption of the pyramidal tract and upper motor neurons. See the rationale for item 8.

11. (2) A long-term goal is to establish locomotion, and muscle training is a means of achieving this objective.

12. (4) The habilitation process must be individualized and realistic for the child in accordance with his abilities.

13. (4) All factors will affect the success of Buddy's treatment program.

14. (4) These are typical of organic brain disease. Hypoxemia-ischemia results in abnormal brain activity, especially affecting the behavior modalities.

15. (4) All these are related to Buddy's poor muscle control and inability to communicate his needs adequately.

16. (1) Rest before physiotherapy sessions promotes muscle relaxation, and ensures that less resistance is present during the sessions.

17. (2) This is due to the extreme hypertonicity of Buddy's muscles.

18. (2) Reduction of stimuli promotes muscle relaxation. Even minor distractions can increase muscle hypertonicity.

19. (3) Failure to master muscular activities in the past may discourage Buddy from attempting new motor skills.

20. (4) The nurse must keep in mind that Buddy has spastic but weak muscles that he cannot keep under control. These measures assist him to achieve success with self-feeding.

21. (3) This results from the inability to control spastic muscles.

22. (2) Applesauce is a semisoft food that is easier to fill on a spoon than the other foods listed. It is also easier to manage orally.

23. (4) All these measures are appropriate to assist in development of hand-to-mouth skill, an important first step to self-feeding.

24. (3) Since many baby foods are now vitamin-fortified, vitamin deficiency may not be as great a problem as impaired chewing from disuse of masseter and temporal muscles.

25. (2) This is useful in determining if there is a pattern to Buddy's voiding times. Later, this can be utilized in initiating bladder training.

26. (3) These measures facilitate optimal bowel functioning. Enemas, particularly tap water enemas, are contraindicated because they do not foster bowel control and can cause water intoxication.

27. (4) Taking into account Buddy's spasticity and impaired fine motor development, these measures facilitate the learning of self-dressing techniques.

28. (3) Buddy's mental retardation, hearing loss, and spasticity of muscles used for articulation all preclude normal language development. Competition with normal children would lead to failure and feelings of worthlessness.

29. (4) Normal emotional growth requires healthy interpersonal interaction and a positive self-esteem.

30. (2) This is important in working with Buddy and his parents. Although CP is nonprogressive, it is not regressive.

31. (3) CP is nonprogressive. Deterioration would occur only if the habilitation process were interrupted.

32. (3) This is important in order to foster feelings of worth.

33. (4) All these actions are appropriate in the care and support of the child and his family.

34. (1) The demands on the parents' time, emotional energy, and physical stamina are enormous. The actions indicated in 2 and 4 might be helpful in accomplishing no. 1.

Burn

1. (3) The anterior trunk constitutes 18 per cent of body surface area according to the estimate used from Evan's rule of nine. A more current method estimates the figure to be 13 per cent.
2. (2) Using Evan's rule, the leg is considered to take up 15 per cent of total body surface area.
3. (2) The definition of a second degree burn is destruction of the dermis to a varying extent; the appearance of the area is red to pale ivory, with blistering and pain.
4. (3) Open wounds are very prone to infection, and treatment should focus on prevention of infection. Burns do not hemorrhage.
5. (4) All the listed structures are destroyed in a third degree burn, which is subdermal and is called a full-thickness burn.
6. (2) Third degree burns have to be grafted as they cannot heal on their own. Owing to the destruction of nerve fibers, third degree burns are initially less painful than first and second degree burns.
7. (4) All these actions are appropriate. The wounds need to be debrided and cleansed to promote healing and prevent infection. Normal saline is used to irrigate the wounds as it decreases electrolyte depletion, which would be seen if plain water were used. The soap should not have a hexachlorophene base as neurologic damage (seizures) could result.
8. (2) The weight is the most accurate method of evaluating the fluid loss or burn shock, and will be needed to estimate the amount of fluid replacement required.
9. (2) Some form of tetanus prophylaxis is routinely given after a major burn, as most burns are "dirty" or occur in "dirty" circumstances.
10. (4) *C. tetani* has all these characteristics.
11. (4) All these are burn complications. Renal failure is a danger when hypovolemic shock occurs. Cardiac failure is often seen in the acute phase, when fluid overload is a danger. Gastrointestinal ulcers, especially Curling's ulcer, are found in 25 per cent of patients with burns. Septic shock is a danger when wounds become infected, and can lead to septicemia. Contractures are common in burn patients, and are due to immobilization and healing of the burns.
12. (1) This is the most appropriate initial nursing action and will prevent infection. The other actions are not appropriate at this time.
13. (1) Morphine is used for analgesia or pain relief.
14. (2) Constipation is a major side effect of morphine.
15. (3) Morphine is a narcotic and potentially addictive.
16. (4) All the symptoms listed are clinical indications of hypovolemic shock seen in burns, due to third space fluid shifts.
17. (4) All are essential to prevent the likelihood of shock. Replacing the fluid losses due to fluid shifts is most essential. Pain and hypothermia can enhance shock.
18. (3) Fluid loss via the burn itself (serous oozing) and plasma shifts from the vascular compartment to the burn both lead to potential shock and the need for large amounts of intravenous fluids. The child is placed on NPO (nothing by mouth) to prevent vomiting and aspiration as gastrointestinal activity is decreased. Marked decrease in urinary output, not diuresis, is typical after a burn.
19. (3) The size of the burn or percentage of total body surface area burned is proportional to the amount of fluid loss from the vascular compartment. This percentage estimate is used in calculating fluid replacement.
20. (2) Increasing hematocrit is seen when plasma continues to flow to the burned area with no corresponding shift of blood solids. The urinary output is less with the decreased renal perfusion that occurs in hypovolemic shock.
21. (3) These would all be possible in the first 48 hours or the resuscitative phase. The decreased circulating blood volume, inadequate fluid replacement, and resultant decreased renal perfusion could lead to decreased urinary output and impending renal failure. Also, burn exotoxins could cause renal tubular damage, oliguria, and renal failure. Infection would be seen much later.

22. (4) All these would be necessary to evaluate urinary output accurately: a patent system (without "kinks"), no leakage, and hourly measurements.

23. (2) Owing to the fluid shifts to the burned area and decreased peripheral circulation, I.M. or S.Q. pain medications would be poorly absorbed. Intravenous administration of analgesics is the best and most effective method for pain relief.

24. (3) The sympathetic response to a major burn causes decreased peristalsis, which leads to vomiting, abdominal distention, and gastric dilation.

25. (2) Bubbling rales are symptomatic of pulmonary edema and overhydration. Water intoxication results from cellular overhydration, and a symptom of this is muscle twitching or tremor.

26. (3) Congestive heart failure may be seen 48 hours after a burn, when fluid that shifted into the burn area is reabsorbed back into the vascular system.

27. (1) The signs of septicemia are those listed.

28. (2) Topical antibiotics such as Sulfamylon are used to prevent local wound infection.

29. (4) Whirlpool treatment is a common method of removing topical burn creams, increasing circulation to the burned area, and cleansing the wound.

30. (3) With underhydration, there is less fluid available for cooling the body. Local or systemic infection could cause an increase in temperature.

31. (3) Burns do not hemorrhage. A massive septicemia could cause marrow depression; however, there are no indications of widespread sepsis. Direct heat injury and hemolysis are the most likely cause of Rudy's anemia.

32. (2) Anorexia is a symptom of toxemia.

33. (3) Loss of recently gained skills such as bowel control are often seen with the hospitalized preschooler; the child regresses to cope with anxiety.

34. (2) Eschar is black, necrotic tissue that forms after a full-thickness burn. It has to be removed to allow for the granulation of tissue.

35. (3) No analgesic can completely eliminate pain, and the child has to be told this truthfully. The nurse should reaffirm that she will be present to support and comfort him. Not allowing the child to watch only increases anxiety and pain perception.

36. (4) Play therapy with dolls or puppets will help Rudy to deal with his injuries and feelings. Answers 1 and 2 would interfere with his treatment and are not appropriate. No. 3 is incorrect, as 3-year-olds don't verbalize their feelings that freely.

37. (1) Showing Rudy evidence of improvement is the best approach. Not allowing him to look at his own burns or showing him pictures of other burned children would increase his fear and anxiety. No serious burn heals without scarring.

38. (3) Answers 1 and 4 are inappropriate as they promote regression. No. 2 is impractical. No. 3 is the best as it plans for painful procedures to be done at times distant from meals, and therefore promotes better nutrition.

39. (2) Protein needs are increased by 2 to 3 times the normal daily requirement to promote wound healing.

40. (3) This position promotes extension, and prevents contractures, of hips.

41. (2) *Pseudomonas* is one of the most common infective organisms with burns; *Staphylococcus* and *Proteus* also cause infections in burn wounds.

42. (4) Complete isolation technique (reverse or protective isolation) is used with burn patients. It includes gown, mask, gloves, and careful handwashing.

43. (1) Third degree burns have to be grafted for healing to occur; this also helps prevent infection, which would occur with any large, open wound.

44. (2) All eschar and necrotic tissue must be eliminated prior to grafting and granulation of tissue, or the graft will not take. Answers 1 and 3 are important, but are not the main reasons why grafts are done.

45. (1) Grafts from self (autografts) are permanent, and the incidence of rejection or sloughing is less than for homografts. Homografts (grafts from other humans) are temporary grafts that are eventually rejected by the recipient.

46. (2) A bed cradle is most appropriate; it allows air to reach the sites, but still promotes warmth and privacy.

47. (3) The diet required for wound healing should be high in protein and calories to meet metabolic needs; vitamin and mineral requirements are increased, especially vitamin C.

48. (4) All the choices are appropriate for a 3-year-old as they provide support, comfort, and stimulation which is important after the period of isolation.
49. (3) Dakin's solution is a 10 per cent aqueous sodium hypochlorite solution.
50. (2) Dakin's solution is bactericidal in that it disrupts bacterial enzyme systems. It also interferes with the formation of thrombin.
51. (2) Involving the child in the procedure and allowing him some control promotes acceptance and helps decrease his discomfort.
52. (2) Prevention of contractures in this rehabilitative phase is most important. Answers 2 and 4 are incorrect as they disrupt graft healing. At discharge, pain should be minimal and there should be no need for morphine.

Juvenile Diabetes Mellitus

1. (4) Juvenile diabetes mellitus is the result of the decrease or cessation of pancreatic insulin production.
2. (3) Insulin has the functions noted in a, b, and c.
3. (3) Diabetes is an hereditary, genetically-determined disease.
4. (2) Heredity is a predisposing factor to the development of diabetes. Expression of the clinical manifestation probably requires the genetic abnormality to be present in both parents. It may be a recessive gene. Some researchers claim a viral etiology.
5. (2) a, b, and c reflect the prolonged hyperglycemia, and resultant hypertonic dehydration and starvation.
6. (2) Normal blood glucose ranges between 60 and 100 mg. per 100 ml. of blood. There might be slight variations of this range in different health care agencies.
7. (2) This is the correct description of the usual glucose tolerance test, which is a measure of the rate of clearance of glucose from the blood.
8. (3) Owing to the lack of insulin, glucose could not be transported across the cell membrane, and therefore glucose levels remain elevated.
9. (2) Blood cholesterol rises in diabetes mellitus. This is thought to be the result of the general increases in lipid mobilization.
10. (2) The renal threshold for glucose is 165–200 mg. per 100 ml. of blood. Glucose levels higher than this are not absorbed and are excreted in the urine.
11. (3) See the rationale for item 10. Sources vary from 165–200 mg.
12. (3) Prolonged hyperglycemia causes fluid to be drawn from the tissues into the vascular system and then excreted, resulting in polyuria.
13. (3) Increased amounts of urine often lead to enuresis. Glucose is not irritating and it is too soon for degenerative neural changes. Regression is a possible cause, but increased urinary volume is much more likely.
14. (1) Regular (crystalline) insulin has a duration of action of 5–7 hours. Lente is an intermediate-acting insulin with a duration of action of 24–28 hours.
15. (3) In acidosis, the hydrogen ion is increased and the blood pH lowered.
16. (1) Ketones are organic acids that produce excessive quantities of free hydrogen ions, causing a fall in pH. The kidney attempts to compensate for the increased pH by increasing tubular secretion of hydrogen and ammonium ions in exchange for fixed base, and therefore the base bicarbonate is depleted.
17. (3) The normal range for serum pH is 7.35–7.45.
18. (3) Choices a, b, c, and d all reflect prolonged hyperglycemia (diabetic acidosis), which leads to hypertonic dehydration and the symptoms listed.
19. (1) Nausea, vomiting, and abdominal pain are usually associated with diabetic acidosis and with its attendant electrolyte imbalances, particularly hyponatremia.
20. (4) All of these occur with the dehydration and breakdown of fats associated with starvation.
21. (3) This is the best and most accurate test.
22. (4) One of the most common precipitators of acidosis is a viral or bacterial infection.
23. (3) Increased temperature elevates the basal metabolic rate, increasing the cellular need for nutrients and insulin.

24. (1) Dehydration, with resultant ketosis and acidosis lead to cerebral depression and coma.
25. (2) Hypertonic dehydration is the basis of diabetic ketoacidosis. A sign of dehydration is sunken eyeballs.
26. (3) The double-voiding technique as described provides the most accurate urinary analysis in the diabetic.
27. (3) Starvation leads to breakdown of fats and ketone production.
28. (1) Close monitoring of urinary glucose and ketones is essential and should be done frequently.
29. (3) Kussmaul breathing is characteristic of diabetic ketoacidosis, and results from the losses of sodium, potassium, and magnesium that force the body to buffer excess ketones via the respiratory system.
30. (3) The fall in the pH stimulates the respiratory buffer system, and carbonic acid is broken down. The carbon dioxide is excreted by the hyperventilation characteristic of metabolic acidosis.
31. (2) The carbon dioxide combining power of plasma is related indirectly to bicarbonate concentration.
32. (1) Regular insulin is used initially with diabetic acidosis because of its quick onset of action (30–60 minutes).
33. (3) 250 ml./8 hrs. = 31 ml./hr.

$$\frac{31 \text{ ml./hr.}}{60 \text{ min.}} \times 60 \text{ gH/ml.} = 31 \text{ gH/min.}$$

34. (2) Negative acetone would indicate adequate nutrition and cessation of fat breakdown. Many authorities prefer a trace of glucose to avoid hypoglycemia.
35. (3) Alterations in diet and exercise patterns, and repeated infections, can all lead to episodes of diabetic acidosis and poor control of repeated diabetes.
36. (3) a, b, and c promote normal growth and development, and acceptance of the disease. d would decrease independence — most children are administering their own insulin, etc., by age 8–10 years.
37. (2) Emotional stress may lead to acute increases in insulin requirements and to ketoacidosis.
38. (2) Rapid growth changes in childhood lead to continuing adjustment of insulin needs. The major single determinants of insulin requirements are body size and level of sexual maturation.
39. (4) Most diets eliminate concentrated sweets, and foods should be chosen from the basic four food groups.
40. (3) Carbohydrates provide 4 calories per gram; fat, 9 calories per gram.
41. (4) Urine should be tested before each meal and at bedtime.
42. (3) Too much insulin, too little food, and an increase in exercise all lead to hypoglycemia or insulin shock. Infections would lead to hyperglycemia or ketoacidosis.
43. (3) Hypoglycemia and epinephrine release lead to symptoms a, b, c, and d. Symptom e is seen with hyperglycemia.
44. (4) Peak action of Lente, an intermediate-acting insulin, is 8–12 hours after administration, and hypoglycemia frequently occurs then.
45. (1) Juvenile diabetes is characterized by an absolute lack of insulin, and injectable (exogenous) insulin has to be used.
46. (1) As children with diabetes may be smaller in height and weight than their peers, insulin may play a part in growth and sexual maturity.
47. (3) Children with diabetes are more prone to infections and resulting complications. Infection can lead to ketoacidosis.
48. (2) Foot infections are common with diabetics, and children, with their rapid growth, would be prone to skin breakdown if given poorly fitting shoes.

Nephrosis

1. (2) Infections are a possible etiologic factor and often cause exacerbations of nephrosis.
2. (3) Nephrosis is known to lead to chronic glomerulonephritis and possible renal failure.

3. (4) Symptoms of nephrotic syndrome include pallor, lethargy, irritability, anorexia, edema, diarrhea and oliguria.

4. (3) Hematuria, azotemia and hypertension are more characteristic of acute glomerulonephritis, and usually are not seen with nephrosis.

5. (2) Pathologic changes take place in the epithelial aspect of the glomerular basement membrane.

6. (4) Ascites and the enlarged abdomen diminish the movement of the diaphragm and the depth of respirations, so that the respiratory rate increases.

7. (4) Nephrotic edema is due to hypoalbuminemia and decreased osmotic pressure of the blood.

8. (2) Periorbital tissue (owing to low tissue pressures) often is the tissue that becomes edematous first, particularly after prolonged dependent position (sleep).

9. (3) Ascites in this case is due to accumulation of fluid in the abdomen, and not to pathologic changes in the liver.

10. (2) An accompanying infection would account for increased WBC count, as this count is usually within normal limits or only mildly elevated with nephrosis.

11. (3) Polymorphonuclear lymphocytes in the child normally constitute 45–50 per cent.

12. (3) Increased sedimentation rate is indicative of an inflammatory process.

13. (3) Albumin, globulin, and fibrinogen are the three major components of the plasma protein.

14. (1) Cholesterol, a monohydric alcohol, is partially composed of fatty acids and is found in animal fats and oils.

15. (1) Granular and hyaline casts are seen in the urine.

16. (4) Otto's titer was 12, which is within normal limits; it would have been greater than 250 units if a streptococcal infection had occurred.

17. (4) Steroids such as prednisone are used in nephrosis. It is postulated that they have an anti-inflammatory effect on the renal glomeruli, although the exact mechanism is unknown.

18. (3) Steroids depress the WBCs and inflammatory response, and may mask signs of infection.

19. (4) These are all side effects of steroids.

20. (4) Cushing's syndrome includes all of these plus a "buffalo hump."

21. (1) Penicillin interferes with cell wall formation in bacteria.

22. (3) Prednisone and steroids depress WBC formation and make the patient susceptible to infection.

23. (2) Hypertension due to fluid retention is common with steroid administration. In children, this side effect is rarely observed.

24. (3) Diuretics such as the thiazides can be used to decrease the massive edema.

25. (1) Thiazide diuretics often lead to hypokalemia, of which muscle weakness is a symptom.

26. (3) Intake and subsequent output are used to evaluate kidney function.

27. (3) Daily weights are used to evaluate edema and fluid retention.

28. (3) Weights should be taken at the same time each day on the same scales, with the child wearing clothing of similar weight.

29. (2) The edema of protein malnutrition presents some symptoms similar to those observed in nephrosis, and may be difficult to detect.

30. (1) Furosemide (Lasix) is a potent, rapid-acting diuretic.

31. (2) Onset of action of furosemide is from 30 (I.V.) to 60 (oral) minutes after administration.

32. (4) Side effects of furosemide include hyperglycemia, diarrhea, paresthesias, nausea and vomiting, blood dyscrasias, and dermatitis.

33. (1) Owing to the hypoalbuminemia, the diet may have increased protein; salt and fluids may be restricted to decrease edema.

34. (1) A 4-year-old will probably eat better when he can choose foods he likes to eat. The other choices are inappropriate for a preschooler.

35. (1) The edema and hypoalbuminemia of nephrosis can make Otto prone to skin infections. c and d are not seen with nephrosis.

36. (4) All except a would help to maintain skin integrity. Scrubbing fragile skin would lead to breakdown.

37. (4) Owing to the edematous, friable skin, gentle skin care is a necessity. The skin

should be kept clean and supple. Prevention of pressure sores is important. The scrotum, if edematous, needs support to prevent skin breakdown.

38. (2) Elevating Otto's head will help decrease edema through gravity. Eyes may need irrigation to prevent collection of exudate.

39. (1) For a 24-hour urine collection from a 4-year-old, the nurse should make certain he is aware of the need to save all urine. The first urine should be discarded, and then the collection started. Disinfectant is not a preservative. All urine is sent to the laboratory.

40. (2) Albumin, serum and urine, and serum cholesterol levels are monitored to evaluate recovery.

41. (2) Playing "house" or "doctor" is appropriate for a 4-year-old and allows an outlet for anxiety and energy. Checkers is not appropriate for the preschooler, and the skipping rope, etc., would be too demanding of energy.

42. (4) Motor skills of the 4-year-old include running, climbing, and jumping, and he has a vocabulary of about 900 words.

43. (4) By 30 months of age, children have all their deciduous or primary teeth.

44. (4) Nephrotic children are very prone to infection and should be kept away from those with infections.

45. (4) Edema can lead to distortions and changes in body image in the 4-year-old with nephrosis.

46. (1) Hemorrhage is a common complication following a renal biopsy, and Otto should be kept immobile for 12 hours.

47. (2) The kidney is extremely vascular, and hemorrhage and shock can be complications.

48. (4) The parents should be given information on medication and the side effects of steroids. The need for continued medical supervision should be emphasized, especially since exacerbations are common with nephrosis.

49. (4) The patients should be taught to give prednisone early, around 7:00 A.M., to replicate normal biorhythms. By the time children go home from the hospital, steroids have been decreased.

50. (2) Steroids tend to mask infection, and the child is also more susceptible as a result of the therapy.

Tetralogy of Fallot

1. (1) If rubella is contracted in the first trimester when embryo-organogenesis is occurring, this virus can cause maldevelopment of critical organs such as the heart, brain, and eye (the classic rubella triad).

2. (1) By 8 weeks' gestation, all major organs are formed.

3. (3) Prior to this reduction of hemoglobin, no cyanosis is observed in persons with normal hemoglobin.

4. (3) The old cliché, "you can't see the forest for the trees," is typical in these situations. Daily contact with a person often makes the obvious obscure.

5. (1) The exact mechanism for clubbing is unclear, but it is presumed that peripheral Pa_{O_2} is lower than normal. To compensate for the low peripheral Pa_{O_2}, proliferation of capillaries and tissue overgrowth occur.

6. (4) Inadequate tissue oxygenation results in anaerobic catabolism, and accumulation of lactic acid and other ketones. This results in a decrease of energy available for muscle activity.

7. (3) This toy selection conserves Timothy's energy, and is less detrimental to social and physical development than the other suggestions.

8. (4) Parents of cardiac children tend to overprotect them by allowing behavior unacceptable in a well child and excessively limiting their activity. Parents of such children, or of any chronically ill child, should be encouraged to provide appropriate discipline to help them mature.

9. (4) Erythrocytes contain hemoglobin to carry oxygen to the tissue cells. The body tries to compensate for oxygen lack by increasing production of hemoglobin for O_2 uptake and transport to the tissues.

10. (2) Polycythemia reflects an increased ratio of cells to plasma.

11. (2) The stenotic pulmonary artery cannot transport normal amounts of blood from the right ventricle. Thus, the right ventricle must contract with greater force to

overcome the resistance to flow, and in time the result is ventricular hypertrophy.

12. (3) The cardiac muscle (myocardium) responds to increased cardiac load by increasing the size of each cell (hypertrophy) rather than increasing the number of cells (hyperplasia).

13. (2) The pulmonary stenotic resistance to forward flow of blood to the lungs and the systemic blood return to the right ventricle result in an increased right ventricular pressure that exceeds left ventricular pressure. Blood then flows from the right ventricle to the left through the ventricular septal defect. This flow is turbulent, and causes the murmur heard during ventricular systole.

14. (3) For example, if Timothy has been told by his mother that he will not get any "shots," he may become quite agitated when he subsequently receives an injection. Eventual mistrust of his parents will also ensue.

15. (4) If it has been determined that Timothy's parents have been overly protective, these reactions will occur. See the rationale for item 8.

16. (4) Before consenting to undergo an invasive procedure, patients have a right to receive information in a format they can understand. Consent is a legal document ensuring the patient's instruction about the procedure and its inherent risks. Since Timothy is a minor, his parents must give their consent.

17. (3) A 5-year-old child's thinking is concrete and tangible. Play is an excellent way to help Timothy make associations between ideas.

18. (4) It is important to be honest with the child so that he will not become mistrustful.

19. (3) Phenobarbital is a barbiturate that previously was given to sedate a child the evening before surgery. However, it may produce paradoxic excitement and hyperactivity in children.

20. (2) The usual dose of phenobarbital is about 6 mg./kg./day in three divided doses. The normal weight for a 5-year-old is 35–45 pounds (16–20 kg.). Timothy's weight would have been below average.

21. (2) Promethazine is an antihistamine that suppresses some symptoms evoked by an antigen-antibody response. It has also been found to be useful in the control of postoperative vomiting.

22. (2) Promethazine suppresses the symptoms common to an allergic reaction, but does not interfere with the actual antigen-antibody response.

23. (3) Meperidine is a narcotic analgesic that has a depressant effect on the CNS. It also is a smooth muscle relaxant, and therefore is used in conjunction with promethazine.

24. (2) Thorazine is a phenothiazine derivative that blocks receptor sites in the brain for dopamine and/or norepinephrine. Its antiemetic ability possibly is due to depression of the chemoreceptor trigger zone in the medulla.

25. (2) Although a cardiac catheterization is performed under sterile technique, infection may still occur. Antibiotics are given prophylactically to minimize the chance of infection.

26. (1) General anesthetics have a depressant effect and can alter cardiac rhythm, cardiac output, and ultimately Pa_{O_2}.

27. (4) Insertion of the catheter via the femoral vein is appropriate in children as it permits a right-sided catheterization. In addition, children frequently have septal defects that allow for entry into the left side of the heart.

28. (2) Cardiac defects are identified by determining flow pattern of blood, oxygen saturations, and pressures in cardiac chambers and vessels, and by measurement of stroke volume and cardiac output.

29. (4) The listed symptoms are typically observed in a hypersensitivity reaction.

30. (3) Angiocardiography provides the following information: oxygen saturation within the great vessels and heart chambers; pressure gradients within the heart chambers and vessels; cardiac output; and any cardiac defects.

31. (4) Important postcatheterization nursing responsibilities are to observe for the development of infection, phlebitis, vessel obstruction, bleeding, cardiac tamponade or perforation, cardiac arrhythmias, and reaction to the dye.

32. (3) See the rationales for items 25 and 31.

33. (2) The abnormalities listed are the four defects associated with tetralogy of Fallot. The severity of the condition is estimated from the Pa_{O_2} and hematocrit, and usually is proportional to the degree of pulmonary stenosis.

34. (4) These preoperative procedures will prepare Timothy for his postoperative care, elicit better cooperation from him, and help allay his fears.
35. (4) The preschooler can be helped to deal with reality through a play experience. See the rationale for item 17.
36. (3) It is essential that the nurse prepare the parents for the complex postoperative care that Timothy will require in the intensive care unit. Otherwise they will be very anxious and apprehensive about his welfare, and their fears may be communicated to Timothy.
37. (3) It is important to maintain consistency in Timothy's care to help him deal with the fear he is bound to experience postoperatively.
38. (3) Lowering the cellular metabolic rate, and thus oxygen consumption, facilitate cardiac repair.
39. (2) The use of the cardiac bypass allows for a short, temporary interruption of cardiac function, and facilitates the surgical procedure.
40. (2) A postoperative complication of the surgery can be cardiorespiratory arrest. These items are necessary to effect cardiopulmonary resuscitation.
41. (3) These observations are important to assess evidence of postoperative low cardiac output. This complication is the result of hypothermia and cardiac bypass causing peripheral vasoconstriction. Palpation of weak peripheral pulsations can give evidence of this syndrome.
42. (4) Probably Timothy would have an anterior incision that was sprayed with collodion; therefore, any bleeding should be obvious. Observation of the linen is a "double check."
43. (4) The thoracic suction and drainage should be a closed system. Raising the collection system above the level of the chest would cause the drainage to flow back into the pleural cavity. A break in the system could cause air to be sucked into the pleural cavity.
44. (4) Renal shutdown is a complication of open heart surgery that causes tissue ischemia, especially in the kidney itself, where red blood cell hemolysis is likely to occur.
45. (1) Major surgery of this nature can be emotionally exhausting. Regression may be permitted temporarily as it allows for psychologic withdrawal and rest.
46. (2) Prevention of infection is important, and suctioning helps to keep the airway clear and prevent aspiration.
47. (1) Humidity keeps airways moist, facilitates oxygen transfer, and prevents "drying" of the trachea and bronchi.
48. (3) The Pa_{O_2} is normally 100 mm. Hg and the Pv_{O_2} is normally 40 mm. Hg. A Pa_{CO_2} of less than 35 mm. Hg indicates 2 respiratory alkalosis, and a Pa_{CO_2} of greater than 40 mm. Hg indicates respiratory acidosis.
49. (2) These mechanisms would result in a low Pv_{O_2} as a result of hypoventilation or hypoperfusion. The low Pv_{O_2} may result from increased uptake of oxygen by the tissues.
50. (4) The pressure made by oxygen gas in solution in the arterial plasma is normally about 100 mm. Hg. The Pa_{O_2} is not a measure of the oxygen attached to the hemoglobin inside the erythrocytes.
51. (4) These symptoms of upper airway obstruction are due to tracheal narrowing. Increased respiratory effort plus inadequate ventilation and perfusion result in a decreased Pa_{O_2}.
52. (3) Stress, anxiety, and temporary confusion produced by recovery from the surgical procedure and environmental changes may cause Timothy to pull at tubes.
53. (2) Overhydration increases cardiac work, and the newly repaired heart may not be able to pump the extra fluid.
54. (1) The central venous pressure measures right-sided heart pressure and provides information about fluid status.
55. (3) Underhydration would alter the solvent-to-solute ratio. The blood might become hyperviscous, resulting in sluggish flow and occlusion of vessels.
56. (2) The body attempts to reverse hyperthermia (fever) through increased ventilation, sweating, and blood flow to the skin. Tachycardia develops to meet the tissue demands for oxygen. All these events may be stressful to the repaired heart.
57. (3) Entering the thoracic cavity causes lung collapse (pneumothorax). Chest tubes

and suction assist postoperative re-expansion of the lungs. Serial chest x-rays are taken to monitor the re-expansion.

58. (4) These are all complications primarily of cardiac bypass and increased erythrocyte hemolysis.

59. (1) A child with cyanotic heart disease has delayed growth and development, easy fatigability, and chronic hypoxemia. He presents as sickly and provokes overprotection by the parents. Successful surgical repair greatly improves his physiologic status and results in increased tolerance of activity. If Timothy's parents have been overprotective, they may have difficulty coping with his increased abilities and independence.

Tonsillectomy

1. (1) Recurrent otitis media is a complication of frequent tonsillitis. Hypertrophied adenoids block the nasal passages and cause mouth breathing.

2. (2) *Streptococcus*, the common infective organism causing tonsillitis or pharyngitis, leads to rheumatic fever and acute glomerulonephritis in childhood.

3. (3) Polio occurs most frequently during the summer and early fall.

4. (2) A 5-year-old should be prepared before hospitalization; the best ones to do this are his parents, the people he trusts the most and who know him the best.

5. (2) The best explanation for a 5-year-old is a simple one and should focus on what the child will see and feel. It should also include the fact of getting better and going home. Words like "snip" and "cut" are anxiety-producing and inappropriate. Children at this age are not interested in detailed equipment explanations.

6. (2) A normal diet is usually appropriate for the day before surgery, and then only liquids on the actual day. The child should be on NPO (nothing by mouth) for 6 hours prior to surgery to prevent vomiting. The liquid breakfast may consist of a glass of orange juice, and then NPO after 6:00 A.M. if surgery is scheduled for the afternoon.

7. (3) CBC count and urinalysis are routine prior to any surgery. Often a tonsillectomy is a child's first surgery, and bleeding and clotting times need to be determined.

8. (3) Normal RBC count in a 5-year-old is 4.7–6.1 million per cu. mm.

9. (2) Normal clotting time is 5–8 minutes.

10. (1) Normal bleeding time is 1–6 minutes.

11. (3) A routine urinalysis includes examination for glucose, albumin, casts, RBCs, WBCs, pH and specific gravity.

12. (1) Agglutination of the RBCs is reflected in the erythrocyte sedimentation rate.

13. (1) Loose teeth need to be checked, as endotracheal intubation can knock a tooth out and lead to its possible aspiration. At age 5, Quincy has begun to lose his deciduous teeth.

14. (2) Tonsillar and adenoidal tissue are lymphatic tissue, the primary function of which is to filter microorganisms.

15. (2) The normal 5-year-old can receive up to 0.3 mg; 0.1 mg. is usually used with an *infant*. Dosages are calculated on body surface or weight:

$$.01 \times 19.1 \text{ kg.} = .19 \text{ mg.}$$

Clark's rule:

$$\frac{\text{wt. in lbs.}}{150} \times \text{ adult dose } =$$

$$\frac{42}{150} \times .4 = .112 \text{ mg.}$$

Young's rule:

$$\frac{\text{age (in years)}}{\text{age (in years + 12)}} \times \text{ adult dose } =$$

$$\frac{5}{17} \times .4 = .118 \text{ mg.}$$

16. (2) Atropine decreases mucus production and vagal stimulation.
17. (2) The nurse should always prepare the child before administering an injection, but not in exhaustive detail. The medication has to be given before leaving the unit. As the child will probably be unable to remain immobile, another person is usually needed to help hold him.
18. (3) All except e provide security and comfort; a continuous conversation is inappropriate and may increase wakefulness and anxiety. The nurse's presence and a few quiet words will be more comforting.
19. (4) Quincy should have his head turned to the side to help prevent aspiration if vomiting occurs. The prone position decreases aspiration of vomitus and blood.
20. (3) Signs of hemorrhage include restlessness, pallor, increased pulse, and decreased blood pressure. Increased bleeding from the tonsillar site causes frequent swallowing.
21. (3) Increased secretions and the reluctance to swallow them can lead to aspiration of secretions. Suctioning should be gentle so as not to disturb the clots.
22. (4) Describe the experience or procedure in terms the child already understands. Answers 1 and 2 are completely inappropriate. The lateral Sims and not the knee-chest position is appropriate. Many practitioners prefer to administer Tylenol elixir instead of aspirin.
23. (1) Cold is used to constrict the blood vessels and decrease bleeding and pain.
24. (2) Normal activities are appropriate, but Quincy may need additional rest. A liquid diet is advisable until the sore throat has decreased. The surgery has also made him more prone to throat infections in this immediate postoperative period, and he should be kept from children with infections until his throat is completely healed.
25. (4) Characteristics of the 5-year-old include aggressive physical activity; fantasy; obedience to authority figures; fear of pain and mutilation; and regression as a method of coping with anxiety.

Epilepsy

1. (4) An 8-year-old should be communicated with; the presence of the parent is useful in helping to establish rapport with the child.
2. (1) Hypoxia during delivery can lead to neurologic deficits and seizures in the child later. Seizures tend to be hereditary, and the family history is useful in diagnosing the problem.
3. (4) Birth anoxia, meningitis, lead poisoning, intracranial hemorrhages, cerbral trauma, and icterus can all lead to organic brain changes and seizure activity in children.
4. (4) Socorro is smaller than her peers. The average height of an 8-year-old is 50 inches, and average weight 62 lbs.
5. (3) Erikson calls this the age of industry: the child is learning to compete and produce in competition with his peers. The other three choices reflect developmental tasks achieved at earlier ages.
6. (2) This choice is open-ended and does not place values upon liking or disliking school. It is also a direct question and uses simple, understandable terms. The fourth choice is poor in that it denigrates the child and her achievements.
7. (1) Overprotection is common among parents of children with a chronic illness. Seizures are frightening and can embarrass the child and family, and others who come into contact with the child.
8. (1) The usual aftermath of a seizure is drowsiness or confusion and loss of memory; sleep may also follow.
9. (4) Hyperventilation can precipitate seizure activity in petit mal.
10. (3) Hyperventilation increases the amount of carbon dioxide expired.
11. (4) This reduction of carbon dioxide leads to a decrease in hydrogen ion concentration, an increase in pH, and respiratory alkalosis.
12. (3) The explanation of the test should be truthful and in words the child and family can understand.
13. (2) Answer 2 is correct. The exact mechanism of action is unknown.
14. (1) Trimethadione causes drowsiness, but to a lesser extent than does phenobarbital.

15. (4) Side effects of trimethadione include blood dyscrasias, nausea, fatigue, photophobia, skin rashes, and insomnia. Jaundice is not a frequent side effect.

16. (4) A major point about seizure medications is that they need to be taken continuously and at specific intervals. If the child is school-age, arrangements must be made for administration during school hours if needed. An 8-year-old should not need to crush a tablet before swallowing it.

17. (3) Paramethadione can also be used with this type of seizure. Choices 1 and 4 can be used with all seizures, and choice 2 more often with grand mal seizures.

18. (4) See the rationales for items 2 and 3.

19. (3) Instructions should be given in small, acceptable amounts and using the appropriate medical terminology. The family may be reluctant or may not know the questions to ask, so information needs to be volunteered.

20. (1) A blinking light, even in the form of television patterns, has been demonstrated to precipitate seizure activity.

21. (2) Choices 1 and 3 contain inaccurate information. Fatigue has been shown to precipitate seizure activity.

22. (4) Certain activities that need concentrated attention (e.g., riding a bicycle in traffic or working with a dangerous tool) could be very dangerous for an epileptic.

23. (4) All the behaviors noted are seen with grand mal seizures.

24. (3) Loosening clothing, prevention of aspiration, protection from injury, and promotion of a patent airway are appropriate measures. Once the seizure has started, nothing should be forced into the mouth.

25. (3) Anxiety concerning mental ability is normal. In children with controlled epilepsy, there does not appear to be a decrease in mental abilities.

Leukemia

1. (2) Leukemia is a cancer or neoplastic disease of unknown etiology.

2. (3) Leukemia is characterized by dysfunction of the marrow and the proliferation of immature leukocytes.

3. (4) Normal hemoglobin is 11–16 grams/100 ml. For an 8-year-old it is usually 14 grams or greater.

4. (3) Leukemia (due to the bone marrow invasion by lymphocytes) leads to decreased red blood cell production and anemia.

5. (3) The bone marrow is unable to produce sufficient red blood cells. See the rationale for item 4.

6. (3) Hematocrit is defined as the ratio of red blood cells to the volume of whole blood, and is expressed as a percentage.

7. (3) The normal hematocrit for a child is 42–52 per cent.

8. (1) Anemia results in decreased oxygen transport and fatigue.

9. (2) The main function of neutrophilic granulocytes is phagocytosis.

10. (3) The normal value for neutrophils is 60 per cent for a child over 2 years of age.

11. (4) Platelet production is decreased as a result of bone marrow invasion. Clotting and hemorrhage may occur.

12. (4) Cancer causes hypermetabolism manifested by hyperthermia and weight loss.

13. (1) Other symptoms of leukemia include fever, bone pain, anorexia, fatigue, and weight loss.

14. (3) The leukemic child is susceptible to infection because the lymphocytes are immature and cannot perform phagocytosis effectively.

15. (1) The liver, spleen, lymph nodes, and heart become infiltrated with leukemic cells and cease to function properly.

16. (1) The iliac crest is usually used for bone marrow biopsy. The sternum may be used, but usually is not in children owing to the danger of pneumothorax.

17. (1) The purpose is to improve the severe anemia and avoid fluid overload.

18. (4) Cardiac failure occurs in anemia owing to decreased viscosity of blood, increased heart rate, and inadequate myocardial oxygenation.

19. (2) ABO incompatibility causes agglutination of the red blood cells.

20. (3) Renal shutdown is the most significant response and can cause death from kidney failure.
21. (4) Symptoms of a transfusion reaction include urticaria, chills, back pain, headache, nausea, and hematuria.
22. (4) Stopping the transfusion is essential to prevent further reaction; normal saline should run through a separate I.V. tubing in order to maintain a patent I.V. if further fluids or medications are needed. If one ran normal saline through the blood tubing, one would give more of the blood to the patient.
23. (3) Mike will be able to judge his own activity level, depending on fatigue or interest. He will stay in bed if he feels sick.
24. (4) A normal diet is best, usually with increased fluids. A soft diet may be appropriate if gums are bleeding.
25. (3) Anorexia and buccal ulceration are common side effects of the cancer chemotherapy; the hypermetabolism is seen with all cancers. However, since Mike is on prednisone, he may have an increased appetite alternating with anorexia.
26. (2) The principal use of chloral hydrate is as a hypnotic for sedation and depression of the sensorimotor areas of the cerebral cortex.
27. (1) Side effects of chloral hydrate include nausea, vomiting, gastric irritation, and skin rashes.
28. (3) Weight may decrease gradually owing to hypermetabolism and to the nausea, vomiting, and anorexia associated with the chemotherapy.
29. (2) Ampicillin also disrupts cell wall synthesis, but is effective against a broader spectrum of gram-negative and -positive bacteria than is penicillin G.
30. (1) The action of 6-mercaptopurine is interruption of the mitotic cycle of the cell, in this case blocking nucleic acid synthesis.
31. (3) Hyperuricemia develops when the leukemic cells are destroyed and uric acid is released.
32. (4) All rapidly-reproducing cells are inhibited by 6-mercaptopurine, including normal cells such as skin and hair.
33. (3) Gastrointestinal ulcerations are common, from buccal ulcerations to ulceration throughout the GI tract. Nausea and vomiting are common side effects also. In cancer chemotherapy the line between treatment and toxicity is very fine.
34. (2) The 6-mercaptopurine may cause severe bone marrow depression and consequent leukopenia, which affects the body's resources to fight infection.
35. (3) It is believed that prednisone causes the destruction of primitive lymphocyte-like cells in leukemic bone marrow.
36. (4) If remission occurs during the initial course of therapy, the leukemic child is treated on an outpatient basis. With relapses or severe infections, the child is hospitalized.
37. (2) Alopecia occurs in 50 per cent of patients treated with cyclophosphamide since hair cells, like cancerous cells, reproduce rapidly, and thus are affected similarly by this drug.
38. (2) Hope for a cure is always present and is particularly evident when remissions occur.
39. (1) The question should be handled honestly, and answers 2, 3, and 4 would all increase anxiety. Knowing that the leukemic patient is prone to infection, answer (1) is the best and deals with Mrs. MacLeod's concern. Parental guilt feelings about failure to identify symptoms earlier are very common.
40. (1) The best approach is to allow the mother to ventilate her feelings and detail her reasons for her guilt. The other choices close the conversation and do not promote further discussion.
41. (3) Infection, bleeding, fatigue, and pain are major nursing problems in the terminal phase. Mike is too ill to want other children around; he withdraws within himself, and needs his parents and family the most.
42. (2) Frequent rinsing and cleansing, especially with a mild mouthwash, is recommended. Brushing, even with a soft toothbrush, may cause additional bleeding and pain.
43. (1) Effective protective isolation is one of the major means of preventing infection. However, since leukemic children become infected from their own bodies, and the psychosocial effects of isolation are so severe, many institutions have eliminated isolation as routine care.
44. (3) Mike's multiple physical and psychosocial problems make coordination of the efforts of team members essential.

45. (4) Vincristine has the following side effects: constipation, neuromuscular toxicity, alopecia, paresthesias, and foot drop.

46. (1) Massive septicemia and bleeding are the most common causes of death in childhood leukemia. The terminal event is often intracranial hemorrhage.

47. (3) Choices a, b, and d are correct.

48. (3) Verbalizing their grief, resentment, and anger is necessary to the parents' acceptance of Mike's impending death. Choices b and d would do little to help them deal with it.

49. (2) The time span between diagnosis and death allows the grieving process to begin.

50. (3) The child may passively accept death, depending on his knowledge and understanding. The school-age child focuses on the physical discomforts rather than on the impending death.

51. (3) Avoidance of the dying patient is common because health professionals perceive the death as a failure of their life-sustaining ability.

52. (1) The most helpful action would be to allow Mike some control over his care and environment. Encouraging him to express his concerns and fears would be helpful also; the questions should be nondirective and open-ended. The nurse should not assume that Mike has the usual fears; they may be quite different from those of a typical 8-year-old.

53. (2) Support for the family is essential as Mike becomes comatose, and the nurse's presence is supportive to both the child and his family.

54. (2) A nurse must be aware of her own philosophy and feelings concerning death in order to support the child and family effectively.

Rheumatic Fever

1. (4) Rheumatic fever is classified as a collagen disease because it is characterized by damage to the ground substance of connective tissue.

2. (2) It is believed that the changes in the collagenous tissue are due to a hypersensitivity reaction to the streptococcal antigen.

3. (3) The tissue mainly affected in rheumatic fever is the connective tissue.

4. (4) The structures usually involved are the heart and its valves and the joints.

5. (2) Joint pain may be an indication of previous episodes of rheumatic fever, and is often called "growing pains." Pallor, epistaxis, and abdominal pain also may be noted.

6. (4) The pathologic changes in the joint include inflammatory and proliferative changes.

7. (2) The pulse remains persistently elevated even when Clifford is afebrile; the sleeping pulse is also characteristically high.

8. (1) The characteristic rash of rheumatic fever, erythema marginatum, is erythematous and macular.

9. (1) The normal range of an antistreptolysin-O titer is 12–100 Todd units. An elevation above 200 indicates a recent streptococcal infection.

10. (2) The major symptoms of rheumatic fever include carditis, migratory polyarthritis, chorea, subcutaneous nodules, and erythema marginatum.

11. (3) The most common sequelae of rheumatic fever are valvular damage and cardiac failure.

12. (1) Bedrest is an essential component of the treatment of rheumatic fever.

13. (3) Penicillin is given to counteract streptococcal infection and prevent further bacterial growth.

14. (1) The salicylates are analgesics and anti-inflammatory, and are especially effective for joint pain.

15. (2) See the rationale for item 14. Aspirin decreases the temperature and relieves joint pain and swelling.

16. (3) Side effects of aspirin include gastrointestinal irritation, tinnitus, prolonged clotting time, and purpura.

17. (1) The joints are extremely painful and the bed cradle provides comfort. Usually there are no residual effects from the joint involvement.

18. (3) Range of motion and heat application cause further pain; careful positioning is the best nursing intervention.

19. (3) Prolonged bedrest leads to skin breakdown. The skin is edematous, wet with perspiration, and warm because of fever.
20. (2) A decrease in C-reactive protein indicates a decreasing inflammatory process.
21. (3) The erythrocyte sedimentation rate is evaluated to indicate the presence of an inflammatory process; it decreases as that process abates.
22. (2) Most children with rheumatic fever have difficulty understanding why they have to stay in bed when the acute symptoms have abated.
23. (4) The other choices are scare tactics or untrue. The nurse needs to acknowledge the difficulty for Clifford of staying in bed, but also should emphasize the need to promote full recovery.
24. (4) Signs of congestive heart failure include dyspnea, edema, pulmonary rales, cough, increased and weak pulse, and diaphoresis.
25. (4) All of the noted secondary sex changes take place in the male during adolescence.
26. (3) Erikson's theory postulates that trust, autonomy, initiative, and industry are all developmental tasks that should be accomplished by adolescence.
27. (4) Ego control and moral development take place earlier in childhood; adolescence focuses on development of identity and sense of self.
28. (4) All of these are developmental tasks to be accomplished during adolescence.
29. (4) Detachment and boredom are tactics used by adolescents to control or hide anxieties about illness.
30. (1) An open-ended question promotes further discussion.
31. (3) Pulmonary edema is the result of excessive fluid in the interstitial spaces and alveoli of the lungs. The presence of this fluid interferes with ventilation and diffusion of gases.
32. (2) A cardiac murmur is an abnormal heart sound caused by valvular lesions or stenosis.
33. (3) This choice gives correct information in understandable terms, and focuses on how it will affect Clifford and his treatment.
34. (2) Digitoxin slows the heart rate and increases the force of contraction.
35. (1) Digitalis accumulates within the body and has varying rates of excretion. This tendency to accumulate predisposes some patients to toxicity.
36. (4) Symptoms that may indicate digitoxin toxicity include arrhythmias, heart block, bradycardia, nausea, vomiting, visual disturbances, diarrhea, and disorientation.
37. (2) Decreased serum potassium sensitizes the myocardium to the effects of digitalis and is a major cause of digitalis toxicity.
38. (3) A low sodium diet is used in cardiac failure to decrease sodium retention and resulting edema.
39. (2) Furosemide is a potent diuretic, the main action of which is to increase the renal tubular excretion of sodium and water.
40. (3) Discharge instructions should include the importance of nutrition, rest, prevention of infection, and knowledge of symptoms of rheumatic fever and cardiac failure.
41. (2) Since repeated episodes of rheumatic fever may occur, tending to follow the same symptomatology as the previous ones, Clifford would have repeated cardiac involvement and an increased risk of residual cardiac damage.
42. (3) As Clifford is being discharged on digitoxin, he and his parents should be aware of the signs of digitoxin toxicity, one of which is bradycardia, and how to detect them.
43. (3) Prophylactic medications, particularly antibiotics, often are not continued routinely as the patient feels well and can see no need to take them. this is particulary true in the case of rheumatic fever once the acute symptoms have abated.

Lead Poisoning

1. (2) The most common source of lead is paint and paint chips.
2. (4) Other sources of lead are lead containers or dishes made with a high lead content. Paints used for the older houses usually found in slums often had a heavy lead base.
3. (3) Pica is thought to be caused by unmet oral needs, problems in the mother-child relationship, nutritional deficiencies, and physiologic stresses.

4. (4) Lead encephalopathy causes cerebral edema, increased intracranial pressure, seizures, coma, and death.

5. (4) Lead interferes with normal cellular function by inhibiting certain enzymatic reactions that normally provide cellular energy for substance transport across membranes.

6. (1) Decreased intake of iron and calcium leads to increased absorption and retention of lead.

7. (4) See the rationale for item 4. Increased intracranial pressure occurs, and one of its initial symptoms is increased irritability.

8. (4) The anemia of plumbism (lead poisoning) is microcytic and hypochromic. The red cells have "stippling" and a shorter-than-average life span.

9. (2) A sign of increased intracranial pressure is papilledema.

10. (3) Other symptoms of lead poisoning are abdominal pain, weakness, lethargy, anorexia, altered muscle coordination, vomiting, and constipation.

11. (3) Lead is deposited in the long bones along the epiphysis. Bone x-rays are done in the diagnostic workup for confirmation of lead poisoning.

12. (1) An x-ray examination will be made of the abdomen to check for recent ingestion of paint chips.

13. (2) Grand mal convulsions are found with lead encephalopathy.

14. (2) Neurologic effects of lead and the impact of hospitalization on the toddler lead to the loss of some developmental skills, starting with those most recently acquired.

15. (2) Siblings within the same family often have lead poisoning also. After this has been evaluated, actions (legal or otherwise) should be taken to remove the source if it can be identified.

16. (2) The toddler is very susceptible to separation anxiety. The initial reaction is to protest by crying, screaming, and whining.

17. (4) The presence of a familiar toy from home will help during this phase. Physical touch and comfort is also most effective at this age.

18. (3) An 18-month-old child can sit and walk, and has finger-thumb control. Cooperative play and bladder and bowel control occur at about 3 years of age.

19. (4) These are all normal responses to hospitalization at Peter's age.

20. (2) At 18 months a child would see this action as abandonment. The preschooler and school-age child would view it as punishment.

21. (2) Because of Peter's neurologic irritability, due to the lead poisoning, excess handling and stimulation should be avoided.

22. (3) The main objective of therapy is the elimination of lead as quickly as possible to prevent permanent damage.

23. (1) Permanent neurologic damage is a common complication that may be manifested in seizures, mental retardation, hyperactivity, learning disabilities, and motor incoordination.

24. (4) Lead is primarily eliminated via the kidneys.

25. (3) E.D.T.A. precipitates lead by combining with it.

26. (4) Lead can cause permanent tubular damage. Initial signs of drug toxicity and renal damage are albuminuria and hematuria.

27. (1) Side effects of B.A.L. include hypertension, vomiting, and tachycardia.

28. (2) The action of penicillamine is to chelate lead and promote its excretion in the urine.

29. (2) One of the actions of diazepam is to depress the duration of electrical after-discharge in the limbic system.

30. (4) Side effects of diazepam include drowsiness, ataxia, diplopia, nausea, and jaundice.

31. (2) Withdrawal and regression are common in hospitalized children.

32. (4) The child becomes angry and often ignores or rejects the parent as a method of punishing her.

33. (1) The toddler has decreased growth needs, his food intake is decreased, and Peter may be considered a "picky" eater as a result of his anorexia.

34. (3) This allows Peter some control. Choices 1, 2, and 4 are inappropriate for an 18-month-old child.

35. (4) Coffee contains caffeine, which increases neurologic excitability. Candy has a high glucose content and is bad for the teeth. Nuts are often allergenic foods and can be aspirated. Chocolate contains fat and sugar.

36. (4) The main side effect of ferrous sulfate is to turn the stool dark green to black.
37. (4) Food decreases absorption of iron, and so the best time to give the medication is between meals.
38. (2) Oral needs are very prominent at this age. Also, the pica that Peter exhibited might cause him to continue eating non-nutritive substances that could contain lead.
39. (3) Most cities have building code laws that require the use of paint with low lead levels. The local health department should follow through on any building violations.
40. (1) Lead poisoning has side effects involving the neurologic, renal, and hematologic systems. The hematologic problem is anemia, not clotting.
41. (2) A major developmental task of the toddler is learning to handle his body and increase his gross and fine motor skills.
42. (3) Lead prevention laws deal with the amount of lead allowed in paint, particularly on children's toys and cribs.

Failure to Thrive

1. (2) A normal infant child doubles his birth weight by six months and triples it by one year.
2. (4) In many cases of failure to thrive the major problem is the mother-child relationship.
3. (3) Decreased sensory and environmental stimulation leads to children who fail to thrive. These children may have bald spots as they often are left to lie in bed all the time.
4. (4) Organic causes of failure to thrive include congenital anomalies, chronic respiratory problems, and endocrine disorders.
5. (3) Urinalysis, BUN, and specific gravity provide information concerning basic renal function. An intravenous pyelogram may be done to determine if congenital abnormalities are present.
6. (2) Mental and physical retardation are seen with a, b, and c.
7. (3) a, b, c, and d are infectious processes or metabolic alterations that produce increased caloric expenditure.
8. (2) Cystic fibrosis leads to fat malabsorption in the small intestine. Celiac disease is an intolerance to gluten. Disaccharidase deficiences mean that complex sugars cannot be digested in the small intestine. Pylorospasm and peptic ulcer are stomach conditions, and do not affect the digestive processes.
9. (4) Symptoms of psychosocial problems in the infant may be seen in eating disturbances, sleeping problems, crying, and excessive body movements.
10. (4) Mothers of failure-to-thrive children often have psychologic and social problems of their own.
11. (4) The maternal history may reveal such factors as unwanted pregnancy and difficult labor.
12. (4) The first three choices reflect knowledge and perception of her family and problems. No. 4 shows rationalization and insensitivity to the infant's cues.
13. (3) It is important to obtain a detailed assessment of the child's behavior and habits from the parents and also to observe the mother-child interaction, during feeding and at other times.
14. (3) Infantile colic is seen in the infant with abdominal distention, pain, and crying. Option 1 describes diarrhea; option 2, intussusception; and option 4, pyloric stenosis.
15. (4) Causes of infantile colic include overfeeding, swallowed air, anxiety, and intestinal allergy.
16. (3) Vitamin A deficiency decreases resistance to infections.
17. (2) It is important to allow Patty to become familiar with the nurse before she touches or examines the child. This is particularly true in the case of an infant who is not relating to others appropriately.
18. (3) Self-stimulation, seen either in continous body movements or in handling or holding of body parts, is often seen in children who are isolated and lack sensory stimulation.

19. (4) Symptoms of malnourishment in infants are a large head, thin dry skin, lethargy, and muscular atrophy.
20. (3) The average weight of a normal 9-month-old child is 18–19 lbs.
21. (4) The average length of a normal 9-month-old child is 70 cm.
22. (1) The normal 9-month-old child can creep, using hands and knees.
23. (1) Trust is being developed in the first year; autonomy begins at about 1 year of age.
24. (2) The first words, usually spoken at about 9 months, include "da-da," "ma-ma."
25. (3) Malnutrition is basically a protein deficiency.
26. (4) Bleeding, costochondral beading, and pain are seen with vitamin C deficiency.
27. (3) Enfamil contains 5.2 mg. of Vitamin C per 100 ml. of solution. A higher dosage would be preferred for treatment of a malnourished infant.
28. (2) Vitamin B complex deficiencies lead to irritability.
29. (4) Most infant formulas meet the daily requirements for all these, and are now iron-fortified.
30. (4) Symptoms of thiamine deficiency include anorexia, apathy, fatigue, convulsions, cardiac failure, and polyneuritis.
31. (1) Lack of hydration of interstitial and subcutaneous tissue causes poor skin turgor.
32. (2) With malnutrition, loss of fat tissue is usual.
33. (2) Anxiety with strangers is initially seen at 7–8 months.
34. (2) At 9 months the normal child attempts to feed himself.
35. (4) Avoidance of eye-to-eye contact, lack of social smile, inappropriate response to people, and rigid, tense body movements indicate an abnormal social response.
36. (4) Tactile, visual, and auditory stimulation are important. Toys, mobiles, and cuddling are examples of ways to provide this stimulation.
37. (2) Lack of eye-to-eye contact between mother and child is usually seen in a disturbed mother-child relationship.
38. (4) A 9-month-old can eat all the listed foods.
39. (4) The primary objective is to help the mother develop a more appropriate, normal relationship with her child.
40. (4) Infants and children who fail to thrive are often abused.
41. (2) Dealing with the parents' stresses and anxieties are a major component of therapy for a failure-to-thrive child.
42. (3) Followup by the public health nurse is essential.

3 MEDICAL-SURGICAL NURSING

Coronary Heart Disease

1. (3) Cessation of movement lowers the oxygen demand of skeletal muscles, resulting in a decrease in heart rate and in myocardial oxygen demand. If the narrowed coronary vessels are able to meet the lowered demand, the ischemic pain will be relieved.

2. (4) In cardiac ischemia, myocardial metabolism shifts from aerobic to anaerobic glycolysis, producing large quantities of lactic acid. Accumulation of lactic acid in tissues produces pain.

3. (4) Myocardial oxygen consumption increases in direct proportion to increase in exercise. The sclerotic coronary arteries are unable to dilate sufficiently to provide increased blood volume and the additional oxygen needed by the myocardium.

4. (2) a, Although the mechanism is not fully understood, emotions frequently trigger angina, presumably through sympathetically induced coronary artery vasoconstriction. b, Following a heavy meal, an increased volume of blood is shunted into the splanchnic circulation. c, The initial reaction of peripheral tissues to markedly lowered environmental temperature is sudden vasodilation with increased peripheral blood flow. This causes increased cardiac output, and the increased cardiac workload provokes angina.

5. (2) The angina associated with myocardial ischemia is often referred to surface areas of the neck and left arm because all three structures receive pain fibers from the same segments of the spinal cord.

6. (2) Chest pain frequently induces anxiety because of widespread awareness of the potential hazards of heart disease. Denial, a mental mechanism, is often utilized to minimize this anxiety.

7. (2) Unaccustomed strenuous exercise performed under conditions of prolonged cold exposure raises peripheral oxygen demand, cardiac output, and myocardial workload severely, thereby increasing the danger of myocardial infarction in a person with embarrassed coronary blood supply.

8. (4) The nitrate ion relaxes the smooth, circular fibers of the arteries and arterioles, resulting in vasodilation.

9. (3) Nitroglycerin is available in 0.3-, 0.4-, and 0.6-mg. tablets. A dosage of 0.6 mg is frequently administered for individual attacks of angina; tolerance may occur as a result of chronic usage.

10. (1) Nitroglycerin is a vasodilator that increases myocardial exercise tolerance, and is capable of either relieving or preventing angina caused by exercise.

11. (4) Chest pain can trigger coronary artery spasm, thus increasing the degree of coronary insufficiency. Nitroglycerin, which is nonhabituating, should be taken as often as needed to prevent spasm.

12. (2) Nitroglycerin is volatile and can be affected chemically by light and heat. Tablets will deteriorate unless kept in tightly sealed containers in a cool and dark environment.

13. (1) The onset of action of nitroglycerin is more rapid and its vasodilator effect is stronger when the drug is absorbed from the oral mucosa rather than from the gastric or intestinal mucosa.

14. (3) Sublingual administration of nitroglycerin assures its rapid absorption. The drug then enters the systemic venous circulation, following this route to the heart and then to the coronary arteries, where it quickly produces smooth muscle relaxation and coronary vasodilation.

15. (2) Headache, or a feeling of pulsating fullness in the head, is the most common side effect of nitroglycerin. It is thought to result from dilation of cranial blood vessels, a corresponding increase in intracranial pressure, and irritation of sensitive areas around the venous sinuses.

16. (2) There is some difference among patients in regard to the dosage of nitroglycerin needed to relieve angina. If the ordered dosage is ineffective and no side effects are evident, it is possible that the dosage is insufficient.

17. (2) Although pentaerythritol tetranitrate, a long-acting vasodilator, is not as effective as nitroglycerin in relieving angina, it is often successful in increasing the interval between attacks.

18. (1) a, One method of reducing cardiac workload is to decrease body weight, thereby reducing the mass of tissue to be perfused by the left heart. c, Through stimulation of the sympathetic nervous system, nicotine produces increase in heart rate and coronary vasoconstriction. This combination of events may provoke anginal attacks when coronary atheromatosis is present.

19. (2) During rest, blood flow through skeletal muscles averages 4–7 ml. per minute per 100 gm. of muscle. During exercise, the blood flow through skeletal muscles often increases twenty-fold, to satisfy the muscles' increased need for nutrients and oxygen.

20. (3) Although this remains unproved, regular, mild physical exercise is believed to enhance the growth of collateral coronary vessels. This development may be stimulated by increased ventricular workload and myocardial oxygen demand.

21. (2) The aim of treatment is to reduce the discrepancy between myocardial oxygen demand and the ability of the coronary circulation to meet that demand. Since the caliber of the coronary arteries cannot be changed, myocardial oxygen consumption should be reduced.

22. (4) The most common cause of coronary artery occlusion is gradual buildup of atheromatous plaque beneath the intimal lining of the vessel, and clot formation over the roughened intimal surface. Slowing of blood flow favors intravascular clotting. Coronary flow is more rapid during exertion than during rest.

23. (4) a and b, Infarcted muscle, incapable of contraction, causes impaired ventricular contractility that leads to decreased cardiac output and shock with pallor and diaphoresis. c and d, As stroke volume decreases and left ventricular pressure increases, the pressure is referred backward to the pulmonary circulation, causing transudation of fluid from pulmonary capillaries into alveoli. This interferes with oxygen-carbon dioxide exchange, producing hypoxia, breathlessness, and anxiety. Nausea and vomiting may result from vasovagal reflexes originating in the area of the damaged myocardium and terminating in the smooth muscle of the gastrointestinal tract.

24. (2) Electrical impulses generated by the sinoatrial node initiate waves of depolarization that spread through the myocardium, stimulating it to contract. The electrical current generated by depolarization and repolarization of the myocardium is conducted to the body surface, where it can be sensed by electrodes and measured by a galvanometer.

25. (1) The finding in serial EKG's of ST segment elevation, followed by ST segment depression, T wave inversion, and Q waves, in conjunction with typical changes in serum enzymes, would confirm a diagnosis of myocardial infarction. Accurate diagnosis makes definitive treatment possible.

26. (3) Owing to increasing lack of blood flow, nutrients and oxygen needed for proper cell functioning are diminished. Deprived cells will lose their chemical and structural integrity, and will disintegrate.

27. (1) Although many factors can cause cell death (e.g., interruption of blood supply, bacterial or chemical toxins, extreme heat or cold, ionizing radiation), the most frequent cause is interruption of vital blood supply due to occlusion of a coronary artery.

28. (3) a, Myocardial infarction may reduce the force of ventricular contraction, leading to pump failure, with subsequent pulmonary and systemic venous congestion. c, Since necrotic muscle cannot transmit electrical current, normal impulse transmission between atria and ventricles is apt to be blocked. A hyperirritable ventricular muscle may initiate independent and chaotic rhythms, resulting in ventricular fibrillation. d, If the necrotic myocardium perforates, blood from the adjacent heart chamber flows into the pericardial sac, compressing the heart and interfering with its contractility. e, Either ventricular fibrillation or severe pump failure, causing cessation of coronary blood flow, can result in cessation of all electrical and motor activity, or cardiac arrest.

29. (4) The fissured or ulcerated intima overlying a roughened atheromatous plaque provides a nidus for cellular aggregation and intravascular clot formation.

30. (4) The activity restriction and enforced dependence required for treatment of a myocardial infarction are in opposition to the stereotypic male role in our culture. A man who has enjoyed the strong competition of business and professional life may view a myocardial infarction as a threat to manhood, independence, and social status. On the other hand, a man who has been uncomfortable in the competitive role may see illness as a socially acceptable way to retire from the fray.

31. (2) Severe pain may provoke reflex constriction of collateral coronary vessels that may have developed, thereby further reducing blood supply to the acutely injured muscle.

32. (4) Morphine decreases hypothalamic and limbic system responses to pain stimuli.

33. (3) Therapeutic doses of morphine cause cutaneous blood vessels to dilate. The vasodilation may trigger the release of histamine into surrounding tissue, markedly increasing local blood flow and producing itching.

34. (2) Morphine depresses the respiratory center in the medulla oblongata.

35. (3) Morphine reduces the responsiveness of brain respiratory centers to increases in pCO_2, and depresses cells responsible for regulation of respiratory rhythmicity.

36. (1) Administration of oxygen raises arterial pO_2 levels sufficiently to increase oxygen tension in the ischemic area of myocardium that surrounds the infarct, thereby minimizing the extent of tissue necrosis.

37. (2) An oxygen flow rate of 6 liters per minute through a nasal catheter is comfortable and provides from 30–40 per cent of oxygen in inspired air, which is usually enough to provide a paO_2 of 100 mm. Hg in most patients.

38. (4) Oxygen supports combustion. In an oxygen-rich environment, matches and cigarettes ignite more easily, burn faster, and extinguish with greater difficulty, thereby increasing the patient's risk of physical injury.

39. (4) For the first 7–10 days following a myocardial infarction, absolute bedrest should be provided to decrease strain on the infarcted area of myocardium while cellular necrosis, liquefaction, and fibrosis are taking place. All activities are restricted because they cause increased cardiac workload at a time of decreased cardiac reserve.

40. (3) Pulse deficit is the difference between apical and radical pulses. Therefore, both measures must be known in order to calculate pulse deficit.

41. (1) A variety of arrhythmias may develop as complications of myocardial infarction. Multiple irritable foci of nodal tissue in the myocardium emit impulses at high-than-normal sinus rates. Control of heart rate by first one then another of these foci, together with inability of the atrioventricular node and the ventricular muscle to respond to several foci at one time, cause ventricular contractions to vary in rate and force from minute to minute. Weaker ventricular contractions do not produce a peripheral pulse wave, so that the radial pulse also tends to vary from minute to minute.

42. (2) Weak ventricular contractions do not eject enough blood into the aorta to create a peripheral pulse wave.

43. (4) The steps in the blood-clotting reaction can be diagrammed thus: Thromboplastin complex + prothrombin complex + calcium = thrombin. Thrombin + fibrinogen = fibrin. Fibrin + cells = clot. Heparin blocks clot formation chiefly by inactivating thrombin, thereby preventing conversion of fibrinogen to fibrin.

44. (2) Experimental evidence suggests that prolonged hyperlipidemia is a causative factor in atherosclerotic cardiovascular disease, which is the most common cause of coronary artery occlusion. Heparin reduces the lipid concentration of serum, and this arrests or slows atheromatous arterial degeneration.

45. (4) An already existing clot will not be dissolved by warfarin; however, by blocking the clotting reaction, warfarin can prevent further propagation of an already existing clot, and thus ensure that still functioning collaterals are not obstructed.

46. (4) The clotting reaction can be diagrammed thus: Thromboplastin complex + prothrombin complex + calcium = thrombin. Thrombin + fibrinogen = fibrin. Fibrin + cells = clot. Warfarin blocks intravascular clotting by preventing formation of prothrombin in liver cells.

47. (2) Since warfarin acts by blocking prothrombin formation in the liver, regular prothrombin time determinations are needed to monitor the effectiveness of the prescribed dose of the drug.

48. (3) The most dangerous toxic effect of warfarin is hemorrhage from any of several sites. Bleeding from the kidney or bladder may present as microscopic rather than gross hematuria. Microscopic hematuria causes the urine to have a cloudy appearance.

49. (3) Several enzymes normally present in myocardial cells (e.g., serum glutamic acid, creatinine phosphokinase, lactic dehydrogenase) are released into the systemic circulation in greater-than-normal quantities whenever a large number of myocardial cells undergo necrosis. Increased serum levels of these enzymes can be helpful when one is drawing conclusions about the likelihood of myocardial cell death.

50. (1) The supine position, with head raised slightly and arms supported on pillows, is most comfortable and best promotes chest expansion and venous return from upper and lower extremities.

51. (2) Denial, or negation of an intolerable external reality, is a common and temporarily useful means of coping with the overwhelming anxiety produced by a sudden onset of life-threatening illness.

52. (4) This response is the only one that both acknowledges the patient's desire for independence and also defines the activity limitation imposed by his illness and by his physician's treatment orders.

53. (2) Mr. Powers' dyspnea may cause him to breathe with his mouth open, thereby decreasing the accuracy of an oral temperature reading. Changing his position so as to permit rectal thermometer insertion would impose additional and unnecessary strain on his heart. Measurement of his axillary temperature need cause him no exertion or discomfort, and would yield more accurate information about his general body temperature than would placing a hand on his brow.

54. (2) Only absolute bedrest would provide the conditions needed to maximize myocardial healing and minimize the complications of infarction. Without rest, none of the other elements would be equally protective.

55. (2) This response is the most accurate because it describes what is known of the pathophysiology of myocardial infarction, but refrains from unfounded prognostications concerning Mr. Powers' future.

56. (3) Small, soft, bland feedings would be easy to digest, and thus a considerable asset to a patient in whom portal circulation is impaired.

57. (3) Death of an area of myocardium, by decreasing contractile efficiency of one or both ventricles, can lead to cardiac pump failure, which would be manifested by tachycardia, hypotension, and cardiac dilation. When the heart can no longer eject blood forcibly, the chambers do not empty with each contraction, pressure builds up in each ventricle, and increased pressure is reflected backward to either the pulmonary venous circulation in the case of the left ventricle, or the systemic venous circulation in the case of the right ventricle.

58. (4) The physician could detect all the symptoms of congestive heart failure listed. Through percussion of the cardiac borders, he could determine whether the heart was larger than normal. Through auscultation of the heart, he could determine whether an arrhythmia were present and, if so, its general type. Through auscultation of abnormal heart sounds, he could identify organic or functional valvular disorders. Through auscultation of the lungs, he could detect the rales associated with pulmonary edema.

59. (3) Several factors contribute to the maintenance of mean arterial pressure, i.e., cardiac rate, the contractile power of the myocardium, the elasticity of arterial and arteriolar walls, the volume of circulating blood, and the viscosity of the blood. The one most altered by Mr. Powers' disease is the contractile power of the myocardium. Owing to the infarcted area's incapability of contract-

ing, the organ as a whole becomes less efficient, thus causing a drop in blood pressure.

60. (1) As the left ventricle fails, it fails to empty with each contraction, blood accumulates, and pressure increases in the left ventricle, the left atrium, and the pulmonary venous circulation. When pulmonary capillaries become congested, increased pressure in these thin-walled vessels pushes fluid from the blood stream into the alveoli, which results in interference with gas exchange and dyspnea.

61. (3) Many deaths following myocardial infarction are the result of arrhythmias. Ventricular fibrillation is by far the most severe, because it is life-threatening and requires immediate treatment. Continuing cardiac monitoring will identify premature ventricular contractions and ventricular tachycardia, so that treatment can be instituted to avert ventricular fibrillation and cardiac arrest.

62. (4) All five arrhythmias can occur. Myocardial ischemia leads to the development of irritable foci of nodal tissue in atria or ventricles, which may initiate the idiopathic and eccentric impulses responsible for atrial flutter, atrial fibrillation, nodal rhythm, and premature ventricular contractions. An infarction involving the septum can destroy the bundle of His or left or right bundle branch, producing heart block.

63. (2) Atrial flutter results when a hyperirritable focus in the atrial wall emits impulses at a regular rate of 250–350/minute and takes over as cardiac pacemaker. Because the refractory period of the atrioventricular node is longer than that of the atrial muscle, the atrioventricular node will respond only to every second or third impulse from the atrium. The impulses that are conducted to the ventricle generate a QRS complex. Thus, there are twice or three times as many P waves as QRS complexes in atrial flutter.

64. (1) Normally the impulse from the sinus node takes less than 0.20 seconds to traverse the atrioventricular node. Injury to the atrioventricular node due to ischemia, rheumatic fever, or digitalis intoxication slows passage of the impulse through the atrioventricular node, increasing the length of the PR interval beyond 0.2 seconds, and constituting primary heart block.

65. (4) In second-degree heart block every second, third, or fourth atrial impulse is blocked from transmission to the ventricles. The finding of twice as many P waves as QRS complexes would indicate blockage of every second atrial impulse, which constitutes second-degree heart block.

66. (2) Premature ventricular contractions, the most common of all arrhythmias, are caused by an irritable focus in ventricular muscle that generates an impulse slightly in advance of an expected impulse from the sinoatrial node. The ventricle responds to the ectopic impulse, but since the impulse originated in the ventricle rather than following the normal pathway, there is no preceding P wave and the QRS complex is distorted. Since the ventricle is refractory when the next impulse from the sinus node reaches the ventricle by way of the bundle of His and the bundle branches, there is a compensatory pause following the abnormal QRS complex.

67. (4) Within four to six minutes following cessation of cardiac function the brain and other central nervous system tissue will die owing to oxygen lack. Therefore, in the event of a cardiac arrest, the nurse must re-establish effective cardiac contraction by natural or artificial means, while summoning medical aid to treat the cause of the arrest. The steps of cardiopulmonary resuscitation include: opening the airway; breathing for the patient; and using external compression to force blood from the heart into the arterial system. A sharp blow to the precordium may shock the heart sufficiently to make it resume contraction.

68. (2) Cyanosis is manifested by the blue-gray color of the skin, which is due to anoxemia. The amount of reduced hemoglobin, rather than the lack of oxygenated hemoglobin in blood, determines the presence and depth of the cyanosis. Five grams of reduced hemoglobin per 100 ml. of blood will cause cyanosis to be visible.

69. (1) a, When the capillary hydrostatic pressure exceeds the osmotic pressure of plasma proteins, there will be transudation of fluid from the capillary into surrounding interstitial spaces. c, Reduction of renal blood flow secondary

to decreased cardiac output and arterial blood pressure causes a greatly reduced glomerular filtration rate. Aldosterone and antidiuretic hormone production increase reflexly in response to decreased circulating blood volume. The combination of decreased glomerular filtration of sodium and increased tubular resorption of sodium leads to elevation of serum sodium, retention of water, expansion of circulating blood volume, and transudation of retained fluid into tissue spaces.

70. (3) Edema formation will be most marked in dependent tissues because the movement of fluid from vessels to tissue spaces will be augmented by the force of gravity.

71. (4) In the supine position, the skin of the back is the most dependent portion of the body and the most likely site for accumulation of edema fluid. Edema, by compressing the skin capillaries, interferes with proper nutrition of the tissue, so that a low-grade cellulitis develops. Further trauma from pressure, friction, or bacterial growth can cause breakdown of the already inflamed skin.

72. (3) Bigeminy, or coupling, a regular irregularity in which a regular heart beat is followed by an ectopic contraction in a consistent fashion, is a common symptom of digitalis toxicity. Bigeminy results from the increased myocardial irritability caused by the drug.

73. (2) Although furosemide inhibits reabsorption of sodium from proximal and distal tubules as well as from the loop of Henle, it is its action on the loop of Henle that renders it a highly effective diuretic.

74. (4) Although the diuretic effect of furosemide derives from its ability to increase urinary excretion of both sodium and potassium, sodium is excreted in greater quantities than potassium; hence, potassium is said to be spared.

75. (3) Orthostatic hypotension is most common. It results from excessive diuresis, sudden dehydration, and reduction of blood volume which occur when furosemide is given in high dosage or in conjunction with restricted salt intake.

76. (3) Since the edema of congestive heart failure results primarily from sodium retention, the main goal in treating the edema of congestive heart failure is to increase the excretion of sodium. Therefore, the urine concentration of sodium is the best index of furosemide's effectiveness.

77. (2) Central venous pressure, the pressure at the junction of the superior vena cava and the right atrium, is an indicator both of the right heart's pumping capacity and of the speed and/or volume of venous return.

78. (4) Central venous pressure measurement is done to determine the pressure of blood in the right atrium. The measuring device (manometer) must be standardized for each patient by placing the zero line of the manometer at the level of the right atrium, or in the midaxillary line, or 10–12 cm. from the posterior body surface in the fourth intercostal space.

79. (1) The fact that pressure in the veins is much lower than that in the arteries explains why venous pressures are measured in cm. of water and arterial pressures in mm. Hg. Mercury is a heavy metal, and requires more force to move it than is needed to move an equivalent quantity of water. The central venous pressures are low following hemorrhage or dehydration; normal in pure left heart failure; either normal or low in peripheral circulatory failure or shock; and tending to be high in right heart failure and constrictive pericarditis.

80. (1) Since right heart failure is followed by congestion of the superior and inferior vena cava, with accompanying pressure rise, central venous pressure measurements may be useful in making the differential diagnosis of right heart dysfunction.

81. (1) In order to effect relaxation and a sleep-inducing effect from an H.S. sedative, the patient's elimination and comfort needs should be met before the drug is administered. Safety precautions require that overhead lights be extinguished only after the nurse has ensured that the right drug is given in the correct dose to the specified patient.

82. (3) Slow blood flow predisposes to the settling out of cellular elements. Inflammation roughens the lining of the vein, providing a spot conducive to cellular congregations. Constriction of the vein increases the fixed surface to

which settled elements can adhere in thrombus formation. Increased, rather than decreased, blood viscosity predisposes to clot formation, because the greater the proportion of cellular elements in blood, the more likely is it that they will settle out when blood flow is slowed.

83. (4) In thrombophlebitis, inflammation of the vein wall occurs first, followed by cellular elements settling on the roughened intima. Next, platelets rupture, thromboplastin is released, and clotting occurs.

84. (2) Knee rolls are contraindicated because placement of a firm support under the knee would compress the popliteal vein, impeding blood flow, and predisposing to venous stasis and phlebothrombosis.

85. (4) Phlebothrombosis occurs most commonly in the veins of the lower extremities, owing to venous stasis. Because venous valves permit only unidirectional blood flow, alternate tightening and relaxing of leg muscles several times a day decreases venous stasis by "milking" blood from the lower extremities toward the heart.

86. (1) Cholesterol is a major component of atheroma, and high intake of cholesterol has been found to correlate with high incidence of coronary artery disease.

87. (2) Mr. Powers should avoid: (1) high cholesterol intake in order to decrease atheromatous plaque formation in the coronary arteries; (2) excessive caloric intake because obesity increases the risk of coronary artery disease; and (3) excessive sodium intake because it could precipitate congestive heart failure in a person with decreased cardiac reserve.

88. (3) This response most strongly reinforces reality and supports self-determination by suggesting that: (1) the patient's recent illness indicates a need for change in certain aspects of his life; (2) since he knows more than anyone else about his previous life style and habit patterns, he can best decide what changes must be made to speed recovery and maintain health; and (3) Mr. Powers is able and willing to make the life changes called for by his recent illness and treatment.

89. (4) Since the nurse's instruction regarding medical followup should be congruent with that given by the physician, the nurse should not initiate the teaching until it has been determined what information or direction the patient has already been given concerning followup.

Rheumatoid Arthritis

1. (4) Salicylates produce antipyretic and analgesic effects through depressing portions of the central nervous system, i.e., the temperature regulating center in the hypothalamus and subcortical areas for relief of moderate pain.

2. (3) The salicylates have an anti-inflammatory effect that is due, apparently, to reduction of capillary permeability and suppression of antigen-antibody reactions.

3. (4) Proponents of the psychogenic theory of disease causation believe that some forms of psychologic stress may precipitate an attack of rheumatoid arthritis. Since Mrs. Turk's comments allude to an unresolved family conflict, this information should be recorded.

4. (4) Debris absorbed into the circulation from local joint inflammation produces some of the systemic symptoms of inflammation, i.e., increased temperature, pulse, and respiratory rate.

5. (4) A rule of thumb for approximating normal systolic pressure is that it should be approximately 100 plus the individual's age. The upper limit of the normal diastolic pressure, regardless of age, is 90–100 mm. Hg.

6. (4) Rheumatoid arthritis, a chronic, debilitating disease, results from faulty immunologic mechanisms. It is characterized by symmetric and progressive joint destruction, widespread systemic changes arising from diffuse vasculitis, and resulting granuloma formation. The rough brittle nails and subcutaneous nodules are related to vasculitis; joint crepitation to destruction of joint structures; and hypertrophy of lymph nodes and spleen to immunologic disturbances.

7. (2) Since rheumatoid arthritis, a crippling disease, is characterized by muscle weakness and joint ankylosis, good alignment of the spine, shoulders, hips, and extremities is important to prevent deformity.

8. (2) The joint changes of rheumatoid arthritis include chronic inflammation of synovial membrane, destruction of articular cartilage, and proliferation of granulation tissue within the joint space. As a result of exposed articular surfaces and joining of eroded structures by fibrous bands, abnormal shortening, angulation, and ankylosis tend to deform and immobilize involved joints.

9. (4) The anorexia and weight loss probably result from depression of the hunger center in the hypothalamus by toxic inflammatory products. Mrs. Turk's weighty family responsibilities, coupled with the continuous standing required by her job, would aggravate the severe pain caused by arthritic joint damage. All four factors in combination could contribute to an appearance of wasting, debilitation, and chronic illness.

10. (4) The antigen-antibody reaction of rheumatoid arthritis causes enzymes to be released from the synovium. These result in inflammation of the joint structures and cause transudation of fluid into the joint space, distention of the capsule, and swelling, pain, and limitation of motion.

11. (1) The widespread vasculitis, responsible for many of the systemic changes in rheumatoid arthritis, produces a myositis, which results in flexor spasm in both upper and lower extremities.

12. (3) A normocytic, hypochromic anemia is typical of rheumatoid arthritis and is believed to result from a combination of nutritional inadequacy secondary to anorexia and marrow depression by toxic inflammatory products.

13. (2) Although the antigen responsible for joint tissue changes in rheumatoid arthritis is unknown, some sort of altered protein-polysaccharide complex, similar to that found in the bacterial cell wall, is thought to be the offending agent.

14. (2) This action is the only one likely to facilitate sleep without compromising the patient's welfare in some way. Any drug is potentially dangerous, and limiting her visitors may exacerbate family tensions.

15. (3) Rheumatoid arthritis, a collagen disease involving connective tissues, causes structural change of synovial membranes, cartilage, and tendons.

16. (1) The joint changes in rheumatoid arthritis progress through several stages including inflammatory changes, granulation tissue invasion, degeneration of the articular cartilage, erosion of the exposed bone, and formation of fibrous tissue adhesions between denuded bone.

17. (4) Blood consists of 55 per cent liquid plasma and 45 per cent cellular elements (erythrocytes, leukocytes, and platelets) suspended in the plasma. Centrifuging blood results in the cells, which are heavier than the plasma, being propelled to the bottom of the tube. The percentage of the total blood column which is composed of packed cells can be measured, and is known as the hematocrit.

18. (3) A hierarchy of different types of leukocytes exists, including the granulocytes, of which there are three types (acidophils, basophils, and neutrophils), and agranulocytes, of which there are two types (monocytes and lymphocytes). A differential white blood count measures the relative numbers of the various types. Knowledge of deviations from the normal of specific types is useful in making a differential diagnosis.

19. (1) The reason is unknown for the differential rates of movement of the several types of leukocytes from the blood vessel into the tissues during the inflammatory reaction. However, it is true that neutrophils and macrophages are usually first to move from the vessel (during the early or acute stage of infection), and that lymphocyte, monocytes, and plasma cells move into the tissues later (during the chronic phase of inflammation).

20. (3) The red blood cell sedimentation rate is the speed at which red blood cells settle out of suspension to the bottom of the tube of blood to which an anticoagulant has been added. The sedimentation rate increases during the acute stage of inflammation, probably owing to an increase in circulating fibrinogen, and decreases with the resolution of inflammation; thus, it is a

valuable indicator in evaluating the progress of illness or response to treatment.

21. (1) Granulation tissue derived from inflamed synovium attaches to the articular cartilage in the joint, interfering with its nutrition and causing it to erode. The exposed underlying bone undergoes absorption.

22. (2) Apparent narrowing of the joint space on x-ray examination results from loss of articular cartilage and proliferation of granulation tissue between previously articulating joint structures.

23. (1) During the stage of acute synovitis, enzymes produced by the inflamed synovium erode articular cartilage in the joint. Physical activity increases both the synovitis and cartilage destruction, thus, bedrest should be maintained until temperature reduction and symptom abatement indicate a lessening of rheumatic activity.

24. (2) From cholesterol, the adrenal cortex produces two classes of steroids: corticosteroids (of which cortisone is one) and adrenal androgens.

25. (4) Prednisone, a synthetic glucocorticoid, prevents or decreases the effects of local inflammatory reactions by inhibiting capillary dilation, fluid transudation, white cell diapedesis, phagocytosis, fibrin deposition, capillary proliferation, and collagen deposition.

26. (1) Prednisone, like other naturally occurring glucosteroids produced by the adrenal cortex, causes sodium retention and edema by a direct effect on the kidney tubule.

27. (1) Ascorbic acid, or vitamin C, is a water-soluble vitamin that facilitates carbohydrate metabolism and collagen tissue formation.

28. (2) Ascorbic acid is essential for production of collagen, a strong, fibrous protein, which forms the framework of such connective tissues as bone, dentin, cartilage, ligament, and tendon. Adequate intake is therefore essential for proper growth of bone and teeth, and proper healing of soft tissue wounds and fractures.

29. (3) Diazepam produces tranquilizing, muscle relaxant, and anticonvulsant effects. Rheumatoid arthritis, characterized by spasm of extensor muscles that can lead to severe distortion of the limbs, is treated with diazepam to relieve skeletal muscle spasm and prevent deformity.

30. (2) Diazepam has sedative and hypnotic, as well as muscle relaxant and anticonvulsant, effects. It is particularly apt to cause drowsiness in elderly persons.

31. (1) Normocytic, hypochromic anemia, one of the accompanying conditions of rheumatoid arthritis, is treated with oral ferrous sulfate. The iron is required for the synthesis of hemoglobin to correct the anemia.

32. (4) Anorexia, nausea, constipation, and diarrhea are all possible toxic effects of ferrous sulfate, resulting from irritation or necrosis of the gastrointestinal mucosa.

33. (4) Additional vitamin B_1 improves impaired appetite and carbohydrate metabolism, producing an increased food intake and more efficient utilization of carbohydrate as an energy source. Additional vitamin B_2 improves metabolism of amino acids and carbohydrate, enhancing their use for energy and body tissue building. Additional vitamin C improves production of collagen. Additional vitamin A increases the body's resistance to infection by improving the integrity of epithelium. Increased protein intake facilitates weight gain and repair of inflammatory and degenerative joint changes. Increased caloric intake facilitates weight gain.

34. (3) Antimalarial agents chloroquine; anti-inflammatory agents like phenylbutazone and indomethacin; and gold sodium thiomalate have all been used with limited success in some patients whose joint symptoms did not respond to salicylate therapy.

35. (3) The normal red blood cell count for a female is 4.5 million/mm.³ of blood. Mrs. Turk's red blood cell count is 88 per cent of normal; her hemoglobin concentration is 70 per cent of normal. Therefore, her hemoglobin concentration is decreased to a greater extent than is her red blood cell count.

36. (4) Increased red cell sedimentation rates, such as those typical of rheumatoid arthritis, result from the increased amounts of fibrinogen in the blood; this

enhances rouleaux formation, or "piling" of cells upon one another, which then speeds their settling out of suspension.

37. (3) The normal white blood cell count is 5000–10,000/mm.³ of blood.

38. (1) Neutrophils normally constitute from 50–60 per cent of total white blood cells.

39. (4) The rheumatoid factor is an autoantibody or a macroglobulin that circulates in the plasma and serves a protective function by localizing antigen-antibody complexes, thus decreasing tissue injury.

40. (1) Atrophy of muscles, subcutaneous tissues, and skin over involved rheumatoid arthritic joints is probably due to ischemia secondary to vasculitis.

41. (4) Treatment during acute synovitis with joint effusion includes absolute bedrest. The fact that Mrs. Turk is febrile, underweight, poorly nourished, and subjected to prolonged bedrest predisposes her to decubiti over the scapulae, elbows, sacrum, and os calcis.

42. (2) Erosion of cartilage and bone; weakening of tendons, ligaments, and joint sac; and imbalance of opposing muscles produce subluxation of unstable joints. Subluxation of metacarpophalangeal joints with displacement of extensor tendons, combined with muscle contractures, tends to pull the hand from the midline toward the ulna. Hyperextension of the proximal interphalangeal joint with ankylosis produces a "swan neck" deformity of the proximal interphalangeal joint.

43. (2) Muscle weakness, stiffness, and imbalance can result from Mrs. Turk's prescribed inactivity and predispose her to flexion contractures of the major joints. If optimal body alignment is maintained, any contractures and ankyloses that do occur will leave involved joints in positions of maximal function.

44. (3) Maintaining the position of maximal function ensures that, if the joint became ankylosed, the position would facilitate the activities of daily living.

45. (2) The position of the hand and arm in holding a glass of water will best accommodate the greatest number of feeding, dressing, grooming, and self-help activities.

46. (1) Flexion deformities are more apt to occur than extension deformities because, in general, flexor muscles tend to be stronger than extensors.

47. (2) Flexor muscles of the wrist are capable of exerting more force on contraction than are wrist extensors.

48. (2) According to the interpersonal theory of psychiatry, each individual "learns" how to express his sexual role and "learns" to be dependent or independent through interaction with significant others. Our earliest role models for demonstrating methods of coping with illness and disability are our parents, siblings, and parent surrogates.

49. (2) Acute synovitis can cause joint pain and tenderness so severe that even the weight of bed linen causes severe discomfort in involved extremities. This can be avoided by supporting the linen on a bed cradle.

50. (2) Mrs. Turk's reaction to the pain, distortion, and immobility associated with her illness is likely to be depression, which together with pain produced by movement would discourage her from initiating the active exercises. The nurse should firmly and repeatedly direct her to exercise the involved joints in order to minimize residual deformity and loss of function.

51. (3) Application of heat to involved joints by repeated immersion of each part in a warm paraffin bath relieves muscle spasm and decreases joint pain.

52. (4) Passive exercise improves circulation by the milking effect on vessel walls of alternate contraction and relaxation of adjacent muscles. Increased circulation decreases muscle atrophy by improving nutrient supply to, and wast removal from, muscle tissue. Passive exercises prevent muscle shortening and preserve range of motion by relieving spasm and preventing ankylosis.

53. (4) In rheumatoid arthritis, the amount of joint pain is approximately proportional to the degree of inflammatory change in joint tissue. By exercising a rheumatoid joint up to, but not beyond, the point of pain, it is possible to prevent contractures without causing unnecessary mechanical damage to inflamed structures.

54. (4) If the theory that rheumatoid arthritis patients tend to repress hostility is correct, the unexpressed anger might generate unconscious guilt, for which painful treatment might be perceived as punishment. However, "punishment" also provokes anger that, if unexpressed, can create a vicious circle of events. Consequently, the nurse should continuously reinforce the notion that the objective of exercising the joints is to minimize deformity and maintain function.

55. (2) All passive-aggressive behaviors, such as delaying, withstanding, withholding, and avoidance, may be covert or hidden expressions of hostility.

56. (2) Joint pain and limited motion in upper extremity joints make eating so difficult that more than usual time and energy are needed to consume a meal. The patient with rheumatoid arthritis suffers malnourishment of many body tissues owing to widespread vasculitis and persistent anorexia. Sufficient time should be provided so that Mrs. Turk can eat all her food without undue fatigue or frustration.

57. (1) Paraffin should be heated slowly in a double boiler over an electric, rather than a gas, burner, because it can easily be ignited by an open flame.

58. (2) The incidence of disabling spinal and hip deformity is high in patients with rheumatoid arthritis. Consequently, Mrs. Turk should be instructed to sleep supine on a firm mattress with a bedboard, so as to keep her body in proper alignment during the many hours (10–11) that she should spend each day in sleep and rest.

59. (4) a, Cortisone's anti-inflammatory effect retards wound healing. b, The high incidence of peptic ulceration, which rises with increasing cortisone dosage, can be decreased by administering the drug with meals. c, Cortisone is more apt to precipitate serious psychosis in persons with a previous history of emotional instability. d, Cortisone promotes gluconeogenesis, which results in hyperglycemia and glycosuria in some patients.

60. (4) Decreased mobility in intervertebral and hip joints makes it difficult to touch fingers to feet. A long-handled shoe horn, slip-on shoes, and long-handled reaching tongs facilitate self-dressing and feelings of independence. A patient with limited lower and upper extremity motion cannot safely sit down in the bottom of the tub and then rise to full standing position again. Therefore, a rubber-footed stool or chair, which can be placed in the tub and braced against tub sides, makes it possible for a patient with knee, hip, intervertebral, or shoulder stiffness to take a shower rather than a bed bath or basin bath; this facilitates the application of moist heat to involved extremities to relieve muscle spasm and pain. Decreased mobility of knee joints makes it difficult to sit and to rise from a sitting position, so that a built-up toilet seat facilitates self-care in elimination. Limited mobility of intervertebral, hip, and knee joints makes it difficult to maintain balance through rapid postural adjustments. Use of a walker should prevent falls due to loss of balance.

Bronchiectasis and Segmental Lung Resection

1. (2) Inhalant allergens, such as ragweed pollen, sensitize the nasal mucosa and precipitate hay fever attacks.

2. (3) Histamine is released by body tissues upon injury. Wherever liberated, it causes capillary vasodilation and increased capillary permeability, resulting in localized edema.

3. (3) Bronchiectasis is characterized by cylindric or saccular dilation of sections of the bronchial tree. Sacculation causes pooling and infection of bronchial secretions, with progressive destruction of smooth muscle and elastic tissue in bronchial walls.

4. (3) Bronchial pneumonia is an acute infection of lung parenchyma. If slowly or imperfectly resolved, it may result in chronic bronchitis, with progressive scarring and obstruction of bronchial segments and poor drainage of secretions from distal air passages, leading to the development of bronchiectasis.

5. (2) b, Prolonged bronchial obstruction causes secretions to be retained and to become dehydrated, thickened, and secondarily infected. d, Chronic infection weakens bronchial walls by destroying cilia, destroying smooth muscle and elastic fibers, and distorting normal architecture with fibrous scar tissue.

6. (3) Replacement of ciliated with nonciliated epithelium eliminates the sweeping action of cilia that normally removes mucus and debris from the bronchial tree. Segmental constriction of the bronchial tree with circular bands of fibrous tissue interferes with the flow of gases and secretions through the air passages. Destruction of smooth muscle and elastic fibers in the bronchial wall prevents the normal peristalsis that aids in removal of secretions. Anastamoses between branches of the bronchial artery and the pulmonary artery shunt blood from the systemic to the pulmonary circulation, thereby increasing pulmonary artery and pulmonary capillary pressures, and increasing right heart workload.

7. (3) When heart rate is regular, counting the pulse for one minute yields an accurate measure of heart rate.

8. (4) a, The depth of inspiration yields information about the amount of chest movement that is possible. b, The sounds on inspiration and expiration provide information about the amount and type of secretions in the air passages and the degree of bronchial constriction present. c, Rhythmicity indicates information about the mechanism(s) of primary importance in controlling respiratory movement (increase in carbon dioxide vs. lack of oxygen). d, The magnitude of chest and abdominal movement may indicate the presence of respiratory decompensation or congestive heart failure. e, The length of inspiration relative to that of expiration indicates the degree of bronchial obstruction present.

9. (3) Secretions that accumulate in dilated segments of the bronchial tree tend to become secondarily infected with microorganisms that are pus producers, and therefore are typically mucopurulent in type.

10. (2) The copious mucopurulent sputum tends to separate on standing, with the heavier elements settling to the bottom: a frothy top layer of sticky bubbles, which later combines with a middle layer of watery, saline-containing liquid and a lower layer of heavier pus cells and mucus plugs.

11. (1) Change from supine to upright position causes secretions pooled in the dilated bronchial segments during sleep to shift to adjacent undilated segments, stimulating the cough reflex and resulting in expectoration of large volumes of secretions.

12. (2) b, Both foreign materials in the bronchotracheal tree, and irritation or distention of the duodenum or stomach, inititate impulses that are carried by the vagus nerve to the cough and vomiting centers in the medulla. Thus, initiation of the cough reflex at the same time that the stomach is distended or hyperirritable may precipitate concomitant vomiting. d, The Valsalva maneuver, or forceful expiration against a closed glottis, commonly occurs during coughing. It causes increased intrathoracic pressure, resulting in decreased venous return to the right atrium and decreased left ventricular output, which could cause cerebral ischemia. Thus, paroxysms of coughing in a person with decreased cardiac reserve or impaired cerebral circulation could cause transient syncope.

13. (2) a, Retained infected secretions cause inflammation of lung parenchyma distal to the dilated segment of bronchus. c, Progressive inflammatory destruction of the bronchial wall may result in erosion of a bronchial artery with moderate-to massive-hemoptysis. e, Atelectasis and parenchymal scarring, by increasing resistance and pulmonary artery pressure, may increase right ventricular workload to the point of producing right heart failure. This latter is secondary to lung disease, and is referred to as cor pulmonale.

14. (3) Change of position causes pooled secretions to be redistributed to more dependent portions of the lung. Movement of secretions over sensitive bronchial walls stimulates coughing.

15. (4) Pooled bronchial secretions tend to become secondarily infected. The bronchiectatic patient should cover his mouth and nose in order to prevent contamination of his environment by the droplet spray that accompanies forceful expulsion of air and secretions from the bronchial tree through oral and nasal passages.

16. (2) When bronchial secretions are secondarily infected with anaerobic pathogens, the breath has a particularly foul odor, which may decrease the patient's appetite for food.

17. (1) Dyspnea is a subjective state characterized by feelings of breathlessness and apprehension. The prolonged muscular work necessary to maintain ventilation under conditions of decreased respiratory reserve may be the primary cause for the sensation of distress that is associated with breathlessness.

18. (2) The patient is apt to be most comfortable in semi-Fowler's position, with the arms elevated on pillows, because it permits maximal chest wall expansion with least muscular effort, and fosters gravity drainage of secretions to lung bases, leaving the upper and middle lobes available for gaseous exchange.

19. (3) One mode of treating hay fever is to administer antihistamine to antagonize the capillary dilator and bronchoconstrictor effects of the histamine liberated by antigen-antibody reactions.

20. (4) As a result of an unknown effect on the central nervous system, most antihistamines produce sedation and somnolence.

21. (2) The sedation and somnolence produced by antihistamines may so dull perceptions and slow reflex activity as to interfere with the rapid eye-mind-hand coordination required for safe driving.

22. (4) Mr. Kaufman has a low-grade fever, characteristic of chronic inflammatory reactions. It is probably due to the infected pooled bronchial secretions.

23. (3) The patient is most apt to suffer from inadequate food intake resulting from a combination of dyspnea, cough, and anorexia.

24. (4) The nasal mucosa appears pale and edematous in allergic rhinitis.

25. (3) Emphysema is a chronic lung condition in which obstruction of terminal bronchioles causes air trapping in the alveoli. As more and more air is trapped, intrapleural pressure becomes less negative and the chest becomes fixed in the position of inspiration: i.e., the ribs elevate, the diaphragm descends and flattens, and the anteroposterior diameter of the chest increases.

26. (3) Resonance is the full or resounding tone elicited when percussing the body surface over a hollow or gas-filled structure, such as normal lung tissue. The finding of decreased resonance suggests a decrease in the proportion of air-filled alveoli, as seen in pneumonitis, when some of the alveoli are filled with inflammatory exudate.

27. (3) Rales, or abnormal breath sounds heard on inspiration and/or expiration, are produced by the passage of air through secretions or constricted air passages. In bronchiectasis, the pooling of thickened secretions in dilated segments of the tracheobronchial tree results in auscultation of persistent, coarse, wet inspiratory rales, particularly in the posterior lung bases.

28. (1) "Clubbing" of digits refers to the bulbous swelling and rounding of the terminal digit. It is frequently seen in adults with chronic obstructive lung disease, and results from hypertrophic bony changes secondary to anoxia of peripheral tissues.

29. (3) Chronic sinusitis is common in bronchiectatic patients. It is hypothesized that aspiration of infected sinus contents may be a causative factor in the development of bronchiectasis.

30. (2) Either venous or capillary blood can be used for counting blood cells. However, capillary blood must be free-flowing and obtained from warm, noncyanotic skin that does not require vigorous squeezing to obtain the sample; otherwise, false results may be obtained.

31. (3) Simple disinfectant solutions will not destroy the serum hepatitis virus.

32. (4) A routine urine examination includes testing for all the cited characteristics, because it can be performed quickly and inexpensively on a small urine sample, and yields valuable information for diagnosis and management of many diseases.

33. (4) If a refractometer is available, a drop of urine is sufficient for determination of specific gravity. If a hydrometer is employed, from 6–10 ml. of urine must be available.

34. (3) At the end of deep inspiration the chest is fully expanded, permitting maximal exposure of all chest structures to x-rays, and optimal penetration of varying densities within the field of radiation, i.e., bone, soft tissue, fluid, and air densities.

35. (1) Vital capacity is defined as the maximal volume of air that can be completely expired following the deepest possible inspiration. It also can be considered as the measure of an individual's ability to take in the deepest possible breath.

36. (3) Bronchoscopy consists of inspection of the interior of the tracheobronchial tree with a long, slender tube containing a light source and a series of mirrors. This can be used to visualize the trachea and mainstem bronchi, and to examine the mucosa for inflammation, ulceration, or tumor. If the patient is being prepared for a bronchogram, a radiopaque dye can be introduced through the bronchoscope into the tracheobronchial tree. Suction can also be applied through the bronchoscope to remove mucous plugs, improve ventilation, and obtain stagnated secretions for microscopic examination.

37. (2) The bronchoscope may produce sufficient trauma to cause laryngeal edema and possible airway obstruction after the tube is removed. Shortness of breath and laryngeal stridor are warning symptoms of laryngeal edema.

38. (2) A local anesthetic is applied to the pharynx and larynx in preparation for passage of the bronchoscope. Because the anesthetic destroys the normal gag reflex, no food or fluid should be taken for four hours following the procedure so that aspiration of foreign substances into the lower airway does not occur.

39. (3) Passage of the bronchoscope interferes with air passage into and out of the lung, making the patient anxious and increasing his discomfort during the procedure. He will be more relaxed and better able to cooperate if he practices breathing in and out through his nose with his mouth open while preparing for the examination.

40. (2) Since the radiopaque dye used to outline the tracheobronchial tree will not reach the smaller branches if they are filled with secretions, postural drainage should be initiated to remove secretions from the lower air passages.

41. (3) During passage of the bronchoscope it would be possible accidentally to dislodge false teeth and bridges and force them into lower airway passages.

42. (3) Penicillin, an antibiotic with wide-spectrum, bactericidal effect, is useful against bacteria typically found in infected bronchial secretions.

43. (4) Allergy to penicillin is fairly common and causes such diverse symptoms as fever, skin rash, hives, stomatitis, angioedema, and hematuria. Anaphylactic shock may also occur. Since angioedema of respiratory passages and anaphylaxis are potentially lethal, penicillin should never be given to a person with known sensitivity to the drug.

44. (4) Saturated solution of potassium iodide is an expectorant that liquefies tenacious bronchial secretions so they can be removed more easily by coughing or by postural drainage.

45. (2) Since it is being given to liquefy pulmonary secretions, additional water should be administered to ensure adequate hydration of the tissues.

46. (3) Dyspnea is associated with apprehension and anxiety, both of which may interfere with sleep. Pentobarbital is a central nervous system depressant with sedative effects of intermediate duration.

47. (3) Elimination and personal hygiene needs should be met before comfort measures are given to prepare the patient for sleep. The room light should be left on while the pentobarbital is administered to permit proper checking of drug order, patient identification, and drug preparation and dosage.

48. (1) In bronchiectasis, infected bronchial secretions cause bronchial tissue damage. Repair and/or replacement of damaged tissue requires adequate dietary intake of essential amino acids.

49. (4) Chronic sinus and bronchial infections cause hyperpyrexia, which results in elevation of the rate of cellular metabolism.

50. (3) The following is the protein content of the foods listed: 3 oz. of canned tuna — 24 grams; 1 cup of red beans — 15 grams; 1 cup of creamed cottage cheese — 31 grams; 1 cup of whole milk — 9 grams.

51. (3) The following is the protein content of the foods listed: ½ cup of sweet potatoes — 2 grams; ½ cup of green beans — 1.2 grams; ½ cup of peas — 4.5 grams; ½ cup of corn — 2.5 grams.

52. (1) The following is the caloric content of the foods listed: ½ cup of sweet potatoes — 67 calories; ½ cup of green beans — 22 calories; ½ cup of peas — 54 calories; ½ cup of corn — 85 calories.

53. (3) The following is the caloric content of the foods listed: 1 cup of whole milk — 160 calories; 2 slices of fried bacon — 100 calories; 3 oz. of broiled hamburger — 185 calories; 1 medium-sized baked potato — 90 calories.

54. (3) The following are the caloric and protein contents of the foods listed: 1 boiled frankfurter — 155 calories and 6 grams of protein; ½ cup of cottage cheese — 120 calories and 15 grams of protein; 1 cup of baked custard—385 calories and 13 grams of protein; 1 poached egg — 80 calories and 7 grams of protein.

55. (4) a, Oral hygiene before meals eliminates the unpleasant breath odor that depresses appetite in bronchiectatic patients. b, Removal of the sputum cup eliminates a stimulus causing aversive conditioning to food. c, Smaller, more frequent meals prevent gastric distention, which tends to stimulate emesis during paroxysms of coughing. d, Helping the patient to eat during periods of dyspnea conserves his energy and increases the likelihood that he will consume all food served to him.

56. (3) b, Increasing water intake, even without giving an expectorant, helps to liquefy bronchial secretions so that they move more easily as the patient changes position, and thus stimulate cough. c, A reduction of temperature and metabolic rate improves nutrition and speeds healing because a smaller proportion of Mr. Kaufman's caloric and protein intake is then needed to fuel hypermetabolic cells.

57. (2) Thoracentesis is the procedure for removing infected exudated in empyema; postural drainage is the procedure for removing infected secretions in bronchiectasis.

58. (4) By positioning the patient so that his large bronchi, trachea, pharynx, and mouth are each more dependent than adjacent more distal segments of the airway, and all are more dependent than secretions pooled in dilated bronchial segments, the secretions can be stimulated to flow out of the air passages.

59. (3) Mr. Kaufman is prone to dizziness because, during drainage, he is predisposed to paroxysms of coughing that may induce syncope owing to the Valsalva maneuver mechanism.

60. (2) One hour before a meal the stomach is empty of food and secretions, so there is little danger that cough will induce concomitant vomiting. It also allows sufficient time for the treatment and for subsequent coughing, expectoration, and cleansing mouth care before eating.

61. (3) In this position, the lower and upper air passages are more nearly perpendicular to the floor, thus aiding gravity drainage of bronchial secretions from the lung. However, the pressure of abdominal viscera against the stomach may induce vomiting, and interference with venous drainage from the head may produce headache, so the position may have to be modified in susceptible patients.

62. (3) When the bronchial secretions begin to flow out of the lung and coughing is initiated, Mr. Kaufman will need a container to expectorate into and tissues to cleanse his mouth. A call bell should be at hand so that he can summon help if he should feel faint or in danger of falling.

63. (4) Deep inspiration is necessary to move air beyond the obstructed segments of bronchi, and coughing is required to raise intrapulmonary pressures sufficiently to forcibly eject air and secretions from dilated segments of the tracheobronchial tree.

64. (4) a, The nurse should help Mr. Kaufman to assume the correct position in order to reinforce the purpose and principles of the method while demonstrating the most effective position for drainage, available comfort measures, and advisable safety precautions. d, The nurse should remain with the patient throughout the treatment in order to observe his reaction to and tolerance of the procedure, since the position used can be extremely taxing to those with decreased cardiac reserve or cerebral circulation. e, The nurse should help Mr. Kaufman to assume normal position following postural drainage, because some patients tend to lose their balance as a result of orthostatic hypotension.

65. (4) Increased intrapulmonary pressures and perivascular scarring produce increased resistance to pulmonary circulation, with consequent increase in right ventricular workload, which may lead to right heart failure in a patient with diminished cardiac reserve.

66. (2) Bleeding occurs in bronchiectasis as a result of erosion of a bronchial artery. The sudden, deep inspiration that occurs during paroxysms of coughing may pull blood and infected secretions from the bleeding site into other sections of lung. If the blood clots quickly, it may not be removed by subsequent coughing. Because blood is an excellent culture medium, and bacteria are present in great number and variety in infected bronchial secretions, aspiration pneumonia is apt to develop quickly in a debilitated patient.

67. (4) Since the combined factors of obstruction and dilation of diseased bronchial segments predispose to chronic inflammation and structural damage, which leads to still further scarring and dilation, bronchiectasis tends to be self-perpetuating. Thus, if the disease is limited to certain segments or lobes of one lung, segmentectomy or lobectomy may be the most effective treatment.

68. (1) The solution that is placed in a closed chest drainage bottle serves as a one-way valve to seal off atmospheric air and prevent its entry to the pleural space through the chest drainage tube. Aseptic technique must be used in preparing and maintaining the closed drainage system, in order to prevent introduction of pathogens into the pleural space. Thus, sterile water is used to create the seal.

69. (2) a, Blood and serum are excellent culture media, that if not removed from the pleural space, may result in infection. b, When the chest cavity is entered during surgery, the lung collapses because negative intrapleural pressure is lost. When the chest wall is closed at the end of the operation, the intrapleural pressure is equivalent to atmospheric pressure. In order to promote re-expansion of the operated lung so that negative intrapleural pressure is re-established, certain changes must occur. Air must enter the lung through the tracheobronchial tree, to extend lung parenchyma and force air and fluid out of the intrapleural space through the chest drainage tube with each inspiration. At the same time, air must not be permitted to re-enter the intrapleural space through the drainage tube when the lungs deflate during expiration.

70. (3) After the closed chest drainage system has been established, each respiration by the patient pushes more and more air from the interpleural space, gradually reducing the intrapleural pressure from 0 mm. Hg (normal atmosphceric pressure at sea level) to −4 mm. Hg to −10 mm. Hg (normal negative pressures within the intrapleural space). The immersion of the long glass tube (connected to the chest catheter) in the sterile water permits passage of air and fluid out of the pleural space, and it also serves as a water seal to prevent back flow of air and fluid to the pleural space during expiration.

71. (2) In order to monitor the patient's condition and to prescribe necessary fluid replacement without overloading the cardiovascular system, the surgeon must know the exact amount of drainage lost from the pleural space. Marking the time and fluid level on the drainage bottle makes later fluid calculations possible.

72. (2) Because intrapleural pressures vary with inspiration and expiration, fluid rises a few centimeters in the tube on inspiration and falls on expiration. This oscillation indicates that the drainage tube is patent and the drainage apparatus is functioning properly. Moderate bubbling of air from the bottom of the long glass tube up through the liquid indicates that air is being forced from the intrapleural space as desired.

73. (4) All events listed would eliminate the one-way seal, permitting air to enter the intrapleural space and deflate the lung.

74. (1) Two large forceps (or clamps) would be needed to double-clamp the chest catheter if the water seal were to be broken, in order to prevent re-entry of air into the pleural space.

75. (4) Fowler's position would facilitate accumulation of secretions in the lower portion of the pleural cavity, permitting maximal expansion of the upper and middle lobes of the lung.

76. (3) Coughing, by sharply increasing intrapulmonary pressure, aids in lung re-expansion. The patient is more apt to cough deeply and frequently if he can do so without extreme discomfort.

77. (1) This device provides more adequate lung aeration through the intermittent application of positive pressure (i.e., greater than atmospheric pressure) so as to force oxygen into alveoli and flush carbon dioxide from residual air spaces.

Intermittent positive pressure breathing can be used to decrease respiratory insufficiency, improve coughing efficiency, increase removal of secretions, and administer aerosol medications.

78. (2) Patients with respiratory allergies often suffer some degree of bronchospasm in response to emotional stress and/or specific allergens. Bronchospasm impairs normal drainage of lung secretions. Isoproterenol is a sympathomimetic drug that acts on beta receptors, relaxing smooth muscles in the bronchial wall and thereby relieving bronchospam.

79. (3) Shoulder muscle contractures and shoulder ankylosis are possible complications of prolonged immobilization of the upper extremity. Passive, followed by active, exercises of the right arm and shoulder help to prevent both complications.

80. (3) Reduction of body iron and protein stores due to blood loss and decreased food intake could impair normal blood production for some time following surgery, which in turn would impair cellular oxidation and metabolism. Impaired nutrition during the intraoperative and postoperative phases of treatment would reduce body stores of certain trace elements that are thought to be part of essential enzyme systems. The long-range effects of anesthetic agents on the liver, lungs, kidney, and central nervous system may impair metabolism of fat, protein, and carbohydrate for weeks or months. All these factors could predispose Mr. Kaufman to weakness and decreased resistance for some time following surgery.

Appendicitis and Appendectomy

1. (4) In evaluating Don's history the nurse should recognize the classic symptoms of appendicitis and the potential need for emergency surgery. She should prevent the ingestion of food, fluid, or medication by mouth. An infirmary nurse would be unlikely to administer an enema without a physician's order, and in any case should recognize that an enema should never be given to a patient with undiagnosed abdominal pain because of the obvious danger of intestinal perforation and peritonitis.

2. (3) Although the appendix is attached to the tip of the cecum, which is usually located in the right lower quadrant of the abdomen, the cecum or the appendix can be rotated so as to be pointed in any direction from its cecal attachment. The location of the appendix determines the location of appendiceal pain, which may manifest itself as back or flank pain, suprapubic pain experienced during urination, or rectal pain stimulated by examination or defecation.

3. (4) The nurse should determine: a, how much Don understands about his diagnosis and probable treatment, in order to decide what further information he needs about his forthcoming surgery and postoperative care; b, where he lives (since he is a minor and it will be necessary for one of his parents to give consent for the operation) and how close he is to various family members (in order to assess the amount of psychologic support he is likely to receive from each during his present illness); c, the extent of his previous experience with surgery, in order to gauge his probable expectations concerning this hospitalization; d, his smoking and drinking habits (in order to predict the ease of his anesthetic induction and the possible anesthetic risk) and his eating habits (to establish his nutritional status); (e), his religious and social affiliations, so as to check which persons other than his family should be notified of his progress.

4. (3) Anxiety stimulates the vasomotor center in the medulla and the sympathetic nervous system, initiating sympathetic vasoconstrictor impulses to vessels throughout the body, with elevation of the blood pressure.

5. (1) Following occlusion of the appendiceal lumen by any stricture or substance, continuing secretion of appendiceal mucus and growth of microorganisms in the retained secretions produces distention of the appendix. When appendiceal distention produces sufficient pressure to interfere with venous drainage of the organ, vascular congestion of the appendiceal wall ensues and inflammation extends to the nearby cecum, interfering with propulsive peristalsis.

6. (4) Of the five specific types of white blood cells in the peripheral blood, neutrophils are the most numerous, usually constituting from 50–70 per cent of the total number.

7. (2) White blood cells have the following capabilities: diapedesis (the ability to squeeze through the pores of the blood vessel walls, so as to migrate from capillaries into the tissues); ameboid movement (the ability to move through the intercellular spaces by protruding a pseudopodium from one end of the cell, and then drawing the remainder of the cell body toward the pseudopodium); chemotaxis (the tendency to move toward degenerative products of inflammation and cell necrosis); and phagocytosis (the ability to engulf and digest dead tissue and foreign bodies). A neutrophil can phagocytize from 5 to 20 bacteria before it becomes inactivated and dies.

8. (1) Rebound tenderness following application and quick release of manual pressure over some area of the abdomen away from the suspected site of inflammation is the result of stimulation of sense receptors in inflamed parietal peritoneum overlying the inflamed appendix. If there is chemical irritation of the appendix and overlying peritoneum without rupture of the appendix, pain will be felt in the right lower quadrant. If the appendix has ruptured, spilling bowel content and producing generalized peritonitis, pain will be felt diffusely throughout the abdomen. Total absence of bowel sounds would suggest paralytic ileus due to diffuse peritoneal irritation. If inflammation and/or necrosis of the cecum had caused complete bowel obstruction, the bowel would first become hyperactive, with increased frequency of bowel sounds, and then there would be a change in the character of sounds: prolonged rushing sounds, followed by high-pitched "tinkling" sounds, and finally no bowel sounds whatsoever.

9. (3) Assumption of the side-lying position, with the right knee bent, relieves tension on rigid and tender abdominal muscles, thereby decreasing discomfort.

10. (4) Behavior as in a, c, and e may indicate the use of denial in handling overwhelming anxiety concerning his illness. Behavior as in b suggests an extremely narrowed field of attention, probably the result of extreme anxiety. Behavior as in e may be the result of regression provoked by an overwhelming threat to physical or psychologic integrity.

11. (3) The objective of preoperative skin preparation is to reduce the number of bacteria that could be carried into body tissues and cavities during the operative procedure. Bacteria can be removed from the intact skin surface by cleansing with an antiseptic soap a cationic detergent such as benzalkonium chloride, or an iodophor such as povidone-iodine. A sterile basin will be needed to hold the antiseptic solution. Sponges are needed to apply the antiseptic, since mechanical removal is more effective than chemical disinfection in removing bacteria from the skin. The operative site should be shaved with a sharp, new blade, since bacteria tend to adhere to the hair shaft. Sponges are also needed to paint the prepared skin with antiseptic, so as to remove any bacteria or debris transferred to the site during the shaving procedure.

12. (4) The area of skin prepared for surgery should always be much wider and longer than the expected line of incision, in case intraoperative complications make it necessary either to extend the primary incision or to perform additional incisions for exploratory, drainage, or resuscitative purposes. By preparing the area from nipple to groin and from bedline to bedline, a midline incision for exploration, a flank incision for drainage, or a thoracotomy incision for resuscitation are made possible, in addition to the right lower quadrant incision that would probably be employed for appendectomy.

13. (3) A variety of microorganisms normally populate unbroken skin. Any of these organisms can become pathogenic if introduced into subcutaneous tissues. Normal skin bacteria are concentrated in hair follicles, on hair shafts, and in moist skin areas. The purpose of shaving the operative area is to remove the hair as a source of microorganisms, and to denude the skin so as to facilitate chemical and mechanical cleansing.

14. (3) *Micrococcus pyogenes* is a normal inhabitant of the unbroken skin.

15. (3) A bladder that is distended could easily protrude into the surgical field during pelvic or low abdominal surgery, thus becoming vulnerable to accidental

injury during an operative procedure; it could easily be perforated by a retractor, lacerated by a scalpel, and so on. It is important to ensure that the bladder be empty, small, and out of the way during surgery, the patient therefore should be encouraged to void immediately before the operation.

16. (3) The most common toxic effect of penicillin is hypersensitivity, which may cause a variety of manifestations: fever, erythema, purpura, urticaria, maculopapular rash, glossitis, arthralgia, angioedema, or anaphylaxis. Preoperative complications should be avoided, and one way to do this is to question the patient regarding any penicillin allergy.

17. (4) Don should be taught to perform all these measures, which are self-protective activities for the immediate postoperative period, designed to avoid the more common postoperative complications. Deep breathing and coughing exercises help to expand collapsed lung tissue and prevent postoperative pneumonia. Turning from side to side decreases pressure injury to the skin of the back and helps to prevent postoperative atelectasis. Alternate flexion and extension of ankle, knees and hips helps to prevent phlebothrombosis and pulmonary embolism.

18. (2) Don should be told preoperatively that he may experience right lower quadrant pain after recovering from anesthesia, and that he should inform the Recovery Room nurse so that the prescribed analgesic can be administered. Thus, Don will be more likely to turn, cough, and deep breathe if he can do so without extreme discomfort. He should be told that he will receive postoperative intravenous infusions, so that he will not interpret their use as evidence of unexpected complications or unfavorable progress. He should be instructed in the use of the positive pressure ventilator so that, if pulmonary complications develop postoperatively, he will be able to cooperate and realize maximal benefit from treatment.

19. (2) A signed consent from a mentally competent adult must be obtained for any surgical procedure. Surgery for a minor under 18 years of age must be consented to by an adult relative. If the latter cannot be present, his or her consent can be obtained by phone, telegram, or letter.

20. (1) The surgeon is legally responsible for securing written consent for the operation because it is he who will disrupt the patient's physical integrity. However, it is the nurse's responsibility to protect the patient from unwanted physical injury (as from a surgical procedure to which he had not consented) by checking to see that a signed or properly authorized consent for surgery has been obtained and is affixed to the patient's chart.

21. (1) The patient, or the guardian of a minor or incompetent adult, cannot reasonably consent to a surgical procedure until he has been given a full explanation of what will occur during surgery and what complications or losses he may suffer as a consequence of the procedure. Since the surgeon is the most knowledgeable in this respect, he has greatest responsibility for conveying this information to the patient. The nurse is responsible for determining whether the patient has understood the information and has freely consented to undergo the procedure described.

22. (2) Since emergency surgery provides little time for the repeated supportive interactions so necessary for trust-building between patient and physician, it is important that the nurse demonstrate, by every word, tone, and facial expression, her own confidence in and respect for the surgeon who will perform the operation.

23. (4) Meperidine is a synthetic central nervous system depressant. It alters the affective reaction to pain, in part by producing sedation and euphoria; has a spasmogenic effect on the stomach and intestine, causing a decrease in propulsive peristalsis; and has a respiratory depressant effect that results from a decreased responsiveness of medullary respiratory centers to carbon dioxide. Repeated use of meperidine results in tolerance to many of its effects, and produces habituation and physical and psychologic dependence upon the drug. Since its duration of action is shorter than that of morphine, the need to take meperidine repeatedly and at short intervals makes the habit of drug-seeking very easy to acquire during meperidine usage.

24. (1) Most persons react to impending surgery with strong anxiety. This causes increased sympathetic nervous system activity, i.e., tachycardia, elevated

blood pressure, and muscular tension, which is physically taxing to the patient; it also complicates anesthesia induction, necessitating larger than usual doses to reach the stage of surgical anesthesia. Meperidine, therefore, is given preoperatively, both to relieve anxiety and to decrease the amount of anesthetic needed during surgery.

25. (3) Because many of the agents used for inhalation anesthesia are irritating to mucous membranes, they tend to increase secretion of saliva and mucus. In order to prevent aspiration of secretions during intubation, atropine, a parasympathetic depressant, is usually given preoperatively in 0.4- to 0.6-mg. dosages.

26. (4) The effect of meperidine is to alter the patient's state of consciousness so as to decrease alertness. Don is likely to fall asleep within minutes after the drug is given. Some patients, however, experience untoward effects such as CNS excitation, tremor, or convulsions, which involve a danger of falling. Don's bed rails should therefore be elevated to guard against this possible danger.

27. (3) During transportation from the infirmary to the operating room, Don should be prevented from falling or from extending his arms over the cart edges by elevating the side rails or by securing him to the cart with a strap over his hips and another over his thorax and arms.

28. (4) Anesthesia provokes severe anxiety in many persons since it is characterized by complete loss of control over body movements, consciousness, and vital functions. It is natural to equate this temporary loss of autonomy and self-determination with death, the ultimate and permanent loss of control over physical functioning.

29. (1) An endotracheal tube is inserted into the patient's trachea by way of his mouth or nose, and is maintained there for the purposes of removing secretions and facilitating ventilation. Anesthesic agents may produce severe toxic or allergic effects, such as laryngospasm, bronchospasm, vomiting, and excess mucus production. These complications could lead to asphyxia, cardiac arrest, and death. With an endotracheal tube in proper position, and connected to a closed gas system, aspiration of saliva or vomitus is impossible, and obstruction of larynx or trachea by edema or spasm is prevented.

30. (4) Cyclopropane is an extremely potent anesthetic gas with a relatively pleasant odor that is minimally irritating to respiratory mucosa. It permits rapid and pleasant induction, can be used to produce any desired level of anesthesia, and in deeper levels will produce sufficient muscle relaxation to eliminate the need for neuromuscular blocking agents. Its margin of safety between anesthesia and lethal concentrations is wider than that of most other anesthetic agents in common use.

31. (2) Cyclopropane depresses the response of medullary respiratory centers to carbon dioxide concentrations. Laryngospasm or bronchospasm may develop during induction. A variety of arrhythmias may be produced by cyclopropane, of which sinus bradycardia, atrial fibrillation, nodal rhythm, ventricular extrasystole, and bigeminy are most common.

32. (2) Stage I of anesthesia, analgesia, begins with administration of the anesthetic agent and lasts until consciousness is lost. During the analgesic stage the patient may appear inebriated or drowsy.

33. (1) Cyclopropane has the ability to depress excitable tissues in several portions of the central nervous system. As a general CNS depressant, it tends to decrease nervous tissue excitability through the following continuum: analgesia, sedation, hypnosis, general anesthesia, autonomic effect, and coma. Thus, the "higher" centers are depressed before the "lower" centers.

34. (4) Stage II, delirium, extends from loss of consciousness to the beginning of surgical anesthesia. Excitement and involuntary activity may occur during Stage II. Typically, skeletal muscle tone increases, breathing is irregular, the pupils may dilate, blood pressure and heart rate increase, and the patient may thrash about actively.

35. (3) Patients' subsequent accurate reporting of comments made by operating room personnel while anesthesia is being induced has demonstrated that the ability to move, speak, and feel pain is lost before the ability to perceive auditory stimuli.

36. (1) Cyclopropane is explosive and flammable throughout its usual anesthetic dose

range. Therefore, it must be administered by means of an anesthetic machine, or a "closed" system of tanks, machines, tubes, valves, bags, and masks. All components of a "closed" system are composed of electrically conductive materials, so as to reduce spark production and prevent explosion.

37. (3) In Stage IV, respiratory paralysis, the vital respiratory and circulatory centers in the medulla are seriously depressed; the patient demonstrates no respiratory movement; there is diminished cardiac activity; and the pupils are fully dilated and fixed. Preparations should be made to administer cardiopulmonary resuscitation at this stage, or cardiac arrest will quickly follow.

38. (3) The pupils begin to dilate, and continue to do so, in Stage III of anesthesia. By the time the patient enters Stage IV, the pupils are fully dilated and incapable of reacting to light.

39. (1) Both kinking of the appendix and blockage of the appendix by a fecalith interfere with drainage of appendiceal secretions, leading to distention of the organ, infection of retained secretions, and extension of inflammation through the appendiceal wall to the overlying peritoneum.

40. (4) Appendiceal secretions usually contain *Escherichia coli* and other pathogens. When drainage of these secretions is blocked, such organisms multiply rapidly, invade the wall of the appendix, and produce acute inflammatory changes.

41. (4) *Clostridium histolyticum,* a normal inhabitant of the intestine, produces a proteolytic enzyme that rapidly breaks down gangrenous tissue, like that of an appendix with an obstructed blood supply.

42. (2) When an actively inflamed appendix ruptures without having been walled off by omentum or adjacent loops of bowel, the contents of the necrotic appendix are discharged into the peritoneal cavity, and the bacteria, which had multiplied rapidly in retained appendiceal secretions, begin to multiply in peritoneal fluid.

43. (4) The purpose of the postanesthesia unit is to enable specially trained personnel to provide continuous care to the immediately postoperative patient until he has completely recovered from the effects of the risk of such life-threatening complications as anoxia, asphyxia, shock, hemorrhage, respiratory arrest, and cardiac arrest. All the equipment listed is needed to combat these complications. A flowmeter is required to permit oxygen administration in order to reverse or prevent tissue anoxia secondary to the anesthetic. Suction apparatus is needed to aspirate potentially troublesome oropharyngeal and tracheobronchial secretions, thereby maintaining an open airway. Mechanical airways (oropharyngeal, endotracheal, or tracheostomy tubes) are necessary to prevent airway obstruction and facilitate ventilation in patients with obtunded reflexes and/or excessive secretions. The positive pressure ventilator delivers various gas mixtures into the patient's airway under greater than atmospheric pressure, in order to decrease high pCO_2 or increase low pO_2 levels. The CPR cart is needed to treat respiratory and cardiovascular emergencies promptly and effectively.

44. (1) While Don is under the influence of the anesthetic agent, his jaw and tongue will be relaxed. It is possible for the relaxed tongue to fall back into the throat, producing airway obstruction. For this reason, the oropharyngeal airway should be left in place until Don awakens sufficiently to respond to simple commands and until his swallowing reflex has returned.

45. (3) Swallowing movements indicate that the pharyngeal reflexes have returned, so that the patient is in less danger of aspirating oropharyngeal secretions. Ability to respond to simple commands shows that he is sufficiently alert and oriented that he is not likely to fall or to dislodge the tubes and dressings. Stabilization of vital signs and central venous pressure at acceptable levels indicates that he is not bleeding, nor in respiratory, cardiac, or circulatory failure. These findings demonstrate that Don is no longer prone to the most serious postoperative complications, and can now be safely maintained on close, rather than continuous, nursing attention.

46. (4) Injury to pharyngeal, laryngeal, and tracheal tissues during insertion of the endotracheal tube, and irritation of those same tissues by accidental or unavoidable movement of the tube during use, may lead to inflammation, edema, or infection of the traumatized tissue following tube removal. Inflammation of

pharynx and larynx result in sore throat and hoarseness. Edema of larynx or trachea may be severe enough to obstruct the airway. Use of an oversize tube, or overinflation of the cuff on the endotracheal tube, may produce tracheal erosion and collapse. Mechanical damage and edema of the trachea, together with the effects of certain anesthetic agents, may produce laryngospasm, or spasmodic contraction of laryngeal muscles, with partial or complete obstruction of the airway.

47. (2) Low Fowler's position favors lung expansion and restricts inflammatory exudate, if any, to the lower abdomen, where it can be more quickly absorbed than would be possible if it were distributed widely throughout the entire peritoneal cavity.

48. (2) The formula for calculating the number of drops per minute necessary to administer the ordered intravenous infusion in 8 hours is:

$$\text{Drops per minute} = \frac{\text{Total vol. to be infused} \times \text{drops/ml.}}{\text{Total time of infusion in minutes}}$$

The directions on each intravenous tubing set indicate the number of drops necessary to administer 1 ml. of fluid through the tubing (tubing from one company may deliver 1 ml. in 10 drops; tubing from another company may deliver 1 ml. in 15 drops). Thus:

$$\text{Drops per minute} = \frac{\text{Total vol.} \times \text{drops/ml.}}{\text{Total time in minutes}} = \frac{1000 \text{ ml.} \times 15}{480 \text{ min.}} = 31 \text{ drops/min.}$$

or

$$\text{Drops per minute} = \frac{\text{Total vol.} \times \text{drops/ml.}}{\text{Total time in minutes}} = \frac{1000 \text{ ml.} \times 10}{480 \text{ min.}} = 21 \text{ drops/min.}$$

So, to infuse the ordered solution in 8 hours would require a flow rate of 31 drops per minute with tubing of one brand, and 21 drops per minute with tubing of another brand.

49. (2) Normal saline solution, or a solution of sodium chloride that is isotonic with blood, contains 0.9 of 1 per cent of NaCl. A solution of this concentration will neither crenate nor shrink blood cells, nor cause them to swell, so it will interfere as little as possible with normal blood cell physiology.

50. (2) Spasm of the internal bladder sphincter may result from the spasmogenic effect of certain drugs used perioperatively, such as morphine or meperidine.

51. (3) This action approximates the conditions usually associated with normal micturition without subjecting the patient to unnecessary hazard. Application of heat or pressure to a recently operated abdomen might cause mechanical or inflammatory injury. Ingestion of large amounts of fluid would be apt to produce nausea.

52. (3) The normal urinary output per day varies from 1000 to 2000 cc. (ml.), with an average of 1500 cc. (ml.).

53. (3) If a limp or soft suction tube is to be used, immersion of the tube in ice before insertion stiffens it, making it easier to swallow, and less likely to kink or curl in the lower pharynx or upper esophagus.

54. (3) Optimal gaseous exchange is required to prevent anoxia of vital brain, heart, kidney, and liver tissue, all of which may have been dangerously stressed by the toxic effects of anesthesia. Improved tone of intestinal muscle is needed to restore propulsive peristalsis, which could have been hampered by appendiceal, cecal, and peritoneal inflammation. Acceleration of blood flow in the extremities decreases the possibility of phlebothrombosis and pulmonary embolism, to which immobility and dehydration predispose any patient following major surgery.

55. (2) Only protein can supply the essential amino acids that are necessary building blocks of the granulation tissue needed to close the surgical incision.

56. (3) Vitamin C is essential to capillary proliferation, which is the first step in formation of granulation tissue, and to production of collagen, the ground substance of fibrous scar tissue.

57. (4) Proper surgical aseptic technique requires that the nurse wear clean face mask and sterile gloves while cleansing Don's incision and re-dressing it with sterile gauze pads.

58. (4) Ether would be most effective in removing adhesive from the skin.

59. (1) Since Don was not experiencing pain, vital signs were normal, and the wound was in good condition, there was no indication for calling the physician. Before repeating the dose of the sedative-hypnotic given at bedtime (if ordered) the nurse should administer comfort measures, such as position change and backrub, to see whether these relax the patient enough to fall asleep naturally.

60. (2) Cathartics, like enemas, should never be given for undiagnosed abdominal pain. If such pain is due to inflammatory bowel disease, such as appendicitis, the increased peristalsis provoked by the cathartic might cause bowel perforation and peritonitis.

Peptic Ulcer and Gastric Resection

1. (3) According to research, persons who are genetically predisposed to secretion of large amounts of gastric acid and pepsin also tend to demonstrate psychic conflict between persistent infantile wishes to be loved and cared for and a simultaneous need to repudiate such wishes out of a sense of shame and pride.

2. (3) In persons who are genetically predisposed to ulcer development, those interpersonal events that exacerbate their basic intrapsychic conflict contribute to ulcer production by excessive stimulation of the parasympathetic nervous system.

3. (3) Stimulation of the parasympathetic fibers of the vagus nerve results in increased secretion of digestive juices, increased tone of smooth muscles of the stomach and intestine, and increased rate and amplitude of peristalsis.

4. (2) A peptic ulcer is a sharply circumscribed loss of tissue in the lining of those parts of the gastrointestinal system that are exposed to the acid and pepsin of gastric juice, which include the lower esophagus, the stomach, and the first portion of the duodenum.

5. (4) The pain of peptic ulcer tends to occur 2–3 hours after a meal because at that time the stomach is empty of food and the highly acid gastric juice is, therefore, undiluted.

6. (3) Milk and crackers are usually successful in relieving the pain of peptic ulcer. Soda crackers, being alkaline in composition, help to neutralize the hydrochloric acid in gastric juice. Milk protein, like all protein, has an acid-buffering ability. It also has a demulcent or soothing effect because it tends to coat the irritated gastric mucosa. Milk fat inhibits gastric secretions.

7. (4) As a result of wide individual variations in the amount of melanin in the skin, the color of skin is an unreliable index of the degree of anemia. Unless the hand has been held in an awkward position or has been exposed to extreme cold or heat, the nail beds or palms will reveal anemia when there has been a significant reduction in the blood's hemoglobin content.

8. (2) Prolonged vomiting produces generalized dehydration. The symptoms of dehydration include poor tissue turgor; i.e., when the skin of the chest or arms is pinched and lifted away from underlying tissue, it remains elevated for several seconds before returning to its original position.

9. (2) Anemia can be defined as a decrease in the concentration of hemoglobin in the peripheral blood. Hypochromic or iron deficiency anemia develops when the supply of iron in the body is inadequate to support red blood cell production as a result of inadequate dietary intake of iron, malabsorption of iron from the gut, or chronic blood loss. The daily loss of small amounts of blood over a protracted period, as may occur in a patient with recurrent peptic ulcer dis-

ease, tends to deplete body iron stores, and so it is a common cause of hypochromic anemia.

10. (3) The presence of hemoglobin in a stool specimen is interpreted as an indication of bleeding from the upper gastrointestinal tract, such as would occur in a bleeding peptic ulcer. A peroxidase, such as hemoglobin, is capable of catalyzing the oxidation of the test substance guaiac by peroxide, thereby producing various shades of blue, depending on the amount of hemoglobin in the test material.

11. (3) The usefulness of a peroxidase test for occult or hidden blood in stool is impaired somewhat by the fact that dietary meat contains hemoglobin and myoglobin, which yield positive guaiac test results for 3–4 days after ingestion of the meat. The withholding of meat from the diet for 72 hours before collection of a stool specimen increases the usefulness of the guaiac test as an indicator of upper gastrointestinal bleeding.

12. (1) The value of x-ray examination as a diagnostic tool depends upon the fact that substances of different densities block the passage of x-rays to different degrees. A plain x-ray film of the gastrointestinal tract will show only faint shadows, with occasional fluid levels or gas collections. The lumen of the tract can be better visualized by x-ray when filled with a radiopaque substance, such as barium sulfate. The latter is the inert salt of a heavy metal that can be ingested or injected into the upper or lower tract to outline the walls of the alimentary tube, to reveal excavations, protrusions, deformities, and abnormalities of propulsion.

13. (4) Plain barium sulfate, which may be used, has a bland or chalky taste. The oral mixtures used for upper gastrointestinal film series are frequently flavored with mint or wintergreen.

14. (4) After the barium mixture is ingested, the patient is positioned and turned so as to facilitate flow of the thick mixture through the upper alimentary tract. He is maintained in a sitting position while the barium mixture is swallowed so as to facilitate its flow through the esophagus, then positioned on his left side to encourage its flow into the stomach, and then turned to his right side to permit flow from the stomach into the duodenum. Several x-ray films are taken of each organ as the barium bolus passes through it.

15. (3) Gastric hypersecretion and hyperacidity are two factors that contribute to production of a peptic ulcer. Following a 12-hour fast it should be possible to aspirate no more than 50 ml. of pale gray, translucent, slightly viscid gastric secretions from the stomach. In suspected peptic ulcer disease, analysis of gastric content is undertaken to determine the basal gastric secretion, or the response of the stomach to those endogenous stimuli that are present in the fasting state, such as psychogenic influences mediated by the vagus nerve and such hormones as gastrin and adrenocorticoids. For this purpose the patient must undergo the 12-hour fast and forego all medicine affecting gastric secretion for 24 hours.

16. (1) A variety of substances have been used as test meals to stimulate gastric secretion; among them are the Ewald test meal.

17. (2) Hypersecretion and hyperacidity are characteristic of peptic ulcer disease.

18. (2) By definition, hypochromic anemia is an anemia in which hemoglobin synthesis is deficient. Since hemoglobin consists of iron, protoporphyrin, and globin, reduced availability of any of these components results in hypochromic anemia. Hypochromic red blood cells typically are smaller than normal, with an increase in the area of central pallor.

19. (2) The body's iron stores represent a balance between iron absorbed and iron lost from the body. There is no evidence in Mr. Gunderson's history or physical findings to suggest a problem with food and iron absorption. His symptoms are those of peptic ulcer disease, which is a common cause of progressive depletion of iron stores.

20. (3) Patients with peptic ulcer disease display increased gastric secretion of hydrochloric acid. Normally, an adequate blood supply and a protective coat of mucus protect the gastric mucosa from injury from hydrochloric acid in the gastric juice. Under normal conditions, the application of an irritant to the gastric mucosa is followed by an outpouring of mucus. It is theorized that, in the peptic ulcer patient, impairment of mucosal blood supply or reduction in

protective mucus renders the gastric mucosa more vulnerable than usual to erosion by the excessive acid present in gastric secretions.

21. (2) A duodenal ulcer, which typically develops within 3 cm. of the pylorus on either the anterior or the posterior duodenal wall, may, upon penetration through the mucosa and muscularis, erode the gastroduodenal artery and produce massive hemorrhage. In 1–2 per cent of cases penetration occurs rapidly and the ulcer perforates into the abdominal cavity. Obstruction of the pylorus may result from inflammatory edema associated with an actively eroding pyloric ulcer, or from contraction of circumferential scar tissue deposited following the healing of a recurrent duodenal ulcer.

22. (1) Large meals cause discomfort during the stage of acute ulceration. In patients with active peptic ulcer disease, the hourly administration of milk and cream will lower intragastric pH to a greater degree than will the administration of three regular meals per day.

23. (1) A diet of milk and cream contains large amounts of cholesterol: 3 oz. of milk contain 34 mg. of cholesterol; 3 oz. of cream contain 80 mg. of cholesterol. Research has shown a higher-than-normal incidence of atherosclerosis in patients who have received large amounts of milk and cream over long periods for treatment of peptic ulcer.

24. (1) Gastric antacids, or agents that neutralize and remove acid from gastric contents, are of two types: systemic and nonsystemic. A systemic antacid like sodium bicarbonate is capable of producing metabolic alkalosis because the cationic portion of the molecule forms a soluble compound on combination with gastric acid, and so can be absorbed into the blood to disturb the acid-base balance of body fluids. Aluminum hydroxide gel is a nonsystemic antacid because the cationic portion of the molecule forms an insoluble compound in combination with gastric acid, and so cannot dissociate in the intestine and be absorbed into the blood to alter the acid-base balance of body fluids.

25. (3) Aluminum hydroxide gel is formed when aluminum hydroxide and aluminum oxide are combined with water. The resulting preparation is insoluble in water, so it coats and protects the ulcer from further irritation by acid gastric juice. An astringent is a substance that shrinks and toughens tissues by exerting a slight protein-coagulating effect. When aluminum hydroxide reacts with hydrochloric acid, the resulting compound, aluminum chloride, has an astringent effect that affords still further protection to the eroded mucosa.

26. (2) Propantheline bromide is a synthetic cholinergic blocking agent thought to block impulses at the parasympathetic ganglia, as well as at the smooth muscle and gastric gland receptor sites. It produces parasympathetic effects similar to those of atropine without causing the CNS side effects of atropine and other naturally occurring anticholinergic alkaloids. Propantheline thus is used for its antispasmodic and antisecretory effects.

27. (3) All anticholinergics produce the following side effects: dry mouth, due to inhibition of saliva secretion; blurring of vision, due to mydriasis; and urinary retention, due to reduction in tone of the urinary bladder.

28. (3) Although the barbiturates are known to depress synaptic impulse transmission at several points in the central nervous system, cells in the reticular activating system of the midbrain and medulla are especially sensitive to depression by the barbiturates. Since this multineuronal, polysynaptic pathway is responsible for nervous activation in the wakefulness-sleep cycle, it is apparent that any drug that depresses the reticular activating system decreases wakefulness and predisposes the individual to sleep.

29. (2) Most of the drug is transformed by the liver to inactive metabolites and therefore phenobarbital should be administered with caution to patients with chronic liver disease.

30. (2) The symptoms of barbiturate toxicity are the result of extreme depression of the central nervous system; depression of the medullary respiratory center occurs early and produces shallow rapid respiration, with decreased minute volume, hypoxemia, and respiratory acidosis. If respiratory center depression persists for even a short time, atelectasis, pulmonary edema, and bronchopneumonia are apt to develop in short order.

31. (4) The typical patient with peptic ulcer disease is torn between strong dependency needs and a powerful drive toward self-sufficiency as a means of main-

taining self-pride. It is the stress of these opposing drives, expressed through increased parasympathetic activity, that predisposes to ulcer formation. Presumably, the degree of Mr. Gunderson's physiologic stress could be decreased if he were able to reduce his demands upon himself.

32. (4) The nurse should encourage Mr. Gunderson to explore the long-range importance of each of his former activities and decide which to retain and which to eliminate in order to reduce stress. By responding in a nondirective and reflective manner to his worries and concerns, the nurse can facilitate ventilation of feeling and objective problem solving. Controlled studies have shown that rest and adequate sleep are beneficial in treatment of peptic ulcer. If Mr. Gunderson can identify those situations that provoke or aggravate his ulcer symptoms, he can avoid potentially stressful circumstances.

33. (2) The foods in a Sippy diet are chemically and mechanically bland. Fried foods are mechanically irritating to gastric mucosa and chemically irritating in that they stimulate gastric secretion.

34. (3) Cooked, refined, whole-grain cereals, such as rice; pureed vegetables and cream soups, such as cream of pea soup; and milk products, such as cottage cheese, are allowed on a strict ulcer diet. All these foods are mechanically and chemically bland.

35. (3) Patients on a liberal ulcer diet may be given refined and finely ground cereals such as Cream of Wheat; cooked vegetables with low fiber content, such as baked potato; pureed vegetables, such as strained spinach; and boiled, broiled, or roasted low-fiber meats, such as chicken.

36. (4) Eating habits and dietary patterns acquired over many years are not easily relinquished. To be most effective, dietary instruction should be given in a series of brief, spaced encounters, with opportunities for repetition, questioning of key information, and simultaneous exposure of the patient and supportive family members to key dietary concepts and principles. Since Mr. Gunderson was removing himself prematurely from prescribed treatment out of concern for his business interests, it is likely that he would have paid little attention to the scanty information given him about food preparation, and would have no opportunity to correct misunderstandings or be given needed encouragement. Also his wife was not included in the dietary instruction.

37. (2) Peptic ulcer patients are advised not to drink coffee or tea because caffeine stimulates gastric secretions.

38. (1) The fact that Mr. Gunderson did not follow his prescribed ulcer diet or abstain from drinking coffee, although he continued to suffer ulcer symptoms and was repeatedly given dietary instruction by his physician, suggests denial of his illness. This might represent an inability to accept the role of invalid.

39. (3) Hemorrhage occurs in 15–20 per cent of ulcer patients. If vomiting develops, the vomitus will contain bright red blood. If blood remains in the stomach and is acted upon by acid gastric secretions, the blood in the vomitus will have a coffee-ground appearance. A large gastrointestinal hemorrhage, by reducing circulating blood volume suddenly and decreasing left ventricular output markedly, can reduce blood pressure to shock levels.

40. (3) An acute gastrointestinal hemorrhage invariably makes the patient very anxious. Some of this anxiety can be alleviated if a nurse, preferably one familiar to him, remains at his side throughout the initial physical examination. This will indicate her awareness of his anxiety and of the seriousness of the situation, and show that she is available to care for him and explain the procedures. After gastric suction siphonage is begun, the drainage bottle should be concealed from the patient's view so that he will not be upset by the amount of his blood loss.

41. (3) Both pain and anxiety tend to increase the respiratory rate. Massive gastrointestinal hemorrhage markedly decreases blood volume and lowers the oxygen-carrying capacity of the blood. In response to tissue anoxia, compensatory tachycardia and tachypnea develop. Although metabolic acidosis does produce increased respiratory rate, there is no reason to suppose that Mr. Gunderson has metabolic acidosis. Rather, loss of acid gastric secretions through prolonged vomiting would lead to metabolic alkalosis.

42. (4) Hydrochloric acid and smaller amounts of sodium and potassium chloride are lost with the gastric juice that is removed through suction siphonage. As more

and more hydrogen ions and chloride ions are lost from the stomach, more bicarbonate ions enter the circulation, rendering body fluids more basic.

43. (2) Although, theoretically, Mr. Gunderson has been under medical therapy for one year, he has not cooperated with the treatment regimen. There is no reason to suppose that he will do so in future, nor any certitude that if he were to cooperate his bleeding would not recur. Intractability of an ulcer to treatment is one indication for surgical treatment.

44. (3) The gastric glands in the fundus of the stomach secrete the gastric juices. A typical gastric gland consists of three types of cells, each of which produces mucus, pepsin, or hydrochloric acid. When food enters the gastric antrum, distending it, the hormone gastrin is released by the gastric mucosa and is carried by the blood to the gastric glands, where it stimulates the production of acid by the parietal cells as much as eightfold. Removal of the lower half of the stomach eliminates the gastrin mechanism for stimulation of gastric acid secretion.

45. (2) Because the common bile duct and the pancreatic duct both empty into the duodenum, and since the digestive juices carried by these ducts and produced by the small intestine wall are essential to digestion of the three major foodstuffs, the duodenum is not removed when a subtotal gastrectomy and gastroenterostomy are performed.

46. (1) Stimulation of the dorsal motor nuclei of the vagus nerves produces impulses that are carried by the vagus fibers to the gastric glands, where they cause secretion of large quantities of pepsin and hydrochloric acid. Stimulation of the vagus nerves also causes mucosal cells in the gastric antrum to secrete the hormone gastrin, which in turn stimulates the gastric glands to increased production of highly acid gastric juice. Section of the vagus nerves (vagotomy), by interrupting vagal impulses to gastric parietal cells and to the antrum, decreases hydrochloric acid production.

47. (2) A high abdominal incision is used in gastric surgery. Therefore, during the immediate postoperative period, Mr. Gunderson will experience considerable pain on deep breathing and coughing because marked descent of the diaphragm will compress surgically traumatized tissue. This will subject him to increased risk of atelectasis and pneumonia, owing to his understandable reluctance to breathe deeply.

48. (3) As a result of capillary oozing from the site of anastomosis, some dark red drainage may appear in Mr. Gunderson's gastric drainage for the first few hours following surgery. The appearance of a large quantity of bright red blood would suggest hemorrhage from the operative site. Yellow-green coloration would signify the presence of bile, which also would be abnormal. It would be unreasonable to expect clear and colorless gastric drainage for several days after surgery, as postsurgical inflammatory changes alone would result in production of pink and/or yellow exudate.

49. (1) Since the surgeon would have positioned the nasogastric tube during surgery so as to avoid any injury to the suture lines, the nurse should irrigate the nasogastric tube postoperatively. She should use only the prescribed fluid and prescribed force, as application of undue force against the suture line by catheter or irrigating solution may loosen sutures or dislodge clots, and reinstitute bleeding.

50. (3) Mucus and tissue shreds, decomposing clots, and other debris, if adherent to the suture line, could interfere with healing. Until fibrous connective tissue has firmly joined the surgically opposed gastric and jejunal walls, the anastomosis could pull apart, spilling gastric and intestinal content into the peritoneal cavity. Until vessels cauterized or ligated during surgery are completely obliterated by fibrous tissue, clots could be dislodged or ligatures released, and active bleeding resumed. With a nasogastric tube in place, such bleeding could be detected soon after occurrence.

51. (4) A patient with a nasogastric tube is usually plagued with a dry mouth, because mouth breathing is favored and because, without oral food intake, he lacks the primary stimulus to salivary secretion, chewing. Frequent oral hygiene, using soft sponges or applicators soaked in a mixture of glycerine and lemon juice, will increase the patient's comfort markedly. Glycerine has a demulcent or

soothing effect on mucous membranes; lemon juice stimulates salivation and relieves the sensation of thirst.

52. (3) Low Fowler's position permits lung expansion with least effort; increases coughing effectiveness and vital capacity; prevents reflux of gastric content into the lower esophagus (the cardiac sphincter is prevented from closure by presence of the nasogastric tube); and prevents pressure of lower abdominal viscera against the surgically traumatized stomach, duodenum, and jejunum.

53. (1) Mr. Gunderson's behavior represents both poles of the intrapsychic conflict experienced by the typical ulcer patient: on the one hand he has an overwhelming need to be cared for; on the other hand, pride requires that he reject both that need and the person who satisfies it.

54. (3) Manipulation of Mr. Gunderson's small bowel during surgery would have impaired normal peristaltic activity for some time following the procedure. Return of normal bowel sounds, which usually occurs on the second or third postoperative day, would signify that normal peristalsis had resumed, and that air and fluids would again begin to move along the tract toward the rectum. At this point, the nasogastric tube is usually removed.

55. (3) A clear liquid diet, used for postoperative patients, is an inadequate diet that consists chiefly of water and carbohydrates. Clear liquids are those that contain no solids and no gas-forming substances. Tea, bouillon, and clear gelatin are non-gas-forming.

56. (1) Milk produces gas as a result of the fermentation of milk sugar, lactose, by intestinal bacteria.

57. (4) All are allowable on a soft diet, which is used as a transition diet in conditions that require mechanical ease in eating and digestion. It is an adequate diet in that it contains the recommended daily dietary allowances of the major food groups, but is moderately low in cellulose and connective tissue.

58. (2) When a subtotal gastrectomy is performed, the reservoir function of the stomach is lost. Therefore, shortly after food is swallowed, it is mixed slightly with gastric juice and dumped quickly in largely undigested form into the jejunum. Once there, the undigested carbohydrate in the chyme is rapidly transformed into a hypertonic intestinal content that draws large volumes of fluid from the blood and intercellular spaces. The resultant drop in blood volume produces decreased cardiac output, and signs and symptoms characterizing shock.

59. (3) By eating frequent small meals, Mr. Gunderson can decrease the amount of food that enters his stomach with each meal, thereby reducing the volume of osmotically active particles to be dumped into the jejunum immediately after ingestion. By eliminating liquids from all meals, he can slow the passage of food from the stomach, thereby allowing some hydrolysis to take place in the stomach rather than in the jejunum. By reducing the amount of carbohydrate in the diet, he can increase the proportion of protein and fats, which will be less likely to produce troublesome osmotic effects in the jejunum as they are hydrolyzed less quickly into osmotically active particles. By lying down briefly after each meal, Mr. Gunderson can retard gastric emptying, allowing the oral and gastric digestive juices to mix with the food more adequately and hydrolysis to begin in the stomach rather than in the jejunum.

Pernicious Anemia

1. (4) The chest pain in pernicious anemia is usually anginal in type and is due to myocardial ischemia; the palpitations are the result of tachycardia. Both develop in response to tissue anoxia produced by decreased oxygen-carrying capacity of the blood. The indigestion is a result of secondary atrophy of epithelial cells of the tongue, stomach, and small intestine due to a defect in DNA synthesis, which is also the underlying cause of defective blood cell formation. When blood hemoglobin concentration decreases to the point that myocardial function is impaired, congestive heart failure will develop, followed by dyspnea, orthopnea, and pedal edema.

2. (3) In addition to defective DNA synthesis, vitamin B_{12} deficiency produces a defect in synthesizing myelin, with resulting neuropathy involving first the

peripheral nerves and subsequently the posterior and lateral columns of the spinal cord. Degeneration of peripheral nerves results in loss of position sense and muscle weakness. A footboard is therefore needed to support the weight of the upper bed linen and to maintain the feet in proper alignment to prevent foot drop. Extra blankets are the only safe means of keeping the lower extremities warm in a patient with pernicous anemia, since neurologic damage and loss of sensation make external heating devices dangerous.

3. (1) Dyspnea or difficult breathing, a subjective state of discomfort, is associated with severe anemia and characterized by hyperventilation. This situation represents a compensatory response to anoxia resulting from severely reduced blood hemoglobin concentration.

4. (2) Pernicious anemia is characterized by atrophic changes in the gastrointestinal epithelium, one manifestation of which is a smooth, beefy red tongue. Typically, the tongue is sore, which contributes to the patient's reluctance to eat properly. Creamed chicken is bland, and thus least likely to irritate the tongue.

5. (2) The pale yellow color of Mrs. White's skin undoubtedly indicates a minimal degree of jaundice. In pernicious anemia, lysis of increased numbers of red blood cells releases more hemoglobin than normal into the blood. More heme than normal is converted to unconjugated bilirubin and more unconjugated bilirubin is carried to the liver than can be converted by the liver cell to conjugated bilirubin. Hence, unconjugated bilirubin accumulates in the serum, raising the level of total serum bilirubin and increasing the icterus index to above normal levels.

6. (2) The macrocytic red blood cells seen in pernicious anemia are more fragile than normal red blood cells, and so more easily lyse as the cells squeeze through tissue capillaries. Hence, increased quantities of unconjugated bilirubin are found in the peripheral blood.

7. (4) Jaundice, or icterus, may be defined as yellowish discoloration of the skin, and is due to increased accumulation of bilirubin in body tissues. Because there is great individual variation in the amount of melanin deposition in the skin, the degree of jaundice is easiest to assess by observing the color of the sclera.

8. (4) The smooth, beefy red tongue seen in pernicious anemia is one manifestation of atrophy of gastrointestinal epithelium, which, like the anemia, is due to defective DNA synthesis secondary to a lack of vitamin B_{12}. It is likely that the same genetic defect that interferes with absorption of vitamin B_{12} may also interfere with absorption of vitamins B_1, B_2, and B_6. Mrs. White's sore red tongue may represent a combined vitamin B_{12} and vitamin B_2 deficiency.

9. (3) Vitamin B_{12} deficiency also produces a defect in myelin synthesis. A demyelinating neuropathy can develop, first in the peripheral nerves and later in the posterior and lateral columns of the spinal cord. If pernicious anemia is not treated promptly, and if the neurologic symptoms persist for longer than 12–18 months, the neurologic changes are apt to be irreversible, since the initial inability to synthesize myelin causes gradual deterioration of the axon, followed finally by deterioration of the cell body of the neuron.

10. (4) The demyelinating neuropathy caused by vitamin B_{12} deficiency, if untreated, involves the higher portions of the central nervous system also. Thus, any or all of the psychologic symptoms listed may occur.

11. (1) Most patients with pernicious anemia have a poor appetite, as a result of secondary atrophy of gastrointestinal epithelium and a lack of B complex vitamins. For the patient with severe glossitis and/or stomatitis, frequent oral hygiene may decrease oral discomfort and improve taste enough to increase interest in eating. Cotton-tipped applicators seem to be best suited to provide oral hygiene for a patient with severe stomatitis.

12. (3) In severe anemia, the tissue anoxia resulting from decreased transport of oxygen by the blood causes vessels in peripheral tissues to dilate. This increases venous return to the heart which is followed by increased heart rate and increased cardiac output.

13. (3) Ascending fibers in the dorsal columns of the cord transmit impulses deriving from vibratory, touch, kinesthetic, and pressure stimuli. Ascending fibers in the lateral columns of the cord transmit impulses deriving from pain, temperature, crude touch, and pressure stimuli. Fibers in both dorsal and lateral

portions of the cord become unmyelinated in untreated pernicious anemia. Mrs. White's complaints of numbness (a touch disorder) and tingling (a pain sensation) are the result of degeneration of fibers in the dorsal and lateral columns of the cord.

14. (4) A sore tongue and disordered taste buds contribute to poor eating habits. The demyelination of peripheral nerves, with decreased position sense, numbness, weakness, and spasticity, all interfere with the finely coordinated hand-to-mouth movements involved in feeding activities. Breathlessness, fatigue, and lassitide, resulting from tissue anoxia, together with CNS symptoms cause the pernicious anemia patient to eschew physical activity. Lack of exercise also contributes to failing appetite.

15. (4) During the last few weeks of gestation and after birth, red blood cells are produced in the bone marrow.

16. (3) Both red and white blood cells are derived from undifferentiated mesenchymal cells called "stem" cells, which differentiate into red cell, white cell, and platelet precursors. The hemocytoblast, the red blood cell precursor, is a large cell with a large nucleus. As the hemocytoblast is serially transformed to a mature erythrocyte, the cell and its nucleus become smaller; more hemoglobin is formed in the cell; and finally the nucleus is extruded, leaving the mature erythrocyte without a nucleus.

17. (2) The hemoglobin molecule is composed of a protein consisting of four polypeptide chains called "globin" and an iron-protoporphyrin compound called "heme."

18. (3) When normal red blood cells are discharged from bone marrow into the general circulation, their average life span is 120 days. As the cells age, they become progressively more fragile until they are broken down by the spleen or bone marrow.

19. (4) Most red blood cells are lysed in the spleen when they are forced through the red pulp of that organ.

20. (4) All anemias, whether resulting from decreased production of blood elements, excessive destruction of blood elements, or acute or chronic blood loss, are characterized by decreased oxygen-carrying capacity of the blood.

21. (3) In pernicious anemia, a genetically determined lack of an intrinsic factor normally secreted by gastric mucosa leads to inadequate absorption of vitamin B_{12}, which slows DNA synthesis and interferes most noticeably with replication of rapidly dividing cells of the marrow and gastrointestinal epithelium.

22. (3) Macrocyte means "large cell." In pernicious anemia, the gradual reduction in numbers of red blood cells leads eventually to a severe anemia or decreased oxygen-carrying capacity of the blood. The resulting tissue anoxia triggers marrow release of increased numbers of immature red blood cells into the general circulation. Hence, the peripheral blood shows greatly reduced numbers of red blood cells, a great proportion of which are larger than normal cells.

23. (3) The slowing of DNA synthesis produced by lack of vitamin B_{12} interferes with production of all three types of blood cells in the marrow. Thus, a patient with pernicious anemia demonstrates pancytopenia, or decreased numbers of mature red blood cells, white blood cells, and platelets in the peripheral blood.

24. (2) After birth, blood cell production occurs in the bone marrow. A small sample of red marrow from any one site has been found to be representative of the entire mass of red marrow in the body, regardless of location. In an adult, the sternum, the spinous process of the vertebrae, and the anterior or posterior iliac crest are readily accessible flat bones from which marrow can be obtained by needle biopsy with minimal risk to vital tissues. Because greater force is required to puncture the vertebral process than to puncture the outer table of the sternum, sternal puncture is used more frequently than vertebral puncture.

25. (4) This best expresses in lay terms the purpose of a marrow biopsy, and the salient steps of the procedure as the patient would experience them. Most lay persons would neither comprehend the scientific connotation of the word "tissue" nor be familiar with the usual site for marrow aspiration. They also would not understand the relationship between numbers and types of cells in the marrow and numbers and types of cells in the peripheral blood. The

nurse's deflection of a patient's question by suggesting the issue be discussed with a physician may be unfavorably interpreted as indicating either lack of knowledge by the nurse, lack of consideration for the patient's feelings, or unfavorable prognosis for illness.

26. (2) Tissue oxygenation is the basic regulator of red blood cell production in the bone marrow. When kidneys become hypoxic they release an enzyme into the blood that splits a glycoprotein called "erythropoietin" from one of the plasma proteins. Erythropoietin is carried by the blood to the bone marrow, where it stimulates red blood cell production. Within 2–5 days of the development of tissue oxygen lack and erythropoietin release, increased numbers of red blood cells begin to appear in peripheral blood.

27. (1) This best explains the purpose and procedure for gastric analysis in lay terms, and with reference to those points of procedure with which the patient would be most concerned. It is natural for a patient to dislike the prospect of having a tube inserted through his esophagus. It would increase, not decrease, his anxiety to tell him not to worry. Since most laymen would not understand the relationship between atrophy of gastrointestinal epithelium, lack of intrinsic factor, inadequate absorption of vitamin B_{12}, and marrow production of blood cells, reference to that chain of events would not answer Mrs. White's question satisfactorily.

28. (4) The nasogastric tube is needed for removal of gastric secretion. The metal basin is required so that the patient can expectorate all saliva and nasopharyngeal secretions while the gastric secretions are being aspirated. The bulb syringe will be needed to remove gastric secretions if manual aspiration is to be the method used. The hypodermic needle and syringe are necessary for administration of histamine, employed as a stimulant of gastric secretion. The electric suction machine should be available in case the physician prefers the machine to the syringe for continuous aspiration of gastric secretions.

29. (3) The pharmacologic effects of histamine are to dilate fine blood vessels, constrict the smooth muscles of the bronchioles, and increase secretion of the parietal and chief cells of the gastric mucosa.

30. (2) Histamine is metabolized by intestinal bacteria and is poorly absorbed from the intestine. Severe, rapid absorption of a parenterally administered dose of histamine can cause serious allergic reactions in sensitive individuals. The drug should be given hypodermically, since absorption from this route is slower than by the intramuscular or intravenous routes.

31. (1) In pernicious anemia, malabsorption of vitamin B_{12} leads to defective DNA synthesis. As a result atrophy of gastric mucosa occurs and causes impaired secretion of hydrochloric acid by parietal cells. Therefore, a histamine-fast achlorhydria is characteristic of pernicious anemia.

32. (2) The Schilling test determines whether B_{12} is or is not being absorbed from the gut. Intrinsic factor is needed for B_{12} to be absorbed. In pernicious anemia there is a lack of intrinsic factor. The test involves the oral administration of B_{12} tagged with ^{57}Co. All urine is collected for 24 hours and is examined for the degree of radioactivity of B_{12}. If the urinary excretion of ^{57}Co is more than 8 per cent of the dose given, this is normal and demonstrates that intrinsic factor is normal. If less than 8 per cent is recovered, the person is given another standard dose of ^{57}Co-labeled vitamin B_{12} orally, plus a capsule of intrinsic factor. Again, the urine is collected for 24 hours and tested for the amount of radioactivity. If more than 8 per cent of ^{57}Co-labeled B_{12} is recovered, the diagnosis of pernicious anemia is confirmed.

33. (1) Patients with pernicious anemia experience severe muscle weakness, lassitude, fatigue, and breathlessness. Patient comfort will be increased if nursing care procedures are interrupted from time to time to allow the patient to rest and regain strength.

34. (2) Weakness and lassitude favor immobility in the bedridden pernicious anemic patient. Decreased touch and pain sensation resulting from subacute combined degeneration of the spinal cord render the patient relatively insensitive to the discomforts usually associated with prolonged skin pressure and irritation. Thus, Mrs. White is at greater-than-normal risk of decubitus ulceration over bony prominences of the back and feet.

35. (3) The decreased oxygen-carrying capacity of the blood in anemia produces anoxia of all body tissues. In severe anemia, the combination of decreased blood viscosity and severe tissue anoxia so augments venous return as to increase cardiac output to two or three times normal. Marked increase in cardiac workload under conditions of myocardial anoxia predisposes to congestive heart failure.

36. (4) The psychologic symptoms of vitamin B_{12} deficiency include irritability, suspicion, confusion, and depression. This is due to demyelinizing changes in the cerebral white matter similar to those in the posterior and lateral columns of the spinal cord.

37. (3) Mrs. White has decreased pain and temperature sense in her legs and feet as a result of demyelizing of peripheral nerves and posterior and lateral columns of the cord. She would, therefore, be increasingly subject to burns following the local application of heat to lower extremities.

38. (3) Subacute combined degeneration of the cord renders Mrs. White weak, uncoordinated, unsteady, and unbalanced. Unless the side rails are elevated at night, she may easily lose her balance and fall from bed while in a confused or semi-awake state.

39. (2) As a result of the cerebral demyelinization associated with vitamin B_{12} deficiency, Mrs. White has been confused. Confused elderly patients are apt to become completely disoriented at night when visual clues to their whereabouts are lacking and auditory clues are diminished.

40. (3) Vitamin B_{12} deficiency is due to either lack of intrinsic factor or a defect in intestinal absorption. Since patients with pernicious anemia can absorb orally administered vitamin B_{12} when they are supplied with intrinsic factor, but fail to do so without concomitantly administered intrinsic factor, it is assumed that the cause of pernicious anemia is failure of the stomach to secrete intrinsic factor.

41. (3) The Schilling test demonstrates that the pernicious anemia patient is unable to absorb vitamin B_{12} from the gastrointestinal tract unless intrinsic factor is present in the tract. When not secreted by the gastric mucosal cells intrinsic factor can be supplied in the form of desiccated hog stomach.

42. (4) If Mrs. White's neurologic symptoms are of longer than 18 months' duration, it is likely that demyelinization of peripheral nerves and spinal cord tracts is complete, that both axons and cell bodies of involved neurons are dead, and that neurologic changes are irreversible.

43. (4) Exercise, by improving cerebral circulation, can help to improve morale in a depressed patient. Disuse of a muscle leads to atrophy and loss of contractile strength as a result of decreased circulation to, and nutrition of, the muscle fibrils. Active exercise is required to prevent muscle atrophy and maintain muscular strength and endurance. Normal motion of joints and soft tissues is maintained by movement of the body parts through full range of motion several times each day. Whenever normal range of motion is restricted by disease, enforced immobility, or disuse, the tissues become tight, limiting the arc of motion possible. Passive motion of a joint through full range of motion several times a day will help to prevent contracture deformities by relaxing muscle spasm and preventing fibrous tissue adhesions, but active exercise is required to prevent muscle atrophy and maintain muscle strength.

44. (1) Until parenteral vitamin B_{12} can correct Mrs. White's secondary atrophy of gastrointestinal epithelium, she will continue to be anorexic. In addition, lack of physical exercise eliminates the usual physiologic stimulus for hunger and makes eating unpleasant.

45. (2) This response best acknowledges Mrs. White's expression of feeling, while reinforcing the reality of her need for improved nutrition. Any attempt by the nurse to deny or minimize Mrs. White's fatigue would probably be interpreted as callous disregard for her feelings or lack of understanding of her illness.

46. (2) Adequate intake of all four basic food groups is essential if Mrs. White's long-term nutritional inadequacy is to be corrected. For example, parenteral administration of vitamin B_{12} alone, will not, correct her anemia. Protein and iron, as well as vitamin B_{12}, are required for adequate red blood cell formation. Further, the secondary atrophy of gastrointestinal epithelium has undoubtedly left Mrs. White with a deficiency of other B complex vitamins and trace

minerals. She may also demonstrate psychologic symptoms as a result of neurologic damage associated with her illness. It would not be unusual for a confused and suspicious older patient to develop irrational ideas about the food served to her. The nurse should explore Mrs. White's feelings about food in order to determine whether unrealistic fears are contributing to her disinclination toward eating.

47. (3) Pepsin in most active at pH of 2 and completely inactive at a pH above 5. Typically, a histamine-fast achlorhydria is found in patients with pernicious anemia, so that it is customary to administer a few drops of dilute hydrochloric acid to such patients in conjunction with each meal. In this way the acidity of gastric content is assured, so that pepsin is able to hydrolyze protein during the gastric phase of digestion.

48. (2) The dilute hydrochloric acid given Mrs. White should be further diluted in 150–250 ml. of water and sipped through a glass straw, so as to avoid damaging the teeth through the solvent effect of the acid on tooth enamel.

49. (2) This is the item that would most contribute to Mrs. White's comfort and pleasure without at the same time constituting a hazard. For example, the ingestion of chocolate candy would be apt to suppress her already scant appetite for nutritious food. Her muscular weakness and incoordination would make it difficult or impossible to do embroidery. For as long as complete bedrest is prescribed, it is unwise to bring a confused elderly patient a gift of house slippers.

50. (3) The loss of position sense, which results from demyelinizing of fibers in the peripheral nerves and spinal cord, predisposes Mrs. White to foot drop. Since she is unaware of the position of her feet, they could easily be pulled by the weight of the upper bed linen into a position of plantar flexion, and remain thus because of her lack of pain perception.

51. (3) By properly alligning the patient's feet so that the foot is at right angles with the lower leg several times throughout the day, the nurse can ensure that Mrs. White does not remain in a nonfunctional position in which muscular contractions and ligamental shortening could produce foot drop. If Mrs. White is encouraged to push her feet alternately against the footboard, whatever proprioceptive impulses the diseased neurons can transmit will be stimulated, thus preparing her for retraining in walking.

52. (1) Reticulocytes are the immediate precursors of mature red blood cells, and normally are not seen in peripheral blood in concentrations exceeding 0.5–1.5 per cent of total erythrocytes. The appearance of increased numbers of reticulocytes in peripheral blood would indicate that Mrs. White's marrow had begun to increase production of red blood cells, which is the desired effect of vitamin B_{12} therapy.

53. (3) Since Mrs. White's neurologic changes are probably irreversible, the weakness and incoordination that she evidenced on admission will not have disappeared after three weeks of vitamin B_{12} therapy. Twenty-one days of bedrest have probably decreased her muscular tone and strength despite the active exercises used to prevent muscle atrophy. The combined effects of neurologic defects and prolonged immobility will render Mrs. White especially susceptible to falls on the first few occasions that she attempts to resume walking.

54. (4) Muscle meats are a primary source of the protein, vitamins, and minerals needed to produce blood cells, improve appetite, and restore lost skeletal muscle mass.

55. (2) Mrs. White's nutritional inadequacies are multiple and of long duration. Since maintenance of optimal nutrition is essential to her welfare, she must be instructed in the purpose of both and their importance to her future health.

56. (4) Mrs. White's inability to secrete intrinsic factor is a permanent and irreversible defect. She will continue to be unable to absorb vitamin B_{12} from her bowel, and must continue to receive vitamin B_{12} by parenteral means for the rest of her life.

Cholelithiasis and Cholecystectomy

1. (3) The Thoma glass pipette is a graduated capillary tube divided into 10 parts, above which is a mixing bulb containing a glass bead. The volume of the *red*

blood cell pipette is such as to effect a 1:200 mixture of blood to diluent. The volume of the *white* blood cell pipette is such as to effect a 1:20 mixture of blood to diluent. A piece of heavy-walled rubber tubing with mouthpiece is attached to the upper end of each pipette. A microscope is an instrument consisting of two or more magnifying lenses, with a light source that is used to produce a magnified image of a small object, such as a blood cell. A hemoglobinometer is a device to permit measurement of the concentration of hemoglobin in a sample of blood.

2. (3) A protein pyrogen which is released from polymorphonuclear white blood cells or from tissue cells that have been injured by bacteria is carried by the blood to the hypothalamus, where the pyrogen "resets" the temperature-regulating center for a higer-than-normal temperature. Irritation of the gallbladder wall causes inflammation of the tissues, characterized by an increase in the number of circulating white blood cells.

3. (3) The gallbladder, a long, hollow, pear-shaped, musculomembranous sac located on the undersurface of the right lobe of the liver, with a capacity of 45 ml., stores and concentrates bile. When stimulated by the hormone cholecystokinin, it contracts, thereby expelling bile through the cystic and common bile ducts into the duodenum.

4. (2) Vague digestive complaints, such as postprandial belching and distention, are common in patients with cholecystitis, and are due to reflex disorders of gastrointestinal motility associated with inflammation of the gallbladder and gall ducts and decreased bile supply to the duodenum.

5. (4) When red blood cells are broken down in the spleen, heme is converted by reticuloendothelial cells to unconjugated bilirubin, which is quickly bound to albumin and carried to the liver. This complex is too large to be filtered through the glomerular membrane so it is not excreted in the urine. In the liver, albumin is split from the bilirubin molecule, which is conjugated with glucuronic acid to form bilirubin diglucuronide, which is secreted in the bile. Bacterial action in the intestine converts conjugated bilirubin into urobilinogen, some of which is excreted in the stool, and the remainder of which is absorbed into the blood. Of the urobilinogen that is absorbed, a portion is excreted in the urine, and the rest is returned to the liver for reuse in bile synthesis. Therefore, there is normally no bile, but a trace of urobilinogen, in the urine.

6. (4) Once in the intestine, conjugated bilirubin, which is water-soluble, is converted by the normal bacterial inhabitants of the bowel into urobilinogen. Bacteroides, lactobacilli, and coliform bacteria are common inhabitants of the lower intestinal tract.

7. (3) The kidneys can excrete conjugated, but not unconjugated, bilirubin. Therefore, in severe obstructive jaundice, when unconjugated bilirubin can still be conjugated by the liver cell, but cannot pass in bile to the intestine, large quantities of conjugated bilirubin are returned to the blood through rupture of distended bile canaliculi, and appear in the urine, coloring it brown.

8. (1) When the hepatic or common bile duct is completely obstructed by tumor, stone, or edema, bile produced by the liver cells accumulates in the intrahepatic bile ducts; pressure increases, rupturing the canaliculi, and bile empties directly into the lymph or portal blood leaving the liver. Since conjugated bilirubin can be excreted by the kidney, bile appears in the urine.

9. (1) The onset of symptoms in acute cholecystitis results from vigorous attempts by the gallbladder to empty its content following ingestion of a heavy fatty or fried meal. The presence of fat and peptides in the duodenum causes release of cholecystokinin by duodenal mucosa, which stimulates the gallbladder to contract and the sphincter of Oddi to relax so as to discharge bile into the duodenum. Biliary colic is a severe, intermittent, cramping pain, occurring in waves, which results from acute distention of the biliary tract with bile, pus, or mucus, together with inability to empty the biliary tract despite strong, wringing contractions of the blocked structure.

10. (1) Meperidine is a synthetic CNS depressant with analgesic, sedative, euphoric, and respiratory depressant effects similar to those of morphine, but of shorter duration (2–4 hours). In equi-analgesic doses, meperidine produces less spasm of the biliary tract and less rise in pressure in the common bile duct than does morphine.

11. (3) In order to ensure that each ordered dose of medicine is administered to the correct person, the nurse should ask the patient to state her first and last names. If she were to call the patient by name and wait for an appropriate response, a confused or deaf patient might respond affirmatively even when addressed by the wrong name. Also, it is possible to have two patients with the same surname in the unit at the same time.

12. (4) Atropine, a derivative of belladonna, is a naturally occurring alkaloid that antagonizes acetylcholine, thereby acting primary as a parasympathetic nervous system depressant, but having certain CNS effects as well. Its principal effects include decreased secretion of saliva and gastric juice; decreased motility of the gastrointestinal tract; decreased tone and motility of ureters and urinary bladder; decreased respiratory secretions; relaxation of bronchial and bronchiolar muscles; increased heart rate; pupillary dilation; and paralysis of the muscles of accommodation.

13. (1) The upper arm, over the region of the deltoid muscle, is a preferred site for hypodermic administration of drugs since the site is easily accessible and the underlying bone, blood vessels, and nerves are well protected by a large mass of muscle.

14. (4) It is easier to insert a needle into firmly held tissue than easily displaced tissue. The discomfort associated with needle insertion can be reduced by providing pressure on surrounding tissue, which interferes with impulse transmission through sensory nerves, and distracts attention from the sensation of mild pain by interposing a sensation of strong pressure. The tissue should be lifted away from underlying bone, as injury to the periosteum causes severe pain.

15. (4) Rubbing will cause local vasodilation, fostering absorption of the drug from intercellular spaces.

16. (2) By insertion of the needle at a 45° angle, the medicine can most easily be delivered into the loose areolar tissue below the skin but above the muscle.

17. (2) The colicky pain is the result of strong, episodic, wringing contractions of smooth muscles lining the gallbladder and bile ducts. Atropine, through its parasympatholytic activity, decreases the tone and relaxes spasm of smooth muscles of the gastrointestinal tract and related structures.

18. (2) Dry mouth and dilated pupils are the anticipated pharmacologic effects of the drug, which causes decreased secretion of saliva and blocked response to acetylcholine stimulation by the sphincter muscle of the iris.

19. (4) Physostigmine, an anticholinesterase or parasympathomimetic drug, antagonizes both the parasympatholytic effect and the CNS effects of atropine.

20. (4) This is the one truthful, nonevasive, and supportive response. Sending a concerned relative into another room or directing him to the patient's physician for information constitute an omission of the nurse's responsibility to provide moral support to the patient and family. Although the exact nature of Mrs. Peach's illness is not yet known, her husband should be relieved to learn that she has been given an analgesic.

21. (4) Biliary cirrhosis, or chronic, progressive, fibrotic liver destruction, can be a complication of bile duct obstruction in which liver parenchymal cells are destroyed and replaced with fibrous tissue, with consequent distortion of liver architecture. Inflammatory changes in liver parenchyma interfere with glycogenesis, and decreased glycogen stores render liver cells more susceptible to viral and chemical injury. It is thought that administration of intravenous glucose solution forces deposition of glycogen into liver cells, increasing their resistance to injury by retained bile pigments.

22. (3) Pledgets are needed to cleanse the venipuncture site with antiseptic solution. An armboard is necessary to immobilize Mrs. Peach's arm to prevent her from dislodging the needle or angiocatheter. Adhesive tape is required to immobilize the needle shaft or catheter connector, to label the venipuncture site, and to secure the tubing to the arm so as to eliminate "drag" on the needle. A small basin is needed to collect fluid when the intravenous fluid line is cleared of air.

23. (4) Any of the problems listed may arise during intravenous infusion of fluid. The infusion should be checked at regular intervals and corrected as appropriate.

24. (2) Bacterial infection of the wall of the gallbladder and bile ducts produces inflammatory changes in these tissues, which could increase biliary obstruc-

tion to an even greater degree. Cephalothin (Keflin) exhibits bactericidal effects against many gram-positive and gram-negative organisms. Since many of these organisms have been cultured from acutely and chronically inflamed gallbladders, cephalothin is used to treat Mrs. Peach for gallbladder infection.

25. (2) Intravenous infusion of cephalothin is frequently associated with the development of phlebitis of the vessel used for infusion.

26. (2) This position effects maximal relaxation of the gluteal muscles, and clarifies the landmark to be used in locating the proper site for intramuscular injection, which is a point 2 inches below the iliac crest within the upper outer quadrant of the buttock.

27. (4) When administering a medication by the intramuscular route, a long No. 19–No. 22 needle should be introduced at a 90° angle, so as to inject the medicine deep into the belly of the muscle.

28. (2) Intramuscular medicine should be injected in muscular tissue, and absorbed slowly from the injection site into blood vessels traversing the tissues. A drug preparation suitable for intramuscular administration may be unsuitable for intravenous administration because it is irritating to vascular linings. It is possible, when injecting a drug into a large muscle, for the tip of the needle to enter a blood vessel. After injection, the plunger should be drawn back slightly. If the needle has inadvertently entered a blood vessel, blood will be drawn into the syringe. If this occurs, the syringe and needle should be withdrawn slightly, and the plunger again drawn back slightly to determine whether the needle is still in the blood vessel. If no blood is aspirated, the drug can be injected into the tissues.

29. (3) Tetracycline is a semisynthetic, broad-spectrum antibiotic effective against a broad range of gram-positive and gram-negative bacteria. However, as the count of coliform organisms in the feces declines, any organisms that have acquired resistance to the drug, such as *Proteus* and *Pseudomonas*, may overgrow and cause severe diarrhea.

30. (3) Gallstones may be composed of cholesterol, bile pigments, and calcium salts, either singly or in varying combinations. Most mixed stones are not radiopaque. Stones that are composed principally of calcium salts are radiopaque.

31. (3) When the pyloric sphincter opens and chyme enters the duodenum, fat and peptides in the food mixture cause the duodenal mucosa to produce the enzyme cholecytokinin, which is absorbed into the blood and carried to the gallbladder. It causes the gallbladder muscles to contract, ejecting bile through the cystic and common bile ducts into the duodenum.

32. (4) All are gas-forming foods, as are many high-residue, strongly flavored vegetables and fruits.

33. (2) Stercobilin, an oxidation product of urobilinogen, is largely responsible for the brown color of stools. In severe or complete obstruction of the hepatic and common bile duct, no bile is able to reach the intestine; consequently, no conjugated bilirubin can be acted upon by intestinal bacteria to yield urobilinogen, which cannot then be oxidized to form stercobilin. The feces therefore are not brown, but clay-colored.

34. (3) To halt bile flow from the liver to the duodenum, either the hepatic or the common bile duct must be completely obstructed. Since Mrs. Peach's history and physical findings are those of gallbladder disease, it is reasonable to suppose that she has had this disease for several months or years, and that her recurrent episodes of jaundice and clay-colored stools represent occasions on which stones have passed from her gallbladder, traversed the cystic duct, and lodged for a time in the common bile duct, blocking it completely.

35. (4) Chemical analysis has shown some gallstones to be composed wholly of cholesterol, bile pigments, or calcium salts. Most are a mixture of all three substances.

36. (1) Hypercholesterolemia, which is commonly seen in pregnant patients, those with diabetes or hypothyroidism, or those who ingest a high-fat diet, predisposes to gallstone formation because the liver cell produces cholesterol from free fatty acids and secretes it in the bile. Cholesterol is only minimally soluble in water, and bile is an aqueous medium.

37. (3) Cholesterol occurs in large amounts in egg yolk, and in moderate amounts in

meat fat, whole milk, and milk products. Neither corn oil nor margarine contains cholesterol.

38. (1) Stagnation of bile favors the precipitation of cholesterol, bile pigments, and/or calcium salts from solution in the bile, by encouraging greater-than-normal concentration of the bile.

39. (2) Infection of the gallbladder or ducts causes roughening of the mucosal lining, an outpouring of excess mucus, and sloughing of cells from the mucosal surface. Aggregations of inflammatory debris may serve as a nidus or focal point about which crystals of cholesterol, bile pigment, or calcium may collect.

40. (3) The normal upper limit for direct serum bilirubin is 0.4 mg./100 ml.; for indirect serum bilirubin, 1.1 mg./100 ml.; and thus for total serum bilirubin is 1.5 mg./100 ml.

41. (2) Jaundice does not become apparent until the concentration exceeds 4 mg./100 ml.

42. (3) It probably is obstructive, owing to blockage of the common bile duct with gallstones.

43. (1) An excess of bile acids and bile salts in the blood and tissues causes itching. Sodium bicarbonate is an alkaline sodium salt that is sometimes effective in relieving pruritus when applied locally in weak solution. Its effect is presumably due to its ability to neutralize acidic ions which are eliminated in the sweat.

44. (3) Intermittent jaundice is apt to be the result of gallstones. Sometimes a single irregularly shaped stone produces intermittent jaundice when it shifts its position within the duct, so that the duct is first completely obstructed; then partially obstructed, allowing some bile flow to the duodenum; and then completely obstructed again. Intermittent jaundice sometimes results from passage of one stone after another from the gallbladder into the common bile duct, with each stone totally obstructing the duct during its passage from cystic duct to duodenum.

45. (3) Chocolate, nuts, and bacon are all high in fat content.

46. (1) This response is truthful, reflecting the reality of Mrs. Peach's need for continuing medical supervision, without using a threat to ensure compliance with the treatment plan.

47. (3) The inflammatory changes that take place in the gallbladder wall of a patient with gallstones may progress to empyema, if retained bile becomes grossly contaminated. This could cause gangrene and rupture of the gallbladder. With rupture, bile and purulent material would spill into the peritoneal cavity, producing chemical and bacterial peritonitis. Recurrent common bile duct obstruction, with concomitant bile stagnation and pressure rise in intrahepatic bile ducts, could produce chronic inflammation and fibrosis of the periportal tissues of the liver, or biliary cirrhosis.

48. (1) A cholecystogram, or roentgenogram of the gallbladder, is used to visualize its size and condition and to look for evidence of gallstones.

49. (2) Since pure cholesterol and pure pigment stones are radiolucent, and only 10–15 per cent of gallstones contain enough calcium to be radiopaque, it is customary in preparing a patient for a cholecystogram to administer an iodine-containing dye in oral form. The dye is absorbed from the gut, excreted in the bile, and concentrated in the gallbladder. On x-ray examination, the gallbladder is visualized as a radiopaque shadow, and the stones, if present, will appear as radiolucent defects in that shadow.

50. (4) From 10 to 12 hours are required for the orally administered dye to reach the duodenum, be absorbed into the blood, carried to the liver, excreted in the bile, carried to the gallbladder, and dehydrated sufficiently to outline the gallbladder on the x-ray film.

51. (3) Some persons who are sensitive to iodinated compounds may suffer nausea and vomiting following orally administered dye. The nurse should therefore check to ensure that the dye is retained. If it is lost through vomiting, the gallbladder will not visualize on x-ray examination. Consequently, the radiologist might assume incorrectly either that the liver is incapable of excreting the dye, that the hepatic or cystic duct is blocked, or that the gallbladder is incapable of concentrating the dye.

52. (4) If stones are not obvious in a cholecystogram taken after oral administration of an iodine dye, a fatty meal is given to stimulate gallbladder evacuation so as to enhance detection of low-density, calcium-containing stones, which would be obscured by a heavy concentration of dye in the gallbladder.

53. (3) The iodine dye used for gallbladder visualization is excreted by the kidneys. As a result of irritation of renal tissues by the dye, its excretion is sometimes accompanied by temporary pain in the region of the kidney.

54. (1) In order for oral administration of the iodine-containing dye to outline the gallbladder on x-ray examination, the dye must reach the duodenum, be absorbed into the blood, be excreted by the liver, and be concentrated by the gallbladder. Omission of any of these steps would result in nonvisualization of the gallbladder on the radiograph. Thus, decreased intestinal absorption of dye or inability of the liver to excrete the dye, as in parenchymal liver disease, would render the test inconclusive.

55. (2) Sodium iodipamide is a radiopaque medium used for slow intravenous cholangiography. Following intravenous injection, it is carried to the liver, where it is rapidly excreted. The contrast medium appears in the bile, permitting visualization of hepatic and common bile ducts. Intravenous cholecystography is used when oral cholecystography is not effective.

56. (1) Sodium iodipamide appears in the bile within 10–15 minutes following intravenous injection, so films can be taken 10–20 minutes after the infusion.

57. (2) In iodine-sensitive individuals it is possible for sodium iodipamide to cause anaphylactic reaction, with sudden fall of blood pressure to shock levels, so it should not be given to such patients.

58. (2) Surgery constitutes a metabolic as well as a physical stress upon the organism. Since the liver is a multipurpose organ involved in many metabolic functions, and since Mrs. Peach's gallbladder disease may have predisposed her to liver parenchymal injury, liver function tests should be done to determine her ability to withstand the stress of major surgery.

59. (4) Total and direct serum bilirubin concentrations are tests of liver functions since it is the function of the liver cells to absorb and change unconjugated bilirubin to conjugated bilirubin and excrete it as bile. Since the normal ratio of direct or conjugated bilirubin to total bilirubin is known, this is the mode of measuring parenchymal liver cell efficiency. Alkaline phosphatase, an enzyme produced mainly in bone, is normally removed from the blood by the liver cell and excreted in the bile. In parenchymatous liver disease and biliary tract disease, as well as in various bone diseases, there is apt to be an increase of alkaline phosphatase in the serum. The plasma proteins, i.e., serum albumin and alpha and beta globulin, are synthesized in the liver cell. Albumin synthesis is reduced in liver cell damage, as in hepatic necrosis and cirrhosis. Alpha and beta globulins are increased in liver infections, such as viral hepatitis, and in obstructive jaundice. They fall in patients with hepatocellular injury, such as cirrhosis and hepatic necrosis. Prothrombin is produced in the liver cell. Therefore, a prolongation of prothrombin time is typically seen in hepatitis, cirrhosis, and chronic bile duct obstruction. Serum flocculation tests are nonspecific tests in which plasma proteins that are abnormal in quality or quantity are precipitated by various agents.

60. (3) The van den Bergh test is used to measure the amount of unconjugated (indirect) and conjugated (direct) reacting bilirubin in the serum. Conjugated bilirubin yields a magenta color almost immediately after the addition of Ehrlich's diazo reagent to the serum. For unconjugated bilirubin to yield the magenta color, methyl alcohol as well as Ehrlich's reagent must be added to the serum.

61. (2) Serum alkaline phosphatase is an enzyme produced by many body tissues, including the liver. Normally, most of the alkaline phosphatase in the serum is that produced by bone. In cholestasis, the liver cells or the bile ducts produce and release increased quantities of alkaline phosphatase. Thus, serum alkaline phosphatase levels tend to rise in obstructive jaundice.

62. (2) The normal serum albumin level is 3.5–5.0 grams/100 ml. The normal serum globulin level is 2–3.5 grams/100 ml. Thus, the normal ratio between the two is roughly 2:1.

63. (1) Since all serum albumin is synthesized in the liver cell, and only part of the

serum globulins are produced in the liver cell (gamma globulin is also synthesized in the spleen and lymph nodes), parenchymal liver cell disease decreases albumin production to a greater extent than globulin production.

64. (2) Prothrombin, the precursor of thrombin, is instrumental in converting a precursor to fibrin strands, which entangle the cells in the blood-clotting reaction.

65. (2) The cephalin-cholesterol flocculation test is a nonspecific test of liver function. A positive test indicates only that there has been some quantitative or qualitative change in a serum protein synthesized in the liver.

66. (3) Since any factor that interferes with pulmonary ventilation, gas diffusion, or alveolar perfusion would complicate inhalation anesthesia, a chest x-ray is performed preoperatively to screen the patient for evidence of cardiac or respiratory problems that would indicate the need for further workup.

67. (3) Vitamin K, a fat-soluble vitamin absorbed from the small bowel, requires the presence of bile in the gut. In obstructive jaundice no bile is in the gut, so the vitamin K needed for blood clotting is not absorbed.

68. (2) Hemorrhage is a common, much-feared postoperative complication. Mrs. Peach's prolonged clotting time is undoubtedly due to decreased prothrombin production associated with obstructive jaundice. Vitamin K is being given parenterally to increase the prothrombin level and ensure normal clotting time.

69. (2) Vitamin K is required by the liver cell in synthesizing prothrombin, as well as factors VII, IX, and X. In the absence of vitamin K, the concentration of these four substances falls so low as to interfere significantly with normal blood clotting.

70. (1) Bile salts emulsify fat particles in the intestine and assist the absorption of fatty acids from the gut. When fats are not absorbed adequately from the gut, fat-soluble vitamins, including vitamin K are also poorly absorbed. Little vitamin K is stored in the body, so within only a few days after bile secretion ceases, the patient develops a vitamin K deficiency.

71. (3) Obese patients have increased susceptibility to atherosclerosis and to arteriosclerotic cardiovascular disease.

72. (2) It is desirable that Mrs. Peach remain immobile during the 10–15 minutes required to make the EKG tracings, in order to eliminate skeletal muscle contractions that would create artefacts in the record of cardiac impulse transmission. She will be more apt to lie quietly if she is in a state of emotional and physical relaxation. A full explanation of the purpose and nature of the EKG relieves anxiety and promotes mental relaxation. Placement in supine position and attention to physical comfort predisposes to physical relaxation. An electrolyte-containing jelly must be used on the skin areas to which EKG electrodes are attached, in order to facilitate transmission of low-voltage current from the body surface to the galvanometer.

73. (3) Each anesthetic agent and drug given during the intraoperative period has predictable pharmacologic, and possible toxic, effects that must be watched for during the immediate postoperative period. The nurse should check Mrs. Peach's operative record to learn which anesthetic(s) and associated drugs were given during surgery, the dosage and times of administration of each, and any untoward effects that developed during the intraoperative period.

74. (3) Gallbladder surgery is apt to be lengthy, so there is opportunity for significant blood loss. If preoperative administration of vitamin K has not corrected lowered prothrombin levels, additional blood may be lost as a result of a clotting disorder. Hemorrhage results in a decrease in circulating blood volume and a subsequent fall in systemic blood pressure. Because the oxygen demand of liver cells is high, and because long-standing biliary obstruction may have compromised blood supply to the liver's parenchymal cells, it is important to protect the liver from increased injury due to anoxia during the surgical procedure. By administering blood during surgery, the oxygen-carrying power of the blood can be maintained at a level that protects the liver cells from further injury.

75. (3) During the removal of the gallbladder and the insertion of the T tube, it is common to spill some bile and blood into the peritoneal cavity that cannot be

completely removed during the procedure. A Penrose, or soft rubber drain, left in place in the gallbladder bed and brought through the closed skin incision, provides a channel through which such foreign material can drain to the surface during postoperative healing.

76. (4) The common bile duct is apt to be edematous following surgery as a result of tissue manipulation. In order to prevent postoperative obstruction of the common bile duct by swelling, and to facilitate bile drainage to the body surface until edema subsides, a T tube is placed in the common bile duct, with short arms directed toward the hepatic duct and the duodenum, and the long arm brought through a stab wound in the right upper quadrant and sutured to the skin.

77. (4) The effects of anesthesia or drugs administered during the perioperative period may produce nausea and vomiting. Manipulation of the small bowel during surgery interrupts peristalsis for 2–3 days following surgery, interfering with the normal movement of gas and fluids through the intestinal tract. Vigorous or prolonged vomiting would place a strain on the suture lines, and subject Mrs. Peach to the dangers of aspiration pneumonia and/or electrolyte imbalance. By maintaining nasogastric suction siphonage or 2–3 days following surgery, gastrointestinal secretions can be removed continuously so as to prevent gastric distention, which would decrease respiratory excursions, and prevent vomiting, which could dislodge strategic sutures and drains.

78. (2) Normal saline is preferred to water for irrigating a nasogastric tube because it is isotonic with body fluids, and thus less likely to upset acid-base balance if large quantities of irrigating solution must be used.

79. (2) As a result of the high abdominal incision and tissue manipulation during surgery, the patient experiences severe discomfort on deep breathing during the early postoperative period. To compensate for this, the patient tends to breathe shallowly, to avoid coughing deeply, and to move about as little as possible. Restriction of respiratory movement impedes re-expansion of collapsed alveoli and removal of tracheobronchial secretions; there is thus a tendency for retained secretions to become dehydrated and secondarily infected, and for bronchopneumonia to develop.

80. (3) After recovery from anesthesia, Mrs. Peach will be most comfortable in low Fowler's, since that position facilitates greatest chest expansion with least expenditure of muscular effort, and favors drainage of bile from the T tube, thus decompressing edematous bile ducts.

81. (4) The bile and blood spilled in the peritoneal cavity during surgery is apt to pool behind and above the liver; elevating the bed head about 30° facilitates drainage of these materials from the subphrenic space to the point where the Penrose drain exits the anterior abdominal wall. In this position gravity will assist bile drainage through the hepatic duct to the long arm of the T tube to the skin, thereby decompressing the common bile duct and relieving pressure on the duct suture line.

82. (2) Because the danger of postoperative hemorrhage is greatest immediately following the patient's return to the Recovery Room, and under ordinary circumstances decreases from that point, the wound dressings should be checked every 15 minutes for two hours, then every 30 minutes for two hours, and then less frequently.

83. (4) Pulmonary complications are most apt to develop within the first 48 hours following surgery. The irritating effect of the endotracheal tube, the anesthetic agent, and the oxygen all tend to increase tracheobronchial secretions. Immobilization of the patient during the lengthy surgical procedure predisposes to atelectasis in dependent portions of the lung. Aspiration of secretions is most apt to occur during the immediate postanesthetic period while the glottic and cough reflexes are obtunded by drugs. Thus, it is imperative that Mrs. Peach be stimulated to turn, cough, and deep breathe at frequent intervals during the first 24 postoperative hours, to remove secretions and re-expand collapsed alveoli.

84. (4) Regular oral hygiene will remove accumulated secretions and pathogens from the oral cavity which, if aspirated, would cause bronchopneumonia. Side-to-side or side-to-back changes in position every one to two hours can prevent atelectasis of dependent lung tissue, and encourage perfusion and

aeration of both lungs. Deep breathing and coughing, by increasing negative intrapleural and positive intrapulmonary pressures, facilitates re-expansion of collapsed alveoli. Frequent monitoring of respiratory functions enables the nurse to identify complications and institute appropriate emergency measures rapidly.

85. (3) Moist heat causes dilation of blood vessels, and fosters absorption of excess interstitial fluid and foreign substances from intercellular spaces into tissue capillaries.

86. (3) Bile facilitates fat digestion, absorption of vitamins from the bowel, and neutralization of acidic chyme as it enters the duodenum. If common bile duct edema is severe following surgery, causing excessive bile losses through the T tube, this bile can be recycled by administering it through the nasogastric tube so as not to lose normal physiologic effect during the early postoperative period.

87. (3) Visual and olfactory cues are influential in regulating the flow of digestive juices. Bile has an unpleasant appearance, so Mrs. Peach's comfort during administration of T tube drainage through her nasogastric tube will be increased if her view of the material is obstructed in some way.

88. (4) The gallbladder is not essential to life. Its surgical removal does not interfere with good health, and in most patients causes only mild, if any, physiologic disturbances. Only 25 per cent of those who undergo cholecystectomy have mild symptoms following surgery.

Cerebrovascular Accident

1. (4) The signs and symptoms of intracerebral hemorrhage vary with the site and extent of blood seepage into brain tissue. Severe headache frequently occurs owing either to meningeal irritation or to sudden increase in intracranial pressure. Hemorrhage into the internal capsule can cause unilateral weakness of facial muscles with resultant sagging. If the motor speech cortex or associated fibers are involved, speech will be slurred or the patient will be aphasic. Hemorrhage into the motor cortex or the pyramidal tracts will result in weakness or paralysis of muscles of the arm and leg on the side of the body opposite that of the cerebral lesion. Vomiting occurs with increased intracranial pressure.

2. (1) Mr. Crown's hypertension on admission, together with narrowing and tortuosity of retinal vessels and moderate cardiac enlargement, suggests that he had been hypertensive for several years, which could have damaged blood vessel walls. Weakened cerebral blood vessels are most apt to rupture at the site of arterial microaneurysms, small congenital sacculations that occur at the bifurcations of the circle of Willis.

3. (3) The pulse is typically full and bounding, reflecting both the higher-than-normal mean arterial pressure and the increase in intracranial pressure.

4. (2) If a cerebrovascular hemorrhage does not provoke circulatory collapse, the high pulse pressure produced by the recent rise in systolic pressure results in flushing of the skin, with an increase in skin temperature.

5. (3) Deep coma is characterized by complete insensibility, loss of purposeful motion, incontinence, absent reflexes, nonreaction to painful stimuli, and (often) depressed respirations.

6. (2) During his first few hours of hospitalization Mr. Crown's greatest potential problem is aspiration of vomitus or nasopharyngeal secretions. Thus, the tracheal suction machine is most critical to his welfare.

7. (3) The collar should be loosened in order to facilitate respiration and to assist venous drainage from the head so as to minimize cerebral edema. Padded side rails should be applied to protect Mr. Crown from falls and fractures, since convulsions may occur following intracerbral hemorrhage.

8. (4) Arteriosclerosis, the deposition of atheromatous plaque beneath the intima of arteries with calcification, causes the vessels to become rigid and occludes the smaller vessels that nourish the arterial wall. Ischemia of a vessel wall leads to destruction of elastic fibers of the media, which together with subintimal calcification decreases the vessel's elasticity.

9. (4) Inadequate perfusion of the kidney cortex stimulates the release of renin, a potential vasoconstrictor, which by increasing peripheral resistance raises blood pressure. Sustained sympathetic stimulation causes release of epinephrine by the adrenal medulla, with generalized vasoconstriction and elevation of blood pressure. A pheochromocytoma or tumor of the adrenal medulla, which periodically secretes excessive quantities of norepinephrine, produces episodic elevation of blood pressure to pathologic levels. Mineralocorticoids, hormones produced by the adrenal cortex, lead to sodium and water retention causing an increase in circulating blood volume and in mean arterial pressure.

10. (3) The upper normal limit for diastolic blood pressure has been set at 90 mm. Hg. The normal systolic blood pressure for any individual can be roughly calculated by adding 100 to the age. Obesity and increasing age cause both systolic and diastolic pressures to increase.

11. (4) The force of left ventricular contraction determines the force with which blood enters the arterial system. The elasticity of arteries determines the degree to which arteries can accommodate the increased volume of blood that enters the vessels during ventricular contraction. The amount of narrowing or dilation of arterioles determines the amount of resistance to blood flow through a segment of the circulation. An increase in blood volume stretches the walls of the great veins and the right atrium, exciting stretch receptors that signal the vasomotor center to emit vasodilator impulses, and signal the kidney to increase sodium and water excretion.

12. (3) Blood pressure may be defined as the force exerted by blood against a unit area of blood vessel wall. Since pumping of the heart is intermittent, arterial blood pressure fluctuates from a systolic level of about 120 mm. Hg (pressure in the large arteries when the heart is in systole) to a diastolic level of about 80 mm. Hg (pressure in the large arteries when the heart is in diastole). The mean arterial pressure can be defined as the average pressure in the arteries throughout the entire pressure pulse cycle, or as the average pressure tending to push blood through the systemic circulatory system. Of all pressures affecting blood flow to tissue, mean pressure is of greatest importance.

13. (2) The media of arterioles contain many smooth muscle fibers and few elastic fibers. They are also small enough to offer considerable resistance to blood flow. Since the muscle fibers in the arteriolar walls are under sympathetic nervous system control, arterioles can constrict or dilate markedly, raising or lowering resistance to blood flow; they therefore are more important than other vessels in regulating blood flow to tissues.

14. (4) The pumping action of the heart and constriction of the arterioles are most capable of sudden change in systolic blood pressure. In long-standing hypertension, intracranial hemorrhage may be precipitated by a sudden elevation of blood pressure due to extreme physical exertion or strong emotion, since the effect of generalized arteriolar constriction is to increase the relative blood volume (the volume of blood relative to the capacity of the vascular bed.)

15. (2) Hypertensive damage to the small vessels of the retina results in vascular narrowing; next, twisting of those vessels that elongate in response to prolonged pressure increase; and then rupture of the weakened vessel and seepage of blood between layers of retinal cells.

16. (2) Hypertrophy may be defined as an increase in the size of an organ due to an increase in the size of the cells. In hypertension the prolonged elevation of mean arterial pressure causes increased workload for the left ventricular muscle. Since the heart muscle must contract more forcibly to eject blood into the arterial system against a greatly increased pressure, the myocardium hypertrophies in response to its increased workload.

17. (3) Cardiac output is equal to stroke volume times heart rate. The workload of the heart is equal to the amount of blood pumped out of the heart per unit of time multiplied by the mean pressure in the arterial system.

18. (4) In 80 per cent of patients with cerebral thrombosis, and somewhat fewer patients with cerebral hemorrhage, the cerebral vascular accident is preceded by transient warning signals. When the carotid and middle cerebral arteries are involved, the most common warning signs are blindness in one eye, speech disturbances, confusion, and muscle weakness in one extremity or one side of

the body. When the vertebral and basilar arteries are involved, the most common warning signs are dizziness, syncope, double vision, and numbness.

19. (4) In performing a spinal tap, the physician inserts the spinal needle between the third and fourth lumbar vertebrae. Consequently, the patient should be placed on his side on a hard surface, with the knees pulled up to the chin so as to flex the spine, separate the vertebral processes, and facilitate needle insertion.

20. (4) To ensure maximal spread of the vertebral processes in preparation for spinal needle insertion, the patient's spine must be kept parallel to the bed surface, and the shoulders perpendicular to the spine. To achieve this position, a small pillow should be placed under the head, the upper shoulder should be prevented from falling forward, and a pillow should be placed between the knees.

21. (4) The nurse should prepare the needed equipment on the instrument tray in the expected order of use. After donning mask, sterile gown, and gloves, and disinfecting the skin, the physician will use the 2-cc (2-ml.) syringe and needle to anesthetize the puncture site; the spinal needle and stylet are inserted; the stylet is removed from the needle and a stopcock is attached to the needle hub; a manometer is attached to the stopcock; the cerebrospinal fluid pressure is measured; the manometer is removed; and a sample of spinal fluid is collected in several sterile test tubes.

22. (2) Normal initial spinal fluid pressure, i.e., before collection of spinal fluid specimens, is 70–150 mm. of water.

23. (2) Normal cerebrospinal fluid is clear and colorless. Xanthochromia (a pale pink to pale orange to pale yellow color) of the supernatant fluid may be due to: (1) the presence of conjugated bilirubin, which can diffuse across the blood-cerebrospinal fluid barrier in adults; (2) excessive vitamin A in carotenemia; or (3) hemoglobin from lysed red blood cells following intracerebral or subarachnoid hemorrhage.

24. (4) The normal plantar reflex consists of flexion of the toes and withdrawal of the foot by flexion of the knee and hip. The Babinski response is an abnormal response to plantar stimulation, and consists of slow extension of the great toe with fanning of the remaining toes. It indicates damage to the pyramidal portion of the motor control system, as might occur with hemorrhage into the region of the internal capsule.

25. (1) While Mr. Crown is still comatose, the paralysis of muscles on one side of the face is demonstrated in the paralyzed cheek, which balloons out with each respiration.

26. (4) Fifty per cent glucose, a hypertonic solution, can be administered intravenously to raise the osmotic pressure of the blood so as to draw excess fluid from tissue spaces into blood vessels, decreasing edema in the area surrounding the hemorrhage. This therapy is used only when there is a serious threat to life from declining brain stem function, since the benefit of such treatment is transient.

27. (2) Cheyne-Stokes respirations have a regularly oscillating respiratory rhythm characterized by periods of gradually increasing hyperpnea that alternate with periods of apnea. They are usually seen with neurologic damage at subcortical or brain stem levels.

28. (2) The unilateral facial paralysis and comatose state predispose to mouth breathing, which results in drying of the oral mucosa. The mouth should be cleaned frequently and the tongue, gingivae, and lips lubricated with glycerine to prevent cracking and infection of delicate oral mucosa. Oral infection in a comatose patient increases the risk of aspiration of contaminated material and development of hypostatic pneumonia.

29. (4) Cotton-tipped applicators are less apt to traumatize dried oral mucosa than a toothbrush or a gauze-wrapped tongue blade. An unconscious patient should not have fluid placed into his mouth, because he is unable to swallow and would be apt to aspirate the solution. An alkaline mouthwash applied to the swabs decreases the pH of the mouth, and discourages growth of normal inhabitants and frequent contaminants of the mouth and pharynx.

30. (4) Aphasia and paralysis may render a patient unresponsive to verbal stimuli long after he is again able to perceive conversation from caregivers. The first

step in speech rehabilitation should consist of the opportunity to hear and respond, nonverbally if necessary, to the speech of others.

31. (3) During deep coma the swallowing, epiglottic, and cough reflexes are absent, and the patient is at risk of aspirating oropharyngeal secretions or vomitus and developing aspiration pneumonia.

32. (1) While comatose, the patient should not be placed on his back, and only briefly on the paralyzed side. He should be positioned primarily on the unaffected side, but rotated to lie on the affected side for 15–20 minutes every two hours in order to facilitate drainage of bronchopulmonary secretions and prevent hypostatic pneumonia.

33. (4) Motor, sensory and psychomotor functions return in inverse order to that in which they disappeared when coma developed. Nonspecific responses to painful stimuli, as the most primitive type of responsiveness, are first to reappear; then, purposeful responses to noxious stimuli; the ability to respond to simple commands; orientation to person; opening of the eyes when called by name; recognition of being in a hospital; and ability to identify the year and the month.

34. (2) In hypertensive cerebrovascular disease, intracranial hemorrhage most often occurs from the lenticulostriate artery, a branch of the middle cerebral artery that penetrates the region of the basal ganglia.

35. (2) Intracerebral hemorrhage into the region of the internal capsule causes abrupt onset of flaccid paralysis, which normally lasts for only a few days, followed by spasticity with accompanying increased tendon reflexes.

36. (4) Maximal return of function is achieved usually within 8–9 months following a cerebrovascular accident. However, aphasia, dysarthria, and cerebellar ataxia may improve for a year, and sensory improvement up to two years, following the injury.

37. (2) Following a hemorrhage, the blood that escapes from the ruptured vessel into surrounding brain tissue acts as an irritant, drawing fluid out of nearby intact vessels and causing edema of viable brain tissue adjacent to that destroyed by clotted blood. When, in the course of the normal inflammatory reaction, this edema fluid is again resorbed into the vascular system, some of the symptoms of CNS dysfunction will disappear.

38. (2) Following a cerebrovascular hemorrhage or thrombosis, motor function in the leg and face are more apt to be restored than that in the upper extremities. Muscles of the trunk are infrequently affected following a stroke, because they receive innervation from both sides of the cerebral cortex.

39. (1) Various areas of the cerebral cortex govern language abilities: an area of the frontal lobe controls speech articulation; the sensory cortex of the temporal and parietal lobes govern interpretation of spoken and written language. The above are governed by areas in the dominant hemisphere of the brain. Mr. Crown suffered a right hemiplegia and an expressive aphasia following his stroke, indicating injury to the motor speech area in the cortex or the fibers extending from that area.

40. (2) There are centers in the medulla which, in conjunction with the hypothalamus, control many autonomous nervous system functions, such as regulation of heart rate and respiratory rate. Hemorrhage into the medulla, with destruction of these centers, leads to a steady rise of body temperature and to depression of heart and respiratory rates.

41. (3) After a cerebrovascular hemorrhage, bowel and bladder control usually returns within a few days following return to full consciousness. Since an indwelling catheter predisposes the patient to cystitis and ascending urinary tract infection, and restriction of fluid intake predisposes to dehydration and urinary tract infection, it would be best to offer the urinal at frequent intervals and to direct the patient to empty his bladder. After a short time on such a schedule, bladder sphincter control should return and continence will be restored.

42. (2) Those hemiplegic patients in whom urinary incontinence persists are those who regress to a marked degree during illness. Illness provokes regression to a less mature level of functioning, as an effort to protect the ego against the overwhelming threat of illness. By offering additional support immediately following a cerebrovascular accident, the nurse can decrease the patient's frustration and anxiety, thereby minimizing his need to regress.

43. (4) Bedridden, immobilized patients are highly susceptible to phlebothrombosis of the lower extremities characterized by swelling, redness, heat, and tenderness. These signs should be reported immediately since pulmonary embolism is a life-threatening complication of phlebothrombosis.

44. (4) Aphasia, the inability to use language as symbols, results from an organic brain lesion, and can be of several types: motor or executive; receptive or sensory; and global or total. Mr. Crown's difficulty was a primary deficit in speech production or a motor speech defect.

45. (1) Motor aphasia that results from a cerebrovascular accident usually improves with time, but until speech begins to return the patient tends to repeat a few habitual phrases or words over and over again. The words most often retained are profanities and vulgarities. When words begin to return the patient uses them inappropriately at first, often uttering the antonym for the word intended.

46. (4) The return of motor language skills is hastened by practice in speaking. As soon as Mr. Crown has regained consciousness the nurse should encourage him to speak on every possible occasion, asking him questions, giving him time to formulate an answer, correcting his malapropisms, providing cues for correct language usage, and applauding his efforts to improve.

47. (1) In reteaching Mr. Crown the names of items in daily life, the nurse can use newspaper and magazine pictures and headlines to provide visual cues as she supplies concomitant auditory cues by repeating the proper names for each item pictured.

48. (4) In providing language instruction to a patient with brain damage, the nurse should engage as many as possible of the patient's senses to re-establish psychologic connections between each word symbol and the item it represents.

49. (1) Applying lotion will soften the skin and help to allay any irritation due to friction from the bed linen. Gentle rubbing of the area will increase circulation, which has been impaired by pressure of the mattress against a bony prominence. The side-lying position relieves pressure from the reddened area, and restores normal circulation so that resolution of inflammation can take place.

50. (4) As a result of losses associated with his illness (mobility, sensation, speech, control over emotions, contact with family and friends, control over excretions), Mr. Crown will experience a profound grief reaction characterized by depression.

51. (2) Until speech retraining has effected maximal functioning of Mr. Crown's cheek, tongue, and pharyngeal muscles, he is susceptible to aspiration pneumonia. As a preventive measure, he should be positioned on the affected side to facilitate drainage of saliva from the mouth.

52. (2) Preparation for walking involves re-establishing those neuromuscular pathways disrupted by the cerebral hemorrhage. By pressing his feet alternately against the footboard, Mr. Crown can exercise the muscles of the upper and lower leg that are used in walking, and stimulate the proprioceptive impulses needed to coordinate walking movements.

53. (2) Paralysis of facial muscles and loss of the blink reflex may cause the eyelid on the affected side to remain open, predisposing Mr. Crown to injury of the cornea by a foreign body and drying out of the conjunctiva. Delicate eye structures should be protected by gently irrigating the eye with normal saline solution. This can be followed by instillation of sterile mineral oil or artificial tears solution, closing the lid gently, and covering the eye with a pad held in place with nonallergenic adhesive tape.

54. (2) Paralysis of cheek, tongue, and pharyngeal muscles and loss of the glottic reflex interfere with normal swallowing movements. Before feeding Mr. Crown, the nurse should give him some ice chips to test his ability to swallow and to provide practice in swallowing small quantities of liquid without choking.

55. (3) With return of motor impulses, spasticity of muscles in the affected arm and leg will occur. Because adductor and flexor muscles tend to be stronger than abductor and extensor muscles, there is a tendency for the right arm and right leg to become adducted and for the knee, elbow, and wrist to become flexed. Muscle spasticity also discourages movement, so that the involved extremities

tend to be kept in one position for long periods. If preventive nursing measures are not instituted, contracture deformities will occur.

56. (1) Movement of all joints through full range of motion several times daily stimulates circulation to muscles, joint structures, and bones; discourages collagen deposition in muscles and subcutaneous tissues; and prevents formation of fibrous tissue bands between movable joint structures.

57. (3) A hemiplegic patient who is improperly positioned is apt to develop deformities including footdrop, supination of the foot, and knee flexion. If the leg and foot become "frozen" in this position, the patient will have great difficulty in walking. The nurse therefore should maintain Mr. Crown's legs and feet in proper alignment by ensuring that the knees are in neutral position, the soles are flat and at right angles to the leg, and the toes pointing vertically toward the ceiling.

58. (3) By extending Mr. Crown's legs so that both feet are supported at right angles to the leg by a footboard or box at the bottom of the mattress, footdrop can be prevented.

59. (4) Obstruction of the bowel lumen by a hardened fecal mass stimulates vigorous peristalsis, causing cramping abdominal pain. Irritation of bowel lining by the hardened feces leads to outpouring of inflammatory fluid which, together with increased peristalsis, leads to passage of numerous small, watery stools around the retained fecal mass.

60. (4) The fiber or nondigestible carbohydrate found in vegetables and fruit resists enzymatic digestion and absorbs liquids as the food bolus traverses the intestinal tract, thereby increasing intestinal bulk. Bulk in the large bowel is a stimulant to defecation.

61. (4) Assigning a nurse or a relative to feed Mr. Crown increases his dependence on caregivers, and decreases his sense of autonomy and motivation for recovery. Providing nourishment by intravenous or gastric tube feedings eliminates bulk from the diet, which is needed to re-establish normal gastrointestinal motility. Encouraging the patient to feed himself with special implements provides opportunities for him to exercise many of the hand, arm, shoulder, facial, and tongue muscles that were paralyzed.

62. (3) The quadriceps femoris, a large muscle of the upper anterior thigh that acts to extend and stabilize the knee during walking, can be strengthened during bedrest by quadriceps setting exercises. These consist of pushing the popliteal space against the bed and lifting the heel off the mattress to the count of five.

63. (3) The motor and sensory losses that result from cerebral hemorrhage, and the depression produced by sudden loss of control over one's body and one's life, effect significant changes in body image for the hemiplegic patient.

64. (3) In general, a patient who survives a cerebrovascular accident will experience some return of motor, sensory, and language function. The amount of function regained is determined by the speed with which specific rehabilitation efforts are instituted and the persistence of caregivers in pursuing rehabilitation efforts for the full period during which motor and sensory improvements are possible (two years).

65. (4) Aspiration pneumonia results from ingress of infected material into the lower airway. The normal bacterial inhabitants of the upper airway can be pathogenic to lung tissue. Lack of the glottic reflex and paralysis of pharyngeal muscles favor aspiration of solids and secretions. Pooling of blood in dependent portions of the lung predisposes to transudation of fluid into alveoli.

66. (2) Tracheobronchial secretions tend to drain from higher to lower portions of the respiratory tree on the basis of gravity. Since a right pleural effusion would limit ventilation and gas exchange in the right lung to a significant extent, Mr. Crown would be most comfortable on his right side, which would maximize the efficiency of his left lung.

67. (1) In lobar pneumonia the visceral and parietal pleurae overlying the diseased pulmonary lobe become inflamed as bacteria migrate from lung parenchyma to overlying tissue. On inspiration, the friction of the inflamed pleurae against each other results in pain.

68. (1) Phagocytosis of the bacterial cell by the white blood cell is thought to stimulate production of an endogenous leukocytic pyrogen which, when released from

the white blood cell and carried by the blood to the hypothalamus, resets the temperature regulating center for a higher body temperature, producing fever and chills.

69. (2) The dyspnea in pneumonia results from the obliteration of large numbers of alveoli with inflammatory coagulum, causing a decrease in total lung capacity. The pleural effusion pain is sharp, stabbing, and so severe as to interfere with breathing and coughing, so that the patient grunts with the effort of limiting chest wall expansion to minimize pleuritic pain.

70. (2) Strains of antibiotic-resistant organisms develop in patients who are inadequately treated with certain antimicrobial drugs, and in some weakened individuals in a hospital environment. Mr. Crown's sputum and blood should be cultured to identify the specific organisms responsible for the pneumonia and septicemia, so that the physician can order the antibiotic to which that etiologic agent is most susceptible.

71. (2) Lobar pneumonia, an acute infection producing an acute inflammatory reaction, results in a marked increase in neutrophils typical of acute inflammation.

72. (3) Alterations of sensorium are common in acute infectious diseases characterized by bacteremia and high fever. The delirium seen in acute pneumococcal pneumonia may result either from toxins elaborated by the pneumococci, or from disturbances in nerve tissue metabolism produced by very high temperature.

73. (4) Tetracycline has a local irritant action on the gastrointestinal mucosa, producing dyspepsia and diarrhea in some patients. Since tetracycline is removed from the blood by the liver, its high concentration in that organ may lead to parenchymal liver cell damage and jaundice. Injury to renal glomeruli and tubular cells by the drug can lead to retention of nitrogenous wastes in the blood, or azotemia. Tetracycline can also delay blood coagulation by altering the physicochemical character of the blood lipoproteins, with the result that even minor trauma may produce purpura.

74. (4) Humidified oxygen should be administered to Mr. Crown to prevent drying of respiratory mucosa and dehydration of tracheobronchial secretions, which would predispose to pneumonia.

75. (2) Persistent unproductive cough is exhausting to a debilitated, weakened patient, and painful to one with acute pleuritis. Until the inflammatory coagulum is liquefied in the normal process of resolution, it cannot be removed by coughing. Codeine has a moderate cough-suppressive effect by depressing the cough center in the medulla.

76. (2) 1 grain equals 60 mg.; ½ grain equals 30 mg.

77. (4) Maintenance of body temperature at hyperpyrexic levels (105°, 106°, 107° F.) for prolonged periods causes irreversible damage to sensitive cells in the nervous tissues.

78. (4) During the initial stage of inflammation, when the capillaries dilate and fluid escapes into alveoli, sputum will be watery. When leukocytes leave the capillaries and enter the alveoli, erythrocytes often leave the capillaries at the same time as the white blood cells; thus, the sputum contains small amounts of bright red blood. With time the red blood cells in the exudate rupture, and the hemoglobin released is converted to acid hematin, which is dark red, so the sputum is rusty in appearance. When white blood cells begin to engulf the bacteria, large numbers of white blood cells die, and the exudate becomes yellow in color and malodorous.

79. (3) Herpes simplex virus is present in cells of the mouth and nose of normal persons. Patients weakened by acute febrile infection, such as pneumonia, are susceptible to infection of the oral mucosa by this virus, which produces herpes simplex or "cold sores," which are painful, fluid-filled vesicles at the mucocutaneous junction.

80. (2) The crisis or turning point in pneumococcal pneumonia is that moment when the body's defense mechanisms overcome the invading microorganisms and reverse the course of illness. The fever abates, symptoms of systemic toxicity decrease, and inflammatory coagulum liquefies and is removed by involved lung. When crisis occurs, the vital signs fall rapidly to premorbid levels.

81. (3) If resolution of pneumonia is incomplete, localized aggregations of inflamma-

tory coagulum may become encapsulated in lung parenchyma to produce a lung abscess. Decreased paO_2 levels at a time of increased tissue oxygen demand and increased heart rate may cause heart failure in a patient with diminished cardiac reserve. Adynamic ileus develops as a result of the low oxygen saturation of the arterial blood supply to the small bowel.

82. (2) Prolonged pressure occludes blood vessels of the dermis, causing poor nutrition of skin and subcutaneous tissues, with eventual breakdown, infection, and necrosis of tissue. The nurse can test Mr. Crown's resistance to pressure injury of the skin by observing him for skin discoloration over bony prominences after he has been left in one position for varying periods (4 hours, 3 hours, 2 hours, 1 hour), and then moving him at intervals shorter than that which produces skin reddening.

Mammary Carcinoma and Mastectomy

1. (4) Carcinoma of the breast is most common in the fifth and sixth decades in single or childless married women. Breast-feeding seems to confer a degree of protection against breast malignancy if it is carried out for as long as six months.

2. (4) Infiltration of malignant cells through normal breast tissue and attachment to the fibrous septa of the breast may cause the nipple to retract. Attachment of the tumor to the skin causes wrinkling or dimpling over the lump. Fixation of the tumor to the pectoral fascia may cause flattening or shortening of the breast or deviation of the nipple. A malignant tumor within the ductile system of the breast may give rise to bloody discharge from the nipple.

3. (4) During the last half of the menstrual cycle, progesterone is secreted in large quantities by the corpus luteum, and causes the breasts to swell and become tender during the few days immediately preceding menstruation. Following menstruation, when progesterone production ceases and estrogen production increases progressively, breast swelling and tenderness rapidly disappear.

4. (3) The incidence of breast cancer rises sharply at the age of menopause and continues to increase thereafter. It is most common in single women and in those with a family history of malignancy. Therefore, it cannot be said that nothing is known about the cause of the disease, although the exact etiologic relationship between genes, hormone levels, and breast carcinoma cannot be specified. Without treatment, a malignant breast tumor usually does not regress and exacerbate, but tends to increase steadily in size. Although some malignant tumors seem to begin slowly and insidiously, this is not true of breast cancer.

5. (4) Benign tumors are usually encapsulated. Malignant tumors are unencapsulated, so that cells at the periphery of the tumor easily move and grow into surrounding structures. Benign tumors tend to grow slowly; malignant tumors usually grow rapidly. Benign tumors closely resemble the tissues of origin in regard to architecture, cell arrangement or substances elaborated. In some malignant tumors the cells are so undifferentiated that resemblance to the tissue of origin is slight. Benign tumors do not metastasize. Malignant tumors spread locally by infiltrating into surrounding tissues, and distally by lymphatic transfer of malignant cells to distant sites.

6. (2) Although visual inspection, manual palpation, and x-ray examination may all provide presumptive evidence of a malignant breast tumor, a definitive diagnosis of breast carcinoma can be made only by biopsy and microscopic examination of an excised piece of tumor tissue.

7. (3) Metastasis is the transfer of clumps of malignant cells from a primary tumor to a secondary site in the body via the lymph and blood vessels.

8. (4) Carcinoma of the breast metastasizes to several sites, of which the most common are the other breast, the lung, the brain, the liver, and the bony skeleton.

9. (3) Carcinoma cells usually are detained in the first filter they traverse, or the regional lymph node, so they produce secondary tumors at that point. When carcinoma occurs in the upper outer quadrant of the breast, the axillary lymph

nodes are the first filters to become choked with tumor tissues, causing a palpable axillary lymph node.

10. (1) Mammography is a radiographic examination of the breast, which may be done with or without injection of the ducts of the breast with an opaque contrast medium. It is a useful screening technique that can detect nonpalpable breast carcinomas.

11. (4) At this point it would be inappropriate for the nurse either to deny or affirm the probability that the breast mass is malignant. Response 2 is factually correct, but it ignores the feelings of anxiety behind the question, which presumably is less a request for information than an appeal for understanding and support.

12. (4) The preoperative workup would include a complete blood count to check for evidence of anemia and/or infection. A significant decrease in the number of red blood cells could result in anoxia of vital brain, myocardial, liver, and kidney tissue in the event of a hypotensive episode during surgery. An increase in polymorphonuclear neutrophils would signify an acute inflammation or infection. This would raise the basal metabolic rate, increasing the tissue oxygen need during the critical intra- and postoperative periods, and could serve as a focus from which postoperative wound infection, pneumonia, or septicemia might develop. A chest x-ray was taken preoperatively to identify underlying heart or lung diseases that would increase the hazard of inhalation anesthesia. Since preexisting liver cell damage would render the liver increasingly susceptible to injury by drugs, anesthesia, or intraoperative blood loss, certain liver function tests should be included in the preoperative workup. Blood chemistry examinations for glucose, blood urea nitrogen, uric acid, creatinine, and electrolytes are used to screen for diabetes mellitus, renal failure, and acid-base imbalance.

13. (3) Type A blood contains A antigen on the surface of the red blood cell and anti B antibody (an agglutinin) in the serum. Type B blood has B antigen and anti A antibody in the serum. In type AB blood there are both A and B antigens and no antibodies in the serum. In type O blood there is neither A nor B antigen, but there are anti A and anti B antibodies in the serum. Mrs. Forman has anti B antibodies in her serum. If she should receive either type B or type AB blood, the anti B agglutinins in her serum would react with the B antigen on the donor's red blood cells, causing the donor cells to clump, which would block circulation through such vital tissues as the kidney, liver, myocardium, and brain. Since the red blood cells in type A and type O blood contain no B antigen, Mrs. Forman could safely be given transfusions of either type A or type O blood.

14. (2) The antigen and antibody responsible for ABO incompatibility and the resultant clumping of red blood cells are a red blood cell agglutinogen and a serum agglutinin. Since during transfusion the volume of recipient cells and serum exceeds the volume of donor cells and serum, the donor cells are more apt to be precipitated by agglutinins than vice versa.

15. (4) Prothrombin time determination, a test of liver function, is not done routinely unless there is a history of liver dysfunction. Determination of hemoglobin concentration is a routine part of the "complete blood count" rather than the routine blood chemistry examination. Creatinine, albumin, and cholesterol are included in the latter. Creatinine, a nitrogenous waste product of muscle protein that is normally present in the blood and is secreted by the renal tubule, is one index of renal tubular function. Serum albumin is the most abundant of the serum proteins synthesized in the liver, and thus serum albumin concentration is one index of liver cell function. Cholesterol is a steroid that is the major component of esterified lipids, and therefore is one breakdown product of fat metabolism. Since cholesterol is synthesized chiefly in the liver cell from products of fat metabolism, the serum concentration of cholesterol is an index both of the quantity of animal fat in the diet and of the efficacy of liver function.

16. (3) The skeletal system is the commonest site for distant metastases in breast carcinoma. The thoracic and lumbar spine, skull, ribs, femur, and bony pelvis are the bones most frequently involved. Therefore, in checking Mrs. Forman for possible metastases, her physician would order a full skeletal x-ray survey.

17. (3) In contemporary American culture the female breast has become the symbol of femininity and female sexuality. As a result, both the diagnosis of breast carcinoma and the procedure of mastectomy are especially threatening to the female patient.

18. (4) A radical mastectomy consists of removal of the breast inclusive of the primary tumor, the pectoralis major and minor muscles, and the fat and lymphatic glands of the axilla. In order to cover the skin defect created by removal of so large a mass of tissue, the skin surrounding the excised tissue may have to be undermined to a considerable extent. Therefore, preoperative skin preparation should include cleansing and shaving the neck, the front and back of the left thorax (beyond the midline and to the level of the umbilicus anteriorly), and the entire left arm.

19. (4) Carbon tetrachloride, an organic solvent, is effective in removing nail polish. Colored nail polish should be removed because operating room and recovery room personnel frequently inspect the nail beds for symptoms of reduced blood oxygenation or impaired peripheral circulation.

20. (4) False teeth should be removed to prevent their breakage or loss and to avoid blockage of the airway during anesthesia and the immediate postanesthetic period. Contact lenses should be removed to eliminate breakage or loss and to prevent eye injury from inadvertent displacement of the lens during anesthesia. Ideally, all jewelry should be removed and properly stored for safe-keeping until the patient has fully recovered from the effects of anesthesia. In some institutions, however, patients who insist on wearing a wedding band to the operating room may be allowed to do so if the ring is securely taped to the finger.

21. (3) Sparks of electricity, generated by movement of the nurse's clothing or body parts, would be capable of igniting an explosive anesthetic gas. Therefore, operating room nurses are enjoined to wear conductive shoes, the soles of which are composed of a substance that conducts electric current from the nurse's body to the floor. The flooring tile of the operating room is similarly conductive, in that it contains small wires that conduct electric current from human bodies and electrical equipment to a ground wire in the floors and walls of the building, and thence to the ground underneath the edifice.

22. (4) All the measures listed should be performed. Personal identifying data on the bracelet, chart, and schedule should be compared to ensure that the correct patient is having the correct surgery. Mrs. Forman should be secured to the operating table by fastening canvas straps across the thighs and trunk to prevent her from falling if she should become agitated or hyperactive during Stage 2 of anesthesia, delirium. The chart should be checked to ascertain that the surgeon has obtained a properly signed permit for the operation(s) to be performed and that the proper dosage of the ordered preanesthetic medications has been given according to schedule, so that intubation and induction will be safer and more pleasant. Since the left arm will have to be abducted and supported while the axillary fat and lymph nodes are excised, a padded arm board should be attached to the table, and the arm affixed to the board in comfortable position.

23. (3) Operating rooms often have laminar air flow, which is a continuous supply of fresh, filtered, humidified, and temperature-controlled air circulated from ceiling ducts in such a way that dust, droplets, and contaminants leave the room through exhaust registers located in the walls at floor level. This prevents contamination of the wound and of the operating equipment and supplies. Opening a window would interfere with laminar air flow, and possibly create drafts; these could cause excessive loss of body heat and could produce shivering in the anesthetized patient, which would interfere with surgery and with detection of symptoms of tissue anoxia. Noise should be kept to a minimum to aid quick and accurate communication between operating room personnel, and an open window might admit distracting sounds.

24. (4) The length and nature of the preoperative hand scrubbing procedure vary among institutions. A procedure commonly used is one that establishes the proper sequence for brush cleansing of fingers, hands, and forearms, together with the time to be spent in scrubbing each part. The usual time prescribed for the entire preoperative hand scrub procedure is 10 minutes.

25. (2) At the conclusion of the hand scrub procedure, the skin of the hands and forearms is considered surgically clean or fairly clear of pathogenic microorganisms, and the skin of the upper arms is regarded as grossly contaminated. Since the last step in the hand scrub procedure is to rinse the hands and forearms with copious amounts of freely running water, the hands and arms will be wet when the nurse leaves the scrub sink to move into the operating room. If forearms and hands were carried in the dependent position, water would run from the margin of contaminated skin at the elbow over the clean skin of the forearm and hand, increasing the possibility of contaminating the sterile gloves, gown, or instruments, and consequently the patient's surgical wound.

26. (4) Shaking or waving the arms would disturb laminar air flow, creating eddy currents of air and distributing particulate matter and droplets widely, so such movements should be avoided. It is possible to steam sterilize a paper towel, but subjecting paper to steam under pressure decreases its absorptive ability and renders it more friable. Thus, paper crumbs could be shredded and could fall into the sterile field, contaminating supplies and the surgical wound.

27. (3) The nurse's hair shouuld be entirely covered by a cap before she enters the surgical suite. The face mask should be tied over the cap so that it covers the mouth and nose before the hand scrub procedure is begun, since without a mask the surgically clean arms and hands could be contaminated with droplet spray. After the scrub, the nurse moves into the operating room, dries her hands and arms with a sterile towel, and dons sterile gown and sterile gloves, the wrappers of which have been opened by a circulating nurse. Thus, at the conclusion of the sterile gowning procedure, the cuffs of the sterile gloves extend over the knitted wristbands of the sterile scrub gown.

28. (1) After completion of the preoperative hand scrub and drying of hands and arms on a sterile towel, the hands are considered to be surgically clean, not sterile. Therefore, no part of the scrub gown should be touched which could later come into contact with sterile materials or the patient's wound. The neck of the scrub gown, under usual circumstances, does not contact any of the sterile materials during the operation. Therefore, the gown should be seized by the neckband, lifted up, held at arm's length away from the scrub table, and allowed to unfold to permit insertion of the arms into the sleeves without the outside of the gown front and sleeves touching any contaminated surface.

29. (2) Both the neckband and the back of a sterile scrub gown are considered to be contaminated: the former because it is in close contact with the neck and face, and because the nurse seized it with ungloved hands before putting it on; the latter because she might accidentally back into unscrubbed and ungowned operating personnel.

30. (4) Sterile supplies or equipment may be delivered to the scrub nurse by any of the methods described, because in each instance the circulating nurse touches only an outer wrapper, the handle of a sterile tray, or sterile lifting forceps; the scrub nurse touches only the sterile item requested. Thus, neither the scrub nurse, the scrub table, nor the proferred item is contaminated during transfer.

31. (4) Localized recurrence of malignant tumor growth sometimes occurs in the wound following radical mastectomy. It is possible for malignant cells from the periphery of a tumor to be disengaged from the surgical specimen, adhere to surgical drapes or instruments, and later be implanted along the wound edges during grafting or closure.

32. (4) Since carcinoma of the breast spreads both by local penetration and by metastasis through blood and lymph channels, a radical mastectomy includes removal of the entire breast, subcutaneous fat, muscles of the anterior chest wall, and all ipsilateral lymph nodes.

33. (4) A split thickness skin graft is the type best suited for repairing a defect caused by loss of a large area of skin. It consists of removal of an area of epidermis, together with one half to two thirds of the underlying dermis from a donor site; suturing the graft to the recipient site; and applying firm pressure over the graft so as to maintain contact between the graft and underlying tissue until the graft becomes adherent.

34. (2) Following removal of a split thickness skin graft, the donor site will heal best

in a dry, cool environment. A protective, nonirritating dressing such as a layer of petrolatum gauze over the exposed nerve endings will reduce pain during healing.

35. (1) In order for a split thickness skin graft to become viable, it must remain in continuous contact with underlying tissues until capillaries can grow into the graft from the denuded surface. The suction apparatus should be checked regularly to ensure that any blood or serum that seeps into the space beneath the graft is immediately aspirated.

36. (2) It requires only a few hours for a split thickness skin graft to become adherent to underlying tissues if the graft is maintained in continuous contact with the denuded surface. A pressure dressing is used to control bleeding from the recipient site and to ensure adherence of the graft to underlying tissue.

37. (2) The removal of all lymph nodes from the left axilla will interrupt lymph drainage from the left arm. In addition, the pressure dressing over the graft will encompass the upper arm, further impairing circulation in that extremity. Therefore, following surgery, Mrs. Forman will develop some lymphedema of the left arm and hand.

38. (1) The pressure dressing over the graft will restrict chest movement, predisposing Mrs. Forman to atelectasis and pooling of tracheobronchial secretions. Pain on chest expansion will discourage her from coughing and deep breathing. All these factors will increase her susceptibility to pulmonary complications during the early postoperative period.

39. (1) The breast has an abundant blood supply. During surgery, a great many blood vessels must be cauterized or ligated. The dislodging of a clot or ligature from one of the larger vessels divided during surgery would result in severe blood loss. The nurse should check the vital signs (until they are stable) and the wound dressing every 15 minutes. Thereafter, vital signs should be measured every 30 minutes for 2 hours, and then hourly until the next morning.

40. (3) If the axillary wound were to bleed extensively, the blood would be apt to drain down between the lateral chest wall and the immobilized left arm to pool on the lower sheet under the left shoulder and chest.

41. (3) Elevation of the left arm will counteract to some extent the edema formation due to impaired lymph drainage. Restriction of edema formation will minimize weight gain in the extremity, thereby facilitating the patient's movement in bed, which should contribute to her physical comfort.

42. (4) All listed measures should be taken to protect Mrs. Forman from postoperative pulmonary complications. Turning her from the back to the right side helps to prevent atelectasis in long-dependent segments of the lung, and will favor venous return circulation from the left arm. Supporting the left arm and chest wall while the patient coughs encourages her to breathe and cough deeply enough to mobilize and evacuate secretions from the lower tracheobronchial tree. Placing head and back pillows to encourage chest expansion facilitates the re-expansion of alveoli collapsed as a result of prolonged immobility during surgery. Relieving pain in the operative area by administering the ordered analgesic renders Mrs. Forman more cooperative in the turning, coughing, and deep breathing that she has been instructed to perform. The use of intermittent positive pressure breathing four times a day forces re-expansion of collapsed alveoli in posterior lung segments by increasing intrapulmonary pressures.

43. (4) In a radical mastectomy all the structures down to the ribs and intercostal muscles are removed, and so there is little soft tissue remaining to which to suture the wound edges. Until the skin edges and the split thickness skin graft become firmly adherent to underlying tissue, strong traction on the skin of the anterior chest wall might cause the wound to dehisce. To prevent this, the left arm is maintained in a position of complete adduction for 4–7 days postoperatively by immobilizing it with adhesive tape or Elastoplast.

44. (3) Dehiscence is defined as the act of splitting open. There is a greater incidence of wound dehiscence in elderly, debilitated, obese, or malnourished patients, and in those with malignancies.

45. (2) The system of venous valves permits only unidirectional blood flow through a vein, and thus keeping the hand higher than the forearm, the forearm higher than the upper arm, and the upper arm higher than the shoulder enable gravity

to facilitate venous return flow. Changing the position of the left hand and arm at frequent intervals mobilizes edema from interstitial spaces so that it can be absorbed into venous capillaries. Frequent extension of the fingers, wrist, and elbow increase venous return flow by the "milking" action of muscle contraction and relaxation on vessels traversing the muscles.

46. (4) The loss of a considerable mass of tissue from the left anterior chest wall, the tendency to drop the left shoulder, and immobilization of the left arm with a bandage or sling all tend to throw Mrs. Forman off balance, increasing her susceptibility to falls during her first few attempts to ambulate.

47. (4) When Mrs. Forman is first allowed to sit up in a chair, the increased weight of the edematous left arm may tend to pull her sideways, predisposing to backache. Her comfort will be increased if two large pillows are placed on a side table or on the chair arm, and her left arm supported on pillows in such a manner that she can comfortably sit upright with spine straight and shoulders level.

48. (2) If lymphedema of the left arm continues to be a problem for several weeks or months following surgery, Mrs. Forman may develop the habit of carrying the left shoulder lower than the right, which could create permanent changes in the bony spine and thorax.

49. (2) Considerable finger dexterity and smooth movement of the wrist and elbow are needed to carry out daily living and housekeeping activities. Flexing and extending the fingers, as well as supination and pronation of the hand at frequent intervals during the early postoperative period will help to achieve this. Internal and external rotation and circumduction of the shoulder should be postponed until the incisions are more completely healed.

50. (3) The first three exercises listed all require motion at the shoulder joint, and so discourage contracture deformity of the shoulder, the so-called "frozen shoulder" syndrome. Doing pushups from the prone position would be much too strenuous an activity for a person whose pectoral muscles have just been removed.

51. (2) In order to regain proper balance for walking, Mrs. Forman should be instructed early in the postural adjustments that she must make in order to maintain proper sitting, standing, and walking posture following the loss of a breast and axillary tissue.

52. (1) This response best acknowledges the feelings behind Mrs. Forman's question, while emphasizing the necessity for arm exercises in a clear, direct, and nonthreatening manner.

53. (3) There is a high incidence of cancer in the contralateral breast in patients who have had a radical mastectomy for breast cancer. Therefore, an important aspect of the predischarge preparation is instruction in proper technique for self-examination of the breast.

54. (2) Most patients have some degree of lymphedema following radical mastectomy. Mrs. Forman should be told that the edema in her left arm may gradually decrease and disappear with the growth of new lymph channels to replace those destroyed during surgery. In some patients, however, as a result of postoperative wound infection, imperfectly obliterated dead space in the axilla, or postoperative radiation of the axilla, lymphedema of the arm may persist indefinitely. When this occurs the amount of arm swelling can be limited by wearing a custom-made elasticized sleeve from wrist to shoulder during the waking hours of each day.

55. (4) Rapidly proliferating and relatively undifferentiated cells are permanently injured by lower doses of radiation than are more mature, more slowly dividing nonmalignant cells.

56. (3) The rapidly proliferating cells of the gastrointestinal epithelium are more susceptible than other less rapidly dividing cells to radiation injury, the symptoms of which therefore include gastrointestinal dysfunction. Fasting before and after therapy can help to minimize gastrointestinal symptoms.

57. (3) The chest scar will tend to become less prominent and less highly colored with time. The scar itself and the skin surrounding it can be made more soft and supple by twice daily massaging with cocoa butter or cold cream.

58. (2) In American culture, the female breast and feminine identity are so closely associated that some women have great difficulty accepting their changed

body image following mastectomy. A common early manifestation of this problem is reluctance or inability to look directly at the incision. Later in the recovery period, failure to resolve the normal grief reaction provoked by loss of a breast may cause a woman to avoid social activities or withdraw from close relationships with friends and relatives.

59. (4) In order to feel safe and self-confident about resuming her former social life, Mrs. Forman needs to be told what activities she is able to perform, that family and caregivers expect her to do as much as she is capable of, and that facilities exist to ease her return to accustomed activities.

60. (4) All the methods can be used to treat metastatic breast carcinoma. X-ray examination is used to shrink metastatic tumors and increase the patient's sense of well-being. Gonadal hormones, androgen premenopausally and estrogen postmenopausally, retard the growth of metastatic tumors. Oophorectomy may have a palliative effect on breast carcinoma metastases. When further deterioration makes further palliation necessary, adrenalectomy may increase the patient's comfort for a while longer. Cytotoxic agents have been used to treat patients with malignant tumor metastases. Cyclophosphamide, 5-fluorouracil, methotrexate, and adriamycin in varying combinations have been used with success in treating metastatic breast malignancy.

Prostatic Hypertrophy and Prostatectomy

1. (4) The exact cause of prostatic hypertrophy is unknown, but it is thought to result from an imbalance between pituitary, testicular, and adrenal hormones that coincides with the male characteristic.

2. (4) An enlarging prostate encroaches upon the lumen of the urethra, interfering with urinary drainage. As the prostate increases in size, and increasing quantities of urine are retained in the bladder, urine may back up into the ureter and into the kidney pelvis. This causes the exertion of pressure on the renal medulla and cortex, with eventual destruction of renal tubules and glomeruli.

3. (4) All the symptoms listed may arise. Frequency develops because the hypertrophied gland interferes with bladder emptying, so that urine remains in the bladder following each voiding. Residual urine becomes infected and the inflamed bladder wall is hyperirritable. As the amount of residual urine increases, less time is required between voidings for bladder stretch receptors to become stimulated, generating the desire to urinate more frequently. Urgency develops because urethral obstruction stimulates the vesicular muscle to hypertrophy so that, with the increase in sensory impulses from bladder to cord, the detrusor muscle goes into spasm, producing a sense of urgency. Decreased size and force of the urinary stream is seen when the urethral resistance to urine flow exceeds the power of detrusor muscle contraction. With complete decompensation of bladder muscle, the bladder can neither expel urine forcibly with each voiding nor close the internal sphincter at the end of voiding, so that urine dribbles from the bladder after voiding has ceased.

4. (3) Cleansing the skin around the urinary meatus with an antiseptic solution prior to urine specimen collection decreases the possibility of external contamination of the specimen. A sterile container should be used to collect and transport urine to the laboratory to avoid accidental inoculation of the specimen with pathogens from outside the patient's body. Mr. Ridgely should be instructed to void into first one, then another, receptacle without stopping because the first few milliliters of a voided specimen consist of "urethral washings," or urine that contains the cellular debris and bacterial inhabitants of the urethra. The urine collected in the second container is residual urine from the bladder and should be analyzed for bacteria, pus cells, blood cells, and epithelial cells, which are usual findings in a urinary infection.

5. (3) Because the prostate encircles the urethra just as it leaves the bladder, the flattened posterior aspect of the median lobe rests against the lower 2.5 cm. of the rectum, and can be palpated through the anterior rectal wall with sufficient

clarity to permit assessment of the size, consistency, and surface characteristics of the gland.

6. (2) A nonsterile glove, water-soluble lubricant jelly, and a deftly arranged sheet drape should be used to minimize the patient's discomfort and embarrassment during the rectal examination. Neither a head lamp nor a protoscope are used in digital examination of the prostate.

7. (3) The underlying tissue change in benign prostatic hypertrophy is nodular hyperplasia of the fibromuscular tissue, usually containing some glandular elements. Hyperplasia is an increase in the size of an organ due to an actual increase in the number of cells.

8. (2) The prostate gland is a chestnut-sized, encapsulated, five-lobed organ consisting of glandular, smooth muscle and fibrous tissue that surrounds the male urethra just as it leaves the bladder. Hypertrophy or hyperplasia of the lateral and median lobes causes urinary obstruction by compressing the urethra.

9. (3) When the enlarging prostate obstructs the urethra, the detrusor muscle of the bladder hypertrophies so as to contract more forcibly against the urethral obstruction. With increasing obstruction, a point is reached at which the overstretched bladder muscle outgrows its blood supply and decompensation occurs. Muscle contraction is then too short to expel all urine from the bladder. The amount of urine left in the bladder after each voiding is an index of the degree of detrusor decompensation.

10. (4) All are possible consequences of untreated prostatic hypertrophy. Stagnant urine becomes infected. Toxins elaborated by microorganisms in the urine irritate the bladder lining, producing cystitis. Muscle decompensation causes residual urine to accumulate, distending first the bladder, then the ureter, then the kidney pelvis.

11. (3) Urine may contain organic acids, albumin, sugar, blood, acetone, fat, and epithelial cells, and thus is a good medium for bacterial growth. Urinary tract obstruction causes slowing of urine flow through the tract, so that bacteria that ascend the urethra and enter the bladder have more time to multiply and overcome body defenses to infection.

12. (2) Ingestion of large quantities of fluids increases the volume of urine produced. Increased quantities of more dilute urine constitute a physiologic lavage of the urinary tract, in that offending bacteria and bacterial products are diluted; they thus are less irritating to urinary mucosa and, unless urinary obstruction is complete, are more quickly removed from the body.

13. (4) As Mr. Ridgely's prostate continues to enlarge, it will encroach further and further upon the urethral lumen. With minimal prostatic hypertrophy the amount of residual urine left in the bladder may be small (10–20–30 ml.). With severe prostatic hypertrophy, the amount of residual urine may be as much as 500–1000 ml.

14. (4) The urine of a patient with urinary tract infection typically contains living and dead bacteria, pus cells, red blood cells, epithelial cells, mucous shreds, and occasionally casts. The presence of such particulate matter in the urine causes the specific gravity of the urine to be higher than normal. The distinctive odor of the urine in certain urinary infections results from decomposition of the organic matter being used as an energy source by rapidly multiplying bacteria.

15. (1) Indwelling or self-retaining catheters are constructed with a 5-ml. (regular) or 30-ml. (for hemostasis) inflatable balloon a short distance from the catheter tip. After the catheter has been inserted into the bladder, it is inflated with sterile saline. The distended balloon keeps the catheter from being dislodged from the bladder by accidental traction on the catheter or attached drainage tubing.

16. (2) When more than 1000 ml. of urine remains in the bladder after each voiding, the bladder muscle has stretched thin, and blood vessels in the wall of the bladder are weakened by loss of normal support structures. It is unwise to empty an overdistended bladder completely, because the sudden reduction in intravesicular pressure will result in bleeding from bladder mucosa and collapse of bladder muscle. Decompression drainage is a system whereby bladder muscle tone is maintained because the catheter and drainage tubing are connected so that urine must exit the system against gravity, which prevents

immediate bladder emptying and resultant bleeding, and permits return of muscle control as the dilated bladder gradually returns to normal size.

17. (4) Frequent causes for obstruction in a urinary drainage system are external compression of the catheter or drainage tube by the patient's body or bedframe; reversal of drainage flow by the looping of excessively long tubing; and internal obstruction of catheter and tubing by clots and inflammatory debris. Catheter contamination is a frequent source of bladder infection in a patient with an indwelling catheter. Stagnation of urine encourages microbial growth. When urine within the drainage receptacle contaminates the drainage tubing, microorganisms ascend the tubing and catheter, enter the bladder, and produce infection.

18. (2) By lowering the "Y" connector an inch or two each day, the physician can decrease the pressure against which the bladder must contract to evacuate urine, permitting elimination of more and more urine each day until normal bladder capacity is reached.

19. (2) An operation is a procedure performed with instruments that in some way violates the integrity of the human body. Subjecting a person to such a procedure if he has not given informed consent constitutes assault and battery. Mr. Ridgely's signed consent for cystoscopy indicates that, having been given information about the purpose, procedure, and possible complications of cytoscopy, he is willing to undergo the examination.

20. (1) Lidocaine (Xylocaine) is a potent local anesthetic that can be applied topically or by injection into tissues. Its effect is more prompt, stronger, and longer-lasting than that of procaine.

21. (3) In the elderly, the combination of prolonged immobility, knee flexion, and pressure against popliteal tissues predisposes the patient to stagnation of venous blood flow, pressure injury of venous walls, and possible phlebothrombosis.

22. (4) As the workload of a muscle increases, the muscle fibers hypertrophy so as to contract more strongly, thereby improving work efficiency.

23. (1) The most common source of infection in a patient with obstructive uropathy consists of organisms introduced into the urethra during the course of instrumentation and treatment. Trauma from cystoscopes, sounds, and catheters weakens tissues, leaving them susceptible to bacterial infection. Poor technique permits bacterial contamination of equipment.

24. (4) For Mr. Ridgely's drainage system to remove urine, reduce pressure, and avoid contamination and trauma to the tissues, the catheter, drainage tubing, and collection container must be positioned so that urine can fall freely by gravity and without obstruction from bladder to receptacle whether the patient is supine, sitting, or upright.

25. (4) When possible, a sterile, closed, disposable urinary drainage system should be used for the patient who must have an indwelling catheter. Once the system is established, the connections between catheter, drainage tube, and receptacle should not be broken. Urine should be removed from the receptacle every eight hours, using care not to contaminate the spigot or drainage port. The external urinary meatus and adjacent catheter should be cleansed daily with antiseptic.

26. (1) Mr. Ridgely's urinary tract infection, fever, and prolonged bedrest will have caused increased tissue protein breakdown. A high-protein diet should be given preoperatively to restore nutritional losses and ensure postoperative healing.

27. (2) The purpose of culturing urine is to identify which organism(s) are responsible for a urinary infection, so as to employ antibiotic or antiinfective agents that will be effective against those organisms.

28. (1) The urine must be collected in a sterile container so as to avoid contamination of the sample, which would confuse the diagnosis and needlessly complicate treatment.

29. (2) Urea, the principal end product of protein metabolism, is synthesized in the liver from amino acids, passed into the blood, and excreted in the urine. The level of urea nitrogen in the blood depends on the amount of protein ingested, the amount of urea produced by the liver, and the amount of urea excreted by

the kidney. Urea is excreted by glomerular filtration, with 40% of the urea in the filtrate being resorbed by the tubules. When protein catabolism is normal, an increase of blood urea nitrogen above normal occurs when glomerular filtration rate is reduced to 30–40% of normal.

30. (3) Creatinine is a product released from normal muscle tissue during metabolic activity; it circulates in the blood and is filtered through the glomerulus, secreted by the tubule, and eliminated in the urine. Since the creatinine level is independent of dietary protein intake, it is superior to the blood urea nitrogen concentration as a screening test of renal function.

31. (1) In America, the incidence of arteriosclerotic heart disease (which is second only to hypertensive heart disease as a cause of organic heart disorder) increases with age. An episode of hypotension or anoxia during general anesthesia and surgery would be especially hazardous to a patient with poor coronary circulation. Following recovery from a myocardial infarction, certain characteristic EKG changes may persist for months or years.

32. (4) Following intravenous injection of radiopaque dye, serial x-ray films of the urinary tract at 2, 5, 10, and 15 minutes following dye administration permit visualization of the renal pelvis, ureter, bladder, and urethra, yielding information about the size, shape, and location of these structures.

33. (2) Alkaline phosphatase in an enzyme produced in many tissues, but predominantly in bone. It is elevated in biliary tract obstruction and in conditions characterized by increased osteoblastic activity, such as metastatic bone tumors.

34. (3) Acid phosphatase is an enzyme found in high concentration in prostatic tissue. Elevation of the serum acid phosphatase is seen in patients with prostatic cancer that has metastasized.

35. (3) Sulfonamides exert a bacteriostatic effect upon sensitive organisms by inhibiting an enzyme reaction involved in the formation of pteroylglutamic acid (folic acid) from para-aminobenzoic acid.

36. (2) A transurethral prostatectomy is the removal of prostatic tissue by a succession of small cuts performed under direct endoscopic vision. Although a coagulating current is used during the procedure to seal bleeding vessels in prostatic tissue, a certain amount of bleeding will occur from the operative site during the first few hours following surgery, so the urinary drainage will be blood-stained.

37. (2) The lithotomy or dorsosacral position is one in which the patient lies on his back with hips and knees flexed and legs abducted.

38. (3) An electrode is a metal terminal through which an electrical current can be applied to or taken from the body. In a transurethral resection, an electrode to which a cutting loop is attached is passed through the urethra to cut out small pieces of prostatic tissue.

39. (4) Because electrical current of sufficient voltage generates heat, it can be used to coagulate protein such as body tissue.

40. (3) Since Mr. Ridgely's transurethral resection is performed under spinal anesthesia, he will be fully conscious and aware of his surroundings throughout the procedure. As a result of natural anxiety, he will probably be especially attentive to conversations between members of the operating team.

41. (3) Throughout the resection procedure an irrigating solution is pumped into the bladder and out again to carry away the flakes of resected tissue, blood, and other debris that could obstruct the surgeon's view of the prostate. In addition, distention of the bladder with irrigating solution minimizes the possibility of bladder perforation by the cystoscope or electrodes.

42. (2) Sterile water is hypotonic in relation to body cells and tissues. Cell walls are semipermeable membranes. Osmosis is the movement of a solvent across a semipermeable membrane from a dilute solution to a more concentrated solution. Thus, water would tend to move into blood and tissue cells, causing them to swell and rupture.

43. (4) An electrolyte is a substance that readily dissociates into positive and negative ions in solution, and so is capable of conducting an electrical current. Sodium chloride rapidly dissociates in water into positively charged sodium ions and negatively charged chloride ions. A sodium chloride solution readily transmits an electrical current.

44. (2) Splinting the penis following a transurethral resection prevents movement, which could exacerbate bleeding from the prostatic bed. By inflating the large Foley bag (30 ml.) and pulling it firmly into the prostatic fossa, pressure can be applied to any bleeding vessels in the prostatic tissue.

45. (4) Spinal anesthesia causes hypotension through paralysis of sympathetic vasomotor nerves. If the transurethral resection is lengthy, considerable blood can be lost during resection, with a decrease in circulating blood volume and in blood pressure. It is customary to give a sedative or tranquilizer preoperatively to the patient who is to receive a spinal anesthetic. Several of the drugs used for this purpose, such as pentobarbital and promethazine, reduce blood pressure to a mild or moderate degree. Extreme changes of position, as from the lithotomy to the recumbent position, may, by sudden redistribution of blood volume, cause reduction in blood pressure.

46. (3) Difficulties in visualizing the prostate during surgery may result in failure to cauterize a bleeding vessel in the operative site. Excessive blood loss decreases circulating blood volume, causing the blood pressure to fall to shock levels. Falling blood pressure in an elderly patient with cerebral arteriosclerosis produces cerebral anoxia and confusion.

47. (1) The bladder should be irrigated frequently to remove clotted blood and prevent obstruction of the drainage system, which would cause bladder distention and further bleeding from the operative site.

48. (3) Pressure of the inflated Foley bag against the internal urinary sphincter produces a feeling of urgency. If Mr. Ridgely succumbs to the sensation and bears down to void around the Foley bag, painful bladder spasm will ensue. He should be advised to ignore the sensation as it will decrease in intensity with time.

49. (4) Straining at stool, by increasing pressure within the abdomen and pelvis, may exert pressure against the prostatic fossa, causing necrotic surface tissue to slough and provoke hemorrhage.

50. (1) Enemas, suppositories, and high-bulk diet should be avoided, since they could cause mechanical trauma to the prostate and provoke bleeding. A mild cathartic, such as citrate of magnesia, is a better means of preventing constipation.

51. (4) During a transurethral resection, urethral mucosa is destroyed in the area of the prostate. With healing, fibrosis occurs, which may cause urethral strictures. Postoperative urethral strictures can be treated by progressive dilation of the narrowed segment.

52. (4) Following transurethral resection, a large fluid intake is required to prevent urinary tract infection that would interfere with healing of the prostatic fossa. Heavy lifting and strong exercise must be avoided for 3–4 weeks following surgery or until the prostatic bed is completely healed, otherwise bleeding will begin anew. Constipation must be avoided because straining at stool can cause separation of necrotic tissue from the prostatic bed, with severe hemorrhage as a consequence. Since considerable blood loss can result from sloughing of necrotic tissue, the doctor should be notified immediately if bleeding develops following surgery.

53. (2) Alcohol should be avoided following transurethral resection of the prostate as it would be irritating to the inflamed bed of the prostate and could cause painful bladder spasm.

54. (1) Since 10–14 days are required to complete the inflammatory changes that result in desiccation of the coagulated tissue and desquamation from the surface of the prostatic bed, the eschar may not lift from the wound for that length of time, and when it does excessive bleeding may occur.

Diabetes Mellitus and Leg Amputation

1. (3) Insulin is a hormone produced by the beta cells of the islets of Langerhans in the pancreas. It provides active transport of glucose into tissue cells, facilitates oxidation of glucose within the cell, promotes conversion of fatty acids into adipose tissue, promotes protein synthesis, and promotes glycogenesis. Deficiency of insulin causes diabetes mellitus.

2. (3) In diabetic acidosis, incomplete lipid metabolism produces an increase in serum concentration of the ketone bodies: beta-hydroxybutyric acid, acetoacetic acid, and acetone. Both of the former two yield hydrogen ions on dissociation, thereby decreasing plasma pH. At a pH of 7.2, respirations are stimulated and breathing becomes rapid and deep. The body neutralizes ketones by buffering. Acetoacetic acid is combined with $NaHCO_3$ to form carbonic acid acetoacetate, a weak acid that dissociates into CO_2, which is excreted by the lungs, and sodium acetoacetate, which is excreted by the kidney. Carbonic acid is blown off by the lung as CO_2 and H_2O, so respirations are increased in rate and depth.

3. (1) Patients with diabetic ketoacidosis lose body water through excessive urination, excessive exhalation of water vapor, and nausea and vomiting. Poor circulation and increased concentration of glucose in body fluids and tissues predispose the diabetic to infection of all types. The hypermetabolism of infection may throw a previously balanced diabetic into ketoacidosis. The combination of infection, hypermetabolism, and dehydration causes temperature elevation.

4. (2) In ketoacidosis a lack of insulin blocks glucose absorption and oxidation by tissue cells, so serum glucose concentration rises sharply. In coma due to cerebral hemorrhage, a transient glycosuria may be seen at the time of the hemorrhage, but this glycosuria is less severe than that seen in ketoacidosis, and it clears more quickly.

5. (4) Unavailability of glucose as a cellular energy source leads to hunger and fatigue. High concentration of glucose in the urine results in cystitis, which causes burning on urination. Arteriosclerotic changes in vessels of the eye lead to retinal degeneration, with progressive loss of vision. Circulatory impairment and accumulation of glucose in tissue fluids result in pruritus.

6. (2) Excessive urinary excretion of glucose, ketones, and sodium causes osmotic diuresis, and urinary loss of large amounts of water is reflected in excessive thirst.

7. (1) Lack of insulin interferes with transport of glucose across the cell wall and oxidation of glucose within the cell. When glucose is no longer available as an energy source for cellular metabolism, the body converts tissue protein to glucose for use as an energy source.

8. (4) As serum glucose levels rise, more glucose is filtered through the glomerulus. As the concentration of glucose rises in the renal tubule the osmotic pressure of tubular content increases, so less water is absorbed from the tubule and more water is excreted as urine.

9. (4) All body cells function best at a pH of 7.35–7.45. In ketoacidosis the accumulation of ketone bodies and loss of bicarbonate in the urine cause a decrease in pH to 7.2 and lower, and a concomitant depression of cerebral function, leading to dulling of consciousness, coma, and possibly death.

10. (3) Unavailability of glucose leads to catabolism of body fat as a source of energy. Excessive fat breakdown causes accumulation of ketones in the serum. Both beta-hydroxybutyric acid and acetoacetic acid dissociate in serum to yield hydrogen ions, which decrease the pH and depress the function of nervous tissue.

11. (2) Beta-hydroxybutyric acid, acetoactic acid, and acetone are intermediate products of fat metabolism. In instances of rapid fat metabolism, or situations in which fat metabolism cannot proceed to the end products of carbon dioxide and water, large quantities of ketones or acidic intermediaries accumulate in the serum.

12. (2) The patient in diabetic ketoacidosis is treated aggressively to reverse the acidosis and dehydration as rapidly as possible. One way to assess the adequacy and efficacy of treatment is to observe changes in the volume of urinary output and the concentration of ketone bodies and glucose in the urine, since these quantities provide indirect measures of serum ketones and glucose. A comatose patient is incontinent. To obtain hourly urine specimens for testing, an indwelling catheter should be inserted.

13. (2) A hypodermic syringe is used to distend the balloon of an indwelling catheter because an overdistended balloon will rupture, the amount of sterile water

needed to fill the balloon is specified, and greater accuracy in measurement is possible with a hypodermic than with a bulb syringe.

14. (4) Sterile water should be used to distend the balloon so that, if it should rupture, pathogenic organisms will not be introduced into the bladder. Diabetics have greater than average susceptibility to urinary tract infections.

15. (2) When an indwelling catheter is in place, the external urinary meatus and surrounding skin should be washed several times a day with soap and water to remove tissue debris, secretions, and microorganisms.

16. (2) Mrs. Hershey's 4+ glycosuria and 4+ ketonuria are the result of uncontrolled diabetes mellitus with ketoacidosis, indicating that the high serum concentrations of glucose and ketones have exceeded renal threshold and are being excreted in large amounts in the urine. The numerous bacteria, pus cells, and occasional red blood cells seen in the urine indicate infection in the bladder, urethra, ureter, or renal pelvis.

17. (3) Indwelling catheters generally should not be irrigated unless obstructed, for fear of introducing contaminants into the closed urinary drainage system. The patient will need increased fluid intake to correct her dehydration and combat urinary tract infection. Careful recording of fluid intake and output is needed to assess the adequacy of fluid replacement for former losses and as a guide for intravenous fluid therapy. Serial urine analyses for glucose and acetone will be needed to monitor the adequacy of insulin dosage in controlling carbohydrate and fat metabolism.

18. (3) Glucose is an excellent bacteriologic culture medium, and Mrs. Hershey's urine undoubtedly carried a high concentration of glucose for several days before treatment was begun.

19. (2) The normal range for fasting blood glucose concentration is 60–100 mg. per 100 ml. of blood.

20. (3) Glucose is filtered from the blood in the glomerulus. As filtrate moves through the tubules a certain amount of glucose is resorbed from the filtrate into tubular capillaries, but the amount of such resorption is limited. In general, the renal threshold for glucose, or the blood concentration above which glucose will appear in the urine, is 160–170 mg. per 100 ml. of blood.

21. (3) Carbon dioxide combining power, a measure of plasma bicarbonate, normally is 24–30 volumes per cent.

22. (1) Mrs. Hershey's ketosis resulted from oxidizing body fat for fuel. By administering glucose and insulin intravenously, normal carbohydrate metabolism is facilitated, thereby eliminating the need to use fat as the major fuel source.

23. (2) Treatment for diabetic ketoacidosis consists of the intravenous administration of regular crystalline insulin in sufficient doses to effect proper metabolism of intravenously administered glucose and remaining ketones in body fluids and tissues. Under these conditions, serum concentrations of glucose and ketones are expected to shift swiftly and continuously, and rapid restoration of normal concentrations must be achieved if permanent damage to nervous tissue is to be avoided. Hourly urinalyses for sugar and acetone are performed during the first few hours of treatment to assess the adequacy of insulin dosage and to prevent overdosage.

24. (3) The diabetic patient is unusually susceptible to infection as a result of high concentration of blood glucose in all body tissues, impaired circulation, and decreased macrophage mobility. The presence of an indwelling catheter traumatizes the urethra and bladder, and provides a potential avenue of infection of the urinary tract. The catheter should be removed as soon as the patient is conscious enough to retain urine and to provide a specimen on request.

25. (4) Because each diabetic patient reacts in a highly individual way to the type and dosage of insulin prescribed, and because coexisting diseases may vary the speed of carbohydrate-fat-insulin metabolism in individual patients, serial urinalyses must be performed to determine the hours of the day when Mrs. Hershey's glycosuria and blood glucose concentration tend to be highest. When this is known, the physician can order the type of insulin which, if administered at 6 or 7 A.M. each day, will provide peak action at the time of the patient's highest blood sugar level.

26. (1) Since it is desirable to know what the patient's blood and urine glucose level is

at the hour that the urine is collected, Mrs. Hershey should be instructed to void one half-hour before the scheduled urine collection time. In that way, the urine specimen tested will reflect her current physiologic state, not her condition two or three hours before the sample was collected.

27. (1) Because insulin increases cell membrane permeability to glucose, and catalyzes the phosphorylation of glucose in the liver, it facilitates transport of glucose across cell membranes and fosters conversion of blood glucose to liver glycogen.

28. (2) Insulin is a polypeptide, or protein molecule, which would be digested by the hydrochloric acid and enzymes in gastric and intestinal secretions.

29. (2) The onset of action for regular insulin occurs within one hour following administration. Peak action occurs 2–4 hours after administration. Duration of action is 6–8 hours.

30. (3) N.P.H. insulin, an intermediate-acting insulin, has an onset of action from 2–4 hours following administration, and a peak action within 6–12 hours after administration.

31. (3) The "P" in the designation N.P.H. refers to protamine, as N.P.H. insulin is a modified P.Z.I. suspension with concentrations of insulin, protamine, and zinc so arranged that the onset and duration of action for N.P.H. is intermediate between regular and P.Z.I. The duration of action of P.Z.I. is 36 hours. The duration of action of N.P.H. is 24 hours, facilitating closer control of patients who require fairly large doses of insulin.

32. (3) Since N.P.H. is a mixture or suspension of regular insulin with P.Z.I., the vial should be rotated gently before each dose is withdrawn to ensure uniformity of the mixture.

33. (1) U. 100 insulin contains 100 units of insulin in each milliliter of the mixture. The formula for computing the volume of insulin mixture to be injected is:

$$\frac{\text{Desired dose}}{\text{Available dose}} \times \text{minims per ml.} = \text{number of minims to be injected}$$

$$\frac{60 \text{ U.}}{100 \text{ U.}} \text{ per ml.} \times 15 \text{ min. per ml.} = 9 \text{ minims to be injected}$$

34. (3) As a result of an overdose of insulin, omission of meals, nausea and vomiting, or overexertion, the diabetic patient may develop hyperinsulinism. This causes hypoglycemia, the symptoms of which are headache, weakness, apprehension, irritability, tremor, diaphoresis, and coma.

35. (1) Hyperinsulinism should be treated with prompt intravenous administration of 20–50 ml. of 50 per cent glucose, if the patient is comatose. If she is awake, sweetened orange juice, hard candy, or lump sugar should be given.

36. (4) The pancreatic defect responsible for Mrs. Hershey's lack of insulin is irreversible. She will probably require insulin administration and dietary regulation for the rest of her life.

37. (1) Sulfisoxizole (Cantrisin) is a rapidly absorbed and rapidly excreted sulfonamide. The sulfonamides in general are distributed to all body tissues, and exert a bacteriostatic effect on many gram-positive and -negative organisms as a result of the fact that they block several enzyme systems essential to bacterial growth.

38. (2) One gram is equivalent to 15 grains, so 2 tablets are required to administer the desired dose.

39. (2) One gram of protein yields 4 calories when metabolized. One gram of carbohydrate yields 4 calories. One gram of fat yields 9 calories when metabolized. $(180 \times 4) + (90 \times 4) + (80 \times 9) = 1800$ calories.

40. (3) By dividing Mrs. Hershey's prescribed caloric intake among five rather than three feedings each day, a mid-afternoon and bedtime snack can be provided to eliminate the extremes of blood glucose concentration that occur when three large meals are eaten at long intervals. By thus flattening the curve of blood glucose concentration, better insulin-dietary balance is made possible.

41. (2) An individual's basal caloric requirement, or the number of calories required

to maintain body metabolism in the basal or resting state, is equal to 10 calories per pound of ideal body weight per day.

42. (3) Biochemical studies have revealed that a carbohydrate intake of roughly 1 gram of carbohydrate per pound of body weight is required to prevent catabolism of body fat and protein as energy sources. Since the catabolism of body fat leads to ketoacidosis in the diabetic, no less than this level of carbohydrate intake should be provided.

43. (2) In order to prevent catabolism of body tissue as an energy source, the diabetic diet should provide a minimal protein intake of 0.5 to 0.66 grams of protein per pound of ideal body weight (or roughly 1.0 to 1.5 grams of protein per kilogram of ideal body weight).

44. (1) Of those listed, only the peas are a 7 per cent vegetable (supplying 7 grams of carbohydrate in a 100-gram serving). The others on the list are so-called "A" vegetables, and have negligible carbohydrate content.

45. (4) Of those listed, mashed white potatoes are included on the bread exchange list because a standard 100-gram serving of mashed potatoes contains about 15 grams of carbohydrate. The others on the list are "B" vegetables, and contain 7 grams of carbohydrate per 100-gram serving.

46. (3) Of the alternatives given, only one is listed on the bread exchange. One half-cup of lima beans, like one slice of baker's bread, contains 15 grams of carbohydrate.

47. (1) Carbohydrate quantities are as follows: One small orange contains 10 grams; one cup of strawberries = 10 grams; one cup of applesauce = 20 grams; eight prunes = about 40 grams; one large banana = 20–30 grams.

48. (3) Both 1 oz. of beefsteak and 1 oz. of haddock contain negligible carbohydrate, 7 grams of protein, and 5 grams of fat; 3 oz. of cheddar cheese = negligible amounts of carbohydrate, 21 grams of protein, and 27 grams of fat; two eggs = negligible amounts of carbohydrate, 12 grams of protein, and 12 grams of fat; one cup of cottage cheese = negligible amounts of carbohydrate, 31 grams of protein, and 9 grams of fat.

49. (4) The fat exchange list indicates that 1 teaspoon of mayonnaise is a suitable exchange for 1 teaspoon of butter, because both have negligible carbohydrate and protein and 5 grams of fat. Five small olives, one eighth of an avocado, and 6 small nuts would be suitable exchanges for 1 teaspoon of butter.

50. (3) This response is accurate, nonevasive, and based on knowledge possessed by the nurse. It is not likely that Mrs. Hershey will later be switched from insulin to an oral hypoglycemic agent. The decision to use insulin rather than the latter is based on considerations other than the personal preference of the physician. The nurse cannot know whether Mrs. Hershey or her sister is the more insulin-deficient.

51. (4) Mrs. Hershey should be helped to become as self-sufficient as possible following hospital discharge. Since she suffers no physical or mental handicap or limitation, she should be instructed to test her urine for sugar and acetone; administer her daily insulin dose; plan, prepare, and serve her own diet; provide protective foot care; and recognize and treat the symptoms of ketoacidosis and hyperinsulinism.

52. (4) All these factors should be considered. If Mrs. Hershey is short and overweight, caloric intake should be limited so as to gradually decrease her weight, thereby facilitating dietary control of diabetes. Since she is middle-aged, she will require fewer calories per day than a teenager, but more calories per day than a bedridden 80-year-old. The amount of daily involvement in physical labor and active sports should help to determine her daily caloric requirement. If, before this illness, Mrs. Hershey had exercised good dietary habits, a fairly liberal diabetic diet would probably be prescribed, advocating meal planning with exchange lists. If she were grossly overweight and had given a history of irregular and poorly balanced meals, a rigidly controlled weighed diet would most likely be prescribed until ideal body weight is achieved. If Mrs. Hershey were a member of an ethnic group that eats large quantities of carbohydrate, the physician might restrict her carbohydrate intake less than her fat intake.

53. (2) This response is truthful and to the point. Although it may be true that the physician wants Mrs. Hershey to lose weight, it is imperative that she comprehend the interconvertibility of fats, proteins, and glucose if she is to regulate her diet effectively. It is not a foregone conclusion that Mrs. Hershey will have to weigh her diet; it may be possible for her to regulate it through use of exchange lists. The purpose for decreasing caloric intake is to reduce weight so as to improve diabetic control, not to improve digestion.

54. (1) Because food habits and dietary patterns are conditioned by a number of psychologic, social, and cultural influences, they are exceedingly resistant to change. Breaking a culturally conditioned or family decreed dietary tradition may be seen by the patient or others of importance as an abandonment of group values.

55. (3) To be suitable for self-injection of insulin, a site must be easily accessible to the patient, relatively insensitive to pain, and free of bone, blood vessels, and nerves. Sites listed in a, c, and d meet these qualifications.

56. (3) Repeated injections of insulin into the same site produces inflammation of tissues, which leads to atrophy, induration, or fibrosis of the injured tissue, all of which will interfere with later insulin absorption. To avoid tissue damage, possible sites for insulin administration should be mapped, and the injection site should be rotated daily so that each site is used less frequently than every 2 weeks.

57. (3) Boiling the reusable syringe and needle in a pan of water for 20 minutes before each use will destroy the more common pathogens (but not bacterial spores).

58. (4) The single tablet copper reduction test (Clinitest) is a screening test for urine sugar. It includes combining 5 drops of urine, 10 drops of water, and one Clinitest tablet in a test tube, allowing the solution to boil, and comparing the color of the urine with a color chart. Blue color indicates absence of sugar. Orange indicates 4 + sugar concentration.

59. (4) Diabetics are extremely susceptible to skin infection, as a result of impaired circulation and increased glucose concentration of body fluids. The incidence of skin infection is especially high in those diabetics whose disease is poorly controlled by diet or insulin.

60. (4) Dietary excesses, insulin omission, unhygienic practices, lowered physical resistance, respiratory infection, and severe physical stress of any type are apt to precipitate diabetic acidosis by increasing the disparity between glucose "load" and insulin supply.

61. (1) In diabetic acidosis, dehydration leads to decreased blood volume, with fall in blood pressure and impairment of cerebral blood flow. Additionally, the ketone bodies that accumulate in the body fluids release hydrogen ions, decreasing the pH of the serum. As pH decreases beyond 7.2 there is evident depression of cerebral function, with listlessness, drowsiness, and stupor, deepening into coma.

62. (2) Mrs. Hershey should wear a diabetic identification bracelet or carry a diabetic identification card with her at all times so that, if she becomes suddenly ill while away from home, those who care for her will be immediately alerted to her condition, the amount and type of insulin prescribed, and her physician's name and phone number. She should also carry several pieces of hard candy to relieve hypoglycemia whenever she feels diaphoretic and shaky.

63. (2) Disturbed fat metabolism in the diabetic leads to increased incidence of atherosclerosis. Decreased blood supply renders tissues more susceptible to infection. Proper foot care for the diabetic requires scrupulous cleanliness of the skin and the stockings; use of lubricating lotion to prevent skin fissuring; avoidance of friction, pressure, and traumatic injury; and properly fitted stockings and shoes.

64. (3) Atheromatous changes in large and medium-sized arteries decreases blood supply to vital organs of the body. Impaired coronary flow may lead to progressive myocardial failure or acute myocardial infarction. Improperly perfused tissues suffer increased susceptibility to infection. Infection of anoxic tissues leads rapidly to gangrene. In diabetics, sorbitol and fructose accumulate in peripheral nerves, causing peripheral neuropathy due to segmental demyelinization of the fibers and delayed nerve impulse conduction. Diabetes is characterized by microvascular pathology in the retina. Tortuosity and microan-

eurysms of retinal blood vessels, with proliferation of new vessels over the disc and into the vitreous, lead to retinal degeneration and blindness.

65. (2) A program of moderate exercise should be prescribed for the diabetic patient since exercise, by increasing energy demand, increases catabolism of carbohydrates, facilitating weight control and lowering blood glucose.

66. (3) Either atrophy or hypertrophy of adipose tissue may occur when the same site is used repeatedly and frequently for insulin injection. Atrophy of subcutaneous tissue is evidenced by a loss of tissue mass, with dimpling or recession of overlying skin. Hypertrophy is evidenced by lumpiness or induration of the tissues. Either deformity results in delayed absorption of any drug injected into the affected tissues.

67. (4) Decreased arterial blood flow to a part renders it pale, because skin vessels are less well perfused; cold, as less heat is brought to tissues by the circulating blood; atrophic, since the skin is deprived of the nutrients needed for cellular replacement; and painful, owing to ischemic neuritis.

68. (3) The inflammatory reaction, which is the classic tissue reaction to injury, consists of a brief initial vasoconstriction followed by vasodilation, engorgement, transudation, diapedesis, phagocytosis, resorption, and repair, Arteriosclerotic vessels are inelastic and unable to increase their diameter so as to enhance arterial blood flow to an area of inflammation. At the same time, infection speeds the rate of cellular metabolism, increasing cellular oxygen demand. When oxygen demand outstrips blood supply, gangrene results.

69. (1) Loss of an extremity constitutes a profound change in body image which, as a result of clothing styles, is especially threatening to women.

70. (1) The rate of most chemical reactions increases with rises in temperature. By markedly lowering the temperature of body tissues the metabolic activities by which bacteria grow and reproduce can be decreased, so that bacterial growth is retarded, bacterial injury to tissues is retarded, and dissolution of dead tissue cells is impaired. Local applications of cold serve to decrease pain impulse perception by sensory end organs and impulse transmission through sensory nerve fibers to the brain.

71. (4) The blood vessels of the thigh that are divided during an above-knee amputation are large and capable of carrying a considerable volume of blood. If the ligatures applied to the sectioned vessels should slip during the first few hours or first couple of days following surgery, massive blood loss would result. A tourniquet should be attached to the head of the bed where it can be immediately available if hemorrhage should occur.

72. (4) We all carry a mental concept of our physical body that is a composite of the physical structure observed on looking into a mirror; our conception of the "ideal" body; our beliefs concerning the utility, attractiveness, and worth of our physical structure; the sensations of pain, pleasure, touch, pressure, vibration, and position experienced in relation to bodily function; and the reactions of others to our physical appearance and abilities.

73. (4) An important aspect of each individual's life experience is the conscious perception of the self as object. The concept of physical selfhood grows from interaction with the environment and with others of importance to oneself. The basis for physical selfhood is the sheer weight, mass, and extent of the body. An important aspect is the degree of physical movement of which one is capable, because fight and flight are basic methods of self-preservation. The size of the body and the speed and force of movement contribute to an individual's sense of personal safety, freedom, and status.

74. (2) Answer 2 is correct.

75. (3) Postoperatively the stump should be elevated on pillows for only 24 hours to reduce edema, since prolonged stump elevation predisposes to hip flexion contracture. Cranking up the foot gatch of the bed frame, or suspending the stump from the Balkan frame, likewise predisposes to hip flexion deformity. The safest means for reducing stump edema on the second postoperative day would be to raise the foot of the bed on blocks, because the hips are kept in neutral position by this means.

76. (4) Since arm muscle strength is essential to satisfactory use of crutches, Mrs. Hershey should be helped to increase the strength of the triceps (which ex-

tends and stabilizes the elbow). She can best exercise the triceps by using her palms to push herself upward from a prone position.

77. (1) The joint deformities most apt to occur following amputation are hip joint flexion contracture, stump adduction contracture, knee flexion contracture (with below-knee amputation), and footdrop of the unamputated limb. All can be avoided by correct positioning and regular exercise of the extremity.

78. (4) If a prosthesis is to be used, the tissues of the stump must be molded so that the stump will fit properly into the socket of the prosthesis. Such molding is accomplished by application of an elastic pressure bandage to the stump so as to shape and shrink it to the desired size through application of equal pressure over all soft tissue covering the amputated bone.

Fractured Femur and Internal Fixation

1. (4) The strong muscles of the thigh and hip cause marked displacement of bone fragments following a fracture of the femur. Laceration of vessels at the site of injury causes hemorrhage into soft tissue, with discoloration of overlying skin. If the bone fragements were separated by the injury, there may be abnormal movement between the two fragments on careful manipulation of the part.

2. (4) If soft tissue is interposed between fracture fragments, and the fragments are moved during transportation, there could be further laceration of periosteum, blood vessels, nerves, muscle, and other vital tissues. To prevent further soft tissue damage, the injured leg should be splinted before the patient is moved from the site of his fall.

3. (3) Much of the anxiety associated with injury and illness derives from the patient's loss of control over his life and circumstances. Mr. Marble's fall was sudden and unpredictable, and his injury deprived him of mobility. Anxiety might make him distrustful of a young and apparently inexperienced physician whom he therefore denigrates by calling him "Sonny."

4. (4) To prevent further soft tissue damage by sharp bone fragments, Mr. Marble's pants should be cut open along the leg seam and laid back without moving his leg. The pants can be repaired later, if desired.

5. (3) Following a femoral fracture, blood extravasates into the soft tissues of the thigh from vessels of the periosteum, the bone itself, and muscles surrounding the fracture site. Some of the extravasted blood dissects through deeper tissues into the subcutaneous tissues and skin, which become discolored by pigments released from lysed red blood cells.

6. (2) Any fracture site should be x-rayed in both anteroposterior and lateral projections to investigate the exact nature and full extent of the injury. An anterior or posterior displacement of a fragment might not be visible in an anteroposterior view, and a lateral or medial displacement might not be visible in a lateral view.

7. (4) A tonic spasm is a continuous, involuntary muscle contraction. The muscles of the thigh and hip are large and, on contracting, exert great force on their points of insertion. When a bone is fractured, continuous strong contraction by an attached muscle tends to displace the fragment from accustomed alignment.

8. (4) In an oblique or spiral fracture of the femur, tonic spasm of attached muscles tends to pull the fragments closer together, and the oblique surfaces of the fragments slide over one another, causing the two bones to overlap, so that the limb is shortened.

9. (1) Because the vessels of the thigh are large and carry a large volume of blood, rupture of a good-sized vessel in the periosteum, the medullary canal of the femur, or the muscle surrounding the fracture site may result in the loss of as much as 1 liter of blood within an hour or two following fracture of the femur. The normal circulating blood volume for an adult male is about 5 quarts. Loss of 20 per cent of the circulating blood volume can decrease the blood pressure to shock levels.

10. (2) Following a massive hemorrhage, the decrease in circulating blood volume causes a fall in systolic pressure. The decrease in arterial pressure initiates strong sympathetic stimulation, which releases epinephrine and norepineph-

rine, thereby constricting arterioles in the skin, kidney, and viscera, producing pallor and oliguria. Epinephrine also increases the heart rate, causing rapid, weak, and thready pulse. The anxiety and diaphoresis associated with shock are the result of high levels of circulating catecholamines.

11. (2) Until the fragments of the fractured femur are immobilized by internal or external fixation, the injured leg should be immobilized by splinting every time the patient is moved, no matter how short the distance. Splinting prevents further soft tissue damage and stops the closed fracture from being converted into an open fracture. It also decreases hemorrhage from damaged vessels, and minimizes pain and muscle spasm.

12. (2) However Mr. Marble is to be treated, he will be immobilized for some time and must be kept in good body alignment to prevent lasting deformity. To ensure proper alignment of the spine, he should be placed on a firm, nonsagging mattress. One means of preventing mattress sag is to place a full-length bed board between mattress and springs.

13. (3) No. 1 is a "put down." No. 2 passes the buck. No. 4 jumps to an unwarranted conclusion. No. 3 is a truthful answer, given in good faith.

14. (1) Buck's extension is a form of skin traction, in that a light traction force is applied to the distal fragment of the fractured femur through a pull exerted by a weight attached to adhesive strips affixed to the skin of the leg. In skeletal traction, metal pins or screws are inserted into a bone and weights are attached, so that the traction pull is exerted directly on skeletal structures rather than on skin.

15. (1) The muscle spasms that follow fracture of the femur are exceedingly painful; also by compressing blood vessels, they interfere with circulation of blood and lymph in the part. Light skin traction should be applied to the injured extremity to reduce muscle spasm.

16. (1) Dirt, oil, desquamated skin, and moisture all weaken the attachment of adhesive tape to the skin. The skin of the leg should be washed and dried thoroughly to ensure proper adherence of the tape.

17. (3) Moleskin, which can be cut to preferred widths and lengths, can be used instead of adhesive tape to apply gentle skin traction in Buck's extension. The spreader board provides a site for attachment of moleskin that prevents pressure against the internal and external malleoli. The pulley maintains smooth, even traction on the leg with changes in the patient's position.

18. (4) Traction is effective in reducing a fracture or relieving muscle spasm because pull is exerted on the fractured extremity in two opposing directions. The traction force usually consists of metal weights or sandbags. Counter traction or opposing force may be either the weight of the patient's body or other weights. In Buck's extension, the foot of the bed is elevated to augment the effect of gravity in pulling the patient's body in the opposite direction from the pull exerted by the traction weights.

19. (4) Compression of the peroneal nerve against the upper 3 inches of the fibula by too tight application of the tape or moleskin causes peroneal paralysis, and results in plantar flexion and inversion of the foot.

20. (4) For traction to be effective in relieving spasm, the pulling forces must remain constant and smooth. For the prescribed pull to be exerted, the traction ropes must be free of the bed and bedding, and must run freely in the pulley without contact between the rope knots and the pulley wheel.

21. (4) Hypertensive and arteriosclerotic heart diseases are common in older persons, and increase the risks from general anesthesia and major surgery. Myocardial ischemia produces T-wave inversion. Myocardial injury produces ST segment depression or elevation in certain EKG leads.

22. (2) Pulmonary emphysema is characterized by an increase in the diameter of air passages distal to the terminal bronchioles. It is caused by chronic bacterial bronchiolitis and/or trapping of air distal to infected bronchioles.

23. (1) Decreased elasticity of lung parenchyma and expiratory closure of unsupported respiratory bronchioles cause hyperinflation of alveoli and an increase in residual volume. Bullous areas of the lung distal to fibrosing bronchiolitis may be perfused but poorly ventilated. These two defects combine to produce poor oxygenation of blood.

24. (4) Epithelial cells are continually being shed from the bladder mucosa. One to

three epithelial cells per low-power field in any urine specimen may be expected on the basis of normal desquamation and replacement of bladder epithelium.

25. (3) Casts are cylindric molds of the renal tubules or ducts. They may be composed of fat, red blood cells, white blood cells, or hyaline (a transparent protein material). The type of cast seen indicates the nature of particulate matter present in tubular filtrate.

26. (2) The specific gravity of normal adult urine can vary from 1.001 to 1.035 under a range of conditions but with average adult fluid intake of 1000 to 1500 ml./day the normal specific gravity of the urine would range from 1.010 to 1.020.

27. (4) Care should be taken not to cut the skin during preoperative skin preparation as the laceration could become infected by normal skin bacteria, e.g., *Staphylococcus aureus*, and cause contamination of bone fragments during the operative procedure.

28. (2) Spinal anesthesia is a loss of sensation produced by injection of an anesthetic into the spinal subarachnoid space between the levels of L_2–L_3 and L_5–S_1. This site is used for the injection because the spinal cord extends to the level of L_2.

29. (2) Older patients show decreased tolerance to barbiturates, which frequently cause confusion. Chloral hydrate is a fast-acting CNS depressant that has little effect on respiration or blood pressure when given in therapeutic doses, and which does not suppress REM (rapid eye movements) sleep to the same extent that barbiturates do.

30. (4) In order to maintain proper position of the fracture fragments, after femoral pinning it is necessary to prevent adduction and external rotation of the thigh and acute hip flexion. An effective means is to apply boot casts and connect the casts at the ankle with a cross-bar.

31. (1) In applying a cast to immobilize or support a part, the skin is washed and dried; the part is covered with a protective layer of tubular stockinette of greater length than the intended cast; a thin layer of sheet wadding is wrapped around the stockinette; pieces of felt are positioned over bony prominences to protect the skin from pressure injury; and moistened plaster of Paris bandage is used to encase the part in a cast or mold that, upon drying and hardening, will hold the extremity in desired position.

32. (2) Plaster of Paris bandage should be moistened with water of tepid temperature, or slightly less than blood heat. Warmer water speeds up setting of the plaster; cooler water delays it.

33. (3) Air bubbles will rise from the bandage to the top of the water until the bandage is completely saturated. When water has penetrated every layer of the roller, the bandage should be removed from the water, since the process of crystallization has then begun.

34. (1) Plaster of Paris-impregnated bandage is available in preparations with various setting speeds, from very rapid (2–4 mins.) to rapid (5–8 mins.) to slow (10–18 mins.). Regular plaster of Paris will set or harden in about 10 minutes.

35. (2) A patient with a newly applied cast can easily become imbalanced and fall from bed during turning. To avoid accidents, adjustable side rails should be attached to the bed. The cast will not dry for a day or two. To maintain proper contour of the cast, both boot casts should be supported full length on plastic-covered pillows until dry. A heat lamp should not be used to dry a cast, as too rapid drying will make the cast crack.

36. (2) In any boot or short leg cast, all toes should be visible in order that any circulatory impairment may be seen and to permit movement of the toes.

37. (2) The blood vessels of the thigh carry a large volume of blood. If bleeding were to occur from the operative site, blood would be apt to drain down the side of the thigh under the dressing, and pool under the hip on the lower linen.

38. (3) Obstruction of arterial blood flow causes the skin to be pale and cold as a result of inadequately perfused tissues. Obstruction of venous blood flow makes the tissues cyanotic and edematous, reflecting the increased concentration of reduced hemoglobin and increased hydrostatic pressure in tissue capillaries.

39. (3) The blanching test, a measure of circulatory effectiveness in a casted extremity, consists of brief compression of the thumb or great toe nail (which produces blanching of the nail), followed by quick release of the pressure. By comparing

the speed with which color returns to the nail on the casted and uncasted extremity, one can determine whether the cast has obstructed circulation to any degree.

40. (3) Paralysis and gangrene are possible consequences of circulatory obstruction in a casted extremity. If the patient's physician cannot be contacted when circulatory embarrassment is diagnosed in a casted arm or leg, the cast and underlying padding should be bivalved, or cut completely through on either side of the extremity. The top half of the cast should be removed to free the tissues of pressure, and the extremity should be left in the bottom half of the cast to maintain proper alignment.

41. (3) The peroneal nerve courses just under the skin on the outer aspect of the calf, just below the knee. Compression of the nerve between cast and the head of the fibula may produce peroneal paralysis.

42. (3) The peroneal nerve innervates the dorsiflexors of the foot and toes and the evertors of the foot, and provides sensation to the dorsum of the foot and lateral aspect of the lower half of the leg. Following peroneal nerve compression, numbness and a sensation of pressure on the lateral aspect of the leg develop as a result of ischemic injury to sensory fibers. If ischemia continues, an unpleasant tingling sensation develops as a result of fibrotic changes in the nerve. If the leg is exercised while circulation remains occluded, aching and burning pain develop in the leg and foot as remaining sensory fibers are stimulated by accumulations of lactic acid. Complete paralysis of the nerve results in inability to extend the toes or foot.

43. (3) Since a cast that has set but not dried completely can be molded by strong pressure, the casted extremity should be supported on the open palm while the patient is lifted, so as to prevent finger indentations in the cast surface. The damp cast should be supported full length on pliant, rubber-covered pillows so as to avoid flattening dependent portions of the cast against a hard mattress. A bed board should be placed over the springs to keep the mattress from sagging and the damp cast from bowing under heavier body parts. Since the cast must dry slowly from the inside out, in order to prevent mold growth in the cast interior, the cast should be left uncovered and exposed to room air until the surface is white and shiny, and yields a resonant tone on percussion.

44. (1) Free circulation of warm, dry air around the damp cast enhances water evaporation from the cast surface. Application of heat to a cast surface is apt to burn the skin beneath the cast.

45. (2) While the cast is drying the loss of heat of evaporation leaves the patient feeling cold and clammy. Body heat loss can be minimized by covering the exposed skin while leaving the cast exposed to air.

46. (4) Depending on the thickness of the cast and the heat, humidity, and air temperature of the room, most casts require 24–48 hours to dry completely.

47. (4) The skin of Mr. Marble's leg could be excoriated by compression by finger indentations on the wet cast surface; pressure of unpadded bony prominences against the rigid inner cast surface; irritation by plaster crumbs, food crumbs, and other debris that fall into the cast; and irritation of surrounding skin by the rough plaster edges of an "unfinished" cast.

48. (4) The symptoms of skin excoriation, infection, or pressure ulcers under the cast surface are the signs of inflammation and infection anywhere in the body: swelling, redness, heat, pain, and inflammatory exudate. Thus, the cast may be warm to touch over a localized area of inflammation as a result of heat conduction through the cast materials. Itching of inflamed tissues would signify irritation of sensory end organs by inflammatory exudate and debris. Dampness and discoloration of an area on the cast surface would suggest an outpouring of inflammatory exudate. An offensive odor from the cast interior would indicate purulent exudate or necrotic tissue in the wound.

49. (4) Plaster casts are heavy, inflexible, and awkward to handle, limiting the patient's movement in bed. Immobility predisposes older individuals to circulatory stasis in the skin, lungs, and deep veins. Circulatory stasis is most severe in the more dependent portions of the body. Sluggish capillary blood flow, together with friction over pressure points, produces decubitus ulcers. Pooling of blood in dependent lung capillaries predisposes to transudation of fluid into adjacent alveoli, with development of hypostatic pneumonia. Decreased ve-

nous blood flow in the legs predisposes to phlebothrombosis and pulmonary embolism. Prolonged bedrest causes demineralization of bones and impaired urinary drainage, which in combination predispose to development of urinary tract stones.

50. (4) Slowing of blood flow, injury to vessel walls, and increased coagulability of blood all predispose to intravascular clotting. Aged, immobilized patients, lacking the blood-pumping action of contracting leg muscles, suffer venous stasis in the legs, further increasing their risk of phlebothrombosis.

51. (3) With decreased weight-bearing during long bedrest, increased calcium salts are mobilized from the bone, enter the blood, are filtered by the glomerulus, and appear in the urine. A decrease in muscle metabolism during inactivity results in the production of urine that is more alkaline than normal. Calcium salts are more apt to precipitate out of solution in alkaline urine. When patients lie supine for long periods, gravity no longer aids the flow of urine from the kidney, so that urine stagnates in the kidney pelvis and salts crystallize out of solution.

52. (4) By increasing the daily fluid intake, more dilute urine is produced, so that the tendency for crystallization and precipitation of salts is decreased.

53. (1) Isometric exercise consists of functional activity of a muscle without a change in muscle length. When a muscle is exercised without a change in length, the part is not moved, but the tension in the muscle is temporarily increased. Quadriceps setting consists of pushing the popliteal space against the mattress, and lifting the heel free of the bed to the count of five. Gluteal setting consists of pinching the buttocks together and attempting to move the leg to the edge of the bed.

54. (3) By moving Mr. Marble from bed to supine position on a cart twice a day, pressure can be relieved on the skin of the back and buttocks, and bronchopulmonary secretions that have pooled in dependent (posterior) portions of the lung can be mobilized and removed by coughing. Twice-daily transfer of the patient from bed to a wheelchair enhances urinary drainage from kidneys, ureters, and bladder.

55. (4) When a bone is broken, vessels in the periosteum and bone tissue rupture, and a hematoma forms around and between the fracture fragments. Upon organization, this hematoma develops into a specialized type of granulation tissue called "callus," which consists of cartilage, calcium and phosphate ions, and osteoblasts. Callus is eventually replaced by bone that grows into the area from surrounding periosteum.

56. (4) The skin under a cast is usually covered with a scaly or crusty exudate. Application of an emollient will help to soften and remove the crust.

Cirrhosis of the Liver

1. (3) The liver cell removes the NH_2 group from amino acids in preparation for converting the remainder of the molecule to carbohydrate or fat; removes excess glucose from the blood and stores it as glycogen; stores the fat-soluble vitamins, vitamin B_{12}, and iron. Kupffer cells phagocytize foreign particles and remove them from the blood.

2. (2) The liver stores vitamins A, D, K, and B_{12}.

3. (3) In cirrhosis, a chronic, degenerative liver disease, hepatic cells die and are replaced by bands of fibrous tissue that divide the regenerating liver tissue into nodules.

4. (4) In early cirrhosis there is accumulation of fat globules in liver cells and deterioration of cellular organelles. With time, damaged liver cells die and are replaced with bands of fibrous tissue. Hepatic cells regenerate and are surrounded by fibrous tissue bands, creating nodular masses that disrupt normal liver architecture and compress interlobular arteries, veins, and canaliculi.

5. (3) Cirrhosis is caused by a combination of malnutrition and toxic damage to the liver cell by alcohol.

6. (2) In some nonalcoholic patients, liver cell damage due to acute viral hepatitis, intrahepatic biliary obstruction, and hepatocellular toxins may progress to

fatty infiltration, fibrosis, and nodular degeneration of remaining liver cell mass.

7. (4) Increased fibrosis of liver parenchyma interferes with blood flow through the organ, increasing the pressure in the portal circulation. Increased portal vein pressures cause venous engorgement of the stomach, spleen, and bowel, interfering with digestion and absorption, and causing anorexia and diarrhea. Fibrotic constriction of canaliculi results in inadequate bile supply to the duodenum, with impaired digestion of fats, and flatulence. Liver cell destruction results in decreased glycogen storage, impaired glycogenolysis, and lack of emergency energy stores, which causes easy fatigability.

8. (1) The increased incidence of peptic ulceration in cirrhotic patients may be due to the damaged liver's inability to inactivate the histamine normally present in portal blood. Alcoholism predisposes to pancreatitis, because heavy alcoholic intake causes duodenitis, with edema or spasm of the sphincter of Oddi; obstruction of the pancreatic duct; intrapancreatic activation of proteolytic and lipolytic enzymes; and autodigestion of pancreatic tissue and blood vessels.

9. (3) The color of vomited blood depends on the length of time the blood has been in contact with hydrochloric acid in gastric secretions. If vomiting occurs shortly after the onset of bleeding, the vomitus will be bright red. If there is a delay of a half-hour or more, it will be dark brown to black, with a coffee-ground appearance.

10. (1) Whenever a patient vomits, mouth care should be given to remove food particles, gastric secretions, and blood from the mouth, as these have an unpleasant taste and odor, and can serve as a culture medium for normal bacterial inhabitants of the oral and nasal cavities.

11. (3) The splenic vein, right and left gastric vein, and superior mesenteric vein all empty into the portal vein. The increase in portal vein pressure that occurs in Laennec's cirrhosis is referred backward through the portal system, causing congestion of the stomach, with dyspepsia; congestion of the spleen, with splenomegaly; and transudation of fluid from mesenteric capillaries into the peritoneal cavity, or ascites.

12. (4) The portal circulation is a venous system with capillaries at either end. Venous blood from the stomach, spleen, and intestine is carried to the liver by the portal vein; passes through the liver sinusoids and is acted on by the liver cells; and leaves the liver via the hepatic vein to return to the right heart. In cirrhosis, fibrosis and scarring obstruct blood flow, compressing the softer-walled veins and increasing pressure in the portal circulation.

13. (2) Increased portal vein pressure and decreased serum albumin levels predispose Mr. Kemper to accumulation of ascitic fluid. With massive ascites, increased intra-abdominal pressure may cause umbilical hernia.

14. (3) In semi-Fowler's position the large accumulation of ascitic fluid will exert least pressure on the diaphragm, and so produce least interference with diaphragmatic excursions during respiration.

15. (2) Minute quantities of estrogen and progesterone are produced by the adrenal cortex, in males as well as females. The normal liver oxidizes estradiol and conjugates estrogens, which are then excreted in the bile and urine. The cirrhotic liver cannot oxidize and/or conjugate adrenal estrogens, so that they accumulate in the blood, causing feminizing changes. Spider angiomas are dilated, tortuous, cutaneous arterioles found in the areas drained by the superior vena cava. They are thought to result from estrogen stimulation of arterioles.

16. (2) In cirrhosis, progressive death of liver cells and their replacement with fibrous tissue bands distorts normal liver architecture, compressing intralobular and interlobular vessels. Constriction of central veins, sinusoids, and branches of the portal vein all serve to increase pressure in the portal vein and the vessels that empty into it.

17. (4) Because the cirrhotic patient is troubled with anorexia, he does not usually eat regular, well-balanced meals and is apt to be lacking in protein, vitamins, and minerals. Lack of B complex vitamins often produces peripheral neuritis.

18. (1) Excessive alcoholic intake has several deleterious effects on the gastrointestinal system: morning nausea, vomiting, epigastric distress, abdominal distention, belching, gastritis, and peptic ulcer. Most of these interfere with appetite

and predispose to chronic malnutrition. Since Mr. Kemper's diet is apt to be lacking in meat, milk products, fresh fruit, and vegetables, he is prone to vitamin deficiency diseases.

19. (2) Distortion of liver architecture and destruction of liver cells permits "leakage" of conjugated bilirubin. from the liver cell backward into the sinusoid and the systemic venous circulation. When bile pigments are deposited in tissue cells, pruritus results.

20. (2) The adrenal cortex produces small quantities of estrogen in the male. In cirrhosis the damaged liver cell can no longer oxidize and/or conjugate estrogen, so that estrogen accumulates in the blood, breast tissue is stimulated, and gynecomastia results.

21. (1) Cirrhotic patients may develop anemia due to upper gastrointestinal tract bleeding or inadequate intake of protein and vitamin B_{12}. Massive quantities of ascitic fluid increase intra-abdominal pressure, elevate the diaphragm, and interfere with respiratory excursions. Rapid, shallow respirations result in poor alveolar gas exchange.

22. (1) Serum albumin is synthesized wholly in the liver cell. Alpha and beta globulins are synthesized in the liver cell; gamma globulins are synthesized in lymphoid tissue. In severe cirrhosis, liver cell damage results in a proportionately greater decrease in serum albumin than in serum globulin. The normal albumin-globulin ratio is about 2:1. In cirrhosis the marked depression in serum albumin causes this ratio to move closer to 1:1.

23. (2) Cholesterol, a sterol present in many foods, is absorbed from the intestine into the lymph and is carried to the liver. In addition to that ingested in the diet, a large quantity of cholesterol is formed in body cells. The normal concentration of serum cholesterol is 150–250 mg. per 100 ml. of blood.

24. (3) Cholesterol is fat-soluble and capable of forming esters with fatty acids. Normally, about 70 per cent of the cholesterol in the plasma is in the form of cholesterol esters.

25. (2) As a result of either decreased red blood cell production or increased blood loss, Mr. Kemper would be apt to have an abnormally low red blood cell count. As a result of destruction of large numbers of parenchymal liver cells, a smaller-than-normal proportion of the serum cholesterol would be esterified.

26. (3) Vitamin B_{12} is necessary for synthesis of DNA. Diseased liver cells are unable to store normal amounts of vitamin B_{12}, so DNA replication and red cell production is hampered. Poor appetite and impaired intestinal absorption cause long-term protein and vitamin lack in the cirrhotic, with impairment of red blood cell production. Gastritis, peptic ulceration, and bleeding esophageal varices are also possible sources of bleeding.

27. (2) The principal effect of serum albumin, which is synthesized in the liver, is to maintain the colloid osmotic pressure of the blood. Damaged liver cells are unable to synthesize albumin in normal quantities, so that fluid leaks out of capillaries and accumulates in dependent tissues. Massive ascites may compress the large veins of the abdomen enough to interfere with venous return from lower extremities. Increased hydrostatic pressure in leg veins causes transudation of fluid from capillaries into tissue spaces.

28. (2) Damaged liver cells cannot synthesize prothrombin, so the clotting reaction is interfered with in cirrhosis, and petechiae and epistaxis are apt to result.

29. (1) Purpura, which consists of hemorrhage into skin and mucous membranes, may result from a lack of thrombocytes, of vascular integrity, or of clotting factors. Cirrhotics may have thrombocytopenia due to lack of vitamin B_{12}; capillary fragility due to lack of vitamin C; and lack of prothrombin due to parenchymal cell death.

30. (4) There are several connections between the portal and the systemic venous circulations. Among these are the umbilical, rectal, and esophageal veins. When portal blood flow through the liver is severely obstructed, veins in any one of these three areas may dilate to permit blood from the gastrointestinal tract to circumvent the liver on its return to the heart. Dilated veins of the rectum frequently occur in cirrhosis.

31. (3) When fibrous tissue obstructs blood flow through the liver, portal blood may circumvent the liver, and return to the inferior vena cava by way of gastric veins and dilated esophageal veins.

32. (3) Massive bleeding from esophageal varices or bleeding peptic ulcer causes sudden decrease in blood volume, a lowering of systemic blood pressure, a decrease in venous return flow, and a reflex tachycardia. Loss of 10 per cent of the blood volume is followed by compensatory withdrawal of fluid from intercellular spaces into the vessels, and subsequently a shift of intracellular fluid to the intercellular compartment. This latter move causes intracellular dehydration, and thirst results.

33. (3) Hepatic coma results when excess nitrogenous substances, as ammonia, are absorbed from the intestine and not metabolized by the liver, and so reach the cerebral circulation. Hemorrhage from esophageal varices introduces a large quantity of protein into the intestine that, if digested by gastrointestinal enzymes and acted upon by intestinal bacteria, will yield excessive amounts of ammonia.

34. (4) In cirrhosis the regenerated liver cells have an inefficient relationship to blood supply. In the event of hemorrhagic shock, parenchymal liver cells are inadequately perfused, and hepatic necrosis will result unless transfusions are given to restore blood volume to normal.

35. (1) The liver performs a variety of functions that support total body metabolism. The best means of reducing liver workload is to decrease the rate of metabolic activity in all body tissues by maintaining the patient on total bedrest.

36. (1) The Sengstaken-Blakemore tube is a triple lumen tube with two balloon attachments that provides gastric suction, gastric tamponade, and esophageal tamponade. When the esophageal balloon is inflated, the patient cannot swallow his saliva. While the Sengstaken tube is in place, Mr. Kemper should be kept absolutely quiet in the supine position, to prevent movement of the tube and rebleeding, and to prevent aspiration of secretions.

37. (2) The esophageal balloon can be connected to a manometer and the balloon inflated to a pressure that exceeds portal venous pressure, thereby compressing the bleeding varix and providing hemostasis until a clot can form to seal the ruptured vessel.

38. (2) Rupture of either the gastric or the esophageal balloon would be followed by a fall in pressure on the attached manometer. Rupture of the gastric balloon would permit the entire tube to move cephalad, with possible obstruction of the airway.

39. (3) After the Sengstaken tube is inserted and the gastric balloon is inflated and clamped, the tube is retracted slowly until the gastric balloon is held tightly against the cardioesophageal junction, whereupon the tube is secured to the nares and face to maintain traction on the tube and pressure against the cardioesophageal junction. Constant pressure from the gastric balloon may cause pressure necrosis of the gastric mucosa, with further bleeding.

40. (4) When the esophageal balloon is inflated Mr. Kemper will be unable to swallow his saliva, which will drain into the upper portion of the esophagus and pool above the esophageal balloon. To prevent reflux of these secretions into the pharynx and their aspiration into the lower respiratory tract, they should be aspirated from the mouth, pharynx, and esophagus at regular intervals.

41. (2) Since Mr. Kemper will not be able to swallow his saliva while the esophageal balloon is inflated, an emesis basin should be left at the bedside for him to expectorate into.

42. (3) Any movement of the Sengstaken tube is apt to dislodge clots and reinstitute bleeding. Every effort should be made to maintain the tube in unchanged position until it is removed by the physician. With the tube in place, the stomach is partially distended by the inflated gastric balloon. If fluid is to be given through the gastric tube, it should be given slowly so as not to distend the stomach unduly, which action would be apt to stimulate retching and regurgitation of the tube.

43. (3) Hepatic coma results from disturbed nervous tissue functioning due to excessive blood ammonia levels, hypoxia, and acid-base imbalance. Ammonia is formed in the intestine by the breakdown of protein by intestinal bacteria. Enemas were ordered to rid the bowel of blood proteins released by the bleeding varix.

44. (4) When hepatic failure develops in the cirrhotic patient, inadequate bile delivery to the duodenum causes digestive disturbances, of which nausea, vomiting,

and diarrhea are common manifestations. Loss of fluid and electrolytes through vomiting and diarrhea upsets acid-base balance and raises body temperature. The liver becomes inflamed and swollen, stretching the liver capsule and producing right upper quadrant pain. Transaminase, an enzyme present in high concentration in liver cells, is released into the blood stream in large amounts when there is inflammation or necrosis of parenchymal liver cells.

45. (4) Prednisone, a synthetic glucocorticoid, promotes mobilization of body glucose during an emergency, exerts a strong anti-inflammatory effect, and regulates sodium-potassium-water balance. It also increases the body's ability to resist a variety of noxious stimuli and environmental changes, through mechanisms that are imperfectly understood.

46. (4) Fetor hepaticus is a peculiar musty or mousy breath odor observed in patients in hepatic coma. It results from the elimination of abnormal metabolites.

47. (4) Asterixis, or "flapping tremor," is a characteristic of impending hepatic coma. The tremor is elicited by asking the patient to hold his hands and arms perfectly still while extending them maximally against gravity. Periodically, he will be unable to sustain the position and will involuntarily drop his arms, and then quickly jerk the limb back into position, producing a flapping effect.

48. (2) In a normal adult the daily fluid intake ranges from about 1500 to 2000 ml., depending on body weight, physical activity, caloric intake, and environmental conditions of heat and humidity.

49. (2) A cation is an ion that carries a positive electrical charge. The sodium and potassium ions each carry a single positive charge, having one more proton in their nucleus than electrons in surrounding orbits. Each calcium ion carries two positive charges, having two more protons in its nucleus than electrons in surrounding orbits.

50. (2) The normal range of serum sodium is 135–145 mEq./L. The daily adult exchange of sodium is about 3–6 per cent of total sodium content in the body, and consists of sodium ingested and sodium lost through urine and sweat.

51. (4) Hypernatremia is usually due to a loss of body water, and consequently a relative excess of sodium in body fluids. The symptoms associated with hypernatremia are primarily those of the underlying dehydration: decreased urinary output, dry skin and mucosa, elevated temperature, flushed skin, and intense thirst.

52. (4) Aldosterone, the principal mineralocorticoid secreted by the adrenal cortex, increases resorption of sodium from the ascending loop of Henle and the distal tubule, and increases potassium secretion into the distal tubule. The effect of hypersecretion of aldosterone is sodium retention.

53. (1) The normal serum chloride concentration ranges from 95 to 105 mEq./L. In the adult the average daily exchange of chloride is about 2–7 per cent of the total body content of chloride. Chloride losses usually follow those of sodium, but since chloride can be compensated for by increases of serum bicarbonate, there is not the same loss of body water following loss of chloride as occurs following loss of sodium.

54. (2) The normal range for serum potassium concentration is 3.5–5.0 mEq./L. During glucose metabolism by the cell and during formation of new cells, a large amount of potassium enters body cells, and thus is the major intracellular cation. During strenuous exercise and during broad-scale tissue breakdown, potassium leaves the cells.

55. (4) Hypokalemia may cause nausea and vomiting due to decreased intestinal motility; abdominal distention due to paralytic ileus; weak irregular pulse due to decreased neuromuscular irritability; shallow respirations due to abdominal distention; and muscular weakness due to decreased neuromuscular irritability.

56. (2) Fresh fruits (oranges, bananas), dried fruits (apricots, peaches, raisins), and Coca-Cola all contain significant quantities of potassium.

57. (4) Chronic alcoholics generally have a long-standing history of malnutrition, because their alcoholic intake meets their daily caloric needs and dulls the appetite for protein and vitamin-rich foods. Malnourished tissues are susceptible to necrosis. Inability of damaged liver cells to synthesize albumin results in decreased serum osmotic pressure and subcutaneous edema. Edematous tis-

sues are especially susceptible to pressure injury. Inadequate protein intake and catabolism of body protein as an energy source leads to muscle wasting. Lack of muscular and soft-tissue padding over bony prominences predisposes to decubitus ulceration. Physical immobility causes poor circulation of dependent tissues, resulting in pressure injury to skin of the back and heels.

58. (2) The presence of glycogen within a liver cell protects the cell from injury due to ischemia and certain toxic metabolites. By increasing the serum glucose concentration above the level of current cellular energy needs, hepatic cells that are still functioning can be stimulated to store glycogen.

59. (1) Neomycin, a broad-spectrum antibiotic effective against several gram-negative and -positive organisms, is not inactivated by gastrointestinal secretions and enzymes. Thus, neomycin can be given orally as well as intramuscularly.

60. (1) Neomycin is poorly absorbed from the gastrointestinal tract, so is given orally when it is intended for preparation of the bowel for surgery or for management of hepatic coma, since in these instances it is desirable that the drug remain in the GI tract to suppress growth of intestinal bacteria.

61. (3) Hepatic coma is caused by the toxic effect of ammonia on brain tissue. Ammonia is produced when intestinal bacteria break down protein in the bowel. Following esophageal bleeding, ammonia production from blood proteins can be reduced by killing the intestinal bacteria responsible for ammonia production.

62. (3) The patient in hepatic coma has little functioning liver tissue remaining, so liver glycogen is minimal. If energy needs are not met through external nutrients, body proteins and fat must be catabolized as emergency energy sources. Highly concentrated glucose solutions are administered intravenously to patients in hepatic coma to prevent catabolism of body tissue, and thus avoid increased ammonia production and further brain damage.

63. (3) Debilitated cirrhotics are susceptible to abdominal hernia because poor nutrition and muscle wasting weaken the anterior abdominal wall, and the accumulation of ascitic fluid increases intra-abdominal pressure. Ascitic patients are susceptible to pneumonia because increased intra-abdominal pressure due to ascites restricts diaphragmatic movement, leading to poor aeration and collapse of alveoli in basilar lung segments. Chronic alcoholic patients are subject to peptic ulcer because alcohol stimulates the gastric glands to secrete acid.

64. (2) Ascitic fluid is rich in protein and paracentesis, involving the removal of ascitic fluid, results in the loss of considerable protein in a patient already protein-poor. Paracentesis is not used to treat ascites in the cirrhotic patient unless diuretic therapy is ineffective and the ascites is causing the patient respiratory distress.

65. (3) Giving an anxious patient information about a feared treatment provides him with a measure of control over his situation. Just as uncertainty generates anxiety, knowledge of forthcoming events yields a feeling of control, which may decrease anxiety to a manageable level.

66. (3) After applying a mask and sterile gown and gloves, the physician will use the sterile 2-cc (2-ml.) syringe and needle to anesthetize the skin and subcutaneous tissue of the anterior abdominal wall at the puncture site; use the scalpel to make a small stab wound below the umbilicus; insert the trocar and cannula through the parietal peritoneum; remove the trocar and collect two specimens of ascitic fluid in sterile test tubes; attach a length of rubber tubing to the cannula; and allow the desired quantity of ascitic fluid to flow into a basin or bucket.

67. (2) To avoid puncture of the bladder with the trocar, the patient should be instructed to void immediately prior to the paracentesis.

68. (3) In order that gravity may assist the drainage of ascitic fluid from the peritoneal cavity during paracentesis, the patient should sit upright on the edge of a treatment table with his back supported and his feet on a stool.

69. (2) If too much ascitic fluid is removed or if it is removed too rapidly, fluid may shift out of the blood vessels to replace that withdrawn from the peritoneal cavity, producing hypovolemia, shock, and syncope.

70. (1) To determine the effect of ascitic fluid removal and possible intravascular fluid shifts on Mr. Kemper's cardiovascular dynamics, the nurse should monitor his pulse rate and volume at frequent intervals throughout the paracentesis.

71. (4) Chronic alcoholic-cirrhotic patients are poorly nourished and prone to skin breakdown. The skin may be easily irritated by adhesive tape, and if inflamed may heal slowly. Since only a portion of Mr. Kemper's ascitic fluid will be removed during paracentesis, and following the procedure his intra-abdominal pressure will still be higher than normal, small amounts of ascitic fluid may seep from the abdominal puncture wound for several hours following the procedure. The wound should be dressed with sterile gauze fluffs to absorb the drainage, and the abdominal binder should be applied to hold the dressings in place.

72. (1) With abstinence from alcohol, minimal hepatic fibrosis may persist without progression. If Mr. Kemper continues to drink, the liver cell damage will certainly progress, and portal hypertension, hepatic encephalopathy, and typical complications will ensue within months.

73. (1) One pint of water weighs approximately 1 pound. An effective means of monitoring body fluid retention is to weigh the patient daily at the same time and have him wear the same clothing.

74. (3) Because of his decreased number of functional liver cells, Mr. Kemper is unable to produce enough bile to digest fats normally, so his dietary fat intake should be decreased.

75. (2) In the United States, the average daily sodium intake ranges from 4000 to 7000 mg. Meats, eggs, and milk are all relatively high in sodium content.

76. (1) Sodium diets can be classified as follows: mild restriction — 2400–4500 mg. Na/day; moderate restriction — 1000 mg. Na/day; strict restriction — 500 mg. Na/day.

77. (4) All of the foods listed are high in sodium and must be eliminated from a strict low-sodium diet.

78. (1) Mr. Kemper's indigestion may create an unpleasant mouth odor that contributes to his anorexia. Therefore, his appetite may be improved by providing him an opportunity to brush his teeth and rinse his mouth before meals. Ascites, by compressing the stomach, may contribute to poor appetite. Provision of five small, rather than three large, meals per day may increase food intake, thereby improving nutrition.

79. (1) In severe liver damage, conjugated bilirubin leaks back through the liver cell into the sinusoid, exits the liver through the hepatic veins to the systemic circulation, and is eventually deposited in body tissues, where it causes pruritus.

80. (1) The cirrhotic patient should be given a liberal carbohydrate intake so that proteins and fats need not be used as fuel sources. Catabolism of protein for energy purposes increases the risk of hepatocerebral coma. Lack of adequate bile synthesis interferes with normal fat digestion and absorption.

81. (1) Any factor that increases the metabolic rate, such as infection, increases hepatic workload, which could precipitate liver decompensation and coma in a patient with marginal liver function.

82. (3) In some patients in whom hepatic fibrosis severely obstructs portal blood flow through the liver, a portacaval anastamosis is done to permit blood in the portal circulation to bypass the liver.

Hyperthyroidism and Thyroidectomy

1. (2) Graves' disease is an autoimmune disorder in which an antibody, a serum globulin called "Long-Acting Thyroid Stimulator" (LATS), is developed against a component in the thyroid cell membrane. This globulin, like the thyroid stimulating hormone produced by the anterior pituitary gland, stimulates the thyroid to produce increasing quantities of thyroxine and triiodothyronine.

2. (1) Adenosine triphosphate is the compound in which available energy is stored in living cells. It consists of adenine, one of the two purines in nucleic acids; ribose, a five-carbon sugar; and three phosphate radicals. The terminal phosphate radical is attached to the molecule by a high-energy bond. When the bond is broken and the radical freed, large amounts of energy are released.

3. (3) Thyroid hormone increases metabolism in most cells of the body except the brain, retina, spleen, and lungs. In patients with severe hyperthyroidism the basal metabolic rate ranges from 40 to 60 per cent above normal. An increased rate of cellular metabolism causes a rise in body temperature.

4. (4) Pulse pressure is defined as the difference between the systolic and the diastolic blood pressures. In the normal young adult systolic pressure is about 120 mm. Hg and diastolic pressure about 80 mm. Hg, so the pulse pressure is about 40 mm. Hg. Mrs. Trimble's pulse pressure is 65 mm. Hg, or higher than normal.

5. (3) An increased rate of cellular metabolism causes more rapid utilization of oxygen than normal, and production of greater-than-normal quantities of metabolic end products. Accumulation of metabolic end products such as lactic acid produces vasodilation. Widespread vasodilation lowers the diastolic blood pressure.

6. (1) Excessive thyroid hormone accelerates the metabolic activity of most body cells, and increases cellular oxidation of glucose to carbon dioxide and water. The increased volume of metabolic water produced by increased cellular respiration is eliminated from the body through increased perspiration.

7. (4) Exophthalmos is due to edema and deposition of large quantities of mucopolysaccharides in the extracellular spaces of retro-orbital tissues. If exophthalmos is severe, it may stretch the optic nerve to the point of producing blindness.

8. (3) The patient with Graves' disease also may demonstrate infrequent blinking, failure of convergence as an object is moved toward the nose, and lagging of the lids as the eyeball moves toward the floor on downward gaze.

9. (3) In Graves' disease there is generalized lymph node hyperplasia and lymphocytic infiltration of skeletal muscles and liver.

10. (3) The thyroid gland is composed of spherical follicles lined with cuboidal epithelial cells enclosing a colloidal mass of thyroglobulin. In Graves' disease the epithelial cells increase in number (hyperplasia) and size (hypertrophy).

11. (3) In Graves' disease the increased rate of cellular metabolism results in increased cellular energy demand, which is reflected in an increase of appetite. Thyroid gland enlargement may be so marked as to interfere with swallowing. Anxiety, nervousness, and emotional instability cause tearful outbursts in the hyperthyroid patient. One manifestation of hypermetabolism is hyperperistalsis, with frequent loose bowel movements.

12. (3) In many patients with Graves' disease an experience of acute psychic or physical stress precedes development of thyrotoxicosis. A marital breakup, death of a spouse, surgical operation, severe trauma, or acute infection are common precipitators of thyroid hypersecretion.

13. (3) Hyperthyroidism typically produces oligomenorrhea or amenorrhea, probably by disrupting the delicate ovarian-pituitary balance.

14. (3) Nervousness and irritability are expected consequences of Mrs. Trimble's hormonal imbalance. It is comforting for the anxious and hypersensitive hyperthyroid patient to know that her professional caregivers appreciate the physiologic reasons for her impatience and irritability, accepting those symptoms of her illness with the same equanimity with which they acknowledge her tachycardia, hyperpyrexia, weight loss, and diaphoresis.

15. (1) The hyperirritability of the hyperthyroid patient predisposes to insomnia. In order to decrease upsetting stimuli from the environment, the patient should be placed in a quiet single room removed as far as possible from the mainstream of traffic flow through the unit.

16. (2) In hyperthyroidism the increased rate of cellular metabolism and the marked cutaneous vasodilation render the patient intolerant of heat.

17. (2) The basal metabolism test measures the rate of oxygen consumption in the resting, fasting state. In addition to thyroid disease, the following factors may increase the basal metabolic rate (BMR): anxiety, stress, lack of sleep, food intake within 12 hours, anemia, and hypertension, dyspnea, fever, neoplasm, and certain central nervous system and sympathetic nervous system stimulants.

18. (4) Abnormal iodinated proteins are produced and released by the thyroid gland in Graves' disease, and accumulate in the serum, causing an elevation in protein-bound iodine. The protein-bound iodine test is sensitive and reliable,

but its value as a thyroid function test is limited by the fact that, following ingestion or injection, a wide range of iodinated materials remain bound to serum protein for months or years. Substances that elevate the protein-bound iodine of the serum are: expectorant cough medications containing iodide; iodine-containing skin antiseptics; and iodine-containing radiopaque dyes used in x-ray studies of the gallbladder, kidney, and respiratory tract.

19. (4) Anxiety will elevate BMR in a normal subject. Dyspnea is extremely anxiety-producing. In the course of the test the nostrils are clamped and the patient is instructed to breathe pure oxygen through a mouthpiece. The measurement will be more valid if the test conditions are explained beforehand so that the test situation is as unthreatening as possible.

20. (3) Measurement of BMR requires measurement of oxygen consumption in the resting, fasting state, so food must be held for 12 hours and the patient must have eight hours of restful sleep preceding the test.

21. (1) Fever elevates the BMR by accelerating chemical reactions within body cells. To obtain an accurate measure, the patient must be afebrile.

22. (3) The administration of almost any drug prior to measurement of BMR will alter test results. Nicotine increases the heart rate by sympathetic stimulation and raises blood pressure by epinephrine release. Valid measurement of BMR requires that the patient desist from smoking 12 hours prior to the test.

23. (2) The radioiodine uptake test consists of administration of a minute, measured amount of I_{131} by mouth. Twenty-four hours later a scintillation detector is positioned over the neck to measure the amount of radioactive iodine taken up by the thyroid gland. A normal thyroid gland will absorb from 5 to 35 per cent of ingested iodine within 24 hours. A hyperactive gland will absorb a greater proportion of ingested iodine.

24. (4) Administration of any iodine-containing drug within one to four months prior to radioiodine uptake study would decrease the amount of I_{131} absorbed by the thyroid gland and invalidate the I_{131} test results.

25. (2) The typical staring expression is caused by forward displacement of the eyeballs and decreased blink reflex. The exophthalmos results form deposition of mucopolysaccharides in the retro-orbital tissues. The decreased blink reflex may be the result of forward displacement of the eyeball, swelling of the eyelids, or weakness of the eyelid muscles.

26. (1) Nervousness, anxiety, irritability, and fatigue predispose the hyperthyroid patient to outbursts of anger or tears in the face of even minor frustration. Fine hand tremor, muscular weakness, and loss of visual acuity result in fumbling, clumsiness, and an increasing tendency to drop small objects.

27. (1) Muscle weakness, hypermetabolism, and catabolism of body protein cause easy fatigability for the hyperthyroid patient. Frequent, spaced rest periods should be provided throughout the day to minimize fatigue.

28. (3) The hyperthyroid patient needs some form of occupational therapy to fill time and engage her interests during long hours of hospitalization. Of the activities listed, hooking a rug involves less fine hand and eye movements, so would be better suited for an uncoordinated patient with visual problems.

29. (2) Palpitations, or awareness of one's own heartbeat, may result from tachycardia, increased pulse pressure, or occasional premature ventricular contractions, all of which are common manifestations of thyrotoxicosis.

30. (1) Acceleration of tissue metabolism results in increased quantities of metabolic end products that cause vasodilation. Increased blood flow to body tissues causes an increase in heart rate and in cardiac output. Excessive protein catabolism produces metabolic end products that depress heart muscle. The combination of increased heart rate and decreased myocardial contractility predisposes to heart failure.

31. (2) The BMR has a wide normal range: -20 per cent to $+20$ per cent according to some authorities; -15 per cent to $+20$ per cent according to others.

32. (4) The normal serum level for protein-bound iodine is 4–8 μg./100 ml. of serum. Mrs. Trimble's serum concentration was 15 μg./100 ml., which is higher than normal and well within the range of that seen in patients with untreated hyperthyroidism (7–20 μg./100 ml.).

33. (2) The thyroid's uptake of I_{131} is an index of the proportion of all ingested iodine that is accumulated by the thyroid gland. The normal gland will absorb from

15 to 45 per cent of a measured dose of I_{131} within 24 hours of administration.

34. (4) The normal level of serum cholesterol ranges from 150 to 250 mg./100 ml. It typically is reduced in hyperthyroidism, increased in hypothyroidism.

35. (2) Propylthiouracil blocks the formation of thyroid hormone by interfering with the binding of iodine into an organic compound.

36. (1) Propylthiouracil is capable of producing numerous side-effects, of which the most common are fever, skin rash, lymphadenitis, and agranulocytosis. The last-named is the result of marrow depression by the drug.

37. (1) Lugol's solution, or compound iodine solution, contains 5 per cent of elemental iodine solution and 10 per cent of potassium iodine in an aqueous solution.

38. (4) Propylthiouracil causes the thyroid gland to become more vascular and friable. Increased vascularity of the gland can be counteracted by simultaneous administration of potassium iodide along with the propylthiouracil for 7–10 days immediately preceding thyroidectomy.

39. (3) Iodide preparations may cause burning of the mouth and gastric irritation. To minimize mucosal irritation, Lugol's solution should be well diluted with milk and given through a straw.

40. (3) Chronic iodide poisoning produces a coryza-like syndrome and symptoms of skin and mucosal irritation, such as fever, swollen parotid and submaxillary glands, excessive salivation, and acneform skin rash.

41. (1) Sedatives may be given to facilitate rest in the restless, hyperthyroid patient. Phenobarbital, a barbiturate of moderate duration (6 hours), is a suitable sedative for a hyperactive, excitable patient.

42. (4) Pentobarbital is a shorter-acting (3–6 hours) barbiturate than phenobarbital, and is frequently administered as a bedtime hypnotic to the anxious, hyperactive patient who has difficulty sleeping in the hospital.

43. (1) The short-acting barbiturates, of which pentobarbital is one example, produce a sedative effect within 10–15 minutes after administration.

44. (2) Sixty mg. equals 1 grain; so 100 mg. equals about 1½ grains.

45. (2) Thiamine hydrochloride, or vitamin B_1, is also known as the antineuritic or antiberiberi vitamin.

46. (1) Thiamine is a major component of the coenzyme thiamine pyrophosphate, which mediates the metabolism of pyruvic acid, an intermediate compound in carbohydrate metabolism.

47. (2) When administered intramuscularly, thiamine hydrochloride causes local tissue irritation, producing severe aching pain in the injection site.

48. (3) An increase in BMR increases cellular energy needs; speeds glucose catabolism; and when glycogen stores are exhausted, causes catabolism of body fat and protein as energy sources. A high-carbohydrate diet is given to the hyperthyroid patient to ensure adequate glucose for current cellular energy needs, replace liver glycogen, halt catabolism of body proteins, and foster weight gain.

49. (2) The hyperthyroid patient catalyzes tissue proteins to satisfy increased cellular energy needs. A high-protein intake is needed to provide amino acids from which new tissue proteins can be synthesized. Proteins are needed to provide the eight essential amino acids that cannot be synthesized in sufficient quantities by the human body, and so must be supplied from outside sources.

50. (3) Vitamins are organic compounds found in foods and utilized by the human body as components of those vital enzyme systems that regulate basic metabolic activities. When the rate of cellular metabolism is increased, more than usual amounts of enzymes are needed to catalyze metabolic reactions, so increased vitamins are required to synthesize enzymes.

51. (4) Restlessness, tremulousness, and easy fatigability may make it difficult for a hyperthyroid patient to eat a large meal. Some of the prescribed calories, carbohydrates, and proteins should be provided as between-meal feedings in order to decrease the volume of food that must be consumed at each sitting.

52. (3) Large amounts of sodium chloride are lost in the sweat, which also contains urea, lactic acid, and potassium ions. A hypermetabolic patient eliminates large quantities of these substances through eccrine sweat glands. Since all of

these substances are irritating to the skin, frequent bathing is necessary to prevent skin irritations.

53. (2) Failure of lid closure during sleep leads to excessive drying of eye tissues, with corneal ulceration and infection. In the exophthalmic patient the eyes should be irrigated, sterile mineral oil or artificial tears should be instilled, and the lids should be gently taped shut to prevent injury to the eye during sleep.

54. (3) The hyperthyroid patient is hyperpyrexic, restless, and hyperkinetic, perspiring freely, changing position frequently, and pulling the bed linen this way and that. She is also easily fatigued and in need of restful sleep. The bed should be remade frequently, providing clean, dry, wrinkle-free linen in order to promote relaxation and sleep.

55. (2) Because the hyperthyroid patient is hypersensitive and emotionally labile, discussion of upsetting topics is apt to provoke emotional outbursts, which are often followed by exacerbations of physical symptoms.

56. (3) Hyperthyroid patients who are inadequately treated wth antithyroid drugs before surgery are subject to hyperthyroid crisis or thyroid storm during the immediate postoperative period. Thyroid crisis results from spillage of thyroid hormone into surrounding tissues during surgical manipulation of the gland. Absorption of the excessive hormone leads to markedly increased cellular metabolism postoperatively, with extremely high temperature and heart rate, and growing restlessness, irritability, and prostration.

57. (4) Extreme anxiety about the forthcoming surgical procedure causes excessive stimulation of the sympathetic nervous system, predisposing the patient to thyroid storm.

58. (1) Operative trauma to neck tissues and tracheal intubation during surgery cause sore throat and difficult swallowing for 2–3 days following thyroidectomy. The patient should be told preoperatively that dysphagia is an expected consequence of surgery, so that she will not interpret the symptoms as an indication of a more serious complication.

59. (4) If laryngeal irritation and edema develop following thyroidectomy, oxygen therapy must be initiated to prevent hypoxia. As a result of dysphagia, the patient will require intravenous fluid therapy for 2–3 days postoperatively to maintain proper electrolyte and water balance. An ice collar may be applied to relieve throat pain or swelling of neck tissues during the immediate postoperative period. Continuous steam inhalations may be ordered to humidify inspired air, to soothe irritated laryngeal and tracheal mucosa, and to liquefy tracheobronchial secretions so that they can be removed by coughing.

60. (2) Laryngeal edema, laryngeal hemorrhage, or laryngeal nerve paralysis may all produce respiratory obstruction follqwing thyroidectomy. A tracheostomy set should be kept at the bedside postoperatively in case an emergency airway must be established.

61. (4) If symptoms of hyperthyroid crisis develop postoperatively, oxygen must be administered promptly to meet the greatly increased cellular needs for oxygen and to protect hyperfunctioning myocardial, liver, and kidney tissue from hypoxia.

62. (4) Local irritation of the larynx and trachea by the endotracheal tube and mechanical tissue trauma during surgery cause an increase in pharyngeal and tracheobronchial secretions following thyroidectomy. Frequent suctioning will be required to prevent airway obstruction for several hours after surgery.

63. (3) The four parathyroid glands are attached to or embedded in the posterior surface of the thyroid gland, and may accidentally be injured or removed during thyroidectomy. Such removal would produce hypocalcemic tetany within one to four days postoperatively.

64. (2) Hemorrhage into tissues of the neck could obstruct the airway by exerting pressures on the epiglottis.

65. (2) If hemorrhage from the thyroidectomy wound is external rather than internal, blood may run down the side of the neck under the dressing, and pool on the lower linen under the patient's neck or shoulders.

66. (4) Placing the patient in semi-Fowler's position, with the neck neither flexed nor hyperextended, will facilitate breathing and the swallowing of oral fluids.

67. (2) Swelling of the neck above the thyroidectomy wound might signify either hemorrhage from the operative site or subcutaneous emphysema. Either devel-

opment would indicate a potentially serious airway hazard, and should be diagnosed and treated promptly.

68. (4) The symptoms of thyroid crisis are the symptoms of hyperthyroidism in greatly exaggerated form, such as sudden severe elevation in temperature, pulse, and respiratory rate; air hunger; muscle hyperactivity; and excitement or delirium.

69. (4) The nerve supply to the larynx consists of two branches of the vagus nerve: the superior and inferior laryngeal nerves. The superior branch provides sensation to the laryngeal mucosa and innervates the cricothyroid muscle. The inferior, or recurrent, laryngeal nerve innervates the remaining intrinsic muscles of the larynx. The laryngeal muscles open and close the glottis and regulate the tension on the vocal cords. Edema of or injury to the laryngeal nerve results in hoarseness or a change in vocal timber produced by a change in the tension on the vocal cords.

70. (1) The parathyroid gland synthesizes parathormone, which enhances calcium absorption from the bowel, stimulates osteoclasts in the bone to release calcium ions from bone into the plasma, and decreases calcium salt excretion by the kidney. Calcium in the plasma is biologically active only in the ionic state, when it controls cellular irritability. In hypocalcemia, nerves fire spontaneously, muscles respond to lower levels of stimuli, and muscle relaxation is slowed. Hypercalcemic tetany is characterized by carpopedal spasm, with flexion of the metacarpophalangeal joints, wrist, and elbows, and extension of the legs and feet.

71. (3) In order to eliminate strain on the suture line, the nurse should support Mrs. Trimble's head whenever she is moved so as to prevent extension or flexion of the neck. As soon as practicable, the patient should be taught how to brace her head and neck with her two hands to prevent strain on the incision when turning or sitting up in bed.

72. (1) Although a subtotal thyroidectomy was performed, it is possible that insufficient thyroid tissue remains to permit euthyroid function. Mrs. Trimble will require regular medical followup to detect possible signs and symptoms of hypothyroidism, for which she would be treated with thyroid hormone.

Adenocarcinoma of the Rectum

1. (3) A carcinoma that arises from glandular or lining epithelium and which forms rudimentary gland spaces is called an adenocarcinoma.

2. (2) Mr. Oakes' 4+ stool benzidine reaction indicates the presence of hemoglobin, and therefore of blood in his stool. The most probable cause for his weakness is chronic blood loss through gastrointestinal bleeding, with resulting hypochromic anemia, and decreased oxygen-carrying capacity of the blood.

3. (1) On the basis of Mr. Oakes' medical history (weakness, constipation alternating with diarrhea) and physical findings (4+ stool benzidine, fungating rectal mass), the most probable cause for the constipation is obstruction of the large bowel by a tumor.

4. (4) The tumor itself acts as an irritant to the bowel, stimulating the secretion of mucus and increasing peristalsis, which results in intermittent diarrhea.

5. (2) The benzidine test is a measure of peroxidase activity. Hemoglobin, which is a peroxidase, catalyzes the oxidation of benzidine, the test substance, by peroxide, producing a blue color. A 4+ reaction is strongly positive.

6. (1) "Fungating" means growing like a fungus, i.e., increasing rapidly in size and demonstrating a soft, mushroom-like structure.

7. (2) Most persons find a proctoscopic examination uncomfortable, embarrassing, and unpleasant, so make it as unthreatening as possible, the nurse should explain the procedure and its purpose beforehand. To ensure that the rectum and sigmoid can be well visualized during proctoscopy, the patient should eat a light, low residue supper on the previous evening, and should administer serial enemas on the morning of the examination. When the patient enters the examining room, the nurse should help him to assume the desired position, drape him so that only the rectum is exposed, and remain at his side to reassure him and check on his condition throughout the procedure.

8. (1) Cathartics are not used to prepare a patient for a proctoscopic examination because there is a prolongation of cathartic effect in some patients, with movement of fecal material and fluid into the rectosigmoid when the proctoscope is introduced into the bowel. Generally, two or three tap water enemas, administered slowly enough and in sufficient quantity to distend the bowel, will cleanse the lower bowel without irritating the mucosa.

9. (2) The presence of feces in the lower bowel prevents adequate visualization of the rectum and sigmoid colon. Mass movements of the transverse and descending colon, caused by overdistention, propel fecal material toward the anus. Most of the time the rectum is empty of feces, as a result of the weak functional sphincter that exists at the junction of the sigmoid and rectum. When a mass movement of the descending colon forces feces into the rectum, the defecation reflex is initiated. If this reflex is not opposed by volitional control, peristaltic waves sweep toward the anus, the internal and external anal sphincters relax, and evacuation occurs.

10. (3) The physician uses rubber gloves and a lubricant to perform a digital examination of the anus and rectum. Two-thirds of all rectal carcinomas and 12 per cent of all gastrointestinal carcinomas lie within reach of the examiner's finger, and have a favorable prognosis if removed early. A water-soluble lubricating jelly is used to lubricate the gloved examining finger and the proctoscope or sigmoidoscope prior to its insertion into the anal canal. Long, cotton-tipped applicators are used to remove small amounts of fluid or stool that remain in the bowel following the preparatory enemas. A paper or plastic-lined waste basket is required for proper disposal of used materials.

11. (4) Although the lithotomy position is most satisfactory for digital examination, the knee-chest position is required for adequate proctoscopy because in this position the viscera slide cephalad, creating a negative pressure and making insufflation unnecessary to distend the bowel.

12. (2) When, following mass movement of the transverse and descending colon, a large mass of feces is forced into the rectum, the desire for defecation is felt. Similarly, when the proctoscope is introduced into the rectum, reflex contraction of the rectum occurs and the urge for defecation is felt.

13. (3) Anorexia is a symptom of carcinoma and is due to depression of the appetite area in the hypothalamus. Bleeding results from erosion of the tumor into a blood vessel in the bowel wall. Carcinomas of the rectosigmoid grow circumferentially, producing some degree of bowel obstruction and resultant colicky, lower abdominal pain. As the tumor grows in size and obstruction increases, the colon proximal to the tumor tends to dilate slowly, and fecal material accumulates in the right colon, leading to fecal impaction and marked distention of the right lower quadrant.

14. (2) The incidence of colon malignancy is increased in persons with familial polyposis and chronic ulcerative colitis.

15. (4) Retained barium may harden and cause fecal impaction. In a patient whose rectum or sigmoid colon is partially obstructed by a circumferential tumor, there is increased danger that retained barium may obstruct the intestinal lumen.

16. (2) A generous amount of water-soluble gel is needed to lubricate the proctoscope prior to insertion. Part of this lubricant is deposited around the anus during placement and removal of the instrument. Excess lubricant should be removed from the perianal region following removal of the proctoscope, to prevent soiling of the patient's clothing. To ensure accurate diagnosis and appropriate treatment, the nurse must ensure that the biopsy specimen is properly labeled.

17. (2) Because malignant tumors tend to outgrow their blood supply, tumor tissue is friable. Removal of a biopsy specimen from the rectum may injure vessels in the bowel wall, predisposing to hemorrhage.

18. (2) Because venous drainage from the bowel is carried by way of the portal circulation to the liver, malignant tumors of the bowel frequently metastasize to the liver, and will be evidenced by changes in liver function tests. An elevation of alkaline phosphatase suggests liver metastases. Since many of the agents used for general anesthesia are detoxified or metabolized by the liver,

liver function tests would reveal the patient's risk in undergoing general anesthesia.

19. (3) Fifty per cent of patients with rectosigmoid carcinoma already have extension of tumor growth to regional lymph nodes. Although liver and lung are the most common sites for metastases from colon malignancies, a significant number of such tumors metastasize to bone.

20. (4) The incidence of chronic arteriosclerotic heart disease is high in patients in the seventh decade. Since coronary insufficiency and myocardia ischemia would increase Mr. Oakes' risk of complication during and following general anesthesia, an EKG should be performed preoperatively to provide baseline data against which to compare postoperative EKGs if cardiac dysfunction should develop during the immediate postoperative period.

21. (4) Mr. Oakes' red blood cell count is 4.5 million/mm.^{3}, or about 90 per cent of normal. His hemoglobin concentration is 10/100 ml. of blood, or 66 per cent of normal, so his hemoglobin concentration is decreased to a greater degree than his red blood cell count.

22. (2) Mr. Oakes' red blood cell count is 4.5 million/mm.^{3}, or about 90 per cent of normal. His hematocrit is 38 per cent, or about 69 per cent of normal. Therefore, his red blood cell volume is decreased to a greater degree than the number of red cells, suggesting that the cells are smaller than normal, or microcytic.

23. (2) Microcytic hypochromic anemias are generally the result of chronic blood loss, because gradual depletion of body iron stores through chronic bleeding leads to production of smaller-than-normal red cells, each of which contains less than normal amounts of hemoglobin.

24. (3) A soft-cooked egg contains 160 calories; a cup of chocolate milk, 190; 3-oz. hamburger patty, 185–245; baked potato, 90.

25. (1) "Complete" proteins contain all eight of the essential amino acids in sufficient quantities for optimal tissue maintenance and growth. The protein of eggs, meat, and milk are complete proteins. Those found in wheat, legumes, and gelatin are incomplete proteins in that they are incapable of replacing or rebuilding body tissue.

26. (3) Farina, hard-cooked egg, and cottage cheese are low residue foods; stewed prunes are high residue.

27. (3) Eggs, baked poultry, tomato juice, and baked white potato are all permitted on a low residue diet; milk drinks and concentrated sweets are not allowed.

28. (4) Mr. Oakes' understanding of his pathology, prescribed treatment, and probable prognosis will generate either hope or despair, and influence his willingness to cooperate with the treatment plan. The extent of metastatic spread determines the patient's strength and ability to carry out the activities of daily living. The moral and physical support provided by family and friends influence his will to live. Basic ego strength determines his ability to handle the problems provoked by a diagnosis of malignancy. The attitudes of health team members encourage Mr. Oakes in either healthy or unhealthy responses to his illness and treatment.

29. (4) Most persons equate general anesthesia with death, the ultimate loss of control over volitional activity. A major change in body structure and function that affects elimination disrupts the individual's accustomed view of himself and his relation to significant others. The financial expense of major surgery and hospital care is now so high that few can pay for such care without help from a "third party payer." The patient facing a colostomy fears that loss of control over defecation will create problems of soiling and odor that will alienate friends and family.

30. (2) Mr. Oakes will have greater trust in the ability of the treatment team to meet his needs if they present a unified approach to his problems and concerns. He may seek additional information or helpful understanding from the nurse. In order to provide emotional support, the nurse should ascertain exactly what Mr. Oakes has been told about the diagnosis, prognosis, proposed treatment, possible complications, long-term effects, and alternative courses of action.

31. (2) Of the alternatives given, this is the only one that encourages Mr. Oakes to talk further about his concerns and ventilate his feelings about illness and treatment.

32. (4) In order to give his informed consent for colostomy surgery, Mr. Oakes should be given detailed information as presented in all the responses.

33. (4) A patient with a diagnosis of malignancy fears mutilation, dysfunction, pain, debility, and death. These threats may make him apt to regress markedly, exhibiting extreme dependence on caregivers, and doubting his ability to cope with the problems of illness. The losses suffered, e.g., loss of health, loss of body functions or body parts, and loss of job provoke a strong grief reaction in the patient, the second stage of which is characterized by anger, at himself, his family, his doctors, and unkind fate. Anger may give way to feelings of guilt, for not having sought treatment earlier, for not having lived a better life, and so forth.

34. (2) Phthalylsulfathiazole is a sulfonamide that is poorly absorbed from the gastro-intestinal tract and is used to decrease the bacterial count of the intestine prior to colon resection.

35. (2) Sulfadiazine is absorbed readily and rapidly from the intestine and is distribut-ed throughout all body tissues. Only 5 per cent of a dose of phthalylsulfathia-zole is absorbed from the intestine, so the drug remains in high concentration in the intestine content, and reduces the coliform bacteria count markedly.

36. (4) Neomycin is a broad spectrum-antibiotic that is not inactivated by gastrointes-tinal secretions, and also is poorly absorbed from the GI tract.

37. (3) Neomycin is well absorbed following intramuscular administration, and is widely distributed to various body tissues and fluids. Its chief toxic effects are renal damage and nerve deafness.

38. (3) Neomycin is effective against *Proteus vulgaris*; tetracycline is not.

39. (3) Only this response describes the effects of blood transfusion in positive terms without dodging the patient's question or emphasizing his loss of health and strength.

40. (2) Surgical trauma to the intestine invariably causes slowing of peristalsis, which interferes with passage of chyme through the intestine. Gastric suction is employed during the intra- and immediate postoperative periods to prevent distention of the stomach by fluid or gas.

41. (3) A distended urinary bladder would be susceptible to injury during an ab-dominoperineal resection. Therefore, an indwelling catheter should be insert-ed preoperatively, and should remain in place throughout the procedure and for several days postoperatively.

42. (3) Meperidine is a synthetic CNS depressant with analgesic, sedative, euphoric, and respiratory depressant effects similar to those of morphine.

43. (4) Promethazine hydrochloride, a histamine antagonist, causes sedation and somnolence, and is used to potentiate the CNS depressant effects of narcotics and analgesics.

44. (3) Atropine is a parasympathetic depressant or anticholinergic drug that de-creases secretions, slows peristalsis, and stimulates the vital centers in the me-dulla.

45. (1) Regional lymph node involvement is the most common form of metastasis in colon cancer. In order to eliminate all local extensions and regional metastases, the surgeon will remove the primary tumor, a long segment of colon above and below the lesion, and the entire blood and lymph supply of the bowel segment in which the tumor is located.

46. (2) Even though phthalylsulfathiazole is given preoperatively, it is impossible to remove all bacteria from the bowel content. The colostomy stump will remain clamped for the first few days following surgery to prevent contamination of the skin incision and the peritoneum with fecal drainage. By the second or third postoperative day the wound margins will have healed sufficiently to seal off the peritoneum, and the colostomy stump can be unclamped to permit irrigation of the colostomy.

47. (2) An abdominoperineal resection for removal of a rectosigmoid malignancy is a major and lengthy operation, consisting of two procedures that may be per-formed by two teams of surgeons working simultaneously. Because the surgery involves sectioning of major blood vessels, and results in extensive restructur-ing of pelvic viscera, there is considerable blood loss during surgery and great risk of postoperative hemorrhage.

48. (4) The prolonged surgical procedure, the removal of a large mass of tissue, and the sectioning of numerous veins and arteries results in major intraoperative blood loss. Continuous nasogastric suction results in loss of fluid and electrolytes. Mechanical tissue trauma during surgery causes fluids to shift from the vascular compartment into the bowel lumen and the peritoneal cavity. Exudation from the wound itself constitutes another source of intravascular fluid loss following surgery. Loss of fluid from the vascular compartment decreases circulating blood volume, which results in decrease of systemic blood pressure. Fear and anxiety provoke increased activity of the sympathetic nervous system, causing tachycardia; there is insufficient time between cardiac contractions to permit adequate cardiac filling, so stroke volume decreases, and systemic hypotension results. Certain anesthetic agents have a depressant effect on the myocardium, decreasing muscle contractility, reducing cardiac output, and decreasing systemic blood pressure.

49. (4) Wound hemorrhage, infection, and dehiscence are fairly common following abdominoperineal resection. By maintaining the patient in the side-lying position during the immediate postoperative period, the nurse can check the perineal dressing frequently for serous, bloody, or purulent drainage, and summon the surgeon at the first sign of difficulty.

50. (2) Nearly all patients have difficulty in voiding following abdominoperineal resection. Operative removal of perirectal lymphatics may cause mechanical trauma to the urethra. The indwelling catheter is left in place for a few days to splint the urethra until irritation and edema subside.

51. (4) The patient with colon carcinoma is debilitated and malnourished as a result of the hypermetabolism, tissue necrosis, and anorexia associated with malignant disease. Malnutrition, especially protein and vitamin deficiencies, lower the body's resistance to infection. Anesthetic agents obtund the cough and glottic reflexes, and increase the danger of aspirating vomitus and oral secretions. Prolonged bedrest causes atelectasis in dependent lung segments, and encourages retention and infection of tracheobronchial secretions. All these factors in combination predispose to hypostatic pneumonia. Immobility predisposes to venous thrombosis by eliminating the pumping action of muscles against the venous wall. Malignancy predisposes to phlebothrombosis, perhaps as a result of enzymatic changes in those blood proteins associated with the clotting reaction. Decreased resistance to infection and contamination of the wound with fecal material during surgery predispose to postoperative wound infection. Immobility, due to incisional pain and weakness, together with the weight loss and muscle-wasting associated with malignancy, renders the cancer patient unusually susceptible to decubitus ulcer.

52. (3) Tetracycline is a broad-spectrum antibiotic that exerts a bacteriostatic effect on a wide range of gram-positive bacteria, gram-negative bacteria, rickettsiae, and amebae. Following an abdominoperineal resection the patient is liable to hypostatic pneumonia, ascending urinary tract infection, and surgical wound infection. Since all of these are apt to be mixed infections, a broad-spectrum antibiotic is the drug of choice.

53. (2) This response is most therapeutic because it stimulates the patient to talk further and express his feelings about the diagnosis.

54. (2) This action by the nurse would be least damaging to her ongoing relationship with the patient. If she were to leave the room when the patient first broached the subject of malignancy, he would be unlikely to raise the issue with her in any later conversation. If she denies that the patient has cancer, he will mistrust her when he later is told of the diagnosis. If she refuses to care for the patient again, the nurse will deprive him of a relationship that he has found supportive, as his question to her has indicated.

55. (3) When the clamp was removed from the colostomy stump on the second postoperative day, normal peristalsis would not have returned, and the bowel would have contained a transudate resulting from surgical trauma to tissues.

56. (3) Infection of the perineal wound is common as a result of fecal contamination of the tissue during surgery. To prevent abscess and sinus formation, the perineal wound must be kept clean of bacteria and inflammatory debris while it is allowed to heal by secondary intention. Hydrogen peroxide is used to cleanse

wounds because the effervescence created by the release of molecular oxygen exerts a mechanical cleansing effect that removes tissue debris from inaccessible locations.

57. (3) Because there is copious serosanguineous drainage from the perineal wound, the bulky fluff gauze dressings must be changed frequently. The malnourished cancer patient is subject to skin breakdown, so a T binder rather than adhesive should be used to hold the perineal dressing in place.

58. (3) Because a large amount of tissue is removed during abdominoperineal resection, sitting will be exceedingly painful for some time following surgery. Placing a rubber ring under the hips in the sitz bath prevents direct pressure on the perineal wound and permits free circulation of warm water around the wound. The patient may become faint on sitting upright for the first time, and so a call bell should be placed within reach. Because the nurse must check the patient's condition repeatedly, he should be protected from exposure by appropriate draping with a loincloth.

59. (3) It is a basic principle of adult education that learning of new content is facilitated by the stimulation of as many as possible of the learner's senses during instruction.

60. (3) Instillation of a relatively small amount of fluid (200–300 ml.) into the colostomy opening will distend the bowel sufficiently to stimulate peristalsis and cause stool to be evacuated. With dietary regulation and daily colostomy irrigation, it is usually possible to regulate evacuation so that fecal elimination occurs only once daily, at a scheduled hour.

61. (3) A No. 16 catheter is inserted into the colostomy opening for instillation of the irrigating solution. A small funnel is connected to the catheter for the first irrigation. The solution should be placed in a graduate pitcher so that the exact amount of fluid instilled and returned can be measured and recorded. A kidney basin is needed to collect the irrigating fluid returned from the bowel, since the total amount instilled and returned must be recorded as a basis for accurate fluid management.

62. (3) Warm tap water is best suited for colostomy irrigation because it is the one solution readily available to the patient upon his discharge from the hospital.

63. (3) By irrigating Mr. Oakes' colostomy before giving his bath, the nurse can ensure that any colostomy drainage spilled is immediately removed from his skin, clothing, and bed linen, thereby preventing skin irritation and undesirable odors in the patient's environment.

64. (2) Insertion of the catheter about 5 inches into the bowel permits the irrigating solution to be retained long enough to distend the bowel and stimulate evacuation, but prevents entrapment of fluid in distant segments of the bowel with secondary return of solution hours after the irrigation has been completed.

65. (3) On the first occasion that the colostomy is irrigated it is inadvisable to use more than 500 ml. of irrigating solution, as the bowel is incompletely healed and could be traumatized by marked distention with solution.

66. (3) By eliminating certain irritating or gas-forming foods from the diet, and by irrigating the colostomy daily to stimulate evacuation, many patients with left-sided colostomy can regulate its functioning so that a small gauze pad over the opening is sufficient protection against soiling.

67. (4) The patient tends to adopt the attitudes of his caregivers toward his colostomy and altered gastrointestinal functioning. A nurse who displays an accepting attitude and a hopeful attitude toward the patient's ability to irrigate, dress, and regulate the colostomy teaches the patient that he can cope with his new circumstances. By keeping the dressings and bed linen free of fecal drainage, and by encouraging the patient to assume responsibility for colostomy care, the nurse can facilitate his emotional acceptance of his changed body image and modified hygienic routines.

68. (4) The more self-reliant Mr. Oakes can become in managing his colostomy, the greater will be his self-esteem. The greater his self esteem, the more accepting his friends and family will be of his altered functioning. The more support he receives from significant others, the better will be his chances for rehabilitation.

69. (2) This response would be most effective in exploring the fears and anxieties that have prompted Mr. Oakes' remark.

70. (1) Although a stoma bag need not be worn after the colostomy is regulated, disposable bags may be used until regularity is achieved to prevent accidental soiling of clothing. To ensure adherence of the bag to the abdominal wall, the skin should be washed with soap and water, dried thoroughly, and Karaya powder or a Karaya gum ring applied to the skin where the bag is to be affixed.

71. (2) By irrigating the colostomy at the same time of day at which he was accustomed to move his bowel before the operation, Mr. Oakes should be able to utilize his natural biologic rhythms to regulate colostomy function.

72. (3) Until the colostomy is well regulated Mr. Oakes should avoid highly seasoned and high fiber foods, as they may cause diarrhea through stimulation of the already irritated mucosa. Fried foods and carbonated beverages would predispose to flatus and should be avoided by a patient learning to regulate a new colostomy.

73. (3) After the irrigating solution is instilled, the fluid must remain within the bowel for a few minutes before peristalsis is stimulated. About 20 minutes should be allowed for expulsion of the solution in order to ensure that the bowel is completely empty before the colostomy is redressed. Bowel function will be enhanced if the patient is not rushed during colostomy irrigation, and so 45–60 minutes should be allocated.

74. (2) Stricture of the colostomy stoma may occur because of the contracture of fibrous scar tissue around the healing skin and muscle incisions. To prevent obstruction of the stoma, the patient should be taught to use his gloved and lubricated index finger to dilate the opening on a weekly basis.

75. (3) Once his colostomy has been regulated, Mr. Oakes should be able to eat all foods that agreed with him in the past, omitting only such gas-forming foods as beans, onions, cabbage, cauliflower, and Brussels sprouts.

Subdural Hematoma

1. (3) A number of small veins bridge the space between the dura and the arachnoid. A subdural hematoma is generally due to a mass movement of the brain within the skull, with tearing of these small veins and slow bleeding into the subdural space.

2. (3) Since the brain is enclosed in a rigid, bony vault, a subdural hematoma causes symptoms by compression or displacement of brain tissue, with resulting increase in intracranial pressure.

3. (4) In chronic subdural hematoma the symptoms are similar to those of an intracranial neoplasm, and include: some degree of intellectual impairment, fluctuations in levels of consciousness, hemiparesis, and convulsive seizures.

4. (2) Blood that escapes into the subdural space is initially organized into a clot; later, when the blood cells lyse, it is converted into a liquid of high osmotic pressure that draws fluid from surrounding tissues, thereby rising steadily in volume and increasingly compressing brain tissue. Because a patient with subdural hematoma may demonstrate increasing intracranial pressure, his level of consciousness on admission should be noted as a basis for assessing later changes in cerebral function.

5. (3) When a patient loses or gains consciousness, functions disappear or reappear in predictable order. With descending levels of consciousness an individual loses first an awareness of the date and hour; second, the ability to distinguish his surroundings; third, the ability to identify others in his environment; fourth, the ability to respond appropriately to verbal directions; fifth, the ability to withdraw from painful stimuli and finally, all protective reflexes.

6. (3) In testing a patient's ability to follow simple commands, the task imposed by the nurse should not also require the patient to exercise memory, motor dexterity, or abstract reasoning, as these are different CNS functions and should be tested separately.

7. (1) A purposeful response to pain is withdrawal of the part from the painful stimulus. Dorsiflexion of the foot and flexion of the knee when the sole is pricked with a pin serve to remove the foot from the offensive stimulus.

8. (4) The size of the pupils results from a balance between the sympathetically innervated pupil dilator muscle fibers and the parasympathetically innervated pupil constrictor muscle fibers. In a complete third nerve lesion with loss of parasympathetic pupillomotor fibers, pupillary dilation results from unopposed action of sympathetic nerves. The extremes of pupillary diameter are from about 1.5 mm. to 8 mm. Inequality in the size of the pupils is a common finding in subdural hematoma. An abnormally small pupil on one side indicates irritation of the third cranial nerve on the same side. Sluggish pupillary constriction to light stimulation indicates impaired function of the third cranial nerve. Simultaneous movement of both eyes in the same direction is known as conjugate movement of the eyes. The motor impulses that stimulate conjugate eye movement originate in the midbrain and pons, and travel by way of the third nerve to the extraocular muscles. Direction of gaze should be noted, since weakness of intraocular muscles with disorganization of gaze may indicate hemorrhage into the brain stem as a result of increased intracranial pressure.

9. (2) The third cranial nerve is predominantly a motor nerve that originates in the midbrain and innervates the levator palpebrae superioris, the rectus superior, rectus inferior, rectus medialis, inferior oblique, ciliary, and pupillary sphincter muscles.

10. (3) When a light is directed into one eye from the lateral aspect, the normal response is prompt pupillary constriction of the stimulated eye, immediately followed by constriction of the pupil of the opposite eye to a slightly less degree.

11. (3) The third nerve originates in the midbrain. Third nerve paralysis, with a fixed and dilated pupil, may occur as a result of pressure distortion of the midbrain, and signifies that midbrain decompensation is imminent.

12. (2) Three cardinal symptoms of increased intracranial pressure are headache, vomiting, and papilledema.

13. (4) Muscle weakness, spasms, and rigidity may result from damage to the motor nerve cell in the precentral gyrus of the frontal lobe of the cerebrum, or from damage to the motor fibers from those cell bodies as they course through the brain stem on their way to the spinal cord. A subdural hematoma, which is a space-occupying lesion, will exert pressure on underlying brain tissue, and eventually cause herniation of the brain stem through the foramen magnum.

14. (1) The cerebrospinal or pyramidal tracts carry voluntary motor impulses from cell bodies in the precentral gyrus of the cerebral cortex through the internal capsule, midbrain, pons, and medulla. In the lower medulla most of the motor fibers cross to the opposite side of the cord, to descend in the middle and lateral columns and exit in the spinal nerves.

15. (1) A deep tendon reflex is a muscle contraction that occurs in response to a sudden stretch produced by striking the tendon. Although the deep tendon reflexes do not depend on brain control, the strength of response can be affected by signals from the brain. Since the strength of reflex response may have diagnostic significance, the patient's attention should be distracted when deep tendon reflexes are tested so as to eliminate conscious inhibition or exaggeration of response.

16. (2) The ability to perform rapidly alternating movements, such as hand pronation and supination or foot inversion and eversion, requires coordination and gradation of efforts of opposing muscle groups by the cerebellum. With cerebellar dysfunction, alternating movements are performed slowly and clumsily, if at all.

17. (1) The Babinski reflex, a pathologic reflex that indicates impaired functioning of corticospinal tracts, is elicited by using a sharp object to stroke the sole of the foot from heel to base of the toes, and then medially. The normal response to such stimulation would be plantar deviation of the foot and toes. A positive Babinski reflex consists of dorsiflexion of the great toe and fanning of the remaining toes.

18. (2) The motor cortex gives rise to some fibers that descend to the cord through the

pyramidal tract, and some that descend to the cord through the extrapyramidal tract. These two tracts have opposing effects on muscle tone. The pyramidal tract tends to increase muscle tone, and the extrapyramidal tract tends to inhibit muscle tone. The corticospinal, or pyramidal, tract is the major motor pathway from the cerebral motor cortex to the spinal nerves, and carries impulses for voluntary movement. A positive Babinski reflex indicates dysfunction at some point in the pyramidal tract.

19. (3) Brain scanning consists of the intravenous administration of a radioactive substance, followed by use of a radiation sensing device to record scintigraphic images of the brain from anterior, posterior, lateral, and vertex approaches after a period of two hours. As a result of the normal blood-brain barrier, there is little uptake of radioactive substances by normal brain tissue. Radioactive substances are concentrated in such abnormal tissues as tumors, hematomas, and abscesses.

20. (3) Pressure by a slowly expanding subdural hematoma compresses brain tissue and displaces blood vessels in the hemisphere underlying the clot. By injecting a radiopaque dye into the carotid and taking serial x-ray films of the cranium at frequent intervals, it is possible to detect gross distortions of the cerebral vascular pattern. In patients with subdural hematoma, the branches of the middle cerebral artery are displaced inward on the side of the lesion.

21. (4) The level of consciousness is the most reliable index of neurologic status, because consciousness tends to recede or return according to a predictable continuum. A patient who suffers increasing depression of consciousness will proceed through the following levels or stages: lethargy or obtundation, stupor, light coma, and deep coma.

22. (1) Convulsions are common in patients with subdural hematoma. Temperature should not be measured orally in a patient who is subject to convulsions, lest he injure himself by biting and aspirating a piece of thermometer during a seizure.

23. (3) A slowly expanding mass in the unyielding bony cage of the skull causes a gradual increase in intracranial pressure, with disturbances of vital centers in the medulla; this results in a slowly falling pulse and respiratory rate, with an accompanying rise in blood pressure and a terminal rise in temperature.

24. (2) As the volume of a subdural hematoma increases and intracranial pressure rises, brain circulation is impaired, and the cells of the vasoconstrictor center in the medulla become increasingly anoxic. Under conditions of anoxia, the vasoconstrictor center stimulates increased sympathetic discharge throughout the body, with general vasoconstriction and elevation of blood pressure.

25. (1) The medulla oblongata is continuous with the spinal cord inferiorly, and the pons superiorly. It contains the cardiac, vasoconstrictor, and respiratory centers. If a subdural hematoma continues to increase in volume, the medulla will eventually be forced through the foramen magnum.

26. (3) A common symptom of increased intracranial pressure is persistent and projectile vomiting, often unaccompanied by nausea. With gradual depression of consciousness the epiglottic reflex is obtunded, so that with increasing intracranial pressure the patient is in danger of aspirating vomitus.

27. (4) Although the pattern of seizures generally is stereotyped for each individual, this may change with progression of the brain lesion. Since a hematoma may increase in size and compress additional areas of cortex, all characteristics listed should be recorded. A convulsion may stimulate further bleeding from an injured dural vein, and so the patient's level of consciousness before and after the convulsion should be charted to indicate any worsening of his condition. Urinary and fecal incontinence may occur during the clonic phase of a generalized convulsion.

28. (3) The nurse's primary responsibility in caring for a patient during a seizure is to protect him from injuring himself. Protection can be afforded by loosening constricting clothing from the neck, placing a soft object under the head, permitting as full range of motion as possible without injury, placing a padded tongue depressor or a folded handkerchief between the teeth, and remaining at the patient's side to guide his movements so as to prevent injury.

29. (2) Most narcotics cause depression of the respiratory center in the medulla. Mr.

Conklin's vital centers are already depressed by the increased intracranial pressure.

30. (2) With increased intracranial pressure the cerebrospinal fluid pressure is greatly increased. A lumbar puncture should not be performed on a patient with a choked disc, for fear that quick reduction in spinal fluid pressure might cause herniation of the brain stem through the foramen magnum.

31. (3) The scalp should be thoroughly shampooed and examined for dermatitis, in order to decrease the risk of postoperative wound infections. The surgeon's order regarding preoperative scalp preparation should be followed exactly, as only a small area of the scalp may need to be shaved. The hairline is usually preserved to permit the hair to be combed over the scar for concealment; the head is usually shaved in the operating room rather than in the patient's room; and the hair should be saved for later use in a hairpiece.

32. (2) Following surgery Mr. Conklin will need a bed with side rails, because he may be comatose, confused, and convulsive, and thus subject to falls and injuries. A suction machine should be available to remove oral and pharyngeal secretions, as the patient with depressed consciousness lacks glottic and cough reflexes. A tracheostomy set should be available in case of respiratory tract obstruction.

33. (3) Immediately following his return from the operating room Mr. Conklin should be placed on the unoperated side, to permit drainage of secretions from the mouth without at the same time exerting pressure on the catheter that was left in the right burr hole.

34. (1) If subdural bleeding were to resume following surgery, the increase in intracranial pressure would be rapid and the patient's neurologic status would deteriorate quickly. For the first two to three hours following surgery Mr. Conklin's level of consciousness should be checked every 10 minutes.

35. (2) The neurosurgical patient with obtunded reflexes is predisposed to aspiration and/or hypostatic pneumonia. Mr. Conklin's position should be changed frequently during the immediate postoperative period to prevent retention and infection of tracheobronchial secretions, which would increase the likelihood of his developing hypostatic pneumonia.

36. (2) The organisms normally inhabiting the mouth and throat are one source of lower respiratory tract infections in the stuporous neurosurgical patient. Potentially infective material should be removed by repeatedly cleansing the mouth with cotton-tipped applicators dipped in antiseptic solution, followed by lubrication of the oral mucosa with glycerine to prevent drying and cracking of delicate tissues.

37. (2) Declining levels of consciousness indicate increasing suppression of electrical activity in the central nervous system.

38. (2) The corneal reflex consists of involuntary blinking when the cornea is gently stroked with a whisp of cotton. Unilateral absence of the blink reflex may indicate injury to the first division of the trigeminal nerve. The corneal reflex is frequently absent following brain surgery.

39. (1) If the blink reflex is absent, the eye should be protected from injury from a foreign body by regular irrigation with sterile saline solution; instillation of sterile mineral oil or artificial tears solution; gentle closing of the lid with nonallergic adhesive tape; and a protective shield.

40. (4) Positioning Mr. Conklin on his side helps to move the jaw forward, preventing airway obstruction by the tongue. Encouraging him to cough facilitates removal of tracheobronchial secretions from the lower airway. Frequent suctioning of the oropharynx removes secretions from the upper airway and prevents their aspiration. Changing his position frequently prevents atelectasis of dependent lung segments and pooling of bronchial secretions.

41. (4) When the concentration of carbon dioxide and hydrogen ions increases in brain blood flow, cranial vessels dilate to allow more rapid blood flow to brain tissue. In the patient with subdural hematoma, the increase in intracranial pressure resulting from cranial vasodilation may cause further decline in the level of consciousness.

42. (4) Both hypostatic and aspiration pneumonia are characterized by the filling of alveoli with inflammatory coagulum, which decreases the cross-sectional area of lung parenchyma available for gas exchange. When oxygenation of blood in lung capillaries is so decreased that the blood contains more than 5 grams per

cent of reduced hemoglobin, the patient will be cyanotic. If tracheobronchial secretions accumulate in the lower airway, rales will become audible. If fluid is present in the alveoli, cough will be stimulated. When the $PaCO_2$ level increases beyond a certain point, the respiratory center in the medulla will be stimulated and the respiratory rate will increase. When accessory muscles of respiration are called into play, supraclavicular, substernal, and intercostal retractions will be observed.

43. (3) An increase in temperature speeds the rate of metabolic activities and increases the oxygen need of all tissues. Brain, myocardium, liver, and kidney tissue are more easily damaged by oxygen lack than are other body tissues.

44. (2) To protect Mr. Conklin from postural deformity as a consequence of immobility and cerebral dysfunction, he must be maintained in optimal bed position while comatose. A rolled washcloth should be used to maintain the hand in functional position, i.e., slight extension of the wrist and slight flexion of the metacarpophalangeal and interphalangeal joints. A footboard should be used to maintain the foot in neutral position, at right angles to the leg.

Carcinoma of the Tongue and Radical Neck Dissection

1. (3) Chronic irritation of the following types predisposes to development of oral cancer: excessive use of tobacco and alcohol; injury from ill-fitting dentures or jagged teeth; irritation by hot or spicy foods; chronic infection due to poor oral hygiene.

2. (3) Leukoplakia is a condition characterized by the formation on the tongue or buccal mucosa of heavy smokers of smooth, white, thickened irregular patches that may undergo malignant change.

3. (4) Long-range objectives for Mr. Dyer's care should be directed toward improving his self-esteem and self-sufficiency in meeting physiologic and psychologic needs. With continuing emotional support and effective self-care instruction, most patients with mouth cancer can effectively look after themselves following hospital discharge.

4. (4) Given a diagnosis of mouth cancer, most persons would fear pain, disfigurement, inability to talk, difficulty with eating, interference with breathing, dependence on caregivers, and rejection by family and friends.

5. (3) The nurse's preoperative teaching should be built upon and related to information given Mr. Dyer by his surgeon. This communication would be the most effective in determining what the patient has been told by his physician about all phases of his therapeutic regimen.

6. (2) There is a less acute angle between the mouth and pharynx when the head is hyperextended than when it is held in normal position. Because of the effect of gravity on fluid flow, it is easier to swallow in the upright than in the prone position. Swallowing also facilitates entry of the nasogastric tube into the esophagus instead of the trachea.

7. (4) The standard protein allowance normally is 1 gram of protein per kilogram of body weight per day. For a 70-kg. man, the normal daily protein allowance would be 70 grams. Mr. Dyer was to have a high protein diet preoperatively, so of the choices given, an intake of 100 grams of protein per day would be best suited to his needs.

8. (3) Vitamin C, the antiscorbutic vitamin, is necessary for wound healing because it maintains the collagen component of fibrous tissue and preserves the integrity of capillaries.

9. (3) Citrus fruits, tomatoes, and raw leafy vegetables are all good sources of vitamin C. Milk, eggs, and meat are excellent sources of complete protein.

10. (4) In feeding a patient via a nosogastric tube, the nutrient solution must flow through the feeding tube into the stomach through gravity. Gravity flow is facilitated when the patient is in a sitting position.

11. (2) The nurse should ensure that the tube is correctly positioned in the stomach by placing the external end of the tube under water. If the catheter has inadvertently entered the trachea, air bubbles will appear in the water.

12. (2) If the signs listed occur during the feeding procedure, this indicates that nutrient solution has been aspirated into the lungs. The feeding should be

discontinued and the physician notified so that the patient's condition can be assessed and remedial measures taken.

13. (4) Ionizing radiation therapy is administered to halt mitosis, and is most injurious to tumor cells, which are the most rapidly dividing and least differentiated cells in a tissue.

14. (2) Radiation damages tumor cells by bombarding the molecules of nuclear protein, and dislodging electrons from the outer orbits of key atoms.

15. (3) The skin and gastrointestinal mucosa are both composed of rapidly dividing cells, and so are more affected by radiation than less rapidly dividing cells. Inflammation of skin produces itching. Inflammation of gastric and intestinal mucosa causes nausea, diarrhea, and anorexia.

16. (4) Medicated solutions and powders should not be used because they may contain a heavy metal, which would increase the radiation dosage. Radiation causes skin irritation and predisposes to skin breakdown. To minimize the danger of necrosis, other causes of skin irritation should be eliminated, such as friction from clothing, extremes of heat and cold, sun exposure, and application of adhesive and collodion.

17. (1) A variety of microorganisms normally inhabit the mouth. Malignant tumors tend to outgrow their blood supply and undergo necrosis. Necrotic tissue is an excellent culture medium for pathogenic bacteria. Tetracycline is a broad-spectrum antibiotic that is bacteriostatic against a wide range of gram-positive and -negative bacteria, rickettsiae, and some viruses.

18. (3) Tetracycline is irritating to gastrointestinal mucosa. Also, although it is effective against a great numer of gram-positive and gram-negative bacteria, other microorganisms are relatively resistant to tetracycline and tend to flourish in patients receiving the drug. Thus, diarrhea is a common toxic effect of tetracycline, and may be due either to chemical irritation or to superinfection of the bowel by staphylococci.

19. (2) Nausea is a common symptom of radiation sickness. Trimethobenzamide, an antiemetic, depresses the chemoreceptor zone that triggers the vomiting center in the medulla.

20. (4) In order to provide informed consent for the operation, the patient must have been given detailed information regarding its purpose and nature, and the known and possible consequences. Mr. Dyer's consent for surgery must be written, signed, and witnessed so that there is documentation that such consent was given. The patient must be free from any drugs that would cloud his understanding of the signing of consent. The consent form should indicate the date and time so that it can later be verified that it had not been obtained on the morning of surgery after the preanesthetic medication had been administered.

21. (4) The performance of surgery upon a person who had not freely given his informed consent would constitute assault and battery, because the surgical procedure would be interpreted as an unlawful use of force upon another for the purpose of doing physical harm.

22. (3) If a tracheostomy is created before surgery, anesthesia could be administered via this route, thereby facilitating visualization and instrumentation of oral structures during surgery. If an endotracheal tube was inserted, laryngeal edema could occur. A tracheostomy also constitutes an artificial airway for suctioning and resuscitation if the patient should develop postoperative respiratory problems.

23. (4) Cutting the superior laryngeal nerve results in loss of sensation to the glottis and laryngeal mucosa, and paralysis of the cricothyroid muscle, permitting aspiration of food, fluids, and secretions.

24. (1) Anatomic dead space consists of the conducting airways from the nose and mouth to the bronchioles. Respiratory muscle work is required to move air through these structures. A tracheostomy reduces Mr. Dyer's dead space by a considerable amount, thereby decreasing the workload of respiratory muscle.

25. (4) Anxiety can be minimized in the patient who is to be tracheotomized by explaining all of the factors listed.

26. (2) The patient should be advised to avoid talking until the tracheostomy is no longer needed and can be occluded for brief periods in perparation for remov-

ing the tube completely. During the transition period, with the physician's permission, Mr. Dyer could be taught to occlude the tracheostomy tube with his finger when he wishes to speak.

27. (2) Over 60 per cent of carcinoma of the tongue metastasizes to the neck, usually to the same side as that of the primary tumor. The preferred treatment for any malignant tumor is removal of the primary lesion and the regional lymphatics. Thus, a radical neck dissection was also performed.

28. (3) Over 60 per cent of carcinoma of the tongue metastasizes to the lymph nodes of the neck. Adequate removal of the deep cervical chain of lymph nodes cannot be effected without removal of subcutaneous fat, muscle, and the internal jugular vein.

29. (1) Removal of cervical nodes and channels interrupt lymphatic drainage, so edema of the face would develop postoperatively.

30. (2) In a radical neck dissection, a large amount of tissue is removed and many blood vessels are sectioned. A hemostat should be kept at the bedside to clamp off a bleeding vessel if hemorrhage should occur.

31. (2) Coughing causes considerable discomfort in a patient who has had a radical neck dissection. The nurse can minimize this by supporting the back of the patient's head and neck when he coughs.

32. (4) Following a radical neck dissection it is customary to use a pressure dressing to obliterate dead space in the operated area. The trauma of extensive surgery and the removal of lymphatics is apt to cause edema of neck tissues. The presence of the tracheostomy tube, and the irritant effect of the anesthetic gas, tend to increase the production of tracheobronchial secretions. The swallowing process begins with the tongue pressing against the hard palate in order to force the bolus of food or fluid into the pharynx. Resection of part of the tongue thus interferes with swallowing.

33. (3) The wound catheters and attached suction device are used to remove the copious secretions that accumulate following a radical neck dissection, and thus to ensure contact of the skin with underlying tissue and to enhance healing.

34. (1) A common response to instrumentation of the mouth is increased salivation. Since removal of the tongue makes expectoration of mouth secretions difficult, a gauze wick should be placed in the corner of the mouth and extended to a nearby emesis basin to keep the mouth clear of secretions.

35. (4) Tissue sloughing and the accumulation of serosanguineous drainage in the mouth provide an excellent medium for bacterial growth, so the patient who has undergone oral surgery is troubled by a bad taste and a foul odor to the breath. Hourly mouth irrigations with a salt and soda solution remove exudate, tissue debris, and microorganisms; reduce infection; decrease mouth odor; foster healing; and improve appetite and morale.

36. (1) Following a tracheostomy there is increased production of tracheobronchial secretions that tend to block the airway, are rich in protein, and provide an excellent medium for bacterial growth. In order not to introduce pathogens into the respiratory tree when the patient is debilitated, fresh sterile gloves and a fresh suction catheter should be used on each occasion that the tracheostomy tube is suctioned.

37. (1) The physician may order that 3–5 cc. (ml.) of sterile normal saline or Ringer's lactate solution be instilled into the tracheostomy tube immediately before suctioning, to liquefy secretions and aid in their removal.

38. (3) Occlusion of the open arm of the Y tube causes suction to be applied to secretions within the trachea. In order not to aspirate air from the airway before the catheter is in contact with tracheal secretions, suction should not be applied while the catheter is being inserted. Therefore, the open end of the Y tube should be occluded only after the catheter is in desired position in the trachea.

39. (2) Following oral surgery the presence of exudate and sloughing tissue provide an excellent culture medium for the normal bacterial flora of the mouth to overgrow. The patient with a tracheostomy and increased production of tracheobronchial secretions is predisposed to stagnation and infection of tracheal secretions which, if aspirated to peripheral lung tissues, are apt to cause

pneumonia. In order not to cause cross-contamination and infections, separate sterile catheters should be used to suction the mouth and trachea.

40. (3) Hydrogen peroxide is an unstable compound which, on contact with proteinaceous material, breaks down to form molecular oxygen and water. The effervescence created by the release of molecular oxygen loosens encrusted secretions and tissue debris from the lumen of the inner cannula of the tracheostomy tube.

41. (2) Since the patient may have difficulty in learning to breathe again through the upper airway, tube removal should take place gradually. A large-lumen tube should first be replaced by one with a smaller lumen; next, the lumen should be partially obstructed with a cap, and then completely obstructed for a day. If the patient proves able to breathe without the tube for several consecutive hours, it can be removed.

42. (4) Administration of several small feedings prevents overdistention of the stomach and gut. Gastric distention stimulates vomiting, and predisposes to aspiration of vomitus and secretions.

43. (3) The nasogastric tube should be flushed with 50 ml. of clear water following each feeding to clear the tube of the high protein, high carbohydrate feeding mixture, which serves as a culture medium for bacteria and causes diarrhea.

44. (1) A basic objective is to prepare Mr. Dyer to be self-sufficient as soon as possible after surgery, so as to minimize regression and preserve his self-esteem. His instruction on handling the nasogastric tube should begin the first time he is given a tube feeding.

45. (3) When the feeding tube is removed the patient may experience difficulty in swallowing for the first few meals. He should be given gruel, gelatin, or custard until he learns how to swallow again. As he becomes more proficient in swallowing, semisolid foods and ground meats may be gradually added to the diet.

46. (3) As a result of the deep tissue removal, the remaining blood vessels of the neck lie close to the overlying skin. Shaving with an electric razor decreases the danger of accidental injury to a large cervical blood vessel.

47. (2) The sternocleidomastoid originates from the anterior surface of the manubrium and the sternal end of the clavicle, and inserts into the mastoid process. The action of each sternocleidomastoid is to turn the head obliquely to the opposite side. When both contract together, they pull the head downward and forward. Mr. Dyer's rehabilitation should include exercises designed to strengthen other muscles involved in rotating and flexing the head.

48. (4) Since the eleventh cranial nerve (spinal accessory) is usually sacrificed during radical neck resection, the function of the trapezius muscle is impaired. The exercises described will help to strengthen it.

Cataract Removal

1. (3) A cataract is an opacification of the lens due to chemical changes in the lens protein.

2. (4) As a result of the normal degenerative changes of aging, some degree of lens opacification is present in most persons over 60 years of age. Mrs. Merkel's age and her lack of history of eye trauma suggest that her cataract is degenerative in nature.

3. (3) Vitamin A is instrumental in maintaining the integrity of epithelial tissues. Vitamin B_2 is active in the metabolic reactions involved in energy production and protein synthesis; its lack causes faulty protein metabolism. Vitamin C is responsible for normal metabolism of the amino acids phenylalanine and tyrosine. All the above vitamins maintain the lens in good condition.

4. (1) With senile or degenerative cataracts the process of lens opacification is slow, so that the patient experiences gradual blurring of vision. The degree of visual impairment for each patient depends on the stage of cataract development in each eye and the area of lens opacification.

5. (2) Normally, the refractive media of the eye (the cornea, aqueous humor, lens, and vitreous humor) are all clear, and serve to refract light rays and focus them

on the retina. Opacification of any of these media causes diffraction or turning aside of light rays, creating a glaring effect.

6. (2) Poor insulin control of hyperglycemia causes cataract development through production and accumulation of the sugar alcohol sorbitol, which causes osmotic changes in the lens. Chronic hypocalcemia results in cataract formation as a result of calcium deposition in the lens.

7. (3) Since Mrs. Merkel's eyes will be shielded postoperatively, she should be introduced preoperatively to those persons who will care for her after surgery. Eye contact and visual communication are an important aspect of trust-building between patient and caregivers.

8. (3) Mrs. Merkel's examinations revealed her to be in good health except for a mild hypochromic anemia, and therefore impaired iron absorption is the most likely cause for her anemia. Marrow replacement with malignant cells would produce a normochromic anemia, and there would also be a history of chronic bleeding. Failure to secrete intrinsic factor results in pernicious anemia, which is a hyperchromic, rather than a hypochromic, anemia.

9. (1) When iron preparations are given parenterally, common symptoms of toxicity are skin manifestations such as rash or urticaria.

10. (4) Aged patients are prone to disorientation when deprived of visual cues about their surroundings.

11. (4) The two most serious postoperative complications of cataract surgery are hemorrhage and loss of vitreous humor. Following intracapsular lens extraction, the patient should be kept at complete bedrest for 24 hours to prevent rupture of the suture line, with hemorrhage or loss of vitreous. Coughing, sneezing, blowing the nose, and straining at stool all increase intraocular pressure, and thus place stress on the intraocular suture line. Sips of water by mouth and a full liquid supper will be allowed on the evening of the operative day in order to facilitate hydration and prevent constipation. To prevent postural deformities and phlebothrombosis, Mrs. Merkel's extremities should be passively moved through full range of motion on the evening of the day of surgery and each day thereafter.

12. (2) Only this comment acknowledges Mrs. Merkel's expression of feeling in a manner that will encourage her to ventilate her feelings further.

13. (3) To prevent contamination of eye structures during the surgical procedure, the skin and brows surrounding the eye to be operated upon should be bathed with hexachlorophene, a bacteriostatic substance.

14. (2) The scissors used to cut the eyelashes preoperatively should be coated with petrolatum so that the cut lashes will adhere to the scissors blade rather than falling into the eye, where they could irritate the conjunctiva and predispose to postoperative infection. Gauze pledgets should be used to remove the layer of petrolatum jelly and adherent lashes following each cut of the scissors.

15. (2) Atropine, a parasympathetic depressant or anticholinergic drug, blocks the responses of the sphincter muscle of the iris and the ciliary muscle of the lens to cholinergic stimulation. Hence, atropine dilates the pupil and paralyzes accommodation.

16. (2) Phenylephrine hydrochloride, or Neo-Synephrine, is a synthetic adrenergic drug chemically related to epinephrine and ephedrine. It therefore is a sympathomimetic drug, in that its effects resemble those of sympathetic nervous system stimulation.

17. (3) Neo-Synephrine has both a vasoconstrictive and a mydriatic effect, both of which may be achieved by administering the drug into the conjunctival sac.

18. (4) Tetracaine hydrochloride, or Pontocaine, is a local anesthetic that is applied topically to achieve rapid, brief, superficial anesthesia. One drop of 0.5 per cent tetracaine solution will produce anesthesia within 30 seconds that lasts for 10–25 minutes.

19. (2) Mrs. Merkel's eye was massaged preoperatively to decrease intraocular pressure and minimize the danger of loss of vitreous during the operative procedure.

20. (3) Local anesthetics are preferred for intraocular surgery because they do not cause postoperative nausea and vomiting, which would increase intraocular pressure and place increased stress on the intraocular suture line.

21. (1) An iridectomy is the surgical removal of a portion of the iris. The iris, part of

the highly vascular, highly pigmented middle layer of the eye, is a diaphragm located anterior to the lens and posterior to the cornea.

22. (4) Aqueous humor is produced by the ciliary body, passes between the iris and the lens, and leaves the posterior chamber through the pupil. Part of the aqueous humor is removed from the anterior chamber through Schlemm's canal at the angle of the anterior chamber. The intraocular pressure is determined by the rate of aqueous humor production and the resistance to outflow of aqueous humor from the eye. Removing a section of the iris increases the flow of aqueous humor from the posterior to the anterior chamber, decreasing intraocular pressure and reducing stress on the suture line.

23. (4) An elderly patient is apt to have some degree of cerebral arteriosclerosis and hearing loss, as well as visual impairment. Old people who have both eyes bandaged following eye surgery are apt to become disoriented as a result of sensory deprivation. Bandaging only one eye postoperatively allows the patient to retain some visual cues to prevent the listed complications.

24. (4) Research has shown that persons deprived of sensory stimulation perceive their surroundings inaccurately, are unable to reason clearly, have difficulty in remembering, turn their attention increasingly inward, and exhibit hostility, irritability, depression, and hallucinations.

25. (2) Since vomiting raises the venous pressure in the head and elevates the intraocular pressure, exerting stress on the intraocular suture line, a p.r.n. order for an antiemetic should be available.

26. (2) Since a major aim of postoperative care following intraocular surgery is to prevent hemorrhage, Mrs. Merkel should lie quietly without jarring or turning her head for several hours following the operation. She will be more apt to hold her head still if sandbags are placed on either side of her head, and a nurse or relative is nearby to hold her hand and speak to her from time to time.

27. (1) Mrs. Merkel's age and her sensory deprivation render her liable to falls. Side rails should be applied to the bed until she is completely oriented and her eye dressings have been removed, and should be used at night throughout her entire hospital stay.

28. (3) When the return of venous blood from the head is blocked, the blood vessels in the eye dilate and increase the intraocular pressure.

29. (4) Keeping the mouth open while coughing minimizes the increase in venous pressure in the head.

30. (2) Mineral oil is not digested and not absorbed from the bowel. It is used as a cathartic because it softens the stool and prevents resorption of water. However, it is unsuited for long-term treatment of chronic constipation because it dissolves the fat-soluble vitamins A, D, E, and K, and interferes with their absorption from the bowel.

31. (2) It is thought that the thalamus is responsible for the conscious appreciation of pain, and the cortex for the perception of pain. Since salicylates do not cause mental sluggishness or dulling of consciousness, it would appear that they produce analgesia by blocking pain impulses in the thalamus.

32. (4) Direct trauma or increased intraocular pressure may cause hemorrhage into the anterior chamber of the eye (hyphema) as a result of rupture of fragile capillaries. Postoperative infection may result from contamination of the eye during surgery, or contamination of the dressings by vomitus or oral secretions following surgery. Because a mild degree of iritis occurs following cataract surgery, adhesions may form between the iris and the vitreous face, interfering with the flow of aqueous humor and causing glaucoma. If, as a result of increased intraocular pressure, loss of vitreous should occur during or following surgery, scar tissue could attach to the retina and, with later contracture, exert tension on the retina, causing retinal detachment.

33. (2) The chief dangers for the first week following surgery are the possibility of falling from bed owing to impaired vision, and the risk of direct trauma to the eye by the patient's rubbing it, either intentionally or during sleep.

34. (3) For the first week following surgery Mrs. Merkel should not bend or stoop, which would tend to increase intraocular pressure, and should be helped to brush her teeth, comb her hair, and wash her face.

35. (1) The nurse's objective in caring for a patient with visual impairment should not be to relieve the patient of all responsibility for self-care and self-direction, which would decrease the patient's self-esteem, but to provide temporary reinforcement of impaired ego functions. The anxious, aged patient with visual impairment can test reality vicariously through the interpretations of a trusted primary care nurse.

36. (4) All the items listed would provide helpful sensory stimulation, which Mrs. Merkel has strong need of during this period of visual deprivation. Diversions help the long hours of inactivity to pass more quickly and pleasantly.

37. (1) While Mrs. Merkel's eye is shielded, and visual cues regarding her surroundings are ambiguous or lacking, she will need repeated auditory clues as to her present circumstances in order to avoid confusion and disorientation.

38. (1) Aged patients may be infirm, uncoordinated, or subject to dizziness. For some time following intraocular surgery the eye can be easily damaged by accidental trauma from fingers, handkerchiefs, dust, and dirt particles; thus, temporary glasses will protect the eye from trauma, as well as improve visual acuity, until the cataract glasses can be prescribed 4–6 weeks later.

39. (4) Since the operated eye could be easily traumatized during sleep by contact with bed linen or by unconscious rubbing of the eyes, the eyeshield should be worn during sleep until the intraocular suture line has completely healed.

40. (2) Bending and lifting both increases intraocular pressure, and must be avoided for 4–6 weeks postoperatively.

41. (2) Normally, the changes in the anterior curvature of the lens surface facilitate accommodation for near and far vision. Without a lens the ability to accommodate for far vision is lost.

42. (3) Healing of the surgical wound following lens extraction causes the curvature of the cornea to change continuously for 3–4 months following surgery, so permanent cataract glasses cannot be prescribed until postoperative eye changes have been completed.

43. (2) A cataract lens in a glasses frame magnifies objects by one third. Peripheral vision through cataract glasses is poor because thick lenses cause marked curvature and distortion of detail. Mrs. Merkel must learn to fix her gaze through the center of the lens, and to turn her head slowly when looking to the side.

Glaucoma and Iridectomy

1. (2) Aqueous humor flows forward between the iris and the lens through the pupillary space and into the anterior chamber, from which it is absorbed into the venous circulation of the anterior chamber. Normally, the production and absorption of aqueous humor is balanced to maintain an intraocular pressure at about 20 mm. Hg. With increased production or decreased absorption of aqueous humor, this pressure increases, causing damage to the retinal ganglion cells and the optic nerve.

2. (4) Ninety-nine per cent of cases of glaucoma are of the chronic simple or wide-angle type in which the angle is open, the aqueous humor is in free contact with the trabecula, and the obstruction is located within the drainage apparatus itself. Wide-angle glaucoma is due to an hereditary predisposition to obstruction in the drainage system.

3. (2) In open-angle or chronic simple glaucoma, peripheral vision is gradually lost. With increasing injury to the optic nerve, the patient may experience episodes of foggy or blurred vision. Because rapid and high elevations of intraocular pressure may occur after the patient has imbibed large quantities of fluids, the corneal epithelium becomes edematous, creating rainbow halos around lights.

4. (2) As a result of edema of the corneal epithelium, the cornea may have a cloudy appearance. Increased intraocular pressure causes forward displacement of the iris and atrophy of pupillary musculature, so that the pupil is dilated and contracts slowly on light stimulation. Increased intraocular pressure results in congestion of the iris and conjunctiva.

5. (1) Chronic simple glaucoma is characterized by diurnal variations in intraocular pressure, with peak pressures being reached at night and in the early morning hours, so the patient's visual symptoms tend to be more pronounced on arising.

6. (4) Most authorities agree that severe emotional tension may precipitate a sudden elevation in intraocular tension.

7. (1) Intraocular pressure is determined both by the rate of production of aqueous humor by the ciliary body and by the rate of absorption of aqueous humor by the drainage apparatus.

8. (3) In open-angle glaucoma the increased intraocular pressure is caused by resistance to outflow of aqueous humor by a thickened meshwork, narrowed Schlemm's canal, or constricted aqueous vein.

9. (4) A tonometer is used to measure tension. To measure intraocular pressure the patient is placed in horizontal position; the cornea is anesthetized; the tonometer footplate is applied to the cornea; the plunger is elevated; the attached needle is deflected; and the intraocular pressure is computed from the resultant scale reading.

10. (2) The less the aqueous humor in the eye and the lower the intraocular pressure, the softer is the eye, and the greater is the indentation of the cornea by the tonometer footplate. The greater the volume of aqueous humor in the eye and the higher the intraocular pressure, the harder is the eye, and the less is the identation of the cornea by the footplate.

11. (3) A gonioscope is a specialized type of ophthalmoscope used to examine the angle of the anterior chamber of the eye. During gonioscopy a contact glass is placed on the cornea to magnify and illuminate the cornea, so as to permit evaluation of the chamber angle.

12. (3) For about 15 minutes after tonometric measurements are taken the cornea will be insensitive as a result of the topical anesthetic instilled into the eye. Therefore, the eye must be protected from injury by a foreign body.

13. (3) Injury to the optic nerve by increased intraocular pressure causes loss of peripheral vision. Hence, the physician performs a visual field examination on any patient suspected of having glaucoma.

14. (1) Central vision is preserved until late in the course of glaucoma. Loss of peripheral vision occurs so gradually in open-angle glaucoma that the patient may begin to bump into objects lying just outside his direct line of vision before he realizes that he has any serious sight impairment.

15. (2) In glaucoma, increased intraocular pressure depresses the optic nerve head, causing the disc surface to drop back into a deep excavation. Retinal vessels appear to break sharply at the disc margin where they descend into the cup.

16. (2) The water provocation test consists of flooding the body tissues with water so as to cause increased production of aqueous humor. If, after an eight-hour fast and rapid drinking of 1 quart of water the intravascular pressure rises from 8 to 10 mm. Hg within an hour, there is a strong presumption that glaucoma is present.

17. (3) Pilocarpine stimulates the same autonomic effector cells as those stimulated by the parasympathetic nervous system.

18. (1) Pilocarpine is used in glaucoma for its pupillary constricting effect.

19. (1) Physostigmine and carbamylcholine are also parasympathomimetic drugs.

20. (1) The iris contains both circular muscle fibers, which on contraction constrict the pupil, and radiating muscle fibers, which on contraction dilate the pupil. Pilocarpine stimulates the circulatory muscle fibers of the iris. By constricting the pupil, pilocarpine pulls the smooth muscle of the iris away from the drainage meshwork at the angle of the anterior chamber, thereby facilitating absorption of aqueous humor.

21. (1) Accuracy in the administration of eye medications is of the utmost importance, since instillation of the wrong medication into the eyes of a glaucomatous patient could precipitate an acute eye emergency. Of the precautions listed, the most serious errors and complications can be avoided by rechecking the physician's medicine orders and drug container labels to ensure that the correct durg in the prescribed strength is instilled into the correct eye with the prescribed frequency.

22. (4) By washing the hands before administering eye drops, the nurse can decrease the possibility of introducing pathogens or irritants into the eye. By having the patient tilt his head backward before eye drops are instilled, she can ensure adequate contact of the drug with eye tissues. By depressing the lower lid, she can create a conjunctival sac into which to instill the drug so as not to apply it directly on the cornea. By steadying her hand on the patient's forehead, the nurse can avoid contaminating or injuring the eyelid, cornea, or conjunctiva with the dropper. By dropping the medication on the everted lower eyelid, she can avoid both physical and chemical irritation to the cornea.

23. (3) The enzyme carbonic anhydrase removes water from carbonic acid and facilitates production of aqueous humor. Acetazolamide inhibits carbonic anhydrase, slows the production of aqueous humor, and decreases intraocular pressure.

24. (3) Although side effects are common with administration of acetazolamide, they are rarely serious. The more common ones are lethargy, fatigue, numbness and tingling, anorexia and dyspepsia, and diuresis with potassium depletion.

25. (3) So long as intraocular pressure remains elevated, the retinal ganglia and the optic nerve will be increasingly damaged. A nonfunctioning optic nerve cannot be restored. Without treatment, glaucoma progresses to total blindness.

26. (4) This comment is the only one that will encourage Mr. Iago to elucidate the ideas and feelings that underlie his remark.

27. (3) This response will stimulate Mr. Iago to examine his beliefs and feelings about his illness and present circumstances in greater detail than he may have done thus far.

28. (1) An attack of acute glaucoma may be followed by formation of diffuse, small, white lens opacities. The lens receives its nourishment from the intraocular fluids. When the intraocular pressure is elevated, there is interference with lens nutrition.

29. (4) When walking with a sightless person the nurse should offer her arm, as the visually impaired individual has a better sense of balance and direction when he is led toward his destination by someone who walks slightly ahead of him than when he is grasped by the arm and propelled in the desired direction.

30. (3) Fatigue causes greater susceptibility to emotional upsets and crying, which tend to increase intraocular pressure.

31. (1) In some individuals caffeine causes an increase in intraocular pressure.

32. (2) Local anesthetics are preferred for eye surgery, because the patient is apt to be restless following general anesthesia and may injure the operated eye in actively moving about. Following surgery the operated eye will be covered with a dressing and a shield to absorb any drainage that may be present, to prevent pressure against the globe, and to limit movement of the eye. Eye movement and tissue trauma should be avoided to prevent postoperative hemorrhage and disruption of the suture line.

33. (2) In an iridectomy a small wedge of iris is excised to open the angle of the anterior chamber, and to provide an opening between the posterior and anterior chamber through which aqueous humor may circulate.

34. (2) In cyclodialysis the ciliary body is separated from the sclera so as to create a channel for drainage of aqueous humor into the suprachoroidal space.

35. (2) In order to decrease stress on the operated eye it is desirable to restrict head and eye movements for several days following surgery. Placing a small pillow on either side of the head will remind the patient to lie quietly and to avoid head movement.

36. (2) In order to prevent postoperative hemorrhage and stress on the suture line, the patient should be as nearly immobile as possible during the immediate postoperative period. He should be given a call bell and instructed to summon the nurse for any assistance needed; this will serve to remind him to avoid all exertion until he is otherwise instructed.

37. (4) All the activities listed cause an increase of intraocular pressure, either by increasing venous pressure in the head (coughing, sneezing, turning the head, bending over) or by exerting pressure on the globe (rubbing the eyes or closing the lids tightly).

38. (2) A damaged optic nerve cannot be regenerated. If intraocular pressure is re-

duced and maintained at normal levels, further pressure damage to the nerve will not occur.

39. (4) Chronic simple wide-angle glaucoma is hereditary; there is a familial tendency for thickening of the trabecular network, and all of Mr. Iago's children should have their intraocular pressure measured annually.

40. (2) One of the nurse's responsibilities in health teaching is to reinforce reality in regard to health risks and appropriate methods of disease prevention. Mr. Iago's son knows or suspects that he is at risk where glaucoma is concerned. His laughter may result from anxiety, and his remark to the nurse may be a request for clarification. She can clarify the issue and relieve his anxiety through this response.

41. (4) All the factors listed cause a rise in intraocular pressure, either by increasing venous pressure in the head (tight collar, straining at stool, heavy lifting, emotional stress) or by eyestrain and irritation (excessive reading, or TV viewing in a darkened room).

42. (2) Regular use of the prescribed miotic is essential to protect the eyes from the damaging effects of increased intraocular pressure. For safety's sake, the patient should keep extra supplies of pilocarpine at home and at work.

43. (2) Denial is a defense mechanism by which a painful awareness is repressed or an intolerable thought is rejected, because some aspect of external reality is too painful to be dealt with. Failure to administer the needed miotic after having been taught why drug use is essential might indicate denial of the seriousnes of the eye disease.

Emphysema

1. (1) Normally, during inspiration, the bronchioles dilate, the thorax expands, and the elastic lung tissue expands to accommodate the inspired air. In emphysema, expiration is made difficult by a combination of loss of elasticity of lung tissue, excess mucus, and narrowed bronchioles.

2. (2) The thermoregulatory center in the anterior hypothalamus controls heat production and can be reset for a higher-than-normal body temperature by an endogenous pyrogen. This substance is released from granulocytic white blood cells when they are exposed to bacterial endotoxin or bacterial cell protein.

3. (2) Emphysema is defined as enlargement of air passages distal to terminal bronchioles, with accompanying destruction of alveolar walls. These structural changes cause loss of lung elasticity, increase in airway resistance, and hyperinflation of the lung. In lung areas, where obstructive lesions exist, the cross-sectional area for oxygen-carbon dioxide exchange is reduced, hypoxemia develops, and dyspnea results.

4. (4) Cyanosis, a bluish discoloration of the skin and mucosa, results from an increase in the amount of reduced hemoglobin in the small blood vessels of the area. It can be due to a dilation of venules at the venous ends of capillaries, or a decrease in oxygen saturation of the capillary blood.

5. (4) Cyanosis is usually most marked in the lips, nail beds, and ears. Because excessive melanin deposits may obscure bluish skin discoloration, the oral mucosa in black and Latin patients should be examined for cyanosis.

6. (2) Sixty per cent of patients with obstructive emphysema have chronic bronchitis, with tenacious mucus, spasm of bronchial muscles, and thickening of bronchial mucosa, all of which favor stagnation and infection of tracheobronchial secretions.

7. (2) Alveolar air trapping and increased intra-alveolar pressures cause squeezing of small pulmonary vessels, with elevation of pressure in the pulmonary circulation and increased right ventricular workload.

8. (4) Cor pulmonale, or enlargement and failure of the right ventricle secondary to a disease of pulmonary parenchyma, leads to congestion and increased pressure in the systemic venous circulation. Increased hydrostatic pressure in the veins of the lower extremities causes pedal edema.

9. (4) The emphysematous lung is characterized by chronic inflammation and nar-

rowing of bronchioles, together with generalized dilation of distal air spaces due to rupture of alveolar walls and merging of alveoli.

10. (1) Seventy per cent of patients with emphysema have a history of chronic bronchitis, primarily due to cigarette smoking, air pollution, or irritating occupational exposures.

11. (4) Tobacco smoking causes hypertrophy of glands in the respiratory mucosa, with increased secretion of mucus; destruction of respiratory cilia, interfering with movement of mucus upward from the lower respiratory tree; and a decrease in the secretion of the lipoprotein surfactant, which reduces the surface tension of fluids lining the alveoli and respiratory passages. Normal lung contains many elastic fibers that are destroyed by chronic inflammation.

12. (3) In emphysema the fixed position of the bony chest makes it necessary for the patient to use abdominal and neck muscles to ventilate the lungs. Mr. Hale will be most comfortable in a sitting position, leaning forward, with shoulders elevated, arms akimbo, and hands on knees.

13. (2) When anxiety mounts, a patient's physical symptoms are apt to be intensified. Pain, muscle spasm, nausea, and dyspnea may all be increased by anxiety. Anxiety may intensify breathlessness due to increased secretion of epinephrine, which elevates blood pressure, increases heart rate, and increases respiratory rate.

14. (2) As a result of air trapping in overdistended alveoli, the lungs are overinflated and the bony chest becomes fixed in the position of inspiration, with the ribs elevated and moved forward to a more horizontal position, and a resulting increase in the anterior-posterior diameter of the chest.

15. (3) Rales, or abnormal gurgling heard on chest auscultation, are caused by passage of air through secretions or exudates in the air passages.

16. (1) Vital capacity is the maximal volume of air that can be expired after maximal inspiration.

17. (1) Tidal volume is the amount of air that moves into and out of the lung with each normal respiration. The average for an adult male is 500 cc. (ml.).

18. (2) The air trapping that occurs in emphysema causes increased residual air volume, decreasing expiratory reserve volume, and therefore decreasing vital capacity.

19. (4) Normally, the partial pressure of oxygen in arterial blood is 96 mm. Hg, or 4 mm. Hg less than the normal alveolar oxygen tension.

20. (1) Normally, the partial pressure of carbon dioxide in arterial blood is 40 mm. Hg, which is roughly the same as the normal alveolar carbon dioxide tension.

21. (1) There is an inverse relationship between pH and the hydrogen ion concentration. The normal pH of body fluids ranges from 7.35 to 7.45. Acidosis is characterized by an excess of hydrogen ions in the body. Respiratory acidosis is characterized by a pH of less than 7.35 and a rise in pCO_2, and results from some degree of respiratory failure.

22. (3) In health, body fluids are maintained at a slight degree of alkalinity, between pH 7.35 and 7.45, by a number of chemical buffers (bicarbonate ion, plasma proteins, and hemoglobin) and by renal excretion of hydrogen ions.

23. (1) In emphysema, as a result of alveolar hypoventilation, hypoxemia and hypercapnia develop. Lowered arterial oxygen tension causes the kidneys to produce erythropoietin, which stimulates the bone marrow to produce additional red blood cells, so that a compensatory polycythemia develops. Most patients with emphysema have some degree of chronic bronchitis. A mild leukocytosis is typical of chronic infectious disorders. The normal hematocrit in the male is 40–52 per cent, so 55 per cent is slightly elevated, as one would expect as a result of the higher-than-normal red blood cell count. The normal percentage of neutrophils is 55–70 per cent, so 79 per cent is slightly elevated, as would be expected as a result of the inflammatory process in the lung.

24. (1) Patients with emphysema normally have elevated pCO_2 levels and have lost the usual respiratory stimulus, CO_2 stimulation. The elevated pCO_2 depresses the respiratory center, and the respiratory stimulus is now derived from low pO_2 levels. Although these individuals lack oxygen, it is dangerous to raise their pO_2 levels. If arterial pO_2 level is normal and there is retention of carbon

dioxide, the patient will have no respiratory stimulus and will experience carbon dioxide narcosis, which could cause coma and respiratory failure.

25. (3) In emphysema patients it is decreased arterial pO_2 rather than increased arterial pCO_2 that stimulates increased respiration. Administration of 100 per cent oxygen, therefore, would raise arterial oxygen pressures sufficiently to decrease respiratory rate and depth, allowing carbon dioxide and hydrogen ions to accumulate in body fluids.

26. (1) At the venous end of the tissue capillaries, after the blood has given up oxygen to the cells, the pO_2 of venous blood is 40 mm. Hg.

27. (1) In the normal subject the partial pressure of oxygen in the alveoli is 100 mm. Hg, and the partial pressure of oxygen in the arterial blood as it leaves the lung is 96 mm. Hg.

28. (1) The partial pressure of carbon dioxide in the tissue cells and tissue fluids (60 mm. Hg) is higher than the partial pressure of carbon dioxide in the arterial end of the tissue capillary (40 mm. Hg), so carbon dioxide diffuses from the tissue cells into the blood, and the pCO_2 of venous blood becomes about 46 mm. Hg.

29. (2) In emphysema, the rupture of alveolar walls and coalescence of alveoli into larger-than-normal air spaces constitute a considerable loss of lung parenchyma, with a reduction of cross-sectional area for gas exchange. When less oxygen than normal is taken up by the blood in pulmonary capillaries, and less carbon dioxide than normal is given up from the blood in pulmonary capillaries, the result is a decrease in arterial pO_2 and an increase in arterial pCO_2.

30. (1) Bronchiolitis, or chronic infection of the small air passages in the lungs, invariably precedes emphysema. Inflammation of the mucosal lining of the lower respiratory tract causes thickening of the mucosa, spasm of bronchial muscles, and increased secretion of mucus, all of which cause a restriction of air flow that is most pronounced on expiration.

31. (4) Improving the overall fitness of the emphysematous patient greatly increases his comfort and his ability to remain active. Therapeutic measures can be used to decrease symptoms of respiratory obstruction. A physical fitness program with breathing instructions will increase the patient's exercise tolerance and decrease his fear of breathlessness. Long-range goals should include a return to work and some form of recreational activity in order to maintain the patient's morale.

32. (3) By lowering the rate of tissue metabolism, tissue oxygen demand is reduced, decreasing both cardiac and respiratory workload. A decrease in heart rate may enable an overworked right ventricle to compensate for increased resistance to blood flow through the pulmonary circulation. A decrease in respiratory rate should improve gas exchange by increasing the time of contact between pulmonary capillary blood and alveolar air.

33. (3) Tetracycline is a broad-spectrum antibiotic that exerts a bacteriostatic effect by inhibiting the synthesis of bacterial protein in a wide variety of gram-positive and gram-negative bacteria, the rickettsiae, several of the larger viruses, and some amebae.

34. (1) Tetracycline is irritating to the gastrointestinal tract and can cause stomatitis, nausea, vomiting, and diarrhea.

35. (4) The primary purpose of positive pressure breathing is to force air under pressure beyond focal bronchiolar constriction so as to improve alveolar ventilation.

36. (4) By forcing air past points of bronchiolar narrowing, intermittent positive pressure breathing (I.P.P.B.) improves the intrapulmonary distribution of inhaled air. Improved delivery of air to alveoli results in increased oxygen-carbon dioxide exchange. By forcing air past stagnated tracheobronchial secretions, coughing can be made more explosive, and thickened mucus can be more easily removed. Inflation of the lung by I.P.P.B. provides passive motion for the muscles of respiration, improving the tone of those muscles that the patient has not exercised as a result of poor breathing techniques.

37. (2) This comment is the only one that describes the treatments accurately, that provides enough information to enlist the patient's cooperation, and that avoids undue emphasis on the irreversible pathology.

38. (3) The patient must be instructed to breathe slowly, as the anxious patient tends to overbreathe and may become alkalotic.

39. (1) The patient should be instructed to hold his breath momentarily at the end of inspiration to ensure maximal distribution of aerosolized isoproterenol. To overcome airway resistance and decrease air trapping, he should also be instructed to prolong expiration so as to force increased amounts of air past constricted bronchial muscles and thickened mucosa. Prolongation of both inspiration and expiration requires slowing of the respiratory rate to 8–10 respirations per minute.

40. (1) The ventilator used for I.P.P.B. is pressure cycled.

41. (1) The emphysematous patient invariably suffers some degree of bronchitis, and so has increased tracheobronchial secretions that are apt to stagnate and dehydrate in the narrowed bronchioles. The breathing mixture used in I.P.P.B. must be humidified in order to prevent crusting of secretions that would interfere with their removal during coughing.

42. (4) Isoproterenol is a synthetic catecholamine with predominant beta-adrenergic action. In addition to increasing heart rate and force of contraction, it relaxes arterial and bronchial smooth muscles. Isoproterenol was used in Mr. Hale's treatment to dilate the narrowed bronchi and bronchioles, so as to facilitate removal of tracheobronchial secretions and improve alveolar ventilation.

43. (3) Possible toxic effects of isoproterenol include precordial pain, palpitations, and flushing.

44. (3) Since postural drainage results in the movement of stagnated tracheobronchial secretions, it stimulates paroxysms of coughing that result in the expectoration of large quantities of thickened mucus. To ensure that coughing has subsided before the patient begins to eat, postural drainage should not be performed later than one hour before meals.

45. (2) Drainage of the middle and lower lobes of the lung requires that the patient be placed in a head-down position, which may make aged and severely hypoxic patients dizzy the first time. Therefore, the first few sessions of postural drainage should be limited to ten minutes, and the length of the treatments should be gradually increased according to the patient's tolerance.

46. (2) Scrupulous oral hygiene is needed to remove infected respiratory secretions from the mouth following each postural drainage treatment.

47. (3) In emphysema, alveolar air trapping and increased residual air volumes contribute significantly to faulty gas exchange. Breathing exercises that strengthen the abdominal muscles, plus increased diaphragmatic movement, will improve respiratory efficiency and reduce reliance on accessory muscles of respiration.

48. (4) All the exercises listed will encourage the patient to exhale more completely, and thus decrease residual air volumes and improve gas exchange.

49. (2) As a result of anxiety and regression, some patients with chronic obstructive lung disease become excessively dependent on caregivers. Those with severe dyspnea who experience positive results following I.P.P.B. treatments may become excessively reliant on the ventilator. In such patients, increasing emphasis should be placed on prescribed breathing exercises.

Tuberculosis

1. (2) In primary tuberculosis, an initial granuloma develops, and mycobacteria from the lesion reach the hilar lymph nodes and establish a granulomatous lesion. With mobilization of body defenses, both the lesion and the infected hilar node heal, undergo fibrosis, and calcify.

2. (2) Tuberculin is a protein produced by *Mycobacterium tuberculosis* and isolated from a broth in which the organisms have been cultivated. It contains an antigen that elicits an inflammatory skin response in individuals who have developed hypersensitivity to *Mycobacterium tuberculosis*.

3. (1) Purified protein derivative in solution rapidly adsorbs to glass or plastic and loses potency. For the Mantoux test procedure to be accurate, the tuberculin

testing solution must be freshly prepared and must have been stored in the re-frigerator.

4. (2) The tuberculin test results depend on the development of an allergic skin reaction caused by the administered antigen. The most reliable results are obtained when the tuberculin is injected intradermally.

5. (2) Testing is begun with a small dose of tuberculin to avoid severe allergic reactions, with exacerbations of lymphangitis and systemic symptoms, in those patients with extreme tuberculin hypersensitivity.

6. (3) In the Mantoux test the skin reaction to intradermally injected tuberculin is read 48–72 hours following administration.

7. (3) A positive Mantoux test consists of a visible and palpable induration 10 mm. or more in diameter. An area of erythema may surround the area of induration.

8. (1) A positive tuberculin reaction can be temporarily suppressed by an over-whelming tuberculous infection, such as is seen in massively disseminated or miliary tuberculosis.

9. (3) The area of induration resulting from intradermal injection of tuberculin may not be perfectly circular. In determining the size of the indurated area, the largest diameter of induration should be measured.

10. (2) A negative Mantoux test signifies that the individual has never been infected by *Mycobacterium tuberculosis*.

11. (1) B.C.G. is a strain of *Mycobacterium bovis* that is less virulent for humans. Studies have shown that subjects vaccinated with B.C.G. have significantly decreased incidence of clinical tuberculosis.

12. (4) Since B.C.G. vaccination protects the previously uninfected individual against tuberculous infection, it is given to tuberculin-negative persons who must live or work in a situation where they are certain to be exposed to those with active tuberculosis.

13. (3) B.C.G. vaccination is not given to a person with skin disease of any type, because a possible complication of this vaccine is local ulceration at the vaccination site, and anyone with pre-existing skin lesions would be increas-ingly susceptible to this complication.

14. (3) Tim's conversion to a Mantoux positive reaction indicated that he was tu-berculosis-free until sometime during his first year in school. His negative chest x-ray at the end of the freshman year indicated that his natural defenses had overcome the tuberculous infection and that the primary lesion had healed without cavity formation, but that insufficient time had passed for the primary lesion and the infected hilar node to calcify.

15. (4) Afternoon fever of 102° or 103° F. occurs as a result of absorption of tuber-culous protein from the granuloma into the blood, which causes the resetting of the temperature regulating center in the hypothalamus. Night sweats occur as a result of sympathetic stimulation of the eccrine glands in response to elevated body temperature. Ulceration of the bronchial mucosa by the inflam-matory exudate cause the sputum to be blood-tinged. Widespread hematoge-nous spread of *Mycobacterium tuberculosis* to many body tissues may cause anorexia and weight loss.

16. (1) The only absolute proof of active tuberculous infection is identification of *Mycobacterium tuberculosis* from a culture of appropriate body tissues or secretions. The presence of acid-fast bacilli in a smear of Tim's sputum consti-tutes presumptive evidence of tuberculosis. To corroborate this attempts should be made to culture *Mycobacterium tuberculosis* from his sputum, or if that is not possible, from a morning sample of gastric contents.

17. (1) Tubercle bacilli excreted by one person in aerosolized droplets during cough-ing, sneezing, or talking can be inhaled by another. These organisms can reach the respiratory bronchiole, invade the tissues, and establish a tubercular infec-tion.

18. (2) *Mycobacterium tuberculosis* is characterized by a cell wall of high lipid con-tent (60 per cent), which is responsible for the cell's unusual resistance to strong mineral acids and alkalis, to various dyes, and to drying.

19. (3) Epidemiologic studies have revealed that there is an incubation period of 4–6 weeks from inoculation with tubercle bacilli to the appearance of fever, malaise, and tuberculin hypersensitivity.

20. (3) When mycobacteria invade the tissues they are quickly ingested by neutrophils, which in turn are phagocytosed by monocytes. A zone of lymphocytes surround the monocytes and wall the tubercle off from surrounding tissue.

21. (2) On admission, the patient is hypermetabolic as a result of the inflammatory process in the lung. Rest will reduce basic oxygen need, decrease respiratory rate, and decrease lung mobility so as to foster healing.

22. (1) Since *Mycobacterium tuberculosis* is spread from one person to another by way of aerosolized droplets, Tim should be instructed to cover his mouth and nose with a tissue while coughing and sneezing, and to dispose of contaminated tissues in a paper bag. He should also be taught to wash his hands after handling the sputum-filled tissues.

23. (2) On admission to the hospital the patient will be hypermetabolic, fatigued, malnourished, and emotionally labile. Tim's visitors should be restricted to immediate family members until drug therapy has arrested the systemic symptoms so that he is able to eat and sleep comfortably, and has begun to regain strength.

24. (2) The tuberculosis infection threatens Tim with at least temporary loss of his nursing occupation, army officer status, affiliation with friends, pursuit of favorite recreational activities, and furtherance of career and educational plans. The multiplicity of his losses may trigger a grief reaction.

25. (2) Adequate circulation of fresh air should be used to carry droplet nuclei from the room and to dilute tubercle bacilli, thereby minimizing contamination of persons within the environment.

26. (4) Rifampin, an antibiotic that inhibits the growth of *Mycobacterium tuberculosis*, is eliminated primarily in the bile, and causes liver dysfunction in some subjects.

27. (3) Peripheral neuritis develops in about 17 per cent of patients receiving isoniazid. The incidence is related to the dose administered.

28. (4) Isoniazid depletes the body's pyridoxine stores. Neuritis can be avoided in patients receiving isoniazid by simultaneous administration of 100 mg. of pyridoxine daily.

29. (1) The expectoration of a large quantity of bright red blood indicates that the active tuberculous lesion has eroded into a bronchial artery. Tim should be placed on his right side, both to facilitate drainage of blood from the lung and to splint the right side of the chest so as to minimize bleeding.

30. (4) Morphine relieves anxiety through depression of the sensory cortex and the thalamus. It relieves dyspnea by depressing the respiratory center and thus decreasing the respiratory rate, and it relieves the sensation of breathing discomfort through the hypothalamic depression.

31. (3) On inspiration, blood heavily contaminated with mycobacteria is aspirated into air passages and alveoli distal to the site of hemorrhage. The organisms, thus spread throughout the lung, set up new foci of infection.

32. (3) Codeine depresses the cough center in the medulla.

33. (1) For several hours following pulmonary hemorrhage the patient should be given nothing by mouth. When feeding is resumed, small quantities of cold liquids may be given in order to prevent overdistention of the stomach, which could elevate the diaphragm, shift the position of the lung, and cause rebleeding.

34. (1) Ethambutol blocks growth of *Mycobacterium tuberculosis* by interfering with synthesis of RNA. It may cause optic neuritis, resulting in decrease in visual acuity and loss of ability to perceive the color green.

35. (1) Antituberculosis drugs have proved most effective when administered in a single daily dose so as to achieve a peak concentration of all drugs simultaneously.

36. (2) Until ethambutol was developed, para-aminosalicylic acid (PAS) was the principal companion drug to isoniazid in treatment of tuberculosis. PAS suppresses growth and multiplication of *Mycobacterium tuberculosis* by antagonizing the para-aminobenzoic acid necessary for bacterial growth.

37. (4) PAS causes anorexia due to gastric irritation. Extreme fatigue produces anorexia when the energy expenditure required is greater than the patient's energy

reserves. Anorexia can be a symptom of psychologic depression and can be due to the many losses associated with tuberculosis. For patients who deny the seriousness of their illness, anorexia may constitute a rejection of the prescribed treatment regimen. Anorexia may result if the patient's cultural or individual food patterns are totally ignored during hospitalization.

38. (2) A patient with loss of appetite may eat more readily if his family brings in food prepared at home.

39. (3) Experience has proved that, for tuberculosis without large areas of cavitation, two years of treatment with two drug combinations usually produce permanent healing of the tuberculous lesion.

40. (1) During the period of therapy and until his weight is restored to normal, Tim will be subject to feelings of physical weakness and associated psychologic vulnerability.

41. (4) The prognosis in tuberculosis is primarily dependent on the patient's cooperation with and adherence to the prolonged drug therapy necessary for complete healing. Patient failure to take ordered drugs is the most frequent cause of treatment failure. Obtaining, storing, and taking the medicines will require self-discipline.

42. (1) In order to facilitate healing of damaged lung tissue and restoration of body weight, protein and vitamin C intake must be adequate or slightly increased. To remedy nutritional lacks developed during the period of anorexia, the vitamin and mineral content of the diet must be increased. To replace blood losses, increased iron may be required. To maintain calcium balance, increased calcium may be needed.

43. (1) Infants and very young children are especially susceptible to development and hematogenous spread of tuberculosis, because of their lack of cellular immunity during the first three years of life.

44. (2) In some patients, 2–4 months of drug therapy may be required before the tubercle bacilli disappear from the sputum.

45. (3) Flushing sputum papers down the toilet is a safe means of disposal in areas where the sewage system is equipped to decontaminate bacterial waste. Burning is a secondary choice.

46. (1) Sputum tissues often contaminate the patient's hands with tubercle bacilli. He handles the sputum cup after handling the sputum papers, and thus the outside of the cup is frequently contaminated with tubercle bacilli.

47. (3) Inadequate dosage or omission of doses foster development of drug resistance because the lowered blood concentration of the drug favors survival of a few bacterial mutants, which resist the drug's effects and multiply rapidly during the period of lowered drug concentration.

48. (2) If Tim has difficulty in remembering to take his drugs on a regular daily basis, the nurse should advise him to record on a daily calendar each dose taken, and to post the calendar in a prominent place where he is sure to read it two or three times daily.

Chronic Glomerulonephritis and Hemodialysis

1. (2) Glomerulonephritis is an immunologic disorder that is due either to antibodies specifically directed against the basement membrane of the glomerulus, or to nonrenal antigen-antibody complexes that arise elsewhere in the body and are deposited in the glomerulus during filtration. In either case, the antibody or the antigen-antibody complex causes acute inflammation of the glomerulus.

2. (4) Headache occurs in glomerulonephritis as a result of hypertension, and is due to an increase in cerebrospinal fluid pressure. Inflammatory obstruction of glomeruli causes reduction in glomerular filtration rate with oliguria, sodium retention, increase of extracellular fluid, and edema. Periorbital edema is seen early in the disease as a result of the low-tissue turgor in the circumorbital region. If glomerular inflammation is severe, some capillaries are destroyed, and red blood cells pass into the tubular filtrate and appear in the urine. Flank pain is the result of widespread inflammation of glomeruli.

3. (3) Anemia may develop in acute glomerulonephritis owing to loss of red cells

into the urine from ruptured glomeruli or to marrow depression by nitrogenous metabolic wastes. Ischemia of renal tissues causes secretion of renin, and subsequently angiotensin, a potent vasoconstrictor. If the resulting hypertension is severe, cerebral vessels may rupture or the left ventricle may fail. Uremia is a clinical syndrome, not a complication, consisting of serious disturbances in electrolyte balance as a result of renal failure.

4. (4) Morning headaches are a manifestation of hypertension. Visual difficulties are due to retinal arteriolar degeneration, hemorrhages, and exudates that accompany hypertension. Nausea and vomiting are symptoms of uremia, and result from irritation of the vomiting center in the medulla by excess hydrogen ions. Easy fatigability is common in chronic renal failure since high levels of blood urea and creatinine depress the bone marrow, causing anemia, which results in decreased oxygen-carrying power of the blood and consequent interference with cellular oxidative reactions.

5. (3) Glomerular inflammation increases the permeability of the capillary membrane, with loss of albumin from the blood into the tubular filtrate. When albumin is lost in the urine and serum albumin concentration falls, fluid moves out of the capillaries into body tissues and, generalized massive edema results.

6. (2) By placing the patient on absolute bedrest his metabolic activities are minimized, there are fewer metabolic wastes to be disposed of, and the workload of the kidney is reduced.

7. (3) Methyldopa is a selective sympathetic nervous system inhibitor that lowers blood pressure by decreasing both renal vascular resistance and systemic vascular resistance. It is often used to treat hypertension secondary to renal disease.

8. (3) Methyldopa lowers blood pressure by decreasing vascular resistance through blocking the synthesis of dopamine and norepinephrine.

9. (3) The mental depression results from a decrease in brain concentrations of norepinephrine. The nasal stuffiness is a result of dilation and congestion of blood vessels in the nasal mucosa. The reduction of blood pressure upsets the baroreceptor reflexes in the aorta and internal carotid arteries, which normally compensate for the pooling of blood in the lower extremities on assuming the upright position. When these reflexes do not function properly, postural hypotension results. The salivary glands are stimulated by sympathetic and parasympathetic fibers. By decreasing tissue catecholamines, methyldopa eliminates part of the stimuli for saliva secretion, and dry mouth results.

10. (1) Aluminum hydroxide gel is a nonsystemic antacid, a substance that forms relatively insoluble compounds in the gastrointestinal tract that are not readily absorbed and exert no effect on the acid-base balance of the body.

11. (2) Aluminum hydroxide relieves nausea and vomiting, common symptoms of uremia, through its antacid, adsorbent, and demulcent effects.

12. (4) Aluminum hydroxide is constipating as a result of the astringent effect of the aluminum ion.

13. (4) Diazepam depresses the polysynaptic reflexes of the spinal cord and certain limbic structures, producing both a sedative and a muscle-relaxant effect.

14. (3) A portion of diazapam is excreted rapidly (half-life of 7–10 hours); another portion is excreted slowly (half-life of 2–8 days). Thus, cumulative effects can be observed after several days of drug use.

15. (3) Symptoms of CNS depression, such as drowsiness and lethargy, are common side effects of diazepam.

16. (4) Confusion and lethargy are the result of metabolic acidosis and disturbance of brain function by excess hydrogen ions. Muscular twitching results from decreased serum calcium, increased serum potassium, and metabolic acidosis. Foul breath odor is caused by bacterial breakdown of the urea present in saliva to ammonia. The high concentration of urea in the sweat causes urates to crystallize on the skin.

17. (4) Urea is a compound formed in the liver from ammonia that is derived from the deamination of amino acids. Uric acid is an end product of purine metabolism, and creatinine is a waste product of creatine, which is a constituent of muscle tissue.

18. (2) The blood urea nitrogen concentration is determined by the balance among protein intake, protein catabolism, urea production by the liver, and urea excretion by the kidney. The normal range is 10–20 mg./100 ml.

19. (1) Phosphocreatine is a compound providing high-energy phosphate storage in muscle tissue. When it breaks down, one of the end products is creatinine, which is excreted in the urine, both by glomerular filtration and active tubular excretion. The normal range is 1–1.5 mg./ml.

20. (1) Uric acid is a metabolic waste resulting from the catabolism of nucleoprotein. The normal range is 3–7 mg./100 ml., with lower values for females than for males.

21. (3) Potassium is the major intracellular cation, playing an important role in nerve conductivity and muscle contractility. It is released by disintegrating cells and is predominantly excreted in the urine. The normal range is 3.5–5.0 mEq/L.

22. (4) Since potassium is excreted by the kidney, potassium intoxication may result from acute or chronic renal failure. Elevated serum potassium concentration causes cardiac arrhythmias and eventual cardiac arrest.

23. (2) When a semipermeable membrane separates two solutions having different concentrations of dispersed molecules or ions, an osmotic gradient is established, and those substances to which the membrane is permeable tend to move from the solution where they are more concentrated to the solution where they are less concentrated.

24. (2) In renal failure, as a result of decreased glomerular filtration rate and failure of tubular secretion, fluid is retained, with accumulation of excess extra- and intracellular water; serum potassium level rises, and urea, creatinine, uric acid and ammonia accumulate in the serum. In peritoneal dialysis an isotonic or hypertonic fluid or dialysate is injected into the peritoneal cavity and left in place for 30–45 minutes, during which time excess water, urea, phosphate, waste products, and ions diffuse from the blood across the peritoneal membrane into the injected dialysate, which is then removed from the body.

25. (2) Removal of fluid and electrolytes from the blood lowers the blood pressure. If large amounts of fluid are removed rapidly during peritoneal dialysis, the patient becomes dangerously hypotensive so that the brain, myocardium, liver, and kidney are inadequately perfused. The patient's vital signs therefore should be taken before peritoneal dialysis is begun in order to have baseline data. The bladder should be emptied before the peritoneal catheter is introduced to minimize the danger of puncturing the bladder when the lower abdominal wall is incised prior to catheter insertion.

26. (4) If the dialysate is not warmed to body temperature before introduction into the peritoneal cavity, abdominal pain and chilling will develop during dialysis.

27. (3) Within 30–45 minutes the blood and dialysate will have achieved equilibrium in concentrations of the most important metabolic waste substances and ions to which the peritoneal membrane is permeable. The transfer of water across the membrane is more rapid.

28. (3) Drainage of dialysate fluid through the peritoneal catheter may be blocked by plugs of blood or fibrin. A small amount of heparin added to the dialysate will decrease clot formation in the catheter.

29. (2) Sometimes dialysate fails to drain from the peritoneal catheter because the catheter tip is lodged against soft abdominal viscera. The catheter can be repositioned by moving the patient from one side to the other, or by applying manual pressure to both sides of the abdomen.

30. (3) Peritonitis is the most common complication of peritoneal dialysis, and results from contamination of the catheter during insertion or during instillation and evacuation of fluid. The patient's temperature should be measured at four-hour intervals to identify any temperature elevation, which could signify peritoneal infection.

31. (3) Cardiac arrhythmias may develop owing to either potassium excess or deficiency. They also develop in the patient with decreased cardiac reserve in whom sodium and fluid retention precipitates congestive heart failure.

32. (3) It is possible during peritoneal dialysis to osmotically remove large quantities of fluid rapidly from the intravascular space, causing marked reduction in the blood volume. If the reduction in circulating blood volume is too great to be

compensated for by variations in heart action and vascular constriction, severe hypotension may result.

33. (4) Because the patient remains in supine or low Fowler's position with movement restricted and body weight increased for 12–48 hours, pressure injury to tissues of the back or heels is common. Elevation of the diaphragm by the dialysate solution interferes with respiratory movements, and basal alveoli are poorly aerated. Immobility and shallow breathing predispose to hypostatic pneumonia. Irritation or erosion of delicate abdominal tissues by the peritoneal catheter may cause bleeding into the peritoneal cavity. Deposition of fibrin on the serosa may cause bowel loops to become adherent to each other, interfering with peristalsis. Contamination of the peritoneal catheter as a result of poor aseptic technique in hanging or draining fluids predisposes to peritonitis.

34. (2) Pain is most often caused by instillation of dialysate that is too hot or too cold. Chemical or bacterial inflammation of the peritoneum produces severe abdominal pain, which may be generalized or localized. Incomplete removal of dialysate causes overdistention of the abdomen as subsequent volumes of dialysate are instilled, and can cause stretching of the parietal peritoneum, and resultant pain.

34. (4) The nurse should record the exact amounts of fluid instilled and removed in order to determine the net gain or loss of fluid from the abdomen (and the blood) during each cycle. The time of each cycle's beginning and ending should be recorded, because it may be desirable to compare the net fluid gain or loss with the amount of fluid insertion time for the cycle. The exact composition of each bottle of dialysate should be noted because the hyper- or hypotonicity of the dialysate in regard to certain constituents may have to be changed during the treatment to modify the speed of fluid or electrolyte removal. Vital symptoms must be recorded at intervals to detect cardiac arrhythmias, dyspnea, and severe hypotension, all of which would require immediate intervention. Weight and blood pressure must be checked before and after dialysis to determine the efficacy of dialysis in decreasing blood pressure and eliminating edema.

36. (4) Patients in renal failure have increased susceptibility to infection due to decreased formation of granulocytes as a result of marrow depression by toxic metabolites. Both peritonitis and shunt-fistula infections are common complications of peritoneal dialysis. Both can be minimized by preventing staff with upper respiratory infections from working in the dialysis unit.

37. (4) As a result of renal failure, Mr. Proxmire suffers metabolic acidosis, which produces disturbed thinking and impaired consciousness. All the listed answers should be considered.

38. (1) There are many more candidates for hemodialysis than there are treatment facilities, and in most centers a committee reviews all applicants and approves for treatment those whose physical condition and psychologic status indicate that they should profit maximally from hemodialysis.

39. (2) To institute hemodialysis, access to the blood stream can be obtained through an external shunt consisting of cannulas inserted into a large vein and a large artery that lie close to each other. When the patient is not being dialyzed the two cannulas can be attached to each other, so that blood can flow continuously through the shunt to maintain its patency.

40. (3) Since hemodialysis facilities are few in number, one means of making the treatment available to more patients is to enable them to dialyze themselves at home. To do this the patient must have both hands free to operate the dialysis equipment, and thus the leg rather than the arm should be cannulated.

41. (3) If the arterial and venous cannulas should become disconnected at the Teflon joint between the two, considerable blood loss would result, and it would be awkward or impossible for the patient to reconnect the cannulas. He therefore should have two cannula clamps attached to his person so that he can promptly occlude the two limbs of the shunt to prevent undue blood loss.

42. (2) With an arteriovenous fistula, a surgically anastomosed artery and vein, there is no exterior shunt to be traumatized, entangled, or accidentally disconnected, so the danger of hemorrhage is lessened.

43. (1) Because the two limbs of the external shunt can be accidentally disconnected, hemorrhage is an ever-present danger. The skin exit sites of the cannulas are possible areas for infection if aseptic technique is not used in handling the shunt.

44. (2) The dialysate contains higher concentration of glucose than the blood in order to withdraw excess water from the blood, thereby reducing blood volume and blood pressure. It contains a lower concentration of urea than the blood in order to draw urea from the blood and relieve nervous system symptoms of uremia. It contains a lower concentration of phosphate than the blood to draw phosphate from the blood.

45. (2) As a result of tubular damage the patient in renal failure is unable to excrete potassium, so serum potassium levels exceed normal. Renal failure leads to metabolic acidosis, and higher-than-normal amounts of bicarbonate are used to buffer organic acids and are then excreted in the urine.

46. (1) An anticoagulant must be added to the patient's blood as it enters the dialyzing machine to prevent clots from forming and obstructing blood flow through the coils of the machine.

47. (4) Protamine, a powerful heparin antagonist, is strongly basic, and neutralizes the strongly acidic heparin.

48. (1) In order to prevent infection, the skin exit sites around both cannulas should be cleansed daily with an antiseptic solution; rinsed with sterile normal saline; and covered with an antiseptic ointment and a sterile dressing.

49. (2) Because of the danger of massive blood loss with accidental disconnection of the shunt, no substance should be used to cleanse the skin or the shunt that would lubricate the tubing and cause it to slip loose from the connector.

50. (2) The patient should be taught to flex and extend the wrist, elbow, and shoulder of the cannulized arm at regular intervals throughout the day, to foster blood flow through the shunt and prevent clotting.

51. (3) Heparin is added to the saline used to "wash" the clots from the cannulas in order to prevent further clotting of the tubing, which is apt to occur so long as blood is not moving freely through the shunt.

52. (4) The patient in renal failure has difficulty excreting urea, creatinine, and uric acid, the waste products of protein metabolism, so protein intake is decreased to reduce the amount of nitrogenous waste that can accumulate in body tissues.

53. (3) With a decrease in glomerular filtration rate the patient is unable to excrete sodium normally, and in hypertensive persons edema and complications may result. The kidney is also unable to excrete potassium, so that serum potassium levels increase, and there may be neuromuscular irritability and cardiac arrest.

54. (2) The diet should provide a liberal carbohydrate allowance and adequate fat to provide sufficient caloric intake to prevent catabolism of body tissues as a source of energy. Excessive protein breakdown would increase the amount of nitrogenous wastes to be excreted by the kidney.

55. (1) One cup of cooked lima beans contains 12 grams of protein; 1 tablespoon of peanut butter, 3 grams; 1 boiled egg, 6 grams; 1 cup of whole milk, 9 grams.

56. (3) One cup of cooked red beans contains 16 grams of protein; ½ cup of creamed cottage cheese, 16 grams; 2 slices of whole wheat bread, 4 grams; 3 oz. of fried perch, 16 grams.

57. (1) For the patient dialyzed three times a week, the usual amount of weight gain between subsequent dialyses is 1–2 kg. A patient who does not adhere to prescribed dietary and fluid prescriptions retains much more fluid, and his weight gain may be two or three times the usual amount.

58. (2) Because nitrogenous metabolic wastes depress blood cell formation in the bone marrow, patients with renal failure develop a normochromic anemia. To relieve symptoms of anemia, packed red cells rather than whole blood is administered to avoid overloading the left ventricle and precipitating congestive heart failure.

59. (2) Although the patient in renal failure tends to feel optimistic when hemodialysis is begun, the gradual realization of his utter dependence on the machine frequently provokes severe depression. Concern about finances, unavailability

of donors, and the possibility of hemorrhage from accidental dislodging of the shunt cause severe anxiety in some individuals. When this is prolonged or overwhelmingly painful, they may deny the nature or consequences of their illness and neglect to follow the prescribed treatment.

60. (1) The patient in renal failure who must be dialyzed thrice weekly and who is prevented from enjoying his usual life style is forced to accept an unusual degree of dependency.

61. (4) The process of grieving is a reaction to loss. That which is lost may be the company of relatives and friends; a familiar way of life; a chosen occupation; a favorite hobby; a respected social status; a sense of financial or occupational security; or physical strength and mobility. Studies have shown that the process of grieving consists of several phases: shock, denial, despair, detachment, and resolution.

62. (4) Anxiety concerning the cannulas would be the most stressful, because of the importance of cannula functioning to treatment success and symptom relief.

63. (1) Because dietary habits are developed during the formative years and reinforced by strong psychologic and cultural stimuli, they are especially difficult to alter during periods of psychologic and physical stress.

64. (3) Denial is a defense mechanism by which an individual represses consciously intolerable thoughts, events, or situations. It can be useful on a temporary basis, enabling the individual to function effectively in an otherwise intolerable situation. Problems can develop when denial persists and prevents the patient from effective handling of problem situations.

65. (1) Projection is a defense mechanism that consists of attributing to others those undesirable traits, attitudes, motives, and desires that one wishes to disavow.

66. (3) Since the mental mechanisms are psychologic techniques by which the personality attempts to reduce tensions and compromise between conflicting impulses, the nurse should not strip the patient of a defense but should attempt to understand the need for its use. If the mechanism is harmful to the patient, the nurse may be able to support him so that he can satisfy his needs without reliance upon this defense.

67. (2) The tissue rejection reaction is less severe when a kidney is transplanted from a mother, father, or sibling than when the donor is unrelated, and so relatives are apt to be chosen. Walter may feel a loss of status when his wife replaces him as the family breadwinner, and she may feel that she is abandoning her children by taking a job outside the home. Walter's dietary prescription will require that foods be prepared especially for him. His decreased strength will limit his involvement in sports and family projects. His dependence on the dialysis machine will limit the family's vacation trips. Expenses incurred in his treatment will decrease the family funds available for other projects.

68. (2) Only this response acknowledges Mrs. Proxmire's bid for personal understanding and support, enumerating major issues concerning which she may wish to unburden herself further.

69. (4) The patient who cannot reconcile himself to the prospect of chronic illness may deliberately destroy himself by flouting the physician's orders to restrict protein, sodium, potassium, or fluid.

70. (4) A common method of suicide consists of disconnecting the external arteriovenous shunt and bleeding to death.

71. (4) The cost of a hospital-based dialysis treatment program is about $15,000 to $20,000 per year. Few families, especially those with parents in their twenties and thirties, have sufficient savings to be able to afford this. Since chronic renal failure is irreversible, Mr. Proxmire will have to be dialyzed for the rest of his life if a suitable kidney is not located for transplantation. Even if he returns to work, the lethargy, fatigue, and malaise that result from his metabolic imbalances, anemia, and cardiorespiratory inefficiency will render him less hard-working and conscientious than he would otherwise have been, and thus jeopardizing his job security.

72. (3) Group therapy, through sharing, has enabled dialysis patients and their spouses to adjust to the problems provoked by chronic renal disease. Effective health teaching for Mr. and Mrs. Proxmire may enable them to dialyze Walter

at home, which would result in a considerable financial saving. The Kidney Foundation makes funds available to eligible individuals for the purchase of needed equipment and supplies. Individualizing care should include instruction and counseling for his two children, who should be informed about and involved in their father's treatment without being overburdened or deprived of normal childhood pursuits.

Ulcerative Colitis and Ileostomy

1. (2) Anticolon antibodies have been isolated in some patients with ulcerative colitis. Many experience a relief of symptoms when milk is removed from the diet. Patients tend to be immature, hypersensitive, perfectionistic, and dependent. Often an episode of emotional stress precipitates the onset of colitis symptoms.

2. (4) The colitis patient is: often obsessive-compulsive, in that he controls anxiety through ritually repetitive action; usually hypersensitive and easily wounded by casual slights and minor criticism; often hostile and argumentative in his dealings with others, complaining freely about various aspects of his care; apt to be overly dependent on parents or parent surrogates, and liable to be devastated by loss of these by death, rejection, or abandonment.

3. (1) Most colitis patients are ambivalent about their needs for dependency. They desire the protective care of a maternal figure, but also tend to be guarded in their acceptance of solicitude and sympathy from others because they have been conditioned to expect rejection from those upon whom they become dependent.

4. (1) The colitis patient is malnourished and cachectic as a result of severe anorexia and problems of intestinal absorption. In order to correct nutritional lacks, he is usually allowed to eat whatever he chooses. In order to minimize diarrhea, the patient should not be served foods that caused flatulence or fecal urgency in the past.

5. (2) Frequently an episode of emotional stress precedes the onset of colitis symptoms by 3–4 weeks. The precipitating stress may be due to many factors, e.g., separation from a loved relative, loss of a body part, failure at school or work, or extreme disillusionment of some sort.

6. (4) In colitis there are microabscesses in the crypts of the colon. Bacterial protein from these abscesses is absorbed into the blood and carried to the brain to reset the temperature regulating center in the hypothalamus for a higher-than-normal temperature. Abdominal cramping occurs because of a marked increase in large-amplitude peristaltic waves. The increase in propulsive motility of the bowel and inability of the diseased colonic mucosa to absorb water from the feces results in passage of 15–20 watery stools per day. The increased fluid loss resulting from diarrhea produces increased thirst. The loss of sodium from the bowel and generalized toxicity from absorbed bacterial waste products results in anorexia.

7. (1) The colonic mucosa is friable and bleeds easily. Chronic blood loss produces hypochromic anemia because depletion of the body's iron stores results in formation of smaller-than-normal red blood cells with less-than-normal concentration of hemoglobin.

8. (3) Ulcerative colitis is a chronic recurrent illness. Cycles of inflammation, abscess formation, and healing cause spasm of the muscularis mucosa and fibrous tissue scarring, which results in loss of colon pouches, narrowing of the bowel lumen, and shortening of the gut.

9. (4) Diagnosis of ulcerative colitis requires that the physician rule out amebic colitis since its causative agent also causes severe diarrhea and ulcerations of the colon.

10. (1) Stool specimens that are to be examined for protozoa, ameba, and worms must be kept warm and delivered to the laboratory immediately, in order that the motility of the parasites can be observed under the microscope.

11. (2) Acute inflammation of the mucosa and submucosa causes an outpouring of mucus from the remaining intestinal glands. The hyperemia and friability of

the colonic mucosa causes bleeding from the surface following even minimal trauma. Microabscesses in the crypts of the colon cause exudation of pus into the bowel lumen and excretion of pus in the stool.

12. (3) Both sodium and potassium are lost in large quantities in diarrheal stools. Because aldosterone conserves sodium at the expense of potassium, serum potassium levels are more apt to decline than serum sodium levels.

13. (2) Increased dietary protein intake is needed to replace the protein lost from the bowel surface, and to provide protein for repair of mucosal and submucosal ulcerations.

14. (3) One cup of whole milk contains 9 grams of protein; 1 egg, 6 grams; ½ cup of cottage cheese, 16–19 grams; ½ cup of cooked green beans, 1 gram.

15. (3) One slice of enriched whole wheat bread contains 55 calories; ½ cup of creamed corn, 85; ½ cup of creamed cottate cheese, 120; 1 egg, 80.

16. (3) In a low residue diet the following foods are to be avoided: vegetables, fruit (except juices), coarse cereals, fried or fatty foods, tough meats, milk, and cheese.

17. (3) Fruits, vegetables, and milk are major sources of vitamins and minerals. All three are eliminated from a low residue diet, and so if the diet is to be used for more than a few days, supplemental iron, calcium, and vitamins should be administered.

18. (1) Phenobarbital is a long-acting barbiturate used as a sedative for patients with high anxiety levels.

19. (1) Bismuth subcarbonate is a demulcent that has a soothing effect upon irritated intestinal mucosa, coating the tissue and protecting the cells from irritation by noxious substances. Since diarrhea is caused by increased peristalsis stimulated by mucosal irritation, a demulcent lessens diarrhea by decreasing mucosal irritation. Bismuth subcarbonate also has an astringent effect in that it precipitates protein. When applied to an abraded or ulcerated area it coagulates the surface tissue, preventing further loss of tissue fluid.

20. (2) Bismuth subcarbonate protects the bowel from irritation in part by its ability to adsorb noxious substances and carry them out of the intestine in the stool. Unfortunately, vitamins are adsorbed also, making them unavailable for absorption and creating vitamin deficiencies.

21. (4) Iron-dextran is a complex of ferric hydroxide and dextran in normal saline solution. It is dark brown in color, absorbed slowly from tissue, and may stain the skin brown for 1–2 years. To prevent leakage of the medicine from the muscle into the subcutaneous tissue, a "Z-track" technique is used whereby the skin overlying the intramuscular injection site is pulled slightly to one side before the needle is inserted into the tissues and the injection is given. Following a brief pause to allow for dispersal of the medication, the needle is removed and the stretched skin is allowed to return to its normal position, thereby sealing the needle path between the muscle and skin.

22. (3) Atropine is a parasympathetic nervous system depressant that acts by inactivating acetylcholine, the mediator of nerve impulses across the myoneural junction; it thus depresses glandular secretions, decreases muscle tone and motility of the gut, increases the heart rate, and dilates the pupil.

23. (1) Increase in propulsive motility of the bowel is partially responsible for diarrhea. Atropine is used to decrease intestinal motility and relieve diarrhea.

24. (3) Atropine decreases secretion of saliva, producing dryness of the mouth; dilates cutaneous blood vessels in the blush area; blocks the vagal effect on the SA node, so that heart rate increases; and depresses the respiratory center in the medulla, producing shallow respirations.

25. (1) Neostigmine is a cholinergic drug that can be used as an antidote to atropine. It antagonizes atropine's peripheral effects.

26. (3) Since salicylazosulfapyradine has an affinity for connective tissue, it is used to prevent secondary infection of the raw, ulcerated bowel lining and to lessen friability, bleeding, and irritability of the rectosigmoid mucosa.

27. (3) Salicylazosulfapyridine breaks down in the intestinal tract to acetylsalicylic acid and sulfapyridine, which tend to become concentrated in intestinal tissues rather than be absorbed and widely circulated throughout the body. Sulfadiazine is rapidly and readily absorbed from the intestinal tract and widely distributed to all body tissues and fluids.

28. (1) If the urine is alkaline in reaction, salicylazosulfapyridine produces an orange-yellow discoloration of the urine. It effects no color change in acid urine.

29. (2) All the sulfonamides are potentially toxic drugs, having an effect on every organ system and tissue. Sulfonamides produce hemolysis by causing a deficiency in the erythrocytes of glucose 6-phosphate dehydrogenase (an enzyme needed for the cells' glycolysis reaction). The sulfonamides may cause agranulocytosis by depression of bone marrow activity.

30. (4) If the inflammatory process and ulceration penetrates through the muscularis and serosa as well as the mucosa and submucosa, intestinal contents will leak into the peritoneal cavity, producing a chemical and bacterial inflammation of the peritoneum. The parietal peritoneum is well supplied with sensory nerves, so irritation produces sharp pain. Granulocytes that have phagocytosed bacteria elaborate a substance called "endogenous pyrogen" that, when carried by the blood to the brain, resets the temperature regulating center for a higher-than-normal temperature. Increased tissue oxygen demand created by hyperpyrexia and hypermetabolism produces a reflex tachycardia. Severe peritoneal inflammation halts peristalsis, creating an intestinal obstruction, with diminished absorption of gas and fluid from the bowel, distention of the intestine, reflex rigidity of abdominal muscles, and reverse peristalsis.

31. (1) Ice-cold liquids stimulate an increase in propulsive peristalsis of the small bowel, which would increase diarrhea in the colitis patient.

32. (4) As a result of fluid, sodium, potassium, and chloride losses in diarrheal stools, colitis patients develop electrolyte imbalance. In about 5 per cent of patients the inflammatory process is fulminant, and ulcerations erode into a blood vessel to produce massive hemorrhage. Many patients suffer a migratory arthritis, the severity of which parallels the severity of intestinal symptoms. Severe diarrhea may so irritate friable anal mucosa as to produce anal fissures and fistulas. Ulcerative colitis predisposes to cancer of the colon, the risk increasing with the duration of colitis and with the amount of the colon damaged by the ulcerative process.

33. (4) Malnutrition, weight loss, weakness, and fecal incontinence predispose to formation of decubitus ulcers over bony prominences. To prevent decubiti the patient should be placed on an alternating air pressure mattress and given scrupulous skin care.

34. (4) If the patient's strength permits, a tub bath is preferred to a bed bath because the moist heat of a sitz bath relieves the rectal pain and spasm caused by frequent diarrheal stools, and promotes healing of rectal fissures.

35. (2) The colitis patient is fastidious, hypersensitive, and ashamed of the soiling and foul odors that result from intractable diarrhea. The patient considers himself unclean and fears rejection by others as a result of the unpleasant manifestations of his illness. The prevalence of fecal odors in his environment is one factor that contributes to his anorexia.

36. (3) Mrs. Cavers' excessive dependence and obsessive-compulsive behavior are coping mechanisms by which her personality reduces intrapsychic tension and manages stress. By recognizing the adaptive value of these behaviors, the nurse will be more able to accept the patient's clinging, ritualism, and irritability without criticism or retaliation, and will be more willing to provide the emotional support needed to instill hope and mobilize Mrs. Cavers' desire for recovery.

37. (3) The patient who is thin, weak, and diarrhetic is particularly susceptible to decubitus formation. An air mattress or piece of sponge rubber or sheepskin under the buttocks relieve pressure on bony prominences. Frequent bathing with mild soap and back massage with a lubricating ointment lessen skin irritation and breakdown.

38. (4) In severe colitis, fecal urgency may be so severe that the patient cannot wait for someone to bring him a bedpan or help him to the bathroom. If allowed to keep a bedpan at the bedside he can avoid incontinence, soiling, and skin excoriation. Following each defecation the perianal skin should be gently cleansed with soap and water or medicated disposable cleansing pads to remove bacteria-laden pus and prevent further infection. A thin layer of petrolatum over the perianal skin will reduce irritation of the tissues by repeated stools. Wear-

ing a perineal pad reduces the patient's fear of soiling, and so relieves painful rectal muscle spasm provoked by nervousness and anxiety.

39. (3) Most colitis patients suffer severe anorexia as a result of malaise, depression, and fear of precipitating diarrheal episodes by eating. In order to remedy long-standing nutritional lacks the patient should be encouraged to eat whatever he likes so long as it does not aggravate his symptoms. Home-cooked meals may be better received than hospital-prepared foods simply because they are more familiar.

40. (4) Mrs. Cavers must realize that the ileostomy will be permanent, that the drainage from the ileostomy will be semiliquid, and that she must wear a drainage bag continuously in order to give informed consent for total colectomy and ileostomy. She will be more optimistic about her future if she can talk with a well-adjusted ileostomy patient whose life circumstances parallel her own. She will be more highly motivated to cooperate with the rehabilitation program if the nurse describes in detail the postoperative care and support and demonstrates the supplies that will be used to manage ileostomy drainage.

41. (4) For several days before the colectomy and ileostomy operation the patient is placed on a no-residue diet to decrease the danger of peritoneal contamination during surgery. Intravenous fluids are given to relieve the dehydration and electrolyte imbalances produced by prolonged diarrhea. Transfusions are given to correct the hypochromic anemia caused by chronic intestinal bleeding. Antibiotics that are poorly absorbed from the intestinal tract, such as neomycin, are administered to decrease intestinal bacteria and minimize postoperative infections. Because intestinal manipulation during surgery depresses peristalsis for several days following surgery, a nasogastric tube is inserted to keep the bowel empty until peristalsis resumes.

42. (2) Since the small bowel contents are liquid, the ileostomy will drain almost continuously. Since the drainage from the ileum contains a number of digestive enzymes that can excoriate and erode the skin, it must be continuously collected in a drainage bag.

43. (3) Neomycin is a broad-spectrum antibiotic that is not inactivated by gastrointestinal secretions and is poorly absorbed from the GI tract. It is given orally as a preoperative intestinal antiseptic to lower the concentration of intestinal organisms and thus prevent postoperative infection of the suture lines, all of which are subject to fecal contamination.

44. (3) Before the patient leaves the operating room, a temporary plastic drainage bag is placed over the ileostomy stoma and fastened to the surrounding skin in order to prevent fecal contamination of the abdominal incision before the peritoneal cavity is sealed off by the process of epithelialization.

45. (2) Healing by first intention takes approximately six weeks under usual circumstances.

46. (2) Infection and ulceration of the skin surrounding the stoma would interfere with attachment of the ileostomy drainage bag, leading to further skin excoriation and infection, and possible systemic sepsis.

47. (3) The ileostomy bag should be changed several hours after a meal, when peristalsis is slow, so as to minimize leakage of semiliquid fecal drainage onto the skin surrounding the stoma.

48. (3) Sterile fluff gauze is fitted closely around the stoma to protect the abdominal incision from contamination by fecal drainage. After the ileostomy bag is changed, the incision should be cleansed and the sterile fluff gauze reapplied. Newspapers should be used to protect the bed linen from soiling and to wrap the soiled bag before disposal in a covered waste container, in order to reduce odor in the area. Bandage scissors are needed to cut a hole of the desired size in the double-faced adhesive backing of the ileostomy bag, in order to fit the bag to the exact dimensions of the ileostomy stoma. The lower end of the bag is folded in upon itself and sealed with rubber bands in order to provide a water-tight seal for drainage collection.

49. (4) Karaya gum is a dried, gummy exudate that protects the skin from excoriation by irritating substances while permitting healing of underlying tissues. Because it is sticky it can be used to adhere the ileostomy bag to the abdominal skin. Karaya gum becomes gelatinous on contact with liquid, so it will form a

water-tight seal between the drainage bag and the skin surrounding the stoma.

50. (4) A successfully adjusted ileostomate would be an effective role model for a patient with a fresh ileostomy because the two share a common frame of reference. Mrs. Cavers fears rejection from significant others as a result of changes in body image and odors associated with fecal drainage. A patient having suffered mutilating surgery develops self-esteem in direct proportion to the esteem accorded her by professional caregivers. Anxiety restricts the individual's perceptual field and interferes with learning. Measures that decrease anxiety, increase self-esteem, and decrease distraction will facilitate learning.

51. (2) Through active listening and well-timed restatement of key themes, a skilled nurse can assist a troubled patient to ventilate her feelings about a problem, and thus reduce anxiety and mobilize inner resources for more effective problem-solving.

52. (1) Fecal drainage contains protein, which is coagulated by heat. Cold water should be used to wash the ileostomy bag so as not to coagulate the protein in the drainage material and cause it to adhere to the surface of the bag. Mild soap should be used so as not to denature the plastic or rubber of which the bag is constructed.

53. (3) The bag should be dusted with talcum in order to absorb any moisture remaining on the surface of the pouch, and to prevent adherence of the pouch to itself or to the box in which it is stored.

Bladder Carcinoma and Ureterosigmoidostomy

1. (2) The normal capacity of the bladder is 300–400 cc. (ml.). When about 300 ml. of urine has accumulated, stretch receptors in the bladder wall are stimulated, afferent impulses are sent to the central nervous system, and a desire is generated to empty the bladder.

2. (4) Ideally, there should be no residual urine left in the bladder following micturition. However, even a normal bladder, if overdistended for a time, shows a small, transient, residual urine of 1 oz. or so, but this disappears after a short period. When 60 cc. (ml.) or more remains in the bladder following voiding, early bladder decompensation must be suspected, and it must be recognized that an environment has been created that predisposes to urinary tract infection.

3. (2) Carcinoma or contracture of the bladder neck produces obstruction to the flow of urine from the bladder. Initially, the bladder muscle undergoes compensatory hypertrophy to contract more forcefully and overcome the increased resistance to emptying. As the tumor encroaches more and more on the urethral lumen, the bladder's compensatory ability is eventually exceeded, and the detrusor muscle becomes atonic and incapable of contracting forcibly enough to empty the bladder. Thus, residual urine is left in the bladder at the end of each voiding.

4. (3) Stagnation of urine in any portion of the urinary tract predisposes to urinary infection.

5. (3) The radiopaque dye that is injected intravenously to outline the renal pelvis, ureters, and bladder is an iodine-containing dye capable of producing anaphylactoid shock in iodine-sensitive individuals.

6. (2) Preparation of a patient for intravenous pyelography includes cleansing the large bowel of fecal material so that bowel contents do not interfere with x-ray visualization of the kidney, and withholding fluid for eight hours to produce slight dehydration, and thus to concentrate dye in the urine.

7. (4) Immediately following intravenous injection of an iodine-containing dye many patients experience flushing of the face and a sensation of warmth, which are caused by a brief, intense vasodilation and usually abate within a few minutes.

8. (4) Toxic response to an iodine-containing intravenous dye produces a classic

anaphylactoid or severe allergic reaction, characterized by sudden vascular collapse; severe hypotension; intractable bronchospasm; laryngeal edema; giant urticaria; severe pruritus of face, hands, and feet; incontinence; and unconsciousness.

9. (4) A signed operative permit must be obtained for any major diagnostic procedures that involve entering a body cavity. A thorough explanation of the cystoscopy procedure and equipment should be given beforehand in order to facilitate the patient's cooperation and relaxation during instrumentation, as the primary cause of pain during cystoscopy is spasm of the bladder sphincter. Food is withheld before the procedure because discomfort during instrumentation causes some patients to become nauseated. Fluids are pushed for several hours prior to cystoscopy to ensure that sufficient urine will be excreted from each ureter to provide needed specimens, and to wash out of the bladder any bacteria introduced during instrumentation.

10. (1) Only this explanation is thoroughly honest and provides enough information for the patient to understand the purpose and general method of the procedure. Most patients are awake during cystoscopy, having been given a sedative and analgesic in preparation for the procedure, which is considerably more painful than a pelvic examination.

11. (3) The popliteal artery, which is an extension of the femoral artery, lies in the popliteal space behind the knee joint. Prolonged pressure on this vessel by the metal knee rest of the stirrups predisposes to intravascular thrombus formation. The peroneal nerve lies below the head of the fibula on the lateral side of the leg. Continuous pressure on this nerve by the knee rest could produce paralysis, with loss of ability to dorsiflex the foot or extend the toes.

12. (2) Muscular contraction and relaxation exert a pumping action on the blood within the arteries and veins that lie between opposing muscle bellies.

13. (4) The cystoscope, a flexible metal tube consisting of a telescope and a light source, permits observation of the interior of the bladder under magnification. Thus, the bladder mucosa, ureteral orifices, and bladder neck tumor can be inspected. The condition of bladder muscle can be inferred by looking for trabeculations, which indicate muscle compensation, and diverticula, which indicate decompensation. An inflow/outflow valve on the cystoscope permits distention of the bladder in order to observe evenness of bladder expansion with increased volumes of fluid.

14. (3) As bladder muscle hypertrophies to compensate for increased workload, there is separation of hypertrophied muscle bundles, with evagination of bladder mucosa between the bundles.

15. (2) The bladder muscle hypertrophies in response to increased resistance to urine flow from the bladder.

16. (1) Mechanical trauma from passage of the cystoscope produce inflammation of urethral and bladder mucosa, which may trigger spasms of the detrusor muscle or bladder sphincter.

17. (2) Frank, bloody urine with clots may indicate laceration of the bladder or urethral wall by the cystoscope. If the injury is severe, surgical intervention may be necessary to halt the bleeding. Shaking chills and fever may indicate that bacteria from a previously existing cystitis have entered the blood stream as a result of trauma during instrumentation, creating a bacteremia that should be treated with antibiotics. Complete inability to void may indicate that edema of the bladder neck or urethra is so severe as to cause complete urinary retention.

18. (4) Obstruction of the bladder neck causes retention of urine in the bladder. Stagnant urine tends to become secondarily infected, producing inflammation of the bladder lining. As accumulation of urine distends the bladder, increased pressure is referred backward through the system, and the ureter and kidney pelvis become filled with urine. Pressure of the urine-filled pelvis interferes with the blood supply to renal parenchyma, destroying tubules and glomeruli and producing renal failure, so that nitrogenous wastes accumulate in body fluids. Stasis and infection of urine causes certain salts to precipitate out of solution, forming renal stones.

19. (2) *E. coli, P. aeruginosa,* and *P. vulgaris* are all normal inhabitants of the bowel

and frequent contaminants of the urinary tract through ascending tract infections.

20. (2) Giving Mrs. Pine a liquid diet before surgery ensures that the lower bowel will be empty of fecal material when the ureterosigmoidostomy is performed, thereby preventing fecal contamination of the peritoneum and postoperative suture lines.

21. (1) Neomycin and phthalylsulfathiazole are both effective against gram-positive and gram-negative organisms, and are poorly absorbed from the gastrointestinal system. Both are used to decrease the bacterial count in the large bowel before and after intestinal surgery. Magnesium sulfate is a cathartic of moderate strength that is relatively nonirritating to intestinal mucosa.

22. (2) Magnesium sulfate is a saline cathartic or soluble salt that is poorly absorbed from the intestine. It exerts an osmotic effect, preventing water absorption from the intestine, maintaining fluidity of the intestinal content, increasing intestinal bulk, and stimulating defecation.

23. (4) Neomycin inhibits growth and multiplication of many gram-negative and gram-positive organisms. Gastrointestinal secretions do not inactivate the drug. Since it is poorly absorbed from the GI tract, it is given orally to "sterilize" the intestine prior to bowel surgery.

24. (2) Neomycin-resistant organisms may overgrow when other organisms that are sensitive to neomycin are destroyed. As a result, "superinfections" by resistant organisms may occur and cause diarrhea.

25. (2) Phthalylsulfathiazole, a sulfonamide that is poorly absorbed from the bowel, is used to decrease intestinal flora prior to bowel surgery. Within 3–5 days of drug use the feces are soft and odor-free, and the coliform bacterial count is greatly reduced.

26. (2) Drug toxicity, or systemic symptoms of tissue injury by a drug, requires that the drug be absorbed from the bowel and distributed by the blood to sensitive tissues. Since phthalylsulfathiazole is poorly absorbed from the gut, it rarely causes toxic symptoms.

27. (2) Major behavioral changes are easier to effect when the individual has had opportunity to mentally rehearse them under protected circumstances before the actual changes must be accomplished.

28. (4) Carcinoma of the bladder neck, which causes bladder neck obstruction, is slow to metastasize, but eventually spreads to pelvic and periaortic lymph nodes, liver, spine, and pelvis.

29. (1) In ureterosigmoidostomy, the ureters are attached to the sigmoid colon and the lower colon becomes a reservoir for urine as well as stool. Renal infections frequently follow the procedure because peristalsis increases the pressure in the rectum, causing urine contaminated with coliform organisms to reflux into the ureters and produce an ascending urinary tract infection. Waste products in the urine tend to be absorbed through the intestinal mucosa and to cause systemic electrolyte imbalances.

30. (3) Postoperatively a rectal tube is inserted and left in place for several days to drain urine from the lower bowel, so as to prevent distention of the sigmoid colon and strain on the suture lines. The tube is secured in position with adhesive tape to prevent its accidental removal, since the anastomosis could be damaged by reinsertion of the tube.

31. (2) The rectal tube is connected by a sterile tube to a drainage receptacle. Obstruction of the rectal tube with mucus or feces would cause distention of the bowel with urine, placing strain on the anastomosis and causing urine to reflux into the newly sutured ureters.

32. (1) Pentazocine is a synthetic non-narcotic analgesic that displays sedative, hypnotic, and respiratory depressant effects. It is about one fourth as potent as morphine in causing analgesia, and about one half as potent as morphine in producing respiratory depression. The drug is effective in relieving moderate pain such as that associated with labor and surgical and urologic procedures. Meperidine is a synthetic drug with analgesic, sedative, and euphoric effects similar to those of morphine. Like morphine, it acts principally by altering the individual's affective reaction to pain.

33. (1) Patients with a previous history of drug abuse may develop psychologic or

physical dependence on pentazocine. However, the drug causes little or no euphoria, and even its misuse does not interfere with the patient's normal routines or induce abnormal behavior (unless it is combined with other drugs).

34. (3) One of the toxic effects of pentazocine is respiratory depression, which the narcotic antagonists are ineffective in relieving. Methylphenidate hydrochloride, a CNS stimulate, relieves respiratory depression caused by pentazocine.

35. (2) Macrodantin is a urinary antiseptic that is bacteriostatic or bactericidal against a variety of gram-positive and gram-negative organisms. Bacteria that are sensitive to the drug develop limited resistance to it. Macrodantin is used to treat severe urinary tract infections that have been unresponsive to other drugs.

36. (1) Nitrofurantoin has a low level of toxicity, but may cause irritation of the GI tract. Macrodantin is a macrocrystalline form of nitrofurantoin that is less upsetting to gastrointestinal functioning because of its delayed absorption.

37. (2) Sodium bicarbonate is a systemic antacid that is readily absorbed from the GI tract. Many of the waste products excreted in the urine are acidic, so sodium bicarbonate is given to neutralize excess hydrogen ions, and prevent acidosis from absorption of waste products from urine in the sigmoid colon.

38. (1) Pelvic surgery predisposes to postoperative venous thrombosis in the lower extremities. Patients with malignancy are also susceptible to venous thrombosis. Elastic stockings compress superficial veins, thereby increasing blood flow through deep veins and preventing blood stagnation, one factor that contributes to intravenous clotting.

39. (2) During the immediate postoperative period, while the rectal tube is in place, the perianal skin should be covered with petrolatum to minimize skin irritation by the tube.

40. (2) After removal of the rectal tube, the rectal sphincters will control elimination of urine as well as of stool. Since the sphincters must contract more forcefully to retain fluid than to retain solid waste, the patient should increase sphincter strength by alternately contracting and relaxing the muscle.

41. (3) Coping skills that are developed in solving problems in one sphere of life can often be applied to the resolution of difficulties in another sphere.

42. (1) The sigmoid colon should be emptied of urine every 2–4 hours to prevent absorption of urinary waste products from the bowel. In order to ensure uninterrupted sleep, the patient should insert a rectal tube at night and connect it to a drainage bottle at the side of the bed.

43. (4) Mrs. Pine must empty the bowel of urine every 3–4 hours to prevent development of hyperchloremic acidosis. She should avoid harsh laxatives and foods causing diarrhea, as increased peristalsis will increase rectal pressure and cause reflux of contaminated urine into the ureter, which gives rise to ascending infection. The rectal drainage equipment should be washed after each use to control odor and to prevent the culturing of bacteria on the fecally contaminated tube and container, since the cultured organisms would be reintroduced into the sigmoid in even greater numbers at each bedtime. The perineum should be washed daily to prevent irritation and infection.

44. (4) An enema would greatly increase the pressure in the rectum and would force liquid bowel contents into the ureters.

45. (2) Lethargy and nausea are possible symptoms of acidosis. Excess hydrogen ions interfere with normal function of nervous tissue, producing lethargy, deepening into stupor, then coma. An excess of hydrogen ions stimulates the vomiting center in the medulla. Diarrhea is a possible cause of metabolic acidosis, because the gastrointestinal secretions contain large amounts of sodium bicarbonate.

46. (1) The patient with a ureterosigmoidostomy should be maintained on a normal diet to ensure adequate intake of protein and vitamins needed to maintain body defenses, and of roughage to prevent constipation.

47. (3) The patient with a ureterosigmoidostomy should maintain a fluid intake of at least 3000 cc. (ml.) per day, so as to dilute and remove any intestinal bacteria that may gain entrance to the ureter or kidney pelvis.

Varicose Ulcer and Vein Stripping

1. (2) Varicose veins are tortuous veins, so dilated that filling of the valve cusps with blood no longer occludes the vessel and keeps blood moving in one direction. With valvular incompetence, blood stagnates in dependent portions of the sacculated veins, distending them still further and thinning the venous wall.

2. (2) Varicose veins have multiple causes. An hereditary weakness of the valves may lead to incompetence; pregnancy, abdominal tumors, or obesity compress the large veins of the abdomen, interfering with blood return to the heart and increasing hydrostatic pressure in leg veins; and muscles, fascia, or skin provide inadequate support to the vein wall, allowing the vessel to sag, elongate, and fill with blood flowing in a retrograde fashion past incompetent valves.

3. (2) The greater and smaller saphenous veins are superficial veins of the leg, and lie just beneath the skin between fascial layers. Deep veins of the leg are interposed between muscle groups, so that muscle contraction and relaxation alternately compress and release the veins, "milking" blood through the vessel toward the heart.

4. (3) Obesity and pregnancy compress the leg veins of the trunk, producing chronic obstruction to outflow of blood from the legs. Hereditary predispositions, such as deformity of valves, weakness of the vein wall, or inadequate perivascular supportive tissue, favor retrograde blood flow. Prolonged standing in one place eliminates the pumping effect of muscles in squeezing blood through the veins.

5. (2) Venous valves are delicate bicuspid pockets that open in the direction of blood flow, but prevent backflow when the pockets become filled with blood and distended. Venous blood from the lower extremities is normally held in one low-pressure column after another on its return to the heart. When there is valve flap damage or venous dilation the two cusps do not meet when filled with blood and so retrograde blood flow occurs.

6. (1) Increased hydrostatic pressure in distended veins leads to extravasation of fluid from the capillaries, with local edema formation. Venous congestion and edema increase the weight of the lower extremities, causing a feeling of heaviness and fatigue. Because the vascular system is a circuit, congestion and diminished outflow from veins and capillaries leads eventually to impaired arterial blood supply, and the diminished oxygen, calcium, and nutrient supplies to muscle result in cramps.

7. (3) Those occupations that involve standing for hours in one place predispose to development of varicosities in susceptible individuals, because of the high hydrostatic pressure in lower extremity veins when standing, and the lack of muscle-pumping effect when standing still.

8. (4) Wearing round garters and tight girdles and sitting with the knees crossed all compress superficial veins of the leg or thigh, obstructing blood flow toward the heart and fostering blood pooling in the legs. Sitting for long periods slows venous return from the legs by venous compression secondary to knee and hip flexion. Standing for long periods increases hydrostatic pressure in leg veins, distending the veins and pooling blood in dependent vessels.

9. (4) Exercise cramps in leg muscles, like intermittent claudication, are symptomatic of inadequate tissue oxygenation secondary to decreased arterial flow.

10. (3) The inflammatory reaction surrounding a varicose vein obstructs nutrient blood supply to overlying tissues. The skin becomes dry and thin, with loss of normal subcutaneous tissue, so even minor trauma causes tissue necrosis, and healing is difficult.

11. (3) Venous congestion causes capillary dilation. As the capillary widens and becomes more porous, red blood cells escape into surrounding tissue. Breakdown of the red blood cells and hemosiderin deposition cause brownish discoloration of the skin.

12. (2) Edema and induration of tissues surrounding a varicose ulcer interfere with cellular nutrition, so that the ulcer becomes inflamed and infected and is slow to heal. Burning and itching pain are symptoms of inflammation in the superficial layers of the skin.

13. (4) Purulent exudate at the base of the ulcer indicates that it is infected. In inflammation, capillaries dilate, and fluid and granulocytes emerge from the enlarged pores of the dilated capillaries and enter the tissues, where the granulocytes phagocytose several bacteria and dead tissue cells before dying.

14. (2) Action is taken to culture microorganisms in the exudate in order to identify the exact species of organism(s) present in the wound, and to test each organism's sensitivity to various antibiotics, so that the physician can administer the drug most likely to control the infection.

15. (4) In patients with varicose ulcers the perivascular inflammation, edema, and induration interfere with skin nutrition and healing. Adhesive tape is irritating to the skin and should never be used to secure the dressing over a varicose ulcer.

16. (4) Patients with peripheral vascular disease are extremely susceptible to infection. Serum and dead tissue cells in the base of the ulcer constitute an excellent culture medium. Many of the bacterial strains encountered in a hospital or clinic are antibiotic-resistant.

17. (3) The superficial and deep veins of the leg communicate at two main junctions, and are connected by a number of communicating veins. The normal direction of flow is from the foot through the superficial veins, through the communicating veins, into the deep veins, and then toward the heart. The Trendelenburg test is used to determine the presence of incompetent valves in the superficial and communicating veins by observing the speed and direction of blood flow in the superficial veins.

18. (3) Rapid filling of superficial veins from below while pressure is maintained on the saphenofemoral junction indicates incompetence of one or more communicating veins, with escape of blood from the deep veins into the superficial system. Rapid filling of superficial veins from above on release of pressure at the saphenofemoral junction indicates retrograde blood flow from above due to incompetence of valves in the superficial veins.

19. (3) Radiography of an extremity following intravenous injection of a radiopaque substance permits visualization of the venous system of the limb and helps the physician to identify the venous complication.

20. (4) Healing of venous ulcers requires a reduction in the amount of blood pooled in leg veins so as to decrease the venous pressure in superficial veins. Maintaining a supine position or elevating the legs slightly above the level of the trunk facilitates venous return to the heart, decreasing hydrostatic pressure in leg veins.

21. (3) In order for a varicose ulcer to heal it must be cleansed of all devitalized tissue and exudate. Debridement is the mechanical or chemical removal of foreign material and devitalized tissue from a wound, exposing living tissue at the base of the wound.

22. (4) Many of the bacteria that contaminate skin ulcers are saprophytic, in that they live on dead or decaying organic matter. Most bacteria prefer media of a high water content. Dead tissue and inflammatory exudate at the base of an ulcer constitute a suitable culture medium for many species of bacteria.

23. (1) The objective in cleansing a varicose ulcer is to remove bacteria, exudate, and dead tissue so as to produce clean, red, flat, granulation tissue upon which epithelialization can occur or a graft can be laid. The procedure should consist of mechanical removal of debris (hence the cotton balls) without traumatizing capillary buds in the granulation tissue underlying the purulent exudate (hence the mild soap and lukewarm water).

24. (3) Hydrogen peroxide is an unstable compound that, upon contact with tissues, breaks down readily to form molecular oxygen and water. The bubbling caused by the release of nascent oxygen effects mechanical removal of tissue debris from inaccessible regions.

25. (3) *Staphylococcus epidermidis albus* is a natural inhabitant of the skin and becomes an opportunist when the skin is injured. Some individuals become nasal or pharyngeal carriers of staphylococci. The normal flora of the mouth include both aerobic and anaerobic staphylococci.

26. (2) Tetracycline is a broad-spectrum antibiotic that interferes with growth and

multiplication of susceptible organisms by blocking ribosomal synthesis of the proteins needed by the bacteria for growth and reproduction.

27. (3) Tetracycline is eliminated from the blood primarily by glomerular filtration. Renal dysfunction causes accumulation of tetracycline in the body fluids, which leads to fatty degeneration of the liver.

28. (3) The frequency of antibiotic administration is arranged in accordance with the peak concentration of the drug in the body fluids. When antibiotic doses are not given on time, blood levels are not maintained. When bacteria reproduce, mutant organisms may develop that are more resistant than the parent organisms to the antibiotic. Drug-resistant mutants multiply quickly during periods of low blood concentration of the drug.

29. (4) Tetracycline is potentially irritating to gastrointestinal mucosa. Nausea and vomiting are reduced by administering the drug with meals, since mixing with food dilutes it and decreases its irritant effect.

30. (1) The various microbes that normally inhabit the GI tract exist in equilibrium with each other. When tetracycline-susceptible organisms are destroyed, "superinfections" of tetracycline-resistant organisms may occur causing diarrhea.

31. (1) Allergic reactions to tetracycline produce urticaria (hives) and angioedema (nonpitting edema around the eyes, mouth, and hands).

32. (3) Epinephrine is an adrenergic drug that serves as a histamine antagonist by promoting vasoconstriction.

33. (2) Hydrocortisone is an adrenal steroid with anti-inflammatory effects. Since the inflammatory changes surrounding a varicose vein are responsible for impaired nutrition of the skin and subcutaneous tissues, control of inflammation may facilitate skin healing.

34. (3) Compound tincture of benzoin is a mild irritant that promotes healing and resolution of inflammatory exudate; it also has a protective effect.

35. (1) When wound healing occurs, capillary buds proliferate, bringing increased blood to the area. Fibroblasts migrate into the defect from surrounding tissue and elaborate collagen, a protein fiber that provides the ground substance for healing tissue.

36. (2) An Unna's paste boot is composed of gelatin, a protein product derived from partial hydrolysis of collagen; glycerine, a demulcent with a drying effect; and zinc oxide, a demulcent with mild antiseptic and astrigent action. The boot is applied along the full length of the lower leg.

37. (2) The boot provides support for superficial veins by applying even pressure along the skin of the leg; protects the ulcer from accidental injury; and reduces contamination of the ulcer through the mild antiseptic action of zinc oxide and the mechanical covering over the ulcer.

38. (1) Resting for one half-hour with the legs elevated will empty blood from the superficial veins and lessen edema from the tissues surrounding the ulcer, so that the boot will fit firmly to the normal contour of the leg and foot. A dry, sterile dressing should be placed over the ulcer to absorb exudate from the wound and prevent adherence of the boot material to the wound.

39. (2) Before the varicosed superficial veins are removed, the surgeon must determine that the deep veins are patent and that the valves in the deep veins are competent enough to assist return flow against gravity.

40. (3) The foot of the bed is elevated above the level of the heart in order to foster venous return flow through the deep veins and prevent clotting. The legs are kept fully extended because flexion at the knee or hip would retard venous blood flow, and favor clotting.

41. (2) Ambulation prevents thrombus formation by preventing venous stasis. The deep veins of the leg are surrounded and supported by various muscle groups. Contraction and relaxation of these muscles squeezes the vein wall, pumping blood toward the heart.

42. (4) Mrs. Walker will experience some stiffness and pain on walking following a vein-stripping procedure. To ensure her cooperation with early ambulation, the nurse should explain that walking prevents thrombosis and ensures patency of the deep veins. Since the leg dressings and bandages will interfere somewhat with free movement of the joints, the nurse should assist Mrs.

Walker in getting out of bed and accompany her on the first few walks to prevent falls; to avoid tiring her, walks should be alternated with periods of rest. Since movement may loosen the bandages, and an even application of pressure is required to prevent bleeding from ruptured veins, the bandages should be checked and rewrapped as necessary after each walk.

43. (2) New small varicosities may develop in the first few months following vein-stripping as a result of dilation of venous branches not removed during the procedure. To prevent this development Mrs. Walker may be directed to wear elastic stockings or elastic bandages on the operated leg. These can obstruct deep venous and lymphatic drainage if they are not applied correctly so as to exert firm and equal support along the full length of the leg. The patient should be taught how to apply the stocking or bandages so as to avoid segmental constriction of the limb.

Multiple Sclerosis

1. (3) Although the cause of multiple sclerosis is not positively known, the disease is thought to result from an autoimmune reaction, according to research findings derived from animal experimentation.
2. (4) An acute infectious process precedes the initial attack or a relapse in 10–40 per cent of patients. In many cases a relapse is precipitated by fatigue, physical trauma, or emotional crisis. Symptoms are exacerbated by exposure to cold and excessive chilling.
3. (2) Multiple sclerosis, or disseminated sclerosis, is characterized primarily by numerous scattered areas of demyelinization within the white matter of the cord, brain stem, cerebellum, optic nerves, and cerebrum.
4. (1) Antibodies are gamma globulins formed by the plasma cells. Supporting either the autoimmune or the viral theory of etiology, there is elevation of gamma globulin in the cerebrospinal fluid of patients with multiple sclerosis.
5. (3) More than half of multiple sclerosis patients undergo remission after the initial attack, as a result of partial healing of areas of the brain or spinal cord that have previously undergone demyelination. The usual course of the disease is characterized by a series of remissions and exacerbations; each reappearance of symptoms is more severe and long-lasting, with only partial recovery during each remission, and with resulting progressive neurologic defects.
6. (2) A chronic illness is a disease with a long course and from which there can be only partial recovery. Most chronic illnesses are characterized by exacerbations and remissions. Since adequate supportive therapy during remissions may prevent exacerbations, the patient with chronic disease should be given extended medical supervision and education for self-care.
7. (4) Rehabilitation efforts to minimize disability must be based on residual strengths and abilities. The magnitude of a patient's disability is dependent on his need for the lost function. The self-actualizing individual can use adaptive processes to achieve psychologic stability in the face of severe physical or psychic stress. A loss of function that interferes with life style constitutes a severe psychologic burden. Imposition of a chronic illness on a family already beset with numerous psychosocial problems is threatening to all its members.
8. (3) Nystagmus consists of involuntary, rhythmic, conjugate eye movements in either a horizontal, vertical, or rotary direction. It may be due to injury of the vestibular portion of the eighth cranial nerve or to disorders of the pons, cerebellum, or medulla.
9. (2) The demyelinizing and fibrotic lesions of multiple sclerosis can involve the optic nerves. Forty per cent of patients suffer optic neuritis at the onset of illness, with dark spots in the visual field or double vision. Progress of the lesion may lead to temporary blindness in one or both eyes during relapses.
10. (1) A tremor is trembling of voluntary muscles. Intention tremor is a slow, coarse tremor (less than 6–7 vibrations per second) of the limbs, which is intensified on voluntary movement and ceases at rest.

11. (4) The symptoms of multiple sclerosis are multiple and diverse because the demyelinization can effect many structures in the central nervous system: the cord, brain stem, cerebellum, optic nerve, and cerebrum. In the extremities, cord damage produces motor weakness, together with loss of vibratory, temperature, and position sense. It also causes such urinary symptoms as urgency, frequency, and incontinence. Damage to the medulla causes vertigo and vomiting. Damage to the cerebrum produces euphoria or depression, and gradual impairment of the mental abilities.

12. (4) Once urinary problems develop in multiple sclerosis, they usually persist. Early paresis of the lower extremities usually progresses to terminal paralysis of the legs. In late stages of the spinal form of multiple sclerosis, the patient may develop contractures of the extremities. In the cerebral form, weakness of pharyngeal muscles may develop, causing dysphagia, and in the late stages there may be convulsions.

13. (1) Adrenocorticotropic hormone (A.C.T.H.) is produced by the anterior pituitary in response to a hormone from the hypothalamus called the "corticotropin-releasing hormone."

14. (2) A.C.T.H. stimulates the two innermost zones of cells in the adrenal cortex, which are the sites of glucocorticoid synthesis and secretion. It has little effect on the outermost zone of cells, which secretes aldosterone.

15. (4) The toxic effects of A.C.T.H. are the result of increased secretion of adrenocorticosteroids, which cause sodium retention, with resulting hypertension; peptic ulceration, with resulting bleeding; and increased gluconeogenesis, with elevated serum glucose. Excess adrenocorticosteroids also cause growth of excess body hair and acneform lesions.

16. (2) The inhibition of inflammation by the corticosteroids constitutes a decrease in the body's defense against infection. Neither A.C.T.H. nor adrenocorticosteroids should be given to a patient with healed tuberculosis, for fear of reactivating a tuberculous infection by counteracting the inflammatory changes that wall off the causative organisms in the body.

17. (1) Chlordiazepoxide is a minor tranquilizer that relieves mild-to-moderate anxiety by blocking impulse transmission through the reticular formation of the brain stem.

18. (3) The usual reaction to chlordiazepoxide is drowsiness and lethargy, but in some patients it may cause periods of euphoria or hostility.

19. (2) A.C.T.H. stimulates secretion of adrenocorticoids, which promotes sodium retention and potassium excretion.

20. (2) Cortisol causes increased sodium resorption from the renal tubule, and this in turn causes osmotic resorption of increased amounts of water. Increased sodium and water retention tend to produce edema of peripheral tissues.

21. (3) The portion of the frontal lobe that lies anterior to the motor area has several functions, one of which is the elaboration of thought. Patients with injuries involving this portion fail to show interest when told of their condition and its possible implications.

22. (4) The mourning process consists of shock, denial, anger, depression, withdrawal, and acceptance. An individual's values and interests are acquired over a long period and are difficult to change when a sudden alteration in life style requires their abandonment. With loss of autonomy, there is loss of self-esteem. Defense mechanisms are adaptive measures by which the personality protects itself from disintegration when subjected to extreme stress. Because a chronic disease is long-term, incurable, and characterized by increasing disability, the patient must be able to adjust to increasing dependence on others.

23. (4) Primary symptoms of multiple sclerosis include weakness, incoordination, and awkwardness in performance of fine movements. Since the patient's appetite is better when she he can feed herself, plate guards and utensils with built-up handles should be available so that Beulah can feed herself for as long as possible. Muscle weakness makes it difficult to elevate or abduct the arms, and pillows under the elbows lessen the energy expenditure during self-feeding. Easy fatigability makes it necessary for the patient to rest at intervals throughout a meal. By serving the meal early, she can be given the extra time

required to complete the meal without pressure. Appetite is improved when meals are eaten in pleasant social surroundings, such as in a dining room with other patients.

24. (1) Dependency is a condition in which one must seek instrumental aid or affection from another. To most people, it implies inferior status because one's welfare is controlled by another.

25. (2) Patients with the spinal form of multiple sclerosis frequently develop a spastic ataxic paraplegia, with radial deviation of the hand and footdrop as characteristic contracture deformities.

26. (1) Tension increases the patient's tremor, muscle spasm, and incoordination, and time pressures make the patient more tense.

27. (2) Movement of each joint through full range of motion will minimize muscle atrophy and joint contracture. Extreme physical fatigue can precipitate a relapse in the multiple sclerosis patient whose disease is in remission.

28. (2) Late in the disease, multiple sclerosis patients demonstrate extreme emotional lability. The mental and emotional changes are due to demyelinization and scarring in the frontal lobes of the cerebrum.

29. (2) Beulah is predisposed to joint contractures as a result of the immobility and flexor spasms associated with the disease. There is a continuous process of connective tissue breakdown and replacement in the body. When a body part is immobilized, collagen tissue becomes contracted and then compact and hardened.

30. (4) The mobility of joints and soft tissues requires moving the part through full range of motion several times a day. Active contraction increases the oxygen demand of muscle tissue, which causes reflex dilation of local blood vessels, which in turn causes reflex increase in heart rate and force. The sense of position and movement is derived from joint receptors that are stimulated by motion of the part. A reactive depression is a normal reaction to the development of a major physical disability. Appreciable increases in joint movement and muscle strength tend to lighten the depression.

31. (4) Passive exercise is muscular exercise that requires no effort on the patient's part. The weight of the part being exercised should be fully supported, and pressure should not be exerted on the body of the muscles. The joint above the part should be stabilized, and the part should be carried slowly and smoothly through the fullest possible range of normal movement.

32. (3) Pain provokes muscle spasm in susceptible individuals.

33. (3) Sometimes a muscle has some functional ability although it is incapable of lifting a part against gravity. In this case, the patient should be directed to contract and relax the muscle while the weight of the distal portion of the extremity is supported by the nurse.

34. (4) The multiple sclerosis patient is awkward in performance of fine movements, such as those required in buttoning, hooking, or zippering clothing. Beulah will be able to operate Velcro fasteners, because they can be closed with moderate pressure and opened with moderate traction.

35. (4) The course of multiple sclerosis is characterized by progressive demyelinization of increasing areas of the cord and brain in some patients, but by remissions with partial healing in others. Evidence of spinal cord, cerebellar, visual, and mental functioning therefore should be tested at intervals to determine the speed and direction of neurologic change. The amount of stiffness and weakness of the leg muscles can be assessed by noting the patient's stance and gait and her ability to rise from a sitting position. Strength and coordination of arm and shoulder muscles can be observed in the course of pinching, grasping, and lifting activities. Visual acuity can be tested with a Snellen Chart or by giving Beulah print of different sizes to read. The Romberg test of cerebellar function consists of directing the patient to stand with the feet together, first with the eyes open and then with them closed. A positive Romberg test, or inability to stand erect with the eyes closed, indicates cerebellar dysfunction. If, after having been negative, the Romberg test becomes positive, this indicates extension of the demyelination process to involve the cerebellum.

36. (1) Self-esteem is acquired through speech abilities, physical strengths, vocational skills, and autonomy. It is eroded when these are impaired and the patient

assumes that she is held in less esteem by others. In grieving over her loss of autonomy, Beulah is apt to lash out at those caregivers who symbolize her growing dependency.

37. (3) Bethanechol chloride is a cholinergic agent that promotes contraction of bladder muscle. Since it is not destroyed by cholinesterase, it has a fairly prolonged action.

38. (2) Many of the urinary symptoms of multiple sclerosis are due to loss of tone of the detrusor muscle.

39. (1) As a result of the bronchoconstrictor effect of the cholinergic drugs, they are apt to precipitate an allergic attack.

40. (1) Atropine, an anticholinergic drug, is a pharmacologic antidote to bethanechol. It inhibits the effects of acetylcholine, relaxing smooth muscle.

Systemic Lupus Erythematosus

1. (2) Although systemic lupus erythematosus (SLE) is a disease of unknown etiology, it is thought to be due to altered immune response because of the presence of antinuclear antibodies in the serum.

2. (2) In SLE, as in rheumatoid arthritis, there is polyarthritis characterized by joint narrowing and cystic changes, with deformity of metatarsophalangeal and proximal interphalangeal joints. Patients with rheumatoid arthritis may develop positive LE cell tests and may demonstrate antinuclear antibodies. In SLE, as in scleroderma, there are a variety of antibodies in the serum, diffuse involvement of connective tissue, and fibrinoid degeneration of the walls of small arteries.

3. (4) Fibrinoid degeneration of the small arteries and inflammation of connective tissue can produce pathologic changes in many tissues and organs. Nonbacterial vegetations may occur on the heart valves and provide a nidus for development of bacterial endocarditis. The spleen develops infarcts as a result of concentric perivascular fibrosis around central arteries. Small white areas of retinal degeneration occur secondary to occlusion of retinal vessels. Normochromic anemia, leukopenia, and thrombocytopenia develop as a result of hemolysis and marrow disturbances. Vascular changes in the central nervous system may cause subarachnoid hemorrhage, convulsions, hemiparesis, nystagmus, and organic psychosis.

4. (3) Raynaud's phenomenon is a syndrome characterized by paroxysmal bilateral ischemia of the digits, precipitated by cold or emotional stimuli and relieved by heat, which is due either to excessive sympathetic activity or to some abnormality of the vessel wall.

5. (1) A fairly severe leukopenia is seen in SLE. There is also a higher-than-normal proportion of immature white blood cells in the peripheral blood which are inefficient in phagocytosing bacteria. Gamma globulin is that portion of plasma protein which contains antibodies that offer protection against pathogenic organisms. Even though gamma globulin levels are usually elevated in SLE, they may be lower than normal in the lupus patient who has nephrotic changes.

6. (4) Symptoms are exacerbated in patients with immunologic abnormalities when resistance is lowered by any of several stressors, such as exposure to ultraviolet radiation; trauma, especially surgery; pregnancy; and severe emotional upset. Any of these provoke symptom development by upsetting the precarious balance of the body's defense systems.

7. (4) A number of drugs are capable either of causing SLE or of revealing a hitherto latent immune abnormality. Common offenders are the iodides, heavy metals, anticonvulsants, hydrazides, and procainamide.

8. (4) Cutaneous lesions occur in 85 per cent of SLE patients. A maculopapular rash is common on the face, neck, and extremities. Discoid or scaling lesions occur on skin exposed to the sun, and when healed they produce scarring and hypopigmentation. Healing of discoid scalp lesions is followed by hair loss. Urticaria is common, possibly as a manifestation of immune reaction. Purpura develops as a consequence of thrombocytopenia.

9. (4) In 50 per cent of SLE patients vascular degeneration and connective tissue inflammation affect the endocardium, myocardium, and/or pericardium. Inflammation of the myocardium produces nonspecific ST- and T-wave change, a tachycardia that is disporportionate to fever or anemia, and conduction irregularities. Pericarditis causes either a pericardial effusion or a pericardial friction rub. If the myocarditis or valvular defects are severe enough to cause congestive heart failure, cardiomegaly may be apparent.

10. (4) Depending on the location of the lesion, vascular inflammation in the central nervous system may produce a variety of symptoms: paresthesias from spinal cord lesions; palsy from cerebellar lesions; hemiparesis from lesions in the internal capsule; convulsions from lesions of the motor cortex; and psychosis from lesions of the prefrontal lobe.

11. (1) In a blood sample from a patient with SLE, some neutrophils are found that have ingested nuclear material from another leukocyte that has been injured by an antinuclear antibody. The living leukocyte contains a large purple inclusion body that compresses the nucleus against the cell wall.

12. (4) The LE preparation is not a definitve diagnostic test for SLE because LE cells are not always present in SLE patients, and the LE phenomenon has been observed in a number of other diseases, such as those listed.

13. (4) Renal involvement occurs in about half of the patients with SLE, and consists of a mild glomerulonephritis characterized by fibrinoid thickening of the basement membrane and cellular infiltration of the glomeruli.

14. (2) In the serum of an SLE patient there are large numbers of antibodies antagonistic to nucleoprotein, to DNA, and to nuclear RNA.

15. (1) Acetylsalicylic acid is an analgesic, antipyretic, anti-inflammatory agent that is effective in relieving joint inflammation and joint pain in rheumatoid arthritis and SLE. It also decreases fever by resetting the temperature regulating center in the hypothalamus, and relieves inflammation by decreasing capillary permeability.

16. (3) Chloroquine is an antimalarial drug that also has an anti-inflammatory effect, which is helpful in treating the skin lesions of lupus.

17. (2) Prednisone is a glucocorticoid that suppresses the inflammation of connective tissue seen in lupus.

18. (4) As a result of their anti-inflammatory and electrolyte effects, prolonged therapy with corticosteroids may cause decreased sodium excretion, with fluid retention; interference with inflammation, and delayed healing; hypercoagulability of the blood, with thrombus formation; increased gastric secretion of hydrochloric acid, with peptic ulceration; and changes in the electrical activity of the brain, with psychosis.

19. (1) Propoxyphene is a CNS depressant with mild-to-moderate analgesic effect. It has no anti-inflammatory, antipyretic, antitussive, or antispasmodic effect.

20. (4) Aspirin is a CNS depressant. It resets the temperature regulating center in the hypothalamus for a lower temperature, in response to which the peripheral blood vessels dilate, and heat is dissipated through radiation.

21. (4) Both aluminum hydroxide and magnesium hydroxide are nonsystemic antacids that neutralize gastric acid. Since prednisone increases gastric acid secretion and predisposes to ulcer formation, the antacid was given to prevent this complication.

22. (4) Aluminum hydroxide is an antacid that reacts with gastric acid to form aluminum chloride, which has a constipating effect.

23. (2) Magnesium hydroxide is an antacid in that it reacts with gastric acid to form magnesium chloride, which then acts as a saline cathartic, preventing absorption of water from the bowel, and thus increasing intestinal bulk and stimulating defecation.

24. (4) Cushing's syndrome is an endocrine disorder caused by a chronic excess of glucosteroids. Excess cortisol results in retention of sodium, accelerated protein catabolism, elevation of serum glucose, deposition of excess glucose in fat depots, and an associated excess of adrenal androgens. The sodium retention leads to fluid retention and edema, which contributes to rounding of facial features. Mobilization and breakdown of body protein leads to loss of peripheral supportive tissue with weakening of the skin, causing production of striae; and weakening of blood vessels, causing ecchymoses on slight trauma. Hepatic

gluconeogenesis from mobilized and catabolized body protein causes hyperglycemia and deposition of increased fatty tissue in the upper part of the face, the supraclavicular area, the interscapular area, and the mesenteric tissues. The increase in adrenal androgens causes increased body hair and acne.

25. (2) The glucocorticoids are administered to SLE patients to block inflammation of vessels and connective tissue. Unfortunately, blocking the inflammatory response removes one of the body's principal defenses against infection.

26. (2) Muscle atrophy and weakness may occur in SLE as a result of connective tissue damage. Although for the most part the arthritis associated with lupus is not deforming, in some cases the inflammatory joint changes lead to bony necrosis, subluxations, and muscle contractures. To prevent crippling deformities of the lower extremities in the bedridden lupus patient, a footboard should be used to keep the feet in proper alignment.

27. (4) Both the disease and the corticosteroid therapy increase the patient's susceptibility to infection, so Elvira should be protected from nursing staff members with skin and respiratory infections, the causative organisms of which are apt to be antibiotic-resistant.

28. (4) After about two hours of immobility, ischemia of subcutaneous tissue develops at points of pressure. Repeated ischemic insults to tissue, combined with friction against bed linen and maceration of skin by moisture and bacterial action, lead to ulcer formation. Turning the patient every two hours and the use of soft padding minimizes harmful ischemia. Massaging the skin of the back and heels improves circulation to pressure areas. Gentle bathing removes dirt, moisture, and bacteria. Clean, smooth, dry bed linen miminize friction damage to skin.

29. (3) Paranoid behavior includes extreme sensitivity, suspiciousness, jealousy, defensiveness, and hostility. The application of restraints or side rails, or the removal of objects from the patient's unit, would be apt to reinforce Elvira's paranoia. A private duty nurse would be able to protect her from injuring herself or someone else while, at the same time, allowing her a certain freedom of movement.

30. (1) Erythromycin, like penicillin, is more effective against gram-positive than against gram-negative bacteria and is effective against *Neisseria* and spirochetes.

31. (3) The dying patient typically passes through the following stages: denial, anger, bargaining, depression, and acceptance. The emphasis on youth and vigor in the mass media will be apt to accentuate Elvira's anger. The neglect of spiritual values in contemporary culture may deprive her of the religious supports that enable some patients to accept impending death calmly. The increasing tendency to care for moribund patients in hospitals rather than homes may increase Elvira's depression and loneliness by isolating her from family and friends. News of "miracle" cures may interrupt the grieving process.

32. (4) All problems listed are concomitants of dying. Serious illness provokes anxiety, which in turn leads to regression. As strength wanes and physical functions are lost, the individual suffers a loss of control over many aspects of life, being forced to be dependent on others. Radical alterations in body structure by pathologic processes or surgical procedures render the physical body less and less perfect. Changes in appearance, function, and social role erode the sense of self. As death approaches, more and more friends, family, and caregivers disengage themselves from the patient, increasing her loneliness and sense of abandonment.

33. (4) In passing through the stages listed in no. 31 above, the dying patient will experience many negative feelings. The nurse's task is to assist Elvira's progression through the grief stages, and to facilitate the working through of negative feelings by sustaining her hope at each stage in the process.

34. (3) Maslow's theory of a hierarchy of human needs indicates that, generally, survival needs and stimulation needs have primacy over safety needs, which have priority over affection and esteem needs, which in turn have priority over self-actualizing needs. However, at times of extreme stress, there are apt to be some needs unsatisfied at all levels of the need hierarchy.

35. (4) The dying patient's relatives and the health care workers tend to go through

the same grief stages as the patient. When family or caregivers do not work through the stages in the same sequence or at the same speed as the patient, dissonance develops between the patient and significant others.

36. (3) A nurse may feel especially threatened by the death of a patient of her own age-group for whom she has cared over a long period. The death may represent failure to a nurse to whom the patient's full recovery is the only acceptable outcome of the care process. The nurse, like the patient, may need empathic and nondirective guidance to confront and work through her negative feelings about death.

37. (2) This response emphasizes the primary objective to be met in deciding between hospital and home care (maximizing the patient's comfort), and invites Elvira to explore her needs and feelings in light of that objective.

38. (2) The dying patient does not move in an orderly and sequential fashion through all five stages of the grieving process. Some stages are missed or incompletely resolved, and must be returned to. Because family members and caregivers typically have difficulty accepting expressions of anger and guilt from patients, these feelings are least likely to have been completely resolved. Allowing the dying patient to help plan and administer her own care affords her a measure of control over her situation.

Carotid Atherosclerosis and Endarterectomy

1. (4) In order to identify the exact pathophysiology underlying the patient's chief complaint and to ascribe a probable cause for the symptom, the nurse must identify significant time parameters, such as the onset, frequency, and duration of the symptom; and related circumstances, such as the events that provoke, accompany, or relieve the symptom.

2. (4) All the issues listed relate to possible causes of vertigo. Dizziness is a symptom of concussion and of subdural hemorrhage; is a toxic effect of many sedatives, analgesics, and antitensives; may arise from a loss of visual acuity and consequent loss of positional sense; may be caused by hypotension due to pump failure or cardiac arrhythmias; and is sometimes associated with the aura preceding epileptic seizures.

3. (4) Transient ischemic attacks (TIAs) are brief episodes of cerebral ischemia produced by embolization of plaques or clots from an arteriosclerotic carotid bifurcation. Typical symptoms of a TIA are abrupt onset of dysarthria, unilateral blindness, and numbness or weakness of the face, hand, or leg. Symptoms usually clear within minutes to hours.

4. (3) Each symptom could result from obstruction of a single blood vessel in some portion of the central nervous system. Brief, unilateral, neurologic deficits are strongly suggestive of carotid artery obstruction.

5. (2) If the cerebral blood vessel that is obstructed by embolized plaque or fibrin clot is small, collateral blood vessels may dilate to bring increased blood to the area, and the symptoms of neurologic dysfunction may be relieved within a few minutes of onset.

6. (2) The emboli that occlude cerebral vessels to produce TIAs derive from thrombi formed on the irregular surface of atheromatous plaques at the carotid bifurcation. Eventually a clot of sufficient size may occlude a major cerebral vessel, producing a cerebral infarction.

7. (3) Arrhythmias render cardiac contractions inefficient and interfere with complete emptying of the heart during systole. Stagnation of blood predisposes to clotting, so that mural thrombi form in a weakly contracting heart. If these clots are only weakly adherent to the endocardium, they may break loose and be carried to the brain, where they block blood vessels and cause cerebral infarction.

8. (4) A thick, yellow, fatty material consisting of cholesterol and cholesterol esters is deposited under the endothelium of the vessel and covered with dense fibrous tissue. In time calcium salts are deposited in the plaque, and the vessel hardens. Small blood vessels proliferate and grow into the connective tissue

surrounding the atheromatous plaque. Rupture of one of the small vessels causes bleeding into the plaque, causing it to elevate and protrude into the vessel lumen. Eddy currents around the elevated plaque lead to clot formation on the roughened plaque surface.

9. (1) The presence of atheromatous plaque and associated fibrous material causes atrophy of the elastic and muscle fibers in the adjacent media, decreasing the elasticity of the vessel and causing it to stretch and elongate with the pressure of blood against the wall. The elongated vessel twists upon its axis, assuming a serpentine course.

10. (3) As a result of long-standing mechanical trauma to arterial walls, hypertension may cause atherosclerosis. Familial incidence of hyperlipidemia, diabetes, hypertension, or arteriosclerosis all increase Mr. Keeler's risk of developing arteriosclerosis, indicating that genetic factors predispose to disturbed fat metabolism and blood pressure disorders. The incidence of carotid atherosclerosis is significantly higher in cigarette smokers than in nonsmokers.

11. (3) Diets containing excessive amounts of saturated fatty acids in relation to polyunsaturated fatty acids result in an increase in blood cholesterol levels and foster development of arteriosclerosis. A high caloric intake contributes to obesity, which increases the risk of arteriosclerosis. Highly competitive individuals are more than usually susceptible to coronary atherosclerosis, and possibly to arteriosclerosis of other organs also. Physical exercise increases caloric expenditure, decreases obesity, and thus reduces the risk of hypertension and arteriosclerosis. Diabetes mellitus is characterized by disordered lipoprotein metabolism, with increased synthesis and deposition of cholesterol in medium and small arteries.

12. (3) Normally the retinal arterioles are smaller than the veins in a ratio of 2:3. In hypertension the retinal arterioles, like those elsewhere in the body, are constricted, decreasing the AV ratio to perhaps 1:2. Blood pressure damage to the retinal arterioles may cause them to rupture, with hemorrhage into the retina. A thickened, rigid arteriole tends to compress an underlying softer-walled vein where the two cross in the retina, producing a segmental interruption of blood flow in the vein.

13. (3) Arteriosclerotic obstruction of the carotid bifurcation causes embolization of plaque or fibrin aggregates to the retinal artery, as well as to the cerebral arteries. Occasionally a shiny white piece of plaque can be visualized in a retinal artery during a transient ischemic attack.

14. (2) Severe and progressive obstruction to the carotid artery blood flow causes retinal degeneration due to chronic ischemia.

15. (2) Comparing the retinal artery pressures in the two eyes permits the physician to identify a significantly decreased pressure, and therefore a significantly decreased carotid and retinal artery flow on one side (that of arteriosclerotic or thrombotic occlusion).

16. (1) The facial artery is a branch of the external carotid artery. Skin pallor is one symptom of decreased arterial blood supply to a part.

17. (3) Increased stroke volume, as seen in anemia, thyrotoxicosis, or aortic valve insufficiency, causes overdistention of the aorta with ventricular systole, which in turn produces a visible pulse wave in the carotid artery. Increased force of ventricular contraction, a reflex response of the left ventricle muscle to increased peripheral resistance, results in increased distention of the aorta with ventricular systole, and transmission of the exaggerated pulse wave to the carotid artery.

18. (3) The carotid artery ascends the neck obliquely alongside the internal jugular vein and just below the medial border of the sternocleidomastoid muscle.

19. (4) The carotid pulse can be palpated with Mr. Keeler in the supine position.

20. (4) Variations in pulse rate, volume, contour, rhythm, and pattern have diagnostic significance in a wide variety of pathologic conditions.

21. (2) A normal arterial wall cannot be felt. In arteriosclerosis the vessel wall may have a beady or cord-like character on palpation, as a result of subintimal thickening and plaque formation.

22. (3) The carotid body is a structure near the bifurcation of the common carotid artery that contains chemoreceptors and baroreceptors that reflexly regulate

respiration and circulation. A rise in blood pressure causes the baroreceptors to send impulses that inhibit the vasoconstrictor center in the medulla and stimulate the vagal center, producing vasodilation and decreased heart rate.

23. (2) A bruit is an extracardiac blowing sound heard over a peripheral vessel during cardiac systole, and signifies abnormal blood flow through the vessel.

24. (3) Emphysema is a chronic, obstructive lung disease characterized by overdistention and destruction of alveoli, increased anteroposterior diameter of the chest, and fixation of the diaphragm in the position of inspiration.

25. (2) Resonance is the full, low-pitched sound elicited by percussion over normal lung tissue. When alveoli are overdistended and greater-than-normal amounts of air are trapped in peripheral portions of lung parenchyma, percussion elicits hyperresonance.

26. (4) Decreased volume of blood flow through the carotid artery results in less-than-normal filling of the retinal artery. Ischemia of the postcentral gyrus of the left cortex could result in disturbed position sense of the right arm and leg. Ischemia of the left internal capsule may produce muscle spasticity and hyperactive reflexes in the right arm and leg.

27. (4) Dizziness may result from cerebral, cerebrovascular, cerebellar, sinus, mastoid, or middle or inner ear disorders. With descending levels of consciousness, orientation to time is typically lost before orientation to place and to person. Scalp lacerations and swellings are common signs of head trauma. The Romberg and finger-nose tests are measures of coordination, and therefore of cerebellar functioning. Tenderness or pain on percussion of the sinuses or mastoid process is indicative of infection in the sinus or cancellous bone underneath. Observation of a bulging tympanum, with dark fluid visible through the membrane, is indicative of otitis media.

28. (4) A differential white blood count would have given evidence of an acute inflammatory or infectious disease, such as mastoiditis, brain abscess, or meningitis. A spinal puncture could have yielded evidence of subarachnoid hemorrhage. Electroencephalography could have revealed brain wave patterns characteristic of epilepsy. Cerebral angiogram could have outlined an aneurysm of the circle of Willis. A radioactive brain scan could demonstrate a brain tumor or subdural hematoma.

29. (2) Direct carotid arteriography can be performed by injecting the radiopaque dye into the common carotid arteries low in the neck. By means of a catheter inserted through the femoral artery in the groin and passed in retrograde fashion to the aortic arch, both the carotid and vertebral arteries can be outlined to obtain more comprehensive information about cranial blood supply.

30. (2) The radiopaque substance will outline the vessel lumen on x-ray examination, revealing the site of plaque formation or occlusion and indicating the extent of carotid narrowing. This information is useful in determining whether surgery is indicated, and if so which vessel(s) should be operated upon.

31. (1) In some patients neurologic deficits can be produced or exaggerated by allergic reactions to the radiopaque dye. Rupture of a damaged cerebral vessel and extravasation of dye into brain tissue would produce a cerebral infarct.

32. (2) Hemorrhage from a femeral artery puncture site could result in the loss of a considerable amount of blood in a short time. Keeping the patient supine with the legs extended decreases the possibility of thrombus formation at the femoral artery puncture site. The blood pressure should be measured hourly in order to identify hypotension as a symptom of hemorrhage and shock.

33. (3) In 80 per cent of patients who suffer cerebrovascular accident there is a previous history of warning ischemic attacks.

34. (1) Necessary manipulation of the carotid artery during the endarterectomy procedure may cause a necrotic atheromatous plaque to break loose and embolize to the cerebral circulation.

35. (4) Protamine sulfate is a powerful heparin antagonist. It is strongly basic, and combines with strongly acidic heparin to form a stable salt that has no anticoagulant effect.

36. (3) Hemorrhage produces decrease in circulating blood volume, which causes a fall in systolic blood pressure. Decreased blood pressure stimulates the baroreceptors in the aortic arch and carotid birfurcation, causing sympathetic

stimulation, with constriction of skin arterioles and pallor. When mean arterial pressure drops so low that systemic tissues are inadequately perfused with blood, altered glycolysis takes place in tissues, and lactic acid accumulates in the blood. As acidosis develops, the excess hydrogen ion stimulates the respiratory center in the medulla, causing rapid respirations.

37. (4) The endotracheal tube is irritating to laryngeal mucosa. Following removal of the tube severe laryngeal edema may develop, causing respiratory obstruction. If symptoms of airway obstruction develop, either reintubation or tracheostomy will be necessary.

38. (2) Since all muscles of the larynx except the cricothyroid are innervated by the recurrent laryngeal nerve, hoarseness may be sign of tenth nerve damage.

39. (4) If the carotid suture line should separate, severe hemorrhage and shock would result. Loss of a large amount of blood into tissues of the neck could compress pharyngeal or tracheal tissues, causing asphyxia. Laryngeal edema or laryngospasm could cause asphyxia. Clots can form at the site where the carotid artery is clamped during surgery. Embolization of a poorly organized clot from the carotid would cause a cerebral infarction.

40. (3) The risk of hemorrhage from the operative site is greatest during the first few hours following surgery. The symptoms include restlessness.

41. (3) The degree of change in central venous pressure may be as important as the absolute pressure reading in the evaluation of cardiac function or circulating blood volume.

42. (4) Headache may result from dilation and distention of collateral vessels around an area of infarction. Confusion may result from ischemia of sensory cortex and association areas. Infarction of the motor cortex or the internal capsule may produce facial assymetry, or weakness or paralysis of an extremity. Ischemia of Broca's and Wernicke's areas in the frontal and temporal lobes would destroy motor and sensory language abilities.

43. (1) The caliber of the carotid artery was reduced by the insertion of an inlying bypass shunt to maintain cerebral blood flow while the atheromatous plaque was being removed. Temporary narrowing of the carotid lumen would have caused decreased oxygenation of brain tissue during surgery.

44. (3) Mr. Keeler's respiratory mucosa is already irritated by the use of the endotracheal tube during surgery. Administration of oxygen without humidification causes drying of mucus, with retention and secondary infection of secretions.

45. (4) Oxygen supports combustion. The third prong on a three-pronged plug connects to a grounding wire, and so decreases the danger of spark formation and consequent ignition of combustible materials. At each juncture of an electrical plug with a socket, there is opportunity for leakage of electrical current, with spark formation. Electrical cords lying on the floor are apt to be damaged by personnel traffic and rolling equipment, leading to frayed wires, leakage of electrical current, and sparking. Cigarettes, matches, and other smoking materials burn more rapidly in an oxygen-rich environment. Oil, vaseline, alcohol, and ether are all inflammable.

46. (1) Variations in the thickness of the skin and the amount of melanin deposited in the skin make cyanosis more visible in some patients than in others, and so the nail beds are the best site.

47. (3) The movement of oxygen (inspired alveolar air — pulmonary capillaries — systemic arteries — tissue capillaries — tissue cells) occurs as a result of a pressure gradient. The oxygen tension in arterial blood is somewhat lower than that in the alveolus, but higher than that in the tissue fluid.

48. (2) In the normal person, respirations are regulated primarily by the effects of carbon dioxide and hydrogen ion concentrations on the respiratory center in the medulla. In chronic lung disease, in which gases are not readily exchanged in the lungs, the decrease in oxygen saturation stimulates respirations through excitation of chemoreceptors in the aorta and carotid bodies.

49. (4) It is important to make a neurologic assessment to determine whether there are any changes in sensory or motor function. This assists the physician in making a definitive diagnosis and protects the patient if losses are noted.

50. (2) Normally, if a light is flashed into one eye, both pupils narrow and restrict the amount of light that can enter the eye.

51. (2) The oculomotor, or third cranial, nerve is essentially a motor nerve that innervates four of the six external muscles of the eye, including the smooth muscle fibers of the iris.

52. (1) Inequality of the pupils indicates injury of the oculomotor nerve or increased intracranial pressure.

53. (1) As part of determining the patient's level of consciousness or awareness of self and environment, the evaluator should test the patient's response to auditory stimuli. In a state of somnolence or lethargy, increased verbal stimuli may be required to get the patient to respond to simple commands. The other alternatives listed are all means of testing coordination.

54. (3) In the stage of semistupor the response to pain is purposeful, such as withdrawal from a painful stimulus. In deep stupor the response, if any, is nonpurposeful, consisting usually of general restlessness.

55. (4) The glossopharyngeal and vagus nerves, cranial nerves 9 and 10, are closely connected, arising from the lateral surface of the medulla oblongata. Both innervate the pharyngeal muscles.

56. (2) The functions of the ninth and tenth cranial nerves are tested together. One symptom of malfunction of either is impaired gagging when the pharyngeal wall is stimulated.

57. (3) The patient's level of consciousness tends to decline progressively in a predictable stepwise fashion with increasing neurologic deterioration. First, the "higher" cerebral functions are lost, then the ability to be aroused and to respond to simple commands, and finally, the basic reflexes.

58. (1) Muscle strength can be tested in both extremity and trunk muscles. Generally, only a gross test is performed of the strength and equality of hand grip. The grip strength of the two hands should be compared, because a cerebral embolus with infarction would produce contralateral skeletal muscle weakness.

59. (1) Grimacing is a nonpurposeful response to pain stimulation, which would indicate that the patient is comatose. The other three behaviors described indicate that the patient can be roused and is capable of responding in some degree to verbal stimulation, which would indicate somnolence or stupor.

60. (1) Chronic bronchitis, dilation of respiratory bronchioles, and distention of alveolar walls predispose to stagnation and infection of respiratory secretions Physical immobility, together with infected bronchial secretions, lead to occlusion of dependent alveoli by inflammatory exudate.

61. (2) I.P.P.B. treatment delivers air-oxygen mixtures to the lungs under pressure greater than atmospheric pressure, so as to force oxygen through locally constricted air passages to the alveoli and flush accumulations of carbon dioxide from residual air passages.

Laryngeal Carcinoma and Laryngectomy

1. (2) A tumor in the vocal membrane would alter the consistency of the tissue, impeding free movement on phonation, and would prevent complete approximation of the membranes, producing hoarseness.

2. (2) Cough may result from aspiration through inadequate closure of the vocal membranes due to tumor bulk or cord paralysis. If the laryngeal tumor has metastasized to the pharynx, trachea, or lymph nodes, dyspnea may result from narrowing of air passages, and dysphagia from narrowing of food passages.

3. (3) Laryngeal carcinoma is caused by chronic irritation by cigarette smoke, as well as other noxious substances.

4. (2) Carcinoma of the pharynx causes difficulty in swallowing and a sensation of lump in the throat, due to encroachment on the pharyngeal lumen. Pain radiating to the ear may result from extension of the tumor to the eustachian tube, with accumulation of transudate in the middle ear.

5. (3) Optimal visualization of the larynx is facilitated if the patient is relaxed. Mr.

Raspanti will be more relaxed and less likely to gag if he breathes through his mouth. Directing the patient to say "Eeeee" lifts the epiglottis to expose the larynx, and permits evaluation of cord movement.

6. (1) The opening between the vocal cords is "V"-shaped when the patient is breathing quietly. During speech the cords stretch or slacken, move together and apart, and vibrate in response to the pressure of air.

7. (3) Food and fluids are withheld for eight hours before endoscopy to prevent regurgitation and aspiration during or following the procedure. Eyeglasses should be removed to prevent breakage and injury to the patient. Dentures should be removed to prevent breakage during insertion of the laryngoscope, with aspiration of a tooth or a piece of plastic. A signed operative permit is required for any major diagnostic procedure that involves entering a body cavity.

8. (3) Trauma from the laryngoscope may cause edema of the vocal cords, with loss of voice for a few hours following the procedure.

9. (1) The local anesthetic used during laryngoscopy obliterates the gag reflex for 2–4 hours following the procedure. If the patient were to eat or drink during this period he would be in danger of aspiration.

10. (4) Possible complications of laryngoscopy include laryngeal edema, which could produce respiratory obstruction with shortness of breath, restlessness, and apprehension; hemorrhage, with expectoration of bloody mucus; and perforation of the pharynx or trachea, with pain and swelling of the neck due to subcutaneous emphysema.

11. (3) Incision into the cord for removal of a biopsy specimen usually produces blood-streaked sputum immediately following the procedure. Immobility of the cord fosters closure of the sectioned vessels by clots. Coughing and talking causes vibration of the cords, delaying healing of the biopsy site.

12. (2) The patient may be uncomfortable and anxious following laryngoscopy, and should not be discouraged from expressing his needs and concerns. To discourage him from speaking until the biopsied cord has had an opportunity to heal, Mr. Raspanti should be given writing materials.

13. (2) Since the disfigurement and disability resulting from laryngectomy and radical neck dissection are extreme, Mr. Raspanti must be informed that following surgery he will be left with a permanent tracheostomy.

14. (4) Following surgery the patient will be less anxious if he has been briefed preoperatively concerning significant aspects of postoperative care. He should be taught how to breathe deeply and cough so as to prevent hypostatic pneumonia. He should learn that frequent oral hygiene will be needed to prevent infection of the pharyngeal suture lines. He should be given a tracheostomy tube to examine and handle, and should be shown pictures and diagrams illustrating placement and care for the tracheostomy, gastric feeding, and hyperalimentation tubes.

15. (4) All the items listed are necessary: the nasogastric tube to minimize contamination of the pharyngeal and esophageal suture lines; the tracheostomy tube to provide ingress of air to the lungs following removal of the larynx; the drainage tube, which is placed into the neck wound to remove blood and inflammatory secretions that could compress the trachea, disrupt postoperative suture lines, or delay healing of graft tissues; the indwelling catheter to ensure accurate record of fluid output; the peripheral venous catheter to administer fluid to replace that lost during surgery; the central venous catheter to check the adequacy of fluid replacement and the efficacy of right heart functioning; and the peripheral arterial line to measure blood gas changes as an index to the effectiveness of oxygen and respiratory therapy.

16. (4) A total laryngectomy involves removal of the hyoid bone, epiglottis, thyroid and cricoid cartilage, and two or three tracheal rings; the closure of the pharyngeal opening to the trachea; and the formation of a permanent tracheostomy. Since the vocal cords are absent, and air henceforth must be inspired and expired through the tracheostomy rather than the nares, the patient will be incapable of normal speech; will no longer breathe through the nose and mouth; will lose the normal sense of smell; will be unable to "blow" his nose; and will be unable to lift heavy objects, which requires inspiring deeply and holding the breath against a closed glottis.

17. (3) Free and complete expression of feelings is apt to occur only when the patient has full speech ability. Mr. Raspanti will have more energy to invest toward recovery and rehabilitation after he has ventilated and worked through his negative feelings concerning illness and treatment. He should be encouraged to express himself freely before surgery deprives him of the ability to do so.

18. (3) About 75 per cent of persons after laryngectomy are able to master the skill of esophageal speech, which requires that air be swallowed and expelled slowly so as to vibrate tissue folds at the opening of the esophagus while lips, teeth, tongue, and pharyngeal muscles are used to articulate speech sounds. It is easier to master the skill of swallowing and releasing air before surgery than after because the patient is less distracted by physical concerns and can ask questions more easily.

19. (4) Thirty-five per cent of patients with carcinoma of the larynx have metastases to cervical nodes. To decrease the danger of further extension or metastasis of the tumor, the surgeon removes as many of the surrounding neck structures as the patient can survive without.

20. (3) During the immediate postanesthetic period, until the patient regains consciousness, he should be positioned on his side to facilitate drainage of oral and tracheal secretions.

21. (4) As soon as he is conscious following surgery the laryngectomized patient should have his head elevated about 30° to improve lung expansion and diaphragmatic excursion. This also decreases edema of neck tissues, which would compress the trachea and cause airway obstruction.

22. (4) The trauma of surgery causes edema of soft tissues. A pressure dressing is applied over the neck wound to minimize accumulation of serous fluid or hematomas under the skin flap. Most anesthetic agents and narcotic analgesics have a depressant effect on the respiratory center. The laryngectomy and radical neck dissection is a lengthy procedure. Immobility predisposes to atelectasis of dependent alveoli. Mechanical irritation or trauma of the tracheal mucosa results in increased secretion of mucus by respiratory glands.

23. (3) A large amount of blood on the dressing might signify carotid artery rupture. To prevent exsanguination the nurse should immediately apply direct pressure to the wound and summon the surgeon, because the patient may have to be taken to surgery for ligation of the vessel.

24. (3) The diagnosis of malignancy and the ordeal of mutilating surgery are anxiety-provoking. Loss of speech makes it difficult for the patient to express anxiety and seek reassurance from caregivers. Explaining each aspect of care in advance considerably reduces anxiety.

25. (4) Accumulation of secretions in respiratory passages causes rales or crackling sounds due to passage of air through fluid. Airway obstruction by secretions results in anoxia. Anoxia of cerebral tissues causes anxiety and restlessness. Tissue oxygen lack causes vasodilation, which reflexly increases heart rate and respiratory rate.

26. (3) In suctioning the tracheostomy following laryngectomy, care must be taken to avoid introducing potential pathogens through the tracheostomy into the lower respiratory tree, since the patient with a malignancy has impaired immunologic defenses.

27. (3) A flexible rather than a stiff catheter is preferred, because it facilitates entry into the mainstem bronchi. A clear plastic catheter permits visualization of the secretions being withdrawn from the trachea.

28. (2) Tracheal suctioning is a sterile procedure, and sterile gloves and a sterile catheter should be used. To avoid transplanting pathogens from the mouth to the trachea, separate catheters should be used to suction the two cavities.

29. (2) Tracheal or "deep" suctioning causes mechanical irritation of the trachea, and results in removal of gases as well as secretions from the lower air passages.

30. (2) Stimulation of mechanoreceptors in the tracheal submucosa may produce bronchospasm. Sudden decrease in intrathoracic pressure speeds venous return to the right heart. Anoxia causes increased irritability of the myocardium, with generation of impulses from ectopic foci in the atrial or ventricular muscle.

31. (3) The purpose of tracheal suctioning is to remove excess secretions. As soon as secretions are no longer aspirated through the catheter and rales are no longer

heard on auscultation, suctioning should be stopped. Oxygen-rich mixtures should be administered before, after, and at intervals during the suctioning procedures to compensate for lowered alveolar oxygen concentrations during suctioning.

32. (4) During normal breathing inspired air is humidified by the mucosa of the upper respiratory tract. When inspired air bypasses the upper tract and enters the body through a tracheostomy, the air must be humidified or tracheobronchial secretions will become thick and crusted. When the airway is obstructed by secretions, percussion and vibration of the chest wall help to loosen secretions so as to facilitate their removal. After secretions have been humidified and loosened, elevating the foot of the bed by about 12 inches and turning the patient from side to side every 30 minutes encourage gravity flow of secretions toward the tracheostomy, where they can be removed by suctioning. Instillation of a few milliliters of saline into the trachea will liquefy secretions and aid in their removal by suctioning. The more prolonged and forceful the exhalation, the greater is the expulsive force behind accumulated secretions.

33. (2) The suction catheter acts as a foreign body in the trachea, stimulating an outpouring of fluid from mucosal capillaries.

34. (4) The catheter is inserted without suction to avoid sucking mucosa into the catheter openings as the catheter is advanced. The catheter, which is slightly curved at the tip, should be rotated as it is withdrawn with the suction on, to sweep secretions from all sides of the trachea throughout the distance that the catheter was inserted.

35. (4) Cephalosporin derivatives have a bactericidal effect against a variety of gram-positive and gram-negative organisms.

36. (4) Toxic effects of cephalosporin derivatives include some blood dyscrasias, among which is a transient neutropenia that tends to occur on or about the tenth day of therapy.

37. (2) 1000 ml. × 0.25 = 250 grams; 1000 ml. × 0.0425 = 42.5 grams. 250 grams × 4 cal./grams = 1000 calories; 42.5 grams × 4 cal./grams = 170 calories. Total calories, 1170.

38. (1) Under certain conditions, the administration of a hyperosmolar intravenous solution is capable of causing severe electrolyte imbalance. The most serious might be excesses or deficiencies of sodium, potassium, and calcium, since such imbalances cause disorders of cardiac functioning, muscle contraction, and blood clotting.

39. (2) Hyperglycemia, a possible complication of parenteral hyperalimentation, would cause osmotic diuresis. Daily changes in body weight reflect the balance between anabolism and catabolism. Serum acetone levels increase with catabolism of adipose tissue.

40. (2) Because neck muscles are removed during a radical neck dissection, the patient's head is apt to fall backward or to the side. The back of the head should be supported as he moves to prevent undue strain on the suture line.

41. (1) Mr. Raspanti's physical safety and psychologic comfort depend on his being able to summon help quickly and express his needs effectively. A tap bell and a magic slate will enable the speechless patient to do both.

42. (3) The tracheostomy and the nasogastric tubes are left in place for several weeks following surgery. Mutilating surgery weakens the patient's sense of identity and self-esteem, which can be restored by the resumption of self-care. The indwelling catheter is removed as soon as the patient's fluid and electrolyte balance is stabilized, in order to prevent development of a urinary tract infection.

43. (2) On the third or fourth postoperative day the laryngectomized patient has recovered sufficiently from the physiologic stress of the operation to take stock of his physical and psychologic losses. The impact of mutilation, mutism, and uncertain prognosis produce feelings of sadness, worthlessness, and hopelessness.

44. (1) As a result of the pharyngectomy and creation of a new pharynx, there are extensive skin and deep suture lines to be healed following laryngectomy-pharyngectomy-radical neck dissection-pharyngoplasty. Providing nourishment through a nasogastric tube from the third to the tenth day minimizes contamination of the pharyngeal, tracheal, and esophageal suture lines and prevents undue distention of the newly constructed pharynx.

45. (1) Departures from normal contour and consistency of pharyngeal and upper esophageal tissues as a result of surgical tissue loss and plastic repair will cause dysphagia on the patient's first postoperative attempt to drink liquids. Severe coughing places strain on the tracheopharyngeal suture line.

46. (4) The patient's dysphagia during the early postoperative period is characterized by a feeling of strangling or choking. The respiratory component of this discomfort can be minimized by frequent tracheal suctioning to remove secretions mobilized by coughing.

47. (2) The first step in achieving esophageal speech is learning to take air into the upper esophagus and releasing it in a controlled, sustained stream. Mr. Raspanti should wait for an hour or two after meals to practice belching so that the feeding mixture will have passed out of the stomach and cannot be regurgitated.

48. (2) As a result of damage to motor and sensory nerves during radical neck dissection, the patient may experience numbness of the neck, upper chest, and upper back. Paralysis of the trapezius will limit shoulder motion. Postural deformities resulting from loss of muscle action may stress sensitive joint structures.

49. (3) Muscle tonus is involuntary resistance to stretch. A healthy muscle is continuously in a state of partial contraction or tonus. Muscle tone is maintained through a constant flow of nerve impulses to the muscle. Tone is gradually lost by a muscle that is unused, since the normal flow of nerve impulses to the muscle is reduced. The esophagus is a muscular tube, in which tone is lost postoperatively through lack of use. When the upper esophagus relaxes and food enters the esophagus, fibers of the vagus nerve conduct impulses to the swallowing center in the medulla and back again to initiate esophageal peristalsis. Fiber or roughage provides bulk to the food bolus, stimulating esophageal peristalsis and maintaining tone of esophageal muscle.

50. (1) Some patients require from one to two months to learn esophageal speech. Mr. Raspanti may be fatigued and frustrated by speech training, and discouraged by the fact that esophageal speech sounds are more hoarse and low-pitched than normal speech sounds. His morale will be improved by his family's approval and admiration of his new speech sounds.

51. (4) Until the patient learns to coordinate esophageal air capturing and ejection with articulation movements, he may experience digestive difficulties. Anorexia, dyspepsia, and excessive flatulence result from the air swallowing and increased peristalsis associated with nervous tension.

52. (2) Pain has a protective function. Lack of sensation in any body part predisposes to temperature injury or mechanical trauma of the part.

53. (4) Since the humidifying action of the upper airway is lost in the laryngectomized patient, environmental air must be artificially humidified to prevent crusting of tracheal secretions that could lead to obstruction of the lower respiratory passages. A moistened gauze square may be worn over the tracheostomy to humidify inspired air and prevent aspiration of particulate matter. The laryngectomy tube should be changed daily and the soiled tube cleansed of secretions so as to prevent tracheal obstruction and infection. Smoke-laden environments irritate the tracheal mucosa, causing an outpouring of mucus, and possibly obstructing the tracheostomy tube. Mr. Raspanti should return to work as soon as he is physically able, because the communication demands of a steady job provide strong motivation for mastering esophageal speech.

54. (1) Although many lay persons and public workers are trained to perform cardiopulmonary resuscitation, most of the former would not realize that there is no direct connection between the upper airway and the lungs in a patient with a permanent tracheostomy.

Paraplegia and Skin Graft

1. (2) In any gunshot wound of the back the possibility of spinal injury should be investigated. Damage to the spinal cord is characterized by paralysis of body parts innervated by nerves exiting the cord below the level of injury.

2. (3) Leonard should be immobilized in supine position and not allowed to move

until it is determined whether he can move his toes and fingers. If unable to move either, spinal cord injury is certain, and the patient must be transported to a hospital without flexing or extending his spine or head, in order to prevent further and irreparable cord damage.

3. (2) Four persons are needed to lift an injured adult without moving his spine or head. To effect the move, three of the rescuers should lift the trunk and extremities as a unit while the fourth applies firm traction on the head and neck. The patient should be transferred to a firm, flat support, such as a stretcher or a door, for the trip to the hospital.

4. (3) Trauma victims frequently experience a retrograde amnesia for the events that immediately preceded their injury, repressing the situation in order to deal with overwhelming anxiety.

5. (2) Following severe trauma the spinal cord shows no activity at all for several days or weeks, because of edema and congestion secondary to transmission of pressure waves through cord tissues. During the period of spinal shock there is complete loss of motor, sensory, reflex, and autonomic activity below the level of injury.

6. (2) During the period of spinal shock, superficial and deep reflexes are both absent below the point of injury, because impulses are not being transmitted through the inflamed cord segment.

7. (1) Immediately following transection of the thoracic cord there is flaccid paralysis of the lower extremities, as a result of interruption of efferent impulses through the injured cord segment.

8. (3) Prior to immobilization by spinal fusion, Leonard's spine must be kept immobile and in perfect alignment so as to prevent further damage to the spinal cord and spinal nerves by ragged bone fragments. He therefore should be placed on a Stryker frame.

9. (2) If neither a Circoelectric bed nor a Stryker frame is available, the patient should be immobilized on a regular bed frame with a bedboard and a firm horsehair mattress.

10. (2) During the stage of spinal shock the micturition reflex is obliterated, so that urine accumulates in the bladder, the detrusor muscle is paralyzed, and the bladder becomes distended.

11. (2) Even though spinal shock and urinary retention continue for several days, renal secretion of urine eventually distends the bladder beyond the capacity of the urinary sphincter to retain fluid. At this point, urine overflow or dribbling occurs, while the bladder remains distended because the detrusor is not stimulated to contract.

12. (3) Following resolution of cord edema and congestion, spinal reflexes return and autonomic activity is resumed. Restoration of the micturition and defecation reflexes permits reflex emptying of the bladder and bowel, so that with proper training automatic control of urinal and fecal elimination may be possible.

13. (3) The turning sheet is needed to turn the patient as a unit, so as to avoid straining his spine or the cast and causing further damage to the spinal cord. The overhead frame and trapeze will enable the patient to lift himself up at frequent intervals to relieve pressure on bony prominences. The foot support will maintain his foot in neutral position, at right angles to the leg, to facilitate later rehabilitation efforts.

14. (1) The paraplegic patient has suffered multiple severe losses: loss of feeling, mobility, control, and familiar surroundings and activities. Grieving is the normal reaction.

15. (2) The state of spinal shock is prolonged by the presence of infection anywhere in the body, perhaps because circulating bacteria or toxins perpetuate the inflammatory reaction in cord tissues.

16. (4) Motor paralysis of the legs makes it more difficult for the patient to change position frequently. Sensory loss in the lower portions of the body eliminate the sensations of pressure, friction, and pain that ordinarily alert the individual to pressure injury of skin and subcutaneous tissue. Excessive perspiration in the lower portions of the body, which develops when spinal shock subsides, increases the danger of skin injury due to maceration. With loss of weight there is less soft-tissue padding over bony prominences. The interior of the cast

becomes damp from perspiration and soiled from urine and stool, irritating skin over bony prominences and at the edges of the cast.

17. (1) The patient should be informed in advance about the uncontrolled leg movements that develop when reflex activity returns, so he will not be deluded into thinking that the cord injury is healing and that his paralysis is reversible.

18. (2) Resolution of cord edema and congestion permits impulse transmission between the axons of one neuron and the dendrites of another within the cord substance, so that the deep tendon reflexes (such as ankle jerk and knee jerk) return.

19. (3) With return of reflex activity, reflex spasms occur in the paralyzed lower extremities. The spasms may be flexor or extensor, and result from the heightened sensitivity of the lower cord segment, which has been released from control by higher centers.

20. (1) With the return of reflex activity following resolution of spinal shock, certain "spinal automatisms" occur. These are primitive spinal reflexes that are usually kept inactive by the inhibition of higher centers. Two of these are reflex penile erection and ejaculation of semen on tactile stimulation of the lower abdomen or thigh.

21. (3) High protein intake is needed to provide amino acids for repair of decubiti. High bulk intake is advisable to stimulate peristalsis and prevent constipation. High vitamin intake is needed to increase the resistance of the skin and bladder mucosa to infection. High caloric foods should be given to compensate for depressive anorexia and to prevent weight loss.

22. (4) The elimination of large volumes of urine washes pathogens from the upper and lower urinary tract. A common source of ascending urinary tract infections is contamination of the indwelling catheter at the urinary meatus by growth of microorganisms in accumulated proteinaceous debris. The supine position favors stagnation of urine in the renal pelvis and vesicoureteral reflex of urine. Stagnation of urine fosters calculus formation and urinary infection. The automatic voiding reflex that returns with the reappearance of reflex activity can be stimulated by exerting gentle pressure over the bladder, or by stroking the lower abdomen or inner aspect of the thigh. Disconnection of the components of the continuous urinary drainage system permit introduction of pathogens from the nurse's hands.

23. (4) Fresh fruits and vegetables are high in fiber content. Prune or fig juice increases the acidity of the urine, preventing calculus formation. A regular routine of eating, drinking, and evacuating fosters automatic bowel emptying. Stimulating the anal or rectal wall initiates afferent impulses to the sacral cord, with reflex stimulation of strong peristaltic waves in the descending colon. Digital dilation of the external sphincter helps to initiate the defecation reflex.

24. (4) Prolonged tissue ischemia causes elevation of capillary pressure and death of cells in the ischemic tissue. Shearing force causes abrasion of superficial tissue. Placing the patient on an air mattress, padding bony prominences with lamb's wool, and changing position frequently minimizes ischemia of dependent tissues. Applying lotion to the skin over bony prominences, and keeping lower bed linen dry and unwrinkled, minimizes shearing force against the skin of these parts when the patient moves in bed.

25. (3) Following complete cord transection the blood pressure and temperature of the body parts innervated by the isolated segment of the cord fall, and they respond inadequately to reflex stimulation. Failure of reflex adjustments in vasomotor control following change from the supine to the upright position leads to orthostatic hypotension. Most of the eccrine sweat glands are innervated by cholinergic fibers. During the stage of spinal shock the patient does not perspire below the level of cord injury. Following return of reflex activity, he may perspire profusely in the body parts innervated by the isolated segment of cord.

26. (3) With complete cord transection the only type of bladder control possible is that achieved through reflex activity. Automatic bladder activity consists of periodic involuntary contraction of bladder muscle, through a mass reflex that can be stimulated by pricking or stroking a skin trigger point on the thigh, penis,

scrotum, or lower abdomen. Since the automatic bladder does not usually become distended to beyond 10 oz., and there is rarely more than 3–4 oz. of residual urine following reflex emptying, automatic bladder control is an acceptable form of control for the paraplegic patient.

27. (4) Twenty-five per cent of patients with complete cord transection experience pain in the body areas supplied by the isolated segment of cord. This is probably due to the irritation of a nerve root by scar tissue.

28. (4) Strong reflex spasms result from release of the isolated segment of cord from cortical control. The classic reflex spasm of the lower extremities is the withdrawal or defense reflex, with dorsiflexion of the great toe and ankle, flexion of the knee and hip, and adduction of the thigh.

29. (4) The withdrawal reflex can be elicited by application of noxious stimuli to the foot or leg, or even by minimal stimulation of the skin areas innervated by the isolated segment of cord.

30. (2) Inadequate dosage is thought to favor development of drug-resistant strains, because mutants are able to multiply rapidly during periods of low drug concentration.

31. (4) Normal fluid intake for the adult is about 1500–2500 cc (ml.)/day. 3000 ml./day represents a higher-than-normal fluid intake, which should increase renal blood flow, increase glomerular filtration rate, and prevent crystallization of the drug in the renal tubule.

32. (2) The more dilute the urine, the less is the danger that the drug will precipitate out of solution. Increased fluid intake provides a physiologic lavage of renal tubules and renal pelvis.

33. (1) Exposure of the skin to direct sunlight may precipitate or exaggerate the skin and mucosal irritations that sometimes develop as a result of hypersensitivity reactions to Gantrisin.

34. (3) A common side effect of pentazocine (Talwin) is dizziness, which may result from the fact that large doses of the drug cause an increase in blood pressure.

35. (3) Constipation and respiratory center depression are rare side effects. Although psychologic dependency may occur in patients with a predilection for drug abuse, pentazocine is a narcotic antagonist, and physical dependency is not known to occur.

36. (1) Steady employment enables the individual to be financially and psychologically independent. Acquiring such independence is a major psychologic task of young adulthood which, if resolved satisfactorily, contributes strongly to the individual's sense of autonomy and self-worth.

37. (3) Vitamin C is instrumental in collagen formation and capillary proliferation.

38. (1) Fresh or frozen fruits and vegetables are the best sources of vitamin C.

39. (3) Mechanical barriers, such as pus, blood, or necrotic tissue, prevent the "take" of a graft by interfering with vascular connections between the graft tissue and the underlying wound surface.

40. (3) When body tissues become depleted of protein, the plasma proteins are broken down into amino acids and utilized to build tissue proteins.

41. (3) Diazepam has both central and autonomic nervous system effects. It tranquilizes, decreases anxiety, sedates, relaxes skeletal muscle, and prevents convulsions.

42. (4) Drowsiness, ataxia, and tremor may result from CNS depression. Dizziness probably results from sympathetic depression.

43. (1) Nitrous oxide provides rapid and pleasant induction and recovery.

44. (1) The highest concentration of nitrous oxide that can safely be given a patient is 70 per cent; above this, hypoxia develops.

45. (1) When more than skin has been lost from a wound, fat, subcutaneous tissue, or other structures must be replaced to restore normal contour and prevent repeated breakdown; thus, a pedicle flap is required. The vessels of greatest importance to the successful transfer of a pedicle graft are relatively large vessels in the subdermal plexus. With a pedicle transfer graft the connection with the donor site is not severed until vascular continuity with the recipient site is well established, so capillary continuity is never completely interrupted.

46. (2) Wound drains prevent accumulation of serum or blood under the flap, which

would provide mechanical barriers to capillary and fibrous tissue growth between the recipient site and graft tissue.

47. (1) Some elements of dermis must be left for a skin defect to heal without grafting. A pedicle graft is composed of the full thickness of dermis, plus subcutaneous blood vessels and subcutaneous fat.

48. (4) The application of moderate pressure over a graft obliterates potential dead space beneath the graft. This ensures firm contact between the graft and the granulation tissue of the recipient site, so that capillaries can proliferate into the graft tissue, and oxygen and nutrients can diffuse from the underlying granulation tissue into the graft tissue.

49. (3) Continuous low pressure should be attached to the drainage catheter under a skin flap in order to remove any serum or blood as soon as it appears at the graft-wound interface, thereby preventing coagulation of the serum, which would form a mechanical barrier to capillary proliferation.

50. (4) Halothane, a general anesthetic, depresses both the myocardium and vascular smooth muscle, and decreases sympathetic nervous system activity. Systemic arterial blood pressure, myocardial contractile force, and peripheral arteriolar resistance are all reduced by administration of halothane in anesthetic concentrations.

51. (1) When one end of a pedicle flap is cut from the donor site and rotated to the recipient site, the blood vessels of the subcutaneous plexus are twisted and reduced somewhat in caliber. Venous spasm is a common reaction to mechanical trauma to the venous wall, and decreases the speed of blood flow through capillaries proximal to the narrowed vein. Sluggish capillary flow leads to greater-than-normal deoxygenation of the blood, with increased concentration of reduced hemoglobin, and cyanosis of tissues.

52. (3) Rough handling and sudden movement of extremities often trigger flexor and extensor spasms of the parts innervated by the isolated segment of cord. Sudden violent flexor spasms of the knee and hip would stress the sutures by which the graft is attached over the greater trochanter ulcer site.

53. (4) Infection interferes with graft "take" by interposing a barrier of pus and tissue debris between the graft and recipient site. Pressure compresses skin vessels, producing tissue ischemia. A liberal supply of oxygen and nutrients is required for wound healing. High protein, high vitamin, and high caloric intake facilitate wound healing by preventing tissue catabolism and fostering formation of collagen and capillaries in the healing wound. Exudate contains protein, which will clot.

54. (2) Although moderate pressure over a skin graft ensures proper contact of graft tissue with the recipient site, extreme pressure occludes blood vessels, depriving the tissue of oxygen and nutrients needed for wound healing.

55. (4) The capillaries that grow into graft tissue from the recipient site are extremely friable and relatively unsupported by connective tissue during the first week of healing.

56. (1) Denial is an unconscious defense mechanism by which the threats of reality are negated so as to avoid awareness of defects, deficiencies, and dangers.

57. (2) Cultural conditioning associated with toilet training creates a sense of shame concerning elimination behavior and handling of external genitalia.

58. (1) Itching is a form of pain sensation. Some paraplegics are able to experience pain in areas innervated by the isolated segment of the cord.

59. (4) The most common cause of death in the paraplegic is generalized sepsis secondary to a urinary tract infection or an infected decubitus. Self-care instruction should stress the need to inspect the skin of the back, buttocks, legs, and feet daily for evidence of pressure injury.

Arteriosclerotic Obliterative Disease and Femoral-Popliteal Bypass Graft

1. (3) The incidence of arteriosclerosis is increased in patients with diabetes mellitus as a result of deranged fat metabolism and hyperlipidemia. In hypertension, pressure injury of the arterial wall leads to deposition of hyalin beneath the

intima and narrowing of the vascular lumen. Nicotine is a sympathetic nervous system stimulant, causing vasoconstriction, tachycardia, and elevated blood pressure.

2. (3) In diabetes a lack of insulin causes decreased utilization of glucose by tissue cells, increased mobilization of fat from adipose tissue, deranged fat metabolism, increase in serum cholesterol levels, and deposition of cholesterol beneath the intima of arterioles and arteries.

3. (3) With the deposition of yellow fatty plaques below the intima of an artery or arteriole, the endothelial lining of the vessel is elevated and roughened. With narrowing of the vascular lumen, blood flow is slowed and platelets settle out, adhering to the roughened intima overlying the plaque. The platelets rupture, releasing thromboplastin, which catalyzes the conversion of prothrombin to thrombin, which converts fibrinogen to fibrin, which enmeshes blood cells to form a clot.

4. (4) Intermittent claudication, skin pallor, decreased skin temperature, and diminished dorsalis pedis, popliteal, and femoral pulses are usually apparent for some time before the peripheral pulses completely disappear.

5. (1) Intermittent claudication is cramping muscle pain that occurs with exercise and is relieved by rest. It indicates inadequate oxygen supply to contracting muscle.

6. (4) As a result of chronic arterial insufficiency, the skin of the feet and legs is malnourished and becomes thin, atrophic, and dry. The nails grow slowly, and become thickened and dry. Hair is sparse or absent on the toes and the dorsum of the foot as a result of poor skin nutrition. Thick calluses develop on the weight-bearing portions of the foot, and the skin of the toes and heels may become deeply fissured and infected.

7. (2) Rest pain is a serious symptom because it indicates that the arterial blood supply is insufficient even to meet the basal metabolic needs of tissues.

8. (2) Rest pain tends to be more severe at night, and may be relieved by placing the leg in a dependent position, since gravity enhances blood flow into the extremity.

9. (2) The common femoral artery, which is a continuation of the external iliac artery, arises at the inguinal ligament in the groin, where it lies only a few millimeters below the skin.

10. (3) The posterior tibial artery runs down the back of the leg and, after sending off the large peroneal artery to the lateral aspect of the leg, enters the bottom of the foot by running behind the medial malleolus.

11. (3) Lanolin is an emollient used to soften and moisturize dried, thickened skin so as to prevent cracking. Arteriosclerotic obliterative disease causes lowered skin temperature of the legs and feet, and predisposes to pressure sores over the heels and lateral malleoli. When the disease is severe the weight of the upper bed linen may increase the tendency for decubitus ulcer formation.

12. (4) In order to give informed consent for ateriography, the patient must understand the nature of the procedure and its possible consequences, which include: allergic reaction to the dye; dislodgement of a calcified plaque by passage of the catheter; thrombus formation over the arterial puncture site; perforation of a weakened arterial wall by the catheter tip; and major hemorrhage from the puncture site following the procedure.

13. (2) Most of the radiopaque iodine-containing dyes used in angiography are eliminated by the kidneys, and many of the preparations have an osmotic diuretic effect.

14. (4) The pedal blood pressure should be equal to or higher than the brachial artery pressure. Arterial blood pressure can be measured with a cuff or a mercury strain gauge plethysmograph in both thighs, lower legs, and feet. A gross blood pressure difference in the two limbs would suggest arterial disease in the limb with lowest pressure. The degree of pressure reduction in the thigh and lower leg would indicate the location and degree of arterial obstruction. In arteriosclerotic peripheral vascular disease, an exercise test would reveal a slowing of blood flow as calculated from the rate of disappearance of radioactive xenon injected directly into the calf muscle. The adequacy of arterial circulation in an extremity can be inferred by measuring skin temperature

changes in the involved extremity in response to enclosing the trunk in a heating cabinet, or immersing two uninvolved limbs in a warm water bath. A decrease in the amount of treadmill exercise required to produce claudication would indicate increasing arterial obstruction even if the physical appearance of the limb remains unchanged. Systolic bruits can often be heard over the femoral artery of a patient with arteriosclerotic obliterative disease, as a result of turbulent blood flow over atheromatous plaques.

15. (3) In the arterial system of an extremity there are collateral channels and vascular anastomoses that can carry arterial blood around a segmental occlusion.

16. (3) Relaxation of smooth muscle fibers in the arterial wall increases the vascular lumen. Certain adrenergic blocking agents are capable of relaxing smooth muscle spasm, but arteriosclerotic vessels are generally incapable of dilation. Following administration of a vasodilator, uninvolved arteries elsewhere in the body dilate, decreasing blood volume in the arteriosclerotic vessels and accentuating tissue ischemia in the involved extremity.

17. (2) Friction and maceration due to excessive moisture are apt to cause skin ulcers in an arteriosclerotic limb. This can be prevented by placement of cotton between the toes, and wearing wool stockings, which are more absorbent than cotton. The dye in colored hose can be irritating in hypersensitive persons.

18. (3) Many patients with intermittent claudication can walk farther without incurring pain after engaging in a regular program of moderate exercise. Regular walking up to, but not beyond, the point of pain increases the collateral circulation to an extremity.

19. (3) The dietary sources of cholesterol include egg yolk, organ meats, shellfish, and milk products.

20. (3) Most commercial sinus remedies and many commercial "cold" mixtures contain a vasoconstrictor, such as Neo-Synephrine, which would narrow collateral vessels in the involved extremities, further increasing tissue ischemia.

21. (4) Exposure to cold environments causes vasoconstriction of the feet and legs. The active ingredient of most corn remedies is salicylic acid, which dissolves the hardened outer layer of skin. Surface ulcerations heal slowly in patients with decreased arterial blood flow. Poorly perfused tissues are extremely susceptible to injury by excessive heat or friction and, once injured, are slow to heal. Sitting with the knees crossed exerts pressure on the popliteal artery, decreasing blood flow to the lower leg.

22. (3) As a result of elevated glucose concentration in body fluids and poor arterial circulation, diabetics are especially susceptible to infections of the feet and legs.

23. (4) Sudden, sharp pain in the leg would suggest complete occlusion of a major artery by a thrombus or embolus, probably necessitating surgical removal of the clot in order to salvage the limb. Dusky blue discoloration or darkening of the skin of the toe or foot suggests onset of gangrene. Numbness of the foot or leg may develop immediately following arterial occlusion as a result of ischemic neuritis. Drying and atrophy of ischemic skin leads to fissuring and infection. Decrease in arterial blood flow to a part causes pallor and coldness of peripheral tissues. Gradual increase in pallor would indicate progression of arteriosclerotic changes. Sudden onset of pallor would suggest thrombotic or embolic occlusion of an artery.

24. (4) Mr. Walker's symptoms of pallor, coldness, and rest pain of the right leg are indicative of severely decreased arterial flow. The most serious and most likely complication of arterial obstruction is gangrene, or massive tissue necrosis.

25. (2) Ninety per cent of patients who have had diabetes for at least ten years suffer peripheral neuritis, with decreased vibratory and fine touch sensation, which may progress to near-total anesthesia.

26. (4) Deep venous thrombosis, venous stagnation, and edema of the leg are apt to develop following femoral-popliteal repair. The purpose of elastic stockings is to compress superficial veins so as to increase flow through deep veins and prevent blood pooling and thrombosis. To be measured for elastic stockings, the patient should be placed in supine position with the leg slightly elevated, so that the leg will be free of edema when the measurements are taken.

27. (3) Following femoral-popliteal bypass surgery the patient is usually directed to

perform isometric muscle contractions, in order to stimulate blood flow through the graft and the arteries of the leg, and thus prevent intravascular thrombus formation.

28. (4) Iodine is one of the most effective chemical disinfectants available against a variety of bacteria, viruses, fungi, and spores and over a wide range of pH; it is unaffected by the presence of organic material.

29. (2) Since there is danger of scratching the skin during the preoperative shave, the razor and blade are apt to become contaminated with the patient's blood. Use of a disposable razor and blade prevents spread of the serum homologous hepatitis virus through contaminated equipment.

30. (2) The danger of hemorrhage from the femoral and popliteal artery suture lines is greatest during the first 2–3 days following surgery. Rough handling in moving a patient may provoke a startle reaction, with sudden movement of the extremities and tension on the vascular suture line. In a patient who has not fully recovered from the effects of a general anesthetic, the baroreceptor reflexes do not function efficiently. Subjecting such a patient to sudden changes in position may precipitate circulatory collapse.

31. (2) The oropharyngeal airway prevents the tongue from falling backward to obstruct the airway. The airway should be left in place until the patient begins to push it out of his mouth when he regains consciousness.

32. (3) A semicomatose patient should be placed on his side to facilitate drainage of secretions from the mouth and nose. Mr. Walker should be turned to his left side so that his right leg can be elevated on pillows, to minimize the edema that is common following femoral-popliteal repairs. The leg should be extended to prevent slowing of blood flow through the graft and other leg vessels, thus decreasing the danger of thrombus formation.

33. (1) The anesthesiologist who accompanies Mr. Walker to the Recovery Room will have detailed first-hand information about the type of surgery performed, the secondary diagnoses, the medicines and fluids given during the immediate preoperative and intraoperative periods, the length of the operation, the amount of blood loss, and the patient's general condition during surgery.

34. (2) One of the most serious complications following femoral-popliteal bypass surgery is thrombosis of the graft, which would obliterate the popliteal and dorsalis pedis pulses. If formerly palpable pulses disappear, the anastomosis may have to be re-explored.

35. (3) Changing the patient's position every 30–60 minutes causes redistribution of mucus in the lower respiratory tree, which stimulates cough and removal of the secretions. In the side-lying position, excursions of the dependent chest wall are limited by the firm surface of the mattress. Decreased chest expansion predisposes to collapse of dependent alveoli. A shunt is a bypass, or direct communication, between the venous and arterial circulation. Because of the effect of gravity, dependent portions of the lung are apt to be more adequately perfused than superior portions. When there is perfusion of inadequately ventilated alveoli, a portion of pulmonary blood is poorly aerated or unaerated before being returned to the left heart.

36. (3) The patient with obtunded gag reflex who is nauseated is apt to aspirate vomitus, unless positioned in a side-lying position so that vomitus can drain from the mouth easily.

37. (4) The capillary blanching or filling test consists of pressing a thumbnail against the patient's fingernail or toenail and then quickly releasing it. The normal response is blanching of the tissue under the nail with pressure, and return of a normal pink color when pressure is released.

38. (2) The fully conscious individual is oriented to person, place, and time, respectively. He will first be oriented to person, so can give his own name and recognize familiar persons in the environment; and then becomes oriented to place, so can remember that he is in the hospital and give its name.

39. (2) Deep inspiration lowers the intrathoracic pressure, which facilitates venous return to the right heart. Coughing loosens pooled respiratory secretions and impels them upward from the lower air passages toward the pharynx and mouth, so that they can be expectorated.

40. (1) For the first few hours after the bypass graft is inserted there is a reactive

hyperemia in the operated limb as a result of capillary dilation in chronically oxygen-deprived muscle and skin. Immediately following surgery, vasospasm may occur in the operated limb as a result of mechanical trauma during the operation, and this makes it difficult to palpate the dorsalis pedis pulse.

41. (2) The ejection of blood by each left ventricular contraction distends the aorta, creating a pulse wave that is transmitted throughout the arterial system, and is palpable at the radial artery slightly before it is palpable at the dorsalis pedis artery.

42. (4) Pulse rate may be indicative of cardiac pump efficiency, basal metabolic rate, hemoglobin concentration, or blood volume. Pulse rhythm is indicative of myocardial conductivity. Pulse volume may be indicative of myocardial contractile force, blood volume, or cardiac valvular efficiency. Pulse variability may indicate myocardial efficiency or drug toxicity. The speed with which the pulse wave rises and falls yields information about arterial elasticity.

43. (3) Edema frequently develops in the leg following femoral-popliteal repair. Extreme edema can embarrass arterial blood flow by compressing capillaries and arterioles.

44. (3) A slowing of blood flow permits cells to settle out of suspension, rupture, and initiate the clotting process.

45. (2) The risk of hemorrhage is greatest during the first day or two following bypass grafting. With massive hemorrhage there is sudden reduction in circulating blood volume, and consequent reduction in blood pressure.

46. (3) With internal bleeding from the vascular anastomosis, a clot could form in the perivascular tissues that could compress the vessel, causing arterial occlusion and ischemia of distal tissues. Poor capillary refilling on the toenail blanching test would indicate ischemia of the foot.

47. (3) The disappearance of a previously existing pulse suggests thrombotic occlusion of the vessel or graft.

48. (4) Adhesive tape is irritating to the skin and skin lesions heal with difficulty in patients with impaired arterial blood flow.

49. (1) The pathologic process in Mr. Walker's leg arteries is unchanged. Nicotine has a vasoconstrictive effect. Obesity accelerates atheromatous vascular degeneration.

50. (3) Intermittent claudication results from an imbalance between the oxygen demand of muscle tissue and the volume of arterial blood supply. Pain can be decreased by either decreasing the former or increasing the latter.

51. (4) Cold causes vasoconstriction.

52. (4) Increasing general body temperature will produce reflex vasodilation of collateral vessels in the extremity.

53. (2) Heat raises the metabolic rate of tissues and increases oxygen demand.

54. (2) Lanolin ointment softens and moisturizes the skin, preventing fissuring due to excessive drying of the skin and subcutaneous tissues.

Viral Hepatitis

1. (2) The liver is able to sequester large amounts of blood from the peripheral circulation, so its weight varies from 1.0 to 1.5 kg.

2. (1) The celiac artery arises from the front of the abdominal aorta just below the diaphragm, and divides into the common hepatic, left gastric, dorsal pancreatic, and splenic arteries.

3. (2) The splenic vein, carrying venous blood from the spleen and pancreas, joins with the superior mesenteric vein, carrying blood from the small intestine and the right colon, and with the left gastric vein, carrying blood from the stomach and esophagus, to form the portal vein.

4. (2) The normal arterial pO_2 is 95 mm. Hg. The normal venous pO_2 is 40 mm. Hg. About 1100 ml. of portal blood enters the liver each minute. About 350 ml. of arterial blood enters the liver each minute through the hepatic artery. The mean arterial pressure in the aorta is about 100 mm. Hg. The mean arterial pressure in arteries as small as 3 mm. in diameter is about 95–97 mm. Hg. The

pressure continues to decrease as the blood flows through the capillaries, venules, and portal vein.

5. (1) The mixture of hepatic arterial and portal blood in the sinusoid flows toward the center of the lobule, enters the central vein, joins with blood from other lobules to be carried to the hepatic vein, and empties into the inferior vena cava.

6. (4) In hepatitis, liver cells die and are replaced by fibrous scar tissue. Regeneration of new liver tissue occurs, but normal liver architecture is destroyed and the new liver cells have an inefficient relationship to the arterial and venous blood supplies, so the new parenchymal cells are poorly oxygenated and unable to carry out their metabolic functions efficiently. Failure of the damaged liver to produce serum globulin decreases resistance to infection. Hepatic fibrosis obstructs portal blood flow through the liver, increasing pressure in the portal circulation and causing venous engorgement of the stomach and bowel, which predisposes to vomiting, impaired absorption, and diarrhea. Prolonged vomiting results in significant loss of hydrogen and chloride ions, producing alkalosis. Prolonged diarrhea results in significant losses of potassium and bicarbonate ions, causing hypopotassemia and acidosis. Renal changes associated with hepatocellular damage cause poor sodium excretion by the kidney, increased potassium losses through the tubule, and increased formation of ammonia, some of which is absorbed from the tubule and enters the systemic circulation. Ammonia is toxic to nervous tissue, producing disturbed mentation and clouding of consciousness.

7. (4) The splenic, left gastric, and superior mesenteric veins join to form the portal vein. The inferior mesenteric vein empties into either the splenic or the superior mesenteric vein. Venous blood from the rectum, sigmoid, and descending colon is carried by the inferior mesenteric vein to the splenic vein, and thence to the portal vein. Venous blood from the stomach and esophagus is carried by the left gastric vein to the portal vein.

8. (2) The sinusoids surround parenchymal cells and are lined with epithelial cells, which permit movement of substances back and forth between the blood in the sinusoid and the liver cell. In other body tissues, nutrients, electrolytes, oxygen, and carbon dioxide are exchanged between the tissue capillaries and the interstitial fluids bathing the cells.

9. (3) Branches of both the hepatic artery and the portal vein supply blood to the sinusoids.

10. (2) Some monocytes drop out of the circulation, become fixed to the tissues, and perform phagocytic activities from their fixed positions. The Kupffer cells are one example of a fixed-tissue macrophage.

11. (4) Bile consists of water, bile salts, bilirubin, cholesterol, fatty acids, lecithin, and small amounts of electrolytes. The function of bile salts in the small intestine is to break fat globules into minute particles so as to increase the surface area of fat to be acted upon by lipases.

12. (4) Acute viral hepatitis can be caused by either of two viruses: type A, or infectious hepatitis virus, which is usually spread by fecal-oral transmission; and type B, or homologous serum hepatitis virus, which is usually spread by parenteral transmission.

13. (2) Although SH virus can probably be spread by the fecal-oral route under conditions of poor sanitation, the usual mode of spread is through the blood. Needles and instruments contaminated with the blood or serum of infected individuals have been responsible for causing serum hepatitis.

14. (3) Hepatitis A virus produces short incubation hepatitis (15–60 days). Hepatitis B virus produces long incubation hepatitis (50–150 days).

15. (2) Bromsulphalein and indocyanine green are dyes used in excretion tests to estimate the extent of liver function. The BSP test is more sensitive than the ICG test. The dyes are administered intravenously, removed from the blood by the parenchymal cells, and excreted in the bile. Increased retention of the dye in the blood after a given period is indicative of obstructive or hepatocellular disease.

16. (2) The characteristic lesion in viral hepatitis A or B is liver parenchymal cell degeneration and necrosis, with inflammatory cell infiltration and cell regeneration.

17. (2) SGOT and SGPT are more highly elevated in acute hepatitis than in obstructive jaundice, in contradistinction to alkaline phosphatase, which is more highly elevated in obstructive jaundice than in acute hepatitis. SGPT is an enzyme that catalyzes the reversible transfer of an amino group from glutamine to pyruvic acid. It is found in relatively high concentrations in liver tissue and relatively low concentrations in myocardial and other tissues. It is released into the serum in large quantities as a result of necrosis of parenchymal liver cells. The normal serum concentration of SGPT ranges from 6 to 36 Karmen units per milliliter. Patients with viral hepatitis and other types of hepatic necrosis show marked elevation of SGPT (500–4000 U.). SGPT is only moderately elevated (300 U.) in intrahepatic cholestasis and cirrhosis. SGOT and SGPT are maximally elevated in the late prodromal and early icteric stages of hepatitis.

18. (1) GGT is markedly elevated in biliary tract obstruction, slightly elevated in myocardial infarction, and normal in necrosis of skeletal muscle.

19. (4) Intrahepatic obstruction occurs during the icteric stage of infectious hepatitis. Edema and necrosis of the parenchymal liver cells disrupt the bile canaliculi, which become dilated and filled with bile plugs. If bile flow through the canaliculus is completely obstructed, bile does not find its way to the intestine, but leaks back through damaged parenchymal cells into the sinusoids and appears in the systemic circulation.

20. (3) In hepatitis, parenchymal liver cells are edematous and necrotic. Necrotic liver cells are unable to remove free bilirubin from the serum and conjugate it with glucuronic acid. Inflammatory obstruction of canaliculi causes conjugated bilirubin to leak back through damaged parenchymal cells into the sinusoid, to be carried to the systemic circulation. Infectious hepatitis virus may cause cellular damage to kidney as well as hepatic tissue, producing a functional renal failure with progressive oliguria, azotemia, hyperkalemia, and hyponatremia.

21. (4) Glucuronyl transferase is the enzyme that catalyzes the conjugation of free bilirubin with glucuronic acid in the liver cell.

22. (1) An antigen is a protein or protein-polysaccharide complex that provokes formation of gamma globulin antibodies by the B lymphocytes. For a substance to be antigenic, it must have a high molecular weight — at least 8000 or greater.

23. (2) An antibody is a high-molecular gamma globulin having a specific amino acid sequence that gives it the ability to adhere to and interact with the antigen that induced its synthesis.

24. (1) A virus is a submicroscopic infectious agent consisting of nucleic acid in association with a protein. The virus molecule is an obligate parasite, so can replicate only within a living cell.

25. (4) In many patients infectious hepatitis may present as an influenza-like illness with fever, sore throat, enlarged lymph nodes, migratory arthritis, urticaria, and right upper abdominal pain.

26. (2) SH virus is spread chiefly by parenteral means, but it may be excreted in the stool, so fecal-oral means of transmission are possible. Hands are the greatest source of cross-infections for all pathogens spread by interpersonal contact. Handwashing is the single most effective means of preventing the spread of infection.

27. (1) Constipation, pulmonary infections, thrombophlebitis, and decubitus ulcers are common complications of prolonged bedrest. Increased fluid intake increases the water content of the food bolus, thereby increasing intestinal bulk and stimulating propulsive peristalsis; liquefies lung secretions, causing them to move more freely with changes in position, which stimulates cough and encourages removal of secretions; and increases general body hydration. An increase in circulating blood volume increases mean arterial blood pressure, which is the driving force behind blood flow. Increased skin turgor improves the skin's ability to withstand pressure injury.

28. (3) Research has indicated that high carbohydrate, high protein diet is protective of liver tissue. A high protein intake is required to provide the amino acids needed for liver cell regeneration to replace necrotic liver tissue. High carbohydrate intake is needed to force deposition of glycogen in liver parenchy-

mal cells, as glycogen stores seem to increase the cell's resistance to damage by the SH virus.

29. (2) In infectious hepatitis the diet should be moderate-to-low in fat content; fried foods should be avoided. During the obstructive phase of infectious hepatitis, little bile is secreted into the small bowel, so fat emulsification and absorption is limited.

30. (3) From 1800 to 2500 ml. of fluid are required daily by a normal, nonsweating, healthy adult at rest in order to provide for normal urinary excretion and to replace fluid lost by insensible perspiration. The febrile patient with an acute inflammatory illness requires a fluid intake above normal to maintain cellular hydration in the face of evaporative water losses, and to maintain sufficient renal blood flow and pressure to rid the body of increased metabolic wastes resulting from the infectious process.

31. (3) The icteric phase of hepatitis is that period early in the illness when a yellowish discoloration of skin and sclera is apparent. Icterus occurs when the level of serum bilirubin is so high that either free or conjugated bilirubin appears in the extracellular fluid.

32. (2) The normal plasma concentration of total bilirubin is about 0.5 mg./100 ml. of plasma. The skin begins to appear icteric when the serum bilirubin reaches about three times normal, or 1.5 mg./100 ml. of serum.

33. (3) Most hepatitis patients experience a few nonspecific symptoms such as fatigue, nausea, abdominal discomfort, rash, and arthralgia from 7 to 10 days before the appearance of jaundice, pruritus, and dark urine.

34. (4) In the aged, tissue anoxia due to circulatory impairment is the factor that leads to damage of epithelial cells, release of proteases and peptidases, and development of the itching sensation. In patients who perspire profusely, the excessive concentrations of sodium, chloride, urea, lactic acid, or potassium ions in the sweat may damage epithelial cells, releasing proteases, and initiating the itch sensation. The neural control of skin blood vessels is mediated through the sympathetic nervous system. Emotional stress may provoke sympathetic overactivity, with constriction of skin vessels which, if prolonged, may lead to tissue anoxia, with release of the chemical mediators that trigger the itch sensation. The dry skin of the aged patient is more than usually sensitive to irritation by strongly alkaline soaps. Acidosis is characterized by an accumulation of excess lactic acid in body tissues, which may damage epithelial tissues, releasing the proteases that initiate the itch sensation.

35. (2) Drying of the skin can be responsible for pruritus, so treatment consists of infrequent bathing and liberal use of emollients. Since scratching damages the epidermis, releasing histamine and proteases that initiate the itch sensation, the nails should be clipped short to discourage scratching. Hot, dry air has a drying effect on the skin and initiates mild itching sensations to which the patient may respond by scratching. A properly air-conditioned and humidified environment minimizes itch sensation. A given itch stimulus results in much greater subjective perception of itching in a patient who is tired, upset, or bored than in one who is well rested, comfortable, and engaged in a pleasurable activity.

36. (1) Cholestyramine has an affinity for bile acids, so when given orally it combines with and increases the fecal excretion of bile acids, and thus relieves pruritus in jaundiced patients.

37. (4) In infectious hepatitis, jaundice becomes most severe about two weeks after the onset (of jaundice), then gradually subsides and disappears over a period of six weeks.

38. (2) The hepatitis B antigen consists of two parts: a core antigen and a surface antigen (HB_cAg and HB_sAg), and each promotes formation of a corresponding antibody. Although a dose of pooled gamma globulin protects exposed subjects against hepatitis A, pooled gamma globulin does not generally confer protection against hepatitis B because it usually does not contain significant hepatitis B antibody. If a preparation of pooled gamma globulin can be found that contains a high concentration of antibodies against hepatitis B core antigen, however, administration of that mixture would probably confer protection against homologous serum jaundice.

39. (4) Chlorpromazine causes obstructive jaundice in 4 per cent of patients, probably as a result of a hypersensitivity reaction involving hepatic parenchymal cells. Chlordiazepoxide has produced jaundice and hepatic dysfunction in patients on long-term therapy. Large doses of tetracycline may cause fatty infiltration of liver cells and hepatic dysfunction. Barbiturates increase the activity of hepatic enzyme systems responsible for the biotransformation of various organic compounds. Some patients suffer severe hepatic damage due to hypersensitivity to phenobarbital. Methyldopa causes cholestasis and jaundice in a small percentage of patients.

40. (2) The normal liver cell utilizes vitamin K to synthesize prothrombin. In fulminating hepatitis all of the parenchymal liver cells are edematous or necrotic, and thus unable to synthesize prothrombin even when vitamin K is given parenterally.

41. (2) Prolonged confinement is extremely stressful for a young adult accustomed to an active life and considerable geographic mobility. Skin discoloration is extremely stressful because of the tendency of the young toward self-consciousness in respect to physical appearance. A nurse may feel guilty about acquiring an infectious disease through possible neglect of proper aseptic technique.

42. (3) The most effective means of reducing hepatic workload is to decrease the activities of all other body tissues, since the volume of the liver's regulatory, protective, and metabolic activities is directly proportional to the body's muscular and glandular activities. A high carbohydrate, high protein, high vitamin diet is required to facilitate regeneration of hepatic cells damaged by the virus. Increased fluid intake is needed to foster resolution of the inflammatory reaction in liver cells, and to replace fluid lost due to fever and diaphoresis. Emotional stress must be minimized if the patient is to achieve the mental and physical rest necessary for resolution of the acute inflammatory reaction.

43. (2) When a would-be donor is found to be HB_sAg positive, liver function tests and a liver biopsy should be performed to determine whether the individual has associated liver disease or is a carrier of the disease. The healthy carrier should be prevented from donating blood.

44. (4) Since hepatitis B is spread primarily through parenteral means, but occasionally through the fecal-oral route, efforts must be made to identify victims and carriers of hepatitis B virus and to avoid contact with their blood, serum, feces, and secretions.

45. (1) Some of the gamma globulins are synthesized in normal liver cells. Until liver cell regeneration is complete, serum globulin concentration is apt to be decreased, causing increased susceptibility to infection.

46. (2) Hepatitis A and hepatitis B are caused by different, immunologically distinct viruses.

Polycystic Kidney and Renal Failure

1. (3) Glomerular filtration rate is decreased when hypovolemia develops as a result of severe fluid loss through hyperpyrexia, vomiting, and diarrhea. Fever, anorexia, and nausea are symptoms of influenza.

2. (1) A flat plate of the abdomen reveals enlarged or displaced kidneys that contain areas of varying densities.

3. (3) Much of the discomfort associated with cystoscopy results from the painful bladder spasms provoked by introduction of the cystoscope. Progressive muscular relaxation and deep breathing exercises will decrease smooth muscle tension and minimize discomfort.

4. (1) Passage of the cystoscope through the neck of the bladder, and distention of the bladder with water, provoke the desire to void by stimulating the sensory limb of the micturition reflex.

5. (4) The patient is placed in lithotomy position with his legs in stirrups during cystoscopy. Removal of the legs from stirrups at the end of the procedure causes rapid redistribution of circulating blood volume. Since the barorecep-

tors respond less rapidly to a falling blood pressure than to a rising blood pressure, orthostatic hypotension may result.

6. (3) Fluid is withheld for eight hours prior to the study to create relative dehydration to facilitate concentration of the dye in the kidney. Food is withheld because some patients develop nausea and vomiting following dye injection. Cathartics or cleansing enemas are used to remove gas and fecal material from the bowel, so as to afford better x-ray visualization of the kidney and lower urinary tract. Ben should be asked about previous reactions to iodine-containing drugs, because some patients with iodine allergy develop anaphylactoid shock following intravenous injection of iodine compounds.

7. (7) Intravenous administration of iodine produces sudden, brief vasodilation. A mild, short-lasting sensation of warmth, a flushing of the face, or a salty taste in the mouth may be experienced upon intravenous injection of the dye.

8. (4) Anaphylaxis is an acute allergic reaction to ingestion of a foreign protein to which the body tissues have become sensitized. The antigen-antibody complex causes release of histamine, which produces widespread vasodilation, loss of fluid and protein from the vessels, diaphoresis, urticaria and itching, fall in blood pressure, and transudation of fluid into pulmonary alveoli and joint spaces.

9. (3) One tenth of the water in the blood that is circulated to the glomerulus is filtered and and passes into the tubule. Of the 120 ml. of water filtered each minute by the glomerulus, approximately 119 ml. are resorbed as the filtrate passes along the tubule, so the urine concentration test is a test of the efficiency of tubular function.

10. (1) Water is passively resorbed from the renal tubules, whereas most solutes in the tubular filtrate are resorbed by the mechanism of active transport. In hyperhydration, renal tubular cells actively and selectively absorb solute so as to maintain normal serum concentration of each substance and leave most of the water in the tubules to be excreted in the urine. In dehydration, tubular cells eliminate as many metabolic waste products as possible, while at the same time resorbing as much water as possible through means of a countercurrent mechanism of continuous sodium recycling between interstitial fluid and tubular lumen. The standard concentration dilution test measures the ability of the kidney to vary water excretion with the state of body hydration.

11. (4) Normal adults on normal diets with normal fluid intake produce urine of a specific gravity of about 1.016–1.022 during a 24-hour period. Ben's urine specific gravity after taking no fluids for 24 hours should range from 1.020 to 1.035.

12. (3) Phenolsulfonphthalein is a red dye excreted by the renal tubules. The rate at which the dye appears in the urine is dependent on the rate of renal blood flow and the rate at which fluid moves through the tubules, pelvis, and ureter to the bladder. Severe renal disease impairs both renal blood flow and tubular secretion, and reduces excretion of the dye.

13. (2) Normally, 30 per cent of the injected phenolsulfonphthalein is excreted within 15 minutes following intravenous injection. Excretion of less than 30 per cent indicates reduction in renal blood flow. Determination of the amount of dye excreted per unit of time requires knowledge of both the urinary concentration of the dye and the exact amount of urine excreted.

14. (2) As filtrate accumulates and stagnates in the dilated tubules, it becomes secondarily infected. The fluid-filled cysts compress adjacent renal parenchyma, compressiong blood vessels and embarrassing blood supply to the organ.

15. (2) Elevated blood pressure causes headache through increase in intracranial pressure and tension on pain-sensitive structures adjacent to cerebral arteries. Dizziness may result from nervous tissue anoxia secondary to cerebral artery vasoconstriction.

16. (3) With decreased glomerular filtration, nonprotein nitrogen, urea, and creatinine accumulate in the serum. Urea is excreted in sweat, saliva, and intestinal fluid. Mouth bacteria convert some of the urea in saliva to ammonia, causing decreased salivation, a metallic taste in the mouth, and irritation and ulceration of oral and gastric mucosa.

17. (2) The edema of congestive heart failure is due to a combination of sodium and

water retention and increased hydrostatic pressure in the veins; edema of cardiac origin is thus gravity-dependent. The edema of chronic renal failure is due to albuminuria, hypoproteinemia, decreased colloid osmotic pressure of the plasma, and transudation of excess water into interstitial spaces; the edema of renal failure is thus generalized.

18. (1) In the normal kidney, hypoxia of renal medullary tissues causes release of erythropoietin which, when carried to the bone marrow, stimulates red blood cell production. With destruction of renal parenchyma in end-stage kidney disease, erythropoietin production is decreased, and fewer red blood cells are produced by the marrow.

19. (2) Erythropoietin stimulates production of all blood cells formed in bone marrow: red blood cells, granulocytic white blood cells, and platelets. Decreased erythropoietin production by a diseased kidney results in decreased thrombocytes as well as decreased red blood cells.

20. (2) The ammoniacal odor in uremia is due to bacterial conversion of the urea in saliva to ammonia. Ammonia irritates the mucosa, causing ulcers that tend to become infected. Frequent cleansing of the mouth with alkaline mouthwashes decreases oral infection and relieves the ammoniacal breath odor.

21. (2) Potassium is excreted from the body by secretion into the urine through distal tubular cells. When urine output falls below 500–1000 ml./day in renal decompensation, serum potassium levels increase.

22. (3) The bicarbonate ion is an important extracellular buffer against sudden changes in hydrogen ion concentration, in that it combines with hydrogen ions when they are in excess concentration in body fluids, or releases hydrogen ions when they are deficient. The normal plasma bicarbonate level is 24–28 mEq./L. Ben's plasma bicarbonate level was decreased, reflecting his metabolic acidosis.

23. (4) Renal tubular failure leads to retention of hydrogen ions, ammonium ions, and phosphate ions. Excess hydrogen ions in the blood interfere with normal nerve function, producing lethargy, mental clouding, depression, and drowsiness deepening into coma. Renal retention of phosphate leads to a decrease in blood calcium levels, with muscle twitching and convulsions.

24. (2) Anoxia of renal parenchyma causes release of the enzyme renin, which reacts with circulating angiotensinogen to release angiotensin, a potent vasopressor and stimulator of aldosterone production. Long-standing hypertension weakens the walls of cerebral arteries, so that sudden elevation of blood pressure may cause cerebral hemorrhage. In uremia, urea is present in all body fluids. Uremic pericarditis, which is due to irritation of the pericardium by urea present in pericardial fluid, may be characterized by a fibrinous pericardial exudate or an outpouring of pericardial fluid. Either hypertension, by increasing left ventricular workload, or pericardial effusion, by mechanical interference with myocardial contraction, may precipitate congestive heart failure.

25. (4) Excess hydrogen ions in body fluids interfere with normal brain metabolism, producing irritability and confusion. Anemia, due to marrow depression, and malnutrition, due to anorexia, produce easy fatigability in uremic patients. Acidosis and electrolyte imbalances cause demyelinization and axonal degeneration of peripheral nerves, with progressive numbness, tingling, and burning of the lower extremities. Ammonia causes irritation of the gastrointestinal mucosa, with anorexia, nausea, and vomiting.

26. (3) The normal pH of the serum is 7.35–7.45. A pH lower than normal indicates an excess of hydrogen ions. The normal plasma bicarbonate level is 24–28 meq./L. A decrease in pH together with a decrease in plasma bicarbonate indicates metabolic acidosis.

27. (2) The carbon dioxide and water produced by tissue metabolism combines to form carbonic acid, which dissociates into hydrogen ions and bicarbonate ions. In the normal lung, hydrogen ions and bicarbonate ions recombine to form carbon dioxide and water. The carbon dioxide diffuses into the alveoli and is removed by exhalation, as is part of the water.

28. (3) In uremia the concentration of urea is elevated on all body fluids. The enzyme urease present in bacteria converts urea to ammonia. Free ammonia is highly toxic to cells, causing protein denaturation and cell death.

29. (3) Potassium, the main intracellular cation, is excreted from the body through secretion by renal tubular cells. Muscle and nerve membrane potential depend on the ratio of intracellular to extracellular potassium ion concentration. Neuromuscular irritability is increased in slight hyperkalemia and reduced in severe hyperkalemia. Irritability of myocardial cells leads to cardiac arrhythmias. Severe hyperkalemia produces severe muscle weakness. The tubular secretory mechanism is related to the mechanism for hydrogen ion secretion. When the potassium to be secreted is high it prevents removal of surplus acids from the body, producing hyperkalemic acidosis, with peripheral nerve dysfunction and paresthesias.

30. (3) When the diseased kidney is unable to excrete urea, the concentration of urea in all body fluids increases. The excretion of urates by the sweat glands leads to crystallization of urates on the skin.

31. (3) Urea or ammonia in either the pericardial or the pleural fluids cause irritation of the serosa (pericardium or pleura), with production of fibrinous exudate and friction rubs.

32. (3) Furosemide is a sulfonamide with a rapid and strong diuretic effect, which is due to decreased sodium resorption in the proximal tubule and ascending loop of Henle.

33. (2) The onset of diuresis occurs 30–60 minutes following administration of furosemide. The duration of effect is about four hours.

34. (2) Furosemide also causes a high rate of chloride excretion, and so may cause hypochloremic alkalosis. Alkalosis is characterized by neuromuscular irritability, with muscle weakness and cramps, and disturbances of nerve impulse transmission, with numbness and tingling.

35. (3) Methyldopa inhibits dopa decarboxylase, an enzyme that catalyzes the conversion of dopa to dopamine, which is a precursor of epinephrine.

36. (3) Methyldopa causes nasal stuffiness, due to the vascular dilation that occurs following removal of the norepinephrine effect.

37. (4) Phosphates are retained by the patient with chronic renal failure. Phosphate concentration is inversely related to calcium concentration, so phosphate retention causes a decrease in ionized serum calcium and bone demineralization. Aluminum hydroxide gel (Amphojel) interferes with absorption of phosphates from the intestine, and so provides an alternate route for phosphorus excretion.

38. (1) Surplus protein is catabolized to produce heat and energy. Amino acids are deaminated by the liver, and the nitrogen is converted first to ammonia then to urea, which is normally excreted by the kidney. The damaged kidney cannot eliminate urea in normal quantities and so it accumulates in body fluids, causing acidosis and electrolyte derangements. Limiting dietary protein intake causes a decrease in urea production.

39. (2) Marked dietary protein restriction may be ordered when blood nitrogen levels are highly elevated. On a 30-gram protein diet, meat, fish, milk, and milk products are omitted.

40. (2) If the dietary caloric intake is too low to support cellular metabolism, body protein will be catabolized as an energy source, creating a surplus of urea and other nitrogenous wastes to be excreted by the kidney.

41. (4) The 1000-mg. sodium diet requires that no salt be added during cooking or at table; that only one slice of buttered bakery bread be eaten per day; and that all processed meats, canned meats, canned vegetables, condiments, cheese, and bakery products be avoided.

42. (2) Salt and sodium nitrite are used in preparing smoked meats. Condiments and relishes contain salt and monosodium glutamate. Peas and lima beans are salted in preparation for freezing.

43. (4) Baking powder contains sodium acid carbonate. Sodium propionate is a commonly used food preservative. Monosodium glutamate is a commonly used flavor enhancer. Sodium citrate is a common ingredient of cough mixtures.

44. (3) Potassium is an ingredient in most foods. It occurs in high concentration in all foods on the list but vegetable oil.

45. (3) In peritoneal dialysis the dialysate is instilled into the peritoneal cavity and the peritoneum is used as the dialyzing membrane, allowing small molecular solutes to filter from the blood into the dialysate on a concentration gradient.

Some albumin, which is a relatively small molecular weight protein, may pass through the peritoneal membrane during dialysis and be lost in the dialysate. Albumin does not pass through the pores in the cellophane membrane used in the hemodialyzer. The patient with chronic renal disease may already suffer from hypoalbuminemia, and so further loss of albumin should be avoided if possible.

46. (2) Diffusion is the tendency of particles in solution to move about until they are distributed equally throughout the solution. When separating two solutions of differing osmotic concentrations, a semipermeable membrane will permit passage of certain smaller molecules from areas of greater concentration to areas of lesser concentration so as to equalize concentration of the substance on either side of the membrane.

47. (3) Original sources of information are more reliable than secondary sources.

48. (1) A written consent is required for any diagnostic or therapeutic procedure that involves entering a body cavity and has potential for complications. Ben can give informed consent only if he understands exactly what the procedure consists of and what complications may arise.

49. (2) Hypovolemia and shock may result from too rapid removal of fluid during dialysis. Ben's blood pressure and pulse rate should be measured before dialysis begins, to obtain baseline data against which to compare blood pressure and pulse measurements during treatment. He should be weighed before and after dialysis to determine the amount of fluid removed during the procedure.

50. (3) Since the shunt necessitates a break in the skin through which pathogens may enter the cannulated blood vessels, the tubing and the skin surrounding the exit wound should be disinfected daily, and covered with antibiotic ointment and a sterile dressing. The distal loop of the shunt should be left uncovered so that it can be checked regularly for patency.

51. (2) Separation of the shunt tubing from the plastic connector would produce rapid and major blood loss. Two cannula clamps should be affixed to the patient's person to be immediately available to occlude the tubing if the two limbs of the shunt should accidentally become disconnected.

52. (3) The shunting of blood from an artery to a vein creates increased force and velocity of blood flow in the vein, with development of a palpable thrill over the venous limb of the shunt.

53. (1) If Ben is severely uremic at the time of dialysis, osmotic disequilibrium may develop during treatment owing to changing concentrations of fluid, electrolyte, and waste. These symptoms usually abate a few hours after dialysis has been concluded, when the patient has adjusted to lower concentrations of the involved ions and molecules.

54. (2) If molecules and fluid are removed too rapidly from the vascular compartment, the decrease in blood volume can cause precipitous decline in mean arterial pressure, with inadequate perfusion of the brain, myocardium, liver, and kidney.

55. (2) Sudden decline in blood pressure would produce hypovolemic shock. Rapid weak pulse could indicate hemorrhage, shock, or congestive heart failure.

56. (4) If the dialyzer coil were to break and the blood loss were undetected, Ben could rapidly become exsanguinated. Edematous and malnourished patients are especially susceptible to ischemia and skin breakdown over pressure points. Nervous and gastrointestinal disorders are common symptoms of the disequilibrium syndrome that can develop as a result of fluid-electrolyte-waste imbalances during dialysis. Instruction regarding potassium, protein, and fluid restriction should be repeated several times to ensure that Ben understands the purpose of each dietary restriction and is completely familiar with details of the prescribed diet.

57. (4) Hypovolemia causes a decline in mean arterial pressure and brain ischemia. Inadequate oxygenation of cerebral tissues causes anxiety, restlessness, and dizziness. Reflex stimulation of the medullary cardiac center produces tachycardia. Reflex stimulation of the sympathetic nervous system causes diaphoresis.

58. (1) If Ben's blood pressure drops suddenly as a result of hypovolemia, his head should be lowered to minimze cerebral anoxia and the physician should be

summoned. It may be necessary to change the composition of the dialysate so as to decrease the speed of fluid removal, or to administer normal saline intravenously so as to restore functional blood volume.

59. (4) The osmotic disequilibrium created by more rapid removal of urea from the blood to the dialyzer than from the brain to the blood results in movement of water from the blood vessels into brain tissue. Increased intracranial pressure causes headache due to stretching of sensitive tissues around brain arteries; restlessness and confusion due to impaired cerebral functioning; convulsions due to irritation of motor cortex; and vomiting due to stimulation of the emetic center in the medulla.

60. (4) Comparison of pre- and postdialysis weights will indicate the total fluid loss during dialysis. Comparison of pre- and postdialysis blood chemistry values will reveal the efficacy of dialysis in lowering potassium, phosphate, urea, and creatinine. The needle puncture site should be disinfected and covered with a sterile pressure dressing to prevent hemorrhage. Long hours of immobility could have led to skin damage over bony pressure points, especially if the skin was wet with perspiration. If Ben was nauseated during the procedure as a result of osmotic disequilibrium, he may have vomited or omitted a meal. Adherence to the prescribed diet is an important aspect of care for the patient with chronic kidney disease.

61. (4) Constriction or compression of the arm through any means decreases the speed of blood flow through the arteriovenous fistula, and predisposes to thrombobus formation by the blood cells that settle out of suspension. Mechanical trauma to the wall of the fistula causes inflammation and roughening, with rupture of thrombocytes and initiation of the clotting reaction.

62. (2) Denial is a mental mechanism by which the reality of one's circumstances is negated so as to prevent personality disintegration as a consequence of overwhelming threat.

63. (3) Impotence frequently develops in the patient with chronic renal failure as a result of generalized toxicity and impaired neurologic function.

64. (4) The multiplicity and magnitude of problems faced by the patient in chronic renal failure creates major stress in all spheres of daily life. Although Ben must ultimately solve his own problems, he would profit from professional counseling assistance as he grapples with the progressive nature of his illness; the high cost of treatment; the decrease in physical strength; the loss of libido and potency; and the major changes required in habits of diet, drinking, activity, and mobility.

65. (1) As a result of differences in physical status and variations in social and psychologic support systems, not every patient in renal failure is a suitable candidate for renal transplantation. In order to set realistic long-term treatment goals for Ben's care following hospital discharge, the nurse must know whether he is to be dialyzed for the remainder of his life or has been placed on an eligibility list for kidney transplant.

Pancreatitis and Pancreatic Pseudocyst

1. (1) A large intake of alcohol stimulates increased hydrochloric acid secretion by the gastric glands. The resulting hyperacidity of duodenal contents stimulates increased secretion of secretin and pancreozymin, with increased production of pancreatic enzymes and increased volume of pancreatic juice. Occasionally a gallstone migrates from the common bile duct, becomes impacted in the ampulla of Vater, causes reflex of bile into the pancreatic duct, and produces bile activation of pancreatic enzymes.

2. (2) Pancreatitis develops in patients with kwashiorkor, a condition of severe protein deficiency occurring in the presence of sufficient caloric intake.

3. (3) Corticosteroids and chlorothiazide sometimes produce pancreatitis, presumably as a result of an allergic reaction of pancreatic tissue to the drug.

4. (3) Trypsinogen is the inactive precursor of trypsin, a proteolytic enzyme which, when released within the pancreas, lyses pancreatic cells, causing pancreatic necrosis and liquefaction. With extensive autodigestion of glandular tissue

and blood vessels, the pancreatic capsule is eventually perforated, and activated enzymes escape into the peritoneal cavity.

5. (1) The pancreas is located behind the peritoneum. Severe inflammation of pancreatic tissue causes exudation of fluid into the retroperitoneal space. Chemical irritation of the posterior layer of the parietal peritoneum results in pain that is referred to the back and shoulder.

6. (4) Epigastric pain may result from a bleeding peptic ulcer, which would also cause hematemesis and melena. Right upper quadrant pain may result from common duct stone, which would also cause fatty food intolerance, belching, and jaundice.

7. (1) Alcohol stimulates the parietal cells of the stomach to increased secretion of hydrochloric acid. Highly acid chyme results ultimately in increased amounts of pancreozymin, which stimulates increased production of pancreatic enzymes. Alcohol causes duodenitis, with edema or spasm of the sphincter of Oddi, thereby blocking the drainage of pancreatic juice from the pancreatic duct into the duodenum. The combination of increased production of pancreatic juice and obstruction of flow to the duodenum raises pressure in the pancreatic duct, causing edema and fibrosis of pancreatic parenchyma.

8. (2) With severe vomiting and retching, intraluminal pressures in both the duodenum and stomach are raised to a high level. Increased duodenal pressures may cause reflux of duodenal chyme and bile into the pancreatic duct. Bile activates enzymatic precursors of trypsin and lipase.

9. (3) Necrotic pancreatic tissue may become infected by bloodborne bacteria, producing a gram-negative bacteremia. Gram-negative bacteria produce endotoxins that are an integral part of the bacterial cell wall, and are released when the bacterium dies and the cell wall ruptures. These endotoxins cause white blood cells to elaborate a pyrogen that resets the temperature regulating center in the hypothalamus for a higher-than-normal temperature.

10. (3) Rebound tenderness is defined as abdominal discomfort elicited on sudden removal of the palpating hand.

11. (1) Rebound tenderness results from the sudden change in tension on the inflamed parietal peritoneum that occurs on release of hand pressure; thus, the symptom indicates inflammation of the parietal peritoneum.

12. (3) Paralytic ileus is the condition of inadequate or absent propulsive peristalsis occurring within all or a part of the small intestine. Complete absence of bowel sounds suggests paralytic ileus due to diffuse peritoneal irritation.

13. (1) As the pancreatic inflammatory process becomes chronic, there is heavy deposition of calcium in damaged pancreatic tissue, so that x-ray examination reveals localized or diffuse calcifications in the region of the pancreas.

14. (4) The normal leukocyte count is 5000–10,000 cells per cubic millimeter, with about 60 per cent neutrophils, 3 per cent eosinophils, 0.5 per cent basophils, 30 per cent lymphocytes, and 5 per cent monocytes. Leukocytosis is defined as an increase in the leukocyte count above the upper limits of normal. Most infections due to pyogenic bacteria produce a polymorphonuclear leukocytosis.

15. (1) Inflammation is the body's normal reaction to injury by which various cellular and humoral elements serve to restrict the activity of an injurious agent. The classic inflammatory reaction consists of an initial brief vasoconstriction, followed by arteriolar and capillary dilation; transudation of fluid and white blood cells through the enlarged pores of the dilated capillaries; phagocytosis of bacteria and tissue debris by polymorphonuclear leukocytes; absorption of exudate and debris into the blood; and migration of fibroblasts into the area to repair the tissue defect.

16. (2) Amylase is an enzyme that breaks starch down into glucose. The normal mechanism for entrance of pancreatic enzymes into the blood is not known. In pancreatitis, enzymes escape from the pancreas into the peritoneal cavity and surrounding tissues, and are absorbed into the veins and lymphatics. Blood amylase is excreted through the kidney. The normal serum amylase concentration, as determined by the Somogyi method, ranges from 60 to 100 U./100 ml. of blood.

17. (3) In acute pancreatitis, serum amylase concentration rises within a few hours of onset of the disease, and then returns to normal levels within 2–5 days following onset of pancreatic inflammation. Typically, urine amylase levels increase

a few hours after the elevation of serum amylase, but urine amylase usually remains high for some time after serum amylase has returned to normal levels. The normal concentration of urine amylase ranges from 35 ro 260 Somogyi U./hour.

18. (2) The mechanism of pathogenesis of pancreatitis is not fully understood. One theory suggests that increased intraduodenal pressure, rather than obstruction of the pancreatic duct, is responsible for initiating pancreatitis. Serum amylase is elevated in several disorders other than pancreatitis: acute cholecystitis, intestinal obstruction, intestinal perforation, and ruptured ectopic pregnancy are all characterized by elevated serum amylase levels.

19. (4) Within 8 hours of onset of acute pancreatitis, serum amylase concentration increases. Within 2–5 days following onset of illness, serum amylase levels may return to normal; urine amylase levels tend to increase a few hours later than the serum amylase levels, but remain elevated much longer.

20. (4) In pancreatitis, serum lipase activity increases in proportion to serum amylase elevation, but subsides more slowly and over a longer.period. Unfortunately, the test for serum lipase activity is lengthy, so does not yield results quickly enough to direct treatment decisions during the early stages of acute pancreatitis, when prompt surgical intervention may be needed to avert hemorrhage and shock.

21. (4) The production of pancreatic enzymes is governed by both hormonal and vagal control. When acid-containing chyme enters the duodenum, pancreozymin and secretin are released by the duodenal wall and carried in the blood to the pancreas, where pancreozymin stimulates secretion of enzymes and secretin stimulates secretion of water and bicarbonate. Nasogastric suction removes the principal stimulus for pancreatic enzyme production.

22. (1) In the process of giving direct care to patients, the nurse's hands are brought into contact with many different pathogens, many of which are antibiotic-resistant. A venipuncture provides an avenue for direct transmission of pathogens from the nurse's hands to the patient's blood stream, which is an excellent medium for bacteriologic growth.

23. (1) In starting an intravenous infusion for an acutely ill patient who is likely to require repeated intravenous infusions, it is advisable to select the most distal vein for the venipuncture site, and to preserve more central veins for life-saving fluid therapy during later, more critical phases of illness.

24. (1) Holding the hand over the edge of the bed increases hydrostatic pressure in the veins of the hand, and distends the veins so that they can more easily be entered with a needle. Application of a warm moist pack to the dorsum of the hand causes vasodilation, rendering the vein more visible and more accessible to needle puncture.

25. (3) An air embolism may result from accidental injection of air intravenously (usually more than 200 ml. must be injected before untoward results are seen). To prevent this, the fluid tubing should be cleared of air before the skin is punctured.

26. (3) When a patient is in immediate need of fluid replacement and there is no reason to suspect congestive heart failure or renal failure, an isotonic solution can safely be given at a rate of 1–2 cc. (ml.)/minute (60–120 ml. per hour) until the physician can be contacted for a specific flow rate order.

27. (4) The patient with severe anemia has tachycardia and reduced cardiac reserve as a result of myocardial anoxia. Sudden increase in circulating blood volume may precipitate congestive heart failure in the severely anemic patient. In chronic arteriosclerotic heart disease, the coronary vessels are narrowed and the myocardium is chronically anoxic. A sudden increase in circulating blood volume would raise systolic blood pressure, increasing the peripheral resistance against which the left ventricle must pump blood. The left ventricle will be unable to contract more forcefully to compensate for increased peripheral resistance because of diffuse myocardial fibrosis secondary to chronic anoxia. Chronic obstructive lung disease predisposes to cor pulmonale, or right ventricular hypertrophy and failure due to increased pressure in the pulmonary circulation. A rapid increase in circulating blood volume may increase pulmonary blood pressure still further and provoke right heart failure in the patient with chronic lung disease. The patient in renal failure may be hypertensive or

edematous: if hypertensive, too rapid infusion of intravenous fluids may raise blood pressure still higher, causing congestive heart failure or cerebral hemorrhage; if edematous, too rapid intravenous infusion of fluid may increase hydrostatic pressure in the veins and capillaries, causing greater transudation of fluid from the vessels into the interstitial spaces. The patient with cirrhosis develops ascites and dependent edema due to hypoalbuminemia and obstruction to venous blood flow to the heart. Rapid intravenous infusion of large quantities of fluid could overload the venous circulation, and increase both ascites production and edema of dependent tissues.

28. (3) A needle or angiocath may be dislodged or pulled back from its original position in a vein by traction on the fluid tubing. That portion of a needle or angiocath which lies outside of the body tissues is apt to be contaminated by normal bacterial inhabitants of the skin or pathogens from urine, stool, or wound exudate. By pushing a dislodged needle or catheter back into a vein, the nurse would be apt to inject pathogens directly into the patient's blood stream.

29. (4) Broken fragments of a needle or catheter could be carried by the venous blood flow to the vena cava, through the right heart, and to the pulmonary circulation, where the fragment would occlude a pulmonary artery or branch vessel. Placing a tourniquet around the upper portion of the extremity obstructs venous return flow so that the vein can be incised and the fragment removed.

30. (2) There are numerous instances of drug and chemical incompatibilities with which a pharmacist is more apt to be familiar than either the physician or the nurse. Fluid containing glucose and protein constitute an excellent bacteriologic culture medium. The air in a hospital unit is heavily contaminated with pathogenic organisms. Fluid mixtures for intravenous administration should be prepared under septic conditions in a closed room under a laminar-flow, filtered air hood, in order to prevent contamination of the fluid mixtures by those microorganisms that are endemic to hospitals (many of which are antibiotic-resistant).

31. (1) In acute pancreatitis the activation of enzymes within the pancreas causes necrosis of pancreatic tissue and erosion of blood vessels. Loss of enzymes and blood into the peritoneal cavity causes a chemical peritonitis, with a great outpouring of peritoneal fluid. One of the pancreatic enzymes, kallikrein, catalyzes the release of the potent vasodilators, kallidin and bradykinin. The combination of widespread vasodilation and loss of fluid from the vessels into the peritoneal cavity causes marked reduction of blood pressure to shock levels.

32. (3) The pain of pancreatitis is more intense when the patient is lying supine than when he is sitting, or lying on his side with his spine flexed.

33. (4) The pain of pancreatitis is too severe to be relieved by aspirin or codeine. Morphine causes spasm of smooth muscles, so is apt to cause spasm of the sphincter of Oddi, increasing pressure within the duct of Wirsung and perpetuating autodigestion of pancreatic tissue by retained enzymes.

34. (3) Severe reduction in mean arterial pressure is apt to develop as a consequence of decrease in blood volume or decreased force of myocardial contraction. Continuous loss of body fluid through vomiting and nasogastric suctioning, and major loss of intravascular fluid into the peritoneal cavity or into the bowel lumen, decreases circulating blood volume. Once shock has developed, the arteries of the pancreas become even more constricted than those elsewhere in the splanchnic circulation. Extreme pancreatic ischemia results in activation of more trypsin and release of a myocardial toxic factor that is a direct depressant of the myocardium, decreasing cardiac contractility by 50 per cent. The decrease in ventricular force causes further decrease in blood pressure, and shock deepens.

35. (1) When the increased trypsinogen produced by the pancreas and accumulated in the obstructed pancreatic duct is activated, the increased amounts of trypsin in turn activate other enzyme precursors. One enzyme, elastase, digests the elastic fibers in the arterial media, weakening the vessel wall and predisposing to vascular erosion and hemorrhage.

36. (4) The digestion of fats normally occurs predominantly in the small bowel,

whereby bile salts cause emulsification of dietary fats. Fatty acids, one of the products of emulsification, are normally absorbed from the jejunum and carried eventually into the general circulation, to be catalyzed for energy purposes or stored in adipose tissue. With impairment of fat digestion and fat absorption, undigested fat residue is excreted in the stools, which become bulky, frothy, foul-smelling, and greasy.

37. (3) The intrapancreatic activation of lipase leads to fat necrosis in the pancreas and adjacent tissues, and liberation of free fatty acids. Calcium ions than react with the free fatty acids to form calcium compounds, lowering blood calcium levels.

38. (1) The normal serum calcium concentration is 9–11 mg./100 ml. of serum.

39. (3) Hypocalcemia causes increased neuromuscular irritability. Mild-to-moderate hypocalcemia is revealed by Chvostek's sign, which is contraction of the ipsilateral facial muscles upon brisk tapping over the facial nerve in front of the ear.

40. (2) Low serum calcium concentration produces tetany, which is a condition of severe muscular hypertonia accompanied by spasm and tremor.

41. (3) Necrosis of pancreatic tissue and erosion of blood vessel walls causes escape of blood into the peritoneal cavity. The seepage of blood into the abdominal wall can cause blue-green discoloration of the skin in the flanks or in the periumbilical region.

42. (3) When a large collection of pancreatic juice, liquefied cellular debris, and purulent exudate breaks through the capsule of the pancreas and becomes walled off by an inflammatory membrane and the serosa of nearby viscera, the result is a fluid-filled bag known as a pancreatic pseudocyst.

43. (4) The inflammatory and fibrotic changes in the pancreas may destroy the islets of Langerhans, producing diabetes. Severly necrotizing pancreatitis may erode into the adjacent duodenal wall, causing perforation and hemorrhage, and further accentuating the peritonitis and shock resulting from acute pancreatic damage. Activated trypsin and lipase in the peritoneal cavity cause chemical peritonitis of segments of the small bowel, interrupting normal peristalsis and causing transudation of fluid from the inflamed bowel wall into the lumen of the gut. Chemical irritation of the mesentery by pancreatic enzymes in the peritoneal fluid may cause phlebitis, then thrombosis of the mesenteric vein. Accumulations of pancreatic secretions and necrotic cellular debris in the peritoneal cavity become infected by staphylococci and coliform bacteria, to form peritoneal abscesses that may erode into and destroy various abdominal viscera.

44. (4) Pancreatic pseudocysts cause problems by causing pressure on surrounding organs; becoming secondarily infected; rupturing into an adjacent viscus; or eroding a blood vessel and causing severe hemorrhage.

4 PSYCHIATRIC-MENTAL HEALTH NURSING

Anxiety Reaction

1. (1) Primary anxiety evoked by the plethora of external and internal stimuli induces a total feeling of painful tension in the infant. Earlier, Freud emphasized frustration of sexual instincts as the producer of anxiety.

2. (4) The function of anxiety is to warn the person of impending danger. Unlike a drive for hunger or sex, anxiety is produced initially by external causes and not from internal tissue conditions. Later, the individual's previous experiences together with his internal sensations provoke his anxiety.

3. (1) Anxiety is most easily provoked in infancy because the ego has only begun to develop. As a consequence of physiologic growth, frustrations, conflicts, and external threats, the individual experiences anxiety and is forced to learn new methods of reducing tension. Freud thought that the personality was fairly well formed by the end of the fifth year of life, and thus enabled to manage anxiety.

4. (4) Signal anxiety is a learned pattern of response in anticipation of a traumatic event that allows the individual to react with anxiety prior to the event. The statements listed show how this anxiety is protective.

5. (2) Freud described three types of anxiety: reality, neurotic, moral. Reality anxiety is fear of real danger in the environment. Moral anxiety is fear of conscience. Neurotic anxiety is the fear that instincts will get out of control and result in punishment of the individual. Neurotic anxiety is more a fear of punishment than of the impulse expression that results in punishment from the world (parents, authorities, friends).

6. (2) Anxiety reaction (or neurosis) occurs when the ego is unable to regulate drives or impulses. If the ego development is supported early in life and environmental factors do not overly intensify the drives, the ego is able to maintain control of drives and impulses.

7. (2) Fear is a recognized, external threat of danger. Signal anxiety is produced intrapsychically (perhaps "unconscious recalling"). Individuals become aware of tension but are not immediately aware of its origin.

8. (4) Attempts at physiologic differentiation between fear and anxiety have been unsuccessful. Some researchers have postulated that norepinephrine is secreted in response to external threat (fear), and epinephrine in response to internal threat (anxiety). However, these hormones alone would not produce all of these symptoms.

9. (2) Frustration leads frequently to aggression. Eva's anger could derive from her father's leaving and from being overcontrolled by her mother. Palpitations and disturbed respirations are quite typical of an anxiety syndrome. The symptoms abate when the stresses are relieved.

10. (4) Each symptom must be evaluated to assess whether or not its origin is physiologic. If a physical cause is not found, a psychosocial assessment is completed to diagnose the syndrome.

11. (4) The community mental health nurse is interested especially in determining the extent to which Eva can care for herself. If Eva cannot, the nurse next assesses whether the support available to help her is adequate. Based on these two assessments, any need for hospitalization is established. The other assessments would follow.

12. (2) Neurotic individuals have a good ability to discuss reality, but their reactions to it may be disproportionate to the stimuli intensity.

13. (1) According to Sullivan, anxiety is a product of interpersonal relationships. Originally it is transmitted from mother to child, and later in life by threats to one's security.

14. (3) To avoid anxiety, the individual adopts protective measures over his behavior; i.e., punishment can be avoided by conforming to his parents' wishes. These security measures form the self system, and anxiety is controlled un-

less these situations of punishment or threat (maybe due to inconsistency in the environment) cannot be avoided.

15. (1) Absence of anxiety (euphoria) occurs as fears dissipate. Euphoria is an exaggerated sense of well-being accompanied by carefree behavior.

16. (2) Panic is extreme anxiety, with "blind fear" of disapproval and marked disorganization of behavior.

17. (4) Anxiety is minimized or controlled by defense mechanisms, adaptive modes of behavior (including compromise), re-evaluation of the milieu, and fantasy. Overuse of any of these becomes maladaptive.

18. (3) An example of sublimation is someone who becomes a surgeon or psychiatrist not for altruistic reasons, but rather to heal by special powers or to satisfy curiosity and a quest for omnipotence. Sublimation does not result in complete satisfaction.

19. (1) For example, a person may fail to see something that is in plain sight because perception of it is repressed; a person may become sexually impotent because of fear of sex impulses. Repressed content or impulses may be symbolically displaced (rebellion against father displaced to other authority figures).

20. (2) When our reality experiences are too painful we reconstruct the world in fantasy as we would like it to be. We deny reality and escape time and space; thus, "facts" are what we wish them to be.

21. (4) Introjection is the fantasied reincorporation of an object or person into the person's own ego or superego. A widow may unconsciously attempt to "regain" her dead husband by displaying some of his remembered characteristics.

22. (2) When large amounts of impulses, fears, or thoughts are repressed, the ego expends much energy in keeping thoughts in the unconscious. If the ego becomes weakened, this repressed material "threatens" to become conscious, and anxiety (a signal of impending danger) results.

23. (4) Eva repressed many of her thoughts and feelings, probably never was able to please her mother, and felt both unworthy and angry. As her ego was overtaxed (by her fears, father leaving, impending marriage, impending separation from her mother), anxiety increased to the point of rendering her confused and helpless.

24. (3) Channeling anxiety to an organ or resorting to ignoring reality are maladaptive. Insulating the conflict places a burden on the ego, but effectively reduces anxiety. Developing a phobia can reduce anxiety only if the feared "thing" or object is infrequently encountered. Sublimating conflict through socialization and work would be most effective in anxiety reduction.

25. (3) Eva's conflict consisted of wanting to leave home as her father did, but feeling compelled to remain at home with her mother out of a sense of duty.

26. (1) The symptoms in anxiety reaction are almost classic and include palpitations, dyspnea, and unbearable tension. However, these symptoms manifest themselves for a variety of underlying reasons.

27. (3) Secondary gain is "reward" from the milieu for exhibiting symptoms. This "reward" tends to prolong the manifesting of the symptom. Eva didn't receive this secondary gain. The primary gain from symptoms is, of course, reduction of anxiety.

28. (2) Chlordiazepoxide has muscle-relaxant and anticonvulsant properties. It is habituating.

29. (1) It is the inability of the ego's use of defense mechanisms to reduce anxiety that contributes to the development of a crisis. In a crisis the individual's receptivity to help is increased.

30. (1) When crises are handled well, the individual's mental stability is maintained and there is return to the precrisis level of functioning or better; and vice versa.

31. (1) Crisis intervention properly instituted prevents a temporary decompensation from becoming permanent disability. An example of secondary prevention is caring for an alcoholic during delirium tremens. Tertiary prevention applied to an illness is the rehabilitation phase.

32. (4) The impact of illness of any type on a community can be great. The impair-

ment is not only in loss of life and loss of financial gain, but in failure to reach potential in education, family integrity, inventiveness, and security.

33. (4) The goals of crisis intervention are to help return the individual to precrisis state, to assist him in coping with life situations, and to help him avoid hospitalization. The goals were attainable for Eva for the reasons listed.

34. (1) Assessment of the precipitating event(s) and amount of disruption in the life is a first step in crisis intervention. Her father's leaving, perhaps his returning, and the continued nagging by her mother for Eva to marry were disruptive to Eva. A change of environment and development of more independence seem indicated.

35. (4) Eva had the potential to respond well to crisis intervention for the reasons listed here and in item 33. The main approach to therapy for Eva is to help her relate the crisis event to her current feelings.

36. (1) If anxiety and tension are not so extreme that confusion results, persons in crisis are more receptive to guidance than persons with low anxiety levels and well developed, maladaptive defense mechanisms.

37. (4) The initial steps in Eva's crisis therapy would be to focus her anxiety, relate it to the precipitating event, encourage her to express her feelings and strengthen those of her plans for coping that are adaptive.

38. (2) The symptoms first started when her father left, and recurred when she was about to leave the family home.

39. (1) Eva says that her mother is "really a very good woman . . . you know what I mean?" The best answer is to tell her you don't know what she means (1), and give her an opportunity to tell you. Reflecting (2) would not be wrong. Stating what you think Eva is implying (3) is premature. Challenging her on her thought (4) directs the conversation to talk about the mother.

40. (3) After Eva makes a comment about how she felt after her father left, it is *best* to follow with asking her to expand on that feeling (3), and then associating it with current feelings. Asking what her mother did (2) is inappropriate now, and what Eva did (1) is less significant than what she felt. The nurse probably does not understand Eva's feelings (4) at this time.

41. (3) The best response is to ask Eva to tell you her feelings and associate them with the crisis.

42. (4) The nurse should ask Eva to expand her comment until she can express her feelings, and then associate them with current feelings. Later, she could be helped to develop new methods to prevent her feelings from being immobilizing.

43. (3) We frequently express our feelings in physical symptoms, but this action is seldom conscious. When Eva says "I *have* to express myself that way," it would be *most* helpful for the nurse to determine if Eva can say which feelings she needs to express. The nurse could then help Eva express feelings and associate them to the current crisis.

44. (2) Eva ultimately must gain facility in making her own decisions based on what she wants, the goals she has set, and the defensive maneuvers necessary to control anxiety.

45. (1) Patients who experience an episode of confusion or mental illness are at times reluctant to return to the same place of work. Usually this reluctance is unwarranted. Again, the principle here is to help Eva develop ability to make her own decisions and to discuss dependence on others.

Obsessive-Compulsive Reaction

1. (4) Conflict is defined as the coexistence of two opposing goals or motivations. These incompatible needs produce anxiety, and behavior becomes hesitant, vacillating as seemingly maladaptive (i.e., neurotic). Thus, conflict has a major role in the etiology of neuroses.

2. (2) Obsessions and compulsions are classified as neurotic because the individual, in contact with reality, recognizes that the idea or behavior is irrational.

3. (4) Highly specialized and ritualized behavior is most characteristic of

obsessive-compulsive reaction. The purpose of the behavior is to ward off the anxiety engendered by underlying conflict.

4. (1) An obsession is a persistent, conscious desire or idea recognized as irrational by the individual. Obsessions are conscious expressions of unconscious, conflicted wishes.

5. (3) In accordance with a persistent idea, a defensive act is carried out despite some conscious rejection by the individual.

6. (2) Behavioral rituals help to avoid inexplicable anxiety that would arise if the impulse was not followed.

7. (3) Although the behavior is recognized as unrealistic, the compulsive acts are carried out on pain of anxiety if they are not performed. Persons with many modes of self-expression can withstand conflict to a greater extent than those whose repertoire of responses is limited.

8. (4) The rituals of the obsessive-compulsive person are seen as magical manipulations, the intent of which is to decrease intrapsychic tension.

9. (4) Psychologic guilt derives from dread of loss of love or of retributive punishment for forbidden thoughts or deeds. Aggression ensues when drives or goal attainment are thwarted.

10. (1) Sullivan's theory on the development of obsessive-compulsive neurosis appears, at first, to be different from a conflict-oriented etiology suggested earlier. However, the use of the word combination may be conflict-based. Doubting one's effectiveness in childhood only increases the anxiety and the need for more rituals or word combinations as an adult.

11. (1) Dolly's mother lectured her (platitudes and moralizing) on how to behave, but never taught her principles by which to operationalize her behavior. This must have been frustrating and anger-producing for Dolly, but there was no suggestion that she could express her hostility.

12. (2) Erikson suggested stages of psychosocial development to parallel Freud's stages of psychosexual development (oral, anal, oedipal, latent, adolescent, adult). "Autonomy versus shame and doubt" corresponds roughly with Freud's anal phase.

13. (2) Freud suggested that obsessive-compulsive individuals are fixated or regressed to the muscle-training and anal phase of psychosexual development.

14. (4) These behaviors (typical of obsessive-compulsive individuals) are also observed in the psychosexual anal stages of personality development.

15. (2) Compulsive rituals can be "upsetting" to the individual, the family, and a hospital unit. Routines must be altered to allow time for the repetitive behaviors and to ensure prevention of suicide. Obsessive-compulsive persons know, at some level, that the rituals do not remove problems but do manage anxiety.

16. (3) Through conversation and observation, the nurse can establish how much time is spent in compulsive acts. If the underlying conflict is intensified following hospitalization, the ritualistic behavior will increase, and vice versa.

17. (3) Fixation is the persistence of the behavior characteristic of one phase into the next phase of psychosexual development; this "holding over" implies arrested development. Regression is the resumption, under stress, of behaviors typical of an earlier phase.

18. (3) A phobia is a morbid dread of something. It is generally unconscious, and may be immobilizing if the individual must be exposed to the dreadful object. Dolly's compulsive acts are designed to combat (or undo) what she fears.

19. (2) Reaction formation is a common defense mechanism in obsessive-compulsive reaction. The conflict can be reduced by expressing consciously only one of a pair of ambivalent attitudes or goals.

20. (4) Isolation is also a way to express only one part of a conflict. In isolation, feelings (e.g., anxiety) are defensively separated from the act or impulse.

21. (3) Undoing combats anxiety development by repetitive actions designed to offset some other act or impulse.

22. (2) Ambivalence is the existence of incompatible feelings or attitudes toward another person or situation. Isolation, reaction formation, and undoing each deal with one part of the pair of ambivalent thoughts or feelings.

23. (2) Smearing is typically a behavioral holdover from the anal (Freud) or autonomy versus shame and doubt (Erikson) stages of personality development.

24. (2) Repression is an unconscious defense mechanism whereby painful, anxiety-producing thoughts are kept out of conscious awareness. Dissociative reactions and conversion reactions are examples of neuroses in which repression is a prominent feature.

25. (3) Displacement, symbolization, and condensation (many concepts are symbolically represented as one) all contributed to Dolly's obsession that she was contaminated or "dirty."

26. (1) When we recognize our impulses as unacceptable we try to mask them by a multitude of acceptable processes, including displacement and symbolization.

27. (1) The superego, acting as conscience, prohibits the ego from direct forms of id expression. Acting as an ego-ideal, the superego channels behavior along that of persons with whom the individual identifies. Dolly apparently expected herself to achieve a high standard of behavior, perhaps much like that of her moralizing mother.

28. (4) All the concepts listed and many more are important components of psychoanalytic therapy.

29. (4) Resistance in psychoanalysis is the refusal to accept insight into the unconscious. This is demonstrated by the patient's rejection of interpretation.

30. (4) The five behaviors listed are the main forms of resistance in psychoanalysis. The choice of behaviors varies with the patient.

31. (3) Libido is associated with the instincts of the id. Interpretation of libido as desire for sexual relationship is a limited definition.

32. (1) Insight (understanding of behavior) in itself requires ego strength, and further ego strength is required to enable the patient to act constructively on these insights.

33. (4) Acting out is a defense pattern in which a patient expresses conflicts in behavior rather than acquiring insight through verbal communication. The acting out always is relative to unconscious transference to the therapist. Countertransference refers to the analyst's unconscious feelings toward the patient.

34. (4) To enable Dolly to gain insight she must first be helped to free blocked emotions, i.e., those feelings isolated from impulses.

35. (4) The statements listed describe most of the interpretations made in any psychoanalytic situation. This knowledge of interpretations should help nurses direct their interventions.

36. (2) Suicidal thoughts or acts are thought to be an internalization of hostile feelings.

37. (3) Patients frequently discuss only thoughts or situations, rather than their reactions or feelings to people and events.

38. (1) If the expression of only one of a pair of her attitudes or feelings provides Dolly with secondary gain (attention from others in addition to helping to control the anxiety), she may be less willing to accept insight into her unconscious.

39. (3) Asking Dolly a reflective question allows her to express what she thinks about the psychiatrist. Although this questioning may elicit a "no" response, the nurse can follow up with additional comments.

40. (4) If Dolly has had a number of diverse experiences, she is more apt to be able to find gratification from several behavioral styles. Knowledge of the underlying conflict facilitates planning an approach to relieve at least one part of the conflict.

41. (4) The literature describing the personality of most nurses includes references to all the characteristics listed. Obviously, not all nurses exhibit all of these behaviors.

42. (2) The nature of the conflict and any secondary gain from the symptoms are out of Dolly's conscious awareness. Trying to force a change in behavior prior to achievement of insight by Dolly is nonproductive.

43. (2) Behavior modification therapy is the application of learning principles to change of maladaptive behavior. Supportive psychotherapy is a treatment approach in which the personality is strengthened, and insight into the

unconscious conflicts is not imposed. Milieu therapy is treatment through specific changes in environment.

44. (1) Increasing self-esteem is a goal for any patient. When anxiety is high, self-esteem is lowered.

45. (4) The rituals are unconsciously designed to relieve anxiety generated by conflict.

46. (2) Reminding Dolly to begin her rituals early in order that she may retire at a predetermined time is an inviting option; however, this suggestion is based on logic and implies control over the rituals. In a way, for the nurse to remind Dolly to begin her rituals would be encouraging sick behavior. Determining the cause of the increase in anxiety at bedtime is the key to the nurse's intervention.

47. (1) Activity is a good method for relief of tension created by anxiety.

48. (3) When limits must be drawn on carrying out compulsive acts, the limits must be consistently enforced and carried out efficiently. Long explanations and coaxing usually result in more emotional upset.

49. (2) Intellectual explanation would result in the patient's feeling more inadequate and criticized for failure to meet the standard of behavior set for her.

50. (3) Without criticizing or punishing Dolly for her rituals or controlling behavior, the nurse may directly point out that she is contributing to the other patients' negative reaction to her, and that it is unrealistic to expect the "world" to adjust to Dolly's rituals.

51. (3) Unless the underlying conflicts can be identified and insight achieved, Dolly will not be able to relinquish her compulsive rituals. She already recognizes that her rituals are unrealistic, and yet continues them.

52. (3) It is important for Dolly to participate in activities and not to be criticized. The intent of her comment is not clear, so the nurse's reply is an attempt to clarify the communication. Patients who are obsessive-compulsive should be relieved of as many decisions as possible.

53. (2) The set of defenses that Dolly uses prevent her from experiencing fully her emotions, especially guilt and hostility.

Psychotic Depressive Reaction

1. (1) Depression is an extremely important and frequently occurring phenomenon. Difference between neurotic and psychotic depression is quantitative. Dependency needs have been cited as a major psychodynamic force in the development of depression. Therefore, as dependent persons, depressed individuals are vulnerable to frustration. Since their needs for reassurances and nurturing are great, they never get enough and their needs are chronically unmet.

2. (2) Electroshock therapy (EST) induces grand mal seizures by application of electrical current to the skull, hence, the term electroconvulsive therapy (ECT). This procedure is used principally in treatment of depression because it is thought that depressed persons view it as deserved punishment for their guilt. EST produces a memory loss that reduces awareness of painful memories.

3. (4) Metabolism of neural tissue amines, such as serotonin and norepinephrine, has been reported as abnormal in selected areas of the brain in persons who are depressed. For this reason, monoamine oxidase (MAO) inhibitors (Marplan and Parnate) have been used in the treatment of depression.

4. (2) Most of us are reluctant initially to acknowledge mental illness in a family member. Illness is usually disruptive, to some extent, of family life.

5. (2) Insomnia is the single most significant physical symptom of depression. Anorexia, weight loss, and fatigue are frequently occurring physical symptoms. The ego strength is further weakened by lack of sleep. Extreme sleep deprivation can produce affective or schizoid distortion. Sleep produces rapid amelioration of these symptoms.

6. (4) Constipation is one other symptom of a general apathy or slowing down of the psyche and soma.

7. (4) Assessments by the nurse of Mrs. Cowert's general health and interacting behavior, of the amount of observation Mrs. Cowert needs, and of her own reaction to the patient serve as a basis for planning and evaluating nursing interventions.

8. (1) Although Mrs. Cowert has dependency needs, it is unrealistic to adjust the entire milieu for her benefit and perhaps at the expense of the need gratification of other patients.

9. (2) Making Mr. Cowert feel guilty or referring him to talk with the psychiatrist are not helpful to him at this time. It is important to understand as much as possible what made Mrs. Cowert ill. Diluting and distributing the reason for this illness is useful.

10. (1) Mr. Cowert will continue to be a main source of gratification of his wife's dependency needs. He probably feels guilty in that he thinks he contributed to his wife's illness. It is important for him and the treatment team to understand and explore the motivations behind his behavior.

11. (4) Trust is a learned behavior, usually learned in the first year of life. If one never learns to trust, it is difficult to develop in interdependent relationships.

12. (2) In addition to having decreasing ego strength and an oral personality, persons who develop psychotic depression frequently have a strong punitive superego. The superego is somewhat equivalent to the conscience and conveys, "You better not do that because it is wrong."

13. (1) Libido is the energy associated with the id instincts. In common use this term is used to refer to sex drive or desire for sexual relationship.

14. (4) Functioning of a healthy ego assists the personality in mastering the environment through mediation of motor control (e.g., gait), sensory perception, memory storage, affective response (feelings), and thought processes (thinking, comprehensions).

15. (3) Bellak and Small described eight ego functions: adaptation to reality testing: sense of reality; control of drives; object relations (distance between self and others); thought processes; defensive functions; autonomous functions (perception, comprehension, thinking, language); and synthetic function (ability to unite, make whole).

16. (1) Ego development begins at birth and grows rapidly during the first year of life. Ego growth may continue throughout life if adequate support is available to the individual.

17. (2) Reality testing is differentiating internal from external reality, and it involves perception, judgment, and intelligence. Sensory isolation produces disturbances in reality testing ability of the ego.

18. (3) Defense mechanisms are unconsciously employed by the ego to selectively monitor internal and external stimuli. Mrs. Cowert regressed until she wasn't able to perform her usual activities. She internalized her anger (introjection) because expression of intensive anger may bring rejection from those on whom she depends. The cause of the anger is real or symbolic loss to which she is vulnerable because of her excessive dependency needs.

19. (1) Symbolically incorporating a loved or hated object or person is introjection. Sometimes, people display characteristics of the introjected person. Attributing one's feelings to another is projection.

20. (4) The superego is that portion of the personality that functions as conscience and prohibits the ego from direct forms of instinct expression. The superego develops by internalization of behavior of those individuals with whom the person wishes to identify.

21. (2) Guilt is conscious or unconscious dread of loss or punishment for impulses or deeds thought to be forbidden. Psychologically one feels deserving of the blame. Depression is frequently characterized by guilt.

22. (4) Freud's description of the factors basic to the development of depression is similar to that already discussed. After the ambivalent relationship with the love object and strong superego are developed, an actual or symbolic loss allows depression to ensue.

23. (4) These factors are related to the relative strengths of the parts of the personality: id, ego, superego. Of special significance in Mrs. Cowert's depression is the fact that she had not handled loss well in the past.

24. (2) In mourning the individual recognizes the lost object or person. This recognition does not occur in melancholia. However, in mourning one usually does not engage in self-recrimination.

25. (4) Ambivalence often involves the coexistence of love and hate for the same person. Mrs. Cowert probably both loved and hated her cruel mother and her untrusting husband.

26. (4) The sequence of events that permits the manifestation of depression is as follows: loss occurs, anger develops, and is internalized. If the individual notes and communicates his/her feelings openly, diagnosis is relatively easy, but if the depression manifests only in physical symptoms its recognition is more difficult.

27. (4) Self-blame, disillusionment with self, and self-depreciation are typical thoughts of the person with retarded depression.

28. (4) It is important *not* to convey to Mrs. Cowert that her opinion of herself is correct, and thereby increase her feelings of unworthiness.

29. (2) Because of Mrs. Cowert's ambivalent feelings (love and hate) toward her mother, she may think that she was responsible for her mother's death and/or her father's absences from the home.

30. (2) Descriptions by patients of unstructured drawings on cards are analyzed to obtain insight into the patients' thought processes.

31. (4) The Thematic Apperception Test consists of a set of pictures suggesting life situations from which the patient constructs a story. Interpretation of these stories reveals information about the patient's personality.

32. (3) This antidepressant is a tricyclic compound similar to Elavil. The exact mechanism of action is not known.

33. (4) The side effects of the tricyclic antidepressants are varied, but usually are controlled by dose reduction. Dryness of the mouth, tachycardia, and constipation are only a few of those that could occur.

34. (1) The nurse-patient interpersonal relationship is formed with two main objectives: to allow expression of anger and guilt feelings, and to improve self-esteem. Depressed patients do not function well in a stress-filled, rapid-paced environment. Selected routines must be altered to accommodate the patient while ensuring proper physical care (drinking, eating, grooming, and eliminating). Therefore, rigid insistence, humble entreaty, and gentle bantering are not useful. An *attitude* of firm kindness perhaps suggests that the nurse is strong enough to tolerate expressions of anger, and loving enough to accept the patient who has hostile feelings.

35. (4) Sanding furniture is a menial task that allows expression of aggression.

36. (2) Depressed patients may seek menial tasks as an expression of their need for self-punishment. The nurse should allow patients to participate in these activities without questioning their motives.

37. (2) Withdrawal is sometimes a way to express hostility or to prevent impulsive aggressive acts. The reason withdrawal is effective is that it reduces the interaction with others and prompts them to be more attentive to the withdrawn person.

38. (4) Patients who have a retarded depression (as opposed to an agitated depression) experience a general slowing of physical and mental processes. The nursing interventions listed are therapeutic during periods of deep depression.

39. (4) The patient's grooming, eating, drinking, eliminating, and communicating (verbal and nonverbal) are all general indicators of the depth of depression.

40. (4) All the behaviors listed are important, but observation of mood change is a key nursing assessment.

41. (3) Depressed patients most frequently attempt suicide when they experience abatement of their depression. An episode of what may be termed "elation" should be viewed as a "red flag." This type of change may be an indication that decisions have been made to attempt suicide and a method to this end outlined.

42. (3) Dependent persons continually seek directions about what to do, think, and/or feel. They need support and protection.

43. (2) Trying to reason away the delusional thinking is assuming erroneously that the patients can control their thoughts and are capable of logical reasoning.

It would be inadvisable to encourage Mrs. Cowert to give a detailed description of her delusions.

44. (3) Reducing the burden of making simple decisions, and actively helping to meet Mrs. Cowert's nutritional needs, is indicated. The nurse should remember that refusing to eat has significant meaning. It is a way for the patient to express anger at herself (Mrs. Cowert) and toward others.

45. (4) Nursing interventions are planned to meet patients' needs and to encourage as much learning and independence as possible. Associating the identified need with the need gratifiers is therapeutic.

46. (4) Patients eventually bring out the best and worst behavior in us (nurses). All of us have experienced the feelings listed while interacting with patients. How we handle these feelings is more important than the fact that we experience them.

47. (4) The list constitutes a standard set of expected behaviors for depressed persons. In a therapeutic milieu it is possible to have needs met, to be free of fear of retaliation for hostile feelings, and to learn new solutions to old problems.

48. (3) When patients frequently make self-deprecating comments they unknowingly risk the danger of the staff's becoming insensitive to these thoughts. If the feelings behind these thoughts are not explored and insight gained into the purpose of the behaviors, it is unlikely that the self-esteem will improve. It is important not to make any comment that would decrease further the patient's self-esteem.

49. (1) The feeling tone conveyed by Mrs. Cowert when criticizing her psychiatrist probably was anger. If so, the nurse verbalized the implied criticism.

50. (1) The interpretation of the significance of Mrs. Cowert's criticism of the psychiatrist is that she had identified with him. Identification is the patterning of oneself, on the basis of love and/or hate, after the characteristics of another.

51. (3) Feeling humble is not considered part of a positive self-concept, although humility does allow the individual to make a more bearable impact on others than does arrogance.

52. (4) The patient may not "be ready" to be well even if she is making progress toward mental health. Asking the patient to maintain this level of grooming may be a burden. Telling her to put on lipstick and powder indicates that she didn't do enough to please you. Matter-of-factly, yet kindly, commenting on her behavior is most helpful at this time. Spending more time with Mrs. Cowert during this day is indicated.

53. (1) The family is a primary group, other groups are considered secondary. "Artificial" and "intimate" are not official terms used to classify groups.

54. (2) The family is an interactional unit or system in which the behavior of each family member is affected by that of every other.

55. (4) Mrs. Cowert in a family therapy setting would be referred to as the identified patient, indicating that her illness gives a message about the pathology (disturbed psychosocial relationships) of the whole family unit.

56. (2) Singling out a person as the cause of the family's problem is called "scapegoating," a phenomenon that family therapists deal with frequently.

57. (2) The goal of family therapy is to assist members to formulate alternative interaction styles that are healthier for all, and to decrease blame and guilt. The goal is not to allow unchanneled expression of aggression toward other members.

58. (4) Sometimes reality is "too painful" and we, at least temporarily, need to avoid facing our feelings and problems directly. Disturbed communication results when avoidance becomes a pattern.

59. (4) Children may experience the same feelings as adults. Seeing the illness of a person on whom you rely for gratification of many of your own needs is extremely frightening and alarming. Anger at the person for getting ill and blaming oneself for contributing to the illness are common sequelae to mental illness of a family member or close friend.

60. (2) Following an episode of depression, patients can manage if the stress level remains stable and low enough that the pressure of life does not immobilize them. If depression occurs and medications are not taken they are less able to cope and, without additional support, may again require therapy.

Manic Reaction

1. (4) Assessments of the nurse serve as data for formulation of the nursing care approach to patients. Protecting the patient and others is a major consideration.

2. (2) Physical restraint serves to further increase aggression and decrease self-esteem. Individual introductions would be too stimulating for Mrs. Clapper. An orientation to the environment is most appropriate at this time.

3. (2) During an acute manic state, patients are physically active and need room to move about and express some of the "pressure" contained within the body.

4. (3) When disturbing situations disorganize the normal channels of aggression, the individual may lose control of impulses and initiate acting out of aggression.

5. (2) Menopause, failure of her protégé, and suspicion of her husband's infidelity could have been disruptive to Mrs. Clapper's sense of security, and interpreted by her as a loss of love.

6. (2) Elation is a mild word for the intensity of feeling that some persons in a manic state express. The underlying feeling, however, is aggression.

7. (1) It is thought that manic and depressive episodes are two variations of a similar illness. Some patients who have a manic reaction also have a history of a depressive episode.

8. (3) The interaction pattern of persons with manic reactions is dependent and possessive because these individuals typically fear loss of a significant person or of self-esteem.

9. (2) Intense frustration leads almost automatically to aggression. Hostility usually is preceded by suspicion, and emerges after some rumination. Being rude, demanding, derogating, argumentative, and sarcastic are examples of hostile behavior.

10. (1) Real, threatened, or imagined loss of, or rejection by, significant others results in lowered self-esteem and an increase in anxiety.

11. (4) At times, use of tranquilizers is the best way to calm patients so that interpersonal communication is possible.

12. (1) Although it is quite possible that most patients are frightened by the behavior of persons in a manic state, patients are usually more tolerant of psychotic behavior than are personnel.

13. (4) It is paradoxical that when we fear rejection we perform behavior that provokes the feared loss. Such behavior shows a temporary loss of control.

14. (1) The psychodynamic formulation of Mrs. Clapper's manic episode is similar to that of a psychotically depressed person.

15. (3) Denial of reality allows us to avoid momentarily "seeing" ourselves as we are. Victoria's denial became a pattern whereby she defended her ego by denying the feelings, especially anger, that she experienced.

16. (4) The behaviors listed are all typical of persons in an acute manic state. At times, such behavior is slightly entertaining if personnel fail to acknowledge the underlying hostility that it veils.

17. (4) The speech is an expression of the intense feeling and intrapsychic conflict that she is experiencing.

18. (2) During the early phase of a manic reaction, patients are easily distracted and have a short attention span.

19. (1) Victoria is expressing a negative, critical thought that probably is best answered by silence. It would be impossible to forbid her this expression or to interpret it to her at this time, and inappropriate to return the name-calling.

20. (3) Delusional thinking is observed frequently in persons experiencing a manic reaction. The delusions typically are grandiose, since the intent is to offset a low self-esteem.

21. (2) Chlorpromazine (Thorazine) is a major tranquilizer that is used for management of psychotic states. Minor tranquilizers are chlordiazepoxide (Librium) and diazepam (Valium). Some therapists prefer to initiate therapy with chlorpromazine because it acts more rapidly than lithium carbonate.

22. (4) All the side effects listed may occur from chlorpromazine administration. The extrapyramidal side effects (i.e., ataxia), may be treated by reducing the

dose. Hypotension and dry mouth are due to the cholinergic blocking action of the drug.

23. (4) Lithium carbonate calms the patient and controls acute symptoms, but it takes about a week for the drug to be effective after initiation of therapy. All the side effects listed except nephrotoxicity occur early in therapy.

24. (2) The recommended oral dose is 600 mg. t.i.d. in the acute phase and 300 mg. t.i.d. for maintenance. This dosage results in an appropriate blood concentration of 0.8–1.2 mEq. per liter.

25. (1) Mutual advantageous give and take implies an interpersonal relationship in which each participant feels a noncompetitive sharing or compatibility.

26. (1) Knowledge of previous reactions to selected events is a very useful indicator of probable reactions to current situations. Danger exists in this approach if nurses do not assess behavior exhibited currently, and inadvertently "lock" the patient into old behavior patterns.

27. (4) The behavioral objectives listed are proper components of a nursing approach to any patient in a manic reaction. Manifesting reliability, acceptance, and firmness is the key to improving Victoria's ability to relate to others on a healthier plane.

28. (4) The other patients aren't paid a salary to protect Victoria, and so may be less inclined to tolerate her behavior and may physically or verbally "fight back."

29. (3) In most states people do not lose their civil rights when admitted to a unit designed to treat persons who are mentally ill. If the patient is deemed mentally incompetent (not as easy as one might think), power of attorney may be given to another.

30. (3) Note that being antisocial or not being oriented to time, place, or person does not constitute grounds for institutionalization: probably a good thing.

31. (2) Behavior of the manic person usually puts the staff in a defensive posture. To prevent this, it is useful to clearly establish the limitations on behavior based on the patient's needs. The patient needs to express hostility, to be protected, and to feel security derived from knowing what to expect; hence, the necessity of consistently applied limits.

32. (4) It is unrealistic to call the therapist at 1:00 A.M. unless this is part of a preplanned, preannounced treatment approach. The problem here is how to say "no" at the outset and not have an angry patient working up everyone in the unit. The first step is to ascertain why she is awake, demanding a pass. Persons in a manic state do not respond well to direct commands but are easily distracted.

33. (4) The three indicated approaches are therapeutic. Initially the medication dosage may be increased, and later gradually decreased. Limiting the behaviors and giving her attention are indicated. Manic individuals need someone who can remain objectively calm or neutral in the midst of the chaos that can be generated in an acute manic state. The nurse's role is to provide a stabilizing force.

34. (2) Energy outlet is a necessity, but when this energy is expressed by frantic pacing in the unit the danger of exhaustion exists. Channeling of energy through constructive activity is very helpful.

35. (4) Almost any activity is suitable, if it is safe; i.e., does not require judgment in maintaining safety for self or others. Darts would be disastrous, but jogging in an enclosed tract or gym would be therapeutic.

36. (2) Victoria shows no fear of others, weakness, or lack of coordination, but her easy distractibility may prevent her from participating for any length of time in the activities planned by the occupational therapist.

37. (4) Insomnia increases the danger of exhaustion and irritability. The listed activities have been found to be helpful in encouraging sleep in patients.

38. (2) Patients are needy and require someone to convey to them "You are important to me." In spite of our best effort and vows not to, we repeatedly find ourselves being angered by patients, staff, or administration. It is not therapeutic to accept all the patients' behavior, and unrealistic to think we can meet all their needs.

39. (2) The feelings behind the words are more important. It is important to clarify the intent and to be certain you understand the patient's communication.

40. (4) The right approach but very hard to carry out. Patients sometimes have an uncanny sense of our Achilles heel (our vulnerable spot).

41. (3) Victoria needs to express her negative emotional feelings (anger, aggressive hostility, hate) without fear of retaliation. These expressions do need to be channeled.

42. (3) Erikson proposed psychosocial stages to parallel Freud's psychosexual stages of personality development. Identity vs. role confusion is comparable to adolescence; intimacy vs. isolation is decided in early adulthood (about 20–40 years of age); and integrity vs. despair is an issue in the later years of life.

43. (3) All the responses except identifying with a peer group of the same sex are tasks of the young adult. Identifying with a peer group of the same sex is a task of the adolescent years.

44. (4) Since the life expectancy has increased in most countries, it can be assumed that the Clappers potentially have an additional 20 years to participate together in those activities listed.

45. (3) According to Sheehy, being "locked in" is realizing that you've reached your peak and don't have options available to you that would allow a change to a more rewarding life style. Safe but stifled.

46. (3) Women in the young adult years, according to Sheehy, are described as having several potential modes of behavior. The achiever who defers nurturing is one who in pursuit of a career delays marrying and having children. Unlike Victoria, most women in this category pursue careers until about age 35, take stock of their lives, make a basic shift in emphasis, become more outgoing, and perhaps marry.

47. (4) Our own view of ourselves is a determinant of the richness or paucity of our middle years, because so frequently we get the response that we project or anticipate. We've all heard the phrase "he asked for it."

48. (4) The Clappers' adjustments in middle age are comparable because of the stigma of being childless and the stigma of mental illness. In some societies the former stigma is as great as the latter.

49. (4) True feeling of love for another is not negated by mental illness. If Mr. Clapper loves his wife more than he dislikes her, he will make an effort to help her regain a level of mental health.

50. (4) A dependent, childless, manipulative woman facing menopause usually needs extra support. If Henry loves Victoria and patiently reminds her to take her medications, the prognosis is good for both of them. These issues would be addressed in family therapy sessions.

51. (4) The paradigm or model for crisis intervention includes all the techniques listed.

Schizophrenic Reaction

1. (2) Controversy over the precise etiology of schizophrenia still rages, but there is some agreement that social and biologic factors contribute to its development.

2. (4) A chemical etiology of schizophrenia has gained popularity in recent years. It is thought that abnormalities in the synthesis of the catecholamine (dopamine-norepinephrine-epinephrine) pathway predispose to the development of schizophrenia. The data are not conclusive.

3. (1) Bateson's double-bind interaction theory describes a situation in which the child (context) is fixed in an intense emotional relationship with a parent or another (metacontext) by the contradictions between word and deed. This type of situation makes it impossible for the child to discriminate properly or even ask for clarification, because questioning is viewed by the parent as a threat to the needed relationship.

4. (2) According to Bateson, when there is discord between the primary context and the metacontext, schizophrenia develops. In Dr. Gold's case this conflict is illustrated by his parents' verbal encouragement to do well and not be a

disappointment to them, and his mother's limiting his socialization and insisting that he study at home rather than at the university library.

5. (1) Disturbed communication in family interactions and atmosphere contribute to the development of schizophrenia. Needs are not met owing to the inconsistency in family interacting.

6. (2) Confusing, contradictory, inconsistent communications in Dr. Gold's early family life possibly did not allow the development of a healthy ego or of defense mechanisms.

7. (4) As for any group of people, assessment of schizophrenic patients by the nurse will show variation in symptoms or illness. These symptoms in schizophrenic patients involve disorders of feeling expression, thought content, affect, perception of reality, and general levels of behavior.

8. (2) An interpersonal relationship with a schizophrenic person is developed slowly over a period of time because he usually is withdrawn and nontrusting, and communicates symbolically. Dr. Gold needs to interact with patients, but also to learn to trust one person and to build up his own self-esteem. Requesting that the other patients call him "Irv" is not helpful to him. It would be best to allow the individuals involved to work out the terms of addressing each other.

9. (4) Psychopathology of what is collectively called schizophrenia typically includes the items listed. Deterioration in communication that is already disturbed leads to further decrease of ego strengths. This results in more regression and finally loss of identity and inability to perceive reality.

10. (4) The main function of the ego is to test reality or, as listed here, synthesize. Synthetic function of the ego, as defined by Bellak and Small, is the ability to form wholeness or "gestalten"; it therefore is the ability to maintain the functions necessary for adaptation in life (withstand stress, solve problems, and develop coping mechanisms).

11. (1) Each of us has positive and negative parts of our personality, and each are inevitably expressed. We can't predetermine in childhood to express only the positive, nor can we develop a healthy ego by free expression of all drives. The ego is developed primarily in the first year of life, but continues growth throughout life. As conflict is encountered, the infant is found to develop a differentiated personality to cope with this conflict and to recognize himself as an individual; thus, the ego begins to emerge. The mother is a source of satisfaction and dissatisfaction. The resolution of conflict results in strengthening of the ego.

12. (4) As a reality orientation becomes the primary motivator of behavior, rather than the id or pleasure principle, individuals can do all the things listed.

13. (2) Overgratification, prolonged and consistent meeting of all perceived or anticipated needs, does not allow the individual to experience and resolve sufficient conflict to result in ego growth.

14. (3) Hartmann postulated that the autonomous functions of the ego (perception, object comprehension, thinking, productivity, language, and some motor development) do not develop through conflict resolution. Therefore, in schizophrenic patients, some of these functions may remain proficient.

15. (2) Basic trust vs. basic mistrust is the first of eight stages of man's psychosocial development outlined by Erikson. The infant's task is to learn trust of self, trust of others, and trust in the environment.

16. (4) Compare the list in item 9 with the list in item 16.

17. (3) Mrs. Gold had withdrawn her indulgence of her husband's needs and had become critical, and perhaps rejecting, of him.

18. (3) Scapegoating and reinforcing deviant behavior patterns are to be avoided in family therapy. A situation in which one family member is identified as "sick" (schizophrenic) is an indication of the "illness" of the family as a unit. The distorted perceptions of reality and of needs should be identified, and alternative modes of gratification sought.

19. (2) The magnitude of Dr. Gold's withdrawal can be marked on a continuum on which each of us also falls. The purpose of the withdrawal is to evade demands of a painful environment and to limit interactions with people.

20. (3) Dr. Gold was always shy, which in itself is not any more abnormal than is being aggressive. It is a matter of the extent to which we are functioning at

our potential, and of what is our satisfaction with or liking of ourselves and our performance in various avenues of our lives. Because he had insufficient human support, Dr. Gold was unable to maintain a sense of satisfaction and stability as demands on him increased.

21. (1) Regression is a major defense mechanism of the ego that can be observed in operation every day.

22. (4) These features could be rewritten as the classic four A's of schizophrenia: associative looseness (loss of logical thinking); affect (blunting and distortion of affect); ambivalence; and autism (overinvestment in self, preoccupation with fantasy, denial of reality).

23. (1) Denial of internal and external reality contributes significantly to the development of symptoms observed in schizophrenia.

24. (2) Since Dr. Gold developed paranoid features in his schizophrenia (fear that colleagues had instigated a plot to discredit his research, fear of being sued for malpractice), the use of projection is evident. Projection is operational unconsciously in the development of delusions.

25. (1) In order for projection to function, denial of one's own thoughts, motives, and feelings must first be employed.

26. (1) Distortion of reality leads to disharmony of thought and feeling, and therefore to flatness of affect.

27. (4) Narcissism, in psychoanalysis, is equivalent to original self-love. It is a term derived from Narcissus, who fell in love with his own reflected image.

28. (3) Delusions and hallucinations, as bizarre as they may be, are necessary to the patient's psychic economy in that they serve a protective function for the faltering ego.

29. (3) Although delusional thinking represents a distortion of reality and inability to differentiate between thoughts and external reality, it nevertheless reveals a residue of the individual's experiences.

30. (2) Thoughts of persecution and influence are paranoid delusions characterized by ideas that one is being slandered or controlled. The deluded patient tends to blame others for "causing" his own conduct. The purpose of the delusions is to reduce the internal threat to ego integrity.

31. (3) Phenothiazine tranquilizers are thought (the mechanisms of action are not clear) to affect those parts of the nervous system listed. "Extrapyramidal" refers to those nerve tracks outside the main collection of motor nerve fibers arising in the brain and passing down through the spinal cord to the anterior horns. The phenothiazine tranquilizers have largely replaced the rauwolfia alkaloids (i.e., reserpine) because they act faster and cause less serious side effects.

32. (3) Trifluoperazine (Stelazine) is a phenothiazine tranquilizer that, in some patients, causes extrapyramidal reactions (i.e., tremor, akinesia).

33. (2) Benztropine mesylate has an atropine-like action, and is used along with levodopa to treat Parkinson's disease.

34. (4) Auditory hallucinations mean that the patient hears voices that do not exist externally or result from external stimuli, but rather arise from internal stimuli. Hallucinations are projected conflicts, and as such contain an element of frustration and anxiety.

35. (3) Delusions such as ideas of reference overcompensate for feelings of isolation through fantasies of being the focus of universal attention (hence, Dr. Gold's reference to Russian scientists).

36. (2) Further depersonalization by Dr. Gold would indicate further disintegration of his ego and more interest in self.

37. (4) Provision of a warm human experience is *not* to imply a rapidly developed, interpersonal relationship oozing with acceptance and sanction. Schizophrenic patients typically are withdrawn and rejecting of people.

38. (1) The nurse-patient relationship with schizophrenic patients begins with short, specific periods of time in which the nurse may sit quietly beside the patient, or occasionally attempt to draw him into some type of general response.

39. (2) Therapeutic and social relationships differ, and the aim of a therapeutic relationship is to meet needs of selected clients. If, however, the nurse should become extremely anxious while interacting with a patient, it would be ad-

visable for her to retreat, seek the reason for her anxiety, and return to the patient later.

40. (4) The characteristics listed are all aspects of a therapeutic relationship. Communication is the key to success in the relationship.

41. (1) At times, in our face-to-face encounters (interviews) with patients, we neglect having a specific purpose or plan. Note that an interview is more than an exchange of information.

42. (3) Patients, perhaps like us, appreciate having their communications of ideas and feelings understood in the way in which they were conveyed or intended.

43. (2) Communication does *not* require that opinions are modified, only that there is a reciprocal exchange of information.

44. (1) Extremely regressed patients with poor ego strength may be ataxic or have poor motor control. Interpersonal contact, at times, can be facilitated for patients such as Dr. Gold by participation in activities that do *not* require complex decision-making or close physical contact.

45. (1) During the very early contacts with Dr. Gold, when he was incoherent, this comment would have been useless; however, after a relationship with a modicum of trust is established, pointing out anxious behavior can result in identification of people, situations, or thoughts that are causing the anxiety.

46. (4) All the actions listed are blocks to communication.

47. (4) After the nurse consciously recalls that Dr. Gold's "crazy," bizarre, incoherent behavior has a purpose, the focus shifts to helping, encouraging, leading, and assisting him. The hoped-for result is a decrease in anxiety, less need to withdraw, and a stronger ego; specifically, a higher opinion of self-worth.

48. (1) Anxiety, according to Sullivan, results from our interactions with significant others, and causes a reduction in self-esteem.

49. (2) Sullivan's description of the etiology of schizophrenia is congruent with his hypothesis that anxiety is interpersonally engendered. As in the formulations of other theorists, schizophrenic behavior has as its purpose the avoidance of anxiety (or protection of the ego).

50. (3) Sullivan stated that, as the anxiety level increases, the breadth of one's span of interest narrows, and if the anxiety is extreme enough, focus is entirely on the self (this response was referred to earlier as "narcissism").

51. (4) When a person does not wish to talk with other people it usually is because he is angry with them or one specific person in the group. In this case, the nurse simply honored the request of Dr. Gold and sat with him. If this situation occurs in subsequent interactions, the nurse could select a proper time to explore what is causing the anger. Also, it is possible that Dr. Gold does want to talk because, by his comment, he focused attention on his talking.

52. (2) Again, this response is useful only after the nurse-patient relationship is well established. It would be an inappropriate question to put to a withdrawn person who is rejecting of people, because it may place pressure on him to talk and thus increase anxiety.

53. (4) The vagueness of Dr. Gold's comment makes it difficult to know what he is trying to convey. The nurse's reply invites him to clarify his comment, and tells him that it was not fully understood but that the nurse desires to know what he intended to communicate. He possibly is saying, "How do I know that I can trust you?" People want to be understood.

54. (1) Dr. Gold asked the nurse a question that presents a temptation to offer advice. The general rule here is first to determine what he wants to do. Asking him to describe how he offended his patients in the past is contraindicated. Asking his what he might do other than private practice is an indirect "no" answer to his question. A discussion of what he wants to do, and the advantages and disadvantages of his plan, would be helpful.

55. (4) The focus of the nurse's reply is on Dr. Gold's feeling of anger. It is of little value to guess the wife's reason for renting his office, or the manner in which he found out about it. Humans find it difficult to remove stressful thoughts from their consciousness on command.

56. (2) The cause of anxiety is not immediately obvious to the individual expressing it, but Sullivan says anxiety occurs when the self-esteem is threatened.

57. (4) It is quite conceivable that we are not maximally effective with all patients. We experience plateaus where no progress is evident. The steps outlined show how to evaluate whether or not a different approach is indicated.
58. (4) All the reasons listed contribute to Dr. Gold's good progress. It is useful to remember that many patients are discharged and function at a high level of health in the community.
59. (3) These factors reflect chronic symptoms and little real chance for change in the environment that contributed to this illness.
60. (3) It is crucial that patients be prepared long in advance for the termination of the relationship. No one feels satisfied when a significant person leaves abruptly.
61. (4) Departure is sometimes necessary even though you love the person. Separation initiates anxiety and anger.
62. (1) At the onset of a nurse-patient relationship it is therapeutic to establish the appropriate temporal limits of the interaction.
63. (4) All the statements listed are general goals for psychotherapy. It is satisfying when a patient tells you he is "well" and no longer needs psychotherapy, and when you can argue with him without reservation.

Adolescent Adjustment Reaction

1. (2) Adolescence is a period of conflict and perhaps turmoil in which individuals establish a sense of identity. It is a period of physical and emotional metamorphosis that occurs between puberty and young adulthood.
2. (1) Puberty is a period of rapid physical change in which individuals become capable of reproduction.
3. (4) During puberty the individual may feel estranged from himself as the child he has known. This estrangement results from rapidly changing body image, self-concept, sexual role, and social status.
4. (4) Ego strength is not a well-defined term, but is used to refer to a conglomeration of mental and personality traits. The changes of puberty take place so rapidly and with such variety that the ego strength is decreased because of the concurrent demands on the ego to test reality; to control drives and thoughts; to employ defense mechanisms; to re-establish object relations and autonomous functions; and especially to form a new sense of self-identity (synthetic function of ego).
5. (4) Adolescence is a time of looking inward to ascertain who one is, and of seeking to locate one's "place" in the environment. All the tasks listed fall into the looking inward or searching outward categories.
6. (3) During adolescence there is a resurgence of sexual objectives and a drive toward independence. This combination allows adolescents to seek a love object or a sexual partner outside the family.
7. (3) Freud theorized that normal resolution of the oedipal conflict results in identification with, and internalization of values of, the parent of the same sex. Resolution of this identification during adolescence is essential to a healthy personality.
8. (4) The features listed in this item for a healthy individual are essentially the same as the mental characteristics of ego strength: tolerance, forgiveness, acceptance of substitutes, persistence, ability to learn, and vitality.
9. (2) Inconsistency, rage, and intensity are observed frequently in adolescents. The individual who consistently throughout adolescence shows no emotional instability is either extremely secure or is not effectively dealing with the conflicts posed by physical and emotional changes of this period.
10. (1) Adolescents vacillate between peaks and valleys of their emotions. Also, they experience a decrease in ego strength because of the diversity and volume of demand placed on the ego at this time. What results not infrequently is labeled "crazy." When "moody," they are withdrawn; when "high," they may appear manic. Conflict, prevalent during adolescence, is the basis of neurosis.
11. (3) Withdrawal, denial, intellectualization, and regression are defenses commonly employed by adolescents. Preoccupation and confusion are signs of regression

and withdrawal from reality. Ben's retreat from close contact with members of the gang and immersion into religious and charitable acts are examples of denial and sublimation. In Ben's case, talking with the minister's daughter about becoming a missionary could be interpreted as intellectualization, rather than gaining of insight into his sexual thoughts and feelings of sinfulness. There was no indication that Ben experienced a conversion reaction (e.g., paralysis).

12. (3) Initial efforts to be like his peers (gang) and unlike his parents heightened Ben's homosexual feelings, not an uncommon experience in adolescence because of oedipal identifications. His defenses were to control these homosexual, and later heterosexual, impulses.

13. (2) Associating himself, perhaps erroneously, with the minister's daughter (college senior) was an attempt to deny his homosexual and "sinful" feelings: to associate with what he perceived as "good" to offset his self-perception of being "bad."

14. (2) Intellectualization is a way to talk rather than risk experiencing one's feelings. Most defense mechanisms operate out of unconscious awareness, so Ben would not have been aware of the value of his intellectualizing.

15. (4) Regression is the resumption under stress of behaviors that were more satisfactory to the individual in an earlier stage of development. Recall briefly how we tend to dress and groom on a day when we're "falling apart" or "letting it all hang out."

16. (4) Self-denial, asceticism, is keeping a restraint or "iron hand" on oneself. The rigid, undeviating behavior is designed to control expression of impulses.

17. (2) Although Ben's fanatically religious behavior may have appeared to be conformity to parental standards, it was more likely an attempt at rigid self-control of the upsurge in sexual impulses. Adolescents typically don't rush with enthusiasm to the temple or church.

18. (4) Holdover of oedipal conflicts and increased sexual drive result in experimentation with homosexual behavior and masturbation. Feelings of inadequacy and fear that adult responsibilities cannot be accepted lead to exhibitionism and hypochondriasis. Frustration generally results in aggression.

19. (3) Ambivalence is a hallmark of adolescence, and a major manifestation of it is in the struggle with dependence versus independence. Adolescents want adult privileges, but are apprehensive about their ability to assume adult responsibilities.

20. (2) Establishing an ego identity is basic to forming heterosexual relationships, selecting an occupation, and refining the superego.

21. (2) The crisis of self-identification or diffusion is precipitated by rapid physical development and heightened sexual awareness. Finding out who one is in the context of past experiences and current meaning to others is ego identity. Ego identity is not conforming totally to parents or peers and, as described, it must be in the context of one's social environment.

22. (3) Identity diffusion or role diffusion occurs in adolescence when doubt about one's sexual identity or occupational identity lingers. This diffusion results from trying to be too many things to too many persons; i.e., not making one's own decisions or not identifying one's "own thing."

23. (3) Refinement of the superego continues throughout life, but establishing one's own set of values is a task in adolescence. Experimentation is essential to ascertaining what one truly wishes to value permanently. However, we tend to set standards compatible with our own values or those of persons with whom we are identified.

24. (2) Aggressive and sexual drives are intricately linked. Doubt about sexual identity can lead to delinquent behavior. Frustration of sexual desires can cause anger.

25. (3) Frustration with not being able to express or understand his feelings increased Ben's aggression. There was no indication that his parents had rejected him or that his superego was weakened. Although not specifically mentioned, Ben may have had some unexpressed concerns about his future.

26. (1) With his peers Ben could have participated in a group as a member, leader, and/or facilitator. Refinement of social skills and communication abilities were

perhaps best accomplished outside the peer group. He could have shared vicariously the experiences of anyone he encountered.

27. (4) The advantages to Ben of participating in a peer group are those listed. These can be categorized as role-playing and diffusing the intensity of feelings.

28. (3) Membership in a peer group or gang doesn't automatically stop interest in parents and other adults. Adolescents can be quite helpful to each other by exchanging thoughts and feelings.

29. (4) All the behaviors listed would be therapeutic for Ben at this time. The behaviors helpful to adults are also those that are helpful to adolescents.

30. (4) As in most cases, a consistently implemented treatment plan is most therapeutic. Each person listed contributes ideas or assessments to be considered when formulating the plan.

31. (2) If the nurse described is emotionally mature and secure in his/her own completion of the tasks of adolescence, he/she could be helpful to Ben during this episode. This person, however, should not be the only one to interact with Ben.

32. (2) Football is an active sport in which aggression can be expressed and energy expended. It is considered perhaps as a more masculine domain than the other activities.

33. (3) A general rule in interacting with adolescent patients is not to interpret the possible meanings of their behavior, and not to encourage them to express too many thoughts and feelings early in the relationship, because they may become frightened or anxious by their expressions. They become concerned about the ramifications and sometimes experience a decreased ability to control impulses. There is nothing so repulsive to adolescents (or adults!) as pious expressions from others about how successful they were in the area of our failures.

34. (1) It is not helpful to threaten retaliation for or to reward such behavior. Most of us feel anger, maybe to the point of murderous rage, when someone spits on us. The most helpful response in a treatment setting is to express verbally the anger and unacceptability of the act.

35. (2) Anger is always best handled by talking it out or working it out constructively. Impulsive acting out, displacement of, or internalization of anger unfortunately results in punishment of oneself rather than the provoking agent.

36. (1) The nurse's attitude of genuine interest in Ben, and the discussion of topics in which Ben has knowledge or expertise, is infinitely more helpful than being nosey or placating his thoughts, feelings, or behaviors.

37. (2) The object language of adolescents is a most valuable cue to their ego strength. If we assess an individual's unconscious motivation, personality, or superego strength by external appearances, we are routinely in error.

38. (2) Although nurses can be helpful temporarily by being a mother figure or by "mothering" activities, this method of relating is in opposition to ultimate goals to be reached during adolescence. Explicit details of sexual fantasies about other patients can be titillating, but they are nontherapeutic for the adolescent.

39. (2) If Ben is labeled as weird or crazy, it is unlikely that he will obtain the peer support and adult guidance that he needs. We all enjoy interacting with well-adjusted people (when we can find them), but not all persons have had experiences and supports that allowed development of a high degree of mental health.

40. (2) Ben, like the rest of us, will manage if given a little help along the way. Knowledge and understanding of the tremendous pressures on youth in our society, and how parents can help, may increase the support Ben receives from his parents.

Drug Addiction

1. (4) The estimate of the number of heroin users in the United States is variable, ranging from 200,000 to 500,000; the latter figure is believed to be more

accurate. The rate of drug addiction in the U.S. is lower today than it was in the 1920s.

2. (2) The problem of drug addiction in youth is well-known and alarming. It is now common in grade, middle, and high schools.

3. (1) The potential addict finds in the drug a release from tension, and satisfaction of a longing for artificial elation or peace. Most drug addiction does not occur as a result of medical therapy and it does not improve motor skills. Most addicting drugs impair perception and motor skills.

4. (4) Physicians are in a high-risk group for drug addiction, because the practice of medicine is a high-stress occupation and the availability of drugs is commonplace. ˙

5. (3) Heroin is taken by sniffing or injection, which usually leaves a mark called venous tattooing. Icterus, nystagmus, and enlarged liver have many causes. Hepatitis occurs from viral contamination during injection.

6. (4) The motives for self-administration of drugs are numerous, and include those listed. Most texts list escape from reality or release from tension as a major cause.

7. (1) The exact mechanism by which amphetamines stimulate the central nervous system is not known, but it probably acts by stimulating the reticular activating system.

8. (2) An amphetamine abuser takes the drug to prevent fatigue and produce euphoria. It usually is not taken for pain and would be contraindicated in persons with insomnia or nervousness. During an amphetamine high there is a false sense of great physical strength, clear thinking, and no need for sleep. After the "high" (period called "crashing"), there is extreme lethargy and profound depression.

9. (1) In recent years amphetamines were used to facilitate weight reduction but the complications were so great that their use in the treatment of obesity is now rare.

10. (2) The slang terms for Methedrine are "speed" or "crystal." Other amphetamines are Benzedrine and Dexedrine. The usual dose of the amphetamines is 5 to 30 mg. daily; an abuser takes 75 to 100 mg. per day or more.

11. (3) Dependency on heroin is high both physically and psychologically. The physical dependence potential in marijuana is unknown; it has moderate psychologic addicting properties.

12. (4) The natural opiates include opium, morphine, and codeine. The semisynthetic opiates include heroin, hydromorphone, and oxycodone (the latter drug is marketed with other drugs under the trade name Percodan). The synthetic narcotics related to opium are meperidine (Demerol) and methadone.

13. (3) Heroin has many slang names: smack, Big H, horse, thing, Brown, Chinese red, scag, junk, Mexican mud.

14. (2) Cocaine is a stimulant that is injected or sniffed and is commonly called coke, gold dust, or snow. Mescaline is an hallucinogen; the slang terms for it are bean, button, or cactus.

15. (2) LSD commonly produces hallucinations. Marijuana and amphetamines rarely do except in extremely high doses.

16. (3) Pushers do sell cut or dilute forms of drugs, but Wade's higher dosages are due to increased tolerance that develops over time. This tolerance, however, is rapidly lost and becomes a factor in opiate overdose.

17. (3) Addiction to opiates is not known to alter intelligence. In larger doses these drugs produce a feeling that all is well, and as a result ambition and productivity are lowered. Overdose results in altered respirations, convulsions, and coma. Withdrawal symptoms occur when the addict is deprived of the drug for 12–14 hours.

18. (4) The eventual effects of the habit are impaired ethical sense and social deterioration, as a result not of the direct effect of the narcotic but rather of the social consequences of the addicted life.

19. (4) As addiction increases, less attention is paid to work and health. If this results in loss of work and deprivation of supply, the addict is vulnerable to overdose when the drug is taken, and resorts to crime to obtain the needed supply. Social deterioration often results.

20. (4) Heroin administration by injection predisposes the addict to the conditions listed and to hepatitis, usually type B viral.

21. (4) The withdrawal symptoms that arise first are yawning, lacrimation, rhinorrhea, sneezing, and perspiration. As these become more pronounced, anorexia, dilated pupils, tremor, and gooseflesh occur.

22. (4) About a day and a half after the withdrawal of the drug the symptoms peak, and incontrollable twitching and cramping of the muscles in the legs, abdomen, and back are obvious. The blood pressure and pulse rise, and the patient may experience both vomiting and diarrhea. It is obviously dangerous to withdraw opiates in addicted persons without administering a narcotic antagonist and/or methadone.

23. (4) The preferred treatment is to relieve the affective state that provoked the addiction. This method is not always possible, so others are instituted (e.g., methadone). The addict is given methadone to produce a physiologic state that permits him to be socially functional. Methadone is enlisted in dosages of 10–20 mg. daily, and gradually increased over a period of four weeks until the desired effect is achieved.

24. (3) Some researchers think that methadone is as addicting as heroin, but the effects on the body are not as harmful.

25. (1) Two extremes in approach to treatment of addiction have been suggested as effective: prison and voluntary hospitalization. Investigations suggest that 25 to 69 per cent of those who complete a methadone program follow abstinence from drugs.

26. (4) All the symptoms listed are side effects of methadone use. An abrupt overdose of methadone causes oversedation, urinary retention, or abdominal distention.

27. (1) Since naloxone must be administered more than once a day per injection, it is not as useful as methadone (24–36 hours) or methadyl acetate (48–60 hours), which are longer-acting. All of these drugs suppress the withdrawal symptoms in heroin addicts.

28. (4) Although it is true that Wade's desire to alter his drug behavior and its consequences is most influential in this change, he cannot do so until he feels some degree of self-reliance and self-confidence. The key person in enabling the change in life style is the addicted individual; others encourage and support the move toward abstinence.

29. (3) Wade probably developed a stimulus (anxiety, stress, problems)-response (take drugs)-type pattern to cope with life. Two approaches can then be employed to help decrease stress and/or anxiety and to alter his response to stress. Improving his ability to cope, and decreasing drug administration, is often followed by employment and general personality strengthening.

30. (3) Physiologic dependence (withdrawal symptoms) cease within a week to ten days, but psychologic dependence may continue indefinitely.

31. (4) Persons addicted to drugs may chronically neglect their health, and so attention to personal hygiene and nutrition is essential. A protective, accepting atmosphere is therapeutic and includes restriction to the unit, limitation of telephone use, continuing observation, and searching of belongings on admission and of visitors' parcels.

32. (4) Inability to handle feelings significantly contributes to addiction development. Heroin produces a false sense that "all is well."

33. (3) Escape from responsibility and rejection of authority are rather typical of drug addicts. Wade's initial efforts in carving out his turf in the unit will be filled with manipulation. However, he later may become overly dependent on the nurse, a situation to be avoided.

34. (4) A matter-of-fact, straightforward application of minimal standards for conduct is helpful. It is important not to sanction unacceptable behavior, but it is equally important not to retaliate for such behavior.

35. (2) Avoidance of a dependent, mothering relationship is accomplished by making the patient feel secure and self-reliant. Drug addiction may impair one's ability to relate in a close, interpersonal relationship, but does not destroy one's appreciation of sex (used in its broadest application).

36. (3) Teenagers often begin taking drugs to be included in their "in group." Because

of Wade's living situation (married, age 22), his peer group would be different from that of the adolescent. Society's expectation of Wade would also differ from that of an adolescent. It is important for him to participate in group psychotherapy, to help him relate to peers and to begin self-examination.

37. (4) If the psychodynamic etiology of Wade's drug addiction was nongratification of oral dependency needs, pipe-smoking would be one means of providing oral satisfaction. The other activities listed are not viewed as gratifying oral needs.

38. (3) Early in the hospitalization Wade must be oriented to specific rules of conduct. He should understand that the reasons for these procedures are to establish a routine and to avoid misunderstanding what is expected of him. The self-image is not altered just by observing others. Diversion through activity is useful if the patient first understands what is expected of him. Knowledge of why we do a certain thing does not always help us change the behavior.

39. (4) It is the nurse's responsibility to know what provokes or contributes to drug abuse (including those factors listed), and what methods are available to facilitate prevention of drug addiction; viz., teaching, education, and recognition of early signs of drug experimentation.

40. (4) The actions expected of the community health nurse in preventing drug abuse may seem overwhelming, but it is well to remember the pervasiveness of the problem, which may be evidenced in our own families, neighbors, and co-workers.

Alcoholism

1. (4) Addiction is more than a habit or wish for something. It is physiologic and psychologic dependence on a chemical substance.

2. (2) When the blood alcohol concentration is 80 mg. per 100 ml of blood, judgment is impaired. An individual is considered intoxicated when the concentration is 150 mg. of alcohol per 100 ml. of blood. The frontal lobes (feeling of well-being, weakening of will-power) of the brain are affected first, and then other parts of the brain: parietal lobes (distorted sensation, speech disturbances); cerebellum (disequilibrium, incoordination); occipital lobes (double vision, loss of distance perception); thalamus and medulla (depressed respiration, stupor, or death).

3. (1) Tolerance for alcohol develops with continued "intake." Alcohol is absorbed directly into the blood (it is not digested), and is metabolized by oxidation in the liver at a standard rate. Mr. Peabody focused on his own "pain," and experienced drinking as a pleasurable escape from reality. His need for such an experience was probably greater than that of his friends.

4. (3) Tolerance increase means a declining effect of the same dose when repeated over time. As a result, it is necessary to increase the dose to obtain the original effect. Ability to resist the more harmful effects is a measure of the impact on brain functioning. Some researchers think that the destructive effect on the liver is cumulative.

5. (4) The prolonged frustration of never quite measuring up to self- or other imposed demands is contributory to alcohol intake as an effort to experience a feeling of well-being. The psychogenesis of alcoholism is complex and variable from individual to individual. These etiologies include cultural influences, childhood experiences of deprivation of emotional support, mothering by an overindulgent-overprotective parent, absence of parent(s), and an inconsistent environment. Underlying all of these is frustration because the infantile dependency demands become too great to be met, and because an adult passive-dependent person is unable to express his needs adequately.

6. (4) The symptoms listed are the initial, observable physical signs. Delirium tremens is an acute psychotic state that may develop in the chronic alcoholic (one who has been drinking for four or five years) following alcohol deprivation.

7. (2) Persons experiencing an episode of delirium tremens do have tremors, but these are only one feature. As tremor, restlessness, irritability, aversion for

food, and insomnia continue, illusions and hallucinations begin and increase in intensity.

8. (2) Hallucinations of delirium tremens are most often visual. Auditory hallucinations are second in frequency. Other types may occur but do so less often.

9. (3) The hallucinations during delirium tremens usually are fleeting and terrifying. They are viewed as real and worthy of consideration. Alcoholics try to escape imaginary objects or to remove nonexistent insects from the skin.

10. (4) The influence of the Alcoholics Anonymous program lies in its ability to provide new superego standards for the individual. Performance is judged only by ability to control drinking. The responsibility for such control is shared.

11. (4) Everyone is affected by alcoholism, especially, the alcoholic. The speculation of each involved person about missed opportunities and lost potential can often be quite painful.

12. (4) These physical changes are produced either by direct effects of alcohol on organs or as a consequence of malnutrition. Both of these can contribute to brain deterioration, but cirrhosis, gastritis, and pancreatitis are caused by the direct effect of alcohol on these organs. Malnutrition is compounded by organ damage (stomach, pancreas, intestines, liver), by alcohol's high caloric value (7.1 calories per gram), and by decrease in the social value attributed to eating.

13. (4) Korsakoff's psychosis develops following prolonged vitamin B deficiency, which causes cerebral and peripheral nerve degeneration. Therefore, the symptoms listed develop.

14. (2) The individual maintains a good grasp for the present (what is in sight), but loses ability to recall the past. His confabulations, in part, conceal his amnesia.

15. (4) The pattern described develops over time, and is perpetuated by the anxiety and craving for alcohol that is experienced when alcohol is withdrawn.

16. (4) The ego's development is poor because of parental role confusion, over-protection, and conflict. The individual becomes a passive-dependent adult, unable openly to express his needs and internalize his hostilities. Thus, the superego functions by regulating self-esteem through self-condemnation, or by conforming to the ego ideal.

17. (4) The cyclical nature of the alcoholic's drinking is well known. Anxiety and uncertainty about one's behavior when intoxicated cause ego frustrations to mount. Alcohol, at this point in chronic alcoholism, only offers relief from unbearable tensions.

18. (4) Because of a weak ego Mr. Peabody would be unable to postpone need gratification, would show dependence on others, and would experience feelings of inferiority. Because of his previous experiences he could be entertaining, but unable to form strong interpersonal relationships.

19. (4) In addition to the physical and psychosocial trauma to the alcoholics themselves, families and communities are deprived of their abilities. Many alcoholics provide economically for their families. They do cause embarrassment to their families, but this is not the most serious effect of alcoholism.

20. (3) Prejudice and anger are directed toward the alcoholic because many people think that the alcoholic has the choice whether to drink or not to drink.

21. (3) Since humans enjoy experiencing "pleasure" and alleviating "pain," the accessibility of alcohol in a stressful society contributes to its being a major health and social problem. Over half of the adults in the United States drink alcohol regularly, as do about one fourth of the teenagers.

22. (1) Alcoholism is linked to much criminal behavior, but in itself is an attempt at adjustment. It is not simply a moral problem.

23. (3) The vast majority of alcoholics have been found to have an underlying character trait of the passive-aggressive personality. Other alcoholics are compulsive, depressive, paranoid, or antisocial personalities.

24. (2) It is desirable to help Mr. Peabody rely on people rather than on alcohol. However, the dependence should not be total, and is best directed toward control of drinking behavior and reestablishment of social and economic viability.

25. (2) Dictatorial authority is never therapeutic. Those in authority over Mr. Peabody in the past, especially his parents, haven't been too helpful. The staff needs to be aware that he may project his own superego standards upon them, and the program is then perceived as punitive. If this occurs, unrecognized by the staff, Mr. Peabody may drop out of the treatment program.

26. (2) The nurse should continually seek to define the specific reason for Mr. Peabody's alcoholism, and be alert for withdrawal symptoms. Not all alcoholics are cured. They do, on occasion, keep promises.

27. (3) There would be no reason to administer sedatives, other than to help control withdrawal symptoms. Mr. Peabody was not depressed, so there was no indication for antidepressant therapy.

28. (3) The nurse must make a therapeutic contact with the patient in order to assist with his therapy. The response by the nurse facilitates this contact. In the general hospital, nurses traditionally do not smoke in patients' rooms; however, in a mental health setting, smoking in conferences and dayrooms may not be forbidden, and in some settings is encouraged.

29. (2) When Mr. Peabody defiantly states that the nurse can't control his behavior (drinking) he is correct, but perhaps is conveying "I wish someone would make me stop drinking." The nurse's response is a "no-fight" position that confronts him, conveys the expectation that he will stop drinking, and challenges him to declare a nondrinking goal. The nurse also could have asked, "Do you want to stop drinking?"

30. (4) The experience of being with other similarly afflicted persons seems to make alcoholics accept and benefit from group psychotherapy. They frequently have personalities that do not "wear well" over time in a one-to-one relationship.

31. (2) The size of the group is less significant than a goal and leadership, and size only influences the type of activity in which the group can engage. Varied backgrounds may enhance the group work. Continuous contact may end in strife.

32. (2) The goals in Mr. Peabody's treatment were directed toward enabling him to gain control of his drinking. This is best achieved by helping him communicate his needs, tolerate frustration, and develop solutions to problems other than drinking.

33. (1) Group therapy involves adapting to members' changing needs as they arise.

34. (4) The role of the therapist in group psychotherapy is to stimulate behavioral responses from members that will assure progress toward their goals. The methods for accomplishing goal attainment are listed.

35. (4) In group psychotherapy, transferences are made to members and/or leader(s). Transference to a variety of role types is possible.

36. (2) Anger is a very common emotion. Ventilation of feelings in the group setting is helpful, and group members encourage and contradict each other in this expression. Frustration mounts, leading to aggression. Alcoholics tend to internalize hostile feelings; these often are expressed during the course of therapy.

37. (4) The dependent alcoholic with a low self-esteem requires interest expressed toward him as a person of worth. Comment on improvement in grooming is ego building.

38. (4) Leaders in a therapeutic group must strike a healthy balance between assuming all power and direction setting for the group, and allowing the members to wander aimlessly or to be led destructively by a member. This balance is achieved by employing the behaviors listed.

39. (3) The responsibility for group progress is primarily that of the therapist. However, throughout the course of any group therapy, leadership is assumed by the therapist(s) and any of the members. A strong, supportive member can facilitate group progress as effectively as the identified leader (therapist).

40. (2) Excretion of acetaldehyde is blocked by Antabuse. The person who drinks alcohol within 12 hours after Antabuse ingestion (0.5 to 1 gram) feels heat in the face, his skin becomes purple-red, and tachycardia develops. Dyspnea, headache, nausea, and vomiting follow.

41. (2) If the members do not participate (verbally or nonverbally), the group never becomes cohesive, and movement toward any goal is impeded.

42. (3) The point of group therapy is that members more strongly identify who they

are, and accept or change their self-image. If members feel accepted, and give and receive feedback, group cohesiveness develops and progress toward goals can be significant.

43. (3) The goal of group psychotherapy is not to furnish psychoanalytic insight, but rather to provide corrective experiences and identification with others. The underlying hypothesis of group therapy is that the alcoholic's problems usually develop in a social context, and thus can best be modified in a group (social) setting.

44. (3) Members must have anxiety at a manageable level and must feel accepted by the group in order to participate in and benefit from group interaction. Submissive and hostile members typically do not feel accepted.

45. (3) The roles of antagonist (negative, attacking, seeking own goals) and conciliator (placating, soothing) are thought to be disruptive of group progress. The instrumentalist (summarizes, directs) and expressionist (expresses overt thoughts and feelings and encourages others to do the same) both further the work of the group.

46. (4) After the nurse has been able to initiate a therapeutic contact, the varied activities listed are carried out. The nurse interacts with alcoholic persons by showing concern, confronting and communicating understanding of the alcoholic's plight, and warning of the physical dangers of protracted drinking.

47. (1) Roles may change as the group progresses toward its goal; even the leader does not always lead. Nurses' roles in the group are not altered by mood swings, topics discussed, or patient membership.

48. (3) It might be advantageous to make alcohol less accessible but the alcoholic remains potentially an out-of-control drinker for life. It would be artificial not to mention alcohol or not to remember the life of alcohol addiction. The behaviors listed as correct are designed to meet needs for social involvements that disrupt old patterns and provide pleasant new experiences.

49. (1) It is impossible to control the thoughts of another person or to protect him from disappointment. Since the temptation to drink is ever-present to an alcoholic, advice on how to avoid it may be meaningless.

50. (3) In helping an alcoholic to overcome drinking behavior it is essential to involve the family and, as appropriate, the employer. It is important that the employer be encouraged to act consistently and to let Mr. Peabody know what is expected of him.

Chronic Arteriosclerotic Brain Syndrome

1. (3) An organic psychosis is to be distinguished from mental changes associated with normal aging and can occur at any age if sufficient neuropathology is present.

2. (4) The causes of organic psychosis are multiple. Arteriosclerosis and alcoholism are the two main causes.

3. (4) Impairment in memory, orientation, and judgment are classic changes, and comprehension of events and ability for abstraction is diminished. The affect prominent in the individual may become more pronounced.

4. (1) Early life experiences of exploring one's body and differentiating self from mother, as well as exploration of space and growing awareness of time, lead to orientation in these spheres.

5. (3) As brain cells die, memory is impaired and disorientation occurs. The earliest and most frequently occurring disorientation is to time.

6. (1) Keeping a light burning will help Lydia orient herself in space, and the clock and calendar will help orient her to time. Schedules are of no value if she cannot focus on time properly. Lydia probably has established her own routine. Requiring her to recite names would be demeaning. Stimulation by family, friends, and neighbors is helpful in maintaining orientation and interest.

7. (2) The memory patterns for past events are well established, but recent events are

forgotten. Chemicals necessary for placing a thought in the memory may not be available in sufficient quantity.

8. (4) Owing to the death of brain cells, lessened physical energy, and diminished contacts with people, impoverishment of ideation occurs in most aged individuals.

9. (1) Once the brain cells have died, regeneration is not possible. In an acute organic brain disorder, the abnormality may be due to trauma, pressure of a neoplasm, inflammation, or vascular impairment.

10. (1) The personality manifested in arteriosclerotic brain damage is as varied as the premorbid personality patterns of the individual affected.

11. (2) Provision of safety and consistency, in an environment with which Lydia has, or can gain, some familiarity, is indicated. The goal is not to reconstruct the personality, but to help Lydia and others to cope with her overt behavior.

12. (2) Most people learn certain skills that become automatic, such as dressing oneself and engaging in polite social interaction. These skills are not lost unless confusion is present. If Lydia is exposed to news of current events, she could discuss them with considerable insight. Again, this depends on the amount of brain deterioration.

13. (2) Vitamin B is water-soluble and is not stored in large quantities in the body, so deficiencies soon cause impairment of function. Thiamine (B_1), pyridoxine (B_6), and pantothenic acid deficiency contribute to neuritis and other neurologic disturbances.

14. (4) All of Lydia's behaviors resemble what we would do if we were involuntarily placed in a new environment.

15. (3) The response by Lydia's family is a direct, clear presentation of the truth in the situation. The reason given for their actions may initially make her angry, but later may be a comfort to her.

16. (4) Disorientation combined with the unfamiliarity of the environment predisposes Lydia to regression. Also, most persons regress with physical illness.

17. (1) Following denial of their waning physical and intellectual abilities, persons with arteriosclerotic brain syndrome next project their hostile feelings onto others in their surroundings. Some evidence of paranoid thinking may be observed.

18. (3) Lydia is prone to fluctuations in mood (due to chemical and neural pathway changes in the brain), but not to becoming withdrawn or hostile. She is not apt to develop strong, affectionate ties to the nursing home personnel at this time.

19. (4) It is very difficult to ascertain clearly those aspects of behavior that are due to brain tissue changes, and those due to anxiety, insecurity, or threat to the self-esteem. The nurse should carefully observe patterns of behavior, and especially the temporal relationship of behaviors and events.

20. (3) Memory impairment relates to recent events, so it is most likely that, while looking for the candy, Lydia forgot the original purpose in doing so.

21. (2) Reminding Lydia that her friends are waiting in the reception room allows her to decide whether she is able to continue the visit and tell her friends that she forgot they were there, and if so to choose her room or the reception room to resume the meeting.

22. (4) The assessments listed are to enable the nursing home personnel to establish a baseline of physical strength (cerebrovascular damage, intellectual ability) and personality (attitude toward physical decline, life experiences). This will assist in planning Lydia's care, providing for her safety, and predicting possible future needs.

23. (2) As the ego strength is weakened and overchallenged, Lydia becomes less able to control emotions and impulses, and her thinking is less rational. The result is that the premorbid personality tendencies are exaggerated. Declining brain capacity is not followed routinely by regression.

24. (2) An out-of-context comment of this kind frequently catches us by surprise. A factual comment such as: "Lydia, you've forgotten; you decided to sell your car because you don't drive anymore" is almost always the best response. Exploring the comment is inappropriate, as is ignoring it. To remind Lydia of a loss (driver's license) and failing physical capacity may be truthful, but perhaps a little blunt.

25. (2) Hoarding is accumulating a supply to keep in reserve for future "taking in": a reflection of a feeling of insecurity, not an antagonistic or ungenerous gesture.

26. (3) At times we attribute more significance to a situation than is warranted. Lydia is saying simply that she is glad an old friend hasn't forgotten her.

27. (3) Only (1), avoiding the fact that Lydia's mother is dead, is contraindicated. To help orient Lydia, it is preferable first to answer her question with a direct "no," and second to say when her mother died.

28. (1) The social graciousness of aging individuals (i.e., Lydia) is admirable. Again, the confrontation with reality and a promise of a social time together are appropriate responses. Her friend avoided ingratiation (4) or denial of reality (3) and (2).

29. (1) The nursing home personnel should be able to keep Lydia safe and to prevent decubiti or major infections. After assessment of the amount of cerebral damage and the impracticability of Lydia's living alone, the family should be advised of any progression in brain damage.

30. (3) Her son's response is designed to clarify what Lydia is saying and to allow further exploration of her thoughts of dying. The son could have said first, "What are you telling me?" He does not know what people will say about her, and Lydia obviously does care about this.

31. (2) Those persons with the strongest ego, best physical health, and most diverse interests seem to experience less regression and deterioration in aging.

32. (4) Nurses and other members of the health team too frequently direct their efforts to maintaining the status quo. Many aged persons are capable of developing new interests and friends, and planning for the future.

33. (4) Aged persons have needs both similar to and different from those of any other age-group. The nurse's task is to assess those needs most in want of gratification.

Obesity and Behavior Modification

1. (1) Obesity is said to exist if the individual is 10 per cent above normal weight for sex, age, height, and body build or as described in distractor no. 1.

2. (1) Obesity is rarely caused by hormonal imbalance or metabolic deficiency. Excess intake causes the vast majority of cases of obesity.

3. (3) Proponents of the behavior modification theory view obesity as a method of coping. The condition of being obese should be discussed separately from that of overeating, to gain an understanding of underlying needs and impulses.

4. (1) Excessive intake of food is not related to hunger intensity, metabolic need, or food satiety. Stress, anxiety, social pressure, and poor eating habits are highly contributory to the development of obesity.

5. (2) The hypothalamus, a center in the brain, also helps regulate secretion of pituitary hormones, temperature, and osmolality of the blood.

6. (1) Cushing's syndrome is due to overactivity of adrenal glands resulting in overproduction of cortisone. Cortisone is a glucocorticoid or carbohydrate-regulating hormone.

7. (4) A host of factors control one's eating behavior. Those listed have the most influence.

8. (2) Increase in number of cells is called "hyperplasia." Increase in size of cells is called "hypertrophy." The reason for hyperplasia of fat cells in an obese infant is not understood, and not all researchers agree with this finding.

9. (3) Obesity especially predisposes to diabetes mellitus and acute myocardial infarction. There is no evidence that malignancy and obesity are related.

10. (2) The body image is shaped primarily during adolescence. Fat adults have commented that they are surprised each time they view their fat, naked body.

11. (1) Internal cues (feeling full, feeling satiety) and external cues (no more food, another person saying, "that's enough") cause us to stop our food intake. The contributory factor in obesity development is an inability to differentiate physiologic hunger and emotional need.

12. (3) Maggie's obesity was due to psychosocial forces, so behavior modification for her would be directed toward changing eating and other social behaviors.

13. (4) Eating is a complex social behavior or process that involves more than oral intake of food. The goal is to alter behavior rather than achieve a specific amount of weight loss.

14. (4) Self-control is more than an internal process (1) and (3), and more than an external threat (2). The responses to behavior are both positive and negative, depending on which behavior is to be reinforced.

15. (2) Before initiation of a program to help Maggie shape new eating behaviors, a baseline assessment of what stimulates and/or deters eating should be established. Although the nurse should identify reinforcers to guide her own behavior, she should not point out these reinforcers to Maggie. Staff are speculating when they comment on whether or not Maggie will lose weight.

16. (2) Behavior modification therapy is not designed to psychoanalyze personality constructs. This technique attempts to alter the environmental (social) response to behavior, and thereby change the pattern of behavior.

17. (4) Basic assessments prior to initiation of a plan for change of eating are listed. Details are important. Do you eat when happy, sad, lonely? In kitchen or living room? Sitting, standing, or lying? Only at meals? Late in the evenings? When not hungry?

18. (4) How many times have we heard parents say to children, "Clean up your plate!" or "Don't waste food"? The keys to obesity prevention are: put less on the plate; consume it slowly in small bites; eat at the dining table only at meals; and be selective of food consumed.

19. (4) The key assessment is whether or not losing weight continues to be a positive reinforcer for Maggie. Sometimes, after a person loses a lot of weight, "friends" tell her how terrible she looks (not positive reinforcers!).

20. (3) A positive reinforcer usually does not result in an increase in antecedent behavior. An increase in behavior that occurred prior to the implementation of the reinforcer may not be desired.

21. (1) Most people have some way to reward themselves for what they consider a job well done. Eating, as a reward, can be overdone and self-defeating.

22. (2) Developing new social behaviors is the goal for Maggie. She already consumes large amounts of protein and snacks, both of which contribute to obesity.

23. (1) Sitting to eat (slowly) with others and decreasing stimuli for eating are desirable behaviors. Rapid eating is contributory to the development of obesity.

24. (1) Positive reinforcers for Maggie are those stimuli that alter the eating behavior: e.g., Maggie's desires to be pain-free and to be employed.

25. (2) There is a natural reduction of weight during the night, since energy is expended in maintaining body functions and food consumption is nil. Weight is gradually gained throughout the day, and thus would be noted by Maggie when recording her weight four times a day.

26. (4) Two of the listed tips are crucial to weight reduction. Buy foods requiring preparation (working for food seems to decrease the desire to eat, and serves to remind the patient that food consumption is about to take place; too much eating is automatic), and never buy snack foods (it is easier to resist in the grocery store than at home, and most snack foods require no preparation).

27. (1) Weight loss is physiologically safe when 1 kg. (2.2 pounds) is lost per week. Less than this is not sufficiently reinforcing. Weight loss in obese persons is more rapid during the initial weeks of dieting than later in the program.

28. (3) Placing the utensils on the plate for two minutes initially during a meal gives patients an early experience of control over one aspect of eating, and teaches them that food consumption as a behavior can be broken into components.

29. (2) Stimuli, both in and out of our conscious awareness, can provoke eating. To reduce such stimuli, Maggie was instructed just to eat at mealtime — not read the paper, watch television, call the neighbor, or sort the mail.

30. (3) Crocheting is an activity that requires active use of the hands, and completing a vest should be manageable and rewarding. Going to bed early or keeping the children up avoid the problem and are unrealistic. Attacking a new needlepoint pattern may prove too stressful and may provoke eating.

31. (4) Irritability is the most frequent symptom of too severe a weight loss, and this behavior doesn't encourage much positive reinforcement.

32. (1) Weight reduction is facilitated by support from family and friends. One favorite son refused to come home for a visit until his father lost a mutually agreed amount of weight. It is not likely that Maggie's pain will return if she continues moderate weight reduction. In spite of past failures Maggie can lose weight, if needs that stimulate overeating are met. Many patients reach a plateau or even regain some weight, but still keep their weight gain at a minimum.

33. (3) There are a number of "advantages" to obesity that make it difficult for some persons to reduce. An individual with anorexia or cachexia is treated as a sick person. Obesity is not viewed as an illness, perhaps because in some societies it is the norm.

Suicide and Suicide Prevention

1. (4) There is no agreement on why a person takes his own life or what makes the person who commits suicide different from us. Durkheim (Durkheim, E.: Suicide. New York, The Free Press, 1951) in 1897 was the first to attempt a scientific explanation of suicide: (a) altruism (e.g., hari-kari); (b) egoism (e.g., the individual has too few relationships and too little external demand for living); and (c) anomie (e.g., a catastrophic event in one's life provokes suicide).

2. (4) Although the actual causes of precipitating events are numerous, all persons who commit suicide or have suicidal ideation have an intense, underlying sense of deprivation of love, and a deep sense of personal rejection. Any of the factors listed in (2) can be a motivating force for suicidal attempt; those factors in (1) may be what the individual fantasizes will be solved by the suicide. The fantasies can be categorized as fantasies of identification, reunion, rebirth, or escape.

3. (4) Overdose by barbiturates and minor tranquilizers is the major method of death by suicide in women and physicians. For this reason, some therapists have recommended that such drugs be individually wrapped, making ingestion of the large quantity required to kill oneself considerably more difficult than merely taking a handful out of a bottle.

4. (4) The statistics regarding the incidence of suicide are confusing because they are changing. It seems that more women than men attempt suicide, but women are less successful in their attempts.

5. (4) Men attempt more violent methods of suicide and are more successful than are women. In the United States, suicide is most frequent among men, aged, unmarried (single, divorced, widowed), and isolated. In American adolescents it is the second largest cause of death, perhaps because they feel isolated, rejected, and unloved. Suicide is the tenth leading cause of death in the U.S.

6. (4) Suicide is not inherited, but family members whose parents threatened to commit suicide may later attempt suicide themselves. Most persons "warn" others that they have suicidal thoughts, and these are to be considered as serious threats. Persons from all socioeconomic levels commit suicide. Risk of successful suicide is actually low in those who have made a previous attempt.

7. (4) Ambivalence toward life and death is strong in persons who suffer from suicidal thoughts. As a consequence, the opportunities for prevention are good if others (family, friends, or health professionals) detect both subtle and obvious clues, and respond when help is requested either directly or indirectly. For example, the potential suicide may become more isolated or withdrawn, or may show changes in eating, sleeping, or sexual habits. Approximately one half of those who commit suicide have visited a physician recently.

8. (3) The precise reason for most suicides occurring between 6:00 P.M. and midnight is not known. It is conjectured that such individuals have had nonrewarding, ego-weakening experiences throughout the day, and the evening is dark and perceived as more lonely and rejecting.

9. (4) Most people have the assumption that life is better than death. Suicide, however, is an act designed to terminate an intolerable existence. If alternatives are difficult to discern, anxiety increases, self-esteem decreases, and crisis develops. Without direct help the aggression is directed inward in the suicidal act. It is a way to act out a solution.

10. (1) Bonnie Sue's alcoholism and careless grooming may not have been acceptable to her friends and colleagues, especially if when drinking she increased her criticism of her colleagues for their "lack of commitment to excellent patient care." The results are rejection, isolation, and less help with problem-solving.

11. (2) The most common question following suicide of a friend or family member is, "Why did she do it?" For some survivors this question is translated into, "What role did I play in this suicide?"

12. (4) Bonnie Sue in her suicide note communicated what she perceived as her colleagues' insensitivity to her needs and to patients' needs for care and attention. This perception would lead to feelings of frustration-aggression and revive old feelings of unworthiness (and of having been ignored by her aunt).

13. (2) Guilt is a common objective motivating suicide and a common response to suicide. Guilt is conscious or unconscious dread of loss or retributive punishment for impulses forbidden in childhood. Only a nugget of truth needed to be in Bonnie Sue's accusation of her colleagues to make them feel guilty following her death.

14. (4) Psychologists hypothesize that most of us have entertained a fleeting thought about some self-destructive act. Such thoughts usually are quickly "pushed" from consciousness. Another's suicide perhaps makes us realize how vulnerable we could become without love, acceptance, and ego strength.

15. (4) After the decision to commit suicide is made, depression is lessened and renewed energy seems to be available to such individuals. They act as though they were "moving away" (some patients become even more withdrawn), and give away cherished possessions.

16. (2) Suicide notes are not irrelevant and contain some information about the painful existence that no longer can be endured. The exact meaning behind the content of these notes is not well understood, and perhaps never can be.

17. (3) Each loss (a,b,c,d) taken individually seems so minor, but collectively the impact on Bonnie Sue's already weakened ego was unbearable. Change in routine can be perceived as a loss.

18. (3) Bonnie Sue's initial care following the death of her mother seemed adequate until she "upstaged" her cousin and was ignored. Giving her to her aunt for care may have been viewed later as a rejection by her father. If he unrealistically held her responsible for the death of her mother, this may have prevented him from giving her as much affection and love as she needed.

19. (2) Conveying blame overtly or covertly adds to the feelings already haunting the survivors. None of us is powerful enough totally to control or be responsible for the behavior of others.

20. (4) The child whose parent commits suicide must deal with all of these at some juncture in life. The age of the child at the time of the parent's suicide varies the response.

21. (4) These feelings and reactions are very much the same as those we experience following any loss over which we have no control. The extent to which the child feels that he had influence, real or imagined, over the death varies the intensity of his feelings.

22. (4) Any behavior in which we engage with knowledge of its harmful effects on our body can be considered "suicidal." The list is long.

23. (1) Durkheim's egoistic-type persons who commit suicide have too few contacts with the community in which they live. Consequently they are isolated, and the demand from others for them to live is insignificant.

24. (1) Suicide is more frequent among single, widowed, and divorced men than among married men. This, however, may be due to the degree of isolation that unmarried men experience in contrast to that felt by married men.

25. (4) In order to receive help, people must first establish contact with the helping

agent. A major obstacle is that families and friends of those threatening or initiating an act of suicide do not know whom to call or where to find help.

26. (3) Prevention of suicide could be much more effective in view of the fact that 66 per cent of persons with suicidal thoughts communicate their intentions in advance. Such a communication is a cry for help.

27. (4) This statistic conveys that, of whites who are successful in suicide, the vast majority have attempted suicide previously. Another way to put it is that most white persons are not successful at their first suicide attempt.

28. (1) Why this rate is so high is not known. The speculation is that it reflects the high degree of stress on young males in late adolescence or early young adulthood, and alienation from their usual support system.

29. (2) This statistic can be taken to mean that, in blacks, the more frequent the suicide attempts, the less is the chance of suicide. A word of caution in interpreting statistics: remember there are exceptions to the general trend.

30. (4) The 1600 calls per month is equal to about 53 calls per day, or an average of one call every 27 minutes. These data apply to only one suicide prevention center in San Francisco, and do not reflect calls made to other agencies, nor a national average. It is interesting, however, to compare the one per 27 minutes call rate with the projected statistic that there is one suicide in the United States every 24 minutes.

31. (4) These data are crucial to the person giving help designed to prevent suicide. The phone conversation in itself provides some contact with another human being; it may be sufficient to delay an attempt.

32. (3) The intent of initial telephone contact with persons planning suicide is to avert the attempt and the suicide. Assessment of the precipitating factors can be pursued later if the individual will participate in supportive therapy. The more clearly the plan for suicide is formulated, the greater is the danger of it actually occurring.

33. (4) If the person who finally makes a telephone call seeking help is unwittingly rejected, the volunteer has defeated the purpose of the Suicide Prevention Center. The tone of voice is very important in these communications.

34. (3) After assessment of the client's strengths and coping abilities, nurses can ascertain whether or not they can reassure patients by telling them, for example, "you have the strength within you to endure this stress." They also assess the number of repeat contacts indicated. Clients' collective needs are so immense that it is impossible, and usually not therapeutic, to relieve them of their responsibilities.

35. (2) Nurses are not always successful: a fact we learn to tolerate. Individual nurses in individual situations feel more responsible or guilty when a patient commits suicide. Not all suicide is preventable.

36. (4) When selected family members are perceived as troublesome, rude, or not "measuring up," it is convenient insidiously to allow isolation of these persons to develop. Family members can be helpful to persons with suicidal ideation by involving them in family decisions and activities. The feeling of being isolated is a cause of suicide.

37. (2) Problems frequently do not abate, so nurses should approach the client with the intent of improving ability to tolerate stress or altering the response to this stress (situations, people, own health). In this way, hope can be conveyed to the patient who cannot see any solution.